Dermatology in Public Health Environments

Renan Rangel Bonamigo
Sergio Ivan Torres Dornelles

Editors

Dermatology in Public Health Environments

A Comprehensive Textbook

Volume 2

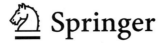 Springer

Editors
Renan Rangel Bonamigo, MD, PhD
Dermatology Service of Clinical
Hospital of Porto Alegre
Federal University of Rio Grande do Sul
Porto Alegre, Brazil

Health Secretary of Rio Grande do Sul
Porto Alegre, Rio Grande do Sul
Brazil

Graduate Pathology Program of
Federal University of Health
Sciences of Porto Alegre
Porto Alegre
Brazil

Santa Casa Hospital of Porto Alegre
Porto Alegre
Brazil

Sergio Ivan Torres Dornelles, MD, MSc
Health Secretary of Rio Grande do Sul
Porto Alegre, Rio Grande do Sul
Brazil

ISBN 978-3-319-33917-7   ISBN 978-3-319-33919-1   (eBook)
https://doi.org/10.1007/978-3-319-33919-1

Library of Congress Control Number: 2017960817

Printed on acid-free paper

This Springer imprint is published by Springer Nature
The registered company is Springer International Publishing AG
The registered company address is: Gewerbestrasse 11, 6330 Cham, Switzerland

Foreword

The invitation to present *Dermatology in Public Health Environments* is certainly among the most honorable in the almost 30 years I devoted to public health dermatology. Having known the organizers for long time, I am sure that, in addition to the search for updated knowledge, high scientific rigor, and careful selection of experienced practicing professionals for writing the chapters, it was a work of love for my fellow beings.

Dermatologic conditions are among the most frequent reasons for the seeking health care. They produce suffering, low quality of life, and overburden of services. They also generate direct and indirect high costs. Access to health services is difficult in middle- and low-income countries, but even in industrialized countries access is far from ideal. A less than optimal approach, which is common especially in primary care services, increases costs and complications.

I am certain that this fully illustrated textbook will be very useful for doctors, nurses, psychologists, and physiotherapists, whether they are in training or full professional activity. The multidisciplinary approach reveals the concern for comprehensive care in outpatient clinics, aiming at improving care and reducing costs. Public health concepts that are not always available to clinically active professionals are innovatively presented in part I. Parts II to VI include in-depth information on different dermatologic conditions, and part VII on systemic diseases with frequent dermatologic manifestations. Practical and helpful is the section on signs and symptoms (part IX). Also innovative is part VIII, which covers emerging issues related with environmental problems and those arising from various human activities.

I reiterate my confidence in the importance of *Dermatology in Public Health Environments* (*Bonamigo RR and Dornelles SIT – editors*), and I am sure that both professionals and patients will be grateful for this great endeavor carried out with excellence.

Mauro Cunha Ramos, MSc, PhD, Dermatologist

"If you can look, see. If you can see, repair"

José Saramago (book: Ensaio Sobre a Cegueira)

Preface by Renan Rangel Bonamigo

Publishing a Dermatology book with an emphasis on public health has a great meaning: it demonstrates that the health of a population is intrinsically related to the social conditions into which it is inserted.

Dermatology is a specialty of daily human suffering, and we consider that each professional involved in care can act to minimize this. Furthermore, it is essential that managers of health systems acquire knowledge of the epidemiologic characteristics of the main dermatologic diseases.

We hope that this book will be useful to students and professionals who are interested in understanding patients with a dermatologic problem and, within academic, scientific, and ethical high precepts, seek to help; and that it is also useful for understanding the multiple relationships that exist between public health and the environment, socioeconomic conditions, and priorities determined by governments and nations.

Acknowledgements

Completion of this work would not have been possible without concepts highly valued in public health: collaboration, sharing, and collective construction. Thus, we acknowledge the dedicated and competent work of all authors and co-authors as well as the Dermatology services that provided images from their files. It is also important to highlight the key role played by Susan Westendorf (Springer) and Gabriel Pires in assisting to resolve the various issues that arose throughout the publishing process. In addition, I would like to thank Daniela, Francisco, Pedro, Ademar and Yuçara for their love and encouragement. Special thanks to Professor Lucio Bakos for the academic example.

Dedication

This book is for all those who dedicate their professional lives to Public Health and, to represent them, I dedicate it especially to Yuçara T. Rangel Bonamigo, a Brazilian nurse who worked in Public Health for many years, as an actual humanistic reference.

Porto Alegre, Brazil   Renan Rangel Bonamigo, MD, PhD

Preface by Sergio Ivan Torres Dornelles

Public health are words that elicit the art and science of preventing disease, prolonging life, enabling health and physical and mental efficiency through the community's organized endeavor. This book results from one idea and the opportunity to make available to health care teams an enriching material to help increase the knowledge of dermatologic diseases affecting the population, by aiming higher than the characteristics that help diagnosis, prevention, and treatment. Some chapters in this book address a series of appropriate measures to develop a social structure that possibly provides all social individuals with necessary health care. This team work by Springer, the editors, and authors certifies health accomplishments that enable an outstanding level of knowledge in Dermatology.

It is already known that the scientific research is traditionally based on reliability. In order to keep such virtue intact and unsuspicious in the scientific environment, a reliable work has to allow for the validation of the reported results by accepting what is made known by the specialized literature as a source of new knowledge. Therefore, the so-called scientific community has to follow behavioral standards not only in the research itself but also in the disclosure of the acquired information and knowledge. These standards were strictly followed in this book because the invited authors have undisputedly followed them. For this reason we are extremely grateful for their extensive contribution to this project and commitment to science.

As editors we expect this book to provide easy access to knowledge for all professionals related to public health, and the provision of improved health and comfort to the population.

Acknowledgements

Life provides many moments to say "thank you". This is one of these moments. Teachers, colleagues, students, patients, they all had significantly motivated us to write this book and that is why we must thank them all. We now say "Thank you" and want you to feel honored.

But I send my special thanks to my family, always central when opportunities must be sought. Therefore, the major foundation which guided my steps toward this goal is my family. My parents provided me a wonderful experience during a first phase; three extremely significant people were the highlights during the second phase, my wife Susana, and my sons Lúcio and Marcel. Thank you so much!

Dedication

For this work to have a long reach in time we must dedicate it to those who somehow helped us to write it. So this book is for all my colleagues from the Outpatient Clinic of Sanitary Dermatology (Ambulatório de Dermatologia Sanitária), where I had worked for three decades, a place that taught me how to give comfort to the less favored. But I have to mention that it was a sought after and cultivated idea which enabled us to collect all of this information, whose progenitor was Professor Renan Rangel Bonamigo, well known for his scientific capacity and ethics. To Prof. Bonamigo, the main editor of this book and a scientific partner for over a decade, we should give full credit.

Another name has to be mentioned, that of Professor Roberto Lopes Gervini, since he was one of my most outstanding masters to whom I owe the most considerate thanks in the fields of science and life.

There is also room to honor all patients who trusted us with their faith and hope in our procedures, people who gave us the opportunity to learn all those details that do not belong in the medical literature.

Porto Alegre, Brazil   Sergio Ivan Torres Dornelles, MD, MSc

Contents

Contributors

Luciana Patrícia Fernandes Abbade Department of Dermatology, UNESP, Botucatu, Brazil

Beatrice Abdalla ABC School of Medicine, Santo Andre, SP, Brazil

Hiram de Almeida Larangeira Jr., Federal and Catholic University of Pelotas, Pelotas, Brazil

Marina de Almeida Delatti Service of Dermatology of the Pontifical Catholic University of Campinas (PUC-Campinas), Campinas, SP, Brazil

Lúcio de Almeida Dornelles Grupo Hospitalar Conceição, Porto Alegre, Brazil

Marcel de Almeida Dornelles Hospital Mãe de Deus, Porto Alegre, Brazil

Gilvan Ferreira Alves London University, London, UK
Private Practice, Brasília, Brazil

Maria Araci de Andrade Pontes Dona Libânia Center for Dermatology, Fortaleza, Brazil

Maurício Mota de Avelar Alchorne Nove de Julho University – UNINOVE, São Paulo, Brazil

Alice de Oliveira de Avelar Alchorne Nove de Julho University – UNINOVE, São Paulo, Brazil

Juliano de Avelar Breunig Hospital Santa Cruz, UNISC, Santa Cruz do Sul, Brazil

Renato Marchiori Bakos Federal University of Rio Grande do Sul, Porto Alegre, Brazil

Sidinéia Raquel Bazalia Bassoli Lauro de Souza Lima Institute, Nursing Division, Bauru, Brazil

João Luiz Bastos Department of Health Public, UFSC, Florianópolis, Brazil

Andre Avelino Costa Beber Hospital Universitario de Santa Maria, Dermatology Service, UFSM – Federal University of Santa Maria, Santa Maria, Brazil

Walter Belda Livre Docente of Dermatology at Medical School of the Universidade De São Paulo-USP, São Paulo, Brazil

Regina Maldonado Pozenato Bernardo Lauro de Souza Lima Institute, Nursing Division, Bauru, Brazil

Wagner Bertolini Santa Casa Hospital, Porto Alegre, Brazil

Giancarlo Bessa University Hospital, Luteran University of Brazil, ULBRA, Canoas, Brazil

Mariele Bevilaqua Dermatology Service of Federal University of Health Sciences of Porto Alegre, Porto Alegre, Brazil

Luciano José Biasi Instituto de Oncologia do Paraná, Curitiba, Brazil

Achilea Bittencourt Pathology Department, Complexo Hospitalar Universitario Prof. Edgard Santos, Salvador Bahia, Brazil

Camila Boff Sanitary Dermatology Service of the Department of Health of Rio Grande do Sul State, Porto Alegre, Brazil

Renan Rangel Bonamigo Dermatology Service of Clinical Hospital of Porto Alegre, Federal University of Rio Grande do Sul, Porto Alegre, Brazil

Health Secretary of Rio Grande do Sul, Porto Alegre, Rio Grande do Sul, Brazil

Graduate Pathology Program of Federal University of Health Sciences of Porto Alegre, Porto Alegre, Brazil

Santa Casa Hospital of Porto Alegre, Porto Alegre, Brazil

Ana Eliza Antunes Bomfim Dermatologist, Clinica Duarte, Pelotas, Brazil

Alejandra Larre Borges Hospital de Clínicas "Dr. Manuel Quintela", Montevideo, Uruguay

Eloísa Unfer Schmitt Botton Private Practice, Porto Alegre, Brazil

Catiussa Brutti Hospital Universitário de Santa Maria, Santa Maria, Brazil

Rosana Buffon Dermatologist, Vicenza, Italy

Helena Reich Camasmie Hospital Universitário Gaffrée e Guinle, Rio de Janeiro, Brazil

Fernanda Oliveira Camozzato Brazilian Center for Studies in Dermatology, Porto Alegre, Brazil

Taciana Capelletti Dermatology Service of Hospital Universitário de Santa Maria, Santa Maria, Brazil

André Vicente Esteves de Carvalho Irmandade Santa Casa de Misericórdia de Porto Alegre, Porto Alegre, Brazil

Fernanda Torres de Carvalho Psychology Service of Sanitary Dermatology Service of the Department of Health of Rio Grande do Sul State, Porto Alegre, Brazil

Cecília Cassal Sanitary Dermatology Service of the Department of Health of Rio Grande do Sul State, Porto Alegre, Brazil

Rafaella Daboit Castagna Service of Dermatology, Federal University of Santa Maria, Santa Maria, Brazil

Luciana Castoldi Psychology Service of Sanitary Dermatology Service of the Department of Health of Rio Grande do Sul State, Porto Alegre, Brazil

Caio Cesar Silva de Castro Department of Dermatology, Pontifical Catholic University of Paraná, Curitiba, Brazil

Cristiane Almeida Soares Cattani Sanitary Dermatology Service of the Department of Health of Rio Grande do Sul State, Porto Alegre, Brazil

Andrea Nicola Centanni Hospital de Clínicas "Dr. Manuel Quintela", Montevideo, Uruguay

Felipe Bochnia Cerci Hospital Santa Casa Residency Training Program, Curitiba, Brazil

Eduardo Mainieri Chem Irmandade Santa Casa de Misericórdia de Porto Alegre, Porto Alegre, RS, Brazil

Raíssa Londero Chemello Service of Dermatology, Federal University of Santa Maria, Santa Maria, Brazil

Liliam Dalla Corte Irmandade Santa Casa de Misericórdia de Porto Alegre, Porto Alegre, RS, Brazil

Adilson Costa State Public Workers Welfare Institute, São Paulo, Brazil

Marco Otavio Rocha Couto Hospital Anchieta, Brasília, Brazil

Paulo Ricardo Criado Department of Dermatology, School of Medicine, Sao Paulo University, Sao Paulo, Brazil

Roberta Fachini Jardim Criado Department of Dermatology, School of Medicine - ABC, Santo André, Brazil

Vanessa Santos Cunha Dermatology Service of Hospital São Lucas-PUCRS, Porto Alegre, Brazil

Marcos da Cunha Lopes Virmond Lauro de Souza Lima Institute, Bauru, Brazil

Antonio Macedo D'Acri Federal University of Rio de Janeiro, Rio de Janeiro, Brazil

Lia Natalia Diehl Dallazem Hospital Universitario de Santa Maria, Dermatology Service, UFSM – Federal University of Santa Maria, Santa Maria, Brazil

Patricia Damasco Dermatology, Hospital Regional Asa Norte/Private Office, Brasilia, Brazil

Gerson Dellatorre Hospital Santa Casa Residency Training Program, Curitiba, Brazil

Department of Dermatology, Hospital Santa Casa de Curitiba, Curitiba, Brazil

Janyana M.D. Deonizio Department of Dermatology of Federal, University of Parana – UFPR, Curitiba, Paraná, Brazil

Isabella Doche University of Sao Paulo, Sao Paulo, Brazil

University of Minnesota, Minneapolis, MN, USA

Sérgio Ivan Torres Dornelles Sanitary Dermatology Service of Health Department of Rio Grande do Sul State (ADS-SES), Porto Alegre, Brazil

Erica Rosalba Mallmann Duarte School of Nursing from the Federal University of Rio Grande do Sul (EENF/UFRGS), Porto Alegre, Brazil

Rodrigo Pereira Duquia Santa Casa de Porto Alegre, Porto Alegre, Brazil

UFCSPA, Porto Alegre, Brazil

Letícia Maria Eidt Sanitary Dermatology Service of the Department of Health of Rio Grande do Sul State, Porto Alegre, Brazil

Gabriela Fortes Escobar Dermatology Service of Hospital de Clínicas de Porto Alegre, Porto Alegre, Brazil

Vinícius Medeiros Fava Departments of Human Genetics and Infectious Diseases and Immunity in Global Health Program, McGill University and The Research Institute of McGill University Health Center, Montreal, Canada

Alcindo Antônio Ferla School of Nursing from the Federal University of Rio Grande do Sul (EENF/UFRGS), Porto Alegre, Brazil

Juliana Dumet Fernandes School of Medicine – São Paulo University, Hospital das Clínicas, São Paulo, Brazil

Ygor Ferrão Federal University of Health Sciences, Porto Alegre, Brazil

Anxiety Disorders Outpatient Unit in the Presidente Vargas Maternal and Child Hospital, Porto Alegre, Brazil

Claudia Elise Ferraz Federal University of Pernambuco, Recife, Brazil

Mariana de Figueiredo Silva Hafner Santa Casa de São Paulo Hospital, São Paulo, Brazil

Laura Freitag Private Clinic, Santa Maria, Brazil

Bianca Coelho Furtado Santa Casa Hospital, Porto Alegre, RS, Brazil

Gabriela Czarnobay Garbin Dermatology of Mãe de Deus Center, Porto Alegre, Brazil

Antonio Gerbase Senior Public Health Consultant, Geneva, Switzerland

Bernardo Gontijo Federal University of Minas Gerais Medical School, Belo Horizonte, Brazil

Thais C. Graziottin Hospital Sao Lucas-PUCRS, Internal Medicine/ Dermatology, Porto Alegre, Brazil

Heloísa Cristina Quatrini Carvalho Passos Guimarães Lauro de Souza Lima Institute, Bauru, Brazil

Vidal Haddad Botucatu Medical School, Sao Paulo State University, São Paulo, Brazil

Renata Heck Sanitary Dermatology Service of the Department of Health of Rio Grande do Sul State, Porto Alegre, Brazil

Dóris Hexsel Brazilian Center for Studies in Dermatology, Porto Alegre, Brazil

Hexsel Dermatology Clinic, Porto Alegre, Rio de Janeiro, Brazil

Isadora Hoeffel Dermatology Service of UFCSPA, Porto Alegre, Brazil

Clarissa Barlem Hohmann Dermatologist, Private Practice, Porto Alegre, Brazil

Dagmar Elaine Kaiser School of Nursing from the Federal University of Rio Grande do Sul (EENF/UFRGS), Porto Alegre, Brazil

Mauro W. Keiserman PUCRS, Porto Alegre, Brazil

Ana Elisa Kiszewski Dermatology Service of UFCSPA, Federal University of Health Sciences of Porto Alegre, Porto Alegre, Brazil

Daniel Boianovsky Kveller Federal University of Rio Grande do Sul, UFRGS, Porto Alegre, Brazil

Renan Lage Hospital e Maternidade Celso Pierro – PUC Campinas, Campinas, Brazil

Luiza Nunes Lages Hospital Universitario de Santa Maria, Dermatology Service, UFSM – Federal University of Santa Maria, Santa Maria, Brazil

Rosana Lazzarini Santa Casa de São Paulo School of Medical Sciences – School of Medicine, São Paulo, Brazil

Leandro Linhares Leite Dermatology Service of Hospital de Clínicas de Porto Alegre, Federal University of Rio Grande do Sul, UFRGS, Porto Alegre, Brazil

Neiva Leite Federal University of Paraná, Curitiba, Brazil

Daniel Lorenzini Federal University of Health Sciences of Porto Alegre – School of Medicine, Porto Alegre, Brazil

Fabiane Kumagai Lorenzini Santa Marta Health Center, Porto Alegre, Brazil

Barbara Lovato Dermatology Service of UFCSPA, Porto Alegre, Brazil

Louise Lovatto Hospital Sao Lucas-PUCRS, Internal Medicine/ Dermatology, Porto Alegre, Brazil

Silvio Maffi Orthopaedics, Porto Alegre, Brazil

Ana Paula Dornelles Manzoni Dermatology Service of UFCSPA, Porto Alegre, Brazil

Lúcia Helena Soares Camargo Marciano Lauro de Souza Lima Institute, Bauru, Brazil

José Carlos Santos Mariante Dermatology of Mãe de Deus Center, Porto Alegre, Brazil

Tatiani Marques Lauro de Souza Lima Institute, Bauru, Brazil

Jeovany Martínez-Mesa Faculty Meridional IMED, Medical Faculty, Passo Fundo, Brazil

Giselle Martins Irmandade Santa Casa de Misericódia de Porto Alegre, Porto Alegre, Brazil

Vanessa Lucilia Silveira de Medeiros Federal University of Pernambuco, Recife, Brazil

Doris Baratz Menegon Ambulatory Nursing Service and Coordinator of the Commission for Prevention and Treatment of Wounds at the HCPA, Brazilian Society of Dermatology Nursing (SOBENDE), Porto Alegre, Brazil

Luiza Metzdorf Federal University of Rio Grande do Sul, Porto Alegre, Brazil

Thaís Millán Service of Dermatology, Federal University of Health Sciences of Porto Alegre, Porto Alegre, Brazil

Renan Minotto Santa Casa Hospital, Porto Alegre, RS, Brazil

Helio Miot Department of Dermatology, UNESP, Botucatu, Brazil

Maria Miteva Department of Dermatology and Cutaneous Surgery, University of Miami, Miami, USA

Lara Mombelli Service of Dermatology, UFCSPA, Rio Grande do Sul, Porto Alegre, Brazil

Marina Resener de Moraes Irmandade Santa Casa de Misericórdia de Porto Alegre, Porto Alegre, Brazil

Elisa Moraes Service of Dermatology of the Pontifical Catholic University of Campinas (PUC-Campinas), Campinas, Brazil

Maira Mitsue Mukai Internal Medicine, Dermatology Service, Hospital de Clínicas de Curitiba, Curitiba, Brazil

Karen Reetz Muller Santa Marta Health Center, Porto Alegre, Brazil

Sílvia Nakajima Alfredo da Matta Foundation, Manaus, Brazil

Susilene Maria Tonelli Nardi Adolfo Lutz Institute, São José do Rio Preto, São Paulo, Brazil

Adriano Heemann Pereira Neto Federal Univesity of Rio Grande do Sul, Porto Alegre, Brazil

Angelo Syrillo Pretto Neto Irmandade Santa Casa de Misericórdia de Porto Alegre, Porto Alegre, Brazil

Marcello Menta S. Nico School of Medicine, University of São Paulo, São Paulo, Brazil

Andrea Nicola Hospital de Clínicas "Dr. Manuel Quintela", Montevideo, Uruguay

Sofía Nicoletti Hospital de Clínicas "Dr. Manuel Quintela", Montevideo, Uruguay

Lisia Nudelmann University Hospital, Luteran University of Brazil, ULBRA, Canoas, Brazil

Daniel Holthausen Nunes Federal University of Santa Catarina – HU-UFSC, Florianópolis, Brazil

Márcia Helena de Oliveira Federal University of Pernambuco, Recife, Brazil

Maria Leide Wand-Del-Rey de Oliveira Dermatology Sector, University Hospital Clementino Fraga Filho –HUCFF/UFRJ, Rio de Janeiro, Brazil

Gislaine Silveira Olm Mãe de Deus Center, Dermatology, Porto Alegre, Brazil

Cristina Maria da Paz Quaggio Lauro de Souza Lima Institute, Bauru, Brazil

Gerson Oliveira Penna Osvaldo Cruz Foundation, Fortaleza, Brazil

Antônio Dal Pizzol Irmandade Santa Casa de Misericódia de Porto Alegre, Porto Alegre, Brazil

Luana Pretto Irmandade Santa Casa de Misericórdia de Porto Alegre, Porto Alegre, Brazil

Katia Sheylla Malta Purim Universidade Positivo, Curitiba, Brazil

Fernanda Razera Dermatology of Mãe de Deus Center, Porto Alegre, Brazil

Bruna Guerra Rech Dermatology Service of Hospital de Clínicas de Porto Alegre (HCPA), Porto Alegre, Brazil

Felice Riccardi Irmandade Santa Casa de Misericórdia de Porto Alegre, Porto Alegre, Brazil

Clarice Gabardo Ritter Dermatology of Hospital Nossa Senhora da Conceição, Porto Alegre, Brazil

Vanessa Barreto Rocha Federal University of Minas Gerais Clinical Hospital, Belo Horizonte, Brazil

Gabriel Roman Hospital de Clinicas de Porto Alegre, Porto Alegre, Brazil

Heitor de Sá Gonçalves Dona Libânia Center for Dermatology, Fortaleza, Brazil

Jesus Rodriguez Santamaría Department of Dermatology of Federal, University of Parana – UFPR, Curitiba, Brazil

Alexei Peter dos Santos Irmandade Santa Casa de Misericórdia de Porto Alegre, Porto Alegre, Brazil

Josemir Belo dos Santos Federal University of Pernambuco, Recife, Brazil

Marcel dos Santos Pontifical Catholic University of Campinas, Campinas, Brazil

Sabrina Dequi Sanvido Irmandade Santa Casa de Misericórdia de Porto Alegre, Porto Alegre, Brazil

Debora Sarzi Sartori Service of Dermatology, UFCSPA, Porto Alegre, Brazil

Natalia Sarzi Sartori Service of Rheumatology, Federal Univesity of Rio Grande do Sul, Porto Alegre, Brazil

Maria Antonieta Scherrer Hospital das Clinicas Federal University of Minas Gerais, Belo Horizonte, Brazil

Silvete Maria Brandão Schneider Hospital de Clínicas de Porto Alegre (HCPA), Porto Alegre, Brazil

Karen Regina Rosso Schons Hospital da Cidade de Passo Fundo, (Medicine Faculty of University of Passo Fundo), Passo Fundo, Brazil

Majoriê Mergen Segatto Private Practice, Porto Alegre, Brazil

José Roberto Toshio Shibue Santa Casa de Curitiba, Instituto de Neurologia de Curitiba, Curitiba, Brazil

Perla Gomes da Silva Federal University of Pernambuco, Recife, Brazil

Rebeca Kollar Vieira da Silva Dermatology Service of Federal University of Health Sciences of Porto Alegre, Porto Alegre, Brazil

Roberta Castilhos da Silva Dermatology, University of Caxias do Sul, School of Medicine, Caxias do Sul, Brazil

Jenifer da Silva Santos Dermatology, University of Caxias do Sul, School of Medicine, Caxias do Sul, Brazil

Aline Francielle Damo Souza Irmandade Santa Casa de Misericórdia de Porto Alegre, Porto Alegre, Brazil

Juliana Mazzoleni Stramari Federal University of Santa Maria, Santa Maria, Brazil

Carolina Talhari Department of Dermatology, State University of Amazon, Manaus, Brazil

Roberto Gomes Tarlé Santa Casa de Misericórdia Pontifical Catholic University of Parana – PUCPR, Curitiba, Brazil

Matilde Campos Carrera Thouvenin Federal University of Pernambuco (UFPE), Recife, PE, Brazil

Ana Claúdia Kapp Titski Federal University of Paraná, Curitiba, Brazil

Lidice Dufrechou Varela Hospital de Clínicas "Dr. Manuel Quintela", Montevideo, Uruguay

Rômulo Mateus Fonseca Viegas Division of Plastic Surgery, Fhemig (MG), São Paulo, Brazil

João Batista Blessmann Weber Pontifical Catholic University of Rio Grande do Sul, Porto Alegre, Brazil

Magda Blessmann Weber Dermatology Service of Federal University of Health Sciences of Porto Alegre, Porto Alegre, Brazil

Carlos Alberto Werutsky Nutrology and Endocrinology, Hospital 9 de Julho, São Paulo, Brazil

Marcia S. Zampese Dermatology Service of Hospital de Clínicas de Porto Alegre, Federal University of Rio Grande Sul, Porto Alegre, Brazil

Vanessa Teixeira Zanetti Hospital Santa Casa de Belo Horizonte – SCBH (MG), Belo Horizonte, Brazil

Charifa Zemouri Academic Center for Dentistry Amsterdam (ACTA), Amsterdam, The Netherlands

Part VII

Skin Manifestations of Major Diseases in Public Health

Cutaneous Manifestations in Diabetes Mellitus

Karen Regina Rosso Schons

Key Points

- The most common skin manifestations in diabetes are cutaneous infections, xerosis, and inflammatory skin diseases
- Necrobiosis lipoidica may be viewed as the prototype of a diabetes-associated skin disease
- Granuloma annulare has a marked association with systemic diseases, particularly diabetes and rheumatic diseases
- Acanthosis nigricans has better outcomes with weight reduction and optimal blood glucose control
- Foot ulcerations are one of the most serious and disabling complications of diabetes and are the most common cause of nontraumatic foot amputation
- Patients with diabetes are more prone to infections than healthy individuals

K.R.R. Schons
Hospital da Cidade de Passo Fundo, (Medicine Faculty of University of Passo Fundo),
Passo Fundo, Brazil
e-mail: ka.bras@bol.com.br

General Epidemiology

Diabetes mellitus (DM) is a metabolic disorder affecting various organ systems, including the skin [1]. It involves a relative or complete insulin deficiency that leads to alterations in glucose, fat, and protein metabolism. In type 1 DM, insulin insufficiency results from a gradual, immune-mediated destruction of pancreatic β islet cells [2]. It is characterized by abrupt onset, insulin deficiency, a tendency to progress to ketoacidosis even in the early stages, and a dependence on exogenous insulin for survival [3]. In contrast, in type 2 DM, chronic hyperglycemia mainly results from end-organ (particularly the liver and skeletal muscles) insulin resistance. This condition is accompanied by a progressive, age-related decrease in pancreatic insulin release. A genetic predisposition and a strong association with obesity exist for type 2 DM [2].

DM is a rapidly growing pandemic. Around 415 million people worldwide, or 8.8% of adults, are estimated to have diabetes. If these trends continue, by 2040 some 642 million people, or one adult in ten, will have diabetes. Approximately 5.0 million adults died from diabetes in 2015, equivalent to one death every 6 s [4]. In addition, DM is the leading cause of new cases of blindness among adults [5].

Table 35.1 Dermatologic manifestations related to diabetes mellitus

Specific	Nonspecific	Complications
Diabetic dermopathy	Skin tags	Diabetic foot syndrome
Necrobiosis lipoidica	Rubeosis faciei	Cutaneous infection
Granuloma annulare	Yellow skin	Diabetic hand syndrome
Acanthosis nigricans	Xerosis	
Diabetic bullae	Pruritus	
Scleredema diabeticorum	Psoriasis	
Kyrle's disease	Vitiligo	
	Lichen planus	

Cardiovascular disease, kidney failure, and limb amputation also occur more often as a result of DM than from any other disease in the majority of high-income countries [4].

Complications related to diabetes are the result of metabolic, hormonal, environmental, and genetic factors manifesting in every organ system. The cutaneous manifestations range widely in severity (from mundane cosmetic concerns to life threatening), prevalence, and treatment response [6].

Skin disorders may be present in 30–79.2% of people with diabetes, and can occur as the first sign of diabetes or may develop at any time over the course of the disease [7–9]. The most common skin manifestations are cutaneous infections (47.5%), xerosis (26.4%), and inflammatory skin diseases (20.7%) [10].

The prevalence of cutaneous disorders seems to be similar between type 1 DM and type 2 DM patients, but type 2 DM patients develop more frequent cutaneous infections and type 1 DM patients manifest more autoimmune-type cutaneous lesions [1].

In this chapter, diabetes-related skin disorders are divided into those specifically or nonspecifically related to diabetes. In addition, skin complications associated with diabetes are also discussed (Table 35.1).

Skin Manifestations

Diabetes-Specific Skin Conditions

Diabetic Dermopathy

Diabetic dermopathy, also known as shin spots, is considered one of the most common cutaneous lesions in diabetes, although it is not pathognomonic of DM [1]. It affects as many as 30–60% of DM patients [2].

Etiopathogenesis
The etiopathogenesis of diabetic dermopathy is unknown but probably represents a post-inflammatory lesion in poorly vascularized skin or a manifestation of microangiopathy [11].

Clinical Presentation
Lesions begin as multiple, discrete, erythematous, coin-shaped macules or annular rings and are prevalent on the shins [2]. Of unknown etiology, its progression is variable and it may fade slowly, leaving a pigmented area without atrophy, or it may resolve completely, with new lesions developing contiguously [5]. It is a dynamic process, with lesions at varied stages present at the same time [6]. The occurrence of lesions correlates with retinopathy, nephropathy, and neuropathy [2, 5]. Macules are asymptomatic and are not directly associated with increased local morbidity [2].

Complementary Examinations
Because the histopathology is relatively nonspecific, a skin biopsy is not necessary [6].

Therapeutic Approach
No treatment for diabetic dermopathy is necessary [2].

Necrobiosis Lipoidica
Necrobiosis lipoidica (NL) has been shown to be associated with multiple systemic diseases,

including sarcoidosis, autoimmune thyroiditis, inflammatory bowel disease, ulcerative colitis, and rheumatoid arthritis. However, its most common systemic underlying disease is diabetes [12].

NL may be viewed as the prototype of a diabetes-associated skin disease. Although it is rare, its prevalence in adult patients is approximately 0.3–1.6%, occurring more frequently in women [3–7].

Most patients with NL will be diagnosed with diabetes at some point in their lives, and type 1 DM is more frequently associated with it [6, 9]. The presence of this disorder in diabetic patients is associated with a higher frequency of retinopathy and nephropathy [3]. Nevertheless, glycemic control has no effect on its course [9, 13].

Etiopathogenesis

The cause of NL remains unknown. The leading theory involves microangiopathy as a result of glycoprotein deposition in the vasculature, resulting in the thickening of blood vessels [13].

Clinical Presentation

The presence of NL is mainly based on a clinical diagnosis [8]. Clinically, NL lesions are localized on the lower two-thirds of the legs (pretibial regions) 90% of the time [14]. Lesions typically present as one to three asymptomatic, well-circumscribed papules and nodules with active borders that slowly coalesce into plaques [13]. Plaques are typically yellowish-brown, with elevated, erythematous borders, an atrophic center, and telangiectatic vessels visible through the skin [8] (Fig. 35.1). Their texture may be similar to that of wax [12, 14]. In isolated cases, lesions may affect the upper limbs, scalp, trunk, penis, or face [6, 12]. They may ulcerate spontaneously [12]. The Koebner phenomenon may also occur [13].

Although the majority of lesions do not result in pain, as a result the associated nerve damage up to 25% can be extremely painful, especially if ulcerated [13].

Squamous cell carcinoma is a rare complication that can arise in long-standing NL lesions, presenting also without ulceration [12, 13].

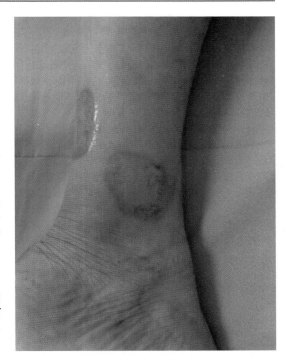

Fig. 35.1 Necrobiosis lipoidica presenting as yellowish-brown plaques with well-delimitated borders and atrophic center (Photograph from the Department of Dermatology Collection, Universidade Federal de Santa Maria, Santa Maria, Brazil)

Differential diagnoses of NL include granuloma annulare, necrobiotic xanthogranuloma, morphea, sarcoidosis, and, in cases of ulceration, tuberous syphilis [9].

Complementary Examinations

The characteristic histologic features are neutrophilic necrotizing vasculitis in the early stages and amorphous degeneration and hyalinization of dermal collagen (necrobiosis) in the later stages [3].

Therapeutic Approach

It should be considered that NL is indolent, and up to 17% of lesions may resolve spontaneously. Therefore, decisions on the treatment of NL are individualized [12].

It is important to note that despite the numerous investigations carried out over the years, no treatment modalities have been shown to be completely satisfactory in treating NL [15].

Nevertheless, the primary treatment is currently the use of steroids, either topical, intralesional, or, rarely, systemic [7, 13]. Steroids should be applied to the active borders of lesions and not to atrophic areas. Steroid use in diabetic patients demands attention in order to prevent glucose dysregulation [13].

In addition to steroids, other treatments are possible, although they have only been successful in some cases or still lack scientific evidence of their effectiveness. Calcineurin inhibitors, topical retinoids, ultraviolet A phototherapy (PUVA) treatment, photodynamic therapy, and cyclosporine are some of the additional options [16]. Pentoxifylline, a potent anti-inflammatory agent with hemorrheologic effects, has been used to improve microcirculatory flow with some favorable results [17, 18].

In nondiabetic patients, baseline blood work should include a fasting blood glucose or glycosylated hemoglobin test to screen for diabetes or to assess glycemic control. If these are not diagnostic of diabetes they should be repeated on a yearly basis, as NL can be the first presentation of diabetes [12].

Lifestyle modifications, such as the avoidance of trauma, are important in minimizing the risk of NL complications [13].

Granuloma Annulare

Granuloma annulare (GA) is a common idiopathic disorder, which occurs twice as frequently in women [19]. Clinical variants include localized, generalized, subcutaneous, micropapular, nodular, perforating, and (rarely) pustular generalized perforating GA [19, 20].

Etiopathogenesis

Although the origin of this condition remains poorly understood, a marked association has been observed with certain systemic diseases, particularly diabetes and rheumatic diseases [3].

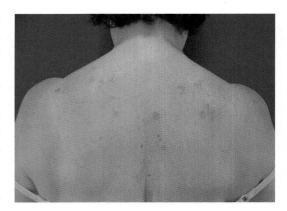

Fig. 35.2 Granuloma annulare: multiple red annular plaques organized around a slightly depressed center (Photograph courtesy of Edison Covatti, Passo Fundo, Brazil)

Clinical Presentation

The most common clinical form is localized GA, which accounts for approximately 75% of all cases [21]. It consists of pale red or violaceous papules that are firm and smooth to the touch. The lesions fuse into single or multiple annular plaques organized around a slightly depressed center [3] (Fig. 35.2). Lesions can occur anywhere on the body, but are more often found on the lateral or dorsal surfaces of the hands and feet. Symptoms are usually absent [20].

Subcutaneous or deep GA presents as a fixed nodule located on the legs, scalp, palms, or buttocks. Other less common variants include disseminated GA, characterized by a diffuse papular eruption, and a perforating form that presents as umbilicated papules with a central crust or scale and transepidermal elimination of necrobiotic connective tissue from the center [3].

Differential diagnosis for GA include other common annular skin conditions such as tinea corporis, pityriasis rosea, nummular eczema, psoriasis, or erythema migrans associated with Lyme disease. The lack of any surface changes to the skin is the key feature that distinguishes GA from these other skin conditions. Less common annular skin conditions (e.g., subacute cutaneous lupus erythematosus, erythema annulare centrifugum) have associated scaling and can be ruled out [22].

Complementary Examinations

Regardless of the clinical presentation, histologically there is dermal or subcutaneous granuloma formation with collagen necrobiosis, mucin deposition and an infiltrate consisting of histiocytes and multinucleated giant cells. Perivascular lymphocytic infiltration is also frequently observed. The histiocytes may be present in an interstitial pattern without apparent organization, or may show a palisading pattern, surrounding areas with prominent mucin [20].

Therapeutic Approach

GA treatment is frequently unnecessary because most of the lesions resolve spontaneously within 2 years of onset [3]. Nevertheless, the appearance of the lesions may require that some patients seek treatment [22].

For localized occurrences of this disease, topical corticosteroids are generally considered the first-line therapy. Depending on the site, high-potency corticosteroids with or without occlusion can be used. For nonresponsive cases, intralesional corticosteroids can be used [23]. Other options for localized disease treatment include calcineurin inhibitors, cryotherapy, or pulsed dye laser treatment. Generalized forms may be treated with one of a variety of systemic therapies, including dapsone, retinoids, niacinamide, antibiotics, antimalarials, phototherapy, or photodynamic therapy, all with only relative therapeutic success [3].

Acanthosis Nigricans

Benign acanthosis nigricans (AN) is most commonly related to endocrinopathies [24]. Obesity is the major underlying disease, often associated with hyperinsulinism, DM, and insulin resistance. Cushing's syndrome, polycystic ovaries, thyroid diseases, hirsutism, Addison's disease, and acromegaly are other endocrine disorders associated with AN [24]. All of these conditions have a significant resistance to endogenous insulin in common [25].

AN also occurs rarely as a complication of an internal malignancy, particularly of the stomach, and secondary to some medications, including nicotinic acid [25] and repeated same-site insulin injections [26].

AN is more common in dark-skinned people and is found more commonly in the adult population, although it can be observed at any age [27].

Etiopathogenesis

Elevated insulin concentrations result in the activation of IGF-1 (insulin-like growth factor 1) receptors on keratinocytes and fibroblasts, leading to epidermal cell proliferation and resulting in the clinical manifestation of hyperkeratosis and acanthosis. Other mediators may also contribute to this condition, such as EGFR (epidermal growth factor receptor) and FGFR (fibroblast growth factor receptor) [28].

Clinical Presentation

Regardless of its underlying disease presentation, AN usually follows the same pattern [25]. Presentation is characterized by symmetric, skin-colored or brownish lesions 1 mm to 1 cm in size [24, 27]. The plaques are palpable with a velvety texture and may have a flat to wart-like appearance [28].

The lesions typically form in large skin folds, particularly in the axillae, posterolateral neck, groin, and abdominal folds. Any other part of the body can also be involved, such as the nipples and phalanges [2, 24, 27] (Figs. 35.3 and 35.4). Associated skin tags are common [2].

Papillomatous growths may be encountered on the eyelids, lips, and oral mucosa, as well as on the esophageal, laryngeal, and nasal mucosa [29], and the palms (tripe palms) and dorsal surfaces of large joints [30]. These generalized forms involving mucosa, however, are more often related to malignancies [27].

Complementary Examinations

Histopathologically the lesions reveal papillomatosis, hyperkeratosis, and mild acanthosis. The dark color is due to the thickness of the keratin-containing superficial epithelium because there is no change in melanocyte number or melanin content [25].

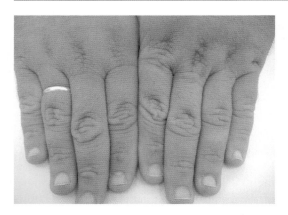

Fig. 35.3 Papillomatous growths on the dorsal surfaces of the hands (Photograph from the Department of Dermatology Collection, Universidade Federal de Santa Maria, Santa Maria, Brazil)

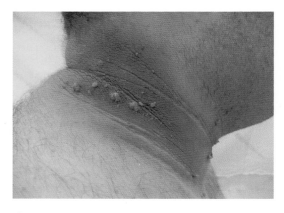

Fig. 35.4 Dark velvety discoloration in acanthosis nigricans associated with skin tags (Photograph from the Department of Dermatology Collection, Universidade Federal de Santa Maria, Santa Maria, Brazil)

Therapeutic Approach

AN has better outcomes with weight reduction and optimal blood glucose control [9, 31]. The use of agents capable of increasing the differentiation and decreasing the proliferation of keratinocytes, such as topical calcipotriene or oral and topical retinoids, may also be useful. Exfoliating agents, such as urea or ammonium lactate, and depigmenting agents can also be of benefit to some patients [31].

Diabetic Bullosis

Bullosis diabeticorum (BD) is considered a rare and relatively harmless skin manifestation related to diabetic patients [32].

Etiopathogenesis

Several hypotheses have been proposed to explain the production of the bullae, such as neurotrophic disturbance, alterations in carbohydrate metabolism resulting in bullae in a manner akin to chemical vesicants, a cationic imbalance due to diabetic nephropathy, immunoglobulin-mediated vasculitis, and ischemia. Nevertheless, the exact etiopathogenesis is still unknown [33].

Clinical Presentation

Spontaneously occurring bullae without pain or any sign of inflammation generally not related to trauma or obvious physical cause are clinical features of BD. Bullae vary in size from a few millimeters to several centimeters and contain a clear, sterile fluid [33]. The main location for BD is on the distal extremities, especially the feet and lower legs, although hands and the forearms may also be involved [34] .Its evolution is self-limited and usually ceases within 2–5 weeks, without scarring. It especially occurs in patients with long-term DM [32–35].

Differential diagnoses can include epidermolysis bullosa acquisita, porphyria cutanea tarda, erythema multiforme, or drug eruption [32–35].

Complementary Examinations

Histopathologic examinations have shown inconsistent levels of skin separation, and no specific signs have been found. Therefore, skin biopsy should be used only in case of continuous eruptions suggesting a chronic skin disease [32].

Therapeutic Approach

Treatment is conservative. The blister must be kept intact in order to cover the lesion and prevent secondary infection. The patient should be instructed to keep the wound clean and protected. Topical therapy is not required [35].

Scleredema Diabeticorum

Scleredema adultorum (SA) of Buschke is a fibromucinous connective tissue disorder. When associated with DM, SA is known as scleredema diabeticorum (SD) [36].

Etiopathogenesis

One proposed hypothesis for the pathogenesis of SD involves the glycosylation of collagen fibers leading to altered degradation. Another implicates hyperglycemia in stimulating fibroblasts and the synthesis of extracellular matrix components [37].

Clinical Presentation

SD is characterized clinically by diffuse, symmetric, and nonpitting induration of the skin, usually involving the neck, shoulders, trunk, face, and arms. Hands and feet are characteristically spared. Differential diagnoses of scleredema include fibrosing disorders such as scleroderma and scleromyxedema [37].

Complementary Examinations

Because of the inelasticity and induration of the thickened skin in scleredema, incisional biopsy is usually recommended to confirm the diagnosis. Histologic analysis shows a thickened dermis with increased deposition of glycosaminoglycans, mainly hyaluronic acid [37, 38]. However, diagnostic imaging may be helpful in accurately evaluating the activity of the disease in cutaneous sclerotic disorders [38].

Therapeutic Approach

There is no standard therapeutic approach for SD. Systemic corticosteroids alone or in combination with cyclophosphamide may facilitate infections and aggravate the diabetic state. The therapeutic

effect of PUVA, prostaglandin E_1, methotrexate, and cyclosporine is uncertain [9]. Glucose control has not been firmly associated with improvement of the disease [37].

Kyrle's Disease

Perforating disorders are a group of unrelated pathologic abnormalities showing the common property of histopathologic transepidermal elimination, whereby the extrusion of altered dermal substances or foreign material through the epidermal channel occurs [39].

Elastosis perforans serpiginosa, reactive perforating collagenosis, perforating folliculitis, and Kyrle's disease (KD) are all classic perforating dermatoses. Clinical and histologic features of these diseases are not uniform and may resemble any of the four diseases [40].

KD is regarded as a genetically determined disease with onset occurring during adulthood, usually between the ages of 30 and 50 years and with a female-to-male ratio of up to 6:1 [41]. Chronic renal failure and/or DM usually accompany this skin disease [40].

Etiopathogenesis

In patients with KD, keratin is the predominant eliminated material. This disorder of keratinization results in the development of dyskeratotic cells at multiple points. These cells have a limited capacity for proliferation. Eventually this results in depleted cells and a consequent defect in the epidermis [42].

Clinical Presentation

KD is characterized by the eruption of asymptomatic, mildly pruritic pinhead-sized papules with silvery scales. These gradually enlarge to form reddish-brown papules and papulonodules with central keratotic cone-shaped plugs, which can be removed with a curette. The papules may be follicular or extrafollicular. Koebner's phenomenon is uncommon, although at times the lesions may be linear [43]. The lower extremities are involved more frequently, but the upper extremities, head, and neck may also be affected [44].

Complementary Examinations

Histologically there are large keratotic and parakeratotic plugs penetrating from the epidermis through the dermis. The plugs cause inflammatory responses and a foreign-body giant cell reaction in the dermis. Mild degenerative changes in the connective tissue with no increase in the elastic tissue may also be noted. KD can remain inactive for years, with a possible clearing of lesions when the associated illness is under control [44].

Therapeutic Approach

Treatment of perforating disorders is difficult. Nevertheless, spontaneous resolution is possible [45]. Prognosis depends on the underlying disease and its response to treatment. In idiopathic cases and treatment-resistant secondary cases, topical steroids and topical and oral retinoids, along with UVB therapy, constitute the first-line therapies [46]. Narrowband UVB also appears to be an effective adjuvant phototherapeutic regimen [45].

Nonspecific Skin Conditions Associated with Diabetes

Skin Tags

Acrochordon or fibroepithelial polyps, commonly known as skin tags (STs), are one of the most common benign skin conditions [47].

Acrochordon is regarded as a sign of impaired glucose tolerance, DM, and increased cardiovascular (atherogenic lipid profile) risk [48]. STs may also play a role in the early diagnosis of metabolic syndrome [47].

Etiopathogenesis

In hyperinsulinemia, insulin is able to activate IGF-1 receptors present on fibroblast and keratinocyte surfaces in a similar way to what occurs in the pathogenesis of AN [49]. Two studies have found the presence of human papillomavirus DNA in STs, at frequencies of 48% [50] and 88% [51].

Clinical Presentation

STs are consisting of skin projecting from the surrounding skin, usually occurring on the eyelids, neck, and axillae [47].

Complementary Examinations

There are no complementary examinations that need to be performed to investigate STs.

Therapeutic Approach

Because they are generally of only cosmetic concern, treatment of STs is not required, and cutting the pedicles of the tags can be performed with microscissors and microforceps [52]. Cryotherapy and electrodesiccation can also be used [53].

Patients with STs also need suitable interventions, such as weight reduction, smoking cessation, and changes in dietary habits [47].

Rubeosis Faciei

Rubeosis, also named rubeosis faciei and rubeosis faciei diabeticorum [54], is a relatively common skin manifestation associated with diabetes that may go unnoticed by patients and physicians [7].

Etiopathogenesis

Hyperglycemia could lead to sluggish microcirculation, which becomes clinically evident from facial venous dilatation; its presence should lead to the evaluation of the patients for other more important microangiopathies, such as retinopathy [7].

Clinical Presentation

Rubeosis presents as a flushing that can be observed more frequently in association with type 1 DM (21–59%). Rubeosis is more prominent in fair-skinned people and usually involves the face, neck, hands, and feet [1].

Complementary Examinations

Rubeosis faciei is a clinical diagnosis and does not demand complementary examinations.

Therapeutic Approach

No treatment is needed, although strict glycemic control can improve the appearance and prevent complications related to microangiopathy in other organ systems [7, 54].

Yellow Skin

Yellow pigmentation of the skin (xanthoderma) may be associated with carotenemia, hypothyroidism, liver disease, and renal disease. The frequency of this phenomenon in diabetic patients is unknown, and the relationship between skin color and blood carotenoid level is controversial [55].

Etiopathogenesis

Not much is known about the relationship of diabetes and yellow skin. Traditionally yellow skin is considered to be related to carotenemia, whereby there are increased β-carotene levels in the blood, but it may also be associated with end products of advanced glycation [56].

Clinical Presentation

Carotenemia is a clinical condition characterized by yellow pigmentation of the skin (xanthoderma) [55]. Carotene deposits are usually most notable in areas with a thick stratum corneum, such as the nasolabial folds, palms, and soles, as opposed to areas such as the conjunctivae and mucosa [57].

Complementary Examinations

Tests for carotene levels can be performed but are generally unnecessary to evaluate yellow skin in diabetic patients.

Therapeutic Approach

No treatment is required, although adjustments to the glycemic level may result in an improvement in the yellow discoloration of the patient's palms and soles.

Xerosis

Rough skin or xerosis, commonly known as dry skin, results from a defect in the stratum corneum. This condition is negatively influenced by winter climatic conditions. DM, as well as other endocrine and metabolic disturbances, is also involved in this condition [58].

Etiopathogenesis

Xerosis is considered to be related to an autonomic peripheral C-fiber neuropathy, and it has been speculated that other factors, such as stratum corneum adhesion and accelerated aging of the skin, may be involved in the development of xerotic skin changes in diabetic patients [59].

Clinical Presentation

Dry skin can affect the extremities, trunk, or even the whole body. Cracking and fissuring of the epidermis can be visible.

Complementary Examinations

No complementary examinations need to be performed to xerosis related to DM.

Therapeutic Approach

Xerosis can be improved to various degrees by emollients, humectants, hydrating agents, and squamolytic agents [58].

Doctors should educate patients about the importance of skin hygiene, including applying fragrance-free creams or lotions within 3 min of bathing to trap moisture within the skin [7].

Diabetic Pruritus

Pruritus is difficult to characterize and define. Various indirect definitions have been proposed that include a sensation which provokes the desire to scratch or an uneasy sensation of irritation in the skin [60].

Itching in people with diabetes frequently can be secondary to many of the skin conditions already mentioned. Nevertheless, chronic pruritus with no primary skin condition is thought to affect a considerable percentage of diabetic patients, with some studies suggesting it affects 3–49% of all diabetics [9].

A large-scale survey of 2,656 diabetic outpatients and 499 nondiabetic subjects was performed between November 2006 and August 2007. The prevalence of truncal pruritus of unknown origin in diabetic subjects was significantly higher than that in nondiabetic subjects [61].

Pruritus is a risk factor for self-injuring behavior in sensory polyneuropathies because itching often induces scratching that can lead to clinically significant tissue damage [62].

Etiopathogenesis

Itches originating in the skin are considered pruritoceptive and can be induced by a variety of stimuli, including mechanical, chemical, thermal, and electrical stimulation [63].

Diabetic polyneuropathy (small fiber neuropathy with damage to myelinated Aδ and nonmyelinated C fibers) and xeroderma (aggravated by age and hypohidrosis in diabetic autonomic neuropathy), as well as certain drugs (glimepiride, metformin, and tolbutamide), have all been implicated in the pathogenesis of diabetic pruritus [9].

Clinical Presentation

Generalized pruritus is considered to be a sign of diabetes. Neuropathic pruritus may cause generalized truncal pruritus and localized itching, particularly in the genital areas of diabetic patients [64].

Complementary Examinations

Skin biopsies are nonspecific and may only help if there is an underlying skin disease suspected as the cause of the symptoms.

One study showed a positive association between postprandial blood glucose and generalized pruritus, suggesting that better control of postprandial glucose might be beneficial to relieve generalized pruritus in diabetic patients [65].

Therapeutic Approach

Symptomatic therapies may include high-dose antihistamines and pain-modulating drugs, such as gabapentin, pregabalin, or antidepressants. Therapy with emollients containing urea and in combination with substances that mitigate pruritus is essential [9].

Psoriasis

Psoriasis is a chronic inflammatory disease associated with several comorbidities. A few decades ago, it was considered to be a disease exclusive to the skin, but today it is considered a multisystem disease. It is believed that 73% of psoriasis patients have at least one comorbidity [66]. There

are reports of a significant association between DM and psoriasis in a large series of patients with psoriasis [48].

It has been suggested that psoriasis is an independent risk factor for the development of type 2 DM, whereby the severity of psoriasis correlates with the diabetic risk [67].

Etiopathogenesis

Immune-mediated inflammatory processes, metabolic biomarkers, and environmental factors could be the potential links between psoriasis and diabetes [68].

There is probably an association between psoriasis and diabetes that is related the actions of T-helper 1 cytokines, which can promote insulin resistance and metabolic dysregulation (i.e., metabolic syndrome) and can promote inflammatory cytokines known to drive psoriasis [67].

Clinical Presentation

Chronic plaque psoriasis (psoriasis vulgaris) is the most common form of the disease and accounts for approximately 90% of the cases. Typical psoriasis lesions are monomorphic, sharply demarcated, erythematous plaques covered by silvery lamellar scales. Extensor surfaces of the forearms and shins, periumbilical, perianal, and retroauricular regions and the scalp are the most common sites for these lesions [69].

Complementary Examinations

Cutaneous psoriasis is a clinical diagnosis, and skin biopsy is rarely used. There are three main histologic features of these lesions: epidermal hyperplasia; dilated, prominent blood vessels in the dermis; and an inflammatory infiltration of leukocytes, predominantly into the dermis [70].

Despite recent advances in the systemic treatment of psoriasis, topical agents represent the primary treatment for a majority of patients with mild to moderate psoriasis, as well as for some with more severe cases of this disease [71].

Therapeutic Approach

Topical therapies such as glucocorticosteroids, vitamin D derivatives, or combinations of both are usually sufficient to manage mild cases of this disease. Topical calcineurin inhibitors are used at difficult-to-treat sites, such as the intertriginous areas or the face. A combination of phototherapy and systemic therapy is needed for patients with moderate to severe psoriasis. Established systemic drugs for the treatment of psoriasis include methotrexate, cyclosporine, acitretin, and, in some countries, fumaric acid esters. Biologics have also been developed and approved for the treatment of psoriasis over the past few years [69].

Vitiligo

Vitiligo, an acquired pigmentary disorder of unknown origin, is the most frequent cause of depigmentation worldwide, with an estimated prevalence of 1% [72]. It is well known that vitiligo is associated with other autoimmune disorders, such as thyroid dysfunction, Addison's disease, insulin-dependent DM, and alopecia areata, showing that vitiligo shares a common genetic etiologic link with these autoimmune disorders. Insulin-dependent DM is found in 1–7% of patients with vitiligo, and conversely, 4.8% of all diabetic patients were found to have vitiligo [73].

Etiopathogenesis

The leading theory of vitiligo's etiology involves an autoimmune cause linked to specific genetic mutations. Although the role of antimelanocyte antibodies in vitiligo is still not well known, high levels of circulating autoantibodies have been found in approximately 10% of patients, especially against tyrosinases 1 and 2 [74].

Clinical Presentation

The most typical skin lesion is an asymptomatic, whitish macule or patch, with regular borders and sharp margins surrounded by normal or hyperpigmented skin [74].

Complementary Examinations

Histologic examination and immunohistochemical studies with a large panel of antibodies generally show an absence of melanocytes in lesional skin, although sometimes a limited number of melanocytes can be observed [72].

Therapeutic Approach

Topical therapy and narrowband UVB are the safest and most effective treatment options in most cases of vitiligo. Topical corticosteroids are still the primary treatment for localized forms of vitiligo because of their wide availability, low cost, and efficacy. Systemic therapy can be attempted in cases of disseminated vitiligo lesions, and in these cases steroids still remain the principal therapy. Surgical therapy could be useful in patients for whom medical therapy has failed [74].

Lichen Planus

Lichen planus (LP) is an uncommon disorder affecting <1% of the general population [7]. Some studies have shown a significant association between LP and increased disturbances of glucose metabolism including DM, glucose intolerance, and insulin resistance [75, 76].

Etiopathogenesis

LP is caused by an autoimmune process mediated by different types of cells and triggered by antigen alterations on the cell surface of the basal layer of the epithelium. In addition, epidermal cells have shown abnormalities in their enzymatic activity, as well as defective carbohydrate regulation in cases of LP, which might be connected with hormones essential for metabolic processes [75].

Clinical Presentation

LP presents as grouped, symmetric, erythematous to violaceous, flat-topped, polygonal papules distributed mainly in the flexural aspects of the arms and legs, and can rarely appear on the trunk. The Koebner phenomenon is common, and the pruritus associated is intense and heals with postinflammatory hyperpigmentation [7].

Complementary Examinations

Histologic examination of the skin or mucosal biopsies is useful to confirm the diagnosis in atypical cases, as well as to avoid inappropriate treatment in cases of severe disease [77].

Therapeutic Approach

Because the cutaneous form of LP may resolve spontaneously, the goals of therapy are to shorten the time between the onset and resolution of the lesions and to reduce itching. Topical glucocorticoids are the first-line treatment. When topical treatments are ineffective, oral glucocorticoid therapy is sometimes used. Other options are phototherapy and oral aromatic retinoids [77].

Skin Complications Associated with Diabetes Mellitus

Diabetic Foot Syndrome

Diabetic foot syndrome is defined as a group of clinical manifestations associated with neurologic abnormalities and various degrees of peripheral vascular disease in the lower limbs of diabetic patients. Ulceration, infection, and/or destruction of the deep tissues can occur [78].

Approximately 30% of diabetics will suffer from metabolic polyneuropathy, which is characterized by symmetric, distal, chronic, insidious onset, and somatic (sensorimotor) and autonomic dysfunction. An inability to detect temperature changes, excessive pressure, and continued traumas develop. Atrophy and weakening of the intrinsic muscles of the foot lead to deformities and abnormal biomechanical loading of the foot. Autonomic neuropathy results in anhidrosis, causing dry skin, fissures, and callused areas with secondary ulceration [79, 80].

The other component of diabetic foot syndrome involves vascular disease. Ischemia reduces the supply of oxygen, nutrients, and soluble mediators that are involved in the skin repair process. Furthermore, hyperglycemia-induced nerve dysfunction leads to the dysregulation of nerve microvasculature and consequent neuropathy [81].

Plantar Ulcers

Foot ulcerations are one of the most serious and disabling complications of DM and are the most common cause of nontraumatic foot amputation [82]. The prevalence of ulcers in the diabetic population ranges from 4% to 25% [81, 83]. Each patient with DM requires a comprehensive foot examination annually to identify risk factors for neuropathy and any evidence of neuropathy or ulceration [81].

Etiopathogenesis

Foot ulcerations are the result of neurologic abnormalities and various degrees of peripheral vascular disease. Both factors work in predisposing patients to ulcers and also making it difficult for ulcers to heal.

Clinical Presentation

The most common locations for foot ulcers are in the projections of the first, second, or fifth metatarsal bone, but may occur in other locations such as the heel and outer edge of the foot or toes. They are painless lesions because surface and depth sensitivity are impaired. Therefore, patients may continually traumatize the ulcerated location, making healing difficult [14].

Measurement of cutaneous pressure perception with the use of Semmes–Weinstein monofilaments is a validated screening test for the potential for neuropathy and ulcers. The loss of pressure sensation at four sites, as detected by the unperceived buckling of a 10-g monofilament, is highly predictive of subsequent ulceration. The four sites include the first, third, and fifth metatarsal heads, and the plantar surface of distal hallux. In addition, vibration testing with a 128-Hz tuning fork applied at a bony prominence is a useful test for peripheral neuropathy. The ankle jerk and patellar reflexes are also examined [81].

In purely neuropathic ulcers the foot is typically warm, pulses are palpable, and there is hypohidrosis. In contrast, in neuroischemic ulcers the foot is cold, pedal pulses are not palpable, and there is atrophy of the subcutaneous muscles and skin appendages [9].

Complementary Examinations

Radiography and other imaging modalities can help in detecting structural changes related to diabetic foot syndrome. Magnetic resonance imaging has high sensitivity and specificity for cases where infection with osteomyelitis is suspected [84].

Therapeutic Approach

The management of a diabetic foot ulcer has better outcomes when a multidisciplinary team is involved [81]. A combination of prevention and infection control, pressure removal thorough relief shoes or devices such as casts or boots, debridement, and dressings are used in combination [78].

Considering that abnormal glucose levels affect the nature of infection and cellular immunity, optimizing glucose control was previously highlighted as crucial for wound healing. Nevertheless, evidence from a recent study was unable to conclude whether intensive glycemic control had a positive or detrimental effect on the treatment of foot ulcers in people with diabetes when compared with conventional glycemic control [85].

The importance of avoiding walking barefoot and potential trauma should be impressed on the patient. Appropriate footwear is essential. The removal of mechanical pressure from a neuropathic foot ulcer is central to the healing of the ulcer. Resting the foot and the use of a nonremovable, total-contact cast is associated with more rapid healing rates [81]. The use of orthopedic innersoles, in accordance with various "offloading" foot techniques using various material features, has also led to good results [14].

The use of moist dressings on clean granulating wounds improves the wound environment. They provide protection against further infection, maintain moisture balance and pH, absorb fibrinous fluids, and reduce local pain. The choice of dressing is further guided by patient requirements and treatment costs [81].

Debridement is the process whereby all materials incompatible with healing are removed from a wound. Several methods are currently used for debridement, including surgery, conventional dressings, larvae, enzyme preparations, polysaccharide beads, and hydrogels. The choice of method should be based on the available expertise, patient preferences, clinical context, and costs [86].

If there are any signs of infection, further investigation should be performed and then followed by the administration of systemic antibiotics according to antibiogram results [9, 81].

There is low- to moderate-quality evidence that suggests a beneficial effect of hyperbaric oxygen therapy when used as an adjunct to standard treatments for diabetic foot ulcers [87].

Charcot Foot

Although Charcot foot does not primarily affect the skin, dermatologists should be familiar with this disorder, as its acute form may imitate erysipelas/cellulitis, deep vein thrombosis, or an acute gout attack [9, 88].

Charcot neuroarthropathy (CN) is an uncommon complication in diabetes that is characterized by severe deformity of the foot and/or the ankle that when not detected early will result in secondary ulceration, infection, and ultimately amputation [89].

Although Charcot foot occurs most often in patients with diabetic neuropathy, other predisposing conditions include alcoholic neuropathy, sensory loss caused by cerebral palsy or leprosy, and a congenital insensitivity to pain [90].

The prevalence of CN in diabetic patients ranges from 0.08% to 8.5%, and most patients who develop CN have had a known duration of diabetes of more than 10 years [84, 89].

Etiopathogenesis

The interaction of several component factors (diabetes, sensorimotor neuropathy, autonomic neuropathy, trauma, and metabolic abnormalities of bone tissue) results in an acute localized inflammatory condition that can lead to varying degrees and patterns of bone destruction, subluxation, dislocation, and deformity [84].

Clinical Presentation

Although Charcot foot is more common unilaterally, it can involve both extremities in up to 39% of cases [89]. The most common presentation is a neuropathic patient who sustains an unperceived injury, continues to walk until a severe inflammatory process leads to osteopenia, distention of the joint, and end-stage foot and/or ankle dislocation [89].

Musculoskeletal deformities in cases of Charcot foot can be very slight or grossly evident, most often owing to the chronicity of the problem and the anatomic site involved. The classic rocker-bottom foot, with or without plantar ulceration, represents a severe chronic deformity and is typical for this condition [84].

All physicians treating diabetic patients should be vigilant in recognizing the early signs of an acute process such as unexplained pain, warmth, edema, or pathologic fractures in a neuropathic foot [84].

The patient often has no recollection of an inciting event or reports only a minor injury. Vital signs are typically stable. The patient may have already been treated for recurrent cellulitis. The edematous limb is often without any open wounds and has increased warmth and erythema, which resolves with the elevation of the foot [88]. If the swelling and rubor persist during this technique, an infectious process is likely to be present.

Complementary Examinations

In the acute stage of CN, venous duplex ultrasonography will likely show negative results for deep vein thrombosis [88].

The erythrocyte sedimentation rate, C-reactive protein values, and white blood cell count are also usually found to be normal [91].

Results from radiography and other imaging modalities may detect subtle changes consistent with active CN or may be normal, emphasizing the importance of early utilization of advanced imaging [84, 88].

Magnetic resonance imaging allows for the detection of subtle changes in the early stages of active CN. It has high sensitivity and specificity for osteomyelitis and has become the test of choice for the evaluation of foot complications in diabetic patients [84].

Therapeutic Approach

The modern approach to treating CN is to diagnose it as early as possible and to institute timely off-loading to avoid adverse outcomes [91].

Total contact casting is well recognized as the gold-standard treatment for CN in general, although it has not become a standard treatment in many diabetic foot clinics because of concerns about complications [91]. Immobilization can be achieved with either a nonremovable or removable cast for an average duration of 14 weeks [88].

Surgical treatment is indicated for chronic recurrent ulcerations and joint instability when patients present with unstable or displaced fracture dislocations. Treatment outcomes and complication rates vary between centers [91].

Cutaneous Infections

Patients with DM are more prone to infections than healthy individuals [6, 9]. Moreover, diabetics exhibit a five-fold increase in complication risks compared with nondiabetics in cases of skin and soft tissue infections [9]. Incidences of infection correlate with mean blood glucose levels [6].

The disturbed skin barrier in diabetic patients and diabetes-induced vasculopathies, together with neuropathies, have been implicated in an increased vulnerability to infections. Recurrent bacterial infections, such as impetigo contagiosa, abscesses, erythrasma, folliculitis, erysipelas, or severe fungal infections, should alert physicians to screen for DM [8].

Treatment options for bacterial infections include the use of local antiseptics or antibiotic agents and, in cases of progressive soft tissue involvement or systemic signs of infection, the use of systemic antibiotics [6, 9].

Patients with diabetes are believed to be particularly susceptible to *Candida* infection because increased glucose concentrations permit the organism to thrive [9]. Thrush, angular cheilitis, candidal balanoposthitis, vulvovaginitis, and paronychia, as well as intertriginous candidiasis, are all common among diabetic patients. In contrast, the increased prevalence of dermatophytosis in diabetic patients is still a matter of controversy [8, 9].

Fungal infection of the nails is also common in diabetes [6]. Up to one-third of diabetics may have onychomycosis, which is a significant predictor of the development of foot ulcers in diabetes [92]. Therefore, treatment must not be neglected in these cases.

Furthermore, foot infections remain the most frequent diabetic complication requiring hospitalization and the most common precipitating event leading to lower extremity amputation [91].

Usually a consequence of an ulceration, the presence of a foot infection is generally indicated by the presence of systemic signs of infection or purulent secretions or by two or more local symptoms (redness, warmth, induration, pain, or tenderness). It is also important to note that local signs of infection can be diminished because of peripheral arterial disease and neuropathy. Osteomyelitis may affect up to two-thirds of patient with diabetic ulcers and may occur without pain [81].

Nasal and eyelid inflammatory lesions in diabetic patients deserve special attention. The possibility of mucormycosis, a rapidly progressive and potentially lethal infection caused by fungus primarily of the genera *Rhizopus* or *Mucor*, must not be ignored. Cutaneous mucormycosis is usually due to skin inoculation or local trauma introducing spores into the dermal layer, where vascular invasion by hyphae can cause infarction and necrosis of tissues. Rhino-orbital-cerebral and pulmonary infections are the most common presentations [93].

Diabetic Hand Syndrome

The term "diabetic hand" is used to characterize complications of DM that occur in the hands. Although the term "diabetic hand" has no precise definition in the literature, Papanas and Maltezos propose defining it as a syndrome of musculoskeletal manifestations of the hand (mainly limited joint mobility, Dupuytren's contracture, and trigger finger) in diabetic patients that is usually associated with long-standing diabetes, suboptimal glycemic control, and microvascular complications. Neuropathic hand ulcers and diabetic hand infections are also cited by the authors as part of the definition of "diabetic hand" [94].

Limited Joint Mobility Syndrome

Limited joint mobility syndrome (LJMS), diabetic sclerosis, the pseudosclerodermatous hand of the diabetic, and diabetic stiff hand are some of the diagnostic terms used in the medical literature referring to diabetic cheiroarthropathy (DCA) [95].

Increased nonenzymatic collagen glycosylation due to chronic hyperglycemia may lead to increased crosslinking between collagen molecules, thereby conferring an increased resistance to collagenases, manifesting clinically as stiffness [94].

Diagnosis is based on the following clinical features: progression of the painless stiffness of hands and fingers (prayer sign), fixed flexion contractures of the small joints of the hands and feet, impairment of fine motion, and impaired grip strength in the hands. As the syndrome progresses, it can also affect other joints [96].

It is important to diagnose LJMS because its presence is associated with the micro- and macrovascular complications of diabetes.

Because of the lack of curative treatment options, the suggested method to prevent or decelerate the development of LJMS is to improve or maintain good glycemic control. Daily joint-stretching exercises aimed at preventing or delaying the progression of joint stiffness may reduce the risk of inadvertent falls and will help maintain quality of life [96].

Dupuytren's Contracture

Dupuytren's contracture (DC) is characterized by palmar fascia thickening, palmar and digital nodules, skin thickening and adherence, pretendinous band formation, and digital flexion contracture. DC affects 16–32% of diabetic patients and is more common among the elderly and those who have had DM for longer periods. It mainly affects the third and fourth fingers, rather than the fourth and fifth fingers, as typically occurs in cases associated with other etiologies [97]. Dupuytren's contracture has been treated with intralesional infiltration of corticosteroids, surgery, and physical therapy [97].

Trigger Finger

Stenosing flexor tenosynovitis typically presents as fingers locked in flexion, extension, or both, more commonly involving the thumb, third finger, and/or fourth finger [97].

The treatment for stenosing flexor tenosynovitis includes a change in activities, the use of nonsteroidal anti-inflammatories, splinting, infiltrations, and, in more severe cases, surgery [97].

Tropical Diabetic Hand Syndrome and Hand Infections

Tropical diabetic hand syndrome is a complication affecting patients with DM that is much less recognized that foot infections.

The syndrome encompasses manifestations that range from a localized cellulitis with variable swelling and ulceration of the hands to progressive, fulminant hand sepsis and gangrene affecting the entire limb [98].

Typically, patients have type 2 DM, are female, present in their fifth to sixth decade of life, and have poor metabolic control. Antecedent trauma (mild abrasion, laceration, insect bites) is often reported [94].

While tropical diabetic hand syndrome is essentially confined to the tropics, hand infections may also occur in the general diabetic population of the Western world. *Staphylococcus aureus* is the most common bacterial isolate, while infections by *Streptococcus, Klebsiella, Enterobacter, Proteus, Escherichia coli*, and various anaerobes may also be found [94].

Early diagnosis and treatment may lead to adequate recovery. Prognosis improves when appropriate blood glucose and insulin control, antimicrobial therapy, drainage, and debridement are performed promptly after diagnosis [99].

Peripheral Neuropathy and Ulceration

Although diabetic foot problems related to peripheral neuropathy are well reported in the literature, we tend to forget the possible involvement of the hands. However, sensory impairment of the hands may occur in patients with severe neuropathy [100].

Screening for hand neuropathies is not a normal practice in most clinics unless patients are symptomatic (e.g., hand numbness or tingling). Such hand symptoms are, however, uncommon, and patients are unaware of neural dysfunction. Marked hand symptoms also seem to be more related to carpal tunnel syndrome than to neuropathy [100].

Hand examinations should not be neglected in patients with severe neuropathy in the feet and/or foot burns. Such patients need to be warned about the danger of hand burns [94].

Education on hand care should be given more attention, particularly in patients with lower extremity neuropathy. Patients in certain occupations (e.g., those that involve handling of hot materials or vibrating machinery) may be at particular risk, and the necessary precautions must be assured in their work environment [94].

Conclusion

DM and insulin resistance are related to a wide range of skin manifestations. Therefore, doctors should be aware of these skin conditions to best assist patients with this metabolic disorder.

Glossary

Acanthosis Hyperplasia of the squamous epithelium.

Acanthosis Nigricans Dark pigmentation with a velvety texture in large skin folds.

Acrochordon Benign pedunculated skin growths usually occurring on the eyelids, neck, and axillae.

Charcot foot Complication in diabetes that is characterized by severe deformity of the foot and/or the ankle that when not detected early may result in secondary ulceration, infection, and amputation.

Diabetic dermopathy Also known as "shin spots," a specific skin condition associated with diabetes mellitus.

Flushing Redness of the skin together with a sensation of local warmth or burning.

Koebner reaction A phenomenon where new lesions appear along a site of trauma or irritation of the skin can. Examples: lichen planus, psoriasis.

lichen planus Inflammatory chronic skin condition of flat-topped erythematous to violaceous papules caused by an autoimmune process,

Macule A change in the color of the skin that is neither raised nor depressed, up to 1 cm in diameter.

Melanocytes Pigment cells responsible for producing melanin. In the human skin they are found in the basal layer of the epidermis and hair follicles.

Necrobiosis Gradual degeneration and death of a cell.

Necrobiosis lipoidica Skin disease marked by one or more tender yellowish brown patches often associated with diabetes mellitus.

Psoriasis An autoimmune skin condition that changes the life cycle of skin cells. The majority of patients presents lesions as clearly defined red and scaly plaques.

Scleredema A dermatologic disorder characterized by hardening and thickening of the skin. When associated with diabetes mellitus is called "scleredema diabeticorum."

Vitiligo An acquired pigmentary disorder of unknown origin characterized by portions of the skin losing their pigment.

Xanthoderma Yellow pigmentation of the skin.

Xerosis Commonly known as "dry skin," results from a defect in the stratum corneum.

References

1. Ragunatha S, Anitha B, Inamadar AC, Palit A, Devarmani SS. Cutaneous disorders in 500 diabetic patients attending diabetic clinic. Indian J Dermatol. 2011;56(2):160–4. Epub 2011/07/01.
2. Pierard GE, Seite S, Hermanns-Le T, Delvenne P, Scheen A, Pierard-Franchimont C. The skin landscape in diabetes mellitus. Focus on dermocosmetic management. Clin Cosmet Investig Dermatol. 2013;6:127–35. Epub 2013/05/23.
3. Baselga Torres E, Torres-Pradilla M. Cutaneous manifestations in children with diabetes mellitus and obesity. Actas Dermosifiliogr. 2014;105(6):546–57. Epub 2014/04/05.
4. IDF diabetes atlas, 7th edition. Available at: http://www.idf.org/diabetesatlas. Accessed 25th May 2015.
5. Urrets-Zavalia JA, Esposito E, Garay I, Monti R, Ruiz-Lascano A, Correa L, et al. The eye and the skin in endocrine metabolic diseases. Clin Dermatol. 2016;34(2):151–65. Epub 2016/02/24.
6. Murphy-Chutorian B, Han G, Cohen SR. Dermatologic manifestations of diabetes mellitus: a review. Endocrinol Metab Clin N Am. 2013;42(4):869–98. Epub 2013/11/30.
7. Duff M, Demidova O, Blackburn S, Shubrook J. Cutaneous manifestations of diabetes mellitus. Clin Diabetes: Publ Am Diabetes Assoc. 2015;33(1):40–8. Epub 2015/02/06.
8. Behm B, Schreml S, Landthaler M, Babilas P. Skin signs in diabetes mellitus. J Eur Acad Dermatol Venereol (JEADV). 2012;26(10):1203–11. Epub 2012/02/22.
9. Gkogkolou P, Bohm M. Skin disorders in diabetes mellitus. J Dtsch Dermatol Ges J Ger Soc Dermatol (JDDG). 2014;12(10):847–63. quiz 64–5. Epub 2014/09/30. Hauterkrankungen bei Diabetes mellitus.
10. Demirseren DD, Emre S, Akoglu G, Arpaci D, Arman A, Metin A, et al. Relationship between skin diseases and extracutaneous complications of diabetes mellitus: clinical analysis of 750 patients. Am J Clin Dermatol. 2014;15(1):65–70. Epub 2013/10/19.
11. Bristow I. Non-ulcerative skin pathologies of the diabetic foot. Diabetes Metab Res Rev. 2008;24(Suppl 1):S84–9. Epub 2008/03/22.
12. Sibbald C, Reid S, Alavi A. Necrobiosis lipoidica. Dermatol Clin. 2015;33(3):343–60. Epub 2015/07/06.
13. Reid SD, Ladizinski B, Lee K, Baibergenova A, Alavi A. Update on necrobiosis lipoidica: a review of etiology, diagnosis, and treatment options. J Am Acad Dermatol. 2013;69(5):783–91. Epub 2013/08/24.
14. Minelli LB, Nonino A, Cantarelli J, Neme L, Marcondes M. Diabetes mellitus and cutaneous affections. An Bras Dermatol. 2003;78(6):735–47.
15. Feily A, Mehraban S. Treatment modalities of necrobiosis lipoidica: a concise systematic review. Dermatol Rep. 2015;7(2):5749. Epub 2015/08/04.
16. Grillo E, Rodriguez-Munoz D, Gonzalez-Garcia A, Jaen P. Necrobiosis lipoidica. Aust Fam Physician. 2014;43(3):129–30. Epub 2014/03/07.
17. Basaria S, Braga-Basaria M. Necrobiosis lipoidica diabeticorum: response to pentoxiphylline. J Endocrinol Investig. 2003;26(10):1037–40. Epub 2004/02/05.
18. Wee E, Kelly R. Pentoxifylline: an effective therapy for necrobiosis lipoidica. Australas J Dermatol. 2015. Epub 2015/11/13.
19. Kovich O, Burgin S. Generalized granuloma annulare. Dermatol Online J. 2005;11(4):23. Epub 2006/01/13.
20. Lukacs J, Schliemann S, Elsner P. Treatment of generalized granuloma annulare – a systematic review. J Eur Acad Dermatol Venereol (JEADV). 2015;29(8):1467–80. Epub 2015/02/05.
21. Hsu S, Le EH, Khoshevis MR. Differential diagnosis of annular lesions. Am Fam Physician. 2001;64(2):289–96. Epub 2001/07/31.
22. Cyr PR. Diagnosis and management of granuloma annulare. Am Fam Physician. 2006;74(10):1729–34. Epub 2006/12/02.
23. Keimig EL. Granuloma annulare. Dermatol Clin. 2015;33(3):315–29. Epub 2015/07/06.
24. Barbato MT, Criado PR, Silva AK, Averbeck E, Guerine MB, Sa NB. Association of acanthosis nigricans and skin tags with insulin resistance. An Bras Dermatol. 2012;87(1):97–104. Epub 2012/04/07.
25. Ahmed I, Goldstein B. Diabetes mellitus. Clin Dermatol. 2006;24(4):237–46. Epub 2006/07/11.
26. Brodell JD Jr, Cannella JD, Helms SE. Case report: acanthosis nigricans resulting from repetitive same-site insulin injections. J Drugs Dermatol (JDD). 2012;11(12):e85–7. Epub 2013/02/05.
27. Kutlubay Z, Engin B, Bairamov O, Tuzun Y. Acanthosis nigricans: a fold (intertriginous) dermatosis. Clin Dermatol. 2015;33(4):466–70. Epub 2015/06/09.

28. Higgins SP, Freemark M, Prose NS. Acanthosis nigricans: a practical approach to evaluation and management. Dermatol Online J. 2008;14(9):2. Epub 2008/12/09.

29. Ramirez-Amador V, Esquivel-Pedraza L, Caballero-Mendoza E, Berumen-Campos J, Orozco-Topete R, Angeles-Angeles A. Oral manifestations as a hallmark of malignant acanthosis nigricans. J Oral Pathol Med: Off Publ Int Assoc Oral Pathol Am Acad Oral Pathol. 1999;28(6):278–81. Epub 1999/07/30.

30. Thiers BH, Sahn RE, Callen JP. Cutaneous manifestations of internal malignancy. CA Cancer J Clin. 2009;59(2):73–98. Epub 2009/03/05.

31. Levy L, Zeichner JA. Dermatologic manifestation of diabetes. J Diabetes. 2012;4(1):68–76. Epub 2011/08/19.

32. Larsen K, Jensen T, Karlsmark T, Holstein PE. Incidence of bullosis diabeticorum – a controversial cause of chronic foot ulceration. Int Wound J. 2008;5(4):591–6. Epub 2008/11/14.

33. Handa S, Sharma R, Kumar B. Bullosis diabeticorum. Indian J Dermatol Venereol Leprology. 1995;61(1):62–3. Epub 1995/01/01.

34. Derighetti M, Hohl D, Krayenbuhl BH, Panizzon RG. Bullosis diabeticorum in a newly discovered type 2 diabetes mellitus. Dermatology. 2000;200(4):366–7. Epub 2000/07/15.

35. Mota AN, Nery NS, Barcaui CB. Case for diagnosis: bullosis diabeticorum. An Bras Dermatol. 2013;88(4):652–4. Epub 2013/09/27.

36. Mohamed M, Belhadjali H, Bechir AB, Moussa A, Zili J. Scleredema adultorum of Buschke with prominent periorbital edema in a Tunisian patient with diabetes mellitus: a case report. Int J Dermatol. 2016;55(2):e100–2. Epub 2015/11/05.

37. Tran K, Boyd KP, Robinson MR, Whitlow M. Scleredema diabeticorum. Dermatol Online J. 2013;19(12):20718. Epub 2013/12/25.

38. Kurihara Y, Kokuba H, Furue M. Case of diabetic scleredema: diagnostic value of magnetic resonance imaging. J Dermatol. 2011;38(7):693–6. Epub 2011/07/07.

39. Lee SJ, Jang JW, Lee WC, Kim DW, Jun JB, Bae HI, et al. Perforating disorder caused by salt-water application and its experimental induction. Int J Dermatol. 2005;44(3):210–4. Epub 2005/04/06.

40. Saray Y, Seckin D, Bilezikci B. Acquired perforating dermatosis: clinicopathological features in twenty-two cases. J Eur Acad Dermatol Venereol (JEADV). 2006;20(6):679–88. Epub 2006/07/14.

41. Nair PA, Jivani NB, Diwan NG. Kyrle's disease in a patient of diabetes mellitus and chronic renal failure on dialysis. J Family Med Prim Care. 2015;4(2):284–6. Epub 2015/05/08.

42. Viswanathan S, Narurkar SD, Rajpal A, Nagpur NG, Avasare SS. Rare presentation of Kyrle's disease in siblings. Indian J Dermatol. 2008;53(2):85–7. Epub 2008/01/01.

43. Sehgal VN, Jain S, Thappa DM, Bhattacharya SN, Logani K. Perforating dermatoses: a review and report of four cases. J Dermatol. 1993;20(6):329–40. Epub 1993/06/01.

44. Ataseven A, Ozturk P, Kucukosmanoglu I, Kurtipek GS. Kyrle's disease. BMJ Case Rep. 2014;2014. Epub 2014/01/17.

45. Gambichler T, Altmeyer P, Kreuter A. Treatment of acquired perforating dermatosis with narrowband ultraviolet B. J Am Acad Dermatol. 2005;52(2):363–4. Epub 2005/02/05.

46. Verma R, Vasudevan B, Kakkar S, Mishra P, Pragasam V, Dabbas D. Kyrle's disease presenting in an extensive distribution along lines of Blaschko. Indian J Dermatol. 2015;60(4):423. Epub 2015/08/20.

47. Wali V, Wali VV. Assessment of various biochemical parameters and BMI in patients with skin tags. J Clin Diagn Res: JCDR. 2016;10(1):BC09–11. Epub 2016/02/20.

48. Vahora R, Thakkar S, Marfatia Y. Skin, a mirror reflecting diabetes mellitus: a longitudinal study in a tertiary care hospital in Gujarat. Indian J Endocrinol Metab. 2013;17(4):659–64. Epub 2013/08/21.

49. Schilling WH, Crook MA. Cutaneous stigmata associated with insulin resistance and increased cardiovascular risk. Int J Dermatol. 2014;53(9):1062–9. Epub 2014/04/05.

50. Gupta S, Aggarwal R, Arora SK. Human papillomavirus and skin tags: is there any association? Indian J Dermatol Venereol Leprology. 2008;74(3):222–5. Epub 2008/06/28.

51. Dianzani C, Calvieri S, Pierangeli A, Imperi M, Bucci M, Degener AM. The detection of human papillomavirus DNA in skin tags. Br J Dermatol. 1998;138(4):649–51. Epub 1998/06/26.

52. Gorgulu T, Torun M, Guler R, Olgun A, Kargi E. Fast and painless skin tag excision with ethyl chloride. Aesthet Plast Surg. 2015;39(4):644–5. Epub 2015/06/06.

53. Allegue F, Fachal C, Perez-Perez L. Friction induced skin tags. Dermatol Online J. 2008;14(3):18. Epub 2008/07/17.

54. Namazi MR, Jorizzo JL, Fallahzadeh MK. Rubeosis faciei diabeticorum: a common, but often unnoticed, clinical manifestation of diabetes mellitus. Sci World J. 2010;10:70–1. Epub 2010/01/12.

55. Julka S, Jamdagni N, Verma S, Goyal R. Yellow palms and soles: a rare skin manifestation in diabetes mellitus. Indian J Endocrinol Metab. 2013;17(Suppl 1):S299–300. Epub 2013/11/20.

56. Lin JN. Images in clinical medicine. Yellow palms and soles in diabetes mellitus. N Engl J Med. 2006;355(14):1486. Epub 2006/10/06.

57. Silverberg NB, Lee-Wong M. Generalized yellow discoloration of the skin. The diagnosis: carotenemia. Cutis. 2014;93(5):E11–2. Epub 2014/06/05.

58. Uhoda E, Debatisse B, Paquet P, Pierard-Franchimont C, Pierard GE. The so-called dry skin of the diabetic patient. Rev Med Liege. 2005;60(5–6):560–3. Epub 2005/07/23. La peau dite seche du patient diabetique.

59. Yoon HS, Baik SH, Oh CH. Quantitative measurement of desquamation and skin elasticity in diabetic patients. Skin Res Technol. 2002;8(4):250–4. Epub 2002/11/09.

60. Tarikci N, Kocaturk E, Gungor S, Topal IO, Can PU, Singer R. Pruritus in systemic diseases: a review of etiological factors and new treatment modalities. Sci World J. 2015;2015:803752. Epub 2015/08/05.

61. Yamaoka H, Sasaki H, Yamasaki H, Ogawa K, Ohta T, Furuta H, et al. Truncal pruritus of unknown origin may be a symptom of diabetic polyneuropathy. Diabetes Care. 2010;33(1):150–5. Epub 2009/12/31.

62. Dorfman D, George MC, Tamler R, Lushing J, Nmashie A, Simpson DM. Pruritus induced self injury behavior: an overlooked risk factor for amputation in diabetic neuropathy? Diabetes Res Clin Pract. 2014;103(3):e47–8. Epub 2014/01/23.

63. Vinik AI. Barely scratching the surface. Diabetes Care. 2010;33(1):210–2. Epub 2009/12/31.

64. Tseng HW, Ger LP, Liang CK, Liou HH, Lam HC. High prevalence of cutaneous manifestations in the elderly with diabetes mellitus: an institution-based cross-sectional study in Taiwan. J Eur Acad Dermatol Venereol (JEADV). 2015;29(8):1631–5. Epub 2014/09/03.

65. Ko MJ, Chiu HC, Jee SH, Hu FC, Tseng CH. Postprandial blood glucose is associated with generalized pruritus in patients with type 2 diabetes. Eur J Dermatol (EJD). 2013;23(5):688–93. Epub 2013/09/05.

66. Machado-Pinto J, Diniz Mdos S, Bavoso NC. Psoriasis: new comorbidities. An Bras Dermatol. 2016;91(1):8–14. Epub 2016/03/18.

67. Azfar RS, Seminara NM, Shin DB, Troxel AB, Margolis DJ, Gelfand JM. Increased risk of diabetes mellitus and likelihood of receiving diabetes mellitus treatment in patients with psoriasis. Arch Dermatol. 2012;148(9):995–1000. Epub 2012/06/20.

68. Li W, Han J, Hu FB, Curhan GC, Qureshi AA. Psoriasis and risk of type 2 diabetes among women and men in the United States: a population-based cohort study. J Invest Dermatol. 2012;132(2):291–8. Epub 2011/10/14.

69. Boehncke WH, Schon MP. Psoriasis. Lancet. 2015;386(9997):983–94. Epub 2015/05/31.

70. Griffiths CE, Barker JN. Pathogenesis and clinical features of psoriasis. Lancet. 2007;370(9583):263–71. Epub 2007/07/31.

71. Wu JJ, Lynde CW, Kleyn CE, Iversen L, van der Walt JM, Carvalho A, et al. Identification of key research needs for topical therapy treatment of psoriasis – a consensus paper by the International Psoriasis Council. J Eur Acad Dermatol Venereol (JEADV). 2016. Epub 2016/03/13.

72. Ezzedine K, Eleftheriadou V, Whitton M, van Geel N. Vitiligo. Lancet. 2015;386(9988):74–84. Epub 2015/01/19.

73. Gopal KV, Rao GR, Kumar YH. Increased prevalence of thyroid dysfunction and diabetes mellitus in Indian vitiligo patients: a case-control study. Indian Dermatol Online J. 2014;5(4):456–60. Epub 2014/11/15.

74. Iannella G, Greco A, Didona D, Didona B, Granata G, Manno A, et al. Vitiligo: pathogenesis, clinical variants and treatment approaches. Autoimmun Rev. 2016;15(4):335–43. Epub 2016/01/03.

75. Seyhan M, Ozcan H, Sahin I, Bayram N, Karincaoglu Y. High prevalence of glucose metabolism disturbance in patients with lichen planus. Diabetes Res Clin Pract. 2007;77(2):198–202. Epub 2007/02/06.

76. Albrecht M, Banoczy J, Dinya E, Tamas G Jr. Occurrence of oral leukoplakia and lichen planus in diabetes mellitus. J Oral Pathol Med: Off Publ Int Assoc Oral Pathol Am Acad Oral Pathol. 1992;21(8):364–6. Epub 1992/09/11.

77. Le Cleach L, Chosidow O. Clinical practice. Lichen planus. N Engl J Med. 2012;366(8):723–32. Epub 2012/02/24.

78. Li X, Xu G, Chen J. Tissue engineered skin for diabetic foot ulcers: a meta-analysis. Int J Clin Exp Med. 2015;8(10):18191–6. Epub 2016/01/16.

79. Blanes JI. Consensus document on treatment of infections in diabetic foot. Rev Esp Quimioterapia: Publ Off Soc Esp Quimioterapia. 2011;24(4):233–62. Epub 2011/12/17.

80. Apelqvist J, Bakker K, van Houtum WH, Nabuurs-Franssen MH, Schaper NC. International consensus and practical guidelines on the management and the prevention of the diabetic foot. International Working Group on the Diabetic Foot. Diabetes Metab Res Rev. 2000;16(Suppl 1):S84–92. Epub 2000/10/31.

81. O'Loughlin A, McIntosh C, Dinneen SF, O'Brien T. Review paper: basic concepts to novel therapies: a review of the diabetic foot. Int J Lower Extrem Wounds. 2010;9(2):90–102. Epub 2010/05/21.

82. Benkhadoura M, Alswehly M, Elbarsha A. Clinical profile and surgical management of diabetic foot in Benghazi, Libya. Foot Ankle Surg: Off J Eur Soc Foot Ankle Surg. 2016;22(1):55–8. Epub 2016/02/13.

83. do Amaral Junior AH, do Amaral LA, Bastos MG, do Nascimento LC, Alves MJ, de Andrade MA. Prevention of lower-limb lesions and reduction of morbidity in diabetic patients. Rev Bras Ortop. 2014;49(5):482–7. Epub 2015/08/01.

84. Varma AK. Charcot neuroarthropathy of the foot and ankle: a review. J Foot Ankle Surg: Off Publ Am Coll Foot Ankle Surg. 2013;52(6):740–9. Epub 2013/08/24.

85. Fernando ME, Seneviratne RM, Tan YM, Lazzarini PA, Sangla KS, Cunningham M, et al. Intensive versus conventional glycaemic control for treating diabetic foot ulcers. Cochrane Database Syst Rev. 2016;1:CD010764. Epub 2016/01/14.

86. Elraiyah T, Domecq JP, Prutsky G, Tsapas A, Nabhan M, Frykberg RG, et al. A systematic review and meta-analysis of debridement methods for chronic diabetic foot ulcers. J Vasc Surg. 2016;63(2 Suppl):37S–45S. e2. Epub 2016/01/26.

87. Elraiyah T, Tsapas A, Prutsky G, Domecq JP, Hasan R, Firwana B, et al. A systematic review and meta-analysis of adjunctive therapies in diabetic foot ulcers. J Vasc Surg. 2016;63(2 Suppl):46S–58S. e2. Epub 2016/01/26.

88. Schade VL, Andersen CA. A literature-based guide to the conservative and surgical management of the

acute Charcot foot and ankle. Diabet Foot Ankle. 2015;6:26627. Epub 2015/03/22.

89. La Fontaine J, Lavery L, Jude E. Current concepts of Charcot foot in diabetic patients. Foot (Edinb). 2015;26:7–14. Epub 2016/01/24.

90. Sommer TC, Lee TH. Charcot foot: the diagnostic dilemma. Am Fam Physician. 2001;64(9):1591–8. Epub 2001/12/04.

91. Petrova NL, Edmonds ME. Acute Charcot neuro-osteoarthropathy. Diabetes Metab Res Rev. 2016;32(Suppl 1):281–6. Epub 2015/10/10.

92. Ameen M, Lear JT, Madan V, Mohd Mustapa MF, Richardson M. British Association of Dermatologists' guidelines for the management of onychomycosis 2014. Br J Dermatol. 2014;171(5):937–58. Epub 2014/11/21.

93. Long B, Koyfman A. Mucormycosis: what emergency physicians need to know? Am J Emerg Med. 2015;33(12):1823–5. Epub 2015/10/11.

94. Papanas N, Maltezos E. The diabetic hand: a forgotten complication? J Diabetes Complicat. 2010;24(3):154–62. Epub 2009/02/17.

95. Cherqaoui R, McKenzie S, Nunlee-Bland G. Diabetic cheiroarthropathy: a case report and review of the literature. Case Rep Endocrinol. 2013;2013:257028. Epub 2013/06/14.

96. Gerrits EG, Landman GW, Nijenhuis-Rosien L, Bilo HJ. Limited joint mobility syndrome in diabetes mellitus: a minireview. World J Diabetes. 2015;6(9):1108–12. Epub 2015/08/13.

97. Silva MB, Skare TL. Musculoskeletal disorders in diabetes mellitus. Rev Bras Reumatol. 2012;52(4):601–9. Epub 2012/08/14.

98. Abbas ZG, Archibald LK. Tropical diabetic hand syndrome. Epidemiology, pathogenesis, and management. Am J Clin Dermatol. 2005;6(1):21–8. Epub 2005/01/29.

99. Ince B, Dadaci M, Arslan A, Altuntas Z, Evrenos MK, Fatih Karsli M. Factors determining poor prognostic outcomes following diabetic hand infections. Pak J Med Sci. 2015;31(3):532–7. Epub 2015/07/08.

100. Coppini DV, Best C. A case of hand ulceration in the diabetic foot clinic – a reminder of hand neuropathy in 'at risk' patients. Diabet Med: J Br Diabet Assoc. 2000;17(9):682–3. Epub 2000/10/29.

Diseases of Thyroid

36

Sérgio Ivan Torres Dornelles,
Carlos Alberto Werutsky, Ana Eliza
Antunes Bomfim, Camila Boff,
and Renan Rangel Bonamigo

Key Points Summary

- Hyperthyroidism and hypothyroidism are disorders with important interaction with the skin
- Iodine intake levels below and above the recommended level are associated with the occurrence of thyroid disorders
- Thyroid hormone deficiency causes thickening, hyperkeratosis, diffuse loss of scalp hair, and nail atrophy
- Generalized myxedema is a severe disease that may occur in hypothyroidism, when mucin is deposited in the skin and other organs resulting in a series of dermatologic and systemic outcomes
- Pretibial myxedema is less frequent, being present in only 5% of cases of Graves' disease. About 90% of pretibial myxedema patients have hyperthyroidism
- Thyroid acropachy is a rare manifestation of thyroid autoimmune disease and can display finger or toe clubbing and edema
- Thyroglossal cyst and cutaneous metastases of thyroid cancer are other diseases associated with the thyroid gland

S.I.T. Dornelles (✉)
Sanitary Dermatology Service of Health Department of Rio Grande do Sul State (ADS-SES), Porto Alegre, Brazil
e-mail: sidornelles@terra.com.br

C.A. Werutsky
Nutrology and Endocrinology, Hospital 9 de Julho, São Paulo, Brazil

A.E.A. Bomfim
Sanitary Dermatology Service of Health Department of Rio Grande do Sul State (ADS-SES), Porto Alegre, Brazil

Department of Dermatology, Clinica Duarte, Pelotas, RS, Brazil

C. Boff
Sanitary Dermatology Service of the Department of Health of Rio Grande do Sul State, Porto Alegre, Brazil

R.R. Bonamigo
Dermatology Service, Hospital de Clínicas de Porto Alegre (HCPA), Federal University of Rio Grande do Sul (UFRGS), Porto Alegre, Brazil

Sanitary Dermatology Service of the Department of Health of Rio Grande do Sul State (ADS-SES), Porto Alegre, Brazil

Graduate Pathology Program of Federal University of Health Sciences of Porto Alegre, Porto Alegre, Brazil

Epidemiology

Thyroid diseases are considered very frequent diseases. Estimates report that hyperthyroidism affects about 2% of the general population, with a 15% increase among the elderly, occurring predominantly in females and in iodine ingestion–deficient regions [1]. Congenital hypothyroidism (cretinism) has an incidence of 1 case per 4000 births; 19% are

© Springer International Publishing Switzerland 2018
R.R. Bonamigo, S.I.T. Dornelles (eds.), *Dermatology in Public Health Environments*,
https://doi.org/10.1007/978-3-319-33919-1_36

sporadic and 5% are genetic. Hashimoto's thyroiditis mainly affects women between the ages of 30 and 50 years, with a female-to-male ratio of 7:1. Postpartum thyroiditis occurs in about 8–10% of women [2]. Hyperthyroidism has a lower prevalence (2% in women and 0.2% in men (English data)) [1]. Regarding Graves' ophthalmopathy in the general population, there are incidence reports of 16 women and 3 men in every 100,000 population per year [3].

Among many dermatologic manifestations, pruritus sine materia seems to be a significant manifestation of thyroidopathies (Artantas et al. [4] report a pruritus prevalence of 2.7% in patients with thyroid disturbances).

The Thyroid and the Environment

Iodine (as iodide) is widely but unevenly distributed in the earth's environment. Most iodide is found in the oceans (about 50 μg/L), and iodide ions in the seawater oxidize to form elemental iodine, which is volatile and evaporates into the atmosphere and returns to the soil through rain, completing the cycle. However, the cycle of iodine in many regions is slow and incomplete, and soils and groundwater become deficient in iodine. Crops grown in these soils will contain low iodine concentrations, and humans and animals consuming food grown in these soils become deficient in iodine [2].

Iodine consists of 65% and 59% of the weights of thyroxine (T4) and tri-iodothyronine (T3), respectively. Thyroid function is crucial for the metabolism of almost all tissues and for the development of the central nervous system in fetuses and children.

Iodine deficiency is the result of insufficient dietary iodine intake, and the physiologic consequence is abnormal thyroid function, hypothyroidism, and goiter [3]. In nearly all regions affected by iodine deficiency, the most effective way to control iodine deficiency is through salt iodization. The World Health Organization / United Nations Children's Fund / International Council for the Control of the Iodine Deficiency Disorders (WHO/UNICEF/ICCIDD) recommends that iodine be added at a concentration of 20–40 mg iodine/kg of salt, depending on local salt intake [3].

A sudden increase in iodine intake in an iodine-deficient population may induce thyroid autoimmunity. It is well established that individual patients with autoimmune thyroiditis may develop hypothyroidism when exposed to excess iodine. Considering the very frequent occurrence of thyroid autoimmunity in the population, it would be expected that a high iodine intake would be associated with a high frequency of subclinical (with elevated serum thyroid-stimulating hormone (TSH) but a free T4 estimate within the reference range) and overt (elevated TSH and a low estimate of free T4) hypothyroidism, and this has indeed been convincingly demonstrated [4, 5].

Four methods are generally recommended to assess iodine intake: urinary iodine concentration, goiter rate, serum TSH, and serum thyroglobulin [4]. The spectrum of disorders that somehow depend on the iodine intake level of the population can be based on the median or range of urinary iodine concentrations, or both. High intake of iodine results in a urinary iodine concentration of 100–200 μg/L. Below these concentrations (50–25 μg/L) insufficient iodine intake occurs, resulting in diseases ranging from cretinism and low IQ to goiter with hypothyroidism or hyperthyroidism. High urinary concentrations of iodine (>300 μg/L) may result in early Graves' disease (GD) [2].

Thus, the thyroid gland contains an advanced set of processes that may enhance or block the use of iodine for thyroid hormone production. Because the processes activated with low and high iodine intakes are different, the type of disease that dominates thyroid pathology in populations may be different depending on the level of iodine intake.

Skin Manifestations of Hyperthyroidism

Hyperthyroidism, or excess circulating thyroid hormone, results from a disturbance in any portion of the hypothalamic-pituitary-thyroid axis. In normal subjects, TSH is made by the pituitary gland and stimulates the thyroid gland to generate and secrete T4 (thyroxine) and T3 (triiodothyronine). In the periphery, T4 is converted into T3 by enzymes mainly in the liver and kidney. T3 (and to some extent T4) then binds to specific nuclear receptors in the tissues (e.g., heart, brain, muscle, and perhaps skin) and mediates the thyroid hormone action [6].

Furthermore, the amount of T4 and T3 secreted by the thyroid gland is regulated by a negative feedback system of the pituitary gland. Specifically, when the body recognizes it has excess thyroid hormone levels, T3 (and T4) binds to the TSH gene regulatory elements in the pituitary gland and inhibits TSH production [7].

Hyperthyroidism is more commonly seen in women than in men (5:1 ratio). The most characteristic (although rare) skin finding in GD is pretibial myxedema, although other more common cutaneous manifestations of hyperthyroidism include warm, flushed, moist skin, with generalized increased sweating [7, 8].

The skin changes, and the hair may become thin and soft; loss of scalp, eyebrow, axillary, pubic, or body hair is common. Hair loss without scarring (alopecia areata) is most often associated with autoimmune disease (GD) [9].

Up to 25% of patients with GD have clinically obvious Graves' ophthalmopathy at the time of the diagnosis of hyperthyroidism [9].

The nails may become soft and friable, and separation of the distal nail plate from the nail bed may occur, producing Plummer's nails [10].

A definitive treatment of hyperthyroidism varies depending on the etiology of the disorder, but usually involves rendering the patient euthyroid with antithyroid drugs (i.e., methimazole or propylthiouracil).

These antithyroid agents can cause pruritic erythematous skin rash, hepatotoxicity, arthralgias, or bone marrow suppression [11].

The implementation of a definitive therapy may include long-term antithyroid agents, radioactive iodine therapy, or thyroidectomy. It requires radioactive iodine from 2 to 3 months to cause hypothyroidism [6].

The skin manifestations associated with hyperthyroidism are classically cleared with treatment of the underlying cause of the hyperthyroidism state as described below [10].

Etiopathogenesis

GD results from stimulation of the TSH receptor through receptor-binding antibodies. Thus, the usual negative report promoted by the T3 and T4 levels of TSH production by the hypophysis is interrupted. The outcome of this abnormal mechanism is excessive T3 and T4 in the peripheral circulation, which entails the clinical manifestations of hyperthyroidism. High levels of T3 and T4 promote the usually seen clinical symptoms of the disease, such as nervousness, anxiety, weight loss, heat intolerance, fatigue, muscle weakness, and palpitations [12].

The dermatologic and ophthalmologic manifestations specific to the thyroid diseases result from the autoimmune effects of antibodies of the TSH, rather than being related to the circulating thyroid hormone levels. In the dermatologic diseases nonspecific to the cutaneous thyroid, alterations are directly related to the circulating levels of T3 and T4 [12].

Clinical Presentation

Dermatologic manifestations of hyperthyroidism vary. The skin is warm, soft, humid, blushed, and tender, and an association with cutaneous pruritus is frequent. Hyperhidrosis may be noticed mainly in the hand palms and feet soles [4].

The hair may become thinner and soft, and hair loss in the scalp, eyebrows, axillae, pubic area, or throughout the body is common.

Complementary Examinations

The blood dosage of free TSH, T3, and T4 levels added to the clinical signs and symptoms of hyperthyroidism seal the diagnosis.

Therapeutic Approach

Treatment includes normalizing the thyroid function, either through medication or the thyroid function ablation [12, 13].

Special Considerations

Graves Ophthalmopathy

Thyroid ophthalmopathy is an autoimmune orbit disease closely associated with GD, although both conditions may exist separately [13].

Around 20–25% of GD patients have ophthalmopathy [14]. The ophthalmopathy develops before the hyperthyroidism presentation in around 20% of patients; concomitantly in 40%; and in 40% of the cases 6 months after the diagnosis [15]. It is worth bearing in mind that the ocular disease may become evident after hyperthyroidism treatment, usually in patients treated with radioiodine [16].

Etiopathogenesis

The most often accepted theory to explain the association between thyroid ophthalmopathy and autoimmune thyroid disease is a possible cross-relationship of sensitized T lymphocytes and/or antibodies against the thyroid and the orbit common antigens [17].

The volume of retro-orbital connective and adipose tissue and the volume of extraocular muscles are increased by cell proliferation, inflammation, and glycosaminoglycan accumulation, mainly hyaluronic acid. Glycosaminoglycan secretion by the fibroblasts is activated by the T-cell cytokines (tumor necrosis factor, interferon-γ), thus showing that T- and B-cell activation is important for the immunopathogenesis of Graves' ophthalmopathy. Glycosaminoglycan accumulation brings about changes in the osmotic pressure which lead to liquid accumulation, muscular edema, and increased pressure inside the orbit. These changes, with the addition of retro-orbital adipogenesis, move the eyeball outside, possibly also interfering in the function of the extraocular muscles and the orbit's venous drainage [12, 13].

Clinical Presentation

The extraocular muscles are the main impaired targets and show increased volume, and together with other important clinical signs determined by inflammatory changes and/or vascular congestion include upper and lower eyelid retraction, conjunctival hyperemia, and preorbital edema [17, 18], as well as sequelae of extraocular mus-

cle hypertrophy translated into visual loss that results from corneal ulceration, secondary to proptosis and optical neuropathy by compression of the optic nerve [17, 19]. Exophthalmos is almost always bilateral and symmetric. The lower rectus muscle is the most often involved muscle followed by the medial rectus, the upper rectus, and the lateral rectus muscles (Figs. 36.1 and 36.2).

Complementary Examinations

The diagnosis is clinical, and imaging methods are indicated when the diagnosis is difficult or an optical neuropathy is suspected [17, 18]. Computed tomography (CT) and magnetic resonance imaging (MRI) are useful to confirm the diagnosis through visualization of the muscle hypertrophy and the orbital fat, and also to assess the critical area of the orbital apex. Often the only finding is increased orbital fat, with resulting proptosis [20].

Therapeutic Approach

Patients are treated according to the degree of disease impairment, always having in mind that most

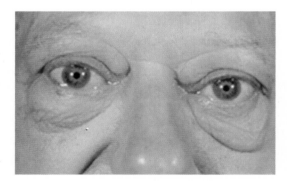

Fig. 36.1 Thyroid ophthalmopathy

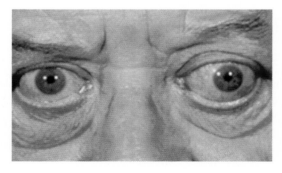

Fig. 36.2 Another aspect of thyroid ophthalmopathy

patients display a mild disease with no progression during the follow-up. Graves' ophthalmopathy patients display hyperthyroidism reversal (when present), symptom relief, and decreased periorbital tissue inflammation [13, 21].

Symptom treatment comprises the use of artificial tears, raised head during sleeping hours, facial support when sleeping, and use of blinders that are often enough for symptom relief. Photophobia and sensitivity to wind or cold air can be reduced with sunglasses [13, 22]. Some studies suggest that use of selenium (100 μg 2×/day, over 6 months) may improve soft tissue edema, besides the implementation of quality-of-life measures, although such results require confirmation [23].

For patients with eye inflammation (red eyes) and increased diplopia and proptosis, a corticosteroid (prednisone 30 mg/day for 4 weeks) course should be started. If large doses are necessary they are intravenously administered. Cases whereby vision is lost, usually preceded by color vision loss, require the patient to immediately undergo corticosteroid therapy (intramuscular dexamethasone 4 mg, or prednisone 100 mg orally) and hospital admission for probable surgical decompression. Rituximab, radiation, and surgical decompression can be also used in select cases [13, 22, 24–26].

Pretibial Myxedema

The cutaneous manifestations of GD may result from excessive thyroid circulating hormone or from the autoimmune nature of GD [27, 28]. The most common clinical findings are ophthalmopathy, acropachy, and pretibial myxedema; the presence of the three findings make up the classic triad of GD, present in only 1% of cases [29].

Pretibial myxedema is a less often seen manifestation, present in only 5% of GD cases and in 15% of cases of patients with GD and ophthalmopathy [30]. About 90% of the patients with pretibial myxedema have hyperthyroidism and 10% are hypothyroid or euthyroid patients, although all of them display laboratory evidence of autoimmune thyroid disease [31]. About 50%

of the pretibial myxedema cases occur after the patient undergoes treatment for thyroidopathy either with radioactive iodine or thyroidectomy [32]. The ophthalmopathy is associated with most of the cases, usually coming before pretibial myxedema occurring within 1–2 years [31]. Its incidence has decreased possibly due to the early diagnosis and treatment implementation for GD. Contrary to what is prompted by its name, it is not limited to the pretibial area, and can reach the ankles and the feet dorsa, and be present in the elbows, knees, upper portion of the trunk and neck [33].

Etiopathogenesis

Pretibial myxedema results from glycosaminoglycan accumulation, specifically hyaluronic acid secreted by cytokine-stimulated fibroblasts. By showing the expression of the TSH receptor proteins by the dermis fibroblasts, the possibility arises that antibodies and/or T-cell-specific antigens start an inflammatory reaction that stimulates glycosaminoglycan production; excessive glycosaminoglycans are deposited in the dermis and the subcutaneous tissue [34–37].

Clinical Presentation

Pretibial myxedema is characterized by a bilateral asymmetric cutaneous thickening, usually with one or more less delimited papules or nodules that can display different diameters [37]. There is color variation from yellowish chestnut to violet, and an "orange skin" aspect due to the cutaneous thickening associated with the follicular prominence is frequently noticed [31, 37]. Lesions are usually asymptomatic although they can be pruritic or even painful [37]. Hyperpigmentation, hyperkeratosis, and hyperhidrosis may also be present. The most frequent sites include the medium and lower third of the pretibial region and, occasionally, the feet dorsa (Fig. 36.3). Other impaired regions are seldom noticed, although there are reports of atypical location, such as the fingers, hands, upper limbs, torso, shoulder, and face, albeit that in most of those reports there was history of trauma, vaccination, local scar, or surgery [31, 32, 37].

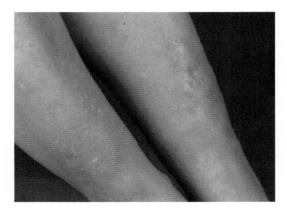

Fig. 36.3 Pretibial myxedema

The lesions usually develop along many months and then stabilize, or, in some cases, spontaneously recede [37]. Rarely the lesions evolve and reach the feet, hands, or legs, in such cases showing a more elephantiasis format [31, 32].

The differential diagnosis can be made with stasis dermatitis, cutaneous mucinosis (in lupus erythematosus, dermatomyositis, scleroderma), amyloidosis, hypertrophic lichen planus, and lipoid necrobiosis [33].

Complementary Examinations

The diagnosis of pretibial myxedema is based on the GD history and clinical characteristics of the lesion (location, nonpitting nature, and badly delimited margins). A biopsy is seldom necessary for the diagnosis, although it can be required when patients display disease-suggestive lesions but with no history of thyroid disease.

Therapeutic Approach

Most of the cases do not require treatment, with resolution occurring some years later. Treatment indications include pruritus, local discomfort, or aesthetic reasons. It is wise, nevertheless, to treat all new lesions so that they do not undergo a chronic process. Treatment encompasses minimization of the risk factors: quitting smoking, weight loss, and treatment of the disturbed thyroid. Improvement in thyroid function does not necessarily improve the myxedema [33]. As initial therapy, medium-to high-potency corticosteroids, with or without

occlusion, are indicated; no improvement after 4–12 weeks of treatment leads to the use of intralesional corticosteroid, mainly for a presentation such as plaques and nodules [38]. Some authors support the use of compression stockings (20–30 mmHg) for lymphedema improvement [33, 37]. There are reports of pentoxifylline used in resistant cases [39]. Other reports mention rituximab and plasmapheresis in severely affected patients [40–43]. Immunoglobulin was effective in a series of noncontrolled cases [44]. When trauma is a precipitating factor of disease recurrence, surgical treatments must be avoided.

Thyroid Acropachy

The exact incidence of acropachy is not known, although estimates refer to 0.1–1% of GD patients [45].

Etiopathogenesis

Acropachy pathogenesis is similar to that of dermopathy. A research study investigated whether fibroblast activation in the periosteum and mucin deposition may be a triggering factor [46].

Clinical Presentation

Thyroid acropachy is a rare manifestation of thyroid autoimmune disease, present in extreme forms of dermopathy, and possibly showing finger or toe edema and clubbing. More seldom seen is acropachy together with distal arthritis [46]. It is part of the acropachy, pretibial myxedema, and ophthalmopathy triad [45].

Three manifestations of acropachy are noticed: finger and toe clubbing (88%); edema, and hardening of the skin of fingers and toes (20%); and presentation of arthritis and periostitis (10%) [46].

The most ordinary form of acropachy is digital clubbing, which occurs in 20% of dermatopathic patients. Digital edema and periosteal reaction in adjacent bone is the total clinical presentation, though less often seen. Thyroid acropachy always occurs in association with Graves' ophthalmopathy and thyroid dermopathy. Involvement of joints is unusual. Acropachy is not usually painful, although some patients have pain and function loss due to severe edema [45, 47].

Complementary Examinations

Skin biopsy shows typical pretibial myxedema findings, including fibroblast activation and glycosaminoglycan deposits [48]. The diagnosis is made with a combination of the thyroid disease history, clinical characteristics typical of ophthalmopathy and pretibial myxedema, and radiographic features of the hands and feet [45]. Fusiform edema of the soft tissues both in the patient's fingers and toes, and subperiosteal bone formation are radiographic findings. Subperiosteal reaction is uncommon in long bones [45–47].

Therapeutic Approach

There is no specific treatment available besides the basal immunologic treatment and management of the associated dermopathy. Painful acropachy periostitis requires use of anti-inflammatory agents [47].

Skin Manifestations of Hypothyroidism

Hypothyroidism, or a deficiency of thyroid hormone, is most often caused by a chronic autoimmune disease (Hashimoto's thyroiditis), but may also result from pituitary tumor or failure, iatrogenic thyroid ablation, goiter, or iodine deficiency [46].

Relatively common causes of primary hypothyroidism also include a prior history of therapy for hyperthyroidism, or a thyroidectomy (partial or total). External radiation given to the head, neck, or chest areas for lymphoma, for example, may also result in hypothyroidism [47].

Patients with hypothyroidism typically have cold, pale skin that is rough, dry, and scaly [10]. The skin may appear yellow because of carotenemia. The most characteristic skin change of hypothyroidism is myxedema, the accumulation of mucopolysaccharides in the skin. Patients seem to have puffiness around the eyes and swelling of the hands. There is often loss of the lateral third of the eyebrows, coarse brittle hair and nails, and generalized hair loss [48].

Cutaneous manifestations of Hashimoto's thyroiditis include acanthosis nigricans, alopecia, melasma, onycholysis, and vitiligo, among others [49].

The assessment of a hypothyroid patient requires a detailed history and physical examination. Many clinicians will also obtain a thyroid sonogram if there is a suspicion for nodules. Serum tests will include TSH initially (with T4 and T3 added if TSH is abnormal or if there is suspicion of central hypothyroidism), as well as measurement of thyroid peroxidase antibodies.

Once the diagnosis is made, the process involves levothyroxine administration, although it will not directly help the autoimmune-mediated aspects of the disease, such as pretibial myxedema and ophthalmopathy [50].

General Skin Manifestations and Generalized Myxedema

Endemic cretinism can result from iodine deficiency in the uterus, although it may result from the transplacental passage of substances that inhibit the production of thyroid hormones by interfering with iodine absorption in the thyroid gland (goitrogens). In 33% of children with congenital hypothyroidism, signs or symptoms of cutaneous abnormality are not found [51].

In Brazil, the bloodspot test ("Teste do Pezinho") is carried out up to the 30th day of life; it is now part of the Sistema Único de Saúde (SUS) (the publicly funded healthcare system) incorporated in 1992 (Portaria GM/MS no. 22, de 15 de Janeiro de 1992), with a legislation that made the test mandatory for all live newborns; it also includes assessment for phenylketonuria and congenital hypothyroidism [52].

Adult hypothyroidism develops insidiously, thus possibly persisting for many years. Adult hypothyroidism is a common type, more frequently occurring in women from 40 to 60 years old [51].

Generalized myxedema is a severe manifestation that may be seen in hypothyroidism, when mucin is deposited in the skin and other organs leading to a series of dermatologic and systemic changes [51].

Etiopathogenesis

There are no exact causes to determine the disease besides its association with low levels of thyroid hormones, associated with relevant dermal accumulations of mucopolysaccharides, mainly hyaluronic acid and chondroitin sulfate [51].

Clinical Presentation

Patients often display early tiredness, a feeling of fatigue, weakness, cramps mainly in the legs, and severe discomfort on cold days. The myxedema is characterized by typical periorbital swelling, thick lips, acral swelling, and widened tongue. Macroglossia may display a smooth and red aspect. The yellowish skin is explained by carotene accumulation in the stratum corneum (as result of the lesser hepatic conversion of β-carotene to vitamin A), and anemia [51, 53]. The carotenemia may be seen in hand palms and soles of feet, and nasolabial folds. Clavicular fat accumulation may be often noticed. The skin is dry, cold, and pale, mainly in the extension areas. Xerosis can be so severe that it may be considered a form of acquired ichthyosis. It becomes pale because of the higher levels of water and mucopolysaccharides in the dermis, which change the light refraction. It also shows a peripheral vasoconstriction that may determine features of cutis marmorata. Hypohidrosis is also noticed. The palms may become significantly drier, possibly mimicking an acquired keratoderma. The skin is diffusely swollen and becomes sturdy when touched. Despite the edematous aspect, the skin is not depressed if pressure is applied upon it. The presence of cutaneous edema may be partially explained by the hygroscopic characteristics of the mucopolysaccharides, although an increase in the transcapillary escape of albumin was shown, possibly resulting in its extravascular accumulation, thus playing a part in this edema. In addition, inappropriate lymphatic drainage can account for the development of exudates in the serous cavities that become visible in the myxedematous state [51–54].

Body and head hair may be dry and brittle. Hair loss results in partial alopecia. Irregular alopecia plaques can be noticed with persistent lanuginous hair. The eyebrows exhibit a characteristic loss of the lateral third bilaterally. Hair growth is slow. Patients with spontaneous or iatrogenic myxedema may also show a greater amount of hair in the telogen phase. This may indicate that the hypothyroidism alopecia is being mediated by hormonal effects [51–54].

The nails show a slow growth and a fragile structure.

In the myxedematous state wound scarring can be impaired, thus determining such a slow process. Purpura may sometimes be noticed as a consequence of the decrease in clotting factor, or loss of vascular support resulting from the presence of mucin in the dermis may be seen [53, 54].

Some reported uncommon observations in the literature can be deduced as actual manifestations of the hyperthyroid state. A manifestation similar to ectodermal dysplasia, possibly inherited in a recessive autosomal manner, was reported by the acronym ANOTHER (alopecia, ungual dystrophy, ophthalmologic complications, dysfunctional thyroid, hypohidrosis, ephelides and enteropathy, and respiratory tract infections) [51].

The systemic manifestations of hypothyroidism are numerous and are not covered in this chapter. It is important to know that mucin deposition also occurs in many organs other than the skin, such as the heart, intestines, and the kidneys, resulting in functional outcomes.

Complementary Examinations

The diagnosis is clinically suspected and confirmed by the low levels of free circulating T4. The TSH serum level is high in primary hypothyroidism and low in secondary hypothyroidism. Myxedema is not seen in secondary hypothyroidism [53, 54].

The anatomopathologic examination shows a mild epidermal hyperkeratosis and development of corneal plugging in the pilous follicles, and small dermal deposits of mucopolysaccharides. In the most noticeable cases edema is seen with separated collagen bundles. In some cases preeminent amounts of dermal mucin can be noticed, mainly perivascular and perifollicular. The number of elastic fibers is decreased [53].

Therapeutic Approach

If the impairment happens in newborns, immediate treatment is crucial for their appropriate mental development. This important treatment begins before the 4th month of life [53, 54].

Whatever the situation, symptoms recede when the therapy employs thyroxine.

Skin Manifestations Related to the Thyroid Gland and Not to Its Function

Thyroglossal Duct Cyst

Thyroglossal duct cyst results from a failed obliteration of the duct developed in the embryogenesis during thyroid migration, and represents the most common median line cyst. Ectopic neoplasias of the thyroid tissues are rare, and rarer if associated with this duct [55].

Etiopathogenesis

In the fourth week of fetal development the thyroid tissue is located in the pharyngeal floor, and through the thyroglossal duct this tissue migrates into its usual position in the thyroid. During the thyroid descent, the gland keeps its connection to the base of the tongue through the thyroglossal duct, and when migration is concluded the duct is obliterated at around the 8th gestational week. This channel persistence is called remnant thyroglossal duct [56].

This congenital remnant is usually noticed as a cyst coated with a secretory epithelium. Both men and women can show this condition, which can be located anywhere in the thyroglossal duct, found in 60% of the cases between the hyoid bone and the thyroid cartilage; 24% suprahyoid; 13% substernal; and 2% intralingual [57].

The diagnosis is made up to 10 years of age in about 30% of the cases; from 10 to 20 years of age in 20%; from 20 to 30 years of age in 15%, and after 30 years of age in 35% of cases. Ectopic thyroid tissue is seen in 62% of cases and is subject to the same pathology of the thyroid itself [56].

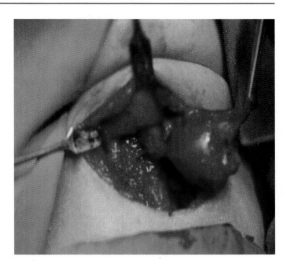

Fig. 36.4 Thyroglossal duct cyst

Clinical Presentation

The clinical presentation shows a nodular lesion of cystic consistency at the medium line of the neck at the level of the thyroid membrane. Cyst infection may happen simultaneously with episodes of airway infection, and signs of local inflammation can be seen (Fig. 36.4). A fistula secondary to the cyst infection may also be apparent [58].

Complementary Examinations

Ultrasonography of the cervical region is the method used to identify the cyst, with an accuracy of 90% [58]. When facing a doubtful diagnosis, an aspiration puncture can be conducted to confirm the presence of thyroid tissue.

Therapeutic Approach

The treatment of choice is cyst removal performed using the Sistrunk technique, comprising removal of the central part of the hyoid bone. If infection is ascertained, the use of systemic antibiotics may be necessary [36].

Thyroid Cancer and Cutaneous Metastases

Thyroid papillary carcinoma accounts for most of the cases of cancers of this type in children, usually occurring as metastases in regional lymph nodes. Papillary carcinoma is made up of Hürthle cells, usually noticed in middle-aged and elderly persons. Among the elderly population, the most common metastases are distant metastases. On the other hand, tumors of undifferentiated cells are characteristic of older people, and may predispose distant metastases besides involvement of regional lymph nodes [56].

Cutaneous metastasis is a rare event [60]. In a series of 724 patients, thyroid metastatic carcinoma accounted for less than 1% of the cutaneous metastases [61], and no thyroid metastasis was noted in a series of 4020 individuals with cutaneous metastases [62].

Etiopathogenesis

Thyroid follicular carcinoma displays metastatic dissemination mainly through hematogenous spread, which occurs in 10–15% of cases of more advanced tumors. The most often affected sites include the bones and the lungs, and less frequently the brain, liver, bladder, and skin.

In 2005 Quinn et al. described four patients with thyroid cutaneous metastasis, three men and one woman, with a medium age range of 64 years, all of whom had invasive thyroid follicular carcinoma [60]. Two of these patients displayed scalp metastases: one in the neck, and another in the sacral skin. In three cases the specific morphology and immunohistochemistry were conducted, revealing that one of these patients showed primarily spinal metastasis of characteristic morphology, although he underwent anaplastic change after treatment. Including these four cases a total of 14 were reported in the literature, with cutaneous metastasis of thyroid follicular carcinoma in most patients: that is, 10 out of 14 patients had primary site histopathology [60].

Clinical Presentation

The morphology of cutaneous metastases is variable. The lesions may manifest as macules, plaques, papules or nodules. They can imitate other conditions, such as alopecia, infections (erysipelas and paronychia), benign cysts (epidermoid or pilar), pyogenic granuloma, and

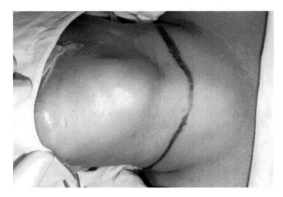

Fig. 36.5 Thyroid papilliferous carcinoma

cutaneous malignant neoplasias (basal cell carcinoma and keratoacanthoma) [63–65].

Cutaneous manifestations common to the thyroid papilliferous carcinoma are nodules in the scalp and neck [63, 66, 67], and lesions in the scar of thyroidectomy [68]. A metastatic tumor at the site of thin-needle aspiration biopsy was also noticed by Tamiolakis et al. [67]. Cutaneous metastases of thyroid papillary carcinoma have also been described on the abdominal wall, arms, buttocks, thoracic wall, face, shoulders, and thighs [60] (Fig. 36.5).

Cutaneous thyroid metastases can occur after an early diagnosis of thyroid cancer, thus making the cutaneous lesion diagnosis easier, as well as being the first identified manifestation of the pathology. Since cutaneous lesions are accessible to clinical examination and patient visualization, they may easily trigger the investigation leading to the primary site of the neoplasia.

Complementary Examinations

Complementary examinations are crucial to the proper identification of the cutaneous metastases because they allow the identification of the lesion's primary site.

Anatomopathologic examination of cutaneous metastases of papilliferous carcinoma and thyroid follicular carcinoma also show characteristics similar to those of the primary site. Immunohistochemistry may be also useful for diagnostic confirmation and exclusion of tumors originating in other organs.

Thyroid papillary and follicular carcinomas express the thyroid transcription factor 1 (TTF-1) and thyroglobulin (a glycoprotein synthesized in the cytoplasm of the thyroid follicular cells, and detected in 95% of papillary carcinomas) [69].

Therapeutic Approach

The therapeutic approach is determined according to clinical staging of the neoplasia. Management includes a partial or total thyroidectomy followed by adjuvant radiotherapy to treat invasion of the cervical region. It can be associated with chemotherapy with isolated doxorubicin, or associated with other chemotherapeutic agents, as well as the use of radioactive iodine. Molecular targeted therapy aimed at specific receptors has shown promising outcomes.

The prognosis for patients with thyroid metastatic papilliferous carcinoma of the skin is usually unfavorable [64, 66]. There are, nevertheless, individuals with thyroid cutaneous metastases who survived many years after the diagnosis [68, 66, 70]. Furthermore, with the advent of molecular targeted therapies, such as tyrosine kinase inhibitors, the prognosis for patients with metastatic disease, and mainly for those with a rearrangement during aberrant transcription of the oncogenesis (RET), is better than the observed prognosis in individuals with thyroid papilliferous carcinoma who underwent treatment before the discovery of these agents [71].

Glossary

Cutis marmorata   Manifests as skin changes displaying violet spots on the trunk and limbs, which can be highlighted by cold temperature.

Diplopia   The condition when an individual sees two images of the same object.

Glycosaminoglycans   Components of the connective tissue. They represent 30% of the body's organic material and can exist as different types, such as chondroitin sulfate for cartilage, bone, or cornea; dermatan sulfate for the dermis and the tendons; and heparan sulfate for the liver, lungs, and aorta.

Hyaluronic acid   A biopolymer made of the glucuronic acid and N-acetylglucosamine. With a viscous texture, it exists in the synovial fluid, the vitreous humor, and the connective tissue of numerous organisms, being an important glycosaminoglycan in articulation composition.

Lymphedema   The accumulation of interstitial fluid rich in proteins of high molecular weight.

Macroglossia   The abnormal growth of the tongue so that it reaches a size larger than the one allowed by the buccal cavity, resulting in impaired phonation and respiratory, suction, and/or swallow function.

Plasmapheresis   An extracorporeal process by which the blood collected from a patient is separated into its plasma and cell element compounds.

Proptosis   Proptosis is characterized by a displacement of the eyeball to the front of one eye, or both eyes.

Proto-oncogene (RET)   RET proto-oncogene activating mutations may result in the development of the thyroid medullary carcinoma. Its research study is useful for the genetic tracking of thyroid medullary carcinoma.

Radioactive iodine   Radioactive iodine treats hyperthyroidism by gradually shrinking the thyroid, ultimately destroying the gland.

Rituximab   A monoclonal chimeric antibody (murine/human) against an antigen that is the protein of the cell surface, CD20

Thyroxine (T4)   A hormone that plays a role in several body functions, including growth and metabolism.

Tri-iodothyronine (T3)   T3 and T4 (thyroxine) are hormones produced by the thyroid gland. They help to control the rate at which the body uses energy, and are regulated by a feedback system.

Thyroid-stimulating hormone (TSH)   TSH stimulates the production and release of T4 (primarily) and T3. As necessary, T4 is converted to T3 by the liver and other tissues.

Thyroid transcription factor 1 (TTF-1)   TTF-1 regulates the transcription of the specific genes of the thyroid, the lung, and the diencephalon. It is used in anatomic pathology as a marker to determine whether a tumor has its origin in the lung or the thyroid.

References

1. Canaris GJ, Manowitz NR, Mayor G, Ridgway EC. The Colorado thyroid disease prevalence study. Arch Intern Med. 2000;160(4):526–34.
2. Lucas A, et al. Postpartum thyroiditis: long-term follow-up. Thyroid. 2005;15:1177–81.
3. Bartley GB, Fatourechi V, Kadrmas EF, et al. The incidence of Graves' ophthalmopathy in Olmsted County, Minnesota. Am J Ophthalmol. 1995;120:511.
4. Artantas S, Gul U, KIliçm A, et al. Skin findings in thyroid diseases. Eur J Intern Med. 2009;20:158–61.
5. World Health Organization/International Council for the Control of the Iodine Deficiency Disorders/United Nations Childrens Fund (WHO/ICCIDD/UNICEF). Assessment of the iodine deficiency disorders and monitoring their elimination. WHO/NHD/01.1. Geneva: World Health Organization; 2001.
6. Zimmermann MB, Jooste PL, Pandav CS. Iodine-deficiency disorders. Lancet. 2008;372:1251–62.
7. Zimmermann MB. Assessing iodine status and monitoring progress of iodized salt programs. J Nutr. 2004;134:1673–7.
8. Bülow Pedersen I, Knudsen N, Jørgensen T, et al. Large differences in incidences of overt hyper- and hypothyroidism associated with a small difference in iodine intake: a prospective comparative register-based population survey. J Clin Endocrinol Metab. 2002;87:4462–9.
9. Burman K. Chapter 41. Hyperthyroidism. In: Becker KA, editor. Principles and practice of endocrinology and metabolism. 2nd ed. Philadelphia: J.B. Lippincott; 1995. p. 367–85.
10. Col NF, Surks MI, Daniels GH. Subclinical thyroid disease: clinical applications. JAMA. 2004;291:239–43.
11. Hollowell JG, et al. Serum TSH, T4 and thyroid antibodies in the United States population (1998–1994): National Health and Nutrition Examination Survey (NHANES III). J Clin Endocrinol Metab. 2002;87:489.
12. Champion B, Gopinath B, Ma G, El-Kaissi S, Wall JR. Conversion to Graves' hyperthyroidism in a patient with hypothyroidism due to Hashimoto's thyroiditis documented by real-time thyroid ultrasonography. Thyroid. 2008;18:1135–7.
13. Jabbour SA, Miller JI. Review article: endocrinopathies and the skin. Int J Dermatol. 2000;39(2):88–99.
14. Cooper DS. Antithyroid drugs. N Engl J Med. 2005;352(9):905–17.
15. Kd B, Mckinley-Grant L. Dermatologic aspects of thyroid disease. Clin Dermatol. 2006;24:247–55.
16. Bahn RS. Graves' ophthalmopathy. N Engl J Med. 2010;362:726.
17. Burch HB, Wartofsky L. Graves' ophthalmopathy: current concepts regarding pathogenesis and management. Endocr Rev. 1993;14:747.
18. Bartley GB, Fatourechi V, Kadrmas EF, et al. Chronology of Graves' ophthalmopathy in an incidence cohort. Am J Ophthalmol. 1996;121:426.
19. Tallstedt L, Lundell G, Tørring O, et al. Occurrence of ophthalmopathy after treatment for Graves' hyperthyroidism. The thyroid study group. N Engl J Med. 1992;326:1733.
20. Cakirer S, Cakirer D, Basak M, et al. Evaluation of extraocular muscles in the edematous phase of Graves ophthalmopathy on contrast-enhanced fat-suppressed magnetic resonance imaging. J Comput Assist Tomogr. 2004;28:80–6.
21. El-Kaissi S, Frauman AG, Wall JR. Thyroid-associated ophthalmopathy: a practical guide to classification, natural history and management. Intern Med J. 2004;34:482–91.
22. Fung S, Malhotra R, Selva D. Thyroid orbitopathy. Aust Fam Physician. 2003;31:615–20.
23. Mafee MF. Orbit: embryology, anatomy and pathology. In: Som PM, Curtin HD, editors. Head and neck imaging. 4th ed. St Louis: Mosby; 2003. p. 529–654.
24. Prummel MF, Wiersinga WM. Medical management of Graves' ophthalmopathy. Thyroid. 1995;5:231.
25. Stiebel-Kalish H, Robenshtok E, Hasanreisoglu M, et al. Treatment modalities for Graves' ophthalmopathy: systematic review and metaanalysis. J Clin Endocrinol Metab. 2009;94:2708.
26. Marcocci C, Kahaly GJ, Krassas GE, et al. Selenium and the course of mild Graves' orbitopathy. N Engl J Med. 2011;364:1920.
27. Wiersinga WM. Immunosuppressive treatment of Graves' ophthalmopathy. Thyroid. 1992;2:229.
28. Bartalena L, Marcocci C, Bogazzi F, et al. Use of corticosteroids to prevent progression of Graves' ophthalmopathy after radioiodine therapy for hyperthyroidism. N Engl J Med. 1989;321:1349.
29. Sridama V, DeGroot LJ. Treatment of Graves' disease and the course of ophthalmopathy. Am J Med. 1989;87:70.
30. Jabbour SA. Cutaneous manifestations of endocrine disorders: a guide for dermatologists. Am J Clin Dermatol. 2003;4:315–31.
31. Kenneth D. Dermatologic aspects of thyroid disease. Clin Dermatol. 2006;24:247–55.
32. Anderson CK. Triad of exophthalmos, pretibial myxedema, andacropachy in a patient with Graves' disease. J Am Acad Dermatol. 2003;48:970–2.
33. Fatourechi V, Pajouhi M, Fransway AF. Dermopathy of Graves disease (pretibial myxedema). Review of 150 cases. Medicine (Baltimore). 1994;73:1.
34. Fatourechi V. Pretibial myxedema – pathophysiology and treatment options. Am J Clin Dermatol. 2005;6(5):295–309.
35. Gopie P, Naraynsingh V. Severe pretibial myxedema. Int J Low Extrem Wounds. 2011;10(2):91–2.
36. Doshi DN, Blyumin ML, Kimball AB. Cutaneous manifestations of thyroid disease. Clin Dermatol. 2008;26:283–7.
37. Shishido M, Kuroda K, Tsukifuji R, et al. A case of pretibial myxedema associated with Graves' disease: an immunohistochemical study of serum-derived hyaluronan-associated protein. J Dermatol. 1995;22:948.

38. Bull RH, Coburn PR, Mortimer PS. Pretibial myxoedema: a manifestation of lymphoedema? Lancet. 1993;341:403.

39. Ajjan RA, Watson PF, Weetman AP. Cytokines and thyroid function. Adv Neuroimmunol. 1996;6:359.

40. Ai J, Leonhardt JM, Heymann WR. Autoimmune thyroid diseases: etiology, pathogenesis, and dermatologic manifestations. J Am Acad Dermatol. 2003;48:641–59.

41. Takasu N, Higa H, Kinjou Y. Treatment of pretibial myxedema (PTM) with topical steroid ointment application with sealing cover (steroid occlusive dressing technique: steroid ODT) in Graves' patients. Intern Med. 2010;49:665.

42. Engin B, Gümüşel M, Ozdemir M, Cakir M. Successful combined pentoxifylline and intralesional triamcinolone acetonide treatment of severe pretibial myxedema. Dermatol Online J. 2007;13:16.

43. Heyes C, Nolan R, Leahy M, Gebauer K. Treatment-resistant elephantiasic thyroid dermopathy responding to rituximab and plasmapheresis. Australas J Dermatol. 2012;53:e1.

44. Antonelli A, Navarranne A, Palla R, et al. Pretibial myxedema and high-dose intravenous immunoglobulin treatment. Thyroid. 1994;4:399.

45. Vanhoenacker FM, Pelckmans MC, De Beuckeleer LH, Colpaert CG, De Schepper AM. Thyroid acropachy: correlation of imaging and pathology. Eur Radiol. 2001;11:1058–62.

46. Fatourechi V, Ahmed DD, Schwartz KM. Thyroid acropachy: report of 40 patients treated at a single institution in a 26-year period. J Clin Endocrinol Metab. 2002;87:5435–41.

47. Bartalena L, Fatourechi V. Extrathyroidal manifestations of Graves' disease: a 2014 update. J Endocrinol Investig. 2014;37(8):691–700.

48. Fatourechi V. Thyroid dermopathy and acropachy. Expert Rev Dermatol. 2011;6:75–905.

49. Weismann K, Graham R. Systemic disease and the skin. In: Champion R, Burton J, Burns D, Breathnach S, editors. Rook/Wilkinson/Ebling textbook of dermatology. Oxford: Blackwell Science; 1998. p. 2703–57.

50. Wang SA, Rahemtullah A, Faquin WC, et al. Hodgkin's lymphoma of the thyroid: a clinicopathologic study of five cases and review of the literature. Mod Pathol. 2005;18(12):1577–84.

51. Thiboutot DM. Clinical review: dermatological manifestations of endocrine disorders. J Clin Endocrinol Metab. 1995;80(10):3082–7.

52. Santos HMGP, Vargas PR, Carvalho TM. Manual de normas técnicas e rotinas operacionais do programa nacional de triagem neonatal. Brasília. Ministério da Saúde. Secretaria de Assistência à Saúde Coordenação-Geral de Atenção Especializada. 1st ed. Brasília; 2002.

53. Wartofsky L. Update in endocrinology. Ann Intern Med. 2005;143:673–82.

54. Heymann WR, Marlton MD. Cutaneous manifestations of thyroid disease. J Am Acad Dermatol. 1992;26(6):885–902.

55. Târcoveanu E, Niculescu D, Cotea E, et al. Thyreoglossal duct cyst. J Chir. 2009;5(1):45–51.

56. Pribitkin AE, Friedman OE. Papillary carcinoma in a tyroglossal duct remnant. Arch Otolaryngol Head Neack Surg. 2002;12.

57. Leonhardt JM, Heymann WR. Thyroid disease and the skin. Dermatol Clin. 2002;20:473–81.

58. Sistrunk WE. The surgical treatment of cysts of the thyroglossal tract. Ann Surg. 1920;71:121–6.

59. Gupta P, Maddalozzo J. Preoperative sonography in presumed thyroglossal duct cysts. Arch Otolaryngol Head Neck Surg. 2001;127:200–2.

60. Quinn TR, Duncan LM, Zembowicz A, et al. Cutaneous metastases of follicular thyroid carcinoma. Am J Dermatopathol. 2005;27(4):306–12.

61. Brownstein MH, Helwig EB. Metastatic tumors of the skin. Cancer. 1972;65:1298–307.

62. Lookingbill DP, Spangler N, Helm K. Cutaneous metastases in patients with metastatic carcinoma: a retrospective study of 4020 patients. J Am Acad Dermatol. 1993;29:228–36.

63. Alwaheeb S, Ghazarian D, Boerner SL, Asa SL. Cutaneous manifestations of thyroid cancer: a report of four cases and review of the literature. J Clin Pathol. 2004;57:435–8.

64. Makris A, Goepel JR. Cutaneous metastases from a papillary thyroid carcinoma [letter]. Br J Dermatol. 1996;135:860–1.

65. Aghasi MR, Valizadeh N, Soltani S. A 64 year-old female with scalp metastasis of papillary thyroid cancer. Indian J Endocr Metab. 2011;15(S2):S136–7.

66. Dahl PR, Brodland DG, Goellner JR, Hay ID. Thyroid carcinoma metastatic to the skin: a cutaneous manifestation of a widely disseminated malignancy. J Am Acad Dermatol. 1997;36:531–7.

67. Tamiolakis D, Antoniou C, Venizelos J, et al. Papillary thyroid carcinoma metastasis most probably due to fine needle aspiration biopsy. A case report. Acta Dermatoven APA. 2006;15:169–72.

68. Bruglia M, Palmonella G, Silvetti F, et al. Skin and thigh muscle metastasis from papillary thyroid cancer. Singap Med J. 2009;50:e61–4.

69. Cohen PR. Metastatic papillary thyroid carcinoma to the nose: report and review of cutaneous metastases of papillary thyroid cancer. Dermatol Pract Conceptual. 2015;5(4):7.

70. Loureiro MM, Lette VH, Boavida JM, et al. An unusual case of papillary carcinoma of the thyroid with cutaneous and breast metastases only. Eur J Endocrinol. 1997;137:267–9.

71. Prescott JD, Zeiger MA. The RET oncogene in papillary thyroid carcinoma. Cancer. 2015;121:2137. [Epub ahead of print]

Dyslipidemias

37

Cristiane Almeida Soares Cattani and Renata Heck

Key Points

- Dyslipidemias may be associated with xanthomas and cardiovascular, pancreatic, and cerebrovascular diseases
- Xanthomas must alert the clinician to dyslipidemias or underlying diseases, especially in children
- Xanthelasma may appear in normolipemic patients
- Tendinous and tuberous xanthomas can be a cutaneous sign of severe familial hypercholesterolemia or systemic diseases
- Management of dyslipidemia involves treating associated disorders and exacerbating factors with a multidisciplinary approach and oral medication
- Early diagnosis of xanthomas and prompt treatment of associated dyslipidemic disorder prevents later systemic complications.

Introduction

Dyslipidemia represents any disorder of lipoprotein metabolism: "dys-" + "lipid" (fat) + "-emia" (in the blood) = disordered lipids in the blood. It confers an increased risk of cardiovascular disease, cerebrovascular disease, pancreatitis, and xanthoma, which are the characteristic skin manifestations in hyperlipoproteinemia (HLP).

Xanthomas consist of the accumulation of lipid-rich macrophages known as foam cells. They do not represent a disease but rather are signs of different lipoprotein disorders. They also may arise without an underlying metabolic defect [1].

Early diagnosis and treatment of dyslipidemias may have a significant impact on the prevention and prognosis of a patient's disease. It can therefore be considered a relevant concern in the public health context.

General Epidemiology

Hyperlipidemia is very common in the general population. Hypercholesterolemia can be defined as a low-density lipoprotein (LDL) cholesterol level greater than 160 mg/dl. It is estimated that more than 100 million people in North America alone have an elevated serum level >200 mg/dl [2].

C.A.S. Cattani, MD (✉) • R. Heck, MD, MSc
Sanitary Dermatology Service of the Department of
Health of Rio Grande do Sul State,
Porto Alegre, Brazil
e-mail: crisalmeidacattani@gmail.com;
reheck2@yahoo.com.br

© Springer International Publishing Switzerland 2018
R.R. Bonamigo, S.I.T. Dornelles (eds.), *Dermatology in Public Health Environments*,
https://doi.org/10.1007/978-3-319-33919-1_37

A high prevalence of dyslipidemias also exists in Brazil. A survey of 49,395 adults living in several Brazilian cities and federal districts showed a dyslipidemia rate of approximately 16.5% [3].

Hypercholesterolemia is therefore fairly common, and most affected individuals have a mild form. However, there are also more severe forms such as familial hypercholesterolemia, an autosomal dominant disease with a somber cardiovascular prognosis. Its prevalence is traditionally 1 in 500, but a recent study in the United States showed an overall nationwide prevalence of 1 in 299 [4].

Although a significant number of people suffer from hyperlipidemia, only a minority will develop cutaneous xanthomas, the exact mechanism of which is not completely understood [2].

Etiopathogenesis

There are two pathways of lipid metabolism: exogenous and endogenous. In the exogenous pathway dietary lipids are absorbed into the intestinal epithelium after been degraded by pancreatic lipase and bile acids to fatty acids and monoglycerides. After absorption, triglycerides are repackaged with cholesterol esters to form the central core of a chylomicron that is surrounded by phospholipids, free cholesterol, and apolipoproteins (ApoA-I, ApoB-48, ApoC-II, and ApoE). These chylomicrons enter the lymphatic circulation and are hydrolyzed by the action of lipoprotein lipase (present in capillary walls) and its cofactor ApoC-II, releasing free fatty acids. These free fatty acids are used as an energy source or stored in adipose tissue.

The endogenous pathway begins in the liver with very LDL (VLDL) synthesis from hepatic triglycerides and circulating free fatty acid. VLDL particles also contain apolipoproteins (ApoB-100, ApoC, and ApoE). Circulating VLDL interacts peripherally with lipoprotein

lipase (LPL), which hydrolyzes VLDL, removing triglyceride content. A residual particle called the VLDL remnant is degraded by the liver after bind ApoB-100 and ApoE receptors. A portion of VLDL remnant interacts with hepatic lipases and is converted into LDL. LDL particles enter the circulation and can be converted to bile acids or used by nonhepatic tissues to produce hormones in cell membrane synthesis, or can be stored.

High-density lipoprotein (HDL) produced in liver and intestine removes the excess cholesterol from peripheral tissues. The cholesterol is esterified to cholesterol esters by the enzyme lecithin:cholesterol acyltransferase (LCAT) after its activation by ApoA-I. HDL transfers the cholesterol esters to LDLs or VLDLs for transportation back to the liver and conversion to bile acids.

Defects in lipoprotein lipase, receptors, apolipoproteins, or cofactors may interfere in the pathway at different times. If the disturbance results in elevation of triglyceride-rich particles, eruptive xanthoma can occur. Xanthelasma, tuberous xanthomas, or tendinous xanthomas occur if the defect results in accumulation of cholesterol-rich particles.

The mechanism of cutaneous lesion formation is not completely understood. Serum lipid seems to infiltrate tissues where they are phagocytosed by macrophages to form lipid-laden foam cells [5].

Clinical Presentation

Xanthomas may present with a variety of morphologies, from macules and papules to plaques and nodules, but the major distinguishing feature of the lesions is the yellow to orange hue.

The morphology and anatomic location of the lesions can suggest the presence of an underlying lipid disorder or a paraproteinemia.

Most cutaneous xanthomas do not appear before adulthood, except in the homozygous form of familial hypercholesterolemia (type II).

Table 37.1 Important types of hyperlipoproteinemias and xanthomas

Type of hyperlipoproteinemia	Type of xanthoma	Laboratory	Systemic manifestations
Type I	Eruptive	Chylomicrons/VLDL ↑	No increased risk
		Triglycerides ↑	Cardiovascular disease
Familial LPL deficiency		LDL ↓	
Familial hyperchylomicronemia		HDL ↓ or normal	
Type II	Plane xanthoma	Cholesterol ↑	Atherosclerosis of peripheral and coronary arteries (premature cardiovascular disease)
Familial hypercholesterolemia	Xanthelasma	Reduced LDL clearance	
Heterozygous	Intertriginous areas		
Homozygous	Interdigital		
Familial defective ApoB-100	Tendinous		
	Tuberous		
	Tuberoeruptive		
	Early appearance (first decade)		
Type III	Plane xanthoma	Cholesterol ↑	Atherosclerosis of peripheral and coronary arteries (premature cardiovascular disease)
Familial dysbetalipoproteinemia	Palmar creases[a]	LDL ↑	
Remnant removal disease	Xanthelasma	VLDL ↑	
Broad beta disease	Tuberoeruptive	Triglycerides ↑	
ApoE deficiency	Tuberous		
	Tendinous		
Type IV	Eruptive	VLDL ↑	Often associated with:
Endogenous familial hypertriglyceridemia		Triglycerides ↑	Type II non-insulin-dependent diabetes
			Obesity
			Secondary hypertriglyceridemia (from medications, alcoholism)
Type V	Eruptive	Triglycerides ↑	Diabetes mellitus
		Chylomicron/VLDL ↑	

LPL lipoprotein lipase, *VLDL* very-low-density lipoprotein, *LDL* low-density lipoprotein, *HDL* high-density lipoprotein
[a]Characteristic

Clinical types of xanthomas include eruptive, tuberous, tuberoeruptive, tendinous, planar (xanthelasma), and verruciform [2].

In 1965, Lees and Frederickson published a system for phenotyping various disorders of lipid metabolism based on electrophoretic migration of the serum lipoproteins present. This is still used today in a modified form.

The clinical presentations of the various changes in lipid metabolism are summarized in Table 37.1.

Eruptive Xanthomas

Eruptive xanthomas are small reddish-yellow papules, from 1 to 5 mm in diameter, arising suddenly in crops over the buttocks, thighs, and the extensor surfaces of the arms, hands, and legs [1] Fig. 37.1.

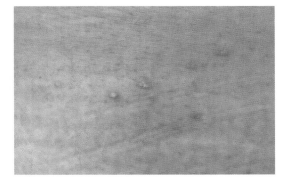

Fig. 37.1 Eruptive xanthoma. Multiple small reddish-yellow papules

They are usually associated with primary or secondary hypertriglyceridemia. Triglyceride levels usually exceed 3,000–4,000 mg/dl.

Eruptive xanthomas usually appear in Frederickson classification type I (elevated chylomicrons), type IV (elevated VLDL), and type V (elevated chylomicrons and VLDL).

Elevated triglycerides may be due to deficient activity of enzymes, as in lipoprotein lipase deficiency (chylomicronemia) or dysfunctional ApoC-II, or in other controlling factors such as impaired insulin activity. Hepatic overproduction of VLDL as a result of a genetic defect that causes an abnormal response to dietary carbohydrates and insulin is defined as Frederickson type IV (endogenous familial hypertriglyceridemia).

Secondary acquired defects in lipoprotein lipase activity, such as those due to uncontrolled diabetes mellitus, often occur in these patients, aggravating the handling of dietary lipids and also leading to elevated chylomicrons (Frederickson type V).

Besides diabetes, hypothyroidism and other conditions such as obesity, pregnancy, and alcohol abuse may impair triglyceride metabolism. This can also be attributed to oral estrogen replacement and other systemic medications (e.g., retinoids, cyclosporine, olanzapine, and protease inhibitor therapy) [1, 2].

In genetically predisposed patients, hypertriglyceridemia induced by isotretinoin therapy seems to correlate with a future risk of metabolic syndrome.

The Koebner phenomenon has been reported to occur with eruptive xanthomas. It emerges frequently, accompanied by tenderness and pruritus (an inflammatory halo may appear in early disease). There are reports of eruptive xanthomas appearing in a patient's old tattoos [6].

Remission of eruptive xanthomas depends on diagnosis and treatment of the underlying primary or secondary disorder in order to lower the triglyceride levels.

Tuberous/Tuberoeruptive Xanthomas

Tuberoeruptive and tuberous xanthomas are often described together because they are clinically and pathologically related. Tuberoeruptive xanthomas appear on extensor surfaces as yellowish or reddish papules or nodules, especially on the elbows and knees. They also may be located in knuckles, buttocks, and other sites (Figs. 37.2 and 37.3).

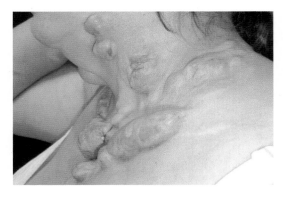

Fig. 37.2 Tuberous xanthoma. Multiple yellowish nodules in cervical region (Courtesy of Dermatology Department of Federal University of Health Science, Porto Alegre)

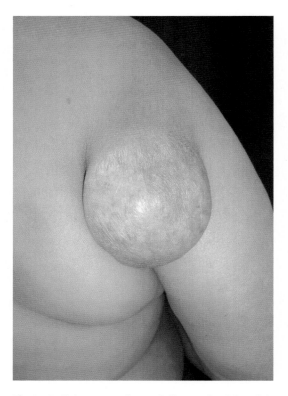

Fig. 37.3 Tuberous xanthoma. Solitary yellowish nodule in axillary region (Courtesy of Dermatology Department of Federal University of Health Science, Porto Alegre)

Tuberous lesions are larger than tuberoeruptive lesions (diameter >3 cm). Both are present in hypercholesterolemic states, with cholesterol and triglyceride serum levels elevated (Frederickson type II and type III).

Dysbetalipoproteinemia (type III) is a genetic disorder of lipid metabolism caused by the presence of an isoform of ApoE, mainly ApoE2, a poor ligand for the high-affinity ApoB-100/E receptor which results in decreased hepatic uptake of chylomicrons and VLDL remnants. Its consequence is high serum levels of cholesterol and triglycerides. In 80% of patients tuberous or tuberoeruptive xanthomas are present. Plane xanthomas of the palm creases (*xanthoma striatum palmare*) may also appear and have characteristic cutaneous features.

Affected patients have an increased risk of developing premature cardiovascular disease, gout, and diabetes.

Unlike eruptive xanthomas, tuberous lesions do not involute as quickly with appropriate therapy [2].

Very rarely tuberoeruptive, planar, and palmar xanthomas have been noticed in severe HDL deficiency (HDL levels <10 mg/dl) or in patients with multiple myeloma and monoclonal gammopathies [7].

Tendinous Xanthomas

These xanthomas are firm subcutaneous nodular lipid deposits that may be found in fascia, ligaments, Achilles tendons, or extensor tendons of hands, elbows, and knees. The appearance of the overlying skin is normal. Ultrasonography can aid the diagnosis by showing hypoechoic nodules or an increase in the anteroposterior diameter of the tendon [8].

Tendinous xanthomas are usually related to markedly elevated levels of cholesterol (>300 mg/dl) [7].

The rate and growth of xanthoma deposition is associated with the duration and severity of LDL levels [7]. Triglyceride and HDL levels are typically normal.

Dysbetalipoproteinemia and hypothyroidism may present with tendinous xanthoma.

However, the most frequent lipid disorder associated with this form of xanthoma is familial hypercholesterolemia (Frederickson type II). This condition is inherited in an autosomal dominant fashion with a high degree of penetrance. Deficiency of normal LDL receptors on cell membranes leads to poor hepatic clearance of circulating LDLs and, therefore, elevated cholesterol levels, with widespread atherosclerosis and premature cardiovascular disease (age <60 years). Xanthomas appear in the first decade of life. Plane xanthomas of the interdigital spaces of the fingers are considered pathognomonic for the homozygous state. Heterozygotes are more common (as mentioned in Epidemiology). Besides tendinous xanthomas, tuberous, tuberoeruptive, and planar xanthomas (including xanthelasma) also may be seen in this disorder.

Another closely related genetic disease is familial defective ApoB-100. Although the LDL receptor is normal, there is a poor affinity of LDL for this receptor because the mutation affects its ligand, ApoB-100. The clinical findings are very similar to those of familial hypercholesterolemia, though less severe.

Rarely, tendinous xanthomas can develop in the absence of a lipoprotein disorder.

Cerebrotendinous xanthomatosis is a rare condition in which despite modest elevations of cholesterol levels there are abnormal cholestanol deposits in tendons and brain tissue, with risk of neurologic disease including cerebellar ataxia and dementia [7]. This disorder results from an enzymatic defect in the bile acid synthetic pathway, leading to the abnormal accumulation of an intermediate known as cholestanol (a physiologic sterol normally found in lower concentrations than cholesterol).

In β-sitosterolemia (phytosterolemia) there is abnormal accumulation of plant sterols with tendinous xanthoma formation and premature cardiovascular disease. Normally, these sterols are eliminated efficiently back to the intestinal lumen by intestinal transporters, but defects in this transport leads to retention of these sterols in the intestinal cell and their secretion on chylomicrons in the plasma space [7].

Plane Xanthomas and Xanthelasma

Plane xanthomas are clinically described as yellow to orange macules, soft papules, patches, or plaques. They can be circumscribed or diffuse and are commonly found in eyelids (xanthelasma), wrists, palms, and intertriginous areas.

They are non-inflammatory, mostly asymptomatic, and their location can help to address the underlying lipid disorder. For instance, intertriginous plane xanthomas that appear in the antecubital fossae or the interdigital spaces are almost pathognomonic for homozygous familial hypercholesterolemia.

Plane xanthomas of the palmar creases (xanthoma striatum palmare) associated with tuberous xanthomas are potentially diagnostic for dysbetalipoproteinemia.

Other systemic diseases may present with xanthomas. In biliary atresia, primary biliary cirrhosis, and conditions with prolonged obstruction of the biliary tree, unesterified cholesterol accumulates in blood, leading to xanthoma formation. They begin as localized beige-orange plaques on the hands and feet, but can become generalized. Patients often present with jaundice, pruritus, and hyperpigmentation of skin.

Plane xanthomas also occur in normolipemic patients (i.e., with normal lipid levels). However, in some cases they have been observed in patients with multiple myeloma, lymphoma, leukemias, and underlying monoclonal gammopathy. In this disorder, monoclonal immunoglobulin G is thought to bind circulating LDL, rendering the antibody–LDL complex more susceptible to phagocytosis by macrophages [9].

Xanthelasma, or xanthelasma palpebrarum, is the most frequent plane xanthoma, characteristic of the eyelids. It can be present even in the absence of a lipid disorder. Elevated LDL cholesterol levels are found in only about one-half of the patients with lesions, but in younger people with xanthelasma and family history of dyslipidemia the lipid profile must be investigated (Fig. 37.4).

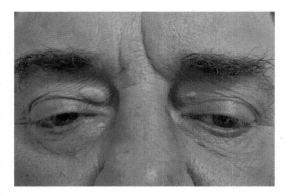

Fig. 37.4 Xanthelasma. Yellow patches on the eyelids

Verruciform Xanthomas

Verruciform xanthomas are planar or verrucous solitary plaques ranging from 1 to 2 cm in diameter. They occur primarily in the oral cavity (mouth) but sometimes in anogenital (including the scrotum) or periorificial sites.

Usually they are asymptomatic and persist for years. This form of xanthoma is not associated with any dyslipidemia but may be seen in lymphedema and in the setting of other diseases such as epidermolysis bullosa, discoid lupus erythematosus, and graft-versus-host disease (GVHD).

Nonmucosal verruciform xanthoma is the characteristic lesion in congenital hemidysplasia with ichthyosiform erythroderma and limb defects (CHILD) syndrome.

Histologically there is usually hyperkeratosis, acanthosis, papillomatosis, and foamy macrophages limited to the submucosa or dermal papillae. Therefore, these xanthomas may be confused with warts and other papillomatous conditions, because the few foam cells beneath the epithelium may be subtle and easy to miss [2, 7].

Xanthomas in Children

In children, xanthomas are uncommon and appropriate investigation is mandatory. If laboratory screening reveals a hyperlipidemia, early intervention must be considered.

The most common dyslipidemias are types IIA, IIB, and IV. Type I and type III HLP are extremely rare in pediatric patients, and type V is uncommon.

As in adults, hyperlipidemias often may be secondary to obesity, hypothyroidism, diabetes mellitus, nephrotic syndrome, or, more rarely, genetic disorders. In these situations xanthomas may develop during childhood [2]. When they occur in children and adolescents (especially tuberous), a more severe form of hyperlipidemia should be suspected [10].

The differential for xanthomas in children includes homozygous familial hypercholesterolemia, β-sitosterolemia, cerebrotendinous xanthomatosis, type I glycogen storage (Von Gierke) disease, and Alagille syndrome. In children Alagille syndrome is an inherited syndrome of biliary hypoplasia leading to elevated serum cholesterol. These patients have a characteristic facies with a prominent forehead, hypertelorism, pointed chin, and nasal dystrophy. Xanthomas may be seen in flexures, elbows, knees, and palms or fingers. Serum cholesterol is elevated when patients are young but can decrease over time. Nearly 12% of patients with this syndrome develops cirrhosis. Treatment consists of medical management. If cirrhosis develops, liver transplantation is indicated, after which xanthomas have been found to resolve [7].

Most cases of type I HLP are caused by congenital deficiency of LPL, congenital deficiency of ApoC-II, or an LPL inhibitor (e.g., an anti-LPL autoantibody).

In one study of patients with LPL deficiency, 80% presented xanthomas before 10 years of age. In contrast, Apo-CII deficiency is usually diagnosed later in life (>13 years old). ApoC-II deficiency rarely presents in infancy [11].

In children, LDL cholesterol concentrations of 130 mg/dl or higher define type IIA HLP. The plasma is clear in this type because LDL particles are not large enough to scatter light, as opposed to VLDL or lipoprotein remnants that are large enough to cause turbidity.

In type IIB HLP, triglyceride levels are elevated to 125 mg/dl or higher, and LDL cholesterol levels are also elevated. If the triglyceride level is typically 300–400 mg/dl or higher, the plasma appears turbid (lipemic).

Hypertriglyceridemia (usually the type IV HLP phenotype) is frequently observed in children with obesity, diabetes, or both conditions. Familial hypertriglyceridemia is rarely expressed in childhood unless another underlying cause of hypertriglyceridemia is present [11].

The differential diagnosis of the various clinical presentations of xanthomas are listed in Box 37.1.

> **Box 37.1 Differential Diagnosis of Xanthomas**
> *Xanthelasma*:
>   Sebaceous hyperplasia
>   Syringoma
>   Adnexal neoplasms
>   Periocular xanthogranuloma
>   Palpebral sarcoidosis
> *Plane xanthomas*:
>   Amyloidosis
>   Pseudoxanthoma elasticum
>   Sarcoidosis
> *Eruptive xanthomas*:
>   Xanthoma disseminatum
>   Disseminated granuloma annulare
>   Sarcoidosis
>   Generalized eruptive histiocytomas
>   Non-Langerhans cells histiocystosis
>   Xanthomatous lesions of Langerhans cells histiocytosis
>   Juvenile xanthogranuloma (micronodular form)
> *Tuberous or tendinous xanthomas*:
>   Cysts
>   Lipoma
>   Neurofibroma
>   Erythema elevatum diutinum
>   Rheumatoid nodule
>   Subcutaneous granuloma annulare

Complementary Examinations

Patients seeking a dermatologist because of xanthomas must be evaluated for an underlying dyslipidemia and referred to the specialist.

Lipid Profile

The standard lipid profile consists of direct measurement of total cholesterol, HDL cholesterol, and triglycerides, with a calculated LDL cholesterol, obtained after a 9-h to 12-h fast.

Metabolic Profile

Since hypertriglyceridemia with low HDL and elevated LDL is indicative of insulin resistance, metabolic screening is recommended with fasting glucose, serum creatinine, hepatic panel, thyroid function tests, and urinary protein [7].

Skin Biopsy/Histopathology

If the diagnosis of xanthomas is in doubt, obtaining a biopsy of the suspicious lesions will reveal accumulations of fat (not cholesterol).

The characteristic histologic finding in xanthomas is the foam cell. This is a macrophage that contains lipid. Dermal infiltrates of lipid are seen in all xanthomas but may vary in the degree of lipid content, the inflammatory infiltrate, the amount and location of the infiltrate, and the presence of extracellular lipid. Laboratory processing must take care not to remove deposits of lipid from the tissue sample and leave artifactual clefting in the histological appearance. Since cholesterol esters are doubly refractile, polarized microscopy is very useful (Fig. 37.5).

Early in lesion development, foam cells are relatively small in number and size. The initial inflammatory infiltrate is mixed, containing both neutrophils and lymphocytes. As increased lipidization occurs as the appearance of the lesion becomes more typical of a xanthoma, but foam cells remain fewer in number when comparing eruptive with other forms of xanthomas.

Extracellular lipids are present in the dermis, which is seen as artifactual clefts filled with a wispy, faint blue-gray material.

Tuberous xanthomas reveal foam cells and cholesterol clefts (fibrosis is often noticed but without a large number of inflammatory cells). Tendinous xanthomas are similar, but with larger foam cells.

Xanthelasmas (the common type of plane xanthoma) can be differentiated by their unique

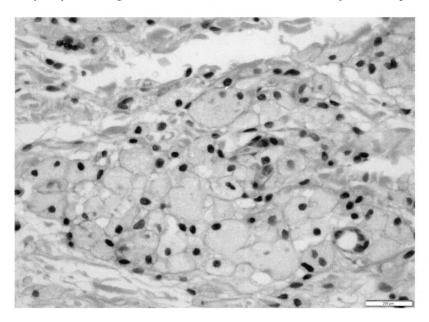

Fig. 37.5 Xanthoma histopathology. Dermal foam cells (macrophages with lipid content) (×400)

histologic appearance: along with foam cells, they may reveal striated muscle fibers, vellus hair, and/or a thinned epidermis (characteristic of the eyelids) indicative of its superficial location. There are no inflammatory cells and minimal fibrosis may be seen [2].

Therapeutic Approach

Management of dyslipidemia involves treating associated disorders and exacerbating factors such as obesity, smoking, and diabetes. It is often necessarily a multidisciplinary approach. Therapeutic lifestyle changes include aerobic exercise, dietary modifications (decreased intake of saturated or *trans* fatty acids), achievement of ideal body weight, and reduced alcohol consumption [2, 7, 12].

When pharmacologic intervention is necessary, statins are the drugs of choice for the initial treatment of dyslipidemia, and have been shown to reduce cardiovascular mortality significantly. Statins competitively inhibit HMG CoA reductase, blocking cholesterol biosynthesis. These drugs mainly act by lowering LDL cholesterol, but also by decreasing VLDL and triglycerides and raising HDL cholesterol levels [13, 14]. The most important adverse effects include elevations in hepatic transaminases and muscle toxicity. A baseline creatine kinase (CK) level should be obtained for reference, but there is no evidence for routinely monitoring muscle enzymes [2, 14]. Concomitant use with cyclosporine, fibrates, macrolides, azole antifungals, and protease inhibitors is contraindicated because of the increased risk of rhabdomyolysis.

Fibrates are the drugs of choice in the treatment of hypertriglyceridemia, and act by reducing hepatic secretion of VLDL and stimulating lipoprotein lipase activity in peripheral tissues. Fibrates are not associated with statins because of the increased risk of muscle toxicity. They can also interfere with warfarin; the anticoagulant dose should be reduced when such an association exists. Available drugs of this class include bezafibrate, ciprofibrate, fenofibrate, and gemfibrozil [13, 15].

Nicotinic acid is one of the oldest drugs used for the treatment of dyslipidemia. It inhibits hepatic synthesis of VLDL and, consequently, LDL levels. There is also an increased activity of lipoprotein lipase, reducing triglyceride levels. HDL levels increase with nicotinic acid. Flushing is a common side effect that limits its use.

The bile acid sequestrants (cholestyramine) bind bile acids, preventing them from being reabsorbed in the intestine. They are effective in the treatment of heterozygous familial hypercholesterolemia but can increase triglyceride levels. The major side effect is gastrointestinal discomfort. Cholestyramine can impair the absorption of coadministered medications such as warfarin, digoxin, levothyroxine, and fat-soluble vitamins, administration of other drugs 1 h before or 4 h after cholestyramine intake being indicated [16].

Ezetimibe inhibits dietary and biliary cholesterol absorption in the intestine without affecting the absorption of fat-soluble drugs. It shows no significant gastrointestinal symptomatology and presents no significant interaction with statins [17].

Drug treatment of dyslipidemia is summarized in Table 37.2.

Lipid disorder correction leads to resolution of xanthomas in many patients. Eruptive xanthomas tend to disappear faster than tuberous or tendinous xanthomas. The latter may require months to years of systemic treatment. Unresponsive xanthomas can be treated with surgery or locally destructive methods [18].

Regarding xanthelasma, many techniques have been described, such as trichloroacetic acid application, cryosurgery, surgical excision, electrocauterization, and laser ablation [19]. Xanthelasma tends to recur despite the technique employed.

Table 37.2 Drug treatment of dyslipidemias

Drug class	Mechanism of action	Effect on lipids	Major adverse effects
Statins	Competitively inhibit HMG-CoA reductase	LDL ↓	Hepatic toxicity
Atorvastatin		Triglycerides ↓	Muscle toxicity
Fluvastatin		HDL ↑	
Lovastatin			
Pravastatin			
Rosuvastatin			
Simvastatin			
Fibrates	Inhibit hepatic synthesis of VLDL	LDL ↓	Muscle toxicity
Bezafibrate		Triglycerides ↓	
Ciprofibrate		HDL ↑	
Fenofibrate			
Gemfibrozil			
Nicotinic acid	Inhibits hepatic synthesis of VLDL	LDL ↓	Flushing
		Triglycerides ↓	
	Increased activity of lipoprotein lipase	HDL ↑	
Bile acid sequestrants	Inhibit intestinal reabsorption of bile acids	LDL ↓	Gastrointestinal discomfort
Cholestyramine		Triglycerides ↑	
Ezetimib	Inhibits cholesterol absorption in the intestine	LDL ↓	Gastrointestinal discomfort

LDL low-density lipoprotein, *HDL* high-density lipoprotein *VLDL* very-low-density lipoprotein

References

1. Pai VV, Shukla P, Bhobe M. Combined planar and eruptive xanthoma in a patient with type IIa hyperlipoproteinemia. Indian J Dermatol Venereol Leprol. 2014;80(5):467–70.
2. Massengale WT, Hodari KT, Boh EE, Nesbitt LT. Xanthomas. In: Bolognia JL, Jorizzo JL, Schaffer JV, editors. Dermatology. 3rd ed. Philadelphia, Elsevier; 2012. p. 1547–55.
3. Gigante DP, Moura EC, Sardinha LM. Prevalence of overweight and obesity and associated factors, Brazil, 2006. Rev Saude Publica. 2009;43(2):83–9.
4. Bruckert E, Hansel B. Familial hypercholesterolemia (Part 1): diagnosis and screening challenges. In: Medscape [Internet]. Accessed 10 Apr 2016.
5. Paller AS, Mancini AJ. Inborn errors of metabolism. In: Hurwitz clinical pediatric dermatology. 4th ed. Philadelphia, Elsevier; 2011. p. 553–7.
6. Gao H, Chen J. Eruptive xanthomas presenting in tattoos. CMAJ. 2015;187(5):356.
7. Schaefer EJ, Santos RD. Xanthomatoses and lipoprotein disorders. In: Goldsmith LA, Katz SI, Gilchrest BA, et al., editors. Fitzpatrick's dermatology in general medicine. 8th ed. New York, McGraw-Hill Companies; 2012. p. 1600–12.
8. Sethuraman G, Thappa DM, Karthikeyan K. Intertriginous xanthomas – a marker of homozygous familial hypercholesterolemia. Indian Pediatr. 2000;37:338.
9. Yamamoto A, Matsuzawa Y, Yokoyama S, et al. Effects of probucol on xanthomata regression in familial hypercholesterolemia. Am J Cardiol. 1986;57:29H–35H.
10. Bhagwat PV, Tophakhane RS, Kudligi C, Noronha TM, Thirunavukkarasu A. Familial combined hypercholesterolemia type IIb presenting with tuberous xanthoma, tendinous xanthoma and pityriasis rubra pilaris-like lesions. Indian J Dermatol Venereol Leprol. 2010;76(3):293–6.
11. Rohrs HJ, Berger S. Pediatric lipid disorders in clinical practice. In Medscape [Internet]. Accessed 10 Apr 2016.
12. Shenoy C, Shenoy MM, Rao GK. Dyslipidemia in dermatological disorders. N Am J Med Sci. 2015;7(10):421–8.
13. Vieira JLC, Vieira PL, Moriguchi EH. Hipolipemiantes. In: Barros E, Barros H. Medicamentos na prática clínica. 1st ed. Porto Alegre, Artmed; 2010. p. 288–303.
14. Rosenson RS, Freeman MW, Rind DM. Statins: actions, side effects, and administration. In: UpToDate [Internet]. WoltersKluwer Health. The Netherlands. Accessed 27 Mar 2016.

15. Rosenson RS, Freeman MW, Rind DM. Lipid lowering with fibric acid derivatives. In: UpToDate [Internet]. WoltersKluwer Health. The Netherlands. Accessed 27 Mar 2016.

16. Rosenson RS, Freeman MW, Rind DM. Lipid lowering with drugs other than statins and fibrates. In: UpToDate [Internet]. WoltersKluwer Health. The Netherlands. Accessed 27 Mar 2016.

17. Sando KR, Knight M. Therapies for management of dyslipidemia: a review. Clin Ther. 2015;37(10):2153–79.

18. White LE, Horenstein MG, Shea CR. Xanthomas. In Lebwohl MG, Heymann WR, Berth-Jones J, Coulson I. Treatment of skin disease. 4th ed. Elsevier; Philadelphia, 2014. p 804–807

19. Goel K, Sardana K, Garg VK. A prospective study comparing ultrapulse CO2 laser and trichloroacetic acid in treatment of Xanthelasma palpebrarum. J Cosmet Dermatol. 2015;14(2):130–9.

Dermatosis and Nutritional Disorders

38

Ana Paula Dornelles Manzoni
and Vanessa Santos Cunha

Key Points

- *Acne*: A low glycemic-load diet can be recommended to patients. The link between milk and acne needs more research before being recommended to acne patients
- *Atopic dermatitis*: Excessively restrictive diets, especially in atopic children, have led to weight loss, poor growth, calcium deficiency, hypovitaminosis, and kwashiorkor
- *Hair disorders*: Caloric deprivation or deficiency of several components, such as proteins, minerals, essential fatty acids, and vitamins can lead to structural abnormalities, pigmentation changes, or hair loss. Combined deficiencies are not uncommon

- *Nail disorders*: A healthy, well-balanced diet composed of an adequate daily intake of vitamins and minerals facilitates nail health in general. The use of biotin has recently shown promise in treating human nail diseases, especially nail brittleness
- *Skin cancer*: A specific diet should not be recommended for skin cancer prevention, because studies have presented conflicting results
- *Vitiligo*: While there may be a relationship between nutritional elements and vitiligo, further research is needed to elucidate the nature of the association and the clinical application

Acanthosis Nigricans

Nutritional Correlation

Obesity is closely associated with acanthosis nigricans, and more than half of adults who weigh 200% more than their ideal body weight have lesions consistent with acanthosis nigricans. Although it is not universally the case, this dermatosis is weight dependent, and insulin resistance is often present in such patients

A.P.D. Manzoni, MD, PhD (✉)
Dermatology Service of UFCSPA, Porto Alegre, Brazil
e-mail: anamanzoni@terra.com.br

V.S. Cunha, MD, PhD
Dermatology Service of Hospital São Lucas-PUCRS, Porto Alegre, Brazil

© Springer International Publishing Switzerland 2018
R.R. Bonamigo, S.I.T. Dornelles (eds.), *Dermatology in Public Health Environments*,
https://doi.org/10.1007/978-3-319-33919-1_38

[1, 2]. Obesity-associated acanthosis nigricans may be a marker for higher insulin needs in obese women with gestational diabetes and has been shown to be a reliable early marker for metabolic syndrome in pediatric patients. The lesions may completely regress with weight reduction [1–4].

Skin Manifestations

Acanthosis nigricans is characterized by symmetric, hyperpigmented, velvety plaques that may occur in almost any location but most commonly appear on the intertriginous areas of the axilla, groin, and posterior neck. The posterior neck is the most commonly affected site in children. Acrochordons are often found in and around the affected areas [3, 4].

Complementary Examinations

The vast majority of cases are due to obesity and/or insulin resistance. Screening for diabetes with a glycosylated hemoglobin level or glucose tolerance test is recommended. Screening for insulin resistance with a plasma insulin level is the most sensitive test to detect a metabolic abnormality of this kind because many younger patients do not yet have overt diabetes mellitus and an abnormal glycosylated hemoglobin level, although they do have a high plasma insulin level.

Therapeutic Approach

No treatment of choice exists for acanthosis nigricans. The lesions are treated for cosmetic reasons only. Correction of hyperinsulinemia often reduces the burden of hyperkeratotic lesions. Likewise, in obesity-associated acanthosis nigricans, weight reduction may result in resolution of the dermatosis. Topical medications that have been effective in some cases of acanthosis nigricans include keratolytics (e.g., topical tretinoin 0.05%, ammonium lactate 12% cream) and triple-combination depigmenting cream (tretinoin 0.05%, hydroquinone 4%, fluocinolone acetonide 0.01%) nightly with daily sunscreen. Calcipotriol, podophyllin, urea, adapalene, and salicylic acid also have been reported, with variable results. Oral agents that have shown some benefit include etretinate, isotretinoin, metformin, and dietary fish oils [1, 3, 4].

Acne

Nutritional Correlation

Many patients believe that diet contributes to acne. Diet as a potential treatment for acne is not new, although over the past 100 years the literature examining diet and acne has been inconclusive. Dermatologists have recently revisited the idea and become increasingly interested in the role of medical nutrition therapy in acne treatment [5]. Research has substantiated the role of specific foods, such as dairy products, particularly milk and its derivatives, as well as dietary patterns, including the high glycemic load typical of the Western diet [6]. The evidence is more convincing for high-glycemic-load diets compared with other dietary factors. To date, no randomized controlled trials (RCTs) have investigated the relationship between frequent dairy or milk consumption and acne [5–7].

A high-glycemic-load diet leads to hyperinsulinemia, which initiates a signaling cascade resulting in increased insulin and insulin-like growth factor 1 (IGF-1) activity and decreased IGF-binding protein 3 (IGFBP-3) activity. IGF-1 is known to stimulate key factors of acne pathogenesis, including keratinocyte proliferation, sebocyte proliferation, and lipogenesis. Milk consumption results in a significant increase in insulin and IGF-1 serum levels comparable with high glycemic food [5–8].

Interventional studies have investigated the effect of low versus high glycemic-load diets on acne. These studies provide compelling evidence that a low-glycemic diet improves acne. Weight loss, however, is a confounding factor [7]. Posterior histopathologic examination revealed reduced sebaceous gland size and decreased expression of sterol regulatory element binding protein 1, a regulator of lipid synthesis, and interleukin-8, an inflammatory cytokine, with a low glycemic diet [9].

Some studies have investigated the association between acne and milk consumption. Acne was positively associated with the frequent consumption of whole milk and skim milk in women and with total, whole, low-fat, and skim milk consumption in girls. In boys, self-reported acne was positively associated with skim milk intake alone [5–7]. Finally, a recent case series reported acne in male patients that was precipitated by whey protein supplementation. These patients experienced resolution of their acne after discontinuing whey protein supplementation [10].

Consumption of salty foods was significantly higher among patients with acne compared with acne-free subjects, making the consumption of salty food a possible participating factor in the development of acne [11].

Some low-quality evidence suggests that tea tree oil and bee venom may reduce total skin lesions in acne vulgaris [12].

Skin Manifestations

Noninflammatory acne is characterized by open and closed comedones. Inflammatory acne originates with comedo formation but then expands to form papules, nodules, and cysts of varying severity (Fig. 38.1) [6, 7].

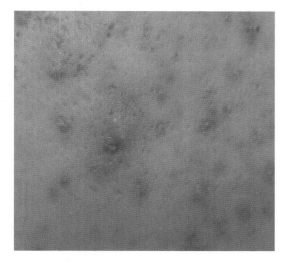

Fig. 38.1 Inflammatory acne (Courtesy of Dermatology Service of UFCSPA)

Eruptive acneiform lesions can be seen in drug-induced acne and when it is related to diet. Clinically it is an abrupt and monomorphous eruption of inflammatory papules, in contrast to the heterogeneous morphology of lesions seen in acne vulgaris [6, 7, 13].

Complementary Examinations

Related to nutritional features, no complementary examinations are necessary.

Therapeutic Approach

Currently the best dietary approach is to address each acne patient individually, while carefully considering the possibility of dietary counseling [13]. Multiple studies have shown the benefit of a low-glycemic-load diet in treating acne, which therefore can be recommended to patients. While observational studies support the link between milk and acne, more research is required before milk-restricted diets can be recommended to acne patients [6, 7, 13].

Acrodermatitis Enteropathica and Zinc Deficiency

Nutritional Correlation

Zinc deficiency is an uncommon nutritional deficiency that can be inherited or acquired. Acrodermatitis enteropathica (AE) classically refers to the inborn error of zinc metabolism that is inherited as an autosomal recessive disorder. Acquired zinc deficiency is more prevalent and may present in the same fashion [14, 15]. Acquired zinc deficiency may be due to inadequate intake, malabsorption, excessive loss, or a combination of these factors. Transient, symptomatic zinc deficiency has been reported in breastfed, low-birth-weight, and premature infants [14, 16–18] (Chart 38.1).

Certain medical conditions and medications can be predisposing factors for zinc deficiency. Some of these medical conditions include cirrhosis, diabetes mellitus, burns, end-stage renal disease, celiac disease, inflammatory bowel disease, and cystic fibrosis [17–19].

Chart 38.1 Correlation of nutrient deficiency and its cutaneous repercussions

Nutrient	Cutaneous repercussion
Biotin	Alopecia, glossitis, keratosis pilaris, periorificial dermatitis, seborrheic dermatitis, and erythroderma
Copper	Depigmented and thinning hair, alopecia, delayed wound healing
Iron	Pallor, koilonychia, glossitis, alopecia
Selenium	Delayed wound healing, psoriasis, skin cancer
Vitamin A or retinol	Xeroderma, acne, brittle hair, and keratotic follicular papules most commonly in the anterolateral surface of thighs and arms, which may spread to the extensor areas of the upper and lower limbs, shoulders, abdomen, dorsal region, buttocks, and neck; phrynoderma
Vitamin B2 or riboflavin	Mucositis, lip and angular cheilitis, glossitis, xerosis, seborrheic dermatitis, scrotal and vulvar eczema, erythroderma, and toxic epidermal necrolysis
Vitamin B3 or niacin	Pellagra, photosensitive dermatitis in symmetric areas, cheilitis, glossitis
Vitamin B5 or pantothenic acid	Purpura, leukotrichia, seborrheic dermatitis, angular stomatitis, glossitis, and burning feet syndrome
Vitamin B6 or pyridoxine	Seborrheic dermatitis, glossitis, oral mucosa ulceration, lip and angular cheilitis, photosensitive pellagra-like lesions
Vitamin B9 or folic acid and B12 or cobalamin	Lip or angular cheilitis; Hunter's glossitis; diffuse, symmetric hair; and mucocutaneous hypo-and hyperpigmentation
Vitamin C or ascorbic acid	Poor wound healing, keratosis pilaris, perifollicular petechiae, ecchymosis, purpura, brittle hair, scurvy (gingivitis, bleeding gums, keratosis pilaris), Sjögren-like syndrome
Vitamin D	Atopic dermatitis, psoriasis, skin infections, acne, autoimmune cutaneous diseases, and skin cancer
Vitamin E	Atopic dermatitis, acne
Vitamin K	Purpura, petechiae, ecchymosis, hematoma
Zinc*	Acrodermatitis enteropathica (alopecia; acral and periorificial symmetric, erosive and eczematous rash); dry, brittle, and thinning hair; delayed wound healing; paronychia; stomatitis; psoriasiform dermatitis; blepharitis; angular cheilitis; vitiligo-like lesions
Protein	Aged appearance; erythematous or hypopigmented lesions most evident in flexure areas; hyperchromic lesions with smooth, fissured, or erosive surface; brittle, slow growing nails; onychomadesis; follicular hyperkeratosis; pale extremities accompanied by edema; dry, brittle, dull, and thin hair, with brownish-red color before becoming grayish-white, flag signal with alternating dark and light stripes in the hair; angular cheilitis; xerophthalmia; stomatitis; vulvovaginitis

*Reference [14]

Skin Manifestations

In AE the main manifestation is erythematous, vesiculobullous, or pustular lesions that lead to dry, scaly, or eczematous lesions distributed around periorificial and acral areas of the body. The borders of affected areas are sharply demarcated with accentuated, craquelé-like scaling and occasional paronychia. Other symptoms are diarrhea, behavioral changes, and neurologic disturbances. In older children, zinc deficiency is characterized by failure to thrive, anorexia, alopecia, nail dystrophy, and repeated infections [18, 19].

Acquired zinc deficiency can have milder clinical features characterized by eczematous or psoriasiform dermatitis accompanied by perlèche. Areas of pressure or rubbing may also be involved. Some plaques appear annular or nummular and may not be as inflamed in chronically undiagnosed patients. Such lesions may become secondarily infected with *Staphylococcus aureus* or *Candida albicans* [14, 18, 19].

Complementary Examinations

Plasma zinc levels should be tested. Specimens should be collected in plastic syringes or acid-washed Vacutainer tubes with no rubber stopper to prevent exogenous contamination that could lead to spuriously normal measurements. Plasma zinc concentrations less than 50 µg/dL are suggestive, but not diagnostic, of AE. Hair, saliva, or urine zinc levels can be obtained but are rarely needed. Because alkaline phosphatase is a zinc-dependent enzyme, reduced serum levels of alkaline phosphatase in the context of normal zinc levels can indicate a zinc deficiency. However, alkaline phosphatase levels are typically not decreased unless the individual has advanced disease. Analysis of maternal breast milk zinc concentrations may help in differentiating AE from acquired zinc deficiency.

Therapeutic Approach

If treated early, most of the symptoms are reversible and usually cause no sequelae. Treatment of AE requires lifelong zinc supplementation, which typically consists of 1–3 mg/kg of zinc gluconate or sulfate administered orally each day. Clinical response is observed within 5–10 days. Serum zinc levels and alkaline phosphatase values should be monitored every 3–6 months [14, 17–19] (Chart 38.2).

Chart 38.2 Correlation of nutrient deficiency and recommended treatment*

Nutrient	
Biotin	Biotin, 10 mg/day orally
Copper	Elemental copper, 0.1–0.5 g, intravenously, 2×/week
Iron	Ferrous sulfate, 500 mg/day orally
Selenium	Sodium selenite, 200 mg/day orally
Vitamin A or retinol	Vitamin A, 50,000–200,000 IU/day orally
Vitamin B2 or riboflavin	Vitamin B2, 10–20 mg/day orally
Vitamin B3 or niacin	Nicotinic acid, 500 mg/day orally
Vitamin B5 or pantothenic acid	Pantothenic acid, 10 g/day orally
Vitamin B6 or pyridoxine	Pyridoxine, 100 mg/day orally
Vitamin B9 or folic acid and B12 or cobalamin	Folic acid, 1–20 mg/day orally Vitamin B12 of 1mg/weekly parenteral
Vitamin C or ascorbic acid	Vitamin C, 500 mg to 1g/day orally
Vitamin D	Vitamin D, 600–800 IU/day orally
Vitamin E	Vitamin E, 400–800 mg/day orally
Vitamin K	Vitamin K, 1–3mg/single dose intramuscularly
Zinc	Zinc, 15–30 mg/day orally
Protein	1.5 g protein/kg orally

*Reference [14]

Allergic Contact Dermatitis

Nutritional Correlation

Approximately 30–50% of individuals who are allergic to natural rubber latex show an associated hypersensitivity to some plant-derived foods, especially fresh fruits. This association of latex allergy and plant-derived food allergy is called latex-fruit syndrome. An increasing number of plant sources, such as avocado, banana, chestnut, kiwi, peach, tomato, potato, bell pepper, and, recently, turnip, zucchini, and cassava, have been associated with this syndrome. The prevailing hypothesis is that allergen cross-reactivity is due to immunoglobulin E (IgE) antibodies that recognize structurally similar epitopes on different proteins. Some forms of eczema will therefore respond to dietary restriction of certain foodstuffs [20–23].

The oral intake of nickel can induce systemic contact dermatitis in nickel-sensitive individuals and depends on the composition of the diet and on factors such as the food preparation process, whether the food is fresh or canned, and/or whether contamination occurred during processing or through kitchen utensils. Food, water, and cooking utensils are all sources of nickel in the diet. Certain foods, such as cocoa and chocolate, soya beans, oatmeal, almonds and other nuts, and fresh and dried legumes are routinely high in nickel content [20, 24].

Food items most commonly mentioned by patients as aggravating dermatitis due to balsam of Peru are wine, candy, chocolate, cinnamon, curry, citrus fruit, tomatoes, and flavorings [20, 24].

Skin Manifestations

A flare-up of a recurrent erythema and vesicular eczema is the most common clinical manifestation [24].

Complementary Examinations

Patch testing is required to identify the external chemicals to which the person is allergic. The greatest quality-of-life benefits from patch testing occur in patients with recurrent or chronic allergic contact dermatitis. Patch testing is cost-effective and reduces the cost of therapy in patients with severe allergic contact dermatitis.

Therapeutic Approach

Therapy involves avoiding any foods suspected of causing contact dermatitis [20].

Atopic Dermatitis

Nutritional Correlation

Food Allergy

Some controversy exists regarding the role of food antigens in the pathogenesis of atopic dermatitis (AD), in relation to both the prevention of AD and the efficacy of withdrawing foods from the diets of persons with established AD. Most reported studies contain methodological flaws. Because of the controversy surrounding the role of food in AD, most physicians do not remove food from the diet. Nevertheless, acute food reactions (urticaria and anaphylaxis) are commonly encountered in children with AD [7, 25].

The National Institute of Allergy and Infectious Diseases Food Allergy Expert Panel suggests consideration of limited food allergy testing (i.e., cow's milk, eggs, wheat, soy, and peanut) if a 5-year-old child has moderate to severe AD and the following: persistent disease despite optimized management and topical therapy, a reliable history of an immediate allergic reaction after ingestion of a specific food, or both. While food allergy is less common in older age groups, when suspected, the choice of food for testing should be made according to the clinical history and to the most prevalent allergies in a given population. Tree nuts, shellfish, and fish become relevant in subsequent childhood years. In older children, adolescents, and adults, pollen-related food allergy should be taken into account; for example, those with birch pollen allergy may develop itching in their mouth with exposure to apples, celery, carrots, and hazelnuts [7, 26].

Prebiotics and Probiotics

The role of prebiotics and probiotics in the diet of patients with AD is controversial. The composition of intestinal bacteria is postulated to affect food sensitization in the gastrointestinal tract and AD pathogenesis [7, 27].

Prebiotics are nondigestible food components, commonly oligosaccharides. There is currently insufficient evidence to determine the role of prebiotic supplementation of infant formula for the prevention of allergic disease and food hypersensitivity. Trials are needed to determine whether this finding persists over a longer period of time, applies to other manifestations of allergic disease, is associated with reductions in allergen sensitization, and is reproducible [7, 27].

Probiotics are live microorganisms currently defined as food supplements with established beneficial effect on human health. More studies of probiotic supplementation have been conducted with *Lactobacillus acidophilus*, *L. rhamnosus*, *L. reuteri*, and *L. fermentum* [7, 29].

The aims of intervention are to avert deviant microbe development, strengthen the immature or impaired gut barrier function, and alleviate abnormal immune responsiveness. However, a recent Cochrane Intervention Review suggests that probiotics are not an effective treatment for eczema and may, in fact, carry a small risk of adverse events such as infections and bowel ischemia [30].

Maternal Diet and Breastfeeding

Maternal diets with the goal of avoiding allergens during pregnancy or lactation do not prevent AD. However, exclusive breastfeeding for 4 months or breastfeeding supplemented with hydrolyzed formula is protective against AD in high-risk infants. For infants at normal risk, breastfeeding does not affect the incidence of AD. It has been reported that restriction of maternal diet during pregnancy and lactation does not affect subsequent AD development. Exclusive breastfeeding for 4 months in high-

risk infants was reported to be protective against AD [7, 27].

Vitamins

Recently, reports in the literature have emphasized the impact of vitamin D on the pathogenesis of AD. Considering the immunologic mechanisms involved in AD pathogenesis, vitamin D may influence that process through its immunomodulatory properties. It is known that the active form of vitamin D ($1,25(OH)_2D_3$) increases the expression of antibacterial peptide, thus preventing cutaneous infections. Some studies have demonstrated the link between vitamin D and Toll-like receptors, cathelicidin production, and the increased susceptibility to bacterial infections. In addition, vitamin D stimulates the synthesis of proteins such as filaggrin, which is essential to the formation of the stratum corneum. Thus, vitamin D deficiency may exacerbate AD by altering the skin barrier and undermining the immune system, leading to a subsequent increase in the risk of infections [7, 14, 31] (Chart 38.1).

Studies have looked at the combination of vitamin D plus vitamin E compared with placebo and found significant improvement in AD, suggesting a potential role for dual therapy. At present, although there is some evidence to suggest the use of vitamin E in AD, more studies are needed to confirm this benefit as well as its value in combination with other vitamins [7, 27, 31].

Skin Manifestations

A number of criteria are commonly used for the diagnosis of AD, namely, eczematous changes that vary with age, chronic and relapsing course, early age of onset, pruritus and xerosis.

Complementary Examinations

Diagnosis of an IgE-mediated food allergy relies on a combination of medical history, skin prick testing (SPT), serum IgE testing, and oral food challenges. Classically, neither the skin prick test nor allergen-specific serum IgE testing is diagnostic because of their limited positive pre-dictive value for clinical allergy [26].

Tests often performed for evaluation include SPT and serum-specific IgE level determination, which assess for immediate/type I hypersensitiv-ity reactions. In cases of extensive eczematous lesions, severe dermatographism, or the recent use of oral antihistamines, specific IgE (sIgE) measurement may be preferable over SPT. With both tests, the negative predictive value is high (95%) and the specificity and positive predictive value are low (40–60%). Negative test results are helpful to rule out food allergy, but positive results only signify sensitization, and require clinical correlation and confirmation to establish the presence of allergic disease and the exact type of allergic response [7, 26].

Baseline sIgE values for cow's milk, peanut, egg white, and seafood have been associated with an increased risk of developing allergies to these foods, while wheat and soybean sIgE levels have not. Higher specific IgE levels and larger wheal sizes (8–10 mm) are associated with a greater likelihood of reaction on challenge. Measuring total serum IgE levels alone, or comparing with allergen-specific levels, is not helpful in deter-mining food allergy [7].

In recent years, atopy patch tests (APTs) have been introduced to assess for type IV hypersensi-tivity/eczematous reactions. Food APTs are not commonly used in the evaluation of patients. These conflicting findings might be explained by the sometimes difficult interpretation of APTs because of nonspecific reactions. In addition, while AD patients are more reactive than healthy controls, the results do not necessarily correlate with disease severity or clinical outcome, and APTs are therefore not currently recommended for routine use [7].

Therapeutic Approach

Food Elimination/Avoidance Diets

A Cochrane review of food allergy in patients with AD showed that an egg- and milk-free diet provided no apparent benefit in unselected par-ticipants with atopic eczema. There appears to be little benefit in eliminating cow's milk from the diet or using an "elemental" (liquid diet contain-ing only amino acids, carbohydrates, fat, miner-als, and vitamins) or "few foods diet" for improving atopic eczema in people who have not undergone any form of testing (for specific IgE to food allergens). There may be some benefit in using an egg-free diet in infants with suspected egg allergy who have positive specific IgE to eggs. This is important, particularly since some children with AD show impaired physical devel-opment, secondary to gastrointestinal involve-ment. Although strict elimination diets may be impractical, there is evidence to show that a strict antigen avoidance regimen may be associated with improvement of refractory widespread AD when conventional treatments have failed [7, 20, 26].

Excessively restrictive diets, especially in atopic children, have led to weight loss, poor growth, calcium deficiency, hypovitaminosis, and kwashiorkor. Proper medical supervision, nutritional counseling from a dietician, and sup-plementation should be included if elimination/avoidance diets are pursued for a prolonged period. Even in those individuals with clinically relevant food allergy, avoidance diets are gener-ally helpful to avoid the effects of IgE-mediated/immediate reactions but are unlikely to affect the course of AD [7, 20].

Prebiotics and Probiotics

Prebiotics are found in vegetables (artichoke, asparagus, bananas, garlic, leeks, onion, toma-toes), grains (barley, rye, whole grains), roots (chicory root, dandelion root, elecampane root), fermented dairy products (e.g., yogurt, butter-milk, kefir), naturally in breast milk, and in some products with added prebiotics (e.g., bread, breakfast cereals, sauces and soups, and dairy products such as yoghurt). Probiotics are mainly found in some yoghurts and can also be con-sumed as capsules, tablets, beverages, and pow-ders [7, 20, 29].

Maternal Diet During Pregnancy and Lactation

The evidence from studies into the role of dietary restriction during pregnancy and lactation has been conflicting. A Cochrane review examining four trials involving egg and cow's milk restriction during pregnancy showed no significant difference in the incidence of AD. Definite conclusions about the effect of breastfeeding in either preventing or delaying the onset of AD are difficult to make. Studies suggest that exclusive breastfeeding for 3–4 months may be beneficial in preventing AD in mothers of infants with a family history of atopy [7, 20, 30].

Vitamins

The specific treatment of vitamin deficiency depends on each case. The general posology is vitamin E, 400–800 mg/day orally and vitamin D, 600–800 IU/day orally for 60 days [14, 31, 32] (Table 38.1).

Autoimmune Cutaneous Diseases

Nutritional Correlation

Eating Disorders

Eating disorders (EDs), including anorexia nervosa and bulimia nervosa, are often associated with autoimmune disease. This fact supports the hypothesis of comorbidity of these disorders and suggests that immune-mediated mechanisms could play a role in the development of EDs. The studies suggest that the link between these facts is based on shared immunologic mechanisms rather than on the shared genetic background, e.g., the shared human leukocyte antigen risk genotype. EDs with correlated cutaneous manifestations include Sjögren's syndrome (SS), scleroderma, sarcoidosis, pemphigus, dermatitis herpetiformis (DH), psoriasis, vitiligo, lupus erythematosus, dermatomyositis, mixed connective tissue disease, and idiopathic thrombocytopenic purpura [33, 35, 36].

Vitamin D

Vitamin D deficiency is clearly correlated with autoimmune cutaneous disease. A high prevalence of vitamin D deficiency was noted among patients with autoimmune diseases, especially systemic lupus erythematosus (SLE). These observations led to the hypothesis that vitamin D deficiency may exacerbate autoimmune conditions. Similarly, patients with SS and scleroderma

tend to have very low vitamin D levels. This may be attributed to characteristics of the diseases, including disseminated skin involvement and renal injury that may interfere with vitamin D synthesis, as well as vitamin D malabsorption in cases of advanced intestinal disease. Moreover, patients with SLE and SS related to severe vitamin D deficiency demonstrated a more severe disease course [14, 34] (Chart 38.1).

Complementary Examinations

Standard laboratory studies that are diagnostically useful when autoimmune cutaneous diseases is suspected should include the following: complete blood count with differential, serum creatinine, urinalysis, erythrocyte sedimentation rate or C-reactive protein, complement levels, liver function tests, creatine kinase assay, spot protein/spot creatinine ratio, antinuclear antibody, anti-dsDNA, anti-Sm, anti-SSA (Ro), or anti-SSB (La).

Serum 25(OH)D is the best test to determine vitamin D status. The circulating half-life of 25(OH)D is 2 weeks. A 25(OH)D level of less than 30 ng/mL is considered vitamin D insufficient. A 25(OH)D level of less than 15 or 20 ng/mL has been used to define vitamin D deficiency. Intestinal calcium absorption is optimized at levels above 30–32 ng/mL. Parathyroid hormone levels start to rise at 25(OH)D levels below 31 ng/mL, which is another marker of vitamin D insufficiency.

Therapeutic Approach

Eating Disorders

It is important to remember the correlation between nutritional and autoimmune diseases when selecting the most appropriate approach and treatment for the patient. In such cases, a multidisciplinary team (e.g., dermatologists, psychiatrists) should treat the patient [33].

Vitamin D

The specific treatment of vitamin deficiency depends on each case. The general posology is vitamin D, 600–800 IU/day orally for 60 days [14, 34] (Table 38.1).

Bullous Diseases

Nutritional Correlation

A variety of dietary factors have been proposed to play a role in the pathogenesis, exacerbation, and therapy of autoimmune and nonautoimmune bullous skin diseases, although in DH the role of food components (gluten) is well established [20, 38].

Pemphigus

A variety of substances (tannins, thiols, phenols, isothiocyanates, phycocyanins) in different foods are believed to have an effect in the induction, maintenance, and exacerbation of pemphigus (including pemphigus vulgaris, pemphigus foliaceus, paraneoplastic pemphigus, and IgA pemphigus), in genetically predisposed individuals. The basis for that belief is the similarity of their chemical structure to that of drugs known to induce the disease. In addition, environmental factors such as the high tannin content in water is believed to play a role in endemic pemphigus among populations in Amazonian Brazil (fogo selvagem) and India. A list of foods containing these substances includes garlic, leek, chives, onion, mustard (thiols), black pepper, red chilies, mango, pistachio, cashews, aspartame, food additives (phenols), mango, cassava, yucca, guarana, betel nuts, raspberry, cranberry, blackberry, avocado, peach, ginger, ginseng, tea, red wine, coffee, spices, eggplant (tannins), mustard, horseradish, kale, cauliflower (isothiocyanates), and *Spirulina platensis* alga (phycocyanins). In some case reports, exclusion of these foods from the diet resulted in disease cessation or improvement, while challenge with the foods caused recurrence. No case reports of pemphigus induced by isothiocyanates have been reported to date, although they are believed to be similar to thiol-containing compounds [20, 28, 37]. The thiol allyl compounds and/or tannins may either be incorporated into keratinocytes, thus leading to simple biochemical acantholysis, or may release sequestered desmoglein antigens from immunologically privileged sites and also interfere with the immune balance, thus leading to antibody-mediated immunologic acantholysis. As occurs with thiol-based drugs, a combined mechanism is also possible [37]. Antigliadin antibodies have been reported in some pemphigus patients. In a recent case report, two patients with new-onset pemphigus were started on a gluten-free diet with subsequent complete remission of the disease. Both patients had serologic markers of gluten-sensitive enteropathy, without signs of celiac disease [20, 28, 38].

Bullous Pemphigoid

No dietary factors have been implicated in the induction of bullous pemphigoid. There is only one case report of nickel-free diet associated with cessation of dyshidrosiform pemphigoid [20, 38, 39]. The presence of antigliadin antibodies in the sera of bullous pemphigoid patients may indicate that some of them have gluten sensitivity. There have been no reports, however, of bullous pemphigoid improving with a gluten-free diet [39].

Linear IgA Disease

In some case reports, gluten restriction in the presence of an underlying gluten-sensitive enteropathy resulted in resolution of linear IgA disease, with recurrence when gluten was reintroduced [20, 38].

Dermatitis Herpetiformis

Research into DH, especially the elucidation of its pathogenesis, has shown that it is not simply a bullous cutaneous disease but a cutaneous-intestinal disorder caused by gluten hypersensitivity. Its association with celiac disease is well established. Exposure to gluten remains the trigger of an, as yet partially elucidated, inflammatory cascade [20, 28, 40].

A gluten-free diet has been shown to result in resolution of enteropathy, a decrease in or the absence of the need for medication, protective effects against the development of lymphoma, and a general feeling of well-being [20]. Gluten is an amorphous protein composed of gliadin and glutenin amino acids, which are found in cereal seeds from the Gramineae family, such as wheat, barley, oats, malt, and rye. They are cereals that contain starch, lipids, and proteins (gliadin, glutenin, albumin, and globulin). Specifically, wheat protein is composed of 68% gliadin and 32% glutamine, and is therefore commonly referred to as wheat gluten. Examples of food products that contain this protein are flour, chocolate milk, which contains malt, processed cheese, beer, whiskey, vodka, mustard, ketchup, mayonnaise, and salami [41]. Recently, it has been hypothesized that patients with DH may be better able to tolerate oats, because of their lower protamine content compared with other cereals. Inclusion of oats in gluten-free diets remains controversial. Because some oats and oat-containing products may be contaminated with gluten-containing cereals, care must be taken when introducing oats into a gluten-free diet [20, 28, 38].

Dietary factors other than gluten may be important in the pathogenesis of DH. Most of the antigens that lead to immune responses are believed to be full-length proteins. Therefore, an elemental diet that contains only amino acids, not full-length proteins, could be beneficial in DH patients because, theoretically, no antigenic stimulation would take place. Disease remission with the elemental diet, as reported in various studies, supports the concept that other antigens may be involved in the pathogenesis of DH [20, 38].

There are two case reports of milk consumption affecting the course of DH, suggesting that milk proteins may serve as DH antigens. A DH patient who was started on a gluten-free diet did not improve until milk and milk proteins were excluded [20, 38].

The symptoms and signs of DH may be exacerbated by topical or oral administration of potassium iodide. When iodides were applied to the healthy skin of DH patients in a potassium iodide patch test study, vesicles appeared that were histologically identical to DH lesions. Potassium iodide and iodine-containing foods (including seafood), as well as thyroid disorders (treated or not treated with iodine), have also been associated with DH onset or flares [20, 38].

Epidermolysis Bullosa

Epidermolysis bullosa patients, especially those with junctional and recessive dystrophic subtypes of the disease, are at significant risk of nutritional compromise. Nutritional profiles of the patients consistently show malnutrition and growth stunting resulting from oral, esophageal, and oropharyngeal problems, such as oral blistering and ulcerations, abnormal esophageal motility, esophageal strictures, dysphagia, dental problems, digestion and absorption problems, anal erosions, fissures, and rectal strictures resulting in chronic constipation, loss of blood and protein through open skin blisters, and hypermetabolism resulting in increased heat loss and protein turnover. Vitamin and mineral deficiencies are common in these patients, particularly iron deficiency, and a refractory anemia that is unresponsive to oral supplements may develop. As with iron, other elements such as zinc, selenium, vitamin E, and carnitine may be deficient. Vitamin D deficiency and lack of physical exercise are two factors that have deleterious effects on bone health, and put patients at risk for low bone mass and fragility fractures [20, 38].

Skin Manifestations

Bullous diseases present typical signs and symptoms, although dietary factors play a role in their pathogenesis or exacerbation. Figure 38.2 shows DH lesions.

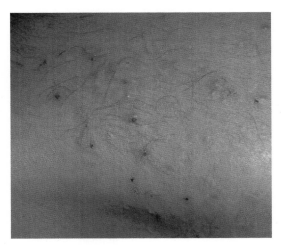

Fig. 38.2 DH lesions: papules, vesicles, erosions, and crusts (Courtesy of Dermatology Service of UFCSPA)

Complementary Examinations

Patients with DH may have malabsorption and nutritional deficiencies of iron, folic acid, selenium, and vitamin B12 as result of inflammation in the intestinal mucosa. Therefore, laboratory tests should be performed regularly to check the nutritional status of such patients. Exclusion of celiac disease is mandatory. IgA anti-tissue transglutaminase antibody is the preferred single test for detection of celiac disease in individuals over the age of 2 years [20, 28, 38].

Epidermolysis bullosa patients are at significant risk of nutritional compromise. The following profiles should be carried out: iron, ferritin, zinc, selenium, vitamin E, and vitamin D (25(OH)D) [20, 38].

Therapeutic Approach

Dietary recommendations should not be overlooked in bullous diseases, and additional studies regarding dietary manipulation and the effect of dietary components are required to better understand the condition and treat patients [20, 38].

Patients with pemphigus should be advised to maintain a balanced diet and avoid foods spiced with garlic, onion, and leek as these culinary plants, belonging to the genus Allium, contain thiol allyl compounds with a proven acantholytic potential. Patients should also be warned against the ingestion of very hot foods and beverages in view of the possible acantholytic effect that the excessive heat may exert on oral and esophageal mucosae. Milk is a nutrient to recommend, because of its high protein content, its easy intake even in the presence of painful oral erosions, and its high level of an oxidative enzyme (sulfhydryl oxidase) that has the potential to neutralize the acantholytic effect of thiol allyl derivatives found in the vegetarian diet [20, 37, 38].

A gluten-free diet is essential in the treatment of patients with DH, since cutaneous and intestinal clinical manifestations are gluten dependent and improve with suspension of its intake. Dapsone remains the primary drug for treatment, but requires monitoring because of its possible side effects, some of which are potentially lethal [28, 40]. The average duration of the gluten-free diet to reduce or discontinue dapsone is 18 months. A long-term gluten-free diet has also been shown to decrease the intensity of skin IgA fluorescence [20, 38].

To date, no clinical trials of iodide-free diets have been carried out in DH patients. Such diets could be considered in patients who consume large amounts of iodide-containing foods (salt, fish) or who do not respond to a gluten-free diet [20, 38].

Depending on their vitamin status, appropriate vitamin supplementation should be given to epidermolysis bullosa patients to optimize their nutrition. Vitamin D and calcium supplementation should be given to young patients in particular in an effort to prevent negative consequences to bone health. Nutritional support is an essential part of long-term management and improves the quality of life by accelerating wound healing, reducing infections, and promoting growth and development. The goals of nutritional support are to address the malnutrition and nutrient and vitamin deficiencies, while alleviating the feeding difficulties and complications that affect the nutritional status in these patients. Chronic constipation frequently contributes to malnutrition and growth failure. A high-fiber diet and adequate fluid intake are important to ease the passage of stools. In infants with epidermolysis bullosa, breast milk is recommended, complemented or replaced by a specially designed formula in cases of poor weight gain. In older children, food texture and consistency should be modified to match individual tolerance [38].

A few case reports have suggested that vitamin E therapy, especially in large doses, may be beneficial in epidermolysis bullosa patients. The action mechanism of vitamin E is believed to involve the reduction of collagenase activity, which results in decreased blister formation [20, 38].

Energy-Protein Malnutrition

Nutritional Correlation

Energy-protein malnutrition (EPM) can be classified as marasmus, kwashiorkor, and marasmus-kwashiorkor. Marasmus refers to a global and chronic deficiency of nutrients resulting from lack of food intake or absorption. Kwashiorkor refers to a disproportionately greater absorption or ingestion of carbohydrates compared with fat and protein intake. Marasmus-kwashiorkor is an intermediate state between them. EPM is uncommon in adults, but has been associated with anorexia nervosa and malabsorptive disorders such as Crohn's disease, cystic fibrosis, and postbariatric surgery. In EPM, the skin becomes dry with scaling and cracking. There may be peeling of patches of skin referred to as the flaky paint sign. This peeling leaves behind a raw surface. Hyperpigmented plaques develop in areas exposed to trauma. The hair becomes thin, sparse, and brittle, and falls out easily. It often loses its normal pigmentation, becoming dull brown or reddish-tinged. If periods of inadequate intake are interspersed with periods of good nutrition, when the normal hair color is restored, horizontal stripes develop in the hair, referred to as the flag sign. Nails may be fissured or ridged. There is atrophy of the papillae on the tongue, angular stomatitis, and cheilosis. As malnutrition progresses, the child becomes weak and hypotonic. The infant or child may appear very quiet, apathetic, restless, or irritable. Older children have a limited attention span [14, 42–44] (Chart 38.1).

Skin Manifestations

From a dermatologic viewpoint, the following manifestations can be found: dry, wrinkled skin giving a more aged appearance; erythematous or hypochromic lesions are seen mostly in areas of friction or flexure, which over time become very evident and hyperpigmented, with smooth, fissured or erosive surfaces. Nails are brittle, slow growing, and with areas of onychomadesis. Areas of follicular hyperkeratosis, and pale extremities accompanied by swelling may also occur. The hair may be dry, brittle, dull, thin, with a red-brownish color before becoming grayish-white. The flag sign depicts alternate dark and light bands in the hair. Angular cheilitis, xerophthalmia, stomatitis, and vulvovaginitis may also be seen [43].

Complementary Examinations

Blood glucose, examination of blood smears by microscopy or direct detection testing, hemoglobin, urine examination and culture, stool examination by microscopy for ova and parasites, serum albumin, human immunodeficiency virus (HIV) test, and electrolytes.

Therapeutic Approach

EPM treatment should be individualized according to the type and severity of the presented manifestations. However, it is essential to correct their cause and supplement the deficient macronutrients [14, 42, 43] (Table 38.1).

Hair Disorders

Nutritional Correlation

Hair follicle cells have a high turnover. Their active metabolism requires a good supply of nutrients and energy. Caloric deprivation or deficiency of several components, such as proteins, minerals, essential fatty acids, and vitamins, caused by inborn errors or reduced uptake, can lead to structural abnormalities, pigmentation changes, or hair loss, although exact data are often lacking. Combined deficiencies are not uncommon, especially in malnutrition [28, 36, 45].

Malnutrition and Weight-Loss Diets

Marasmus is a diet low in calories, whereby amino acids are used to provide energy. The glycogen content of the follicular sheath is reduced, providing less energy for cell mitosis [14].

Kwashiorkor is a result of a low protein intake in a calorically normal diet. It is characterized by reddish, short, dull hair and telogen and dystrophic effluvium. Other conditions involving low protein uptake include infants on special diets, such as in urea-cycle disorders, milk-free diets, gastrointestinal disease, blood loss and blood donation, anorexia nervosa, depression, drug addiction, or malignancy. Protein is the major constituent of hair fibers. Therefore, reduced protein uptake can impair hair growth, even before serum albumin levels are decreased [14, 28].

Diets for weight loss can also lead to hair loss, especially if the daily calorie intake is less than 1,000 kcal and if protein intake is inadequate. Hair loss may be even more profound in diets with a negative nitrogen balance (loss of lean body mass) and be partly due to reduced thyroid activity [45] (Chart 38.1).

Vitamin C

Ascorbic acid is essential for collagen synthesis and crosslinkage of keratin fibers. The reference daily intake for men is 90 mg and for women 75 mg. A deficiency is called scurvy and often occurs in elderly patients, alcoholics, those with mental incapacity, and patients with chronic disease [14, 45].

Zinc

Zinc is a trace element that is required by approximately 300 enzymes, contributing to growth, development, wound healing, immune function, and collagen synthesis, among many other functions. It is essential and must be obtained from the diet. Poor dietary intake of meat and fish can result in deficiency, especially when cereal grains that contain phytate, which chelates zinc and prevents absorption, are a dietary mainstay. Some infant formulas are low in zinc, and in breast milk it is more bioavailable than zinc in formula, culminating with the onset of signs of zinc deficiency, early in life. Zinc may be inadequately absorbed in patients with bowel disease and cystic fibrosis. Increased metabolism or excretion of zinc occurs in a variety of conditions, including alcoholism, malignancy, burns, infections, pregnancy, renal disease, sickle cell disease, collagen vascular disease, and anorexia nervosa. Certain medications, such as diuretics, valproic acid, and penicillamine, can lower zinc levels. The required daily zinc intake for men and pregnant women is 11 mg, and 8 mg for women [14, 28, 45, 46].

Essential Fatty Acids

A deficiency of essential fatty acids can cause changes in hair similar to those seen in zinc deficiency. Essential fatty acid deficiency (EFAD) occurs from decreased intake of linoleic and linolenic acids, long-chain polyunsaturated fatty acids that are important components of the stratum corneum. Linoleic acid is the precursor to arachidonic acid, which in turn is a precursor of prostaglandins, leukotrienes, and thromboxane. EFAD in children is associated with protein-energy malnutrition, low-birth-weight infants, malabsorption, and historically with long-term parenteral nutrition. It may follow surgery in adults [14, 45, 46].

Selenium

Deficiency in selenium, an essential trace element found in soil, can also cause changes in hair similar to those of zinc deficiency. Selenium is a component of at least 35 proteins, many of which are enzymes. An important metabolic system dependent on selenium is glutathione peroxidase, a major antioxidant enzyme. Like EFAD, selenium deficiency can occur in low-birth-weight infants and in patients requiring total parenteral nutrition. It also occurs in locations where the soil selenium content is low [45, 46].

Selenium deficiency has been associated with hair loss after adjuvant chemotherapy with cisplatin. How lack of selenium causes lightening of hair color is unknown. Sulfur-containing compounds such as cysteine and glutathione can shift synthesis of melanin from dark eumelanin to lighter pheomelanin [46].

The reference daily intake for adults is 55 mg. Selenium intoxication from overdosed supplements has been reported [14, 46].

Vitamin A

Vitamin A deficiency is usually discovered in the presence of characteristic ophthalmologic findings, including nyctalopia (night blindness), conjunctival dryness, and, when severe, corneal damage and blindness. Although rare in developed countries, it can occur in patients with malabsorption and in those with EDs. Children are particularly susceptible [45].

Biotin

Biotin (vitamin H) is a cofactor of the carboxylase group of enzymes. These are synthesized as inactive precursors, and become activated when linked to biotin by the enzyme holocarboxylase synthetase. Biotin deficiency can be genetic or acquired. Because it is present in many types of foods and synthesized by bacteria in the gastrointestinal tract, acquired biotin deficiency is uncommon. An important cause of acquired biotin deficiency in children and adults is the antiseizure medication valproic acid. Biotinidase activity was decreased in these patients and was normal in those treated with lower doses of valproic acid who did not develop hair loss. Biotin deficiency has also been reported in patients with Leiner's disease, which, among other findings, is associated with generalized seborrheic dermatitis and failure to thrive. Acquired biotin deficiency in adults occurs in the setting of malabsorption, alcoholism, pregnancy, and unusual dietary habits. In fact, the most frequent cause of acquired biotin deficiency in adults is excess intake of raw eggs. Eggs contain the protein avidin, which tightly binds biotin and prevents its absorption. Cooking denatures avidin, thus inhibiting biotin binding. The reference daily intake for adults is 30 µg [45, 46].

Iron

Iron deficiency is the most common nutritional deficiency worldwide and is associated with developmental delay, diminished intellectual performance, and decreased resistance to infection. The most severe consequence of iron deficiency is anemia resulting from inadequate intake, impaired absorption or transport, physiologic losses, or chronic blood loss secondary to disease. Iron deficiency can be avoided through proper dietary intake. The heme found in meat, poultry, and fish has a higher availability than the nonheme iron found in plants and iron-fortified food, so vegetarians have a recommended daily allowance that is twice normal. The coconsumption of vitamin C enhances iron absorption, while tannins (found in tea and coffee) and phytates (found in bran, cereal grains, flour, legumes, nuts, and seeds) inhibit iron absorption [14, 28, 45].

The mechanism by which reduced iron stores affect hair loss is unknown. Possible mechanisms include the requirement for iron as a cofactor for ribonucleotide reductase, the rate-limiting enzyme for DNA synthesis, or from inhibition of iron-dependent coenzymes such as stearoyl-coenzyme A desaturase. Hair follicle matrix cells are among

the most rapidly dividing cells in the body and may be exquisitely sensitive even to a minor decrease in iron availability, resulting in diminished hair growth in the presence of iron deficiency [45].

Before the development of iron-deficiency anemia, there is a period when iron stores are deficient and hemoglobin levels are normal. Serum ferritin, which is one of the most sensitive and specific markers for iron deficiency, is reduced during this period before the development of anemia. An extensive review revealed that serum ferritin had a greater predictive value than other tests of iron status. Ferritin levels need to be interpreted with caution, because ferritin is an acute-phase reactant and is elevated in inflammatory conditions and chronic disease anemia [28, 45].

Various observational studies on the association between decreased ferritin levels and hair loss have resulted in opposing conclusions. The lack of consensus on the threshold level for iron deficiency and lack of proof that reversing the deficiency reverses the hair loss precludes the statement that iron deficiency is a causative factor in adults with chronic telogen effluvium or diffuse alopecia [28, 45, 46].

The daily reference intake is 8 mg for men and 18 mg for women between 19 and 50 years of age. Different values apply for children, seniors, and pregnant or lactating women [45].

Copper

Copper is crucial for the amine oxidase activity required for oxidation of thiol groups to dithio-crosslinks, which are essential for keratin fiber strength. Some enzymes also depend on copper, such as ascorbic acid oxidase and tyrosinase. In children, a rare autosomal-recessive malabsorption disorder, Menkes kinky hair syndrome (MKHS), may be present. Acquired deficiency is also seen in premature babies, inadequate cow's milk, or parental alimentation, and after prolonged zinc therapy. The reference daily intake for adults is 900 mg [45, 46].

Vitamin D

The role of vitamin D for hair growth is still under investigation. Therefore, obtaining a vitamin D level in telogen effluvium can be helpful. The daily intake for adults is 200–400 IU [45, 46].

Hypervitaminosis

Although excess selenium can cause hair loss, most of what is written about vitamin toxicity causing changes in hair pertains to vitamin A. Hypervitaminosis A is a dangerous condition and can result in liver failure, increased intracranial pressure, and death. The skin is frequently involved in both the acute and chronic forms. Acute vitamin A toxicity is caused by inadvertent consumption of high doses of vitamin A, as was reported in Arctic explorers after a single meal of polar bear or seal liver, or consumption of fish liver. Chronic toxicity results from supplementation exceeding the recommended dose of 5,000 IU daily or inadvertent chronic ingestion [46].

Skin Manifestations

In marasmus the hair is thin, sparse, fragile, and even more easily shed than in kwashiorkor, whereas lanugo body hair may be increased. Children with marasmus appear emaciated and have loss of subcutaneous fat. Alopecia due to telogen effluvium may occur [43, 45, 46].

The cutaneous findings in kwashiorkor are much more apparent. Hair may be brittle and dry, as in marasmus, but may also be soft and fine, with reduced diameter. Hair elasticity is reduced. Eyelashes may be affected, becoming fine and unruly and taking on a broomstick appearance. A characteristic finding in kwashiorkor is lightening of hair color (hypochromotrichia). Sometimes scalp hair exhibits a banded pattern, known as the flag sign. This is due to repigmentation of the shaft during periods of improved nutrition as a result of decreased melanin content in the hair shaft [43, 46].

Hair changes typically seen with vitamin C deficiency include corkscrew hairs, perifollicular hyperkeratosis and hemorrhage, follicular plugging, and curling. These findings are most noticeable on the forearms, abdomen, and legs. Corkscrew hairs are coiled or looped hairs, mainly on the arms, trunk, and legs. They are caused by a decreased number of reduced disulfide bonds, leading to decreased keratin

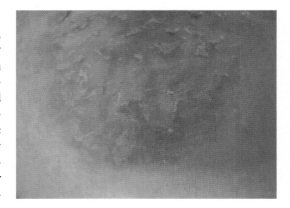

Fig. 38.3 Zinc deficiency lesion (Courtesy of Dr. Renan R. Bonamigo)

crosslinkage, and possibly exacerbated by altered perifollicular connective tissue. Perifollicular hemorrhage appears later and is more common on the lower extremities, anterior forearms, and abdomen. The uniform petechial eruption of scurvy can be mistaken for leukocytoclastic vasculitis, but the presence of corkscrew hairs and the perifollicular nature of the purpura are pathognomonic if recognized. Other symptoms include ecchymoses, bleeding gums, chronic wounds, and infections. Children with scurvy do not always develop the classic cutaneous findings seen in adults, although they may present with skin findings, particularly alopecia [46].

Zinc deficiency can lead to telogen effluvium, thin white and brittle hair, as well as nail dystrophy, a seborrheic and, later, eczema-like or psoriasiform acral and perioral dermatitis (Fig. 38.3), cheilitis, blepharoconjunctivitis, infection, and skin superinfection with *C. albicans* and *S. aureus*. Other symptoms are diarrhea, neurologic disturbances, and growth retardation. Histology shows pale superficial epidermal cells and single-cell necrosis [14, 46].

The clinical features of selenium deficiency are similar to those of zinc deficiency. The cutaneous changes typical of selenium deficiency are often delayed, and deficiency can be subclinical for one to several years. The clinical features of selenium deficiency may occur in infants. Alopecia with pseudoalbinism is common at the time of diagnosis of selenium deficiency, and is considered an early clinical sign [46].

With vitamin A deficiency, the characteristic cutaneous manifestation is phrynoderma. This is a follicular hyperkeratosis with keratin plugs on extensor surfaces, similar to keratosis pilaris. Little has been written on the mechanism by which this occurs. Phrynoderma typically spares the hands, feet, and face. Papules and crateriform nodules have been reported [14, 46].

Surviving infants with the genetic form of biotin deficiency have extensive dermatitis and severe alopecia. Terminal and vellus hair follicles may be lacking on the scalp. In addition, eyebrows, eyelashes, and lanugo hairs may be absent or sparse. There are some case reports of AE-like eruptions [46].

Hypopigmented hair and pili torti are typical in MKHS, as well as the degeneration of brain, bones, and connective tissue, including arterial occlusion, and pale and lax skin. It is associated with copper deficiency [46].

Because the symptoms of chronic hypervitaminosis are insidious, skin changes can be a clue to the diagnosis. They include pruritus, diffuse scaling, desquamation, lip fissures, sore tongue and mouth, brittle nails, nail dystrophy, and diffuse alopecia [14, 45, 46].

Complementary Examinations

Depending of the type and cause of hair loss, complementary examinations should be performed.

Related to nutritional features, the following serum tests are necessary: albumin, zinc, selenium, iron, ferritin, and 25(OH)D.

Therapeutic Approach

Patients often ask if there are any vitamins they can take to help their hair grow and look healthy. However, most vitamins and minerals are obtained from a healthy diet, with the possible exception of iron, and most well-nourished patients do not require supplementation. Exceptions to this occur in patients with malabsorption, chronic illness, congenital heart disease, malignancy, neuromuscular disease, EDs, special diets, and in the elderly [45, 46].

Some clinicians suggest biotin replacement for healthy patients with hair loss. However, there are no clinical trials showing the efficacy of biotin in hair loss, and it is not routinely recommended. The dose recommended varies from 2 to 10 mg per day [45–47].

Although traditionally used in nonspecific hair treatments, zinc supplementation has not been proved to have a beneficial effect on hair growth in patients with normal serum zinc levels. During treatment, zinc levels should be monitored because overdose can lead to copper or calcium deficiency, drowsiness, and headache. The recommended dose for adults is 25–50 mg of elemental zinc and 0.5–1 mg/kg for children [14, 46].

The treatment of MKHS consists of infusions with copper salts [46].

Most authors consider a ferritin level of at least 40 mg/L as adequate in their female patients, while others only require 10 mg/L and some require 70 mg/L. To correct iron deficiency, ferrous fumarate, ferrous lactate, ferrous gluconate, or ferrous sulfate should be taken for several weeks in two to three daily doses [14, 28, 46].

Antioxidants may have long-term effects on hair aging, but are difficult to assess. Taurine, an amino acid, has been shown to promote follicle cell survival in vitro, when combined with the polyphenol catechin and other ingredients. L-Carnitine has been shown to stimulate hair follicle cells in vitro. Components derived from soybeans may also have an effect on hair growth through anti-inflammatory and estrogen-dependent mechanisms, but studies in vivo are lacking and an increased dissemination of hemangioma rubi has been reported. Orthosilicic acid increased hair tensile strength and thickness in some small studies. L-Cysteine supplementation has shown a significant effect in the treatment of diffuse telogen effluvium, avoiding the temporary loss of several thousand hairs. Further studies are needed to expand the evidence regarding the effects of nutritional supplements on hair [45].

There is probably a correlation between alopecia areata and vitamin D deficiency, suggesting that vitamin D deficiency might be a significant risk factor for alopecia areata. More studies with larger numbers of patients are needed to confirm this hypothesis [14, 48] (Table 38.1).

Oral Mucosa Disorders

Nutritional Correlation

The oral manifestations of nutritional deficiency include nonspecific signs and symptoms that involve the mucous membranes, the teeth and periodontal tissues, the salivary glands, and the perioral skin. Owing to the rapid rate of cell turnover in the mucous membranes (3–7 days), the oral cavity may exhibit early signs and symptoms of systemic disease or nutritional deficiency [28, 49].

Water-soluble vitamins that involve the oral mucosa include vitamins B2, B3, B6, and B12, folic acid, and vitamin C. Water-soluble vitamins are not stored in the body in large amounts, so they must be supplied to the body by the diet on a frequent or daily basis. Fat-soluble vitamins that affect the mucosa include vitamins A, D, and E. Minerals relevant to the oral mucosa are calcium, fluoride, iron, and zinc [49] (Chart 38.1).

Vitamin B2

Patients with riboflavin deficiency are at risk for developing edema of the pharyngeal and oral mucous membranes, angular cheilitis, stomatitis, and glossitis [49].

Vitamin B3

Deficiency of this vitamin is referred to as pellagra and may manifest as bright red glossitis, burning mouth, gingival erythema, and dental caries [20, 49].

Vitamin B6

Those at high risk of pyridoxine deficiency include alcoholics and patients taking medications that react with B6 such as isoniazid, L-dopa, penicillamine, and cycloserine. The condition orally presents as glossitis, cheilitis, and gingival erythema [28, 49].

Vitamin B9 (Folic Acid)

Those at high risk of folic acid deficiency include the elderly, alcoholics, and those taking medications that interfere with it, such as methotrexate and phenytoin. Deficiency leads to megaloblastic anemia. Clinical manifestations include burning of the tongue and oral mucosa, a red and swollen tongue, and angular cheilitis [49].

Vitamin B12

The elderly, vegetarians, and those with resected stomach or ileum are particularly susceptible to deficiency of this vitamin. Deficiency of vitamin B12, known as pernicious anemia, presents with megaloblastic anemia, and manifests orally as a red, atrophic, beefy, burning tongue. In addition, vitamin B12 deficiency, along with folic acid and iron deficiencies, is associated with recurrent aphthous stomatitis [14, 49].

Vitamin C (Ascorbic Acid)

Among those at high risk of vitamin C deficiency, also known as scurvy, are alcoholics and individuals with inadequate consumption of fruits or vegetables, the elderly, and infants who consume only cow's milk. Smokers who are deficient in vitamin C are particularly prone to develop periodontal disease. Scurvy presents with hemorrhagic gingivitis with enlarged blue or red gingiva, gingival bleeding, swollen gingiva, and infections. Scurvy also affects dentition, presenting with loose teeth, interdental infarcts, and tooth loss [14, 49].

Vitamin A

Among those at high risk of vitamin A deficiency are patients with malabsorption and fat-absorption disorders, such as celiac disease and short-bowel syndrome. The oral manifestations of vitamin A deficiency include xerostomia (dry mouth), reduced resistance to infections, and impaired growth of the teeth. The oral manifestations of toxicity include cheilitis, gingivitis, carotenemia (orange discoloration of the mucous membranes due to excessive deposition of pigment), and impaired healing. Patients whose livers are compromised because of drug abuse, hepatitis, or excessive ingestion of carrots are at risk of vitamin A toxicity [49].

Vitamin D

Among those at high risk of calcium deficiency are the elderly, women who have had multiple pregnancies, and low-birthweight infants. Vitamin D deficiency may increase the loss of periodontal attachment [14, 49].

Vitamin E (Tocopherol)

Tocopherol is an antioxidant, deficiency of which may be associated with oral cancer. Those at high risk of vitamin E deficiency include premature infants and patients with malabsorption disorders or lipid transport abnormalities [14, 49].

Calcium

Those at high risk for calcium deficiency include premature infants who do not go through the critical intrauterine phase whereby 80% of the body's calcium, phosphorus, and magnesium are absorbed and who also may have malfunctioning kidneys that fail to metabolize vitamin D adequately. Low calcium intake is associated with an increased risk of periodontal disease. Conversely, increased calcium intake has been shown to be associated with decreased risk of periodontal disease and tooth loss, in part due to its role in preventing systemic bone loss [49].

Fluoride

Fluoride makes tooth enamel less soluble and more resistant to demineralization, so its deficiency is associated with an increased incidence of dental caries. However, toxicity causes mottling of the enamel, ranging from mild white flecks to extreme brown discoloration and enamel pitting [49].

Iron

Pregnant women and patients with unusual blood loss or malabsorption disorders are at elevated risk of iron deficiency. Oral manifestations of iron deficiency include atrophy of the lingual papillae, burning and redness of the tongue, angular stomatitis, dysphagia, and pallor of the oral tissues resulting from underlying anemia. Like folic acid and B12, iron deficiency may be associated with recurrent aphthous ulcers [28, 49]. Although the cause of Plummer–Vinson syndrome is still uncertain, this syndrome is associated with iron deficiency along with genetic factors, and presents with angular stomatitis, glossitis, and dysphagia [49].

Zinc

Those at high risk of zinc deficiency include pregnant women, the elderly, vegans, alcoholics, diabetics, and those with HIV/AIDS, inflammatory bowel disease, and sickle cell disease. Excessive consumption of calcium, iron, copper, fiber, phytates, and phosphate salts interferes with proper zinc absorption. Oral manifestations of zinc deficiency include changes to the epithelium of the tongue, an increase in cell numbers, and flattened filiform papillae, ulcers, and xerostomia. Impaired wound healing is one of the most damaging effects of zinc deficiency. Zinc enhances taste and appetite, so deficiency also results in decreased taste sensation, which can cyclically contribute to malnutrition. In AE, the oral mucous membranes may be secondarily infected with *Candida* or *Staphylococcus* [14, 49].

Skin Manifestations

The most frequent oral signs and symptoms of nutritional disorders are angular cheilitis, stomatitis, glossitis, burning mouth, gingival erythema, and dental caries. Individually or in combination, these manifestations could represent early symptoms of vitamin or element deficiency.

Complementary Examinations

Depending of the oral mucosa manifestations, the following serum tests should be considered: folic acid, vitamin B12, 25(OH)D, calcium, zinc, iron, and ferritin.

Therapeutic Approach

Vitamin and element deficiencies should be investigated and treated to resolve the oral signs and symptoms of the nutritional disorders. They will improve once the deficiency is eliminated [14, 49] (Table 38.1).

Nail Disorders

Nutritional Correlation

Several systemic diseases lead to nail changes that dermatologists can visually perceive. However, not all gross changes are secondary to malnutrition alone. Those nail changes attributable solely to malnutrition and other systemic diseases that could manifest secondary to a deficiency in a particular vitamin, mineral, or other trace element (e.g., iron deficiency anemia) are described below [14, 50] (Chart 38.1).

Chromonychia
Chromonychia of the lunula has been reported as a bluish discoloration in copper overload caused by Wilson's disease. Argyria, a chronic elevation of silver salts in the body, has been associated with a blackish-gray discoloration of the lunula and is thought to be photoinduced. Color changes in the nail bed are more diffuse than focal chromonychia of the lunula. Although nonspecific, pallor of the nail bed can be a sign of anemia and an indication that body iron stores may be low. Longitudinal melanonychia of the nail plate secondary to increased melanin production in the matrix has been reported in malnutrition, vitamin D and vitamin B12 deficiencies, and hemochromatosis [50].

Splinter Hemorrhages
Although classically associated with subacute bacterial endocarditis, these are most frequently seen as a result of trauma and have been associated with a number of systemic illnesses. Among the nutrition-related conditions are scurvy (vitamin C deficiency) and hemochromatosis [20, 50].

Terry Nails
Despite its classical association with chronic liver disease, Terry nails may also be seen in malnutrition states, especially in the elderly [50].

Muehrcke Lines
This condition was initially associated with hypoalbuminemia, but this nail change has also been associated with malnutrition and AE [15, 50].

Onycholysis
Onycholysis may be due to exogenous or endogenous causes, with the former representing most of the cases seen in clinics. Some endogenous causes of onycholysis related to nutritional imbalances include iron-deficiency anemia, pellagra, and Cronkhite-Canada syndrome, an extremely rare nonfamilial syndrome characterized by marked epithelial disturbances in the gastrointestinal tract and epidermis. The abnormal mucosal proliferation leads to fluid and electrolyte abnormalities, malabsorption, and malnutrition [20, 50].

Transverse Leukonychia
Although transverse leukonychia is typically associated with deficiency-related states such as AE, pellagra, and low calcium levels, it is also associated with overabundance, such as in the increased blood iron levels that occur in hemochromatosis (Fig. 38.4) [15, 50].

Clubbing
Clubbing can be inherited or acquired. An inherited type of clubbing that falls under the purview of nutritional imbalance includes citrullinemia, a rare autosomal recessive disorder of the hepatic urea cycle that leads to an accumulation of nitrogenous waste compounds and other toxic substances, including citrulline, in the blood. Acquired clubbing secondary to nutritional imbalance may be due to several different combinations of substances and pathologies, including phosphorus, arsenic, alcohol, mercury or beryllium poisoning, hypervitaminosis A, and cretinism caused by iodine deficiency [50].

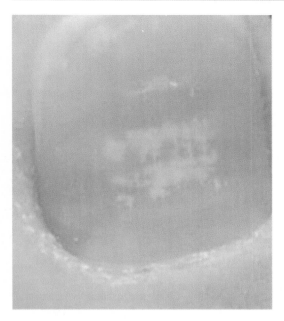

Fig. 38.4 Transverse leukonychia (Courtesy of Dermatology Service of UFCSPA)

Koilonychia

Almost all cases of koilonychia are acquired, although it may be also inherited. It is classically a sign of iron-deficiency anemia and has not been observed in any other type of anemia. However, a few published cases have reported koilonychia in postgastrectomy patients and in patients diagnosed with Plummer–Vinson syndrome. These clinical syndromes have iron-deficiency anemia (e.g., iron malabsorption in postgastrectomy patients and iron-deficiency anemia as one criterion of the Plummer–Vinson syndrome clinical triad) and support the notion that koilonychia is observed only in sideropenic anemia and not in other anemias. Other nutritional states, such as riboflavin deficiency, pellagra, and more commonly, vitamin C deficiency, have been implicated in the development of koilonychia [20, 50].

Hapalonychia

This condition is also known as soft nails and may be associated with occupational diseases, eczematous dermatitis, and certain systemic diseases. Nutritional deficiencies involving vitamins A, B6 (pyridoxine), C, and D, in addition to low serum calcium, have all been implicated in causing hapalonychia [50].

Beau's Lines

Nutritional disorders associated with Beau's lines include protein deficiency and pellagra. Dysregulated blood mineral levels, such as hypocalcemia, chronic alcoholism (another source of malnutrition and malabsorption), and arsenic toxicity, may also play a role in the development of Beau's lines [20, 50].

Onychomadesis

The most common cause of onychomadesis is neurovascular change. Examples would be repeated episodes of decreases in blood calcium levels or a chronic state of hypocalcemia with arteriolar spasm. Such episodes may lead to an abrupt separation of the nail plate from the underlying nail matrix and nail bed, and results in the clinical manifestation of onychomadesis [50].

Onychorrhexis

Mineral imbalances leading to onychorrhexis include iron-deficiency anemia, arsenic poisoning, and zinc deficiency [50].

Trachyonychia

This condition is typically caused by poor or decreased dietary water and food intake, an especially common phenomenon in the elderly. Any of these may contribute to and precipitate the brittle nails and subsequent trachyonychia seen in the elderly [50, 51].

Skin Manifestations

Chromonychia may occur in the lunula, the nail bed, or the nail plate. The word is defined as any color (excluding white) that abnormally discolors a part of the nail unit. Because white is not necessarily considered a distinct color, whitened areas of the nail unit define the term leukonychia.

Transverse leukonychia is distinguished by transverse, opaque white bands that tend to occur in the same relative position in multiple nails. These bands mimic the contour of the lunula and grow out with the nail plate.

Splinter hemorrhages are formed by extravasation of red blood cells from longitudinally oriented nail bed vessels into adjacent longitudinally oriented troughs.

Terry nails are described as any 0.5- to 3.0-mm wide, distal, brown-to-pink nail bed bands with proximal pallor.

Muehrcke lines are characterized by two transverse white bands of pallor. When pressure is applied to the distal plate, the narrow transverse bands disappear, confirming a nail bed change.

Onycholysis is defined as separation of the nail plate from the underlying nail bed.

Clubbing is the term is used when the normal 160° angle between the proximal nail fold and the nail plate exceeds 180°.

Koilonychia is defined as spoon-shaped nail plates. It is thought to result from a relatively low-set distal matrix compared with the proximal matrix that causes nail plate growth to occur in a downward direction as it grows toward the nail bed. When present, it is usually more severe on the index and third fingernails.

Beau's lines are defined as transverse grooves in or depression of the nail plate seen in acute systemic disorders. It is one of the most common signs encountered in clinical practice, but is the least specific. Acute illnesses are thought to cause a temporary arrest of the matrix. If the entire activity of the matrix is inhibited for 1–2 weeks, a Beau's line will reach its maximum depth, causing a total division of the nail plate (i.e., onychomadesis).

Onychomadesis is the term used to describe complete onycholysis, beginning at the proximal end of the nail plate.

Onychorrhexis, or senile nail, describes longitudinal ridges in the nail plate that are most often associated with the aging process.

The term trachyonychia describes rough nail plates with a characteristic gray opacity, brittle (fragilitas unguium) and split free ends, longitudinal ridging, and a rough sandpaper-like surface. Brittle nails and trachyonychia are relatively common in persons older than 60 years. Brittle nail syndrome is a disease characterized by soft, dry, weak, easily breakable nails that show onychorrhexis and onychoschizia [50].

Complementary Examinations

Depending of the nail disorder, the following serum tests should be performed: complete blood count, albumin, iron, ferritin, vitamin B12, 25(OH)D, calcium, zinc, phosphorus, and liver function tests.

Therapeutic Approach

Little information is available on how nutritional supplements affect different nail disorders. It is recognized that if there is a deficiency of any compound, it should be supplemented.

A multitude of regimens exist for treating brittle nails, including buffing and moisturizing, application of essential fatty acids, and the ingestion of vitamin C and pyridoxine, iron, vitamin D, calcium, amino acids, and gelatin. One nutritional supplement that has been investigated and has recently shown promise is biotin, or vitamin H. The use of biotin to strengthen horse hooves in veterinary medicine suggested it could be used to treat human nail disease. One study demonstrated a 25% increase in the thickness of the nail plate in patients diagnosed with brittle nails of unknown cause and treated with biotin (2.5 mg daily) for 6–15 months. Another study showed that biotin was not equally effective in all patients, but a definite trend toward benefit was noted in most of those who took between 1.0 and 3.0 mg daily, with 2 months being the average time before clinically noticeable results. This same study also showed that approximately 10 weeks after biotin was discontinued, nail ridging gradually returned and nail brittleness recurred. The daily requirement of biotin is unknown because it is produced in large quantities by intestinal bacteria. A daily dose of 2.5–3 mg of biotin for approximately 6 months is generally recommended [50, 51] (Table 38.1).

A healthy, well-balanced diet composed of an adequate daily intake of vitamins and minerals facilitates nail health in general. Nails are pure protein, so sufficient protein intake is necessary to ensure healthy nails. Many vegetarians find their nails are first to show the obvious effects of inadequate protein intake [51].

Topical silicon and tazarotene cream 0.1 % have recently been advocated with mixed results for brittle nail syndrome [50, 51].

Necrolytic Migratory Erythema

Nutritional Correlation

Necrolytic migratory erythema (NME) is a rare cutaneous dermatitis that occurs most commonly in patients with a glucagonoma, an α-cell tumor of the pancreas, although it may occur in the absence of a pancreatic tumor (pseudogluca-gonoma syndrome) in the context of other malignancies, liver disease, malabsorption disorders, and inflammatory bowel disease [36]. A number of hypotheses have been proposed concerning the pathogenesis of NME lesions. These include hyperglucagonemia, hypoaminoacidemia, zinc and/or EFAD, liver disease, induction of inflammatory mediators, and generalized malabsorption and malnutrition. It is likely that these theories are not mutually exclusive [20, 36, 38].

It has also been suggested that amino acid deficiency and zinc deficiency contribute to the pathogenesis of NME. Some patients with unresectable glucagonomas have decreased levels of amino acids and show improvement in cutaneous lesions after intravenous administration of amino acids. An improvement in the dermatosis has been observed after zinc supplementation and fatty acid supplementation, suggesting that various nutritional deficiencies may lead to the NME rash. Persistent stimulation of various metabolic pathways by high levels of glucagon may result in hypovitaminosis B and low levels of essential fatty acids and amino acids, thus contributing to the glucagonoma syndrome [20, 38].

Liver disease has been suggested to contribute to NME pathogenesis and lead to low albumin levels, which can produce deficiencies in zinc and essential fatty acids because albumin is their predominant carrier protein in the plasma [38].

Skin Manifestations

The clinical features of the rash include waves of irregular erythema in which a central bulla develops with subsequent erosion and crusting. Central healing occurs, which gives the lesions an annular appearance. The lesions are typically highly pruritic, and predominantly occur at intertriginous sites and areas subject to pressure and friction, such as the perineum, groin, buttocks, lower abdomen, and lower extremities. Stomatitis, glossitis, angular cheilitis, and nail changes may also be seen [38].

Complementary Examinations

Glucagonoma should be investigated, especially with serum glucagon and imaging examinations. Other important complementary examinations include blood glucose, albumin, zinc, liver function tests, erythrocyte sedimentation rate, and C-reactive protein.

Therapeutic Approach

As improvement in the NME rash has been seen after administration of amino acids, zinc, and fatty acid supplementation, deficiency in any of these elements should be corrected [38].

Pellagra

Nutritional Correlation

Pellagra is a systemic nutritional wasting disease caused by a deficiency of vitamin B3 (niacin), which is an essential component of several coenzymes. Besides ingestion, niacin can be endogenously synthesized from its natural precursor, the amino acid tryptophan, a process that requires two other B vitamins, B2 and B6. Pellagra occurs when the intake of niacin and tryptophan are low (primary) or when conversion of the essential amino acid to the coenzyme (secondary) is impaired [14] (Chart 38.1).

At present, pellagra is limited to populations with a compromised dietary intake of niacin and tryptophan or an excessive intake of leucine (a natural antagonist), especially in times of stress or in unique circumstances. These situations include chronic alcohol intake, individuals with significant malabsorption, administration of specific medications, or with a few rare disease entities that affect niacin availability [52].

Skin Manifestations

Classically, patients with pellagra have a syndrome that includes diarrhea, dermatitis, and dementia. The distribution of the cutaneous eruption is typically symmetric and bilateral in parts of the body exposed to sun. The dorsal areas of the hands are the most affected sites, which may present a glove-like distribution; the classic Casal's necklace and neck lesions are also seen. Other skin manifestations linked to niacin deficiency are glossitis and angular and lip cheilitis [52].

Complementary Examinations

Low serum niacin and tryptophan are thought to reflect niacin deficiency and confirm the diagnosis of pellagra.

Therapeutic Approach

Pellagra is often an evolving process, which, if untreated, can lead to progressive deterioration and death over a period of years. Therapeutic response to niacin in a patient with the typical symptoms and signs of pellagra establishes the diagnosis. The recommended intake of 6.6 niacin equivalents per 1,000 kcal daily is accepted for children aged 6 months or older. For infants up to 6 months, it is accepted that breastfeeding by well-nourished mothers supplies adequate

niacin equivalents to fulfill the needs (i.e., 8 niacin equivalents/1,000 kcal) of this age group. A diet high in protein and adequate in calories should be provided in order to prevent and/or treat pellagra. The addition of meats, milk, peanuts, green leafy vegetables, whole or enriched grains, and brewers' dried yeast can enhance niacin intake. The treatment of adult pellagra is nicotinic acid 50–100 mg orally every 6–8 h, not to exceed 500 mg/day [14, 52] (Table 38.1).

Skin Manifestations of Peripheral Vascular Disease

Nutritional Correlation

Peripheral vascular disease (PVD) is a nearly pandemic condition and manifests as insufficient tissue perfusion initiated by existing atherosclerosis acutely compounded by either emboli or thrombi. The atheroma consists of a core of cholesterol joined to proteins with a fibrous intravascular covering. The most important causes of atherosclerosis are high fat levels in the blood, diabetes, and high blood pressure. The disease is typically segmental, with significant variation from patient to patient [53, 54].

Obesity is an important factor in varicose veins. Stasis pigmentation is the result of the escape of red blood cells into surrounding tissues, which results in an inflammatory reaction to the deposited hemoglobin [53, 54].

Skin Manifestations

In PVD the skin may have an atrophic, shiny appearance and may demonstrate trophic changes, including alopecia; dry, scaly, or erythematous skin; chronic pigmentation changes; and brittle nails. Advanced PVD may manifest as livedo reticularis (mottling), pulselessness, numbness, or cyanosis. Paralysis may follow, and the extremities may become cold; gangrene may occasionally be seen. Poorly healing injuries or ulcers in the extremities help provide evidence of pre-existing PVD [53, 54].

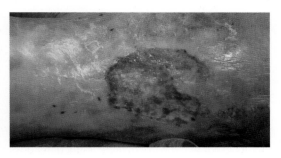

Fig. 38.5 Leg ulcer in a patient with peripheral vascular disease (Courtesy of Dr. Renan R. Bonamigo)

Clinically, in the presence of varicose veins pitting edema usually occurs at the extremities, but varicose veins are not always apparent. There is dark pigmentation and often extensive scaling of the skin. The legs may also be red, warm, and tender because of an inflammatory reaction to the pigment in the dermis. Signs, such as small erosions to very large ulcers, may represent the residue of an underlying eczematous dermatitis, but deep ulcers are uncommon. In most cases, the ulcers occur on the medial ankle or lower calf and usually have a red base of granulated tissue. The subcutaneous tissue may be indurated (Fig. 38.5) [53, 54].

Complementary Examinations

Plain films are of little use in the setting of PVD. Doppler ultrasonographic studies are useful as primary noninvasive studies to determine flow status. Upper extremities are evaluated over the axillary, brachial, ulnar, and radial arteries. Lower extremities are evaluated over the femoral, popliteal, dorsalis pedis, and posterior tibial arteries. One should note the presence of Doppler signal and the quality of the signal (i.e., monophasic, biphasic, triphasic). The presence of distal flow does not exclude emboli or thrombi because collateral circulation may provide these findings.

Therapeutic Approach

At present, therapeutic recommendations include single-agent antiplatelet agents for the prevention of cardiovascular events in patients with asymptomatic and symptomatic disease. These medications should be used in conjunction with efforts to reduce risk factors, including adequate diet with low fatty foods, smoking cessation, and exercise therapy. In the case of obesity, weight reduction is necessary to lower peripheral venous pressure [53, 54].

Phrynoderma and Vitamin A Deficiency

Nutritional Correlation

Vitamin A is a liposoluble vitamin that is vital for retinal photoreceptors and the correct functioning of the immune system, as well as skin keratinization and the process of embryogenesis. Vitamin A intake may be inadequate in patients with restrictive diets and EDs. Although vitamin A deficiency is more common in underdeveloped countries, in developed countries its manifestations can be induced by liver cirrhosis, malnutrition, or alcoholism. Liver disease patients evaluated for liver transplantation often have vitamin A deficiency. Both dietary quality and diversity may deteriorate in economic crises. Nevertheless, vitamin A deficiency remains preventable during economic instability by promoting breastfeeding, providing supplementary vitamin A, fortifying foods targeted at the poor, and encouraging homestead food production that can bolster income and diversify the diet. Early dietary intervention, preferably within the first 1,000 days of life, is important to break the cycle of malnutrition and its undesirable consequences [6, 55].

Vitamin A is also important in cellular differentiation (e.g., growth, reproduction, immune response) and in maintaining epithelial integrity. No nutritional deficiency is more synergistic with infection than vitamin A. The two main mechanisms involved in the prevention of disease are the effect of vitamin A on the immune system and on epithelial integrity. Epidermal vitamin A deficiency may result from a deficit of nutritional vitamin A, exposure to sunlight or any ultraviolet (UV) source, oxidative stress, or chronologic aging. Accordingly, increasing epidermal vitamin A may be beneficial [6, 55].

Phrynoderma has been considered pathognomonic of vitamin A deficiency, but probably represents a nonspecific finding common to cases of nutritional insufficiency, as it has also been associated to fatty acid, vitamin E, and vitamin B2 deficiencies [6, 14] (Chart 38.1).

Skin Manifestations

Phrynoderma is characterized by follicular and keratotic papules that usually affect the anterolateral surface of the thighs and arms. Lesions may overtake the extensor surface of the upper and lower limbs, shoulders, abdomen, dorsal area, buttocks, and neck. Other cutaneous manifestations associated with vitamin A deficiency are xeroderma and thinning, brittle, or corkscrew hair. The correlation between low plasma concentrations of vitamins A and E and the development of acne has recently been speculated [6, 55].

Complementary Examinations

The diagnosis should be suspected in children who are malnourished or in patients with predisposing factors for its development. The following are employed to evaluate serum vitamin A levels:

- The biochemical definition of vitamin A deficiency is a plasma level of 35 μmol/dL or less. Several techniques are available, but high-pressure liquid chromatography is the most reliable. An important factor is that, with protein deficiency, serum vitamin A levels may be decreased despite good vitamin A intake and adequate vitamin A stores.
- Total and holo retinol-binding protein test in the blood tend to correlate with measures of serum vitamin A. These levels can also be decreased in the presence of protein deficiency.

Therapeutic Approach

Oral administration of 200,000 IU of vitamin A at presentation, the following day, and a third dose a week later is recommended. Children younger than 1 year should receive one-half the standard dose, and infants younger than 6 months should receive one-quarter the standard dose. Children with marasmus or kwashiorkor need further nutritional supplementation and monitoring with additional doses of vitamin A at monthly intervals until clinical improvement. Pregnant women should not receive large doses of vitamin A because it may be teratogenic, but a daily dose of 10,000 IU over 2 weeks is safe. In all cases, a diet rich in vitamin A should be advised [14] (Table 38.1).

Porphyria

Nutritional Correlation

Dietary factors have been implicated in triggering porphyria and also as potential photoprotective agents [20, 57].

Porphyria Cutanea Tarda
Porphyria cutanea tarda (PCT) is the most common form of porphyria. A variety of factors have been associated with this disease, namely alcohol, estrogens, polychlorinated hydrocarbons, abnormal iron metabolism, and viral infections, including hepatitis C and HIV. Several dietary factors have been suggested as having a protective role in PCT [20, 38, 56, 57].

Alcohol
The effects of alcohol on porphyrin metabolism and heme biosynthesis enzymes have been investigated in many studies. Alcohol is a frequent factor in triggering and aggravating porphyrin metabolism disorders, both in acute and chronic porphyria. Alcohol is believed to have an inhibitory effect on uroporphyrinogen decarboxylase, either directly (affecting heme biosynthesis) or through an iron-dependent mechanism [38, 57].

Iron
Iron concentrations (total body and hepatic nonheme) are increased in almost 65% of patients, whereas iron depletion by repeated phlebotomy, chelators, or decreased intake is protective. Phlebotomy is effective in patients with normal

body iron stores, suggesting that possible changes in iron homeostasis may contribute to the pathogenesis of PCT [38].

Antioxidants

Deficiency in ascorbic acid (vitamin C) and other antioxidant factors has been proposed to play a role in some patients with PCT. One study showed a significant decrease in α- and β-carotene as well as cryptoxanthin and lycopene in PCT patients. There is conflicting evidence regarding vitamin E [20, 38].

Variegate Porphyria

In acute porphyria, acute attacks can be triggered by stress, menstrual cycle, drugs, chemicals, alcohol, smoking, and fasting, among others. Diet and dietary factors also influence the manifestations of acute porphyria. Fasting or carbohydrate restriction through dieting has been shown to trigger attacks of acute porphyria. This occurs due to increased demand for hepatic heme and an induction in the first enzyme of the heme biosynthetic pathway, aminolevulinic acid synthase, resulting in increased production of heme pathway intermediates. Carbohydrate loading has an inhibitory effect on aminolevulinic acid synthase and has been used as a standard treatment for acute attacks [20, 38, 57].

Hereditary Coproporphyria

As with variegate porphyria, alcohol and fasting can trigger acute attacks, and the avoidance of alcohol and the adoption of a balanced diet are recommended. Carbohydrate loading or glucose loading is beneficial during acute attacks [20, 38].

Congenital Erythropoietic Porphyria

Oral β-carotene has been used as a photoprotective agent with benefit in some patients. Ascorbic acid and α-tocopherol have also been used to quench reactive oxygen species, with some beneficial effects on hemoglobin and erythrocyte levels with long-term therapy [38].

Erythropoietic Protoporphyria

This is the second most common cutaneous porphyria after PCT. A number of dietary factors, most notably β-carotene, have been used as treatment options for the photosensitivity in erythropoietic protoporphyria [20, 38].

A normal diet contains about 40 carotenoids, of which 12 are absorbed in the intestine (α-carotene, β-carotene, lutein, zeaxanthin, β-cryptoxanthin, and lycopene being the most common). β-Carotene has been used for more than 30 years as a photoprotective agent in various photosensitivity disorders and is recommended for the photoprotection of patients with erythropoietic protoporphyria. β-Carotene is believed to quench the singlet oxygen and reactive oxygen species produced subsequent to activation of protoporphyrin by visible light. Dietary sources include yellow and green vegetables, carrots, tomatoes, spinach, sweet potatoes, fruit, and algae [38].

A recent in vitro study analyzed the protective capability of the antioxidants lycopene, β-carotene, ascorbic acid, and α-tocopherol against porphyrin phototoxicity in cell culture experiments. Lycopene provided benefit against protoporphyrin phototoxicity and, in addition, there was an increased protective effect of β-carotene in the presence of ascorbic acid and α-tocopherol, suggesting antioxidant synergy. In vivo studies are required to determine the clinical significance of these findings [20, 38].

Dietary fish oils rich in omega-3 polyunsaturated fatty acids are promising systemic photoprotective agents. There is one case report of an erythropoietic protoporphyria patient who improved with a dietary supplement of fish oils [38].

Skin Manifestations

In cutaneous porphyria there is excessive formation of porphyrins, which photosensitize human skin. With the bullous form there is fragility of exposed skin, blistering, and erosions which lead to scarring, hyperpigmentation and hypopigmentation, and milia (Fig. 38.6). Hypertrichosis and morpheaform areas may also develop on the face and chest. With immediate photosensitivity, severe burning-type pain areas, accompanied by visible edema, develop within minutes of sun exposure. Five main types of cutaneous porphyria

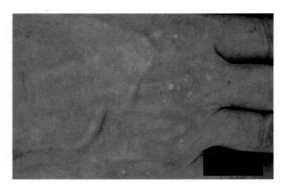

Fig. 38.6 PCT: fragility of exposed skin, erosion, erythema, hyperpigmentation and hypopigmentation, and milia on the hand (Courtesy of Dr. Renan R. Bonamigo)

have been described: PCT, variegate porphyria (mixed porphyria), hereditary coproporphyria, congenital erythropoietic porphyria, and erythropoietic protoporphyria. The latter type presents with acute photosensitivity, whereas the other types show the typical bullous skin changes [57].

Complementary Examinations

Besides the appropriate diagnosis of each type of porphyria, it is important to evaluate the following serum tests: iron, ferritin, liver function tests, and exclusion of hepatitis and HIV infection.

Therapeutic Approach

Avoidance of alcohol is important, both therapeutically and prophylactically, in porphyria patients [20, 38, 57].

There is conflicting evidence regarding the benefits of vitamin E treatment in PCT. Some authors have reported successful treatment with high doses of vitamin E, while others reported no such effect. Similarly, β-carotene has not proved to be useful in treating PCT. More studies are needed to evaluate whether antioxidant supplements can be used as a therapeutic approach to PCT [20, 38].

A recent report evaluated the effects of a high-fiber vegetable and fruit diet in 13 PCT patients. The diet showed a beneficial effect on the severity of skin lesions after 3 weeks. A significant decrease in urinary coproporphyrins was also noted, although there was no significant change in iron levels. More studies are needed to determine whether this diet could be useful in PCT patients [38].

A high-carbohydrate diet is recommended in patients with acute porphyria [20, 38].

The role of oxidative stress in variegate porphyria has not been fully elucidated, and it is unclear whether supplementation with antioxidant nutrients is beneficial for the patients [20, 38].

In hereditary coproporphyria a balanced diet is recommended, and carbohydrate loading or glucose loading is beneficial during acute attacks [38].

The US Food and Drug Administration approved β-carotene for the treatment of erythropoietic protoporphyria in 1975, and it has been widely used since then in these patients and in congenital erythropoietic porphyria. However, the evidence to prove its efficacy has been somewhat contradictory. While a few small studies have supported its use, the only controlled trial failed to show benefits. Although more studies are needed to assess the efficacy of β-carotene, it remains a mainstay of erythropoietic protoporphyria therapy due to its ease of administration and possible beneficial effects. High doses are recommended (120–180 mg/day in adults) to achieve the desirable plasma level of 600–800 μg/dL, and discontinuation of therapy is suggested after 3 months if the therapy is ineffective. Further studies with more patients are needed to assess the effects of fish oils, vitamin C, and vitamin E [20, 38].

Some small studies have attempted to evaluate the role of cysteine, *N*-acetylcysteine, and pyridoxine as photoprotective agents in erythropoietic protoporphyria patients, but the results are controversial [38].

Pressure Ulcers

Nutritional Correlation

The National Pressure Ulcer Advisory Panel defines a pressure ulcer (PU) as an area of unrelieved pressure over a defined area, usually over a bony prominence, resulting in ischemia, cell death, and tissue necrosis. Obese patients may be at particular risk of developing PUs. Malnourished patients given a specific nutritional supplement showed improvement in the size of their PUs in a recent multicenter RCT, although previous trials had not shown the same effects with similar ingredients. Both experimental and control groups were given a high-calorie, high-protein supplement, but the experimental group's supplement also contained high levels of zinc, arginine, and a group of antioxidants: selenium, manganese, and vitamins C and E. The rate of complete healing of PUs did not differ among the groups, but patients who received the extra micronutrients showed a greater decrease in the area of their wounds. Despite this reduction in the size of their PU with the use of supplements, the researchers found no difference in the secondary outcomes of the study, including complete healing or the incidence of infections [53, 54].

Skin Manifestations

The clinical presentation of pressure ulceration can be deceptive to the inexperienced observer. Soft tissue, muscle, and skin resist pressure to differing degrees. In general, muscle is the least resistant and will become necrotic before skin breaks down. Also, pressure is not equally distributed from the bony surface to the overlying skin; it is greatest at the bony prominence, decreasing gradually toward the periphery. A small area of skin breakdown may represent only the tip of the iceberg, with a large cavity and extensive undermining of the skin edges beneath [53, 54].

Complementary Examinations

A complete blood count with differential may show an elevated white blood cell (WBC) count indicative of inflammation or invasive infection. The erythrocyte sedimentation rate (ESR) should be determined. An ESR higher than 120 mm/h and a WBC count greater than 15,000/μL suggest osteomyelitis.

Nutritional parameters should be evaluated to assess adequate nutritional stores needed for adequate wound healing. Useful tests include the following: albumin level, prealbumin level, transferrin level, and serum protein level.

Therapeutic Approach

Nutritional and functional status should be assessed in all patients (hospitalized, obese, or malnourished patients), whereby physicians and health professionals are able to identify individuals at risk of developing PU.

Nonsurgical treatment measures include the following: pressure reduction; wound management (debridement, cleansing agents, dressings, and antimicrobials); and newer approaches, still under study (growth factors, negative-pressure wound therapy, and electrotherapy) [53, 54].

Psoriasis

Nutritional Correlation

The role of nutrition in the treatment of psoriasis has been studied for many years. Most recently, the observation of comorbid conditions associated with psoriasis has stimulated renewed interest in nutrition as a better way to approach the disease [6, 20, 58, 59].

The efficacy of vitamin A and vitamin D derivatives has been well established. As adjuvant therapy, changes in dietary behavior may help augment the effect of well-established treatments. Limitation of alcohol use, adoption of a low-calorie or gluten-free diet, or treatment of comorbid conditions, when applicable to a particular patient, may hasten the clearing of psoriatic lesions in patients undergoing phototherapy or receiving topical or systemic medications. Vitamin B12 and select antioxidants may also provide some benefit. Although many dermatologists often overlook the role of nutrition in the treatment of psoriasis, consideration of nutritional alternatives in select patients may help to enhance care [20, 28, 58].

Weight Loss

Metabolic syndrome is more common among psoriasis patients. An obesity induced proinflammatory state may exacerbate psoriasis symptoms, and psoriasis itself may contribute to weight gain, partially because of social isolation, unhealthy dietary habits, and reduced physical activity. In various clinical studies, weight loss appears to significantly improve psoriasis symptoms and the efficacy of some psoriasis medications, such as biological agents [6, 28, 59].

Alcohol

The relationship between psoriasis and alcohol consumption is complex and multifactorial. Evidence suggests that alcohol triggers and worsens psoriasis and that alcohol abuse is more common among patients with psoriasis [28, 58, 59].

Polyunsaturated Omega-3 Fatty Acid (PUFA)

Arachidonic acid, which is elevated in psoriatic lesions, is converted to leukotriene B4, a potent proinflammatory mediator. PUFAs, such as eicosapentaenoic acid and docosahexaenoic acid, are metabolized to leukotriene B5, a considerably weaker inflammatory molecule. Increased levels of PUFAs are postulated to decrease inflammation and improve psoriasis symptoms. Studies investigating the effect of fish or fish oil supplementation on psoriasis have produced inconsistent results. Several small studies reported improvement of cutaneous lesions and psoriatic arthritis, and a decrease in the side effects of psoriasis medications, after oral supplementation with fatty fish or fish oil [28, 59].

Gluten

Celiac disease and psoriasis are reported to occur simultaneously. For psoriasis patients with celiac-specific antibodies, a gluten-free diet improves psoriasis lesions [20, 28, 59].

Folic Acid

An increased incidence of folic acid deficiency has been reported in psoriasis patients. This observed deficiency may be related to elevated homocysteine levels, decreased intestinal absorption caused by inflammation, and/or increased use by skin epidermal cells. Folate deficiency is also implicated in psoriasis severity. Folate supplementation has been postulated to have an antithrombotic and cardioprotective role in some psoriasis patients. A recent review article, however, found insufficient evidence to support such a hypothesis. Folate supplementation may also be useful for psoriasis patients who have been treated with methotrexate. It was found to diminish adverse side effects of methotrexate therapy, such as hepatotoxicity and gastrointestinal intolerance.

Notably, a reduction in the efficacy of methotrexate with concurrent folate supplementation has also been reported [59].

Vitamin D

The utility of topical vitamin D in the treatment of psoriasis is well established, but the role of oral vitamin D supplementation remains unclear. A correlation between low serum vitamin D levels and increased severity of psoriasis has been suggested. Observational studies have shown the safety and efficacy of oral vitamin D supplementation in the treatment of psoriatic lesions and psoriatic arthritis. Notably, a recent randomized, placebo-controlled trial found no significant difference in the improvement of skin lesions in patients treated with oral vitamin D compared with controls [58, 59].

Selenium and Other Antioxidants

Increased oxidative stress and circulating free radicals may contribute to the inflammatory state of psoriasis. Antioxidants, particularly selenium, vitamin E, and β-carotene, can offset this oxidative imbalance. However, the evidence supporting the amelioration of psoriasis symptoms after antioxidant use is weak. Selenium supplementation has been studied most extensively. Selenium is essential for the normal functioning of glutathione peroxidase and may be found in low levels in patients with psoriasis, particularly those with extended disease duration. Some patients failed to show improvement of clinical symptoms after supplementation with selenium-enriched yeast and combined selenium and vitamin E. Combination antioxidant therapy with selenium, coenzyme Q10, and vitamin E, on the other hand, was associated with rapid clinical improvement and reduction of cell markers of oxidative stress [28, 58, 59].

Inositol and Zinc

A randomized, placebo-controlled, double-blind trial demonstrated a significant improvement in the clinical score of lithium-treated patients taking inositol (6 g/day) versus a lactose placebo for 10 weeks. Zinc supplementation, however, did not produce significant improvement in the psoriasis clinical score in well-designed clinical trials [58, 59].

Taurine

Although early observations suggested that the amino acid taurine was involved in the pathogenesis of psoriasis, a series of studies failed to confirm that excessive or restricted taurine could exacerbate or ameliorate, respectively, the clinical course of psoriasis [58].

Skin Manifestations

Psoriasis is a chronic disease of abnormal keratinocyte proliferation and differentiation, as well as localized and systemic inflammation. The main skin features are sharply demarcated, scaly erythematous plaques, and, occasionally, sterile pustules. The pathogenesis is multifactorial, allowing for multiple therapeutic options.

Complementary Examinations

Psoriasis is associated with overweight/obesity and related cardiometabolic complications. In this context, such diseases should be excluded with blood glucose, lipid profile, echocardiography, and carotid Doppler echography. Other complementary examinations that should be performed include folic acid and selenium.

Therapeutic Approach

Dermatologists should encourage overweight and obese psoriasis patients to attempt weight loss and undertake increased physical activity to improve psoriasis symptoms, comorbid metabolic syndrome, and medication efficacy [6, 28, 58, 59].

Given the prevalence of alcohol use among patients with psoriasis, screening for abuse is advised [6, 20].

Dietary supplementation with polyunsaturated fatty acids, folic acid, vitamin D, and antioxidants can be considered as adjuncts in the management of some psoriasis patients. RCTs have produced conflicting results, necessitating additional studies before definitive recommendations can be made [28, 59].

Screening should be considered for celiac disease, and implementation of a gluten-free diet may improve both conditions if they are present simultaneously [20, 59].

Despite a few promising studies, consistent evidence supporting fatty fish diet or fish oil, vitamin D, folate, and antioxidant supplementation is currently lacking, and additional studies are required before concrete recommendations can be made [59].

Rosacea

Nutritional Correlation

The opinion that food aggravates rosacea has been accepted. Patients are counseled to avoid rosacea triggers and, thus, refrain from such items as spicy foods, alcoholic beverages, and hot, caffeinated drinks. The list of triggers may be more extensive and has been reported to include fruits, marinated meats, and cheeses. With regard to alcohol ingestion in rosacea patients, a survey found red wine as the most likely culprit, followed by distilled spirits, with beer as the least likely to cause symptoms in patients. With regard to spices, cayenne pepper aggravated rosacea 36% of the time, red pepper

34%, black pepper 18%, white pepper 9%, and paprika 9% of the time. In the fruit/vegetable category, citrus items and tomatoes were most often identified as triggers [6, 60].

In addition to particular food types triggering rosacea, the temperature of food and beverages can also be an aggravating factor. For years, patients have been told to avoid hot, caffeinated beverages such as coffee and tea, and although caffeine may aggravate rosacea, there is now quantitative evidence that heat is a true culprit. Therefore, for many patients an iced coffee or tea may be less of a trigger than originally thought [60].

Another novel dietary influence in rosacea patients may be the omega-3 and omega-6 fatty acids. Recently, in the ophthalmology literature, evidence has shown that supplements or foods that contain such fatty acids may help with dry eyes. Some dermatologists have been using flaxseed oil, which contains high levels of omega-3 fatty acid, to help combat ocular rosacea [20, 60].

Skin Manifestations

Rosacea is a common condition characterized by facial flushing and a spectrum of clinical signs, including erythema, telangiectasia, coarse skin, and an inflammatory papulopustular eruption resembling acne [6, 60].

Complementary Examinations

The diagnosis is made clinically.

Therapeutic Approach

Clearly the impact of diet on rosacea is more widely accepted and documented than is the case with acne. Thus, patients with this condition should be encouraged to keep a food diary to help them elucidate possible triggers. With little effort, physicians can encourage such diaries and the avoidance of triggers [14, 60].

Scurvy and Vitamin C Deficiency

Nutritional Correlation

Vitamin C, also known as ascorbic acid, is a water-soluble vitamin required for the synthesis of collagen, L-carnitine, and neurotransmitters. It is also involved in protein metabolism. Vitamin C is a strong antioxidant and has been shown to regenerate other antioxidants such as vitamin E, and also plays an important role in immune function and improves the absorption of nonheme iron. Vitamin C cannot be produced by humans but is readily available in many types of food. Citrus fruits are the best known sources of vitamin C, but red and green peppers, tomatoes, potatoes, and other vegetables are also excellent sources [14, 61, 62].

Vitamin C deficiency leads to scurvy. Humans, unlike other animals, are unable to produce vitamin C and therefore depend on dietary sources. Scurvy has been described since ancient times and is best known for its high incidence in sailors. In the 1700s, addition of citrus fruit to the diet of sailors largely cured scurvy in that group, but there were still incidents of "land scurvy" in populations with abnormal diets. Today, scurvy is extremely rare because of improved food supplies, vitamin-fortified foods, and vitamin supplements, but can occur in populations with poor diets. The main function of vitamin C is in the triple-helix formation of collagen; vitamin C deficiency impairs collagen synthesis and results in the typical signs of scurvy [14, 61] (Chart 38.1).

Skin Manifestations

The first signs are fatigue, malaise, and lethargy. The first cutaneous disorder is keratosis pilaris on the lateral and posterior areas of the arms, buttocks, and thighs. These lesions may become hemorrhagic, particularly in areas of pressure. The main changes in the oral cavity are the presence of edematous, erythematous, and friable gingivae with a tendency to bleeding. Symptoms can mimic SS with xerosis and keratoconjunctivitis. Other findings include conjunctival and gastrointestinal bleeding, ungual linear hemorrhage reflecting the weakness of blood vessel walls, osteochondral changes, and thinning corkscrew hair [14, 61, 62].

Complementary Examinations

Laboratory tests are usually not helpful to ascertain a diagnosis of scurvy. Presentation of an infant with the typical clinical and radiologic picture of scurvy, along with a supportive history of dietary deficiency of vitamin C, is often sufficient to diagnose infantile scurvy. Plasma ascorbic acid level may help in establishing the diagnosis, but this level tends to reflect the recent dietary intake rather than the actual tissue levels of vitamin C. Signs of scurvy can occur with low-normal serum levels of vitamin C. The best confirmation of the diagnosis of scurvy is its resolution following vitamin C administration. Noninflammatory perivascular extravasation of red cells and deposition of hemosiderin near hair follicles with intrafollicular keratotic plugs and coiled hair may be seen in a skin biopsy specimen.

Therapeutic Approach

Upon administration of adequate oral vitamin C, the symptoms of scurvy resolve within 1–12 days. Dosage forms are: males: 90 mg/day; females: 75 mg/day; pregnant women: 85 mg/day, not to exceed 2,000 mg/day (80 mg if <18 years; not to exceed 1,800 mg/day); nursing women: 120 mg/day, not to exceed 2,000 mg/day (115 mg if <18 years old; not to exceed 1,800 mg/day) [14] (Table 38.1).

Anemia, secondary to blood loss, is a common finding in scurvy and is usually associated with folate and iron deficiencies.

Skin Cancer

Nutritional Correlation

The role of diet and nutrition in carcinogenesis and, as a potentially modifiable factor, in cancer prevention is still under debate. The identification of a nutrient supplement with cancer-preventive properties would be a major breakthrough for public health. However, cancer is not a uniform disease and the existence of such a nutrient, or combination of nutrients, has been debated [6, 7].

Nonmelanoma Skin Cancer (NMSC)

Vitamin A
Multiple interventional studies have evaluated the effect of retinol, isotretinoin, or β-carotene on NMSC incidence. Studies found no significant difference in NMSC incidence between intervention and control groups after β-carotene supplementation. The study results for retinol and synthetic retinoids are more varied. Another study revealed no significant difference in time to first NMSC or in total number of tumors in retinol-treated versus control high-risk patients. Conversely, in patients with moderate risk, oral retinol supplementation significantly decreased the hazard ratio for first squamous cell carcinoma (SCC), but did not affect basal cell carcinoma (BCC) risk. Similarly, 10 mg of isotretinoin daily did not affect BCC development. Smaller studies of isotretinoin in patients with xeroderma pigmentosum and acitretin in renal transplant patients identified statistically significant reductions in NMSC incidence in treatment groups. These studies suggest that the impact of retinol and synthetic retinoids on NMSC may be affected by individual patient risk factors and comorbidities [63–65].

Vitamin D
In vitro studies in NMSC lines reveal differential expression and downstream effects of key components of the vitamin D system. Loss of the vitamin D receptor enhances susceptibility to

UV-induced tumorigenesis in mice. Vitamin D inhibits the hedgehog signaling pathway and upregulates nucleotide excision repair enzymes, potentially protecting against NMSC. Despite evidence from animal and in vitro studies, human studies are conflicting. One case–control study found an inverse relationship between vitamin D level and the risk of NMSC. Conversely, other studies identified a significant positive association between plasma vitamin D levels and NMSC risk. Sun exposure may confound these results, because UV radiation simultaneously increases serum vitamin D levels and promotes DNA mutations that are key in the development of skin cancer [7, 64, 66].

Vitamin E

Decreased plasma levels of α-tocopherol were found in patients with actinic keratosis and BCC compared with controls. Inverse associations between vitamin E dietary intake and supplementation and subsequent BCC development were observed. Conversely, two cohort studies found a positive association between dietary and supplemental vitamin E and BCC development, while others were unable to identify an association between vitamin E supplementation or serum levels and subsequent NMSC. In addition, a double-blind, placebo-controlled study found no clinical or histologic difference in response to UVB after 6 months of daily oral α-tocopherol (400 IU) supplementation [7, 64].

Vitamin C

In vitro studies of human keratinocyte cell lines show that ascorbic acid, which is a stable form of vitamin C, decreases UVB-induced cytotoxicity as a free radical scavenger and a potentiator of α-tocopherol-induced antioxidative activity. Vitamin C administration significantly inhibits UV-induced DNA, RNA, and protein synthesis in BCC and SCC cell lines in mice and rats. The photoprotective properties of topical vitamin C have been shown in porcine skin. In humans, studies of vitamin C and NMSC are inconsistent. Inverse relationships between the consumption of foods containing vitamin C, vitamin C supplements, and plasma levels of ascorbic acid with NMSC were identified in three case–control studies. Conflicting results were obtained in two cohort studies that identified a positive association between BCC and the intake of vitamin C rich food or supplements. In addition, three case–control studies and five cohort studies failed to identify a significant association between vitamin C and NMSC [7, 67].

Selenium

Selenium protects against UVB-induced cytotoxicity in human keratinocytes and carcinogenesis in mice. Studies have found a potentially protective role of selenium for NMSC. In a case–control study, the mean plasma selenium level was significantly lower among NMSC cases than controls. Similarly, a cohort study found an inverse relationship between serum selenium concentration and subsequent NMSC. Finally, in a study of eight women treated with topical L-selenomethionine for 2 weeks, a significant increase in the minimal erythema dose after UV irradiation was observed, suggesting a possible photoprotective effect of topical selenium. The only RCT that has investigated the impact of oral selenium supplementation on NMSC found no significant association with the risk of BCC, but, interestingly, elevated risks of SCC and total NMSC. Other studies found no significant association between dietary or plasma selenium and NMSC [7, 68].

For women, there is little evidence for lower or higher nutritional intake of selenium exhibiting a major impact on cancer risk. The only RCT results that have a low risk of bias support concerns an increased risk of NMSC by selenium yeast supplements in women who had already suffered from this disease. For men, there is evidence for an inverse association between higher selenium biomarker levels and cancer risk. However, we cannot exclude the possibility that this effect may well be the result of other factors related to higher selenium biomarker levels than selenium exposure itself. Results from two RCTs have failed to provide evidence that NMSC or prostate cancer can be prevented by selenium supplementation in men. In addition, concerns have been raised about possible toxicities from the long-term intake of supplemental selenium. At present, regular intake of selenium supplements for cancer prevention cannot be recommended to either the selenium-replete or -deficient populations [7, 68].

Low-Fat Diet

A study of patients who were following a low-fat diet found no significant difference in NMSC; therefore, a fat-restricted diet should not be recommended for NMSC prevention [7].

Melanoma

Polyunsaturated Fatty Acids

PUFAs are anti-inflammatory molecules that protect against UV damage. PUFA supplementation decreases skin sensitivity to UV irradiation and cutaneous expression of p53 in animal and human studies. Additionally, in animal and in vitro studies PUFAs were shown to increase apoptosis, promote cell-cycle arrest, and decrease tumor growth. PUFAs can inhibit metastatic melanoma, and when used as an adjunct to surgery promote recurrence-free survival. Some animal studies of PUFA supplementation found increased tumor growth and immunosuppression. These conflicting results of in vitro and animal studies do not elucidate a protective role of PUFAs against melanomagenesis. Clinical data are also conflicting. Studies, including two case–control trials and one prospective cohort study, reported an increased risk of melanoma in patients with higher dietary PUFA intake. In contrast, the incidence of melanoma is low in populations with PUFA-rich diets, including Inuits and cohorts in both Italy and Australia [7, 59].

Alcohol

The role of alcohol consumption in melanomagenesis is complex and involves the interplay of biological, behavioral, and epidemiologic factors. From a cellular standpoint, ethanol induces DNA damage and promotes the production of reactive oxygen species. Hormonal effects of ethanol include promoting prostaglandin synthesis and the secretion of melanocyte-stimulating hormone. Finally, alcohol consumption alters immune function and increases the metastatic potential and growth of melanoma cells. Several large, population-level studies have found a positive association between alcohol consumption and melanoma risk. In fact, a recent systematic review reported a 20% increase in melanoma risk in patients who regularly consumed alcohol. A potential confounding factor is increased high-risk behaviors in alcohol users, including sunburns. Three smaller case–control studies, however, found no association between alcohol consumption and melanoma risk, and one population-level study reported decreased melanoma risk among Swedish women who were also alcoholics [6, 7].

Vitamin D

Polymorphisms of the vitamin D receptor gene may affect melanoma risk. The relationship between serum vitamin D levels, dietary vitamin D supplementation, and melanoma risk, however, remains largely uncertain. Observational studies investigating vitamin D status and melanoma risk provide conflicting results. Two large, prospective cohort studies reported an increased melanoma incidence in patients with higher serum vitamin D levels. Another nested case–control study found no association between serum vitamin D levels and melanoma risk. In addition, one case–control and another cohort study found no association between dietary vitamin D and melanoma risk, while others reported an inverse relationship. Moreover, multiple case–control studies have reported inverse associations between vitamin D levels and poorer melanoma prognosis – namely, an increased Breslow thickness and more advanced stage. Earlier metastatic disease occurred in patients with low serum vitamin D levels, whereas higher vitamin D levels were independently protective against melanoma relapse and death. An RCT found no significant difference in incident melanoma rates in the intervention group (calcium plus 400 IU vitamin D daily) compared with a placebo group. Interestingly, in high-risk patients with a history of NMSC, supplementation resulted in a significantly lower melanoma risk, suggesting a potential role for vitamin D supplementation in this population [63, 64].

Vitamin E

Multiple studies found no association between vitamin E and melanoma risk. Other studies have suggested inverse correlations between melanoma incidence and serum and diet vitamin E levels, supporting a protective role. However, an RCT reported no differences in melanoma incidence in patients receiving long-term vitamin E supplementation (400 IU/day) compared with controls. The safety of vitamin E supplementation is also unclear, since increased all-cause mortality was found in patients receiving high-dose (400 IU/day) vitamin E [20, 28].

Selenium

Selenium is a trace element and antioxidant that relieves the UV-induced depletion of glutathione peroxidase and appears to induce dose-dependent apoptosis and cell-cycle arrest in human melanoma cell lines. In animal studies, oral selenium supplementation resulted in decreased melanoma tumor growth and reduced pulmonary and brain metastases in mice. Human studies, however, are conflicting. In one case–control study, increased environmental exposure to selenium yielded a nearly fourfold greater melanoma incidence than in unexposed controls. Other studies found no significant relationship between selenium levels and melanoma risk. Conversely, metastatic melanoma patients in a case–control study were found to have significantly lower selenium levels than controls [68].

Green Tea Polyphenols

Polyphenols found in green tea, including epigallocatechin-3-gallate (EGCG), possess anti-oxidant, anti-inflammatory, immunomodulatory, anticarcinogenic, proapoptotic, and photoprotective properties. ECGC inhibits melanoma cell invasion and migration. In addition, green tea supplementation during interferon therapy decreases melanoma cell growth in mice, suggesting its possible use as a treatment adjunct. Despite these promising cell and animal studies, a prospective cohort study was unable to find a significant association between tea consumption and melanoma incidence [7].

Resveratrol

Resveratrol is a naturally occurring polyphenolic compound found in grapes, red wine, some berries, and peanuts. Resveratrol and its chemical analogs have photoprotective, antioxidant, anti-inflammatory, and anticarcinogenic capabilities. The introduction of resveratrol in cell cultures and topical application in human skin resulted in increased cell survival, decreased production of reactive oxygen species, and diminished clinical erythema after UV irradiation. Resveratrol induces the apoptosis of human melanoma cells and promotes cell-cycle arrest. In addition, resveratrol may have a role in metastatic disease, because it possesses antiangiogenic properties and inhibits hepatic and pulmonary metastases. Resveratrol can be used as an adjunct to chemotherapy, radiation, and interleukin-2 by sensitizing melanoma cells to these treatments and preventing toxic endothelial cell injury. Although population-level human RCTs are still lacking, one observational study reported decreased skin toxicity in breast cancer patients being treated with external beam radiation after supplementation with a mixture of vitamins and antioxidants, including resveratrol [7].

Lycopene

Lycopene is a carotenoid found in red fruits and vegetables. It is a potent antioxidant and free radical scavenger that protects against UV photodamage. In animal and human cutaneous models, topical application of lycopene before UV irradiation decreases the inflammatory response, diminishes the generation of matrix metalloproteinases, increases the mean erythema dose, and preserves DNA integrity and normal cell proliferation. Similarly, oral lycopene supplementation decreases toxicity from external beam radiation in patients with breast cancer. Finally, lycopene inhibits platelet-derived growth factor BB and melanoma-induced fibroblast migration, which are known to facilitate metastatic disease. From an epidemiologic perspective, the association between lycopene and melanoma risk is unclear. Three case–control studies found no significant association between serum lycopene levels and the risk of subsequent melanoma. When dietary lycopene intake was stratified into quintiles, however, one case–control study found that patients in the highest quintile had a significantly lower melanoma risk [7, 28].

Skin Manifestations

Basal Cell Carcinoma

The characteristic features of BCC include the following: waxy papules with central depression, pearly appearance, erosion or ulceration, bleeding (especially when traumatized), crusting, rolled (raised) border, translucency, surface telangiectasia, and slow growth (0.5 cm in 1–2 years) [68].

BCC occurs mostly on the face, head (including scalp), neck, and hands. It rarely develops on the palms and soles. BCC usually appears as a flat, firm, pale area that is small, raised, pink or red, translucent, shiny, and waxy, and the area may bleed following minor injury. BCCs may have one or more visible and irregular blood vessels, an ulcerative area in the center that often is pigmented, and black-blue or brown areas. Large BCCs may have oozing or crusted areas. The lesion grows slowly, is not painful, and does not itch [68].

Squamous Cell Carcinoma

Approximately 70% of all SCCs occur on the head and neck, most frequently involving the lower lip, external ear and periauricular region, or forehead and scalp. The classic presentation of SCC is that of a shallow ulcer with heaped-up edges, often covered by a plaque. Of course, the presenting appearance of each SCC varies according to the site and extent of disease [68].

Melanoma

Clinician and patient education regarding the warning signs of early melanoma has been achieved successfully through the use of the ABCDE criteria for a changing mole, which are as follows [68]:

- Asymmetry: half the lesion does not match the other half
- Border irregularity: the edges are ragged, notched, or blurred
- Color variegation: pigmentation is not uniform and may display shades of tan, brown, or black; white, reddish, or blue discoloration is of particular concern
- Diameter: a diameter greater than 6 mm is characteristic, although some melanomas may be smaller in size; any growth in a nevus warrants an evaluation
- Evolving: changes in the lesion over time are characteristic; this factor is critical for nodular or amelanotic (nonpigmented) melanoma, which may not exhibit the ABCD criteria above

Complementary Examinations

The essential examination is skin biopsy to confirm the diagnosis of skin cancer and serum 25(OH)D.

Therapeutic Approach

A specific diet should not be recommended for skin cancer prevention, because studies have presented conflicting results [14, 68] (Table 38.1).

Skin Infection

Nutritional Correlation

Vitamin D

Recently it has been shown that vitamin D represents a direct regulator of antimicrobial innate immune responses. The innate immune system of mammals provides a rapid response to repel assaults from numerous infectious agents including bacteria, viruses, fungi, and parasites. A major component of this system is a diverse combination of cationic antimicrobial peptides (AMPs) that include the α- and β-defensins and cathelicidins. Because bacteria have difficulty developing resistance against AMPs and are quickly killed by them, this class of antimicrobial agents is being commercially developed as a source of peptide antibiotics. Recent studies have shown that cathelicidins, in addition to being antimicrobial, are multifunctional proteins with receptor-mediated effects on eukaryotic cells and activity in chemotaxis, angiogenesis, and wound healing. In the skin, there is low constitutive expression of hCAP18 in the basal layer of keratinocytes but rapid upregulation upon inflammation and injury. Because AMPs serve a role in host defense and may act as mediators of other biological processes, their expression is tightly regulated. Moreover, vitamin D induces increases in antimicrobial proteins and secretion of antimicrobial activity against pathogens including *Pseudomonas aeruginosa*. Some studies have demonstrated the link between vitamin D and Toll-like receptors, cathelicidin production, and increased susceptibility to bacterial infections. In addition, vitamin D stimulates the synthesis of proteins such as filaggrin, which is essential to the formation of stratum corneum. Thus, vitamin D deficiency may exacerbate AD by altering the skin barrier and undermining the immune system, leading to a subsequent increase in the risk of infections [6, 7, 14] (Chart 38.1).

Obesity

Obese patients easily become overheated and sweat more profusely because of the thick layers of subcutaneous fat, thus exaggerating areas of inflammation and rashes.

It is widely accepted that *C. albicans* infection is more prevalent in patients with diabetes mellitus because these patients have a significantly higher pH in intertriginous areas. This may be a factor that promotes the susceptibility of patients with diabetes mellitus to *Candida* infection of the skin. Nevertheless, it is noteworthy that some studies have reported that despite half of the patients studied having diabetes mellitus, intertrigo was not a frequent finding. However, the statistical linear trend showed a strong predisposition to intertrigo according to the degree of obesity [36, 53].

Skin Manifestations

Common locations of candidiasis include the genitocrural, subaxillary, gluteal, and submammary areas, and between the abdominal skinfolds. Typically such patients present scaling, erythema with macules, papules, and/or satellite pustules. They may complain of itching or burning over the affected area. *C. albicans* has a predilection for colonizing macerated skinfolds. Accordingly, intertrigo in its various forms is the most common clinical presentation of candidiasis on the skin [69].

Impetigo is the most common bacterial infection. This acute, highly contagious infection of the superficial layers of the epidermis is primarily caused by *Streptococcus pyogenes* or *S. aureus*. Impetigo is classified as either nonbullous (about 70% of cases) or bullous [69].

Complementary Examinations

Gram stain and culture of the pus or exudates from skin lesions, and serum 25(OH)D.

Therapeutic Approach

There is convincing evidence that vitamin D directly regulates AMP gene expression in humans, revealing the potential of these compounds for the treatment of opportunistic infections [14, 64] (Table 38.1).

The statistical linear trend showed a strong predisposition to infection according to the degree of obesity. Hence, weight loss is the best means of reducing this predisposition [36, 53].

Urticaria

Nutritional Correlation

Many patients with chronic urticaria attribute their symptoms to food intolerance. Food products including wheat, dietary fats, and alcohol are thought to play a role in the development of urticarial lesions [20, 28].

Pseudoallergens

The term pseudoallergen is used to describe a stimulus that provokes histamine or cutaneous mast cell degranulation via a nonimmunologic pathway (i.e., not IgE mediated). It has been estimated that 1–3% of patients with chronic urticaria exhibit pseudoallergic reactions. Pseudoallergens include, but are not limited to, artificial preservatives and sweeteners, food dyes, aromatic compounds in some natural foods (e.g., tomatoes, herbs), and phenolic substances (salicylic acid, *p*-hydroxybenzoic acid, anethole, ethyl vanillin, citron oil, and orange oil). Although the existence of pseudoallergens is not universally accepted and remains somewhat controversial, pseudoallergens are postulated to induce or aggravate chronic urticaria in a subset of patients [20, 59].

Pseudoallergen-induced urticaria may be related to increased gastroduodenal permeability or altered histamine metabolism. Several studies found that pseudoallergen-free diets improved symptoms in a small subset of patients with chronic urticaria, including those who were unresponsive to standard treatments [59].

Because patients differ in terms of the specific pseudoallergens that trigger urticaria, symptom diaries and oral food challenges are useful in determining whether an ingredient or additive plays an exacerbating role. Interestingly, after several months of dietary avoidance many patients can return to a normal diet without experiencing reoccurrence of urticaria. In contrast to medications, a pseudoallergen–free diet may be curative rather than symptom suppressing [20, 28, 59].

A variety of artificial pseudoallergens has been identified, primarily in the form of preservatives and dyes (tartrazine, sodium benzoate, BHT, Sunset Yellow FCF, Food Red 17, Amaranth, Ponceau 4 R, Erythrosine, Brilliant Blue FCF) as well as additives such as monosodium glutamate and sweeteners (saccharine). Both humoral and cell-mediated immune responses have been shown to be responsible for inciting urticarial lesions. Artificial food additives are thought to play a greater role in chronic urticaria afflicting children, whereas natural pseudoallergens evoke more sensitivity among adults. Although artificial pseudoallergens have received significant attention, there also is increasing awareness of the role of natural pseudoallergens in urticaria. These include natural food dyes, such as annatto extract, salicylates, and aromatic compounds, found in high concentrations in several types of fruits, vegetables, and spices. Unlike artificial pseudoallergens, quantities of naturally occurring pseudoallergens are difficult to estimate as they vary considerably in each fruit or vegetable depending on its type, age, and place of origin. They include phenolic substances such as *p*-hydroxybenzoic acid, cumaric acid, salicylic acid, natural flavors, and ethereal oils. Natural pseudoallergens pose a challenge in the management of urticaria because of the difficulty of avoiding all foods containing these ingredients. Testing to determine the natural pseudoallergens to which the patient is sensitive can help in developing a dietary regimen. Although complete elimination is not possible, lowering the consumption of certain natural pseudoallergens may help to ameliorate symptoms of urticaria [28, 59].

Gluten

Because some cases of urticaria are immune mediated, it is not surprising that an association between chronic urticaria and celiac disease has been proposed. Chronic urticaria may be a cutaneous manifestation of celiac disease. Alternatively, increased mucosal permeability in celiac disease can facilitate the passage of antigens, provoking urticaria symptoms. In addition, the inflammatory response generated in celiac disease may trigger production of anti-IgE receptor antibodies that inappropriately activate mast cells; this pathogenic mechanism has been implicated in 35–40% of cases of chronic urticaria. In addition, there are several case reports of resolution of urticaria with concomitant celiac disease soon after initiating a gluten-free diet [20, 28, 59].

Vitamin D

Compared with unaffected controls, patients with chronic urticaria have significantly lower serum vitamin D levels. Some studies have shown complete clinical resolution of urticaria after vitamin D supplementation. An RCT found that high-dose (4,000 IU/day) vitamin D supplementation improves chronic urticaria regardless of baseline vitamin D status [14, 59] (Chart 38.1).

Wheat

Wheat-dependent exercise-induced anaphylaxis is part of a larger entity of food-dependent, exercise-induced anaphylactic reactions, whereby ingestion of a specific food before physical exercise triggers anaphylaxis. Symptoms include pruritus, urticaria, angioedema, dyspnea, hypotension, and shock, which are indistinguishable from those in classic IgE-mediated anaphylaxis. Common triggering foods include celery, shellfish, peanut, tree nuts, and tomato. A frequent cause, however, is wheat. The water-salt-insoluble component of wheat, gliadin, is rich in glutamine residues and becomes modified by the intestinal enzyme, tissue transglutaminase (tTG). Exercise, a physical stressor, may be a potential activator of tTG. Exercise may also increase intestinal allergen absorption, provoke abnormal responses of the autonomic nervous system, or lower the threshold for IgE-mediated mast cell degranulation [28, 59].

Alcohol

Alcoholic beverages are a known cause of several hypersensitivity reactions, including the "flushing syndrome" seen in patients of Mongolian descent or drug-induced by disulfiram, from an elevated acetaldehyde level; asthma exacerbation; exercise-induced anaphylaxis; and urticaria and angioedema. Although urticaria is a rare reaction, there are several theories regarding its mechanism, including altered prostaglandin metabolism, acetaldehyde-induced hapten formation and release of IgE, and a non-IgE-mediated anaphylactic release of histamine. Total serum IgE levels are increased with alcohol consumption. In addition, individuals who regularly consume alcohol have increased sensitization to dust mites, grass pollen, and food allergens [20, 59].

Probiotics

Intestinal microbiota plays an important role in the development of food allergy and food allergen-associated urticaria. Probiotics, when given in infancy, may address the root cause by preventing allergic sensitization to foods, which can subsequently manifest with urticaria [20].

Skin Manifestations

Urticaria is characterized by transient, erythematous, raised skin lesions that are typically intensely pruritic. Although usually not life threatening, the skin disorder is difficult to manage and often impairs the quality of life. The classification of urticaria is based on the duration of the symptomatic episode; it is defined as acute if whealing persists for less than 6 weeks and as chronic if it persists for 6 weeks or longer. The pathogenesis is not yet fully understood, and a triggering factor is only identified in 10–20% of cases [59].

Complementary Examinations

In chronic urticaria patients, it is mandatory to perform complementary examinations to exclude diseases that could be associated or be the cause of the symptoms. The following serum tests are recommended: complete blood count, erythrocyte sedimentation rate, C-reactive protein, liver function tests, thyroid-stimulating hormone, anti-thyroid peroxidase antibodies, antinuclear factor, complement, protein electrophoresis, cryoglobulins, 25(OH)D, total IgE, and serology to hepatitis and HIV infections. Urinalyses with culture and stool test are also important.

Therapeutic Approach

Interventional trials support the benefit of a pseudoallergen-free diet and vitamin D supplementation for patients with chronic urticaria. Given its low cost and safety profile, a pseudoallergen-free diet can be recommended to a subset of chronic urticaria patients. Before issuing a recommendation for vitamin D supplementation, appropriate dosage and treatment duration should be determined through RCTs [20, 28, 59].

A gluten-free diet may ameliorate chronic urticaria symptoms in patients who have concomitant celiac disease. However, there are currently no RCTs to support this recommendation [20, 59] (Table 38.1).

Vitiligo

Nutritional Correlation

Vitamin B12

In the literature, studies of the use of vitamin B12 or cobalamin in the treatment of vitiligo have yielded contradictory results. This makes it difficult to determine when cobalamin deficiency should be investigated in patients presenting with vitiligo. Some studies found that vitiligo patients had higher homocysteine and hemoglobin levels and lower levels of vitamin B12 and holotranscobalamin, which is considered the earliest marker of deficiency. The authors suggested that the association may be due to a common genetic background among patients with cobalamin deficiency, hyperhomocysteinemia, and vitiligo. In a study of patients with vitiligo, most patients experienced repigmentation with prolonged oral folic acid and ascorbic acid and parenteral vitamin B12 supplementation. However, another study compared UVB therapy alone and UVB therapy with vitamin B12 and folic acid, and found no significant difference in the repigmentation rates between the two groups [70, 71].

Vitamin D

Low levels of vitamin D have been observed in vitiligo patients and in patients with other autoimmune diseases. Therefore, the relationship between vitamin D and vitiligo needs to be investigated more thoroughly. Vitamin D increases melanogenesis and the tyrosinase content of cultured human melanocytes by its antiapoptotic effect. However, a few growth-inhibitory effects on melanocytes were also reported. Vitamin D regulates calcium and bone metabolism, controls cell proliferation and differentiation, and exerts immunoregulatory activities. Vitamin D exerts its effect via a nuclear hormone receptor for vitamin D and decreases the expression of various cytokines that cause vitiligo [72].

Phyllanthus emblica, Vitamin E, and Carotenoids

Phyllanthus emblica, vitamin E, and carotenoids are compounds showing antioxidant, anti-inflammatory, and repigmentation effects. A study compared two groups of patients, one treated with one tablet of an oral supplement containing *P. emblica* (100 mg), vitamin E (10 mg), and carotenoids (4.7 mg) three times a day for 6 months (group A) and a control group, which instead was not treated with antioxidants (group B). Both groups were simultaneously treated with a comparable topical therapy and/or phototherapy. After a 6-month follow-up, a significantly higher number of patients in group A had a mild repigmentation on the head/neck regions and on the trunk. The number of patients who presented no repigmentation in head/neck, trunk, and upper and lower limbs was significantly higher in group B. Moreover, group B patients showed higher signs of inflammation, more rapid lesion growth, greater worsening of the disease, and more erythema, whereas group A patients showed a greater disease stability. These results suggest that the use of antioxidant supplementation in patients with vitiligo might represent a valuable instrument, but further research is needed [20, 28].

Gluten

In celiac disease and for associated DH, the elimination of gluten has been associated with significant improvement. Since celiac disease is commonly associated with vitiligo, in patients who have both conditions eliminating gluten will be particularly advantageous.

Rechallenging with gluten would be more conclusive and has been recommended, although it is not an option that patients are always willing to pursue.

There is one documented case of rapid repigmentation of acrofacial vitiligo involving the elimination of gluten in an adult patient without concomitant celiac disease. This novel approach certainly needs to be further explored [20, 28].

Iron

Iron is involved in the antioxidant system, and large amounts of iron are sequestered by ferritin. Ferritin is an important acute-phase reactant whose serum level is increased in some autoimmune disorders. Only one report has investigated serum ferritin levels in vitiligo. Immune-mediated and free-radical damage to melanocytes is the most probable pathologic mechanism for vitiligo. Although the exact immunopathogenic mechanisms are still unknown, the autoimmune pathogenesis of vitiligo is supported by data from the literature: detection of circulating antibodies to melanocytes and circulating melanocyte specific cytotoxic T cells in vitiligo patients, and the association with other autoimmune disorders and vitiligo [20, 70].

Skin Manifestations

Vitiligo manifests as acquired white or hypopigmented macules or patches. The lesions are usually well demarcated, and round, oval, or linear in shape. The borders may be convex [1]. Lesions enlarge centrifugally over time at an unpredictable rate and range from millimeters to centimeters in size. Initial lesions occur most frequently on the hands, forearms, feet, and face, favoring a perioral and periocular distribution. Vitiligo lesions may be localized or generalized, with the latter being more common than the former. Localized vitiligo is restricted to one general area with a segmental or quasi-dermatomal distribution. Generalized vitiligo implies more than one general area of involvement. In this situation, the macules are usually found on both sides of the trunk, either symmetrically or asymmetrically arrayed [73].

Complementary Examinations

Serum vitamin B12, iron, and 25(OH)D level are recommended.

Therapeutic Approach

There are few reports in the published literature of dietary intervention as a treatment modality for vitiligo. While there may be a relationship between nutritional elements and vitiligo, further research is needed to elucidate the nature of the association and the clinical application [14, 73, 74] (Table 38.1).

Dermatosis and Bariatric Surgery

Metabolic and nutritional diseases are among the main complications of bariatric surgery (BS). These are secondary to decreased oral intake, as well as alterations in food absorption in the stomach and areas of the small intestine. Patients may also experience diarrhea, nausea, and vomiting, which may trigger fluid and electrolyte imbalance that may persist for more than 5 years after surgery. Typically, patients after undergoing BS show decreased absorption of liposoluble vitamins, iron, vitamins B12, A, D, E, and K, folic acid, and thiamine. Studies have suggested that gastric bypass surgery in patients with psoriasis can result in complete remission. The improvement starts immediately after surgery, before any weight loss. Similarly, in the literature there are case reports of remission of necrobiosis lipoidica after BS. However, there is still much to be elucidated about the true nature of the mechanisms leading to this process [14].

Glossary

Antimicrobial peptides A growing class of natural and synthetic peptides with a wide spectrum of targets including viruses, bacteria, fungi, and parasites.

Cathelicidin Related antimicrobial peptides found in lysosomes of macrophages and polymorphonuclear leukocytes, and keratinocytes. Cathelicidins have a critical role in innate immune defense against invasive bacterial infection.

Essential fatty acid An unsaturated fatty acid that is essential to human health but cannot be manufactured in the body.

Pseudoallergen An antigen that causes allergy-like symptoms, but without identifiable sensitization of the immune system.

References

1. Brickman WJ, Huang J, Silverman BL, Metzger BE. Acanthosis nigricans identifies youth at high risk for metabolic abnormalities. J Pediatr. 2010;156(1):87–92.

2. Scott AT, Metzig AM, Hames RK, Schwarzenberg SJ, Dengel DR, Biltz GR. Acanthosis nigricans and oral glucose tolerance in obese children. Clin Pediatr (Phila). 2010;49(1):69–71.

3. Phiske MM. An approach to acanthosis nigricans. Indian Dermatol Online J. 2014;5(3):239–49.

4. Barbato MT, Criado PR, Silva AK, Averbeck E, Guerine MB, Sá NB. Association of acanthosis nigricans and skin tags with insulin resistance. An Bras Dermatol. 2012;87(1):97–104.

5. Burris J, Rietkerk W, Woolf K. Acne: the role of medical nutrition therapy. J Acad Nutr Diet. 2013;113:416–30.

6. Katta R, Desai SP. Diet in dermatology. J Clin Aesthet Dermatol. 2014;7(7):46–51.

7. Bronsnick T, Murzaku EC, Rao BK. Diet in dermatology: Part I – atopic dermatitis, acne, and nonmelanoma skin cancer. J Am Acad Dermatol. 2014;71:1039.e1–12.

8. Ferdowsian HR, Levin S. Does diet really affect acne? Skin Ther Lett. 2010;15(3):1–2. 5.

9. Kwon HH, Yoon JY, Hong JS, Park MS, Suh DH. Clinical and histological effect of a low glycemic load diet in treatment of acne vulgaris in Korean patients: a randomized, controlled trial. Acta Derm Venereol. 2012;92:241–6.

10. Silverberg NB. Whey protein precipitating moderate to severe acne flares in 5 teenaged athletes. Cutis. 2012;90:70–2.

11. El Darouti MA, Zeid OA, Abdel Halim DM. Salty and spicy food: are they involved in the pathogenesis of acne vulgaris? A case controlled study. J Cosmet Dermatol. 2015; doi:10.1111/jocd.12200.

12. Cao H, Yang G, Wang Y. Complementary therapies for acne vulgaris. Cochrane Database Syst Rev. 2015;1:CD009436.

13. Bowe WP, Joshi SS, Shalita A. Diet and acne. J Am Acad Dermatol. 2010;63:124–41.

14. Manzoni APDS, Weber MB. Skin changes after bariatric surgery. An Bras Dermatol. 2015;90(2):157–68.

15. Iyengar S, Chambers C, Sharon VR. Bullous acrodermatitis enteropathica: case report of a unique clinical presentation and review of the literature. Dermatol Online J. 2015;21(4).

16. Sehgal VN, Jain S. Acrodermatitis enteropathica. Clin Dermatol. 2000;18(6):745–8.

17. Tuerk MJ, Fazel N. Zinc deficiency. Curr Opin Gastroenterol. 2009;25:136–43.

18. Maverakis E, Fung MA, Lynch PJ, Draznin M, Michael DJ, Ruben B, et al. Acrodermatitis enteropathica and an overview of zinc metabolism. J Am Acad Dermatol. 2007;56(1):116–24.

19. Garza-Rodríguez V, de la Fuente-García A, Liy-Wong C, Küry S, Schmitt S, Jamall IS, et al. Acrodermatitis enteropathica: a novel SLC39A4 gene mutation in a patient with normal zinc levels. Pediatr Dermatol. 2015;32(3):e124–5.

20. Lakdawala N, Babalola O, Fedeles F. The role of nutrition in dermatologic diseases: facts and controversies. Clin Dermatol. 2013;31:677–700.

21. Kaplan DH, Igyarto BZ, Gaspari AA. Early immune events in the induction of allergic contact dermatitis. Nat Rev Immunol. 2012;12(2):114–24.

22. Thyssen JP, Johansen JD, Linneberg A, Menne T, Engkilde K. The association between contact sensitization and atopic disease by linkage of a clinical database and a nationwide patient registry. Allergy. 2012;67(9):1157–64.

23. Lachapelle JM. Allergic contact dermatitis: clinical aspects. Rev Environ Health. 2014;29(3):185–94.

24. Fonacier LS, Sher JM. Allergic contact dermatitis. Ann Allergy Asthma Immunol. 2014;113(1):9–12.

25. Simpson ME, Dotterud CK, Storro O, Johnsen R, Oien T. Perinatal probiotic supplementation in the prevention of allergy related disease: 6 year follow up of a randomised controlled trial. BMC Dermatol. 2015;15:13.

26. Sidbury R, Tom WL, Bergman JN, Cooper KD, Silverman RA. Guidelines of care for the management of atopic dermatitis: section 4. Prevention of disease flares and use of adjunctive therapies and approaches. J Am Acad Dermatol. 2014;71(6):1218–33.

27. Simpson MR, Dotterud CK, Storro O, Johnsen R, Oien T. Perinatal probiotic supplementation in the prevention of allergy related disease: 6 year follow up of a randomised controlled trial. BMC Dermatol. 2015;15:13.

28. Kaimal S, Thappa DM. Diet in dermatology: revisited. Indian J Dermatol Venereol Leprol. 2010;76(2):103–15.

29. Fuchs-Tarlovsky V, Marquez-Barba MF, Sriram K. Probiotics in dermatologic practice. Nutrition. 2016;32(3):289–95.

30. Gunaratne AW, Makrides M, Collins CT. Maternal prenatal and/or postnatal n-3 long chain polyunsaturated fatty acids (LCPUFA) supplementation for preventing allergies in early childhood. Cochrane Database Syst Rev. 2015;22:7.

31. Samochocki Z, Bogaczewicz J, Jeziorkowska R, Sysa-Jędrzejowska A, Glińska O, Karczmarewicz E, et al. Vitamin D effects in atopic dermatitis. J Am Acad Dermatol. 2013;69:238–44.

32. Bergstrom KG. Evidence for supplement use in atopic dermatitis. J Drugs Dermatol. 2012;11:1245–7.

33. Raevuori A, Haukka J, Vaarala O, Suvisaari JM, Gissler M, Grainger M, et al. The increased risk for autoimmune diseases in patients with eating disorders. PLoS ONE. 2014;9(8):e104845.

34. Carmel NN, Rotman-Pikielny P, Lavrov A, Levy Y. Vitamin D antibodies in systemic sclerosis patients: findings and clinical correlations. IMAJ. 2015;17:80–4.

35. Schmidt E, Zillikens D. Modern diagnosis of autoimmune blistering skin diseases. Autoimmun Rev. 2010;10(2):84–9.

36. Liakou AI, Theodorakis MJ, Melnik BC, Pappas A, Zouboulis CC. Nutritional clinical studies in dermatology. J Drugs Dermatol. 2013;12(10):1104–9.

37. Ruocco V, Ruocco E, Lo Schiavo A, Brunetti G, Guerrera LP, Wolf R. Pemphigus: etiology, patho-

genesis, and inducing or triggering factors. Facts and controversies. Clin Dermatol. 2013;31:374–81.

38. Fedeles F, Murphy M, Rothe MJ, Grant-Kels JM. Nutrition and bullous skin diseases. Clin Dermatol. 2010;28:627–43.

39. Lo Schiavo AL, Ruocco E, Brancaccio G, Caccavale S, Ruocco V, Wolf R. Bullous pemphigoid: etiology, pathogenesis, and inducing factors. Facts and controversies. Clin Dermatol. 2013;31:391–9.

40. Clarindo MV, Possebon AT, Soligo EM, Uyeda H, Ruaro RT, Empinotti JC. Dermatitis herpetiformis: pathophysiology, clinical presentation, diagnosis, and treatment. An Bras Dermatol. 2014;89(6):865–77.

41. Mendes FBR, Hissa-Elian A, Abreu MA, Gonçalves VS. Review: dermatitis herpetiformis. An Bras Dermatol. 2013;88(4):594–9.

42. Jen M, Yan AC. Syndromes associated with nutritional deficiency and excess. Clin Dermatol. 2010;28:669–85.

43. Balint JP. Physical findings in nutritional deficiencies. Pediatr Clin N Am. 1998;45(1):245–60.

44. Nicklas TA, O'Neil CE. Development of the SoFAS (solid fats and added sugars) concept: the 2010 Dietary Guidelines for Americans. Adv Nutr. 2015;6(3):368S–75S.

45. Finner AM. Nutrition and hair. Deficiencies and supplements. Dermatol Clin. 2013;31:167–72.

46. Goldberg LJ, Lenzy Y. Nutrition and hair. Clin Dermatol. 2010;28:412–9.

47. Harrison S, Berqfeld W. Diffuse hair loss: its triggering and management. Cleve Clin J Med. 2009;76(6):361–7.

48. Mahamid M, Abu-Elhija O. Association between vitamin D levels and alopecia areata. IMAJ. 2014;16:367–70.

49. Thomas DM, Mirowski GW. Nutrition and oral mucosal diseases. Clin Dermatol. 2010;28:426–31.

50. Cashman MW, Sloan SB. Nutrition and nail disease. Clin Dermatol. 2010;28:420–5.

51. Dimitris R, Ralph D. Management of simple brittle nails. Dermatol Ther. 2012;25:569–73.

52. Wan P, Moat S, Anstey A. Pellagra: a review with emphasis on photosensitivity. Br J Dermatol. 2011;164(6):1188–200.

53. Hidalgo LG. Dermatological complications of obesity. Am J Clin Dermatol. 2002;3(7):497–50.

54. Mazzone A, Bellelli G, Annoni G. Mini nutritional assessment and functional status as predictors of development of pressure ulcers in acute setting of care. J Am Geriatr Soc. 2014;62(7):1395–6.

55. Ocón Bretón J, Cabrejas Gómez MC, Altermir Trallero J. Frinoderma secundario a déficit de vitamina A en un paciente con derivación biliopancreática. Nutr Hosp. 2011;26:421–4.

56. Cepeda-Lopez AC, Aeberli I, Zimmermann MB. Does obesity increase risk for iron deficiency? A review of the literature and the potential mechanisms. Int J Vitam Nutr Res. 2010;80:263–70.

57. Schulenburg-Brand D, Katugampola R, Anstey AV, Badminton MN. The cutaneous porphyrias. Rev Dermatol Clin. 2014;32(3):369–84.

58. Ricketts JR, Rothe MJ, Grant-Kels JM. Nutrition and psoriasis. Clin Dermatol. 2010;28:615–26.

59. Murzaku EC, Bronsnick T, Rao BK. Diet in dermatology. Part II. Melanoma, chronic urticaria, and psoriasis. J Am Acad Dermatol. 2014;71:1053. e1–16.

60. Keri JE, Rosenblatt AE. The role of diet in acne and rosacea. J Clin Aesthet Dermatol. 2008;1(3):22–6.

61. Mandl J, Szarka A, Bánhegyi G. Vitamin C: update on physiology and pharmacology. Br J Pharmacol. 2009;157:1097–110.

62. Riess KP, Farnen JP, Lambert PJ, Mathiason MA, Kothari SN. Ascorbic acid deficiency in bariatric surgical population. Surg Obes Relat Dis. 2009;5:81–6.

63. Rivas M, Rojas E, Araya MC, Calaf GM. Ultraviolet light exposure, skin cancer risk and vitamin D production. Oncol Lett. 2015;10(4):2259–64.

64. Piotrowska A, Wierzbicka J, Żmijewski MA. Vitamin D in the skin physiology and pathology. Acta Biochim Pol. 2016;63(1):17–29.

65. Doldo E, Costanza G, Agostinelli S, Tarquini C, Ferlosio A, Arcuri G, et al. Vitamin A, cancer treatment and prevention: the new role of cellular retinol binding proteins. Biomed Res Int. 2015;2015:624–7.

66. Curiel-Lewandrowski C, Tang JY, Einspahr JG, Bermudez Y, Hsu CH, Rezaee M, et al. Pilot study on the bioactivity of vitamin D in the skin after oral supplementation. Cancer Prev Res (Phila). 2015;8(6):563–9.

67. Freitas B, de Castro LL, Aguiar JR, de Araújo CG, Visacri MB, Tuan BT, et al. Antioxidant capacity total in non-melanoma skin cancer and its relationship with food consumption of antioxidant nutrients. Nutr Hosp. 2015;31(4):1682–8.

68. Linares MA, Zakaria A, Nizran P. Skin cancer. Prim Care. 2015;42(4):645–59.

69. Dennert G, Zwahlen M, Brinkman M, Vincenti M, Zeegers M, Horneber M. Selenium for preventing cancer. Cochrane Database Syst Rev. 2013;5:CD005195.

70. Sladden MJ, Johnston GA. More common skin infections in children. BMJ. 2005;330(7501):1194–8.

71. Gonul M, Cakmak SK, Soylu S, Kilic A, Gul U. Serum vitamin B12, folate, ferritin and iron levels in Turkish patients with vitiligo. Indian J Dermatol Venereol Leprol. 2010;76:448.

72. Atas H, Cemil B, Gönül M, Bastürk E, Çiçek E. Serum levels of homocysteine, folate and vitamin B12 in patients with vitiligo before and after treatment with narrow band ultraviolet B phototherapy and in a group of controls. J Photochem Photobiol B. 2015;148:174–80.

73. Al Ghamdi K, Kumar A, Moussa N. The role of vitamin D in melanogenesis with an emphasis on vitiligo. Indian J Dermatol Venereol Leprol. 2013;79(6):750–8.

74. Whitton ME, Pinart M, Batchelor J, Leonardi-Bee J, González U, Jiyad Z, et al. Interventions for vitiligo. Cochrane Database Syst Rev. 2015;2:CD003263.

Smoking, Alcoholism, and Use of Illicit Drugs

Renan Rangel Bonamigo, Catiussa Brutti,
Taciana Capelletti, Rodrigo Pereira Duquia,
and Mauro W. Keiserman

Key Points
- Smoking tobacco is associated with malignancies, besides the worsening of postsurgical scarring process and skin aging
- Smoking is related to the triggering and worsening of dermatoses, such as Buerger's disease, lupus, psoriasis, and hidradenitis suppurativa
- Cutaneous manifestations of alcoholism include those associated with endocrinologic changes, such as hypogonadism and gynecomastia, nutritional deficiencies of the complex B vitamins, and signs of hepatopathy
- Alcoholism is associated with diseases such as psoriasis, porphyria, seborrheic dermatitis, rosacea, urticaria, and contact dermatitis
- Drug addiction is characterized by recurrent use, and causes severe physical and social consequences
- In addition to the vasculopathy caused by levamisole-contaminated cocaine, this drug produces laboratory changes that may clinically mimic some rheumatologic diseases

R.R. Bonamigo, MD, PhD (✉)
Dermatology Service, Hospital de Clínicas de Porto
Alegre (HCPA), Federal University of Rio Grande do
Sul (UFRGS), Porto Alegre, Brazil

Sanitary Dermatology Service of the Department of
Health of Rio Grande do Sul State (ADS-SES),
Porto Alegre, Brazil

Graduate Pathology Program of Federal University of
Health Sciences of Porto Alegre, Porto Alegre, Brazil
e-mail: rrbonamigo@gmail.com

C. Brutti, MD • T. Capelletti, MD
Dermatology Service of Hospital Universitário
de Santa Maria, Santa Maria, Brazil

R.P. Duquia, MD, PhD
UFCSPA, Dermatology Service, Porto Alegre, Brazil

M.W. Keiserman, MD, PhD
PUCRS, Reumathology Service of Hospital
São Lucas, Porto Alegre, Brazil

Tobacco Smoking

Epidemiology

Smoking is one of the main modifiable risk factors for mortality, with a prevalence of 20–30% in developed countries and 10–50% in developing countries [1]. It decreases life expectancy by 15 years, and accounts for death in one-third of tobacco users. The prevalence is higher in men, blacks, persons with less education, and the impoverished, and it continues to grow, mainly among young women.

Worldwide, more than 5.4 million deaths annually are associated with tobacco smoking, besides tuberculosis, HIV/AIDS, and malaria [1]. Tobacco consumption is related to cardiovascular

© Springer International Publishing Switzerland 2018
R.R. Bonamigo, S.I.T. Dornelles (eds.), *Dermatology in Public Health Environments*,
https://doi.org/10.1007/978-3-319-33919-1_39

diseases, chronic bronchitis, lung emphysema, and many dermatologic diseases [2]. Approximately 40% of neoplasias are associated with tobacco smoking, including those occurring in the lungs, mouth, pharynx, larynx, esophagus, cervix, kidney, and bladder.

Etiopathogenesis

Tobacco smoking comprises a volatile or gaseous phase and a particulate or solid phase. The solid phase has about 3,500 elements, including nicotinic alkaloids [2]. There are many mutagens and carcinogens, notably polycyclic aromatic hydrocarbons, nitrosamines, and heterocyclic amines [3] (Table 39.1).

The skin is an organ exposed to cigarette smoke, both directly through contact with environmental smoke and indirectly through toxic substances that travel from the inhaled smoke into the bloodstream [2]. Dysfunction of the

Table 39.1 Toxic components of tobacco

Phase	Components
Solid	Nicotine
	Phenol
	Catechol
	Quinoline
	Aniline
	Toluidine
	Nickel
	N-Nitrosodimethylamine
	Benzopyrenes
	Benzanthracene
	2-Naphthylamine
Gas	Carbon dioxide (CO_2)
	Carbon monoxide (CO)
	Hydrogen cyanide (HCN)
	Nitrogen oxide (NO_2)
	Acetone
	Formaldehyde
	Acrolein
	Ammonium
	Pyridine
	3-Vinylpyridine
	N-Nitrosodimethylamine
	N-Nitrosopyrrolidine

microvasculature occurs as flow decreases at 30–40%, carboxyhemoglobin increases, oxygen decreases, neovascularization decreases, fibroblast activity decreases, vitamin C decreases, and platelet aggregation and blood viscosity increase.

Cutaneous Manifestations

Tobacco smoking may affect many chronic dermatoses and their treatment. Smoking cessation or decrease can be an effective therapeutic measure. Conversely, nicotine has been effective as monotherapy in some dermatologic conditions (there are cutaneous receptors of acetylcholine of nicotinic class). Thus, smoking can be related to the worsening or the triggering of dermatoses, and there are reported improvements of some dermatoses (Table 39.2).

Obliterans Thromboangiitis

More than 90% of patients with ulcers resulting from Buerger's disease are tobacco smokers. While most tobacco components can induce vasoconstriction and exacerbate the disease, nicotine use can be a prospective therapeutic option. There are reports of successful use of nicotine gum [3].

Cutaneous and Systemic Lupus Erythematosus

The relationship between tobacco smoking and systemic lupus erythematosus has been researched in many studies, and some authors have noticed a positive relationship while others have not. A recent retrospective study assessed the relationship between tobacco smoking and lupus, reaching the conclusion that the discoid and tumid variant was clearly associated with smoking, whereas the systemic form did not show such an association [4]. Besides displaying more disease activity, treatment with antimalarial drugs showed decreased efficacy in tobacco-smoking patients [5].

Carcinogenesis

Epidemiologic studies have shown correlations among tobacco smoking and the incidence and aggressiveness of certain types of skin cancer.

Table 39.2 Relation between tobacco/nicotine and skin manifestation

Skin manifestation	Association	Observations
Aberrant wound healing	↑	Unaesthetic scars, infections, suture failure; affects results of flaps and full-thickness grafts
Buerger's disease	↑	90% of patients with ulcerations are smokers
Lupus erythematosus	↑	Discoid and tumid variants
Lupus erythematosus variant systemic	–	Treatment with antimalarial drugs has limited effectiveness in smokers
Squamous cell carcinoma	↑	Particularly associated with increased risk of penile carcinoma and cancers of the vulva, cervix, anus, and oral cavity
Keratoacanthoma	↑	
Malignant melanoma	?	Effect on the incidence is not established; prognostic implications
Psoriasis	↑	Dose-response relationship with the number of cigarettes smoked per day, particularly in the pustular form
Hidradenitis suppurativa	↑	
Acne vulgaris	?	
Atopic dermatitis	?	
Contact dermatitis	?	
Skin aging	↑	Smoker's face; Favre–Racouchot syndrome
Oral melanosis	↑	Active smoking sign
Stomatitis by nicotine or palate leukokeratosis	↑	Active smoking sign
Yellowish discoloration of the facial hair, nails, and fingers	↑	Active smoking sign
Harlequin nails	↑	Smoking cessation sign
Aphthous ulcers	↓	
Behçet's disease	↓	
Pemphigus vulgaris	↓	
Pyoderma gangrenous	↓	
Herpes simplex	↓	Reduces the intensity and frequency of episodes
Rosacea	↓	
Dermatitis herpetiformis	↓	

↑ increased incidence and/or exacerbation; ? controversial reports; – no relation; ↓ decreased incidence and/or improvement

Smoking is an independent risk factor for the development of squamous cell carcinoma (SCC). Particularly, it is associated with increased risk for penile, vulval, cervical, and anal carcinoma, and oral cancer [3]. Regarding the latter, there is greater risk in women smoking unfiltered cigarettes.

In addition, excessive alcohol consumption has a synergistic effect if combined with cigarette use, thus significantly increasing the risk for the development of mouth carcinoma [2].

Keratoacanthoma

There is a connection between keratoacanthoma and tobacco smoking. In a case-control study of 78 patients the smoking prevalence was 69.2% in the group of keratoacanthoma cases, compared with 21.6% in the control group [1].

Malignant Melanoma

Many research studies that fail to provide enough evidence to establish the influence of tobacco smoking on melanoma incidence. However, prognostic implications have been verified [2]. The proportion of male smokers free from the disease 5 years after the diagnosis was significantly smaller than in nonsmoking men. Moreover, smokers were prone to display early metastases and visceral metastases within the first 2 years after the diagnosis [3].

Postsurgical Complications

Cutaneous complications after surgeries include development of unaesthetic scars, infections, suture failure, and harmful outcomes of total-thickness cutaneous flaps and grafts.

These risks were shown to be dependent upon the amount of cigarettes smoked per day. Although the minimum period of tobacco avoidance is yet to be established, some experimental studies and clinical observations suggest that cessation of tobacco consumption 2 weeks before and 1 week after surgery tends to minimize complications of surgical wounds [9].

Other Dermatoses

Psoriasis

Tobacco consumption is associated with the risk of developing psoriasis, and there is a dose-reaction relationship with the amount of cigarettes smoked per day [3], particularly with the pustular form (Fig. 39.1), when the acrosyringium is the inflammation target. Cessation of tobacco consumption leads to a significant improvement, with fewer pustules, and less erythema and scaling. It is known that 95% of these patients are smokers, most of them being heavy smokers [1].

Hidradenitis Suppurativa

Hidradenitis suppurativa (HS, Fig. 39.2), or inverted acne, is epidemiologically associated with tobacco smoking. Chemical components in tobacco activate keratinocytes, fibroblasts, and two kinds of receptors, the acetylcholine nicotinic

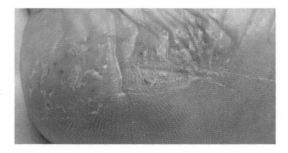

Fig. 39.1 Pustular psoriasis

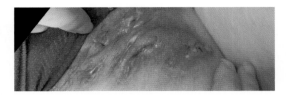

Fig. 39.2 Hidradenitis suppurativa

receptors and the aryl hydrocarbon receptors. These are found in the keratinocytes. Acanthosis, hyperplasia of the infundibular epithelium, and excessive cornification are factors implicated in HS pathogenesis [6].

Acne

Some reports showed a dose-dependent linear relationship between prevalence and severity of acne vulgaris and cigarette consumption, whereas others showed no such association [3].

Atopic Dermatitis

Although tobacco smokers show a total immunoglobulin E (IgE) serum level significantly higher compared with nonsmoking subjects, reports are conflicting regarding effects of tobacco smoking on atopic patients [3]. Mills et al. did not find differences in smoking prevalence between patients with atopic dermatitis and a control group [2].

Contact Dermatitis

There is some controversy regarding the association of the smoking habit and contact dermatitis [1]. Linneberg et al. found a significant association between tobacco smoking and a positive result of contact test for nickel and allergic contact dermatitis [2]. The contact test has to be considered in smoking patients who display hand, face, and neck dermatitis. Besides the standard series, in these cases specific allergens should also be tested, including cocoa, menthol, licorice, formaldehyde, and cigarette components [1]. Nicotinic patches can cause allergic contact dermatitis, or by primary irritation on the application sites, with nicotine being the main involved allergen [3]. A prospective cohort study reported increased severity of occupational hand dermatitis in tobacco smokers [7], but there is no verified association between hand dermatitis and tobacco consumption in any present systematic review [8].

Cutaneous Aging

Tobacco smoking is a significant accelerator of the aging process through multiple mechanisms [1, 3]: free radical development, decrease and increased breakdown of type I and type II collagen synthesis, increased elastic fibers resulting in degradation of elastic material, decreased susceptibility threshold to ultraviolet effects, decreased cutaneous turgor, and induction of metalloproteinase synthesis.

There are characteristic cutaneous signs (Fig. 39.2) related to smoking habit, including the following possibilities [3, 10]:

- "Smoker's face": wrinkles, contour prominence, atrophic greyish aspect, and plethoric frame
- Favre–Racouchot syndrome: multiple and large open comedones located in the lateral and inferior orbital region, consistently associated with long-term solar exposure.

Oral Melanosis

One-third of tobacco smokers display oral pigmentation [3], with melanin gingival pigmentation resulting from increased melanin in the epidermal basal layer [1].

Nicotinic Stomatitis/Palatal Leukokeratosis

This is an area with multiple umbilicated pustules at the two-thirds posterior areas of the hard palate that represent inflamed salivary glands. The condition is more commonly seen in pipe smokers [2].

Yellow Discoloration

Yellow discoloration of mustache, nails, and fingers as side effects of smoking tobacco.

Harlequin Nails

This occurs when tobacco consumption stops and a demarcation arises between a distal pigmented nail and a growing nail [3].

Protective Effects of Tobacco Smoking

A potentially low incidence of some dermatoses in tobacco smokers has been reported. Perhaps because tobacco increases oral mucosa keratinization (among other factors), there are some "negative" associations: (1) ulcers resulting from Behçet's disease apparently improve with tobacco smoking and nicotine; (2) there is a decreased risk for new lesions of pemphigus and pyoderma gangrenosum; (3) tobacco smoking inhibits herpes simplex replication and decreases its cytolytic effect, thus reducing the intensity and frequency of new episodes (but, since the viral oncologic activity is inversely related to its cytolytic activity, tobacco smoking can function as a cancer factor); (4) lower incidence of rosacea among tobacco smokers may result from vasoconstrictive effects; (5) the incidence of positive antiendomysial antibodies among newly diagnosed adults with celiac disease (dermatitis herpetiformis) is smaller in tobacco smokers than in nonsmokers [3].

Alcoholism

Epidemiology

Substance abuse including alcohol and drugs is defined by the American Association of Psychiatry as a maladaptive pattern of substance use clinically leading to significant harm or suffering expressed by one or more than one of the following signs within 12 months:

- Recurrent use resulting in damage,
- Recurrent use in physically dangerous situations,
- Associated legal problems, and
- Recurrent use despite the consequences [11].

Alcohol consumption has an estimated prevalence of 2 billion users and harbors cultural, social, and religious aspects. Its early use is a risk factor for future abuse. It represents up to 4% of deaths in general, and is twice to three times more common in men. Alcohol abuse represents a significant cause of mortality and morbidity and has implications in multiple health conditions [11, 12].

Rehm et al. concluded that ethanol abuse is one of the greatest avoidable risk factors, and actions to reduce the heavy costs associated with ethanol should be urgently implemented [13].

Skin Manifestations

Alcohol is directly toxic to the liver resulting in hepatic steatosis, alcoholic hepatitis, and cirrhosis. Its abuse also accounts for up to 65% of acute and chronic pancreatitis. Although moderate consumption may be protective against coronary disease, heavy consumption can lead to cardiomyopathy, hypertension, arrhythmias, and cerebrovascular hemorrhage. Other medical consequences include increased risk for certain types of cancer, and nutritional deficiencies [14].

Endocrinologic Changes

Hypogonadism
Loss of libido and impotence, testicular atrophy, fertility decrease, and reduced facial hair growth in men.

Hyperestrogenism
Hyperestrogenism consists of gynecomastia, vascular spiders, altered body fat distribution, and loss of body hair. Women seldom show signs of masculinization although they can have mammary atrophy and irregular menses.

Pseudo-Cushing Syndrome
Pseudo-Cushing syndrome may be difficult to distinguish from Cushing syndrome by manifesting full-moon facies, centripetal obesity, loss of proximal muscle mass, buffalo hump, abdominal striae, hypertension, and osteoporosis [14]. Besemer et al. [15] noticed that in most patients biochemical and clinical abnormalities were found, thus mimicking increased activity of the hypothalamic-hypophyseal-adrenal axis. Biochemical changes and regressive hypercortisolism symptoms cannot be normalized unless alcohol consumption is stopped [15].

Nutritional Deficiencies
The cause is probably multifactorial, including inappropriate nutrient ingestion as well as the hepatotoxic effects of alcohol on food metabolism.

Vitamin B1 (thiamine): one of the most commonly seen deficiencies secondary to damaged gastrointestinal absorption. Damaged gastrointestinal absorption presents as cardiac and neurologic complications; patients' skin may appear waxy and their tongue can become thick and reddish.

Vitamin B2 (riboflavin): deficiency results in angular cheilitis, atrophic glossitis, and a facial erythema that resembles seborrheic dermatitis [11].

Vitamin B3 (niacin): pellagra displays a classic tetrad including dermatitis, diarrhea, dementia, and death (if not treated). Dermatitis is characterized by red-chestnut plaques, with eventual vesicles or bullae, on photoexposed skin mainly on the face, arms, and legs (Fig. 39.3). Casal collar is the term used for the lesion plaque around the neck.

Vitamin B6 (pyridoxine): a deficiency also commonly associated with alcoholism, characterized by similar seborrheic dermatitis on the face, neck, shoulders, and perineum. Patients can also show angular stomatitis and glossitis [14].

Vitamin B12 (cobalamin): vitamin B12 deficiency is recognized by hyperpigmentation in "glove" and "boot," whereas folate deficiency can display diffuse hyperpigmentation (Fig. 39.4).

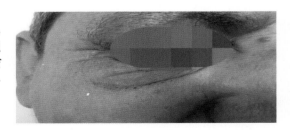

Fig. 39.3 Smoker's face/Favre–Racouchot syndrome

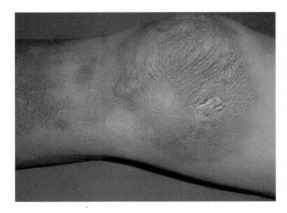

Fig. 39.4 Pellagra

Signs of Alcoholic Hepatopathy

It should be borne in mind that many changes may be secondary to hepatopathy of any etiology and not specific to alcoholic hepatic disease, as shown in Box 39.1.

Psoriasis and Alcohol Use

Many factors are implicated in the pathogenesis of psoriasis, including physical and psychic stress, metabolic factors, tobacco smoking, drugs, infections, and trauma. Extensive evidence shows a link between ethanol abuse and psoriasis [12]. Alcohol abuse is a risk factor for psoriasis, both in men and women, given that many of these patients do not display signs of dependence and also show normal results in hepatic function tests [14].

The distribution of cutaneous lesions in the majority of patients tends to be predominantly acral, involving the hand dorsum and the fingers, resembling a pattern seen in immunocompromised patients, such as HIV patients. This element shows the potential role of ethanol in inducing immune dysfunction with negative immunosuppression [11].

It was shown by a research study that daily ingestion of ethanol higher than 80 g resulted in a more severe psoriasis and a lower reaction to treatment [11]. Moreover, the therapeutic options are limited (methotrexate, acitretin) because of the absolute or relative contraindications [12].

Box 39.1 Cutaneous Signs of Hepatopathy

Gynecomastia

Increased parotid

Decreased pili

Palmar erythema (Fig. 39.5)

Telangiectasia

Jaundice

Ungual alterations

  Terry nails: two-thirds proximal to the ungual fold are white whereas 2 mm distal are pink. Can be seen in 80% of cirrhotic patients [14]

  Hippocratic fingers: alteration of the Lovibond angle between the ungual plaque and the proximal fold greater than 180°, found in 5–15% of cirrhotic patients. It results from increased peripheral blood flow with dilated arteriovenous anastomoses of the fingers and is not due to hypertrophic osteopathy

  Transverse bands (Muehrcke): white bands parallel to the lunula separated by a normally pink nail. Frequently associated with hypoalbuminemia [11]

Solar Exposition and Alcohol

A transversal research study on alcohol consumption and self-referred sunburns, in which adults were asked about alcohol usage in the previous month and history of sunburns in the previous year, concluded that excessive alcohol consumption is associated with higher rates of sunburns, thus making the risk for cutaneous neoplasias higher. The odds ratio adjusted for prevalence and number of sunburns in ethanol consumers was 1.39 (95% confidence interval 1.31–1.48) and 1.29 (95% confidence interval 1.20–1.38), respectively [16].

Some studies have also suggested that basal cell carcinoma in chronic alcoholics tends to show a more infiltrating pattern, especially in immunosuppressed patients. The tumors are more aggressive and display greater destruction and local recurrence [11].

The main ethanol metabolite, acetaldehyde, has been reported as the greatest influential factor in alcohol-related carcinogenesis and mutagenesis [12].

Alcohol use is associated with a higher risk for scaly cell carcinoma of the oral cavity. Its mechanism is still not clear, although it may be multifactorial because of its immunosuppressive effect associated nutritional deficiencies and synergistic effect related to tobacco consumption.

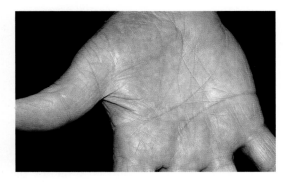

Fig. 39.5 Palmar erythema

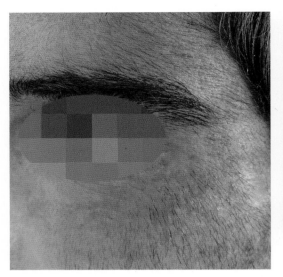

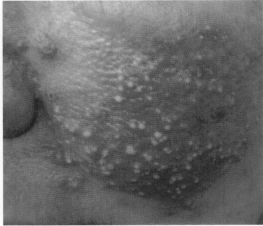

Fig. 39.7 Rosacea

Fig. 39.6 Porphyria cutanea tarda: hypertrichosis and hyperpigmentation

Alcohol and Other Dermatoses

Porphyria Cutanea Tarda

This is the most prolific porphyria worldwide, and is the only type not exclusively inherited. Alcohol has been shown to be the most significant cause of acquired porphyria cutanea tarda (PCT) [12].

The enzymatic fault that accumulates porphyrins which, in turn, induce photosensitivity, leads to cutaneous manifestations predominantly in photoexposed areas, cutaneous frailty, erosions, blisters with milia, and scar development. Other manifestations include hypertrichosis, mainly on the temples, malar region, and mentum, as well as cutaneous hyperpigmentation (Fig. 39.6).

Affected patients must be instructed to avoid exacerbating factors such as alcohol and solar radiation [11].

Seborrheic Dermatitis

An association between alcohol abuse and seborrheic dermatitis was shown in hepatopathic patients and patients lacking nutrition [11].

Rosacea

Rosacea (Fig. 39.7) is exacerbated by alcohol use. The implicated mechanism is vasodilation and the subsequent temperature rise that leads to uncomfortable flushing. Long-term alcohol consumption may result in chronic facial erythema and loss of vasoregulatory control [11, 14].

Urticaria

Although rare, there have been reports of occurrence of immediate manifestations of urticaria/angioedema after consumption of small quantities of ethanol.

Urticariform reactions may be limited to the area of direct contact with ethanol, or may occur systemically after contact through percutaneous absorption or ingestion. Specific IgE in cases of suspected ethanol allergy has not been shown [12, 17]. It is not yet clear whether the urticariform reaction can result from the ethanol itself or from additives therein [11].

Systemic Contact Dermatitis

The exact mechanism of systemic contact dermatitis as regards ethanol (SCDE) is uncertain, but probably results from a hypersensitivity reaction (type IV) involving T-cell activation. Ethanol is widely used in topical products such as hand disinfectants and cosmetics, and also as a vehicle for the topical absorption of transdermal medicines.

A case of SCDE was reported after ethanol ingestion by a patient with fixed erythematous and pruriginous rash, with small skin areas spared on the trunk. The patient reported recurrent alcohol ingestion and previous use of transdermal contraceptives, besides sensitivity to the use of topical preparations with alcohol [18].

Discoid Eczema

Discoid or nummular eczema is found with increased frequency in alcohol abusers [14].

Alcohol and Procedures

Alcohol abuse is a significant risk factor for the following surgical complications [14]:

- Infection of the surgical wound: associated with immunosuppression.
- Suture dehiscence: infection associated with nutritional deficiencies can lead to increased dehiscence.
- Bleeding: resulting from compromised platelet function. Coagulopathy due to deficiency of vitamin K may be present in patients with severe hepatic disease.

Alcohol and Drug Interactions

Alcohol may interact with frequently used drugs in dermatologic therapeutics, such as methotrexate and acitretin, given that the concomitant ingestion of acitretin indirectly increases its re-esterification into etretinate. In addition, flushing may occur after administration of certain drugs, such as disulfiram, metronidazole, griseofulvin, and ketoconazole. Pimecrolimus and tacrolimus, calcineurin topic inhibitors used to treat atopic dermatitis, were reported as resulting in intolerance after topical application associated with ethanol ([12], [19]).

Therapeutic Approach

Genetic, environmental, and psychosocial factors may play a relevant role in alcoholism development. Alcoholism is characterized as a chronic, progressive, and potentially lethal disease involving ethanol dependence and multiple organ dysfunction.

Advising patients to quit smoking and alcoholic beverage abuse must be routine with regard to general skin orientations, together with the standard recommendations to decrease sun exposure, because of the significant morbidity/mortality rate associated with such habits.

Heavy advertising and vested economic interest policies regarding tobacco and alcohol consumption exist worldwide. It has been documented that almost all societies where alcohol and tobacco consumption exists report social and health problems associated with abuse.

Ethanol-associated costs reach more than 1% of the gross national product in medium- and high-income countries, with costs related to social damage making up a significant proportion besides health costs [12].

Use of Illicit Drugs and Drug Addiction

Similar to alcohol abuse, drug abuse (drug addiction) is characterized by the recurrent use in the face of the physical and social consequences [11].

The most commonly used illicit substances include marijuana, heroin, cocaine, crack, ecstasy, LSD, methamphetamines, benzodiazepines, anabolic steroids, and GHB (γ-hydroxybutyrate).

Cutaneous manifestations resulting from drugs, though not being pathognomonic, allow the clinician to identify these patients early, and, possibly after excluding many other etiologic factors, the physician can intervene and make referrals to other specialists [20].

Stigmas Related to the Use of Injectable Drugs

A study reported "track marks" or " skin tracks" along the injected veins in 76% of injectable drug users (IDU). These tracks result from phlebitis with postinflammatory hyperpigmentation. Cutaneous granulomas can develop from months to years after exposition. Ulcerations can also develop from the irritating effect of the drug, repeated trauma, or secondary infection [11].

Cutaneous Infections

Cellulitis, abscess, and impetigo are common among IDUs, who can also show necrotizing fasciitis, septic phlebitis, and gangrene. *Staphylococcus aureus* is the most frequently found agent, followed by the *Streptococcus* species. Infections are the main driver leading drug users to seek medical care [21].

Pruritus and Signs of Excoriation

Pruritus may occur especially with cocaine and methamphetamines. Users can have delusional parasitosis resulting in manipulative lesions and excoriation. Histamine-liberating opioids may cause pruritus that lasts up to 24 h.

Acneiform Eruption

Acneiform eruption has been noted in anabolic steroid abusers.

Damage to the Nasal and Oral Mucosa

Intranasal use of cocaine may result in development of granulomas or septal necrosis, or both. Chronic damage to the nasal mucosa may lead to ischemic necrosis of the cartilage that may evolve to septal perforation.

A well-known effect of methamphetamine abuse is extreme oral disease with dental destruction, known as "meth mouth" [11, 20].

Other Cutaneous and Mucosal Manifestations

The following conditions have been reported to be related to illicit drug abuse: urticaria, angioedema, leukocytoclastic vasculitis, serum disease (amphetamine), maculopapular exanthem, bullous reactions, fixed eruption by drug (heroin), pseudovasculitis/vasculopathy (cocaine: see below), and acute generalized exanthematous pustulosis [11, 20].

Cocaine and Adjuvant Syndrome

It is estimated that more than 17 million people worldwide are cocaine users [22]. Cocaine use causes euphoria and some side effects that include

Table 39.3 Laboratory changes previously described and attributed to the use of levamisole

Laboratory changes described in the literature	
Anemia, leukopenia, or pancytopenia	Rheumatoid factor
Increased creatinine	Anticardiolipin antibodies
Positive P-ANCA and C-ANCA	Hemoglobinuria
Altered FAN and Anti-DNA	Antiphospholipid AB

acute myocardial infarction, tachyarrhythmia, hypertensive crises, and nasal septum perforation, among others [23]. In recent years, changes in patterns of cocaine use have been observed. Purple necrotic lesions on the skin, livedo reticularis, and pancytopenia are often described in association with changes in markers of rheumatologic diseases, such as rheumatoid factor, C-ANCA, P-ANCA, and antinuclear factor (Table 39.3) [24–26]. These changes in clinical and laboratory patterns, which were not previously described among cocaine users, are attributed to levamisole, a medication that has been added to cocaine [25–27].

Cocaine is one of the world's oldest known psychoactive drugs. It is used as a stimulant and is produced from the leaves of the coca plant (*Erythoxylum coca*). Cocaine causes euphoria in the short term. Acute myocardial infarction, hypertensive crisis, heart failure, arrhythmias, and altered mental status are some of the disorders associated with the use of this substance.

In the last decade, cocaine use has been linked to rheumatologic, renal, hematologic, and cutaneous manifestations [24, 25, 28–31]. Over the years the number of reports on this topic has steadily increased. Considering that cocaine has been used for so many years, it was hypothesized that this new profile of diseases found in users was caused by an adjuvant (also called contaminant) which was recently added.

In Brazil and worldwide it is well known that cocaine, as well as other drugs, is often not marketed in its pure form. Many other substances, including talcum powder and medications, were found in analyses of cocaine. In recent decades one of the most frequently added adulterants in street drugs sold as cocaine is the anthelminthic drug levamisole. Approximately 70% of illicit cocaine consumed in the United States is contaminated with levamisole [32, 33].

Levamisole is an immunomodulatory agent that was used to treat various cancers before being withdrawn from the United States market in 2000 because of adverse effects. Potential complications associated with its use include agranulocytosis, skin necrosis, and pseudovasculitis. Levamisole is currently approved as an anthelminthic agent in veterinary medicine [27].

Levamisole is known to cause purpura in 3% of exposed persons. Patients often present with a rapid and progressive development of livedo reticularis, macules, papules, and purpuric plaques followed by hemorrhagic bullae and necrosis. Classically many authors point out purpuric eruption on earlobes; however, lesions may be found in any area of the body (Figs. 39.8, 39.9, and 39.10). Histologically, some cases reveal leu-

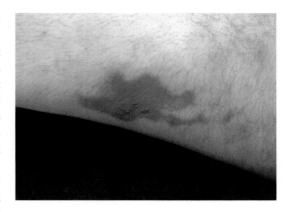

Fig. 39.9 Retiform purpura in a cocaine/levamisole user: reticulated and necrotic center lesion, with "stellate" edges and brighter erythema

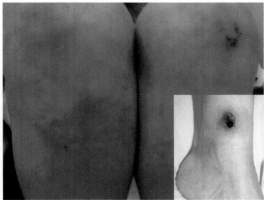

Fig. 39.10 Lesions of livedo reticularis on the knees of a cocaine/levamisole user. Skin necrosis on the right area

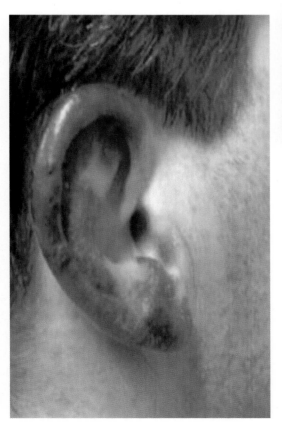

Fig. 39.8 Typical auricular lesion in a cocaine/levamisole user

kocytoclastic vasculitis and small-vessel thrombosis or medium-sized-vessel vasculitis [34].

In addition to the vasculopathy caused by levamisole-contaminated cocaine, this drug produces laboratory changes that may clinically mimic some rheumatologic diseases. Similar to our own cases, some studies have mainly reported positive anti-neutrophil cytoplasmic antibody (ANCA), which often leads to a false diagnosis of autoimmune vasculitis, including polyarteritis nodosa and granulomatosis with polyangiitis (GPA). In addition to this marker, a few cases of individuals with antinuclear factor, anti-DNA, anti-cardiolipin antibodies, and positive rheumatoid factor have been reported [34, 35]. Positive ANCA induced by drugs is common. In the literature there are reports of ANCA positivity with the use of some antibiotics, antithyroid drugs, anti-tumor necrosis factor, and psychoactive agents. Repeated exposure may lead to the formation of autoantibodies in more than 10% of patients, especially after long periods of exposure. The mechanism in the pathogenesis of levamisole/cocaine-induced ANCA positivity is unclear [34, 35].

It has yet to be clarified in the literature whether exposure time or the cumulative dose used is more relevant. The answer is probably multicausal. Depending on genetics and other factors, for some individuals it could be the dose used and for others the exposure time.

Individuals with purpuric lesions, livedo reticularis, acute renal failure, and agranulocytosis with a positive ANCA diagnosis should be excluded from the clinical history of exposure to levamisole and cocaine. Therefore, we recommend the use of ANCA as a diagnostic marker for cocaine use and levamisole. Individuals with these characteristics should be investigated for history of ingested drugs, including cocaine and its derivatives.

The diseases caused by an adjuvant added to cocaine can be grouped into a complex syndrome referred to as autoimmune/inflammatory syndrome induced by adjuvants (ASIA). Four entities are included: (1) postvaccination phenomenon; (2) Gulf War syndrome; (3) macrophagic myofasciitis; (4) siliconosis.

The main environmental factors involved in ASIA are aluminum hydroxide (adjuvant in vaccines), silicone, squalene, and mineral oil used for cosmetic purposes.

Gulf War syndrome is related to multiple vaccinations made in a short time in addition to smoke from oil-well fires or depleted uranium from shells, as well as physical and psychological stress. The majority (95%) of overtly ill deployed Gulf War syndrome patients had antibodies to squalene.

The clinical spectrum of the syndrome that occurs after vaccination include vasculitis, inflammatory myopathy, neurologic syndromes, inflammatory bowel disease, systemic lupus erythematosus, rheumatoid arthritis, autoimmune thrombocytopenia, and other nonspecific autoimmune manifestations.

Silicone, a synthetic polymer, is considered to be a biologically inert substance; however, silicone may mediate autoimmune diseases, mainly scleroderma, although controversy about this issue is ongoing.

It can be observed that the syndrome is described with varied clinical and laboratory (scleroderma and macrophagic myofasciitis) or pleomorphic manifestations (vasculitis). The latter is observed in cocaine/levamisole users. Considering that levamisole is an adjuvant to cocaine, we suggest the inclusion of this new entity in the ASIA group.

In conclusion, drug addiction is a risk factor for sexually transmitted diseases, depression, accidental injuries, criminal violence, and domestic abuse. By recognizing cutaneous manifestations of illicit drug use the dermatologist has the opportunity to intervene, and can have a significant impact on the patient's health [21].

Glossary

Acetylcholine Neurotransmitter released by cholinergic neurons responsible for muscle contraction, learning, and memory, whose action is mediated by nicotinic and muscarinic receptors found at the neuromuscular junctions in the central and peripheral nervous system.

Acneiform eruption Dermatosis related to the development of papules and follicular pustules, with or without comedones, connected to predisposing factors or medicines, located in sites that do not usually show acne, or occurring in life stages other than adolescence.

Carboxyhemoglobin Molecule of carbon monoxide linked to a molecule of hemoglobin. Its development is associated with carbon monoxide toxicity.

Carcinogen A substance, situation, or exposition that can damage the genetic material (DNA), thus initiating or stimulating cancer development.

Cheilitis Lip dermatosis resulting from different causes that manifests as erythemas, scaling, vesicles, fissures, tumefaction, nodules, and so forth.

Comedones Solid development in the pilosebaceous follicles resulting from retained sebum produced by the gland due to acroinfundibulum obliteration by focal keratosis.

Cytolytic Related to cell destruction (cytolysis).

Discoid Semiologic description of lesion feature shaped like a disc.

Glossitis Alterations of the tongue mucosa caused by poor nutrition, infections, and physical, chemical, or drug-induced irritation that are manifested by partial or total loss of the filiform papillae, and smooth and red tongue.

Gynecomastia Increased breast tissue, unilaterally or bilaterally, in men.

Jaundice Yellow color of skin, mucosa, and sclera caused by hyperbilirubinemia.

Keratinization Final phase of the keratinocyte differentiation whereby keratin is formed.

Metalloproteinases Zinc-dependent proteinases that show cleavage activity (gelatinolytic) of the matrix and angiogenic and inflammatory activities, synthesized by many cells including fibroblasts and leukocytes.

Mutagenic Physical, chemical, or biological agent which can cause mutation if exposed to one cell, i.e., damage to the DNA that is not repaired and is passed on to the next generations.

Neovascularization Development of new blood vessels. This process can be physiologic or pathologic.

Nummular Semiologic description of lesion feature as "rounded, resembling coin."

Pathognomonic The characteristic and proper sign of a disease.

Plethoric Red coloration through vascular engorgement in polycythemic patients; increased blood volume.

Rhytids Skin lines and depressions resulting from facial, neck, hand, and arm aging, commonly known as wrinkles.

Steatosis Tissue fat accumulation.

Stomatitis Dermatosis of mucosa of the buccal cavity of multiple etiology, such as infections and nicotine.

Telangiectasia Dilation of dermal small blood vessels.

References

1. Metelitsa AI, Lauzon GJ. Tobacco and the skin. Clin Dermatol. 2010;28(4):384–90.
2. Just-Sarobé M. Smoking and the skin. Actas Dermo-Sifiliograficas (English Edition). 2008;99(3):173–84.
3. Ortiz A, Grando SA. Smoking and the skin. Int J Dermatol. 2012;51(3):250–62.
4. Böckle BC, Sepp NT. Smoking is highly associated with discoid lupus erythematosus and lupus erythematosus tumidus: analysis of 405 patients. Lupus. 2015;24(7):669–74.
5. Chasset F, et al. Influence of smoking on the efficacy of antimalarials in cutaneous lupus: a meta-analysis of the literature. J Am Acad Dermatol. 2015;72(4):634–9.
6. Prens E, et al. Pathophysiology of hidradenitis suppurativa: an update. J Am Acad Dermatol. 2015;73(5):S8–S11.
7. Brans R, et al. Association between tobacco smoking and prognosis of occupational hand eczema: a prospective cohort study. Br J Dermatol. 2014;171(5):1108–15.
8. Lukács J, Schliemann S, Elsner P. Association between smoking and hand dermatitis—a systematic review and meta-analysis. J Eur Acad Dermatol Venereol. 2015;29(7):1280–4.
9. Gill JF, Yu SS, Neuhaus IM. Tobacco smoking and dermatologic surgery. J Am Acad Dermatol. 2013;68(1):167–72.
10. Bologna J, Jorizzo J, Rapini RP. Dermatology. 2nd ed. London: Ed. Mosby; 2010.
11. Liu SW, Lien MH, Fenske NA. The effects of alcohol and drug abuse on the skin. Clin Dermatol. 2010;28(4):391–9.
12. Dinis-Oliveira RJ, et al. Clinical and forensic signs related to ethanol abuse: a mechanistic approach. Toxicol Mech Methods. 2014;24(2):81–110.
13. Rehm J, et al. Global burden of disease and injury and economic cost attributable to alcohol use and alcohol-use disorders. Lancet. 2009;373(9682):2223–33.

14. Smith KE, Fenske NA. Cutaneous manifestations of alcohol abuse. J Am Acad Dermatol. 2000;43(1):1–18.

15. Besemer F, Pereira AM, Smit JWA. "Alcohol-induced Cushing syndrome". Hypercortisolism caused by alcohol abuse. Neth J Med. 2011;69:318–23.

16. Mukamal KJ. Alcohol consumption and self-reported sunburn: a cross-sectional, population-based survey. J Am Acad Dermatol. 2006;55(4):584–9.

17. Wong JW, Harris KL, Powell D. Alcohol urticaria syndrome. Dermatitis. 2011;22(6):350–4.

18. Wolverton W, Gada S. Systemic contact dermatitis to ethanol. J Allergy Clin Immunol. (In practice). 2013;1(2):195.

19. Lübbe J, Milingou M. Tacrolimus Oinment, Alcohol, and Facial Flushing. N Eng J Med 2004;351:2740.

20. Fink B, Landthaler M, Hafner C. Skin alterations due to illegal drug abuse. JDDG: J Dtsch Dermatol Ges. 2011;9(8):633–9.

21. Bergstrom KG. Cutaneous clues to drug addiction. J Drugs Dermatol. 2008;7(3):303–5.

22. United Nations Office on Drugs and Crime, World Drug Report 2015 (United Nations publication, Sales No. E.15.XI.6).

23. Michaud K, Grabherr S, Shiferaw K, Doenz F, Augsburger M, Mangin P. Acute coronary syndrome after levamisole-adulterated cocaine abuse. J Forensic Legal Med. 2014;21:48–52. PubMed PMID: 24365689

24. Jenkins J, Babu K, Hsu-Hung E, Robinson-Bostom L, Kroumpouzos G. ANCA-positive necrotizing vasculitis and thrombotic vasculopathy induced by levamisole-adulterated cocaine: a distinctive clinicopathologic presentation. J Am Acad Dermatol. 2011;65(1):e14–6. PubMed PMID: 21679797.

25. Chung C, Tumeh PC, Birnbaum R, Tan BH, Sharp L, McCoy E, et al. Characteristic purpura of the ears, vasculitis, and neutropenia – a potential public health epidemic associated with levamisole-adulterated cocaine. J Am Acad Dermatol. 2011;65(4):722–5. PubMed PMID: 21658797. Pubmed Central PMCID: 4000158.

26. Streicher JL, Swerlick RA, Stoff BK. Cocaine abuse and confidentiality: a case of retiform purpura in an adolescent patient. J Am Acad Dermatol. 2014;70(6):1127–9. PubMed PMID: 24831315.

27. Lee KC, Ladizinski B, Federman DG. Complications associated with use of levamisole-contaminated cocaine: an emerging public health challenge. Mayo Clin Proc. 2012;87(6):581–6.

28. Chawdhary K, Parke A. Levamisole-induced vasculitis with renal involvement. Conn Med. 2015;79(6):343–6. PubMed PMID: 26263714.

29. Dy I, Pokuri V, Olichney J, Wiernik P. Levamisole-adulterated in cocaine causing agranulocytosis, vasculopathy, and acquired protein S deficiency. Ann Hematol. 2012;91(3):477–8. PubMed PMID: 21773730.

30. Caldwell KB, Graham OZ, Arnold JJ. Agranulocytosis from levamisole-adulterated cocaine. J Am Board Fam Med: JABFM. 2012;25(4):528–30. PubMed PMID: 22773721.

31. Jadhav P, Tariq H, Niazi M, Franchin G. Recurrent thrombotic vasculopathy in a former cocaine user. Case Rep Dermatol Med. 2015;2015:763613. PubMed PMID: 26793396. Pubmed Central PMCID: 4697073.

32. Baptiste GG, Alexopoulos AS, Masud T, Bonsall JM. Systemic levamisole-induced vasculitis in a cocaine user without cutaneous findings: a consideration in diagnosis. Case Rep Med. 2015;2015:547023. PubMed PMID: 26635879. Pubmed Central PMCID: 4618334.

33. Botelho ED, Cunha RB, Campos AFC, Maldanera AO. Chemical profiling of cocaine seized by Brazilian federal police in 2009–2012: major components. J Braz Chem Soc. 2014;25(4):611–8.

34. Strazzula L, Brown KK, Brieva JC, Camp BJ, Frankel HC, Kissin E, et al. Levamisole toxicity mimicking autoimmune disease. J Am Acad Dermatol. 2013;69(6):954–9. PubMed PMID: 24075227.

35. Tichauer et al. Levamisole-induced ANCA vasculitis and cutaneous necrosis. http://www.ePlasty.com, Interesting Case, October 17, 2014.

Hepatitis

40

Gislaine Silveira Olm

Key Points
- The infection caused by hepatitis B and C and its complications are a global health problem
- Several extrahepatic syndromes are associated with these chronic viral infections, including significant morbidity and mortality
- Serum sickness and polyarteritis nodosa are the main cutaneous manifestations associated with infection caused by hepatitis B virus
- Cutaneous manifestations related to infection with hepatitis C include mixed cryoglobulinemia, porphyria cutanea tarda, and lichen planus
- Skin adverse reactions, both local and diffuse, are frequent during the treatment of hepatitis C infection.

Introduction

The World Health Organization estimates that more than 400 million people are infected with either hepatitis B virus (HBV) or hepatitis C virus (HCV), whereas approximately 150 million have chronic hepatitis C. Furthermore, hepatitis accounts for 80% of deaths by hepatic cancer [1].

Viral hepatitis, specifically hepatitis B and hepatitis C, not only cause liver disease but also can present with extrahepatic manifestations, including cutaneous lesions. Among all extrahepatic manifestations of liver diseases, cutaneous manifestations are the most common. In addition, they are easily recognizable and may provide the first clues of liver disease. The spectrum of cutaneous manifestations may vary during the acute and chronic phases of viral hepatitis [2, 3].

Hepatitis B

Epidemiology

HBV is an enveloped DNA virus and a member of the Hepadnaviridae family; it affects the liver, causing inflammation and hepatocellular necrosis. It is estimated that 240 million people are chronically infected worldwide. The main complications of chronic hepatitis B are cirrhosis and hepatocellular carcinoma. About 20–30% of individuals who become chronically infected

G.S. Olm, MD, MSc
Mãe de Deus, Dermatology, Porto Alegre, Brazil
e-mail: gisolm@gmail.com

© Springer International Publishing Switzerland 2018
R.R. Bonamigo, S.I.T. Dornelles (eds.), *Dermatology in Public Health Environments*,
https://doi.org/10.1007/978-3-319-33919-1_40

will develop these complications, and an estimated 650,000 people each year die of chronic hepatitis B [4].

Low- prevalence areas of HBV carriers (0.1–2%) include Canada, the United States, western Europe, Australia, and New Zealand. High- prevalence areas worldwide (10–20%) include Southeast Asia, China, and sub-Saharan Africa. This wide variation of carriers can be explained by different transmission routes and the age at onset of infection. In low-prevalence areas the infection is acquired in adulthood by sexual or parenteral exposure. In high-prevalence settings the infection occurs by intrafamilial spread in the neonatal period or during childhood [5].

Clinical Presentation

The acute infection is symptomatic in only 30% of patients (icteric hepatitis), whereas the other 70% have subclinical or anicteric hepatitis. The incubation period lasts from 1 to 4 months and may be followed by serum sickness–like syndrome with jaundice, right upper quadrant pain, nausea, and anorexia [5].

Cutaneous manifestations of HBV infection are protean and nonspecific. Among patients with HBV infection, 20–30% develop the serum sickness–like disease, and 7–8% the polyarteritis nodosa (PAN) [3] (Box 40.1).

Therapeutic Approach

Antiviral therapies against HBV infection are available; they act to suppress viral replication, prevent the progression to cirrhosis, and reduce the risk of hepatocellular carcinoma and liver-related mortality. However, these treatments fail to eradicate the virus in most patients treated [4].

Seven antiviral agents are now approved for the treatment of chronic HBV infection: two formulations of interferon (IFN)-α (conventional and pegylated) and five nucleoside/nucleotide analogs (lamivudine, adefovir, entecavir, telbivudine, and tenofovir) [6].

Skin Manifestations of Hepatitis B Infection

The cutaneous manifestations of hepatitis B infection are summarized in Box 40.1.

Box 40.1 Skin Manifestations Related to Infection by Hepatitis B Virus

Serum sickness–like syndrome

Polyarteritis nodosa

Papular acrodermatitis of childhood

Serum Sickness-Like Syndrome

First described in 1843 by Graves, the serum sickness-like syndrome is currently considered the most common dermatologic manifestation associated with HBV [7, 8]. The syndrome occurs in the prodromal phase of infection by HBV, and it is estimated that 10–30% of the patients who have acute HBV will develop this transitory syndrome. It is also called "arthritis-dermatitis" and is clinically manifested by polyarthralgias or arthritis with joint swelling similar to that of acute rheumatoid arthritis [2, 7].

Arthritis can be either symmetric and generalized, involving the small joints of hands and feet, or asymmetric, involving the large and monoarticular joints. It is usually extremely painful, although joint injuries are not destructive and damage is not permanent [8].

Skin manifestations are varied. Rash is the most common and may be the only clinical manifestation of acute hepatitis [2]. The rash may be associated with hypocomplementemia; 4% of cases present with angioedema [2, 7].

Histopathology demonstrates leukocytoclastic vasculitis with endothelial edema, fibrinoid occlusion, and hemorrhage [7, 9]. Other skin lesions range from mild rashes to maculopapular, purpuric, or petechial exanthema. Lichenoid dermatitis and erythema multiforme may also occur [2]. In most cases, lesions follow or occur shortly after joint manifestations [8].

Pathogenesis includes the formation of circulating immune complexes including hepatitis B surface antigen (HBsAg), anti-HBs, immunoglobulins, and complement, resulting in skin deposits and causing maculopapular lesions. Immune complexes cause lesions due to the production of C3a and C5 anaphylotoxins, manifested as rash and vasculitis [8].

Serum sickness-like syndrome may persist from days to months, and lasts for an average of 20 days [8].

Polyarteritis Nodosa

The association between HBV infection and PAN was first suggested in 1970 by Trepo and Thivolet [9]. PAN is considered one of the most severe syndromes associated with HBV. It is a rare complication of chronic HBV infection, occurring in approximately 1–5% of patients. However, HBsAg serum positivity is observed in 30–50% of PAN patients [2, 8]. The frequency of new cases of PAN related to HBV has decreased as a result of vaccination and improvements in the safety of blood products [8, 10].

Onset of symptoms, which include fever, malaise, arthralgias, abdominal pain, mononeuritis, polyarthritis, hypertension, and weight loss, occurs weeks to months after HBV infection. There may be progression of PAN with systemic involvement of other organs such as kidneys and gastrointestinal tract, as well as peripheral and central nervous systems. Hepatic manifestations vary from mild to moderate elevations of serum transaminases and cholestasis (rarely) [2]. According to the French Vasculitis Study Group, although the same clinical manifestations are present in patients with PAN related and not related to HBV, PAN patients are generally younger than 40 years and present with peripheral neuropathy (multiple mononeuritis), malignant hypertension, orchitis, cardiomyopathy, and intestinal ischemia [11].

Skin manifestations occur in 10–15% of cases and include palpable purpura in lower limbs that may progress to skin ulcers. Painful, purpuric subcutaneous nodules usually arise in the arterial path of lower limbs, as well as livedo reticularis. Rash and angioedema can also occur in patients with PAN associated with viral hepatitis B [7, 9].

Several hypotheses have been proposed to explain the pathogenesis of extrahepatic manifestations of HBV. The pathogenesis of HBV associated with PAN is a dynamic area of research in which the most current theories are associated with the deposit of immune complexes in the event of antigen excess. HBsAg (3 million kDa) and immune complexes are deposited in the lamina of affected arterioles. However, hepatitis B envelope antigen (HBeAg) (19 kDa) seems to play a predominant role in immune complexes due to its smaller size compared with HBsAg. Antineutrophil cytoplasmic antibodies (ANCA) are rarely identified in PAN related to HBV, unlike the cases of PAN not associated with this virus [2].

Histologically, vasculitis is characterized by fibrinoid necrosis and perivascular inflammation of small and medium-sized vessels. Afterward, mononuclear infiltrate predominates; vessel occlusion, thrombosis, ischemia, and necrosis may occur [8]. Immune responses associated with PAN usually begin within the first 6 months of viral hepatitis B infection [2]. Angiography findings include arterial microaneurysms, stenosis, and occlusion. In most PAN patients, renal angiography shows pathognomonic microaneurysms [8].

The prognosis of PAN related to HBV is bad if not treated, with a mortality rate of 30–50% in 5 years [2]. Conventional treatment of PAN not associated with HBV consists of corticosteroids, immunosuppressive drugs, and plasmapheresis. This treatment may have detrimental effects on PAN associated with HBV because of adverse effects on liver disease and viral replication [8]. The activity of PAN associated with HBV infection decreases after seroconversion for HBeAg and reduction of serum HBV levels. Thus, nucleotide analog antiviral therapy is necessary to treat this form of PAN. In cases of severe vasculitis, immunosuppression and removal of immune complexes with corticosteroids and plasmapheresis are used, followed by prolonged suppression (6–12 months) of HBV by using antiviral therapy [8, 10]. Recurrences are rare in PAN related to HBV, and do not occur when virus replication is terminated and seroconversion is achieved [12].

Papular Acrodermatitis of Childhood

Papular acrodermatitis of childhood (PAC) was first described in 1955 by Fernando Gianotti in Milan, Italy [13]. The following year, Gianotti identified eight cases and published another article with Agostino Crosti [14]. After more than a decade, the relationship between viral infection and PAC was confirmed with the identification of a hepatitis B surface antigen (Australia antigen) in the blood of sick children [15]. In 1976, Ishimaru et al. described an epidemic of PAC associated with HBV in the city of Matsuyama, Japan, and proved the relationship between subtype ayw and HBsAg [16]. Other infectious agents are also related to PAC, including: Epstein–Barr virus, respiratory syncytial virus, cytomegalovirus, and enterovirus [9].

This syndrome affects children from 3 months to 15 years of age, with a peak between 1 and 6 years old. More than 90% of cases occur in children younger than 4 years. There is no predilection for race or gender, and seasonal variant reflects the natural history of the infectious agent. There is an increased incidence in children with personal or family history of atopy [17].

The pathogenesis is still unknown. Nowadays it is recognized that the development mechanism of lesions does not involve a direct local interaction between viral antigens and skin immune cells [17].

Clinically, PAC is manifested by a sudden onset of skin lesions, and in some cases there is prodromal pharyngitis, upper respiratory tract infection, or diarrhea. The most frequent lesions are multiple, pink to red-brown, slightly pruritic papules that may become confluent [7, 17]. Individual lesions present from 1 to 5 mm in diameter with occasional bleeding and, rarely, with scale [17]. Papules tend to be smaller (1–2 mm) the younger the child, with larger lesions (around 5 mm) occurring in older children (Fig. 40.1) [9]. The Koebner phenomenon may occur at an early stage [7]. Papules present symmetric distribution in the face, limbs, and gluteal area, sparing the trunk. They do not affect either the mucosa or the popliteal and cubital surfaces. Rash develops in about 2–3 days, but persists for 15–20 days [7, 9].

Hepatitis, generally anicteric, occurs within 7–14 days after the onset of skin lesions and reaches a peak when papules begin to disappear. The elevation of liver enzymes and hepatomegaly

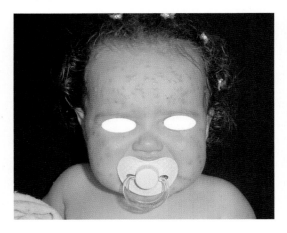

Fig. 40.1 Papular acrodermatitis of childhood (Courtesy of Dermatology Department, Universidade Federal de Ciencias da Saude de Porto Alegre, Brazil)

persists for 2–3 months. Anti-HBs is not detected at the dermatitis stage, but has its peak incidence within 6–12 months later, suggesting that anti-HBs may play an important role in recovery. Inguinal and axillary lymphadenopathy is also common [7, 9].

The histopathology of skin lesions is characterized by perivascular lymphocytic infiltrate with mild endothelial edema [7].

Treatment usually is not necessary because the disease is self-limited and associated with few symptoms. The use of average-potency topical corticosteroids may shorten the duration of lesions. Pruritus, when present, may be treated with antihistamines [17].

Hepatitis C

Epidemiology

HCV is a single-stranded RNA virus of the Flaviviridae family, first detected in 1989. It comprises nearly 10,000 nucleotides whose sequence categorizes HCV into six main genotypes and several subtypes. It is currently the major cause of liver disease and significantly affects the health of a large number of people. Although the estimated number of infected individuals exceeds 170 million, the prevalence of infection varies in different geographic locations [18].

Individuals with exposure to blood or blood products present an increased risk of HCV infection. Intravenous drug users, transplant patients, and health professionals are included in this group. Both sexual and vertical transmission correspond to the minority of cases [9, 18].

Clinical Presentation

Acute hepatitis develops after 4–12 weeks of incubation and is asymptomatic in most cases. Only 25% of cases present symptoms, usually nonspecific, including: fatigue, weakness, anorexia, myalgia, and, rarely, jaundice. Progression to chronic disease occurs in 70–80% of infected patients. Cirrhosis occurs in approximately 20% of cases, and hepatocellular carcinoma in 16% [9, 18].

Extrahepatic manifestations of HCV infection were first described in 1990 and can affect several organs. Forty percent to 75% of patients with chronic HCV infection present at least one extrahepatic manifestation [19].

Approximately 17% of HCV-infected patients have at least one skin manifestation, which may be induced directly or indirectly by HCV. Skin diseases certainly related with chronic HCV infection include cryoglobulinemia, lichen planus (LP), and porphyria cutanea tarda (PCT). In these diseases it is recommended to carry out the testing for HCV infection. Psoriasis, chronic pruritus, and necrolytic acral erythema present possible association with HCV infection. Anecdotal cases are described in patients with chronic rash and vitiligo (Box 40.2) [20].

Therapeutic Approach

Until a few years ago, standard HCV treatment was based on the use of pegylated IFN-α and ribavirin. In 2011, two protease inhibitors, telaprevir and boceprevir, were approved for treatment of patients with genotype 1, to be used in triple combination with IFN and ribavirin. Since 2014, several direct-acting antivirals have been approved, allowing patients to be treated without IFN with high rates of sustained virologic response [21].

Skin Manifestations of Hepatitis C Virus Infection

The cutaneous manifestations of HCV are summarized in Box 40.2.

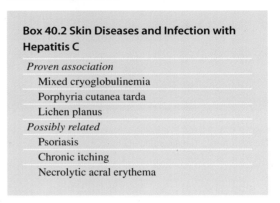

Box 40.2 Skin Diseases and Infection with Hepatitis C

Proven association
- Mixed cryoglobulinemia
- Porphyria cutanea tarda
- Lichen planus

Possibly related
- Psoriasis
- Chronic itching
- Necrolytic acral erythema

Mixed Cryoglobulinemia

Cryoglobulins are anti-immunoglobulins precipitated at low temperatures, and the type of cryoglobulin is used to classify cryoglobulinemia types I, II, and III [9, 18].

Type I is characterized by monoclonal immunoglobulin (Ig), usually IgG or IgM, associated with Waldenstrom macroglobulinemia, multiple myeloma, and chronic lymphocytic leukemia. In cryoglobulinemia type II, there is presence of monoclonal IgM (rheumatoid factor) and polyclonal IgG. Type III is characterized by IgG and polyclonal IgM [2].

The type of cryoglobulinemia most commonly related to HCV is type II. These immunoglobulins may reversibly precipitate at temperatures below 37 °C and form immune complexes with complement, viral antigens and HCV RNA in small and medium-sized blood vessels (arterioles, capillaries, and venules) [2].

Despite the high prevalence of HCV markers in patients with mixed cryoglobulinemia, only 13–54% of patients with chronic HCV infection will develop cryoglobulinemia [9].

The target organs are skin, joints, nervous system, and kidney. Expression of the disease varies from mild symptoms to a life-threatening clinical presentation [22].

The skin is the organ most frequently involved and the most common sign is palpable purpura,

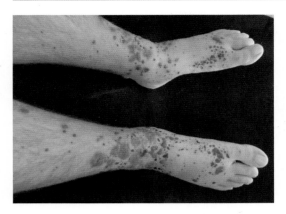

Fig 40.2 Mixed cryoglobulinemia (Courtesy of Dermatology Department, Universidade Federal de Ciencias da Saude de Porto Alegre, Brazil)

which occurs in 70–90% of patients [22]. It begins in the lower limbs and can extend up to the abdominal region, trunk, and upper limbs (Fig. 40.2). Lesions persist for 3–10 days, with late residual brownish pigmentation. Histologically there is unspecific leukocytoclastic vasculitis involving the small vessels with inflammatory infiltrate, and in some cases fibrinoid necrosis and endovascular thrombus. Other manifestations include urticarial vasculitis, livedo, rash, Raynaud's phenomenon, and leg ulcers [22, 23].

The most common symptoms are fatigue, which occurs in 80–90% of patients. Bilateral and symmetric arthralgia are observed in 40–60% of cases and involve, primarily, knees and hands and rarely, elbows and ankles. Arthritis occurs in less than 10% of cases. Neurologic manifestations range from sensory axonopathy to multiple mononeuropathy. The most common form is distal sensory or sensorimotor polyneuropathy. Motor deficit is uncommon and affects mainly the lower limbs, appearing months to years after sensory symptoms [23].

Involvement of the central nervous system (<10% of patients) is characterized by stroke, epilepsy, or cognitive impairment. Kidney changes are reported by 20–35% of patients. The most frequent clinical and pathologic presentation is acute or chronic membranoproliferative glomerulonephritis type I with endothelial deposit. The most common clinical presentation is proteinuria with

microscopic hematuria and variable stages of kidney failure. Other manifestations include xerophthalmia, xerostomia, abdominal pain, and heart and lung involvement [23].

In general, HCV-positive patients have more cutaneous involvement than neurologic involvement [18].

Laboratory findings include a slight increase in transaminases and the presence of rheumatoid factor in 70% of patients [18].

Cryoglobulinemia survival rates at 1, 3, 5, and 10 years are, respectively, 96%, 86%, 75%, and 63% in HCV-positive patients. Mortality is caused by severe infection and advanced liver disease. Factors related to worst prognosis are the presence of severe hepatic fibrosis, and involvement of the central nervous system, kidney, and heart [24].

The therapy for cryoglobulinemia associated with HCV includes elimination of virus, reduced lymphocyte proliferation, and management of cutaneous vasculitis [2]. In mild to moderate disease, pegylated IFN and ribavirin (and protease inhibitor of HCV genotype 1) are the initial choice. In severe cases, a combination of rituximab and pegylated IFN/ribavirin targets the virus and cryoglobulin-producing cells [2, 18].

Porphyria Cutanea Tarda

PCT is characterized by abnormal porphyrin metabolism secondary to a decreased activity of the hepatic enzyme uroporphyrinogen decarboxylase (URO-D) [9].

The familial form is inherited as an autosomal dominant trait and is associated with 50% reduction of URO-D activity throughout the body. The sporadic form is responsible for most cases of PCT and occurs in predisposed individuals. In these individuals, only hepatocytes show a reduction in the activity of URO-D. Alcohol, estrogens, hexachlorobenzene, iron accumulation, and exposure to HCV are extrinsic factors that act as triggers to the appearance of PCT in predisposed individuals [9, 18].

Epidemiologic association between PCT and HCV infection is strong, with rates of 70–90% in southern Europe and 20% in northern Europe, Australia, and England. According to studies, when adjusted for variation and geographic variability, the association between PCT and HCV remains significant, with an average prevalence rate of 50% of HCV in patients with PCT [18, 20].

HCV increases the production of reactive oxygen species, leading to downregulation of liver hepcidin, a key regulator of absorption and metabolism of iron. This contributes to iron overload in addition to other factors, such as genetic predisposition. Thus, there is decreased activity of URO-D [20].

Cutaneous manifestations include vesicles, blisters, erosions, and crusting that usually occur days after exposure to sunlight or trauma. They may result in scarring, miliary cysts, and hyper-/hypopigmentation (Figs. 40.3 and 40.4). Photosensitivity, skin fragility, facial hypertrichosis and sclerodermi-

form plaques may also occur. There is no difference in skin manifestations of PCT between HCV-positive and HCV-negative patients [2, 20].

Increased urocarboxyl porphyrins and heptacarboxyporphyrin in urine, and the presence of isocoproporphyrin in feces, are typical laboratory findings. Increases in liver enzymes, ferritin, and serum iron also occur [18].

Antiviral treatment may improve the clinical manifestations and laboratory findings, especially when preceded by therapeutic phlebotomy. Since iron is also involved in the progression of liver disease associated with HCV, reduction of iron stores due to phlebotomy can improve both conditions [20].

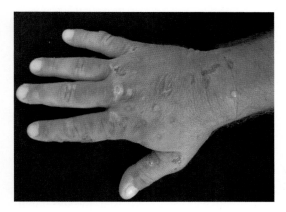

Fig. 40.3 Porphyria cutanea tarda (Courtesy of Dermatology Department, Universidade Federal de Ciencias da Saude de Porto Alegre, Brazil)

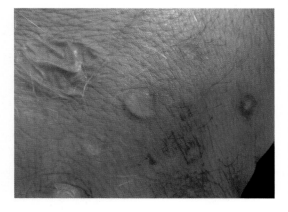

Fig. 40.4 Porphyria cutanea tarda: blisters and vesicles (Courtesy of Dermatology Department, Universidade Federal de Ciencias da Saude de Porto Alegre, Brazil)

Lichen Planus

LP is a chronic inflammatory disease that can affect the skin, scalp, nails, and mucosa. The exact prevalence is unknown, but it is estimated to affect 0.9–1.2% of the general population [25]. The disease is slightly more common in women than in men and occurs at any age, but is more frequent in the fifth decade of life [9].

Several studies confirm that HCV is the main LP-related liver disease [25]. In 1991, Mokni et al. described the first case of LP confirmed by biopsy in a patient with active chronic hepatitis induced by HCV [26]. Since then, the association between LP and chronic HCV infection has been reported in several epidemiologic studies, with contradictory results depending on the design and specific prevalence in each country [9, 20]. In hyperendemic areas such as Egypt, Japan, and southern Europe, the association rate is around 35%, while in northern European countries that have low incidence rate it is 0.5% [20]. Two meta-analysis studies support the association between chronic HCV infection and LP. LP patients have a fivefold higher-risk of HCV infection when compared with controls [27]. The odds ratio for the diagnosis of LP in HCV patients is 2.5. HCV-related oral LP is associated with the HLA-DR6 allele, and the idiopathic forms of LP with the HLA-DR1 allele [25].

Clinically it is characterized by small, planar, polygonal, purple, and pruritic papules. LP affects the extremities (flexor surfaces of the wrists, forearms, and legs) and mucosa. Skin lesions are typically bilateral and symmetric, covered by white, reticulated lines, called Wickham's striae (Fig. 40.5). LP lesions related to HCV are similar to those described in classic LP patients [9, 25].

LP involving mucosa is more frequent in the oral cavity, but can also involve the genital area. Oral LP may be reticular, erosive, atrophic, papular, plaque-like, or bullous (Fig. 40.6) [25]. Oral LP is the clinical phenotype most studied in patients with chronic HCV infection, and the most severe and recurrent clinical variant is the erosive form [20]. Between 1% and 6% of patients with chronic HCV infection have evidence of oral LP, while the prevalence of HCV infection in patients with oral LP is approximately 27% [2].

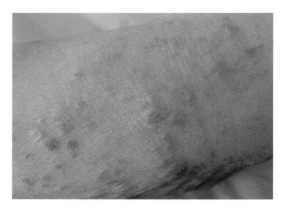

Fig. 40.5 Lichen planus (Courtesy of Dermatology Department, Universidade Federal de Ciencias da Saude de Porto Alegre, Brazil)

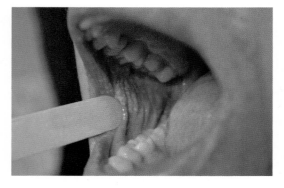

Fig. 40.6 Oral lichen planus (Courtesy of Dermatology Department, Universidade Federal de Ciencias da Saude de Porto Alegre, Brazil)

Histologically, there is lymphocytic infiltrate in the subepidermal band associated with the destruction of keratinocytes in the basal layer, sawtooth epidermal ridges, and pigmentary incontinence [9].

Although the association between LP and HCV is well documented, the pathogenesis remains uncertain. A current hypothesis relates LP to an autoimmune response, mediated by T cells, to a viral protein or a self epitope shared by the virus and present in basal keratinocytes, which are attacked by cytotoxic CD8 T cells [20].

Management of cutaneous LP is similar in HCV-positive and -negative patients. The first-line therapy is topical corticosteroids. In patients with extensive skin lesions, systemic corticosteroids and phototherapy may be used [9]. Contrary to cutaneous LP, oral LP tends to be chronic, with periods of remission and exacerbation. Studies of the use of IFN and ribavirin have shown as much benefit as exacerbation of oral LP in HCV-positive patients. With the direct-action antiviral agents currently available for the treatment of HCV infection, the exacerbation of LP with antiviral therapy is less worrisome. In oral LP the first-line treatment is topical corticosteroids, with a choice of topical calcineurin inhibitors in refractory cases. In cases that do not respond to these treatments, oral corticosteroids and immunomodulators can be used [2].

Skin Diseases with Possible Association with HCV

Psoriasis

Chronic HCV infection and other liver diseases represent some of the many comorbidities that affect patients with psoriasis. The epidemiologic association between psoriasis and chronic HCV infection has been described mainly by clinical studies of population-based hospitals and observational studies in countries with a heterogeneous burden of HCV and psoriasis [20].

Increased risk of HCV infection among patients with mild to moderate psoriasis and psoriatic arthritis was reported in Taiwan, Japan, and Italy, regardless of exposure to antiviral treatment with IFN [20].

Another observational study in the United States did not confirm these findings, probably because of different methodology and the small sample of patients with psoriasis [28]. However, a case–control study of a large number of psoriasis patients by Cohen et al. in 2010 supports previous reports of an association between psoriasis and hepatitis C [29].

A recent study in Japan showed that patients with psoriasis associated with HCV have the following profile: male dominance, relatively late onset of psoriasis, a mean age of 54 years, HCV infection prior to psoriasis in most cases, and association with diabetes mellitus in 35% of patients [30]. In Egypt, one of the areas with the highest prevalence of HCV infection in the world, a study of 100 patients with psoriasis showed a prevalence of 19% of HCV infection while HIV-positive psoriatic patients had more severe psoriasis, needing systemic treatment of longer duration [31]. An abnormal expression of apoptosis regulatory proteins in addition to the HCV infection seems to be related to the severity of psoriasis in these individuals [32].

This evidence supports the role of HCV infection as a trigger for psoriasis in genetically predisposed individuals [20, 31].

Chronic Itching (Pruritus)

Itching is a common symptom in liver diseases, mainly in chronic cholestatic diseases such as primary biliary cirrhosis and primary sclerosing cholangitis [20].

This symptom occurs in about 2.5–23% of chronic HCV patients. The cause is not fully understood, although it may be associated with liver fibrosis, bile duct lesions, and cholestasis [33]. Autotaxin and its product, lysophosphatidic acid, have recently been found in the pathophysiology of itch, as well as in cholestatic liver disease. In chronic HCV infection, autotaxin and lysophosphatidic acid activities are increased, showing a solid correlation with the stage of liver cirrhosis, and its complications and prognosis [20].

In an early infection, itching may be acute and transitory, or persistent in chronic HCV infection. Clinically it may present in two forms: generalized itch in normal skin or itching associated with secondary lesions (papules, nodules, excoriations, or lichenification) [20].

Necrolytic Acral Erythema

Necrolytic acral erythema (NAE) belongs to the family of migratory erythemas, which includes necrolytic migratory erythema, enteropathic acrodermatitis, and other dermatosis secondary to nutritional deficiencies. Clinically and histologically these entities are similar, but present diverse etiology [34, 35].

This dermatosis was first described in 1996, in a cohort involving seven HCV-infected patients from Egypt [35].

NAE symptoms include itching (93% of cases), burning (16% of cases) and/or pain (14% of cases). Erythematous papules, blisters, or erosive lesions are seen at the acute stage. Chronic lesions are characterized by well-defined hyperkeratotic plaques, circled by erythema or hyperpigmentation. In most cases, lesion distribution includes the backs of feet and hands. They occasionally occur in other locations such as legs, knees, and elbows [36].

Physiopathologic mechanisms are not fully understood. The cause of NAE may be multifactorial, whereby liver dysfunction plays a role in the development of cutaneous disease [36]. In some cases, disease remission occurs after oral administration of zinc, although the exact mechanism of this therapeutic response remains unknown [37].

In histopathology, psoriatic epidermal hyperplasia with a variety of other findings has been identified, including dermal inflammation and necrosis of epidermal cells [38].

NAE differs from other necrolytic erythemas because of an acral distribution of lesions and the universal association with HCV infection. It is important to recognize this association because cutaneous manifestations of NAE precede the diagnosis of HCV infection [35].

Adverse Cutaneous Reactions Related to HCV Treatment

HCV treatment with IFN and ribavirin may cause either adverse cutaneous reactions at the site of application or diffuse cutaneous reactions (Box 40.3) [18, 39].

Local cutaneous reactions occur in 12–20% of patients and include erythema, abscess, vesicular-bullous reactions, ulcer, and necrosis [18].

Nearly 25% of patients in treatment with IFN and ribavirin present diffuse cutaneous reactions [18, 39]. Pruriginous cutaneous eruption is the most frequent, occurring in 8–10% of patients. It is characterized by itching, xerosis, and erythematous papules on the trunk and extremities [39, 40]. Transitory alopecia and effluvium have also been described [18, 39].

Two protease inhibitors, boceprevir and telaprevir, have been available since 2011 for the treatment of chronic infection with type 1 HCV genotype, in combination with IFN and ribavirin [40]. This triple therapy increases sustained viral response up to 70%, depending on the characteristics of the virus and the host [41]. During the triple therapy, cutaneous reactions are, in most cases, mild (37%) to moderate (14%) [40, 42]. Lesion patterns are similar to the eruption associated with IFN and ribavirin with no protease inhibitor, but with an increase of frequency (55% versus 33%) and severity (3.7% versus 0.9%). Only 6% of patients in triple therapy present severe cutaneous reactions, and few develop Stevens–Johnson syndrome or DRESS (Drug Reaction with Eosinophilia and Systemic Symptoms) [40].

Box 40.3 Adverse Cutaneous Reactions Related to HCV Treatment

Local	Diffuse
Erythema	Maculopapular exanthema
Abscess	Itching (pruritus)
Vesicular-bullous reactions	Rash
Ulcer and necrosis	Photosensitivity
	Alopecia

Glossary

Cryoglobulinemia Characterized by the presence of cryoglobulins in the serum. This may result in a clinical syndrome of systemic inflammation caused by cryoglobulin-containing immune complexes.

Jaundice Yellowish discoloration of the skin, white of the eyes, and mucous membranes caused by deposition of bile salts in the tissues.

Hepatitis Inflammation of the liver, caused by a virus or a toxin and characterized by jaundice, liver enlargement, and fever.

Polyarteritis nodosa Systemic necrotizing vasculitis that predominantly affects medium-sized muscular arteries and often involves small muscular arteries, resulting in secondary tissue ischemia.

Porphyria Group of diseases in which there is abnormal metabolism of the blood pigment hemoglobin.

References

1. World Health Organization. http://who.int/topics/hepatitis/en. 2016. Accessed 20 Feb 2016.
2. Akhter A, Said A. Cutaneous manifestation of viral hepatitis. Curr Infect Dis Rep. 2015;17:1–8.
3. Ghosn S, Kibbi AG. Cutaneous manifestation of liver diseases. Clin Dermatol. 2008;26:274–82.
4. World Health Organization. Guidelines for the prevention, care and treatment of persons with chronic hepatitis B infection. March 2015. Accessed 20 Feb 2016.
5. Bhat M, Ghali P, Deschenes M, Wong P. Prevention and management of chronic hepatitis B. Int J Prev Med. 2014;5(3):S200–7.
6. Trépo C, Chan HL, Lok A. Hepatitis B virus infection. Lancet. 2014;384:2053–63.
7. McElgunn PS. Dermatologic manifestation of hepatitis B virus infection. Am J Dermatol. 1983;8(4):539–47.
8. Han SH. Extrahepatic manifestation of chronic hepatitis B. Clin Liver Dis. 2004;8:403–18.
9. Jones AM, Warken K, Tyring SK. The cutaneous manifestation of viral hepatitis. Dermatol Clin. 2002;20:233–47.
10. Nishida N, Kudo M. Clinical features of vascular disorders associated with chronic hepatitis virus infection. Dig Dis. 2014;32:786–90.
11. Pagnoux C, Seror R, Henegar C, Mahr A, Cohen P, Le Guern V, et al. Clinical features and outcomes in 348 patients with polyarteritis nodosa: a systematic retrospective study of patients diagnosed between 1963 and 2005 and entered into the French Vasculitis Study Group Database. Arthritis Rheum. 2010;62(2):616–26.
12. Hernandez-Rodriguez J, Alba MA, Prieto-Gonzalez S, Cid MC. Diagnosis and classification of polyarteritis nodosa. J Autoimmun. 2014;48–49:84–9.
13. Gianotti F. Rilievi di una particolare casistica tossinfettiva caraterizzata de eruzione eritemato-infiltrativa desquamativa a foccolai lenticolari, a sede elettiva acroesposta. G Ital Dermatol. 1955;96:678–9.

14. Crosti A, Gianotti F. Dermatosi infantile eruttiva acroesposta di probabile origine virosica. Minerva Dermatol. 1956;31(Suppl):483.

15. De Gaspari G, Bardare M, Costantino D. Au antigen in Crosti-Gianotti acrodermatitis. Lancet. 1970;1:1116–7.

16. Ishimaru Y, Ishimaru H, Toda G, Baba K, Mayumi M. An epidemic of infantile papular acrodermatitis (Gianotti's disease) in Japan associated with hepatitis-B surface antigensubtype ayw. Lancet. 1976;1:707–9.

17. Brandt O, Abeck D, Gianotti, Burgdorf W. Gianotti-Crosti syndrome. J Am Acad Dermatol. 2006;54(1):136–43.

18. Rebora A. Skin diseases associated with hepatitis C virus: facts and controversies. Clin Dermatol. 2010;28:489–96.

19. Ko HM, Hernandez-Prera JC, Zhu H, Dikman SH, Sidhu HK, Ward SC, et al. Clin Dev Immunol. 2012;2012:740138.

20. Gargovich S, Gargovich M, Capizzi R, Gasbarrini A, Zocco MA. Cutaneous manifestation of hepatitis C in the era of new antiviral agents. World J Hepatol. 2015;7(27):2740–8.

21. Zopf S, Kremer AE, Neurath MF, Siebler J. Advances in hepatitis C therapy: what is the current state-what come's nex? World J Hepatol. 2016;8(3):139–47.

22. Saadoun D, Landau DA, Calabrese LH, Cacoub PP. Hepatitis-C associated mixed cryoglobulinaemia: a crossroad between autoimmunity and lymphoproliferation. Rheumatology. 2007;46:1234–42.

23. Cacoub P, Comarmond C, Domont F, Savey L, Saadoun D. Cryoglobulinemia vasculitis. Am J Med. 2015;128:950–5.

24. Terrier B, Semoun O, Saadoun D, Sène D, Resche-Rigon M, Cacoub P. Prognostic factors in patients with hepatitis C virus infection and systemic vasculitis. Arthritis Rheum. 2011;63(6):1748–57.

25. Luckács J, Schliemann S, Elsner P. Lichen planus and lichenoid reactions as a systemic disease. Clin Dermatol. 2015;33:512–9.

26. Mokni M, Rybojad M, Puppin D Jr, et al. Lichen planus and hepatitis C virus. J Am Acad Dermatol. 1991;24:792.

27. Lodi G, Pellicano R, Carrozzo M. Hepatitis C virus infection and lichen planus: a systematic review with meta-analysis. Oral Dis. 2010;16:601–12.

28. Kanada KN, Schupp CW, Armstrong AW. Association between psoriasis and viral infections in the United States: focusing on hepatitis B, hepatitis C and human immunodeficiency virus. J Eur Acad Venereol. 2013;27(10):1312–6.

29. Cohen AD, Weitzman D, Birkenfeld S, Dreiher J. Psoriasis associated with hepatitis C but not with hepatitis B. Dermatology. 2010;220(3):218–22.

30. Imafuku S, Nakayama J. Profile of patients with psoriasis associated with hepatitis C virus infection. J Dermatol. 2013;40:428–33.

31. Youssef R, Abu-Zeid O, Sayde K, Osman S, Omran D, El Shafei A, et al. Hepatitis C infection in Egyptian psoriatic patients: prevalence and correlation with severity of disease. Iran J Public Health. 2015;44(9):1294–5.

32. Gabr SA, Berika MY, Alghadir A. Apoptosis and clinical severity in patients with psoriasis and HCV infection. Indian J Dermatol. 2014;59(3):230–6.

33. Suzuki K, Tamano M, Katayama Y, Kuniyoshi T, Kagawa K, Takada H, et al. Study of pruritus in chronic hepatitis C patients. World J Gastroenterol. 2014;20(47):17877–82.

34. Tabibian JH, Gersteenblith MR, Tedford RJ, Junkins-Hopkins JM, Abuav R. Necrolytic acral erythema as a cutaneous marker of hepatitis C: report of two cases and review. Dig Dis Sci. 2010;55:2735–43.

35. Khanna VJ, Shieh S, Benjamin J, Somach S, Zaim MT, Dorner W, et al. Necrolytic acral erythema associated with hepatitis C effective treatment with interferon alfa and zinc. Arch Dermatol. 2000;136:755–7.

36. Raphael BA, Dorey-Stein ZL, Lott J, Amorosa V, Re VL, Kovarik C. Low prevalence of necrolytic acral erythema in patients with chronic hepatitis C vírus infection. J Am Acad Dermatol. 2011;67(5):962–8.

37. Abdallah MA, Hull C, Horn TD. Necrolytic acral erythema: a patient from the United States successfully treated with oral zinc. Arch Dermatol. 2005;141:85.

38. Abdallah MA, Ghozzi MY, Monib HA, Hafez AM, Hiatt KM, Smoller BR, et al. Necrolytic acral erythema: a cutaneous sign of hepatitis C virus infection. J Am Acad Dermatol. 2005;53(2):247–51.

39. Patrk I, Morovic M, Markulin A, Patrk J. Cutaneous reactions in patients with chronic hepatitis C treated with peginterferon and ribavirin. Dermatology. 2014;228:42–6.

40. Federico A, Sgambato D, Cotticelli G, Gravina AG, Dallio M, Beneduce F, et al. Skin adverse events during dual and triple therapy for HCV-related cirrhosis. Hepat Mon. 2014;14(3):1–3.

41. Falcão EMM, Trope BM, Godinho MM, Carneiro LH, Araujo-Neto JM, Nogueira CAV, et al. Cutaneous eruption due to telaprevir. Case Rep Dermatol. 2015;7:253–62.

42. Montecinos MT, Carrilo JM, Rius MV, Marsol B, PLa AP, Cunill RM, et al. Drug eruptions induced by telaprevir in patients with chronic hepatitis C vírus genotype 1 infection: a prospective study. Actas Dermosifiliogr. 2015;106(3):219–25.

Skin Manifestations Associated with HIV/AIDS

41

Márcia S. Zampese, Gabriela Czarnobay Garbin, and Bruna Guerra Rech

Key Points

- Cutaneous disorders develop in over 90% of HIV-infected persons at some time during the course of the illness; they have been a basic index for the presence and course of HIV infection as well as a challenging task for health care providers because of the severe and recalcitrant nature of such conditions
- Mucocutaneous disease has changed its spectrum after the antiretroviral therapy (ART) introduction. In the pre-ART era major presentations were the opportunistic infections-related skin diseases, whereas the noninfectious skin diseases emerged in the current ART era
- The use of ART in HIV-infected patients results in the immunologic system recovery that can trigger immunopathologic lesions as well as systemic inflammatory reactions, the so-called immune reconstitution inflammatory syndrome

"Ce qu'il y a de plus profond dans l'homme, c'est sa peau.
La peau humaine separe le monde en deux espaces. Cote couleurs, cote douleurs."

Paul Valery

"In the face of AIDS, we must deepen and broaden the philosophy and the practice of health promotion, for it will lead us to the very frontiers of our knowledge of others, and ourselves."

Jonathan Mann

Introduction

In 1981, a new outbreak of opportunistic infections (OIs) and Kaposi's sarcoma was reported among homosexual men in the United States [37, 38]. Thanks to the massive damage to the immune system, this fatal disease was named the acquired immunodeficiency syndrome (AIDS). Shortly after, the syndrome was also reported in hemophiliacs, blood transfusion recipients, injection drugs users, and newborn children of affected mothers [243]. Soon an epidemic of AIDS was noticed among heterosexuals in Africa, mainly

M.S. Zampese (✉)
Dermatology Service of Hospital de Clínicas de Porto Alegre, Federal University of Rio Grande Sul, Porto Alegre, Brazil
e-mail: mzampese@hcpa.edu.br

G.C. Garbin
Dermatology of Mãe de Deus Center, Porto Alegre, Brazil

B.G. Rech
Dermatology Service of Hospital de Clínicas de Porto Alegre, Porto Alegre, Brazil

© Springer International Publishing Switzerland 2018
R.R. Bonamigo, S.I.T. Dornelles (eds.), *Dermatology in Public Health Environments*,
https://doi.org/10.1007/978-3-319-33919-1_41

affecting women [242]. The retrovirus later named human immunodeficiency virus (HIV) was identified in 1983 as the causal agent of AIDS [95]. Two types of HIV are known: HIV-1 is the most common and is found worldwide; HIV-2 is a less virulent variant distributed in West and Central Africa [30].

Both HIV diagnosis and treatment have significantly evolved since the initial recognition of AIDS, and the use of antiretroviral therapy (ART) has led to a dramatic reduction in HIV-associated morbidity and mortality [243]. ART has also modified the patterns of HIV-associated cutaneous manifestations. The variability of these skin and mucosal lesions is related to a multitude of clinical situations: HIV-infected patients without AIDS, patients with advanced AIDS, patients with diffuse inflammatory reaction generated by the effectiveness of ART (known as immune reconstitution inflammatory syndrome (IRIS)), and also adverse effects of ART itself. A complex scenario arises from the interaction between HIV and infected host, and dermatologic disorders can be present at any point of the spectrum of HIV disease. The skin and mucosa can be sensitive indicators of underlying immunosuppression, and mucocutaneous disorders are often the first manifestation of HIV infection and advancing immunodeficiency. Both the World Health Organization (WHO)

clinical staging of HIV/AIDS and the Centers for Disease Control and Prevention (CDC) classification system for HIV infection and AIDS case definition (for adults and adolescents) include 19 and 16 disorders, respectively, that may potentially affect the skin and mucosa [39, 318] (Boxes 41.1 and 41.2). Cutaneous disorders develop in more than 90% of HIV-infected persons at some time during the course of the illness; they have been a basic index for the presence and course of HIV infection, and can be a challenging task because of the severe and recalcitrant nature of such conditions [42, 56, 303, 321]. Since the early description of AIDS over three decades ago, dermatologists have continued to play an important role in recognizing cutaneous markers of HIV infection, treating mucous and skin disorders associated with HIV, and helping to curb the spread of HIV by control of other sexually transmitted infections [303]. The aim of this chapter is to enhance awareness and familiarize healthcare providers with the most frequent cutaneous manifestations associated with HIV and AIDS so that they can recognize the possibility of an underling HIV infection, recommend appropriate testing, and provide timely and suitable management for either disease. We discuss the most frequent mucous and skin disorders associated with HIV/AIDS, which are listed in Table 41.1.

Table 41.1 Skin manifestations and disorders in HIV-infected individuals

Infectious skin disorders	Infectious skin disorders	Noninfectious skin disorders
Viral	*Fungal*	*Xerosis*
Acute HIV infection	Candidiasis	*Seborrheic dermatitis*
Herpes simplex	Dermatophytosis	*Psoriasis*
Varicella zoster virus	Cryptococcosis	*Papular pruritic dermatoses*
Molluscum contagiosum	Histoplasmosis	Eosinophilic folliculitis
Oral hairy leukoplakia	Sporotrichosis	Papular pruritic eruption
Human papillomavirus	*Ectoparasitic infestations*	*Antiretroviral therapy–associated manifestations*
Acquired epidermodysplasia verruciformis	Scabies	Adverse drug reactions
	Demodicidosis	Immune reconstitution inflammatory syndrome
Bacterial	*Protozoal diseases*	*Neoplastic disorder*
Cutaneous bacterial infections	Tegumentary leishmaniasis	Kaposi's sarcoma
Syphilis		
Bacillary angiomatosis		
Mycobacterial infections		

Box 41.1 1993 CDC Revised Classification System for HIV Infection and Expanded Surveillance Case Definition for AIDS Among Adolescents and Adults

CD4+ T-Lymphocyte Categories
Category 1: ≥500 cells/mL
Category 2: 200–499 cells/μL
Category 3: <200 cells/μL
Clinical Categories
Category A
Asymptomatic HIV infection
Persistent generalized lymphadenopathy
Acute (primary) HIV infection with accompanying illness or history of acute HIV infection
Category B
Bacillary angiomatosis
Candidosis, oropharyngeal (thrush)
Candidosis, vulvovaginal; persistent, frequent, or poorly responsive to therapy
Cervical dysplasia (moderate or severe)/cervical carcinoma in situ
Constitutional symptoms, such as fever (38.5 °C) or diarrhea lasting >1 month
Hairy leukoplakia, oral
Herpes zoster (shingles), involving at least two distinct episodes or more than one dermatome
Idiopathic thrombocytopenic purpura
Listeriosis
Pelvic inflammatory disease, particularly if complicated by tubo-ovarian abscess
Peripheral neuropathy
Category C
Candidosis of bronchi, trachea, or lungs
Candidosis, esophageal
Cervical cancer, invasive[a]
Coccidiomycosis, disseminated or extrapulmonary
Cryptococcosis, extrapulmonary
Cryptosporidiosis, chronic intestinal (>1 month duration)
Cytomegalovirus disease (other than liver, spleen, or nodes)
Cytomegalovirus retinitis (with loss of vision)
Encephalopathy, HIV-related
Herpes simplex: chronic ulcer(s) (>1 month duration); or bronchitis, pneumonitis, or esophagitis
Histoplasmosis, disseminated or extrapulmonary
Isosporiasis, chronic intestinal (> 1 month duration)
Kaposi's sarcoma
Lymphoma, Burkitt's (or equivalent term)
Lymphoma, immunoblastic (or equivalent term)
Lymphoma, primary, of brain
Mycobacterium avium complex or *M. kansasii*, disseminated or extrapulmonary
Mycobacterium tuberculosis, any site (pulmonary[a] or extrapulmonary)
Mycobacterium, other species or unidentified species, disseminated or extrapulmonary
Pneumocystis carinii pneumonia
Pneumonia, recurrent[a]
Progressive multifocal leukoencephalopathy
Salmonella septicemia, recurrent
Toxoplasmosis of brain
Wasting syndrome due to HIV

CDC [39]
[a]Added in the 1993 expansion of the AIDS surveillance case definition

Box 41.2 WHO Clinical Staging of HIV/AIDS for Adults and Adolescents with Confirmed HIV Infection

Clinical stage 1 (asymptomatic)
Asymptomatic
Persistent generalized lymphadenopathy
Clinical stage 2 (mild symptoms)
Moderate unexplained weight loss (<10% of presumed or measured body weight)I
Recurrent respiratory tract infections sinusitis, tonsillitis, otitis media, and pharyngitis)
Herpes zoster
Angular cheilitis
Recurrent oral ulceration
Papular pruritic eruptions
Seborrheic dermatitis
Fungal nail infections
Clinical stage 3 (advanced symptoms)
Unexplained[a] severe weight loss (>10% of presumed or measured body weight)
Unexplained chronic diarrhea for longer than 1 month
Unexplained persistent fever (above 37.6 °C intermittent or constant, for longer than 1 month)
Persistent oral candidiasis
Oral hairy leukoplakia
Pulmonary tuberculosis (current)

Severe bacterial infections (such as pneumonia, empyema, pyomyositis, bone or joint infection, meningitis, or bacteremia)

Acute necrotizing ulcerative stomatitis, gingivitis, or periodontitis

Unexplained anemia (<8 g/dL), neutropenia (<0.5 × 10^9 per liter) or chronic thrombocytopenia (<50 × 10^9 per liter)

Clinical stage 4[b] (severe symptoms)

HIV wasting syndrome

Pneumocystis pneumonia

Recurrent severe bacterial pneumonia

Chronic herpes simplex infection (orolabial, genital, or anorectal of >1 month duration or visceral at any site)

Esophageal candidiasis (or candidiasis of trachea, bronchi, or lungs)

Extrapulmonary tuberculosis

Kaposi's sarcoma

Cytomegalovirus infection (retinitis or infection of other organs)

Central nervous system toxoplasmosis

HIV encephalopathy

Extrapulmonary cryptococcosis including meningitis

Disseminated nontuberculous mycobacterial infection

Progressive multifocal leukoencephalopathy

Chronic cryptosporidiosis (with diarrhea)

Chronic isosporiasis

Disseminated mycosis (coccidiomycosis or histoplasmosis)

Recurrent nontyphoidal *Salmonella* bacteremia

Lymphoma (cerebral or B-cell non-Hodgkin) or other solid HIV-associated tumors

Invasive cervical carcinoma

Atypical disseminated leishmaniasis

Symptomatic HIV-associated nephropathy or symptomatic HIV-associated cardiomyopathy

WHO [318]

Assessment of body weight in pregnant woman needs to consider the expected weight gain of pregnancy

[a]Unexplained refers to where the condition is not explained by other causes

[b]Some additional specific conditions can also be included in regional classifications (such as reactivation of American trypanosomiasis [meningoencephalitis and/or myocarditis]) in the WHO Region of the Americas and disseminated penicilliosis in Asia)

Infectious Skin Disorders

Viral Diseases

Acute HIV Infection

Acute HIV infection is also known as primary HIV infection or acute retroviral syndrome. Primary HIV infection refers to the earliest stages of infection, or the interval from initial infection to seroconversion. During this stage, many patients have symptoms of acute HIV-1 illness; they also have very high HIV RNA levels and negative or indeterminate findings in HIV-1 antibody tests.

Etiopathogenesis and General Epidemiology

As with other severe viral infections, HIV-1 infection is associated with an array of clinical manifestations, known as acute retroviral syndrome (ARS), which usually occurs between the first and third week after infectious exposure. ARS is the early manifestation of HIV-1 infection and is associated with high levels of viral replication. The presentation is unspecific, and a mononucleosis-like acute disease occurs in up to 93% of patients [165].

Clinical Presentation

The main clinical findings of ARS include fever, pharyngitis, lymphadenopathy, fatigue, weight loss, and myalgia [55]. The general symptoms may be followed by a transitory morbilliform exanthema or erythematous-scaling papules on the trunk, head, and neck, with centrifugal progression. Oral candidiasis and painful oral and genital ulcers may also develop. Headache, meningismus, and ocular pain are the most frequent neurologic manifestations [31, 165]. Box 41.3 summarizes the most common symptoms associated with ARS. In the prospective study by Braun and colleagues [31], almost one-third of the patients had atypical ARS, from asymptomatic ARS to patients with a wide spectrum of symptoms, usually gastrointestinal and neurologic symptoms. ARS is self-limited, and most of the signs and symptoms disappear in 3–4 weeks. Nevertheless, some patients may present symptoms up to 3 months after exposure [305].

Complementary Examinations

Following HIV infection, serologic markers of the infection appear in a chronologic sequence: viral RNA, p24 antigen, and anti-HIV antibody (Fig. 41.1). About 2 weeks after infection, viremia increases, and then declines to a steady-state level as the humoral and cell-mediated immune responses control HIV replication. This time interval, the serologic "window period," is characterized by seronegative tests, occasionally detectable antigenemia, viremia (as measured by RNA), and variable CD4 lymphocyte levels [54, 59]. Diagnostic tests for primary HIV-1 infection include assays for HIV-1 RNA, p24 antigen, and enzyme immunoassay antibody tests (Table 41.2). Upon encountering high-risk patients with clinical suspicion and a negative or indeterminate HIV-1 antibody test result, confirmation of acute infection requires detection of HIV-1 RNA or p24 antigen, but tests designed for this purpose are not routinely available. A fourth-generation enzyme-linked immunosorbent assay (ELISA) that can concomitantly detect viral p24 antigen and antiviral antibodies is an alternative and more practical strategy [55, 65].

Therapeutic Approach

Given the potential benefits for public and individual health, some treatment guidelines have recommended early ART for patients with acute HIV infection [55, 108, 147]. The introduction of ART before HIV seroconversion decreases the size of the latent viral reservoir, reduces immune activation, and possibly protects against the infection of central memory T cells. Benefits peak during the first weeks after HIV infection, although they are noticeable up to the first 6 months. However, early treatment does not prevent the establishment of the HIV latent reservoir [49, 275].

Herpes Simplex Virus

Human herpes simplex viruses (HSVs) are ubiquitous pathogens with a large reservoir in the general population. HSV-associated diseases are among the most widespread infections; they are incurable and persist in latent form during the host's lifetime. There are two HSV types, HSV

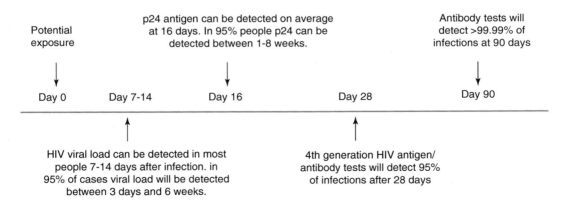

Fig. 41.1 Timeline of HIV serologic markers after exposure

Table 41.2 Tests for HIV-1

Test	Detection		
	RNA/DNA	Antigen	Antibody
PCR/viral load	X	–	–
p24 antigen test	–	X	–
4th generation Ag/Ab tests (p24+ ELISA, ELI, MEIA/ELFA/ECLIA)	–	X	X
1st/2nd/3rd generation Ab only tests (ELISA, ELI, MEIA/ELFA/ECLIA	–	–	X
Rapid tests: finger prick or oral swab	–	–	X
Western blot tests (confirmatory)	–	–	X

Cohen [54, 55], and Constantine [59]
Ab antibody, *Ag* antigen, *PCR* polymerase chain reaction

type 1 (HSV-1) and HSV type 2 (HSV-2), which are closely related but differ in epidemiology [81, 158]. HSV-1 is usually associated with orofacial disease, whereas HSV-2 is related with genital disease; however, lesion location is not necessarily indicative of viral type.

General Epidemiology

Globally, an estimated two-thirds of the population under 50 years old is infected with HSV-1 and 16% with HSV-2, according to WHO global estimates [161, 162]. Taken together, estimates reveal that over half a billion people between the ages of 15 and 49 years have genital infection caused by either HSV-1 or HSV-2 [161, 162]. Genital herpes may be caused by either HSV-1 or HSV-2 but, globally, the large majority of cases are caused by HSV-2; infection is common in both the industrialized and developing worlds, and HSV-2 uncommonly causes infection by nonsexual means [161, 162]. HSV-2 prevalence varies according to the geographic site, age, sex, investigated population, and HIV-1 status [47]. More women than men are infected with HSV-2, and prevalence increases with age, most markedly in the younger ages, slightly declining after 40 years of age [161,

162]. Despite the majority of genital herpes cases resulting from HSV-2, a growing proportion of the anogenital herpes infections has been attributed to HSV-1, particularly among young women and men who have sexual intercourse with other men (MSM) [40]. HSV infection is frequent among HIV-infected patients, with an estimated prevalence of 27%, when the CD4 count is <100 cells/mm^3 [140]; additionally, atypical clinical presentations are more frequent, and a possible spontaneous resolution occurs on a small scale when compared with noninfected HIV patients [199].

Etiopathogenesis

Herpes simplex is an infection resulting from HSV-1 and HSV-2, which are enveloped α-herpesviruses with double-stranded DNA. Both HSV types are distinguished by antigenic differences in their enveloping proteins [21, 199]. HSV infection accounts for a recurrent disease that persists over life, with no cure. Transmission occurs via direct contact with infectious secretions on the mucosae or wounded skin. Most infections are transmitted via asymptomatic viral shedding [21]. The natural history includes first-episode mucocutaneous infection, establishment of latency, and subsequent reactivation. The primary infection via HSV is followed by intense viral replication at the inoculation site. Early infection at the oral cavity results in HSV latency in the trigeminal ganglion, whereas in the genital primary infection the viral latency is located in the sacral ganglion [198].

Inter-relationship Between HSV and HIV

HSV-2 and HIV-1 infections facilitate each other's acquisition, transmission, and disease progression [300]. Epidemiologic data show a relationship between HSV-2 and HIV-1 prevalence. HSV-2 seroprevalence varies from 22% in sexually active adults in the United States to 60% in HIV-1 negative women in the sub-Saharan Africa, and to even more than 80% among HIV-1 infected individuals [151, 313]. The biological background for how HSV-2 increases a host's susceptibility to HIV-1 rests on several interact-

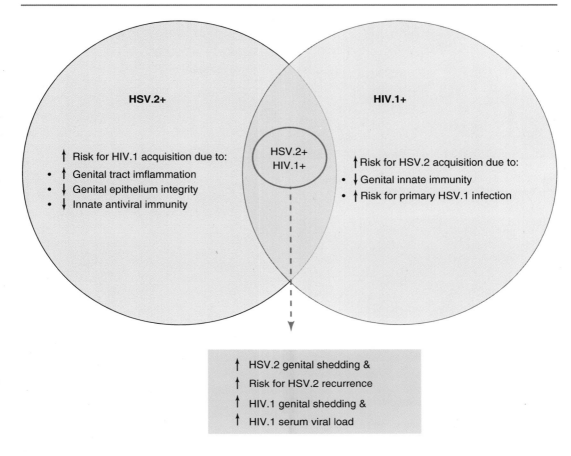

Fig. 41.2 Inter-relationships between HSV and HIV [300]

ing mechanisms: HSV-2 infection increases the concentration of cervical HIV-1 target cells, decreases mucosal innate immunity, and induces a mucosal inflammatory response [300]. The synergistic relationship between HIV-1 and HSV-2 is depicted in Fig. 41.2. HSV-2 infection seems to increase the woman's susceptibility to HIV-1 infection the same way as the opposing situation, that is, HIV-1 positive women display deficient mucosa immunity against the HSV-2 primary infection or reactivation [252]. The HIV-1 and HSV-2 viruses seem to have a synergistic relationship that favors the host's viral shedding: HIV-1-infected women shed more HSV-2 virus, and HSV-2 suppression also seems to decrease HIV-1 viral load in serum as well as HIV-1 shedding in the genital tract [160, 252].

Clinical Presentation

HIV patients with a CD4 count >100 cells/mm^3 show a clinical presentation similar to that of an immunocompetent patient: painful vesicles are grouped under the erythematous base that erupt and make polycyclic lesions with an erythematous halo, usually located in the mouth (Fig. 41.3), genitals (Fig. 41.4), perianal region, and distal parts of fingers. In patients with advanced immunosuppression, the lesions are larger and/or multiple (Fig. 41.5), possibly coalescing and evolving into deep ulcers (Fig. 41.6), with more severe and frequent recurrences; chronic skin lesions may develop an atypical verrucous appearance [140, 141, 209]. Local prodromal symptoms (burning, pruritus, tingling) may occur in recurrences, hours or days before development of lesions [141].

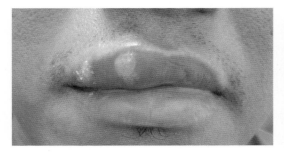

Fig. 41.3 Labial herpes simplex: unilateral grouped vesicles on an erythematous base on upper lip

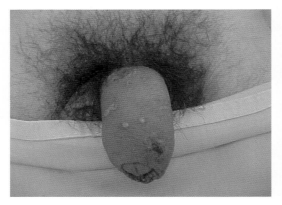

Fig. 41.4 Genital herpes simplex: different stages of lesions, erosion, and crusts on an erythematous base

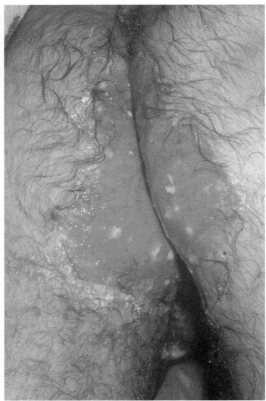

Fig. 41.6 Chronic herpes simplex infection: large ulcers spreading from the perianal area in a severely immunosuppressed HIV patient

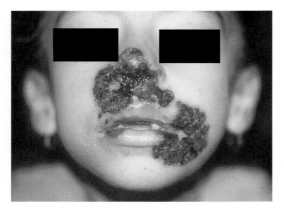

Fig. 41.5 Chronic herpes simplex infection: multiple polycyclic ulcers in a child with advanced AIDS

Complementary Examinations

Despite the low sensitivity and specificity, in typical presentations of HSV infection the clinical diagnosis is plausible, and the anamnesis components

can be helpful: history of unprotected sexual exposure, early episodes of similar wounds at the same site, and associated general symptoms (malaise, fever, lymphadenopathy) [81, 141]. In the presence of atypical clinical presentations, which usually occur in immunosuppressed patients, laboratory tests may be necessary for a definitive diagnosis. These include viral isolation in culture, cytologic smear (Tzanck test), tissue histology, viral antigen detection, viral DNA detection by polymerase chain reaction (PCR) techniques; and type-specific serologic assays [40, 154] (Table 41.3). The Tzanck test is a simple, rapid, and inexpensive tool in clinical practice, although its sensitivity and specificity are reduced. The specimen has to be collected preferably at the base of a recent vesicle or ulcer, stained via the Giemsa, Wright, or Papanicolaou

Table 41.3   Laboratory tests for the diagnosis of herpes simplex infection

Method	Principle	Sample	Sensitivity	Specificity	Advantages	Disadvantages
Viral antigen detection	Immunoperoxidase staining	Swab; smears from lesions; vesicular fluid; exudate from base of vesicle	Middle (80%)	High (90%)	Relatively inexpensive; Rapid Integrity of the specimen not required; Typing possible	Suboptimal sensitivity
	Capture ELISA	Swab; vesicular fluid; exudate from base of vesicle	High (Genital ulcer >95%)	Variable (62–100%)	–	Fresh vesicle; No viral type
	Rapid test device		Unknown	Unknown	Point-of-care testing	–
Virus culture[a]	HSV isolation susceptible cells	Swab; skin lesions; vesicular fluid; exudate from base of vesicle; mucosal sample without lesions	Variable[e]	≈100%	"Gold standard" method; Virus typing; Resistance phenotype testing	Less sensitive than PCR; Specialized laboratories
Molecular biology[a]	HSV DNA detection/quantitation by NAAT (PCR, real-time PCR[b], and commercial assays)	Also blood for molecular biology	High (98%)	High (≈100%)	High sensitivity; Virus detection and typing in the same test; Resistance genotyping; Fast results	Specialized laboratories; Not standardized; Not validated for all samples; PCR: risk of contamination
Cytologic examination	Tzanck smears; Papanicolaou or Romanovsky stain	Skin/mucosal lesions; Biopsies	Low	Low	Inexpensive	Fresh lesion; No distinction between HSV1 and 2, nor VZV
	Detection of infected cells by direct immunofluorescence	Smears; tissue section; smear from base of vesicle	Middle[f]	High (>95%)	Inexpensive; Rapid (<4 h possible); Typing possible	Fresh vesicles; Suboptimal sensitivity; Time-consuming; Not standardized
Serologic tests	Western blot[c]	Serum	≈100%	≈100%	Specific of HSV-1 and HSV-2; Earliest seroconversion: 13 days	Not commercially available
	Monoclonal antibody-blocking EIA[d]		≈100%	≈100%	Distinguish between HSV-1 and 2	Expensive; Not commercially available
	ELISA		93–98%	93–99%	ELISA commercially available	May lack of sensitivity and specificity

Fatahzadeh and Schwartz [81], LeGoff et al. [154], http://doi.org/10.1186/1743-422X-11-83, Levin et al. [158]

CDC Centers for Disease Control and Prevention, *EIA* enzyme immunoassay, *ELISA* enzyme-linked immunosorbent assay, *HSV* herpes simplex virus, *NAAT* nucleic acid amplification test, *VZV* varicella zoster virus

[a]Currently the "preferred" test of CDC (2010)

[b]Real-time PCR: method of choice for skin lesions

[c]Reference ("gold standard") test proposed by University of Washington (USA)

[d]Reference ("gold standard") test proposed by the Central Public Health Laboratory in the United Kingdom

[e]Depending on lesion (vesicular content >90%; ulcer 95%; swab 70%–80%; mucosa without lesion 30%), and also on sample storage and transport conditions

[f]Genital ulcer: 70–90%; asymptomatic: <40–50%

technique, and examined through an optical microscope to identify characteristic virus-induced cytopathologic findings. The Tzanck test verifies the HSV infectious etiology or a herpes zoster etiology; it does not provide a distinction between HSV-1 and HSV-2, nor between HSV and varicella zoster virus infection. The confirmation of the causative agent is obtained through viral culture, which is the gold-standard method, or by PCR-based techniques [40, 154]. Viral culture sensitivity is lower for old, dry, crusty lesions, and in patients with recurrent infection, in contrast to primary lesions [158]. PCR-based testing has the greatest overall sensitivity and specificity. Despite its high sensitivity and specificity, culture and detection by PCR is costly, resulting in limited routine use because of the high prevalence of the virus [40].

Therapeutic Approach

Antiherpetic treatment is beneficial for most symptomatic patients, possibly helping symptom control when used during the infection's early signs and symptoms, or for recurrence suppression. Antiviral agents do not cure HSV infections, but rather modify the clinical course of the disease through the inhibition of viral replication and subsequent epithelial damage [81]. The antiherpetic drugs acyclovir, famciclovir, and valacyclovir are safely used in HIV patients [227, 228]. Acyclovir requires several doses a day because of its short half-life. Famciclovir and valacyclovir have a longer half-life, allowing fewer doses per day, which may ensure better compliance to treatment despite their higher cost. Recommendations for HSV therapy in HIV patients are summarized in the Table 41.4. Long-term suppressive therapy is indicated for patients with severe recurrences, or to minimize the frequency of recurrences or reduce the risk of genital ulcer disease (GUD) in patients with CD4 counts <250 cells/mm^3 who initiate ART [227, 228]. It is worth noting that suppressive treatment does not decrease the HSV or HIV transmission risk in HIV/HSV-coinfected patients [40]. Another important point is that the prevalence of HSV-2 shedding and GUD may increase significantly after ART initiation, possibly related to the

Table 41.4 Treatment of herpes simplex in HIV patients

Orolabial lesions (duration: 5–10 days)
Acyclovir 400 mg PO tid, or
Famciclovir 500 mg PO bid, or
Valacyclovir 1 g PO bid
Initial or recurrent genital lesions (duration: 5–10 days)
Acyclovir 400 mg PO tid, or
Famciclovir 500 mg PO bid, or
Valacyclovir 1 g PO bid
Severe mucocutaneous HSV infections
Initial therapy acyclovir 5 mg/kg IV q8h
After lesions begin to regress, change to oral therapy as above
Continue treatment until lesions have completely healed
Chronic suppressive therapy
Indications:
Patients with severe recurrences, or
Patients who want to minimize the frequency of recurrences, or
To reduce the risk of GUD in patients with CD4 cell counts <250 cells/mm^3 who are starting ART
Treatment:
Acyclovir 400 mg PO bid, or
Famciclovir 500 mg PO bid, or
Valacyclovir 500 mg PO bid
Evaluate ongoing need for suppressive therapy annually
Acyclovir-resistant mucocutaneous HSV infections
Preferred therapy:
Foscarnet 80–120 mg/kg/day IV in 2–3 divided doses until clinical response
Alternative therapy (duration: 21–28 days or longer, based on clinical response):
Topical imiquimod 5% cream three times/week, or
Topical trifluridine[a], or
Topical cidofovir[a] 1% gel, or
IV cidofovir 5 mg/kg IV once weekly

Panel on Opportunistic Infections in HIV-Infected Adults and Adolescents [227, 228]

ART antiretroviral therapy, *bid* twice daily, *GUD* genital ulcer disease, *HSV* herpes simplex virus, *IV* intravenously, *PO* orally, *q8h* every 8 h, *tid* three times a day

[a]Topical formulations of trifluridine and cidofovir are not commercially available; extemporaneous compounding of topical products can be prepared using trifluridine ophthalmic solution and the intravenous formulation of cidofovir.

immune reconstitution inflammatory syndrome (IRIS). ART is not associated with reduced HSV shedding in HIV coinfected adults; it may be prudent to counsel patients during early ART and consider oral acyclovir therapy [169, 297]. Acyclovir resistance may occur mainly in immunocompromised patients, requiring treatment with intravenous drugs such as foscarnet and cidofovir. Both medications are nephrotoxic, requiring hydration and monitoring of renal function. Topical imiquimod, trifluridine, cidofovir, and intravenous cidofovir are alternative therapies.

Varicella Zoster Virus

Varicella-zoster virus (VZV) causes two diseases: varicella (chickenpox) and herpes zoster (shingles). Varicella is the clinical manifestation of the VZV primary infection, whereas herpes zoster (HZ) results from the viral reactivation.

General Epidemiology

Varicella is highly contagious, affecting younger individuals, predominantly children younger than 10 years, while HZ affects preferably adults and elders after their sixth decade, and the cutaneous manifestations lead to higher morbidity. The risk for HZ is higher among the elderly, immunosuppressed patients, and children affected by varicella in their first year of life, or whose mothers were affected by varicella during pregnancy [272]. HIV-infected adults and children, even undergoing ART, are more prone to HZ episodes than the general population, displaying incidence rates ten times higher, resulting in significant morbidity [256]. HZ may occur at any stage of the HIV infection, may be the first clinical manifestation of HIV, or may develop during the IRIS [321].

Etiopathogenesis

VZV is an enveloped large DNA neurotropic virus, an alpha-herpes virus (family Herpesviridae) consisting of a single serotype, with humans as the specific reservoir [158, 272]. VZV causes two forms of clinical presentation: varicella and herpes zoster. The vesicular lesions have high viral concentrations and can result in primary infection in susceptible hosts. The contagious period transitions from vesicle development to crust formation [116]. VZV is cytopathogenic during the productive infection, although it establishes latency after the primary infection (varicella). Following centripetal axonal transport, viral DNA persists in neurons of dorsal root and cranial nerve ganglia, where it can remain quiescent for years. From there the virus can be reactivated and, after centrifugal transport via nerve axons, can cause recurrent infections that represent HZ [272].

Clinical Presentation

Vesicle formation is the hallmark of both types of VZV infection [158]. Varicella starts as a pruriginous vesicular exanthema with disseminating lesions displaying varied evolutionary stages (papules, vesicles, and crusts) (Fig. 41.7), although more prevalent on the face and trunk. In HZ vesicular or bullous lesions can be painful, and their presentation is unilateral and segmental along a cutaneous region innervated by the impaired sensory ganglion (dermatome) [124]. Less frequently, two or more dermatomes may be

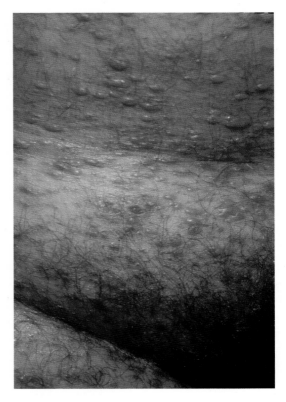

Fig. 41.7 Varicella: varied lesion stages with disseminated hemorrhagic vesicles, blisters, and some crusts

affected. When more than three dermatomes are involved, or more than 20 lesions develop from the early impaired dermatome, disseminated HZ is characterized (Fig. 41.8) [124, 321]. The most affected dermatomes are those corresponding to the thoracic and cervical ganglia, and the ophthalmic branch of the trigeminal nerve (Fig. 41.9).

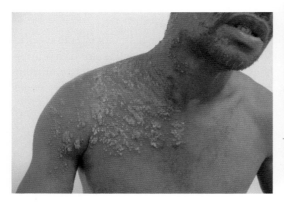

Fig. 41.8 Herpes zoster: severe herpes zoster affecting at least four dermatomes

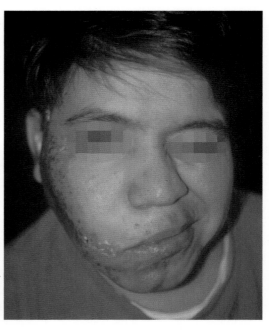

Fig. 41.10 Herpes zoster Ramsay Hunt syndrome: ipsilateral facial paralysis, ear pain, and vesicles in the auditory canal and auricle

In HIV-infected patients, HZ may display atypical lesions, e.g., follicular, ecthyma-like, ulcerated, crusty, verrucous, or hypertrophic. In HIV-infected children the primary infection can be severe and fatal, with systemic dissemination (pneumonitis, pancreatitis, and encephalitis). Extracutaneous involvement can also occur in adults, leading to higher morbidity and mortality. The major otologic complication of VZV reactivation is the Ramsay Hunt syndrome, which typically includes the triad of ipsilateral facial paralysis, ear pain, and vesicles in the auditory canal and auricle (Fig. 41.10) [98]. HZ may also be a manifestation of the immune reconstitution syndrome, developing after the start of ART, usually in patients with increased viral load and decreased CD4 count [124].

Complementary Examinations

Varicella and HZ diagnoses are clinical, mainly based on history and clinical picture; specifically the appearance of the skin eruption and characteristic location, in association with localized pain. Diagnosis verification through laboratory tests are

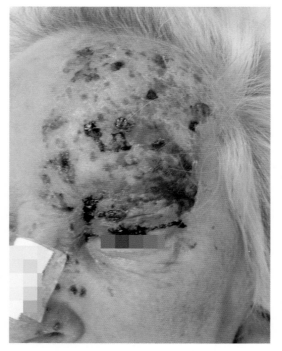

Fig. 41.9 Ophthalmic herpes zoster: unilateral ulcerated lesions and crusts affecting the ophthalmic division of the trigeminal nerve

usually less useful, since most of the tests are time consuming, have low specificity, or are not routinely available. Nevertheless, in selected patients, mainly the immunocompromised, HZ presentation can be atypical and require confirmatory tests for the precise diagnosis [158, 272]. The available laboratory tests include Tzanck smear, direct immunofluorescence, viral culture, PCR, and serology. Tests providing quicker results are the Tzanck smear and direct immunofluorescence; the former does not distinguish VZV from other herpesvirus infections. Immunofluorescence distinguishes both infections and is more sensitive than culture, although less sensitive than PCR techniques. PCR is the most appropriate test because of its high sensitivity and specificity. Culture is highly sensitive, although its time-consuming profile does not qualify the test for timely antiviral therapy [158, 272].

Therapeutic Approach

First-line antiviral therapy is based on antiviral nucleoside analogs (acyclovir, valacyclovir, famciclovir), and comparative trials do not support the efficacy of one over the other. The treatment aims include scarring acceleration, decreasing lesion progression, promoting efficient analgesia and preventing complications, such as postherpetic neuralgia and secondary infections. Early administration may reduce tissue damage, and, consequently, the destruction of affected ganglion cells in HZ can be diminished or even prevented [272]. The oral route is used for mild cases not associated with immunodeficiency. For severe disease, central nervous system (CNS) involvement, disseminated HZ, and HZ associated with impaired immune system, the intravenous route is indicated [158, 272]. Table 41.5 summarizes the antiviral treatment for HZ.

Systemic antiviral treatment is recommended for all HIV-infected patients, including children and pregnant women, regardless of their immunologic status, and even if they present after 72 h [321]. Patients with disseminated HZ should be hospitalized for intravenous acyclovir therapy. VZV/HIV-coinfected patients should be treated until all lesions have healed, which is often longer than the standard 7- to 10-day course [75]. Many approaches can be used for HZ acute pain management, including paracetamol, anti-inflammatory nonsteroidal drugs, tricyclic antidepressants, opiate derivatives, capsaicin, and topical anesthetics [116]. To treat postherpetic neuralgia (PHN; pain lasting longer than 1 month), tricyclic antidepressants or anticonvulsants can be combined with analgesics [124, 199]. Table 11.5 in Chap. 11 lists drugs and doses for the treatment of PHN. For HIV patients with early exposure to VZV, the use of a specific immune globulin over the first 96 h (Table 11.4, varicella zoster immune globulin) is recommended, or oral antiviral treatment over 7 days after exposure [124]. Administration of varicella vaccine is not recommended in HIV-infected patients with severe immunosuppression (CD4 cell percentage <15% or, if older than 5 years, a CD4 count <200 cells/mm^3). Zoster vaccine is not recommended in HIV-infected patients with a CD4 cell count <200 cells/mm^3, and there is no consensus about zoster vaccine for patients with higher CD4 counts [143].

Table 41.5 Antiviral treatment for varicella and herpes zoster

Antiviral drug	Antiviral dose[a]	Administration	Indication
Acyclovir	800 mg 5×/day	Orally	Zoster, varicella in risk patients
–	10 mg/kg q8h	IV	Severe and generalized VZV infections, HZ associated with immunosuppression
Valacyclovir	1 g tid	Orally	Varicella and herpes zoster
Famciclovir	500 mg tid	Orally	
Brivudin	125 mg qd	Orally	
Foscarnet	40 mg/kg q8h	IV	VZV infections caused by TK-negative VZV strains

Dworkin et al. [75] and Sauerbrei [272]
bid twice daily, *IV* intravenously, *q8* every 8 h, *qd* once a day, *tid* three times a day
[a]VZV disease in HIV-infected patients should be treated until all lesions have healed

Molluscum Contagiosum

General Epidemiology

Molluscum contagiosum (MC) is a frequent cutaneous viral infection with an estimated prevalence of 2–8% in the general population. In HIV-positive patients the prevalence reaches up to 33% in patients with a CD4 count <100/mm³ [175]. MC development clearly indicates progression of the HIV-associated disease [209]. Despite the sizable impact ART has made on the prevalence of dermatologic disease, MC remains an important cause of morbidity in HIV-positive populations.

Etiopathogenesis

MC is an infection caused by the molluscum contagiosum virus, a DNA virus member of the *Molluscipoxvirus* genus, in the Poxviridae family [175]. Transmission occurs through skin-to-skin contact with infected persons, including through sexual intercourse, by fomites (towels, pools), or autoinoculation. The incubation period ranges from 7 days to 3 months and transmission occurs as long as there are active lesions [175, 221].

Clinical Presentation

MC presents with white, painless papules with central umbilication (Fig. 41.11). In immunosuppressed HIV patients, this condition tends to be more severe and widespread, and classical lesions can be large (>1 cm), confluent, and disfiguring, particularly when the CD4 count is <200 cells/mm³. Persistent, recurrent, and disseminated lesions with abrupt onset can also occur [209]. The lesions can develop on any body part, although in the HIV patient they mainly affect the genital region and the face [198]. The diagnosis is essentially clinical, based on the morphologic characteristics, although atypical presentations may require histopathologic examination for diagnosis definition [124]. Fungal diseases, such as histoplasmosis and cryptococcosis, are differential diagnoses to be considered in the immunosuppressed patient with molluscum-like lesions [199].

Complementary Examinations

Complementary examinations are usually not required. Investigation of immunodeficiency is

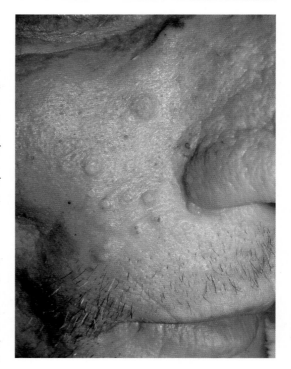

Fig. 41.11 Molluscum contagiosum: pearl-like papules with central umbilication on the face

suggested in atypical presentations. For histologic analysis, the specimen can be obtained by curettage of one or more MC lesions, as well as biopsy. Histologically, MC virus infection is characterized by epidermal hyperplasia with accelerated keratinization and the presence of cytoplasmic inclusion bodies, known as Henderson–Patterson bodies, which displace the nucleus and flatten it against the cell membrane. These inclusion bodies are pathognomonic of the disease [175].

Therapeutic Approach

Given the poor quality of studies and evidence, no specific recommendation can be made for the treatment of MC in HIV-infected individuals other than the initiation of ART [175]. Besides ART initiation that induces immune system recovery, complementary therapy may be necessary for clinical resolution of the lesions. Pharmacologic topical treatment includes retinoids, imiquimod, potassium hydroxide, cantharidin, salicylic acid, and podophyllotoxin.

Nonpharmacologic options consist of destructive techniques and include cryotherapy, curettage of individual lesions, and electrodesiccation [306]. The choice is dependent upon the location and extension of the lesions, skin phototype, resource availability, and the clinician's experience with the technique. Possible complications such as dyschromia and scarring sequelae have to be also considered regarding the therapeutic choice. Topical treatments with tretinoin, podophyllotoxin, and imiquimod can be an alternative when there are many lesions [124, 199].

Oral Hairy Leukoplakia

Oral hairy leukoplakia (HL) is a benign mucous disease related to immunosuppression, indicative of disease progression to AIDS in HIV-positive individuals [101].

General Epidemiology

HL occurs in around 25% of HIV-infected adults, possibly developing at any stage of the HIV infection, although it affects mainly patients with low counts of CD4 and high viral load [198, 255]. The HL/HIV coinfection has epidemiologic significance: HL may be an indicator of HIV infection and predicts HIV disease progression, has been used as a criterion for initiation of ART, has been used in clinical staging and classification systems, correlates with HIV viral load, usually decreases with ART, and recurs as ART fails [101].

Etiopathogenesis

The infection is caused by the Epstein–Barr virus (EBV). In the immunosuppressed patient the viruses proliferate in the epithelial cells of the oral mucosa and the tongue [255]. The pathogenesis of HL is not entirely clear. EBV from saliva, circulating B lymphocytes or monocytes, or latent within-tongue epithelium may replicate under the influence of suppressed anti-EBV cell-mediated immunity, causing typical HL lesions [101].

Clinical Presentation

The clinical appearance of HL involves white or gray plaques of varying size, usually on the lateral border of the tongue or other areas of the oral mucosa, which may show vertical corrugations

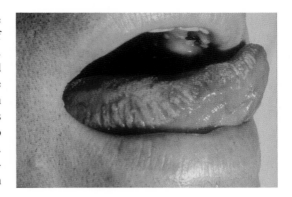

Fig. 41.12 Oral hairy leukoplakia: white linear papules on the lateral border of the tongue

and cannot be rubbed off (Fig. 41.12). They are mostly asymptomatic [101, 232]. The differential diagnosis includes oral white lesions, such as idiopathic leukoplakia, smoking-associated leukoplakia, dysplasia, squamous cell carcinoma, hyperplastic candidiasis, and lichen planus [101].

Complementary Examinations

The histopathologic assessment displays hyperkeratosis, acanthosis with superficial edema, koilocytes on the spinous layer, and absence of inflammation. The definitive diagnosis can be obtained through EBV demonstration through in situ hybridization or PCR [198]. The diagnosis can be verified by EBV identification through in situ hybridization techniques, PCR, and electron microscopy [209].

Therapeutic Approach

HL is usually asymptomatic and has a nonmorbid nature, and generally no treatment is needed. HL may improve or resolve with topical podophyllum and tretinoin [232]. The lesions improve when ART is introduced, leading to recovery of the immunologic status [198, 209].

Human Papillomavirus

Human papillomaviruses (HPV) are a large group of double-stranded DNA viruses widely distributed among humans. HPV-associated diseases include anogenital and other mucocutaneous warts as well as cervical, anal, vaginal, vulvar, penile, and oropharyngeal cancers [231].

General Epidemiology

Infection with cutaneous HPV types is ubiquitous and cutaneous warts are common in children, with a peak incidence during adolescence and declining thereafter. Warts are spread via person-to-person contact or indirectly by fomites [202, 216]. The prevalence of cutaneous common warts in HIV-infected individuals is about 18%, in contrast with 1–2% in noninfected patients [96]. Anogenital warts are a common worldwide public health problem, and sexual behavior is a primary risk factor associated with anogenital and oral HPV infection among men and women, since anogenital HPV is primarily transmitted through vaginal, anal, and oral intercourse [216]. It is estimated that more than 50% of sexually active persons become infected with anogenital HPV during their lifetime, with a peak incidence between the ages of 20 and 24 years old [40]. Despite the introduction of ART, there is evidence that eradication of anogenital HPV infection is especially difficult in patients with a CD4 count <50 cells/mm^3 [182].

Etiopathogenesis

HPV is a group of nonenveloped double-stranded DNA viruses of which at least 150 genotypes have already been identified. HPV is tissue specific, with approximately 40 types known to infect the anogenital region and oral cavity, whereas multiple HPV types are responsible for cutaneous warts [216]. Genotypes are divided into low-risk (nononcogenic) and high-risk (oncogenic), and affect the skin and the mucosae [40]. Low-risk HPV 6 and 11 account for 90% of anogenital warts. High-risk HPV 16 and 18 have oncogenic potential, and underlying immunosuppression is associated with more rapid progression of the premalignant lesions of low and high grades [68, 96]. The interaction between HPV and HIV is complex: HPV causes greater susceptibility to the acquisition of HIV, and HPV/HIV coinfection reduces the HPV clearance. As a result of such counterplay, HIV-infected patients are at increased risk of developing anal and cervical cancers, as well as vulvar and penile carcinomas [254]. Oral and genital warts have been observed in HIV patients receiving ART as part of the IRIS [190].

Clinical Presentation

Warts are benign epithelial skin tumors, usually classified into anogenital and nonanogenital warts. The lesions are mostly self-limited, asymptomatic, or subclinical. The different HPV subtypes are associated with varied clinical presentations. Nonanogenital cutaneous warts are asymptomatic verrucous papules, located at any body part [202]. Common warts (verruca vulgaris) are the most often seen, presenting as papular or nodular, keratotic lesions that display dark points on their surface, corresponding to thrombosed capillary loops (Fig 41.13). They are usually seen on the hands (Fig. 41.14), plantar regions, elbows, and knees. Filiform warts resemble keratotic spicules, usually on the face and neck (Fig. 41.15). Deep plantar warts can be less noticeable and very painful. Flat warts (plane warts or verruca plana)

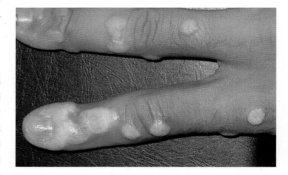

Fig. 41.13 Common warts: hyperkeratotic papules with tiny dark points on their surface, corresponding to the thrombosed capillary loops

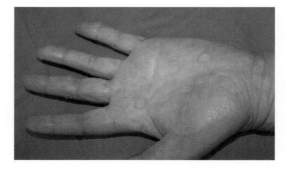

Fig. 41.14 Common warts: yellowish hyperkeratotic palmar papules

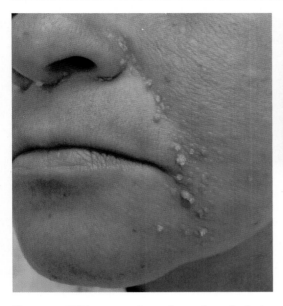

Fig. 41.15 Filiform warts: keratotic papules and spicules on the face

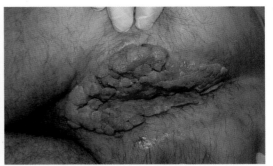

Fig. 41.17 Anal warts: large vegetating plaques in the perianal area

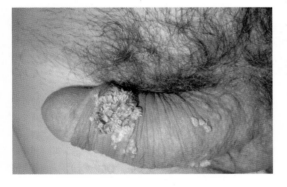

Fig. 41.16 Genital warts: hyperkeratotic papules on the penis with papillomatous lesion in the distal portion

are flat or slightly elevated flesh-colored papules, measuring 1–5 mm wide, frequently numerous on the face and hand dorsum. Anogenital warts, or condyloma acuminatum, are the more common presentation of sexually transmitted HPV infection. HPV causes a multifocal infection of the anogenital skin, lesions being most common at the site of trauma during sexual intercourse, but may occur at any genital or perigenital site [52]. Clinically they are papules, nodules, or plaques, usually asymptomatic (Figs. 41.16 and 41.17).

Complementary Examinations

The diagnosis is clinical, although biopsy can be performed for atypical or treatment refractory lesions. Since anogenital warts can be sexually transmitted, an appropriate screen for other sexually transmitted infections (STIs) is recommended.

Therapeutic Approach

Up to 30% of genital warts will spontaneously regress; however, recurrence is common [216]. Treatment is directed to the visible lesions caused by HPV, and no therapy modalities are curative. Treatment regimens are classified as either patient-applied or provider-administered modalities. Table 41.6 lists the main therapeutic options for external anogenital warts. Therapies for nonanogenital warts are addressed in Chap. 11. There is little evidence to support the unequivocal choice of the best treatment for cutaneous and mucosal warts. All treatments have significant failure and recurrence rates. Data from systematic reviews and economic evaluation of interventions for the treatment of genital warts have suggested that ablative techniques seem to have better primary clearance rates despite their higher cost-effectiveness [148, 299]. The potential advantages and disadvantages of the individual treatments must be considered, and therapeutic choice should be based on location, size and number of lesions, adverse reactions associated with therapy, cost, patient preferences, comorbidities and age; and provider experience. If 3 months of

Table 41.6 Therapeutic options for external anogenital warts

	Treatment	Regimen	Adverse effects	Comments
Patient-applied	Imiquimod[a] 5% **OR** Imiquimod[a] 3.75%	Once at bedtime, three times a week for up to 16 weeks / Once at bedtime, daily, for up to 8 weeks	Local inflammation, itching burning, vesicles, erosions, ulcers, crusting, local sclerosis dyschromia	Not suitable for pregnant women
	Podophyllotoxin 0.5% solution or gel	Twice a day for 3 consecutive days, followed by 4 days of no therapy, for up to four cycles	Local inflammation, erythema, itching, pain, erosions	Total wart area treated should not exceed 10 cm^2 / Total volume of podophyllotoxin should be limited to 0.5 mL per day / Contraindicated for pregnant women
Provider-administered	Cryotherapy (liquid nitrogen)	Weekly or every other week	Pain, local inflammation, bullae, ulcer, necrosis	It can be used in pregnant women
	TCA 80–90% solution	Weekly	Pain, burning	It can be used in pregnant women
	Podophyllin resin solution 10–25%	Weekly	Local inflammation, pain, ulcer	Total wart area treated should not exceed 10 cm^2 / Total volume should be limited to 0.5 mL per day / Contraindicated for pregnant women
	Surgical removal[b]	–	Pain, scarring	–
	Laser (CO$_2$ or Nd:YAG)	–	Pain, scarring	High cost

CDC [40], Clinical Effectiveness Group [52], Kollipara et al. [144], Lacey et al. [148], Park et al. [231], Steben and Garland [293]

TCA trichloroacetic acid

[a]Latex condoms may be weakened if in contact with imiquimod

[b]Either by tangential scissor excision, tangential shave excision, curettage, or electrosurgery

any treatment does not yield improvement, a new therapy should be attempted [40, 144]. Soft nonkeratinized warts respond well to podophyllotoxin and trichloroacetic acid (TCA). Keratinized lesions may be better treated with physical ablative methods such as cryotherapy, excision, TCA, or electrosurgery. Imiquimod is suitable treatment for both keratinized and nonkeratinized warts [52]. HIV patients with impaired cell-mediated immunity may show lower response and higher recurrence rates, eventually requiring combined therapies [52]. Counseling for condom use is highly advisable. Condoms used consistently and correctly can lower the chances of acquiring and transmitting HPV; however, because HPV can infect areas not covered by a condom, condoms might not fully protect against HPV [40]. A vaccine is available for males and females to prevent genital warts. HPV vaccine is recommended routinely for boys and girls aged 11–12 years, as well as for young men through age 21 years and young women through age 26 years who have not previously been vaccinated. HPV vaccine is also recommended for MSM, persons living with HIV/AIDS, and immunocompromised persons through age 26 years. HPV bivalent and quadrivalent vaccines are recommended for girls/women, whereas only HPV quadrivalent vaccine is recommended for boys/men [40, 171].

Acquired Epidermodysplasia Verruciformis

Epidermodysplasia verruciformis (EV) is a rare autosomal recessive genodermatosis characterized by a defect in cell-mediated immunity and increased susceptibility to infections increased susceptibility to specific HPV genotypes infection. There are more than 20 known HPV types associated with EV (EV-HPV) [137, 260]. Acquired epidermodysplasia verruciformis (AEV) is a rare disease observed in patients with impaired cell-mediated immunity and predisposition to HPV infection, mainly described in HIV patients [260, 330]. The main clinical features of AEV are similar to EV: a rash resembling pityriasis versicolor and flat warts (Fig. 41.18a). The rash consists of a widespread papular eruption of reddish to skin-colored, hypopigmented, gray, brown, flat, wart-like lesions mostly involving the sun-exposed areas of the skin. Local trauma may induce the isomorphic (Koebner) phenomenon to produce a linear distribution of papules (Fig. 41.18b). They usually present as multifocal lesions ranging in size from millimeters to centi-meters. In the last decade, several cases of acquired EV have been reported, particularly in HIV-infected patients [137]. It seems that AEV is more frequent in young, vertically HIV-infected patients than in adults infected later in life [164]. In HIV disease, proliferation of lesions is associated with progressive immunosuppression or during IRIS after initiation of ART [131, 308]. Selected EV-HPV strains appear to have a substantial link with oncogenic transformation [131, 308]. Despite this relationship, the role of HPV in the development of AEV lesions and the eventual malignant transformation of these lesions is not known. At present there is no known effective treatment for AEV in HIV patients [330]. Anecdotal reports have shown attenuation of warts with topical glycolic acid [193] or even clearance with topical cidofovir [67]. The detection of high risk HPV types on the skin lesions of HIV-infected children with AEV supports the need for a continuous follow-up, as the long-term cutaneous cancer risk in these patients remains unknown [164, 308].

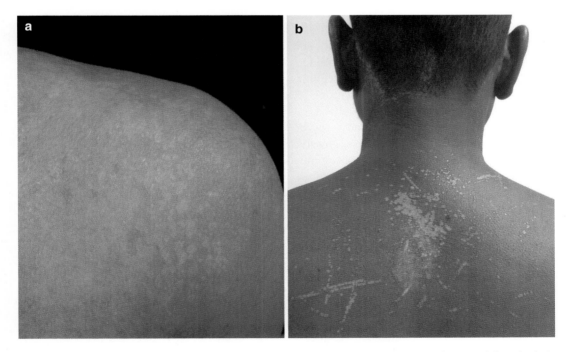

Fig. 41.18 Epidermodysplasia verruciformis. (**a**) Widespread hypopigmented papular eruption resembling pityriasis versicolor. (**b**) Linear distribution of papules induced by local trauma (isomorphic [Koebner]) phenomenon

Bacterial Diseases

Cutaneous Bacterial Infections

General Epidemiology

The most common bacterial infections in HIV-infected patients result from *Staphylococcus aureus* and *Streptococcus pyogenes* [9]. *S. aureus* nasal colonization rate in HIV-infected patients is about 50%, twice the rate observed in non-HIV-infected. Methicillin-resistant *S aureus* infection should also be considered in HIV-infected patients [198, 256, 298].

Etiopathogenesis

The largest amount of cutaneous and systemic bacterial infections observed in HIV patients is multifactorial: frequent nasal colonization by *S. aureus*; cutaneous barrier impairment, and immunologic dysfunction of T and B lymphocytes, neutrophils, and macrophages [198, 298]. Use of venous catheters as well as pruritus, which favor skin microtraumas, also play a role in cutaneous lesion development [298].

Clinical Presentation

The clinical manifestations are varied, and impetigo (Fig. 41.19), folliculitis, furuncle (Fig. 41.20), abscess, ecthyma, and cellulitis are the most often found presentations [9, 298]. The lesions are usually localized on the lower limbs, gluteal region, and scrotum, although they may have a locally aggressive course, eventually evolving into bacteremia and sepsis [209].

Complementary Examinations

Diagnosis is based on clinical findings. Direct examination and culture of smears and tissues, as well as histopathologic study, should be performed as needed [198]. Scrapes from superficial lesions can be examined under a microscope using the Gram technique. Collection of samples from cutaneous lesions and nasal mucosa is recommended for recurrent infections and deeper lesions in order to assess the bacteriologic profile and conduct and antibiogram [96, 298].

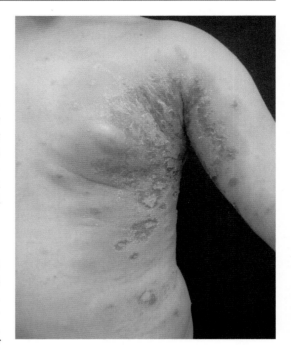

Fig. 41.19 Impetigo: inflammatory superficial weeping lesions covered by orange crusts

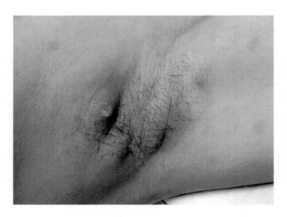

Fig. 41.20 Furuncle: erythematous nodule with spontaneous drainage of purulent secretion on the armpit

Therapeutic Approach

The treatment is similar for HIV-infected and noninfected patients, with a recommendation for therapy maintenance until complete remission. Systemic semisynthetic penicillins or cephalosporins are usually effective for superficial lesions. Abscesses should be drained with surgical incision or needle aspiration, and samples may be used for microbiological assessment

(Gram staining, culture, and antibiogram). For patients with recurrent infections, decolonization of *S. aureus* chronic carriers can be achieved with topical nasal mupirocin [96, 298].

Syphilis

Syphilis is an STI caused by the spirochete bacteria *Treponema pallidum*. A myriad of mucocutaneous and systemic manifestations can be present in different stages (primary, secondary, latent, and tertiary syphilis). Transmission is higher during primary and secondary stages of the infection.

General Epidemiology

Syphilis and HIV overlap and interact in a number of significant ways. They share common risk factors, are sexually transmitted, and can be transmitted vertically to a child or fetus. Syphilis increases the risk of HIV transmission, and HIV infection can alter the natural history of syphilis [240, 294]. While anyone who has sex can contract an STI, sexually active gay, bisexual, and other MSM are at increased risk for STIs; other risk factors for syphilis acquisition include history of early STI, multiple sexual partners, and practices of unprotected oral sex [40, 183, 322]. Rates of primary and secondary syphilis progressively declined from 1990 to 2000 whereas since 2000, an increase in syphilis incidence has been observed worldwide [239, 294].

Etiopathogenesis

In acquired syphilis the disease results from the infection with *T. pallidum* bacteria which penetrate through tiny abrasions during sexual contact. Congenital syphilis is a severe, disabling, and often life-threatening infection seen in infants. A pregnant mother who has syphilis can spread the disease through the placenta to the fetus or at birth. Blood transfusion and indirect transmission via contaminated items or tattoos are rare forms of syphilis transmission [15].

Clinical Presentation

The protean clinical presentations of syphilis earned it the name of the "Great Mimicker." The course of disease comprises primary, secondary,

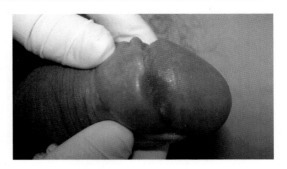

Fig. 41.21 Primary syphilis (chancre): eroded indurated papule, well delimited, with smooth and clean surface

latent, tertiary, and neurosyphilis [235]. In primary syphilis an asymptomatic mucosal or skin lesion (chancre) appears 3 weeks after the initial exposure at the point of contact and usually heals spontaneously after 4–6 weeks (Fig. 41.21). Local lymph node swelling can occur [235]. Typical signs of secondary syphilis are localized or diffuse symmetric mucocutaneous lesions and generalized nontender lymphadenopathy. Lesions are symmetric, slightly erythematous macules and papules (syphilids) measuring up to 10 mm in diameter and are distributed on the trunk, proximal extremities, palms, and soles (Fig. 41.22). Syphilids involving hair follicles may result in patchy alopecia (Fig. 41.23). In some patients, highly infectious papules develop at the mucocutaneous junctions and become hypertrophic in moist intertriginous areas (condylomata lata). General symptoms include fever, sore throat, malaise, weight loss, headache, and meningismus [235]. Latent syphilis is defined as a stage of infection caused by *T. pallidum* in which organisms persist in the body of the infected person without causing symptoms or signs, and has two subcategories. Latent syphilis acquired within the preceding year is referred to as early latent syphilis; all other cases are late latent syphilis or syphilis of unknown duration [41]. Tertiary syphilis is slowly progressive, usually occurring 1–10 years after the initial infection, and may affect any organ. The dermatologic picture is characterized by the presence of soft tumor-like gummas, which are indurated, nodular, papulosquamous, or ulcerative lesions that form characteristic circles or arcs. Besides the

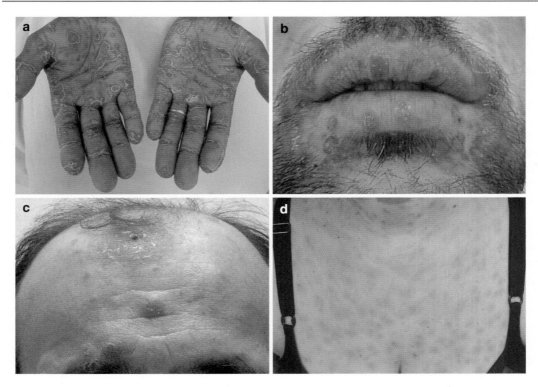

Fig. 41.22 Secondary syphilis. (**a**) Scaling rash on the palms, resembling psoriasis; (**b**) syphilids on the face; (**c**) plaques and nodules in an immunosuppressed HIV patient; (**d**) syphilitic roseola, maculopapular rash on the chest

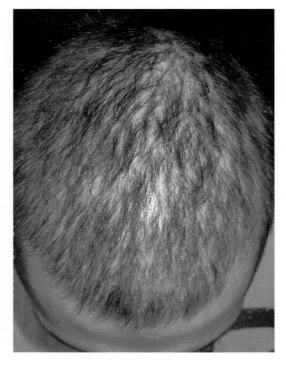

Fig. 41.23 Secondary syphilis: patchy alopecia due to involvement of hair follicles

skin, gummas may appear almost anywhere in the body including the bones [235]. Neurosyphilis may occur at any stage of syphilis, and approximately 35–40% of persons with secondary syphilis have asymptomatic CNS involvement [69]. The natural course of syphilis may be altered in HIV-infected patients, although in most cases the manifestations remain typical. In immunosuppressed syphilis/HIV-coinfected patients, syphilis may have atypical features: a shorter incubation period, a persistent and painful primary lesion overlapping the secondary stage, multiple extragenital primary lesions, high risk for neurologic and systemic involvement, and rapid progression to secondary and tertiary stages [240, 294]. Syphilis/HIV-coinfected patients may develop so-called malignant syphilis, a rare and severe variant of secondary syphilis characterized by large papular, nodular, and ulcerative lesions covered with thick crusts affecting the trunk, the extremities, and even the face [312]. According to a large multicenter retrospective study, concurrent HIV infection increases the risk of developing malignant syphilis by 60-fold [283].

Complementary Examinations

Careful history, sexual risk assessment, and physical examination are valuable information whenever STI patients are evaluated (Box 41.4). Laboratory tools to assess syphilis diagnostic in HIV-infected and noninfected patients are the same. Definitive diagnosis of early syphilis is made through visualization or identification of *T pallidum* spirochetes on dark-field microscopy, through direct fluorescent antibody tests, or with PCR techniques; however, these methods are routinely impractical [18, 294]. A presumptive diagnosis of syphilis is achieved by using serologic tests. Two types of serologic tests are used: nontreponemal (diagnostic) tests including the Rapid Plasma Reagin (RPR) test and the Venereal Disease Research Laboratory (VDRL) test, and the treponemal (confirmatory) tests including the fluorescent treponemal antibody absorption (FTA-ABS) test, the microhemagglutination test for antibodies to *T. pallidum* (MHA-TP), and the *T. pallidum* particle agglutination assay. Nontreponemal tests correlate with disease activity, are reported quantitatively, and are used to monitor treatment response. After treatment, nontreponemal titers typically become negative while treponemal tests remain positive throughout life [18, 40]. Both treponemal and nontreponemal tests can have false-positive results secondary to medications, and autoimmune conditions. Although uncommon, there have been sporadic reports of seronegative syphilis in HIV-infected patients. The false-negative serologic tests are generally due to the prozone phenomenon, which can occur when very high titers of antibodies interfere with the assay, and can be excluded by testing diluted serum [294]. All patients with suspected syphilis should be tested for HIV infection and screened for other STIs. Diagnostic issues are summarized in Boxes 41.5 and 45.6.

Box 41.4 Evaluating Patients for Primary and Secondary Syphilis

Sexual history, risk assessment, and physical exam	
Sexual history, risk assessment (past year):	*Physical examination*
Gender of partners	Oral cavity
Number of partners (new, anonymous, serodiscordant HIV status, exchange of sex for drugs or money)	Lymph nodes
	Skin
Types of sexual exposure	Palms and soles
Recent STIs; HIV serostatus	Neurologic
Substance abuse	Genitalia/pelvic
Condom use	Perianal
History of syphilis prior syphilis (last serologic test and last treatment)	

All patients with suspected syphilis should be tested for HIV infection and screened for other STIs. Repeat HIV testing of patients with secondary syphilis 3 months after the first HIV test if the first test is negative

Box 41.5 Diagnostic Issues in Primary Syphilis

Dark-field

~80% sensitive, varies with experience/skill of examiner and decreased sensitivity as lesion ages.

RPR/VDRL

- A negative RPR/VDRL does not exclude the diagnosis of syphilis; only ~75–85% sensitive in primary syphilis
- Tests must be quantified to the highest titer, and titer on the day of treatment must be used to assess treatment response
- Always use the same testing method (RPR or VDRL) in sequential testing; cannot compare titer from two different tests
- Tests lack specificity (biological false positive); all reactive tests need to be confirmed by a treponemal test for syphilis diagnosis

Therapeutic Approach

Penicillin via the parenteral route is the drug of choice to treat all clinical phases of syphilis [40, 323]. Treatment regimens for syphilis are shown in Table 41.7. No proven alternatives to penicillin are available for treating neurosyphilis, congenital syphilis, or syphilis in pregnant women. Parenteral penicillin G is the only therapy with documented efficacy for syphilis during pregnancy. Pregnant women with syphilis in any stage who report penicillin allergy should be desensitized and treated with penicillin [40]. The Jarisch–Herxheimer reaction is a transitory acute febrile reaction frequently accompanied by headache, myalgia, fever, and exacerbation of cutaneous lesions that can occur within the first 24 h after the initiation of any therapy for syphilis. Antipyretics can be used to manage symptoms [23]. Clinical and serologic follow-up should be performed at 6 and 12 months after treatment [40]. If, at any time, clinical symptoms develop or a sustained (>2 weeks) four-fold or greater rise in nontreponemal titers occurs, a cerebrospinal fluid (CSF) examination should be

Table 41.7 Treatment for syphilis

Clinical stage	Adults and adolescents	Infants and children	Alternative treatment for penicillin-allergic pregnant women[c, d]	Alternative treatment for penicillin-allergic nonpregnant patients
Primary, secondary, and early latent syphilis[a]	Benzathine penicillin G, 2.4 million units IM in a single dose (total 2.4 million units)	Benzathine penicillin G, 50.000 units/kg IM, up to the adult dose in a single dose	Erythromycin 500 mg PO, qid for 14 days	*CDC recommendation* Doxycycline, 100 mg PO, bid
			OR	OR
			Ceftriaxone 1 g IM qd for 10–14 days	Tetracycline, 500 mg PO, qid, each for 14 days
			OR	
			Azithromycin 2 g once PO	*WHO recommendation* Doxycycline, 100 mg PO bid or ceftriaxone 1 g IM qd for 10–14 days
Late latent syphilis[b] and unknown duration	Benzathine penicillin G 2.4 million units IM, 3 doses, 1 week apart (total 7.2 million units)	Benzathine penicillin G 50,000 units/kg IM, up to the adult dose, 3 doses, 1 week apart	Erythromycin 500 mg PO, qid for 30 days	*CDC recommendation* Doxycycline, 100 mg PO, bid
				OR
				Tetracycline, 500 mg PO, qid, each for 28 days
				WHO recommendation Doxycycline, 100 mg PO, bid for 30 days

Table 41.7 (continued)

Clinical stage	Adults and adolescents	Infants and children	Alternative treatment for penicillin-allergic pregnant women[c, d]	Alternative treatment for penicillin-allergic nonpregnant patients
Neurosyphilis	Aqueous crystalline penicillin G 18–24 million units per day, administered as 3–4 million units IV q4h or continuous infusion, for 10–14 days			Procaine penicillin G 2.4 million units IM qd **PLUS** Probenecid 500 mg PO, qid, both for 10–14 days

CDC [40] and WHO [323]

bid twice daily, *q4h* every 4 h, *qd* once a day, *qid* four times a day, *IV* intravenously, *IM* intramuscularly, *PO* per os (oral administration)

[a]Disease acquired in the last 12 months

[b]Any case that do not fall as early latent and those of unknown duration

[c]Table shows WHO recommended regimen; according to CDC guidelines, pregnant women with syphilis in any stage who report penicillin allergy should be desensitized and treated with penicillin

[d]Erythromycin and azithromycin do not cross the placental barrier completely; it is therefore necessary to treat the newborn infant soon after delivery

performed and treatment administered accordingly. If the nontreponemal titer does not decline four-fold after 24 months, CSF examination can be considered and treatment administered accordingly, although initial low titers (<1:8) might not decline [40].

Bacillary Angiomatosis

Bacillary angiomatosis (BA) is a vascular, proliferative form of *Bartonella* infection that occurs primarily in immunocompromised patients.

General Epidemiology

BA is traditionally seen in HIV-infected patients with advanced disease, with CD4 count <100 cells/mm³ [192].

Etiopathogenesis

The infection results from the Gram-negative *Bartonella quintana* and *Bartonella henselae* bacteria. Humans are the reservoir of the bacterium, and the human body louse, *Pediculus humanus corporis*, is its usual vector. Body lice are probably not the only vectors of *Bartonella*. The

transmission of *Bartonella* to humans may also result from cat scratch involving the claw of a cat that is contaminated with *Bartonella*-infected flea feces [73, 86].

Clinical Presentation

There are two distinct *Bartonella*-associated syndromes: bacteremia (in the absence of focal tissue vascular proliferative response) and the tissue infection (BA) associated with angiogenic response. Bacteremia can systemically spread *Bartonella*, mainly to the liver (hepatic peliosis) and the spleen [86]. Angioproliferative lesions are generally cupuliform papules which may also present as nodules or friable and easily bleeding erythematous-violaceous plaques (Fig. 41.24). They may vary in number, from solitary to thousands of lesions, and sized 1 mm to many centimeters. Lesions may also be subcutaneous nodules, masses, or cysts [192]. Vascular cutaneous lesions, such as hemangiomas, pyogenic granuloma, angiosarcoma, and Kaposi's sarcoma, should be borne in mind as the main differential diagnoses.

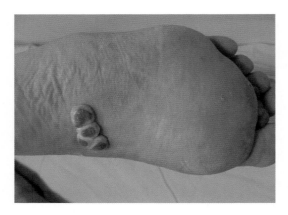

Fig. 41.24 Bacillary angiomatosis: erythematous friable nodules on the foot

Complementary Examinations

Skin biopsy, serologic tests, and peripheral blood culture are the tools available to investigate BA. Histopathologic study of skin or viscera confirms the diagnosis. With the biopsy sample, identification of the pathogen can be performed through culture as well as immunohistochemical and PCR techniques [86, 192]. Histopathology is typical, and shows lobular proliferation of small blood capillaries with large endothelial cells with abundant cytoplasm surrounded by inflammatory infiltrate, which contains many polymorphic nuclear leukocytes and focal necrosis. Optical microscopy provides visualization of *Bartonella* sp. through the Warthin–Starry stain [192].

Therapeutic Approach

All HIV-infected individuals diagnosed with *Bartonella* infection should receive antibiotic therapy. Drug options for cutaneous lesions include oral erythromycin (500 mg four times daily) and doxycycline (100 mg twice daily) for at least 3 months [166]. The intravenous route is appropriate for severe disease. Alternative agents include minocycline, azithromycin, clarithromycin, and ciprofloxacin [166].

Cutaneous Mycobacterial Infections

Mycobacterial infections with cutaneous manifestations are uncommon. Tuberculosis, hanseniasis, and, among the nontuberculous mycobacteria (NTM), the *Mycobacterium avium* complex (MAC), can affect the skin in HIV-infected patients. Treatment depends on the microorganism and the local resistance pattern.

General Epidemiology

Cutaneous manifestations associated with mycobacterial infections are uncommon. Although tuberculosis (TB) is the main opportunistic infection (OI) in HIV-infected individuals, cutaneous TB represents only 1–2% of TB cases [9, 209]. The cutaneous lesions caused by NTM, particularly the *M. avium* complex, are associated with advanced immunosuppression; especially with CD4 counts <50 cells/mm^3 [96].

Etiopathogenesis

The most relevant mycobacteria in the HIV-infected patient include *Mycobacterium tuberculosis* and *M. avium* complex [127]. Cutaneous infections by other mycobacteria, such as *Mycobacterium bovis*, *M. kansasii*, *M. marinum*, *M. malmoense*, *M. ulcerans*, *M. chelonae*, *M. fortuitum*, and *M. abscessus* are less common [96, 124, 209]. Depending on the epidemiologic characteristics of selected populations, some patients may acquire HIV–hanseniasis coinfection (*Mycobacterium leprae*).

Clinical Presentation

Cutaneous tuberculosis: the cutaneous tuberculosis presentation depends on the host immunologic status and environmental factors. The main clinical forms are verrucous tuberculosis, lupus vulgaris, miliary tuberculosis, and scrofuloderma (Dias et al. 2014; [96]). Scrofuloderma is the most common cutaneous form, occurring in skin by direct involvement from an underlying TB focus; and it is characterized by subcutaneous abscesses and nodules, with little inflammation and purulent secretion, mainly in the cervical, clavicular, and inguinal regions (Fig. 41.25). Lupus vulgaris may result from hematogenous dissemination of tuberculosis, or may occur at sites of inoculation or associated with scrofuloderma. The typical lesion is a raised plaque composed of red-brown papules, with "apple-jelly" aspect (Fig. 41.26).

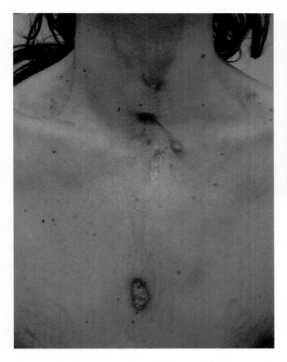

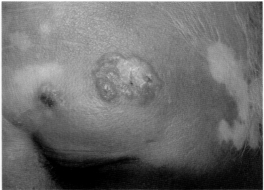

Fig. 41.26 Cutaneous tuberculosis, lupus vulgaris: raised red-brown plaque with "jelly" aspect

Fig. 41.25 Cutaneous tuberculosis, scrofuloderma: subcutaneous abscesses and nodules, with little inflammation and purulent secretion; scarring of old lesions can also be seen

M. avium complex: its clinical presentation is variable and usually the cutaneous condition results from systemic infection. Papules, pustules, nodules, ulcers, abscesses, fistulas, and verrucous lesions may be the clinical expressions of the infection [96, 124].

M. leprae: clinical, immunologic, histopathologic, and virologic features among HIV/hanseniasis-coinfected patients indicate that each disease has progressed as in single infection. However, ART-induced immune reconstitution may trigger potential adverse effects, such as hanseniasis acute inflammatory episodes [9, 237].

Complementary Examinations

Diagnosis confirmation is based on histopathologic study and identification of *Mycobacterium* through PCR and/or culture. Samples can be obtained from a skin fragment or purulent discharge. Complementary diagnostic tools may be necessary for additional systemic investigation,

such as chest X-ray, sputum bacilloscopy, and Mantoux tuberculin skin test. QuantiFERON-TB Gold, a blood test that aids detection of *M. tuberculosis*, can be an auxiliary test, although it does not differentiate active from latent disease [96].

Therapeutic Approach

Treatment regimen depends on the isolated microorganism and the local resistance patterns. For cutaneous tuberculosis, the same therapy as for the pulmonary and extrapulmonary forms is used; in selected cases, a surgical approach may be necessary [124]. For disseminated MAC the optimal therapeutic regimen is not yet established. Treatment should include a minimum three-drug regimen of clarithromycin, rifampin, and ethambutol, until the patient is culture negative, after therapy for 1 year [120, 178]. Management of hanseniasis requires multidrug therapy recommended by the WHO and is covered in Chap. 6.

Fungal Infections

Candidiasis

Mucosal candidiasis has been associated with HIV disease from the initial description of early cases, and is the most common opportunistic fungal infection in HIV-positive patients. Oropharyngeal candidiasis is a marker for immunologic dysfunction and is also a prognostic marker for the development of other subsequent OI in HIV-infected patients [255].

General Epidemiology

Candida species are ubiquitous fungi, and candidiasis is the most frequent fungal OI in association with HIV. Up to 90% of HIV-infected patients will develop oropharyngeal candidiasis at some stage of their disease [24]. Oral candida colonization occurs more frequently in HIV-positive patient in comparison with noninfected ones; it is significantly more common in patients with CD4 cell counts of <200 cells/mm^3, and a low CD4 count also seems to be associated with a higher density of yeast in the saliva of HIV patients [24, 188].

Etiopathogenesis

The genus *Candida* comprises yeast-like fungi that can form true hyphae and pseudohyphae. This genus consists of approximately 200 species, of which about 20 have been linked to human mycosis [57]. The species of clinical interest are *Candida albicans*, *C. parapsilosis*, *C. tropicalis*, *C. glabrata*, *C. krusei*, *C. guilliermondii*, and *C. lusitaniae*. However, several cases of superficial and invasive diseases and emerging species of *Candida* have been described [57, 230]. Less common species are more prevalent among HIV-infected patients, and some strains have showed decreased susceptibility to antifungal agents [206, 219]. Host defects play a significant role in the development of candidal infections. The intact skin constitutes a highly effective barrier to *Candida* penetration, and disruption of the skin allows invasion by colonizing opportunistic organisms. In addition, intravascular devices provide an efficient pathway that bypasses the skin barrier. The major defense mechanisms operating at the mucosal level to maintain colonization and prevent invasion include normal protective bacterial flora and cell-mediated immunity [291]. Candidiasis in HIV patients is strongly related to impaired anti-*Candida* defense mechanisms, both local and systemic, owing to the immunodeficiency [255].

Clinical Presentation

Candida infections can present in a wide spectrum of clinical syndromes, depending on the site of infection and the degree of immunosuppression of the host [291]. Oropharyngeal and esophageal candidiasis are the most common forms in HIV-infected patients, and *Candida* colonization of the oral cavity is a predisposing factor for the development of oral candidiasis in these patients [188]. The pseudomembranous is the most common form of oropharyngeal candidiasis and appears as white plaques, usually asymptomatic, on the buccal mucosa, palate, tongue, or oropharynx. The plaques can easily be rubbed off, a characteristic that distinguishes candidiasis from oral hairy leukoplakia, which presents fixed lesions. Less frequent forms of oral candidiasis are the acute atrophic stomatitis (midline glossitis), which refers to symmetric lesions on the dorsum of the tongue characterized by loss of papillae and erythema, and also the angular cheilitis (perlèche) that is characterized by soreness, erythema, and fissuring at the corners of the mouth [291]. The esophageal candidiasis is an AIDS-defining illness (CDC 1993), usually occurring at a much lower CD4 count and presenting with odynophagia or dysphagia. Candidal intertrigo affects the flexural folds in groins, genitals, armpits, under breasts, and abdominal folds. The pruritic erythematous patches can be seen at moist intertriginous areas, surrounded by slight scales and/or tiny pustules (Fig. 41.27). Candidal balanitis can present as itchy white patches on the glans penis, and the infection can also spread to the perigenital areas. Features of *Candida* vulvovaginitis, are nonmalodorous whitish vaginal discharge, pruritus, dysuria, and dyspareunia [218]. *Candida* vulvovaginitis, even if more frequent in HIV-infected

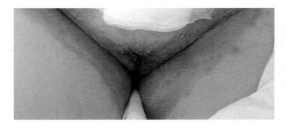

Fig. 41.27 Candidal intertrigo: pruritic erythematous patches in moist flexural folds

women, is clinically similar to that in HIV-negative women and does not appear to be of increased clinical severity [290]. *Candida* are true opportunistic pathogens that can gain access to the vascular circulation and deep tissues through technological devices (e.g., indwelling catheters) affecting high-risk patients who are either immunocompromised or critically ill and causing hematogenous dissemination of the yeast and disseminated candidiasis [291]. Cutaneous features are polymorphic in disseminated candidiasis and include erythematous macules, papules, pustules, and hemorrhagic or ulcerative lesions, or even abscesses.

Complementary Examinations

Typical aspects of most superficial *Candida* infections are quite characteristic to suggest the clinical diagnosis. Diagnosis is confirmed trough the visualization of budding yeast, with or without pseudohyphae, under microscopic examination of scrapings and smears, the addition of potassium hydroxide (KOH) 20%, or Gram stain.

Yeast culture is not usually performed, except for the resistant and recurrent cases. Although other forms of candidiasis should alert the physician to the possibility of underlying HIV infection, thus prompting them for HIV testing, routine screening for HIV is not recommended for women with vulvovaginal candidiasis unless other risk factors are present [292].

Therapeutic Approach

Treatment of candidiasis is variable and depends on the anatomic location of the infection, the patient's immune status, and risk factors for infection; and, in some cases, the *Candida* species as well as the susceptibility of the strain to antifungal drugs (Table 41.8) [291]. Detailed information regarding to the management of *Candida* infections can be found in specific and updated guidelines [57, 230]. Mild forms of candidiasis can be managed with local therapy. Cutaneous candidiasis can be treated with topical antifungal

Table 41.8 Treatment of candidiasis in HIV/AIDS patients

Candidiasis	Drug	Regimen
Cutaneous, mild	Topical antifungal agents[a]	Once or twice per day for 2 weeks or until clearance
Oropharyngeal, mild	Topical GV solution	0.00165%, bid for 7–14 days
	Nystatin suspension	100,000 U/mL, 4–6 mL, 4 times daily, for 7–14 days (swish for at least 2 min and swallow)
	Clotrimazole	One 10-mg troche 5 times daily, for 7–14 days
Moderate to severe; recurrent candidiasis; CD4 count <100/mm³	Fluconazole[b]	200 mg PO on first day, then 100–200 mg daily for 7–14 days
Esophageal	Fluconazole[b]	200–400 mg (3–6 mg/kg) PO daily for 14–21 days
		OR
		IV, 400 mg (6 mg/kg) daily; consider de-escalating to oral therapy as above once the patient is able to tolerate oral intake
VVGC, uncomplicated	Topical antifungal agents **OR**	Nystatin, daily, for 10–14 days **OR**
		Azoles, daily, for 3–5 days
	Fluconazole[b]	150 mg PO single dose
VVGC, compromised host	Fluconazole[b]	150 mg, PO two to three sequential doses 72 h apart
VVGC, recurrent	Induction therapy	Topical Azoles, daily, for 7–14 days **OR**
		Fluconazole 150 mg, PO 2 to 3 sequential doses, 72 h apart
	Maintenance therapy	Fluconazole 150 mg PO weekly for 6 months
VVGC, pregnancy	Clotrimazole or miconazole	Topical, daily for 7 days

Colombo et al. [57], Mukherjee et al. [201], Pappas et al. [230], Sobel [291, 292]
bid twice daily, *GV* gentian violet, *IV* intravenous, *PO* orally, *VVGC* vulvovaginal candidiasis
[a]Azoles, allylamines, butenafine, ciclopirox, and nystatin (no one agent superior to another) [230]
[b]Pregnancy: azoles should not be used during the first trimester

agents such asazoles, allylamines, butenafine, ciclopirox, and nystatin. The Cochrane HIV/AIDS Group evaluated the effects of interventions in treating oral candidiasis in children and adults with HIV infection. The study found no difference with regard to clinical cure between fluconazole and ketoconazole, itraconazole, and clotrimazole. Fluconazole, gentian violet, and ketoconazole were superior to nystatin. Continuous fluconazole was better than intermittent treatment [241]. Gentian violet solution at the concentration of 0.00165% does not stain the oral mucosa, is stable, and possesses potent antifungal activity; additionally it is an affordable option for the treatment of oropharyngeal candidiasis in HIV-infected patients in resource-limited settings [133, 201]. Vulvovaginal candidiasis in HIV-positive women can be treated by conventional methods including the use of maintenance suppressive antifungal therapy [292]. Systemic therapy with fluconazole is recommended for moderate to severe candidiasis, recurrent disease, and for immunosuppressed patients, because of the risk of esophageal candidiasis. In HIV-infected patients, ART appears to reduce the incidence of recurrent oral *Candida* infections and also to protect against vaginal colonization and candidal vulvovaginitis [4, 188, 230].

Dermatophytosis

Dermatophytosis (*tinea*) is a superficial infection caused by dermatophytes, fungi with great affinity to keratin, which proliferates in tissues such as skin, hair, and nails. In HIV-infected patients, immunosuppression may favor frequent exacerbations of dermatophytosis.

General Epidemiology

Dermatophytes are found universally; however, their relative prevalence may vary in different geographic areas according to climatic conditions or host lifestyles ([117]; Segal 2015). Dermatophytes can be transmitted via direct or indirect contact and there are three attributed sources of infection: humans (anthropophilic fungi); animals (zoophilic fungi), and soil (geophilic fungi). Population

mobility, changes in human lifestyle, population aging, and use of antifungal drugs have been responsible for the continuous change in the epidemiology of dermatophytes [211, 277]. The anthropophilic dermatophyte *Trichophyton rubrum* is the most common etiologic agent in dermatophytosis worldwide [211, 277] as well as among HIV-infected patients [60, 138, 258, 284].

Etiopathogenesis

The etiologic agents of dermatophytosis are filamentous fungi in the genera *Microsporum*, *Trichophyton*, and *Epidermophyton* [117, 211]. Keratinolytic enzymes are important virulence factors of some dermatophytes, which possess the ability to utilize keratin from human and animal tissues, or debris from dead animals found in soil [211, 277]. The three genera can infect humans, causing dermatophytosis involving skin, hair, and nails [277]. The term onychomycosis means a fungal nail infection caused by dermatophytes, yeasts, or molds (or a combination of them), whereas tinea unguium refers to onychomycosis caused by a dermatophyte [212]. Predisposing host factors such as disorders of cellular immunity and genetic predisposition, among other factors, play a role in the development of dermatophytosis, especially onychomycosis [211]. The host response to cutaneous fungal infection may be abnormal in patients with HIV. Although dermatophytosis is common in HIV-positive and AIDS patients, the degree of immunosuppression does not seems to correlate with increased risk of this fungal infection [258, 284].

Clinical Presentation

Dermatophyte infections lead to a variety of clinical manifestations: tinea corporis (infection of body surfaces other than the feet, groin, face, scalp hair, or beard hair); tinea manuum (infection of the hands, Fig. 41.28); tinea pedis (infection of the foot, Fig. 41.29); tinea cruris (infection of the groin); tinea capitis (infection of scalp hair); and tinea unguium or dermatophyte onychomycosis (infection of the nail, Figs. 41.29 and 41.30) [212]. Tinea often begins

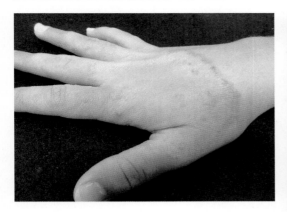

Fig. 41.28 Tinea manuum: erythematous plaque with well-defined edge with scale in the hand

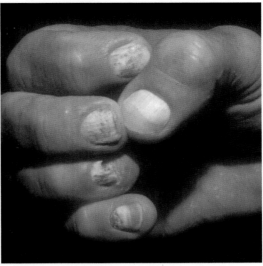

Fig. 41.30 Tinea unguium: dermatophyte onychomycosis affecting all fingernails

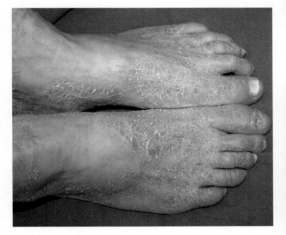

Fig. 41.29 Tinea pedis and tinea unguium: chronic dry, scaling lesions in a "moccasin pattern" on the foot; the patient also has a dermatophyte onychomycosis with nail dystrophy of all toenails

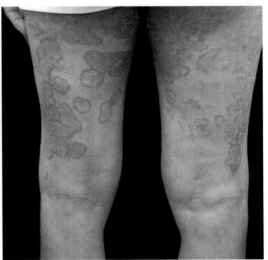

Fig. 41.31 Tinea corporis: multiple erythematous scaling plaques with an annular configuration

as a pruritic, circular, erythematous, scaly patch that spreads centrifugally. Central clearing coexists with an active border, resulting in the characteristic annular shape of tinea corporis (Fig. 41.31). Multiple plaques may coalesce and vesicles occasionally appear. Tinea pedis has three major clinical types: interdigital, hyperkeratotic ("moccasin-type," Fig. 41.29), and inflammatory vesiculobullous. The most common clinical manifestation of tinea capitis, which almost always occurs in small children, is that of scaly patches with alopecia. Although rare cases of tinea capitis have been reported in

HIV-infected adults [163, 207], children with AIDS are the most common cases and can present with severe tinea capitis (Fig. 41.32). Majocchi's granuloma is an example of dermal fungal involvement and is characterized by firm, violet-colored nodules and papules associated to onychomycosis, tinea corporis, or tinea pedis. Majocchi's granuloma may be precipitated by trauma to the skin or follicular occlusion; and

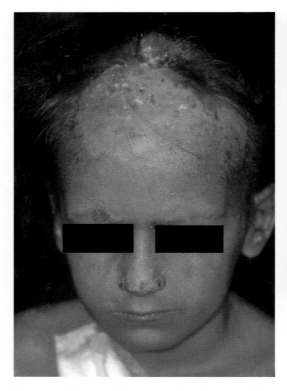

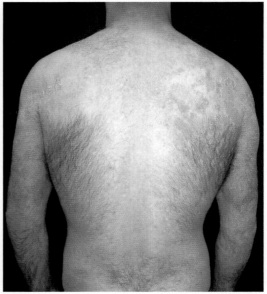

Fig. 41.33 Tinea corporis: anergic form with extensive scaling lesions in an immunosuppressed HIV-infected patient

Fig. 41.32 Tinea capitis: scaly patches with alopecia in a severely ill HIV-infected child

may also be favored by the immune dysfunction in immunosuppressed HIV patients [249]. There are several clinical subtypes of onychomycosis, and immunosuppressed patients with tinea unguium usually show involvement of multiple nails and total dystrophic onychomycosis (Figs. 41.29 and 41.30) ([60]; Surjushe et al. 2007). Dermatophytosis in HIV-infected patients can occur at some point during their illness; and tinea unguium and tinea pedis are the main clinical forms among HIV-infected patients [138, 258, 284]. Introduction of ART and prophylaxis with fluconazole for invasive fungal infection has reduced the incidence of dermatophytosis in HIV-positive individuals. However, dermatophytosis in these patients seems to present more frequently with atypical, multiple, extensive lesions and with little inflammation, called anergic forms (Fig. 41.33) [60, 132].

Complementary Examinations

The diagnosis of a cutaneous dermatophyte infection may be suspected based on the clinical findings. Nevertheless, atypical forms of *tinea* and onychomycosis should be confirmed by mycologic examination. Direct microscopic examination using KOH 20% aids in visualizing hyphae and spores, and confirming the diagnosis of dermatophyte infection [244]. A fungal culture allows the identification of dermatophyte species, and is useful when long-term oral therapy is being considered [113]. Though rarely used, DNA-based methods are effective for identifying mixed infections and quantification of fungal load.

Therapeutic Approach

Most dermatophyte infections can be managed with topical treatments. Effective topical antifungal agents include azoles, allylamines, ciclopirox, butenafine, tolnaftate, and amorolfine [71, 113, 139]. A meta-analysis evaluated the efficacy of antifungal treatment in the context of mycologic cure at the end of treatment and sustained cure. There were no statistically significant differences among the antifungals concerning the outcome of mycologic cure at the end of treatment. For sustained cure, butenafine and terbinafine were each found to be superior to clotrimazole, although the difference in efficacy was not significantly large between antifungal classes [266].

> **Box 41.7 Systemic Antifungals: Indications for Dermatophytosis**
> - Tinea capitis
> - Tinea unguium
> - Tinea involving more than one body region simultaneously (e.g., tinea cruris and corporis, or tinea cruris and tinea pedis)
> - Extensive tinea corporis
> - Tinea pedis with extensive involvement of the sole, heel, or dorsum of the foot or when there is recurring and troublesome blistering
> - Patients who fail topical therapy
>   Sahoo and Mahajan [269]

Oral antifungal therapy is the option for some forms of tinea, for extensive infections, or infections refractory to topical therapy (Box 41.7) [269]. Terbinafine and itraconazole are the preferred systemic agents; griseofulvin and fluconazole can also be effective, but may require longer-term therapy (Gupta 2008; [139, 269]). Table 41.9 shows therapeutic options and regimens for dermatophytosis. According to the Cochrane Skin Group, oral treatments including terbinafine, itraconazole, and fluconazole are at least similar to griseofulvin in children with tinea capitis caused by *Trichophyton* species; the evidence also suggests that terbinafine is more effective than griseofulvin in children with *Trichophyton surans* infection, whereas in children with *Microsporum* infections the effect of griseofulvin is better than terbinafine [48]. For tinea unguium, treatment options include topical and systemic antifungal drugs. Clinical subtype, causative organism, disease severity, treatment side effects, and cost may influence the choice of therapy. Advantages of topical

Table 41.9 Treatment of dermatophytosis

Disease	Drug/regimen	
Limited tinea pedis, corporis, or cruris	Topical antifungal agents[d]	Once or twice per day for 4 weeks or until clearance
Tinea corporis and cruris	Systemic antifungals[e]	Terbinafine 250 mg daily; 3-6 mg/kg/day, for 2–3 weeks
		Itraconazole 200 mg daily, for 1–2 weeks
		Fluconazole 150–300 mg once weekly, for 3–4 weeks
		Griseofulvin microsize 500–1000 mg daily **OR**
		Griseofulvin ultramicrosize 300–375 mg daily, for 2–4 weeks
Tinea pedis	Systemic antifungals[e]	Terbinafine: 250 mg daily, for 2 weeks
		Itraconazole: 200 mg twice daily, for 1 week **OR**
		Itraconazole: 100–200 mg daily, for 2–4 weeks
		Fluconazole: 150 mg once weekly, for 4 weeks
		Griseofulvin microsize 750–1000 mg daily **OR**
		Griseofulvin ultramicrosize 660 or 750 mg per day for 4–8 weeks
Tinea capitis (regimen for children)[a]	Systemic antifungals[e]	Griseofulvin microsize 20–25 mg/kg/day, for 6 to 12 weeks; maximum 1000 mg per day
		Griseofulvin ultramicrosize 10–15 mg/kg/day, for 6–12 weeks; maximum 750 mg per day
		Terbinafine:
		10 to 20 kg: 62.5 mg daily, for 4–6 weeks
		20 to 40 kg: 125 mg daily, for 4–6 weeks
		Above 40 kg: 250 mg daily, for 4–6 weeks
		Fluconazole: 6 mg/kg/day, for 3 weeks **OR** 6–8 mg/kg/week. for 8–12 weeks
		Itraconazole: 5 mg/kg/day, for 2–4 weeks

(continued)

Table 41.9 (continued)

Disease	Drug/regimen	
Majocchi's granuloma	Systemic antifungals[e]	Terbinafine 250 mg daily, for 2–4 weeks
		Itraconazole 200 mg twice daily for 1 week per month for 2 months
		Griseofulvin and daily itraconazole may also be used
Mild to moderate dermatophyte onychomycosis[b]	Topical antifungals	Efinaconazole 10% solution applied to the nails once daily for 12 months
		Amorolfine 5% nail lacquer once-weekly; fingernails for 6 months; toenails for 12 months
		Ciclopirox 8% nail lacquer applied to the nails once daily until nail clearance or up to 12 months
Moderate to severe dermatophyte onychomycosis[c]	Systemic antifungals[e]	Terbinafine 250 mg per day; fingernails for 6 weeks; toenails for 12 weeks
		Itraconazole pulse therapy: 200 mg twice daily for 1 week per month; fingernail for 2 months; toenail onychomycosis for 3 months
		Itraconazole continuous therapy: 200 mg per day; fingernail for 6 weeks; toenail onychomycosis for 12 weeks
		Fluconazole, 150–300 mg once weekly, for 6–12 months or longer[f]

Dias et al. [70, 71], Gupta and Cooper [109], Kelly [139], Piraccini and Alessandrini [244], Sahoo and Mahajan [269], Singal and Khanna [285], Welsh et al. [314]

[a]Fluconazole and itraconazole: alternative therapies, limited efficacy data for tinea capitis
[b]Distal lateral subungual onychomycosis involving ≤50% of the nail and sparing the matrix/lunula
[c]Involvement of >50% of the nail or of the matrix or lunula, proximal subungual or total dystrophic onychomycosis
[d]Azoles, allylamines, ciclopirox, butenafine, tolnaftate, amorolfine
[e]Pregnancy: oral azoles should not be used during the first trimester
[f]Not as effective or as cost-effective as itraconazole and terbinafine

therapy are the minor risk for drug interactions and adverse effects. However, topical antifungals have a limited efficacy if used without nail-plate debridement. A combination of both oral and systemic treatment is often the best choice [244]. Although initial therapy may result in complete or mycologic cure, relapse rates for onychomycosis remain high [109]. Box 41.8 displays topical monotherapy indications for onychomycosis [285].

Box 41.8 Topical Monotherapy Indications for Onychomycosis
- Involvement limited to distal 50% of nail plate, three or four nails involvement.
- No matrix area involvement.
- Superficial white onychomycosis (SWO).
- In children with thin, fast growing nails.
- Prophylaxis in patients at risk of recurrence.
- Patients for whom oral therapy is inappropriate.
  Singal and Khanna [285]

Periodic mechanical removal of the affected nail plate is recommended during the treatment. A nail clipper can be used for remove onycholysis. When several nails are involved and/or there is a lot of thickening, referral to an experienced podiatrist is advisable in order to avoid local injuries [314]. There is no specific guideline available for managing dermatophytic infection in HIV-infected patients and treatment should be individualized and based upon risk-benefit ratio. Due to possible associated comorbidities and drug interactions with several antiretroviral drugs the choice of systemic oral antifungal agent should be cautiously evaluated in HIV patients. Terbinafine clearance is significantly reduced in patients with renal failure and itraconazole should be avoided in hepatic impairment. In comparison with nontreated HIV patients, those under effective ART tend to have less frequent dermatophyte epidermal and nail infections, have infections that clear without specific antifungal therapy, respond better to antifungal therapy, and experience fewer recurrences [132].

Cryptococcosis

Cryptococcosis is an infectious disease with worldwide distribution and a wide array of clinical presentations caused by pathogenic encapsulated yeasts in the genus *Cryptococcus* [184]. Cryptococcal infections are extremely rare in people who are otherwise healthy; most cases occur in immunosuppressed patients, particularly those who have advanced HIV/AIDS.

General Epidemiology

Given the distribution of infections there are differences in the ecology of *Cryptococcus* species. *Cryptococcus neoformans* has been found worldwide, while *Cryptococcus gattii* is endemic in tropical and subtropical areas [45]. HIV infection is the major underlying condition predisposing to the development of cryptococcosis, which presents as a disseminated disease, usually when the CD4 count is <100 cells/mm^3 [11]. Up to 10% of HIV-seropositive individuals with disseminated cryptococcosis develop mucocutaneous lesions [45]. The extrapulmonary cryptococcosis is an AIDS-defining illness (CDC 1993).

Etiopathogenesis

Cryptococcus is a genus of basidiomycetous fungi containing more than 30 species. However, the common pathogenic organisms of cryptococcosis currently consist of two species with a predilection for the respiratory and nervous system of humans and animals. The two species, *C. neoformans* and *C. gattii*, are distinguishable biochemically and by molecular techniques, and there are also important species- and strain-specific differences with respect to geographic distribution, environmental niches, host predilection, and clinical manifestations [184]. Cryptococcosis is acquired through inhalation of basidiospores or desiccated yeast cells from the environment, and rarely by cutaneous route. The infection may be cleared, become latent, cause pulmonary infection, or disseminate, typically to the CNS. The factors that determine whether an exposed person develops symptomatic infection are uncertain but may include the inoculum of fungi (e.g., burden of exposure), virulence factors of the infecting strain, and impairment of cellular immunity [257].

Clinical Presentation

Cryptococcal infection is primary pulmonary, although in immune impaired hosts it can cause systemic illness, mainly affecting the CNS. Cutaneous infections are the third most common clinical manifestations of cryptococcosis [45]. The involvement of the skin is mostly secondary to hematogenous dissemination of the fungus and may act as a marker for disseminated infection, especially in patients with impaired cell-mediated immunity, such as HIV-infected patients. In disseminated cutaneous cryptococcosis the skin lesions can anticipate systemic signs of cryptococcosis and include the typical "molluscum-like" lesions (papules with central ulceration), nodules, abscesses, cellulitis, draining sinuses, ulcers, acneiform lesions, and vasculitic lesions, among others [45, 142, 205, 247]. Primary cutaneous cryptococcosis (PCC) is a distinct epidemiologic and clinical entity with a favorable prognosis even for immunocompromised hosts [213]. Most PCC is associated with local trauma and direct inoculation, and its dermatologic manifestations, usually confined to one body region, are protean and might mimic other cutaneous diseases: a single lesion at the site of infection, solitary nodule, plaque, ulcer, cellulitis, abscesses, and a sporotrichoid pattern have been described [45, 130, 213, 214]. In the case series published by Marques et al., PCC lesions presented more frequently as an infiltrative plaque or tumoral mass with a gelatinous consistency [172]. Cryptococcosis may also occur during IRIS in HIV-infected patients [112].

Complementary Examinations

Definitive diagnosis of cryptococcosis is made by isolation of *Cryptococcus* from a clinical specimen or direct detection of the fungus by means of India ink staining of body fluids [11]. The fungus can be cultured from biological samples such as CSF, sputum, and skin biopsy on routine fungal culture media [184]. *Cryptococcus* can be identified by histologic staining of skin and other tissues. The yeast is best identified by special stains that label the polysaccharide capsule including mucicarmine, periodic acid-Schiff (PAS), and Alcian blue stains [184]. Serologic tests for detection of the cryptococcal polysaccharide capsular antigen can be performed with both serum and CSF using latex agglutination and enzyme immunoassay techniques, whose overall sensitivity and specificity are 93%–100% and 93%–98%, respectively [184].

Therapeutic Approach

Treating disseminated cryptococcosis consists of three phases: induction, consolidation, and maintenance therapy [236]. Table 41.12 shows recommended regimens by the WHO and by the United States Panel on OI in HIV infection [227, 228, 320]. The optimal antifungal regimen for non-

meningeal, nonpulmonary cryptococcosis has not been determined. In general, the suggested therapy is based on extrapolation from literature describing management of immunocompromised patients with mild to moderate pulmonary cryptococcosis in the absence of disseminated infection. Two recommended regimens are displayed in Table 41.10 [227, 228, 320]. Azole antifungals should be avoided during the first trimester of pregnancy. In HIV-infected patients with successfully treated cryptococcal disease, discontinuation of antifungal maintenance treatment is recommended when patients are stable and adherent to ART and antifungal maintenance treatment

Table 41.10 Treatment of cryptococcosis in HIV/AIDS patients

Drug	Regimen	Duration
Disseminated disease (Panel on OI in HIV recommendation)		
Induction therapy		
Liposomal amphotericin B[a] *plus*	3–4 mg/kg daily, IV	For 2 weeks
Flucytosine[a] **OR**	100 mg/kg PO daily in 4 divided doses	
Amphotericin B deoxycholate[a] *plus*	0.7-1 mg/kg daily, IV	For 2 weeks
Flucytosine[a] **OR**	100 mg/kg PO daily in 4 divided doses	
Amphotericin B (either liposomal or deoxycholate) *plus*	As above	For 2 weeks
Fluconazole[b] **OR**	800 mg PO daily	
Fluconazole[b] *plus*	400–800 mg daily	For 2 weeks
Flucytosine[a]	100 mg/kg PO daily in 4 divided doses	
Consolidation therapy		
Fluconazole[b]	400 mg PO daily	For 8 weeks
Maintenance therapy[c]		
Fluconazole[b]	200 mg PO daily	For at least 12 months
Alternative drug: Itraconazole[b,d]	200 mg PO daily	For at least 12 months
Disseminated disease (WHO recommendation)		
Induction therapy (for 2 weeks)	*Consolidation therapy* (for 8 weeks)	
Amphotericin B deoxycholate[a] 0.7–1 mg/kg daily, *plus* flucytosine[a] 100 mg/kg daily in 4 divided doses **OR**	Fluconazole[b] 400–800 mg daily	
Amphotericin B deoxycholate[a] 0.7–1 mg/kg daily, *plus* fluconazole[b] 800 mg daily **OR**		
Amphotericin B deoxycholate[a] 0.7–1 mg/kg/day short course (5–7 days), *plus* fluconazole[b] 800 mg daily for 2 weeks **OR**	Fluconazole[b] 800 mg daily	
Fluconazole[b] 1200 mg/day *plus* flucytosine 100 mg/kg/day **OR**		
Fluconazole[b] 1200 mg/day alone		
Maintenance therapy[d]		
Fluconazole[b] 200 mg daily, for at least 12 months		

Table 41.10 (continued)

Drug	Regimen	Duration
Localized nonmeningeal disease		
WHO recommendation	Panel on OI in HIV recommendation	
Induction therapy	Fluconazole[b] 400 mg daily, for 12 months	
Fluconazole[b] 800 mg daily, for 2 weeks (or 12 mg/kg/day up to 800 mg/day if <19 years)		
Consolidation therapy		
Fluconazole[b] 400 mg daily, for 8 weeks (or 6 mg/kg/day up to 400–800 mg/day if <19 years)		
Maintenance therapy[c]		
Fluconazole[b] 200 mg daily, for at least 12 months		

Panel on Opportunistic Infections in HIV [227, 228] and WHO [320]

Recommendations are listed in decreasing order of preference

Consider to delay initiation of ART by 2–4 weeks after starting antifungal therapy

Route of administration: amphotericin B (IV); flucytosine (oral); fluconazole (oral and IV)

ART antiretroviral therapy, *IV* intravenous, *OI* opportunistic infection, *PO* orally

[a]Monitor renal function

[b]Azole antifungals should be avoided during the first trimester of pregnancy

[c]Efficacy inferior to fluconazole

[d]Lifelong maintenance therapy in patients who do not attain immune recovery under ART

for at least 1 year, and have a CD4 cell count of ≥200 cells/mm^3 (two measurements 6 months apart), or else when patient has a CD4 cell count ≥100 cells/mm^3 (two measurements 6 months apart) and a suppressed viral load for at least 3 months [227, 228, 320]. The optimal time to begin ART and antifungal therapy is not established for forms other than cryptococcal meningitis; considering the risk of IRIS it would seem judicious to delay initiation of ART by 2–4 weeks after starting antifungal therapy [227, 228].

Histoplasmosis

Histoplasmosis, a systemic fungal infection caused by *Histoplasma capsulatum*, is the most common endemic mycosis in AIDS patients. The risk of disease in some HIV-infected populations has declined with effective ART; however, it still causes severe morbidity and mortality in resource-limited settings of endemic areas [210].

General Epidemiology

Histoplasmosis is mainly found in temperate zones worldwide and is more prevalent in certain regions of America, Africa, and Asia. In highly endemic areas, up to 20% of HIV-infected persons will develop disseminated histoplasmosis [177]. Owing to the increase in travel and immigration, histoplasmosis has also been diagnosed in nonendemic areas [1, 177, 215, 226]. The fungus inhabits acidic soils rich in organic matter, particularly with birds and bat excreta, and transmission occurs via inhalation of fungal spores from the soil [317]. Histoplasmosis is considered as an AIDS-defining illness (CDC 1992) [39].

Etiopathogenesis

There are two identified species of dimorphic fungus associated with histoplasmosis: *H. capsulatum* var. *capsulatum*, which is the classic and HIV-associated histoplasmosis agent, and *H. capsulatum* var. *duboisii*, which causes African histoplasmosis [317]. The infection is primarily acquired via inhalation of fungal spores present in nature, which is followed by conversion into the yeast (pathogenic) fungal form at human body temperature [317]. The infection primarily affects the lungs causing localized pneumonitis, followed by hematogenous spread and cell-mediated immune response. Spontaneous resolution usually occurs in 95% of the patients, while in AIDS patients the infection can progress or become reactivated when CD4 levels decrease [257].

Clinical Presentation

Infection may range from asymptomatic presentation to disseminated disease, the latter affecting mostly immunocompromised individuals, particularly those infected with HIV [123]. AIDS patients usually develop progressive disseminated histoplasmosis, a febrile, wasting illness [17]. Mucocutaneous involvement is a common manifestation of disseminated histoplasmosis in HIV-infected patients with CD4 count of <50/mm³. Skin and mucosal lesions can occur with a variable prevalence, uncommon in the United States (<10%), while representing 38–85% of reported AIDS cases in Latin America [62]. A wide spectrum of skin lesions is observed, including disseminated papules, plaques, and nodules with and without crusts, in a diffuse pattern of distribution (Fig. 41.34), more marked on the face. Morphologic variability of lesions seems to be associated with higher CD4 cell counts [62]. Other findings can be seen, such as macules, papulopustules, necrosis, and molluscum-like lesions (Fig. 41.35) [220]. Up to two-thirds of patients experience mucosal involvement, particularly in the oropharyngeal region [257]. Primary skin lesions are uncommon in histoplasmosis. As with other HIV-related systemic mycoses, skin manifestations can be part of histoplasmosis-related IRIS, after starting ART [34].

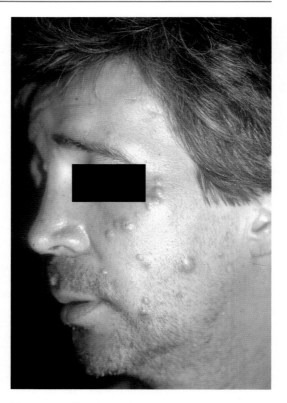

Fig. 41.35 Histoplasmosis: molluscum-like papules on the face

Complementary Examinations

Laboratory observations used to support diagnosis of disseminated histoplasmosis include investigation of anemia, leukopenia, thrombocytopenia, abnormal liver enzymes, elevated lactate dehydrogenase, and ferritin [257]. There are multiple diagnostic tests for disseminated *H. capsulatum* infection, including culture, serology, antigen testing, and direct microscopy. Definitive diagnosis is based on histopathology and/or the isolation of *H. capsulatum* in culture of clinical specimens, such as cutaneous, respiratory, peripheral blood, and bone marrow samples [136]. Limitations of culture are its time-consuming character and the usually low sensitivity (<60–85%, depending on the fungal load, the type of sample, and laboratory skills) [123]. Antibody detection by immunodiffusion or complement fixation has low sensitivity (50–70%) in immunocompromised HIV-infected patients [317]. Enzyme immunoassay methods can detect *H. capsulatum* polysaccharide antigens on several samples (urine, serum, CSF, and bron-

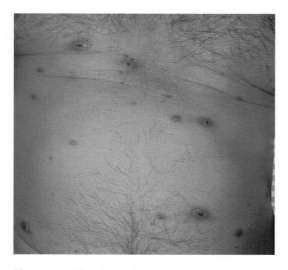

Fig. 41.34 Histoplasmosis: disseminated erythematous papules with central crusts

choalveolar fluid) allowing for a rapid and noninvasive diagnosis [123]. A recent diagnostic meta-analysis on the performance of *Histoplasma* antigens has revealed a high specificity (98%) and sensitivity (81%) for antigen detection in both urine and serum [79]. A simple and less expensive test (not definitive) is the direct microscopy of skin lesions scrapings or body fluids, stained with Giemsa or PAS stain, in order to visualize budding yeasts. Although histopathologic study with specific stains is very helpful, culture is still the gold standard for diagnosis [257].

Therapeutic Approach

Since morbidity and mortality associated with disseminated histoplasmosis remains high in patients who are not under treatment for HIV infection, ART should be initiated as soon as possible to recover cellular immunity. Disseminated histoplasmosis in the HIV-infected host is fatal without therapy [316]. Management includes a phase of induction therapy, followed by long-term maintenance (Table 41.11). The treatment is chosen according to disease severity and immune status. Patients with severe immunosuppression,

Table 41.11 Treatment of histoplasmosis in HIV/AIDS patients

Moderately severe to severe disease	Mild disease
Induction therapy	*Induction and maintenance therapy*[a,b]
Liposomal amphotericin B, 3 mg/kg/day, IV, for 2 weeks or until clinically improved; **OR**	Itraconazole 200 mg PO tid for 3 days, followed by 200 mg bid for at least 12 months
Amphotericin B deoxycholate 0.7 mg/kg daily, IV, for 2 weeks or until clinically improved	
Maintenance therapy[a, b]	
Itraconazole 200 mg PO tid for 3 days, followed by 200 mg bid for at least 12 months	

Panel on Opportunistic Infections in HIV [227, 228], and Wheat et al. [316]
Initiate ART as soon as possible
ART antiretroviral therapy, *bid* two times daily, *tid* three times daily, *IV* intravenous
[a]Do not use alternative agents to itraconazole
[b]Lifelong maintenance therapy with itraconazole in patients who do not attain immune recovery on ART

disseminated disease, organ dysfunction, or pancytopenia are classified as having moderately severe to severe disease and require amphotericin B as the first-choice drug. Patients with mild disease and a single focus of histoplasmosis (other than CNS) have mild to moderate disease and can receive oral itraconazole. Suppressive therapy is mandatory in patients who continue to be immunosuppressed and itraconazole is the preferred oral azole. Monitoring of patients can be attained by checking antigen levels quarterly during therapy to assess treatment response [227, 228, 316]. Antigen monitoring during suppressive therapy is not routinely recommended.

Sporotrichosis

Sporotrichosis is a granulomatous subcutaneous mycosis that has a worldwide distribution and several clinical manifestations. It remains a relevant public health problem in endemic areas, affecting a large at-risk population, which includes HIV-infected individuals. HIV infection aggravates the course of sporotrichosis, leading to a higher incidence of severe disseminated cases and a higher number of hospitalizations and deaths [88, 97].

General Epidemiology

Sporotrichosis is an endemic disease prevalent worldwide in tropical and subtropical areas; and its ecology, epidemiology, and clinical features vary across different geographic regions [43, 250]. The mycosis has a high prevalence in Latin America, especially in Brazil, Peru, and Colombia, and is also endemic in India, China, Japan, and South Africa [5]. Infections are usually sporadic and caused by traumatic inoculation of decaying plant matter, hay, soil, and sphagnum moss, but outbreaks have been associated with traumatic skin injury or with zoonotic spread from infected animals, especially domestic cats [19, 102]. Sporotrichosis may be the initial presentation of HIV infection in 27% of cases [197], and the coinfection is associated with poor outcome [88, 197].

Etiopathogenesis

The *Sporothrix schenckii* complex members, which are dimorphic fungi, cause sporotrichosis.

The virulence-related phenotypes are variably expressed within the multiple cryptic species and might be involved in the wide spectrum of clinical aspects of the disease [5].

Clinical Presentation

A wide spectrum of clinical manifestations is observed in sporotrichosis, ranging from cutaneous, subcutaneous, and disseminated cutaneous forms to pulmonary or systemic presentations (Almeida-Paes 2015). Several factors may influence the clinical presentations of sporotrichosis: the immunologic status of the host, the load and depth of the inoculum, and the pathogenicity of the strain, among others [19]. In cutaneous forms, the infection usually appears after minor trauma. After penetrating through the skin, the fungus converts into the yeast form and may remain localized in the subcutaneous tissue [19]. The initial presentation of sporotrichosis is a papule at the site of injury, which becomes a nodule that usually ulcerates but may remain nodular with overlying erythema or erythematosquamous lesion, constituting the fixed form of sporotrichosis. Weeks after development of the primary lesion, similar lesions may subsequently occur

along the lymphatic path proximal to the original lesion, a characteristic named "sporotrichoid" pattern or "ascending nodular lymphangitis" (Fig. 41.36). The lymphocutaneous form is the most frequent form of sporotrichosis. Osteoarticular and pulmonary involvement accounts for some of the extracutaneous forms [274]. Eventually, the fungi may spread through hematogenous route, characterizing the disseminated cutaneous form, which typically presents as subcutaneous nodules and has mainly been observed among immunosuppressed patients, especially HIV-infected individuals. On rare occasions, inhalation of conidia may lead to a systemic disease. Disseminated cutaneous forms have been observed among immunosuppressed patients, especially HIV-infected individuals [88]. A recent systematic review on published data of HIV-associated sporotrichosis, performed by Moreira et al., found a low median CD4 count (97 cells/mm^3) and 30% mortality rate among 58 patients [197]. Although the skin is the most commonly affected organ, multiorgan dissemination is more frequent in the coinfection, probably due to underlying HIV-related immunosuppression; additionally, a tropism for the CNS occurs

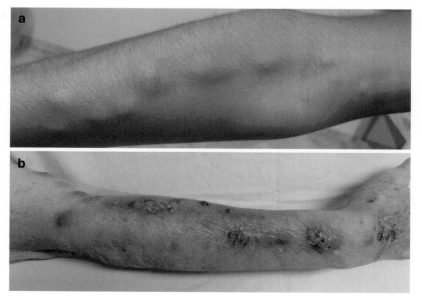

Fig. 41.36 Lymphocutaneous sporotrichosis. Nodules (**a**) and nodulo-ulcerative lesions (**b**) along lymphatic path proximal to the original lesion ("sporotrichoid" pattern or "ascending nodular lymphangitis") in the arm and forearm (Photograph **a** courtesy of Dr. Andre Avelino Costa Beber, Hospital Universitário de Santa Maria, Brazil)

and is almost always fatal [88, 197]. IRIS-associated sporotrichosis accounted for 7.5% of cases, and such AIDS-patients were severely immunosuppressed and had a high HIV viral load at baseline (pre-ART), showing new disease manifestations or reactivation of pre-existing lesions in a median time of 4 weeks after ART initiation [197]. Based on the characteristics of the coinfection sporotrichosis/HIV, some authors have considered *Sporothrix* spp. as an opportunistic pathogen and have suggested the inclusion of disseminated sporotrichosis as an AIDS-defining illness in endemic areas for this mycosis [88, 93, 197].

Complementary Examinations

Culture is the gold standard for establishing a diagnosis of sporotrichosis; it is the most sensitive method and samples include aspirated material from a lesion, tissue biopsy, sputum, or body fluids [19]. Laboratory tools for diagnosis of sporotrichosis also include direct and histopathologic examination aided by special stains. The histology shows a mixed suppurative and granu-lomatous inflammatory reaction in the dermis and subcutaneous tissue, frequently accompanied by microabscess and fibrosis. The organisms, with characteristic "cigar-shaped" buds, may eventually not be visualized even with special stains, such as Gomori methenamine silver and PAS, because of the paucity of yeasts in lesions [19]. Serology is not used routinely in the diagnosis of sporotrichosis.

Therapeutic Approach

The choice of antifungal drug in patients with sporotrichosis is limited, and Table 41.12 lists the available options and regimens. Itraconazole is currently the first-choice treatment for cutaneous and lymphocutaneous forms of sporotrichosis and as suppressive therapy in immunocompromised patients after induction with amphotericin B [19]. Amphotericin B is the preferred agent for initial treatment of disseminated forms, especially in immunocompromised individuals [135]. In the case series reported by Freitas et al., itraconazole was noted to be effective in several sporotrichosis/HIV-coinfected patients who had the

Table 41.12 Treatment of sporotrichosis

	Preferred treatment	Alternative treatment
Disseminated disease	Liposomal amphotericin 3–5 mg/kg/day IV, until improvement	Amphotericin B deoxycholate 0.7–1 mg/kg/day IV, until improvement
	Maintenance therapy[a]: itraconazole 200 mg PO bid, for a total of at least 12 months	
Cutaneous or lymphocutaneous	Itraconazole 200 mg PO daily	Itraconazole 200 mg PO bid[b]; **OR**
		Terbinafine 500 mg PO bid; **OR**
		SSKI PO with increasing doses; **OR**
		Fluconazole 400–800 mg/day PO; **OR**
		Local hyperthermia
	Maintenance therapy: treatment for 2–4 weeks after lesions have resolved	
Pregnant women	*Severe sporotrichosis*	When possible, defer treatment to post delivery
	Liposomal amphotericin 3–5 mg/kg/day IV; **OR** amphotericin B deoxycholate 0.7–1 mg/kg/day IV	
	Lymphocutaneous or cutaneous sporotrichosis	
	Local hyperthermia	
Children	*Severe sporotrichosis*	SSKI with increasing doses equivalent to half the adult dose
	Amphotericin B deoxycholate 0.7–1 mg/kg/day IV	
	Lymphocutaneous or cutaneous sporotrichosis	
	Itraconazole 6–10 mg/kg/day PO, until maximum of 400 mg/day	

Panel on Opportunistic Infections in HIV [227, 228], and Kauffman et al. [135]
Consider to delay initiation of ART by 2–4 weeks after starting antifungal therapy
ART antiretroviral therapy, *bid* twice daily, *IV* intravenous, *PO* orally, *SSKI* saturated solution potassium iodide
[a]Long-term maintenance therapy with itraconazole in patients who do not attain immune recovery on ART
[b]Dose of 400 mg/day PO should be administered for cutaneous forms with a poor initial response to a lower dosage

disseminated form [87]. Although the exact mechanism of action remains unknown, potassium iodide has been traditionally used in the treatment of sporotrichosis with satisfactory results (Casta et al. 2013; [248]). However, its efficacy is not established in immunosuppressed patients. In a saturated solution of potassium iodide (SSKI) one drop is equivalent to 50 mg of SSKI; the recommended dose in adults is 250 mg or five drops of SSKI, with increments of three drops (150 mg)/dose daily until a maximum dose of 30–40 drops (1.5–2.0 g) three times a day, or until the patient experiences unpleasant side effects. In children, the recommended dose is three drops three times a day, increasing by one drop per kilogram per dose to a maximum of 25 drops three times a day [248]. Treatment is limited by side effects including gastrointestinal disturbance, rash, salivary gland enlargement, metallic taste, and thyroid dysfunction [248]. Potassium iodide and itraconazole are contraindicated in pregnant women, and thermotherapy can be used for these patients, with daily application of local heat (42–43 °C) through a hot water bag, a source of infrared, or a similar method until healing of lesions [19, 135]. Sporotrichosis/HIV-coinfected patients should receive suppressive therapy with itraconazole until immune system recovery, and it seems reasonable to discontinue therapy for those who have been treated with itraconazole for at least 1 year and whose CD4 cell counts have remained >200 cells/mm^{3}for at least 1 year [135]. The impact of and the best time for ART initiation during sporotrichosis infection are unknown. Moreira et al. have pointed that ART should be delayed in high-risk patients (CNS disease, low CD4 cell count and high viral load) because of predisposition to IRIS-related meningeal sporotrichosis [197].

Ectoparasitic Infestations

Scabies

Scabies is an infestation of the skin caused by the mite *Sarcoptes scabiei* resulting in an intensely itchy rash with a characteristic distribution pattern.

General Epidemiology

The prevalence of scabies undergoes cyclical fluctuations on a worldwide basis. A recently published systematic review has found a wide range of scabies prevalence worldwide (North America data not available): from 0.2% to 71.4%. In all regions except for Europe and the Middle East the prevalence was greater than 10%. Overall, scabies prevalence was highest in the Pacific and Latin American regions [261]. Scabies affects individuals of different ages, races, and socioeconomic conditions. It is more prevalent in crowded conditions and is primarily transmitted through close personal contact, whereas fomite transmission may occur only rarely [66, 107].

Etiopathogenesis

Human scabies is caused by the mite *S. scabiei* var. *hominis*. The incubation period varies from days to months, and is about 3–6 weeks when the first infection occurs [107]. Pruritus and rash occur as the result of a delayed type-IV hypersensitivity reaction to mite proteins in mite saliva, feces, eggs, and the mite itself. For this reason, signs and symptoms of infestation, such as pruritus and rash, typically develop 3–4 weeks after primary exposure, or 1–2 days after re-exposure [66, 262].

Clinical Presentation

The main symptom of scabies is the intense pruritus, which is accentuated at night and after bathing [107]. The characteristic skin lesions are erythematous dome-shaped 2 - to 3-mm papules, linear excoriations, burrows, and eventually, nodules (Fig. 41.37). The pathognomonic finding is the burrow, a short erythematous pink or white linear papule, resulting from a female mite penetrating and burrowing into the skin (Fig. 41.37). Lesions are most frequently found in the finger webs or on flexor surfaces of the wrists, on the elbows, axillae, buttocks, areolae, and genitalia in adults (Fig. 41.38), or on the face, neck, hands, and feet in infants [107, 173]. Immunosuppressed patients may develop crusted scabies (CS), which is an atypical highly contagious disease caused by hyperinfestation [107]. The initial clinical picture of CS presents erythematous plaques that rapidly evolve to thick crusts, predominating in

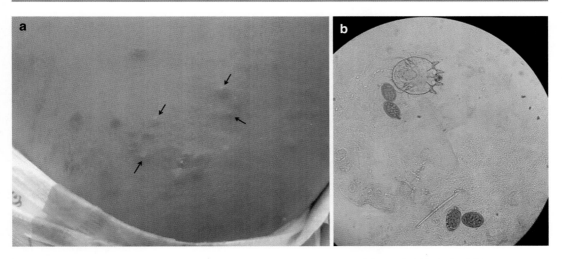

Fig. 41.37   Scabies: pruritic papules and burrows (*arrows*) (**a**); mite, ova, and feces (tiny black dots) (**b**)

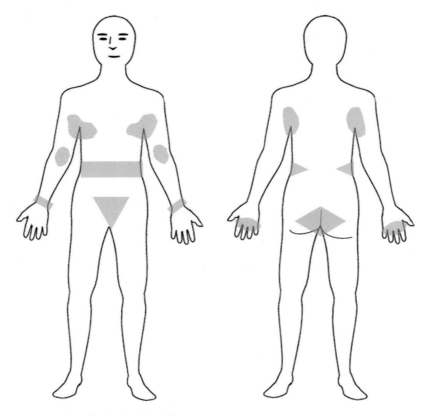

Fig. 41.38   Topography of scabies lesions in adults

the palmoplantar and subungual regions; generalized erythematous scaling eruptions (Fig. 41.39) and scalp involvement may spread leading to erythroderma. Pruritus is mild or absent in CS because of impairment of the host's immune response. The CS/HIV coinfection exhibits a chronic disease with a variable clinical picture; often with psoriasiform appearance and large

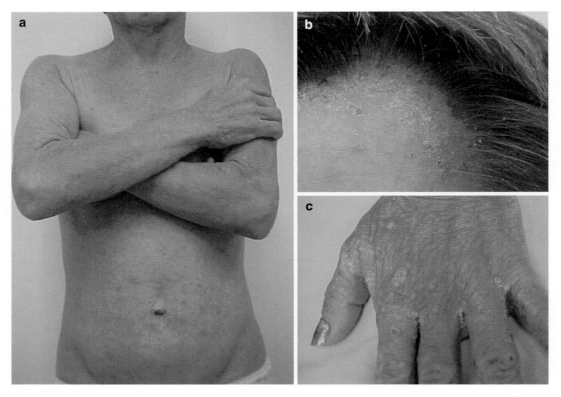

Fig. 41.39 Crusted scabies: disseminated rash (**a**); heavy scaling and crusts on the scalp (**b**) and finger webs (**c**)

numbers of mites in the lesions. Although CS is typically associated with immunosuppressed status, 80% of CS/HIV-coinfected patients reported by Tirado-Sanchez had a CD4 count >200 cells/mm³ [301]. CS/HIV coinfection has also been described as part of the IRIS [82].

Complementary Examinations

The diagnosis is usually established by clinical history, added to the information of similar symptoms among close contacts, and clinical presentation. Dermoscopy can be useful in helping visualization, when a tiny black dot may be observed at one end of the burrow, which is the actual mite [103, 302]. Definitive diagnosis relies on microscopic identification of the mites, eggs, or fecal pellets from scrapings of the skin, which should be taken from nonexcoriated burrows, papules, or vesicles (Fig. 41.37) [262]. Skin biopsy may also be necessary in erythroderma or dubious cases.

Therapeutic Approach

Uncomplicated scabies/HIV-coinfected patients should receive the same treatment regimens as those who are HIV negative. Simultaneous treatment of the patient and close contacts is recommended. The first-line acaricide is topical permethrin 5%. Oral ivermectin is considered a second-line therapy option if treatment with topical permethrin is unsuccessful [107]. Women who are breastfeeding or pregnant and children who weigh less than 15 kg should not be treated with oral ivermectin. Topical permethrin 5% appears to be safe and effective for infants younger than 1 month of age. Cotton mitts or socks on the hands of infants and young children prevent them from rubbing the cream into their eyes and mouth. Topical application of 8–10% precipitated sulfur for 3 consecutive days, although messy and malodourous, is an effective alternative therapy still used because

Table 41.13 Therapies for scabies

	Classic scabies	Crusted scabies[a]
Topical therapy[b]		
Permethrin 5% cream, lotion	Two applications, 1 week apart; **OR** systemic therapy	Once daily for 7 days, then twice weekly until cure; *plus* systemic therapy
Alternative topical therapy		
8–10% precipitated sulfur in petrolatum	Three consecutive nights	
Systemic therapy		
Oral ivermectin	200 µg/kg/dose, two doses 1 week apart	200 µg/kg/dose on day 1, 2, 8, 9, and 15 (22 and 29 for severe infestations)

Mounsey and McCarthy (2013), and UK Scabies Guideline [304]
[a]Keratolytic creams should be used for skin crusts
[b]Apply thoroughly into the skin (except the face), including under the fingernails and toenails; maintain overnight or for 8 h, and washed off

of its low cost and its wide margin of safety in newborns, infants, and pregnant women [200]. Crusted scabies represents a treatment challenge. Dual therapy with oral ivermectin plus topical permethrin 5% is recommended for extended time (Mounsey and McCarthy 2013; [304]). Table 41.13 lists drugs and doses for the treatment of scabies. The pruritus may continue for up to 2 weeks after successful treatment. Oral antihistamines can help to control itching and, after eradication of mites, medium- or high-potency topical corticosteroids can be used (Mounsey and McCarthy 2013). Bedding, clothing, and towels used in the last week by infested persons or their household, sexual, and close contacts should be washed at high temperature (60 °C) and dried in a hot dryer, by dry-cleaning, or by sealing in a plastic bag for at least 72 h [304].

Demodicidosis

Demodex mites are the largest and most complex organisms of the skin microflora and are associated with cutaneous inflammatory disorders such as demodicidosis, also known as demodicosis.

General Epidemiology

It is estimated that 20% of general population harbors *Demodex* mites, while the prevalence in HIV-infected patients ranges from 20% to 95%, and there is a trend of increasing prevalence when the CD4 count falls [145, 325].

Etiopathogenesis

Demodicidosis is an infestation caused by the cutaneous saprophytic mites *Demodex folliculorum* and *Demodex brevis*, which are natural host of the human pilosebaceous follicle. A high concentration of *Demodex* is found in cutaneous areas with numerous sebaceous glands, and eyelashes are a common site of infestation [325]. Their potential to have a pathogenic role in the causation of human skin disorders is still unknown (Chen and Plewig 2014). Altered immune system and/or unusual hypersensitivity against the mite itself could favor the growth of these usually saprophytic agents, thus eventually causing demodicidosis [13, 149].

Clinical Presentation

Clinical presentation is heterogeneous and includes pruritic papules, vesicles, pustules, folliculitis and rosacea-like lesions, plaques, granulomatous and even cystic facial lesions (Chen and Plewig 2014). The rash may be itchy and may also be found on the chest and upper limbs. In HIV-infected patients most demodicidosis cases have occurred in association with CD4 counts of <200 cells/mm^3, and the majority of patients had a facial papulopustular-type rosacea clinical pattern (Fig. 41.40) [53, 326]. Crusted demodicidosis has been described in an HIV-infected female and also in an immunocompetent child, although the severe clinical manifestations in the latter patient could be attributed to local immunosuppression secondary to chronic use of topical steroids [36, 106].

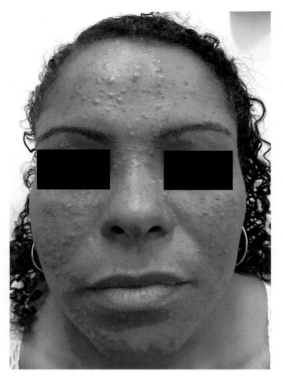

Fig. 41.40 Demodicidosis: facial papulopustular-type rosacea clinical pattern

Complementary Examinations

The diagnosis of demodicidosis depends primarily on the clinical appearance of skin lesions and demonstration of mites on microscopic examination of scrapings (Fig. 41.41). Diagnosis can be made by standardized skin surface biopsy or skin scraping, usually considering abnormal anything more than five mites per cm^2 [46]. As the presence of *Demodex* mites in a specimen is not equivalent to a diagnosis of demodicosis, skin biopsy evaluated in the context of clinical history and appearance is important to confirm the diagnosis [268].

Therapeutic Approach

Treatment of human demodicosis is based on single case reports and is weakly evidence based [46]. Various treatments have been used for *Demodex*-associated skin eruptions, including topical permethrin 5% cream, topical sulfur, oral ivermectin, and oral metronidazole [77]. For mild demodicidosis topical permethrin 5% can be applied to the entire face and other affected areas at night and washed off after 8–14 h, for three consecutive nights on a weekly basis. In cases not responsive to topical

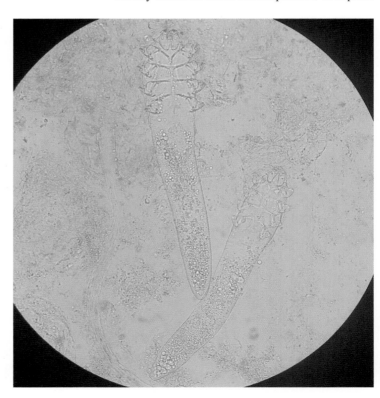

Fig. 41.41 *Demodex* mite (potassium hydroxide preparation of a skin scraping)

treatment, oral ivermectin can be given as two 200-µg/kg doses separated by 1 week. Another possible regimen is metronidazole 0.75% gel and/or oral metronidazole 250 mg three times daily for 3 weeks [125].

Protozoal Diseases

Tegumentary Leishmaniasis

The leishmaniases are among the neglected tropical diseases listed by the WHO. They are caused by species of protozoa of the genus *Leishmania* that are transmitted to humans by phlebotomine sandflies. HIV and *Leishmania* reinforce each other in a deleterious way. The *Leishmania* genus has multiple species that cause cutaneous, mucosal, and/or visceral disease.

General Epidemiology

Leishmaniases prevail in tropical and subtropical areas and in southern Europe, although socioeconomic factors, population mobility, and environmental and climate changes make them also prevalent in nonendemic areas [7, 319]. More than 90% of global visceral leishmaniasis cases occur in six countries: India, Bangladesh, Sudan, South Sudan, Ethiopia, and Brazil. Tegumentary leishmaniasis is more widely distributed, with about one-third of cases occurring in the Americas, the Mediterranean basin, and western Asia from the Middle East to Central Asia [324]. The complex biological system that favors leishmaniasis transmission involves the human host, parasite, sandfly vector, and sometimes an animal reservoir [319]. *Leishmania*/HIV coinfection is considered a serious emerging disease in several regions of the world. The urbanization of leishmaniases and the spread of HIV have led to a geographic overlap of these two infections, and epidemiologic projections estimate a continuous growth of the *Leishmania*/HIV coinfection [32, 319].

Etiopathogenesis

The leishmaniases are a group of noncontagious chronic infectious diseases resulting from macrophage parasitism by protozoan parasites belonging to the genus *Leishmania*, more than 20 species being known. The parasites are transmitted by insect vectors, the phlebotomine sandflies. The infection can result in cutaneous, mucous, and visceral diseases [114]. The genus *Leishmania* is divided into two subgenera: the subgenus *Leishmania* and the subgenus *Viannia*. Tegumentary leishmaniasis is caused by multiple species of both the *Leishmania* and *Viannia* subgenera [319]. The leishmaniases can also be classified according to the source of human infection: in zoonotic leishmaniases the reservoir hosts are wild animals, commensals, or domestic animals; and in anthroponotic leishmaniases the reservoir is human [319]. *Leishmania* and HIV may have enhanced reciprocal effects, especially in relation to the visceral leishmaniasis, as dual infection plays an important role in the pathogenesis, clinical latency, and disease progression of either infection. The immunologic deregulation caused by HIV favors the multiplication of the parasite in tegumentary forms of *Leishmania*/HIV coinfection [6].

Clinical Presentation

Leishmaniases comprise both visceral and tegumentary forms. While tegumentary leishmaniasis (TL) is the most frequent form of the disease, visceral leishmaniasis (VL, also known as kala-azar) is the most severe and life-threatening one [324]. Post-kala-azar dermal leishmaniasis (PKDL) is a cutaneous disease that occurs during or after visceral leishmaniasis associated with viscerotropic *Leishmania* species. TL comprises the cutaneous and mucocutaneous forms, which can be localized, disseminated, or diffuse in distribution and may differ in Old and New World regions (Goto and Lindoso 2012). Based on clinical presentations, cutaneous leishmaniases are classified as localized cutaneous leishmaniasis (LCL), diffuse cutaneous leishmaniasis (DCL), disseminated leishmaniasis, leishmaniasis recidiva cutis (LR), and mucosal leishmaniasis (ML) (Goto and Lindoso 2012). Although some clinical manifestations are more frequently associated with a particular species or subgenus, none is unique to a species [319]. The clinical features of TL are diverse, depending on the *Leishmania* species and host immune response. However, the natural history of the primary lesion is similar. At the site of inoculation a macule appears, followed by a papule, then a nodule that ulcerates and expands to a typical round-to-oval craterform lesion, or evolves as a nodule. Lesions can develop weeks, months, or years after infection, but usually the incubation period ranges from 2 weeks to 3 months. Primary lesions may be single or multiple, and lymphatic involvement manifests as lymphadenitis or lymphadenopathy. The primary lesion may spontaneously heal or may persist as an ulcer, yet some lesions may then evolve into other chronic forms (Goto and Lindoso. 2012; [319]). The main clinical aspects of TL are briefly described in Box 41.9; detailed descriptions can be found in the WHO Report, Control of Leishmaniases [319]. *Leishmania*/HIV coinfection has changed the classical picture of visceral and other forms of the disease, since HIV and *Leishmania* reinforce each other in a deleterious manner. Immunosuppressed status may alter the clinical presentation and treatment response of leishmaniases. In *Leishmania*/HIV-coinfected patients, especially in patients with a low CD4 count (<200 cells/mm^3), TL may show clinical variability, with atypical, multiple, polymorphic lesions and relapsing disease [105, 159, 307]. Cutaneous or mucocutaneous forms can be associated with VL, and visceralization of

DL: disseminated multiple pleomorphic lesions, in two or more noncontiguous areas of the body; acneiform papules; extensive nodular or ulcerated lesions; mucosal lesions are frequent (Fig. 41.43)

DCL: rare and true anergic form; multiple papules, nodules, or tubercles with diffuse cutaneous infiltration and no ulceration; usually no mucosal lesions; do not heal spontaneously; frequent relapses after treatment

ML/MCL: destructive lesions of mucosal tissues of the mouth and upper respiratory tract; occurs years after the onset of cutaneous leishmaniasis (Figs. 41.44 and 41.45)

PKDL[a]: cutaneous disease during or after visceral leishmaniasis associated to viscerotropic *Leishmania* species

TL/HIV: atypical manifestations; macules, nodules, crusted plaques, multiple exudative ulcers, including genitals; oral diffuse infiltration; diffuse cutaneous leishmaniasis with ulcers

Goto and Lindoso [100], Handler et al. [114], WHO [319]
DCL diffuse cutaneous leishmaniasis, *DL* disseminated leishmaniasis (cutaneous), *LCL* localized cutaneous leishmaniasis, *LR* leishmaniasis recidiva cutis, *ML/MCL* mucosal leishmaniasis/mucocutaneous leishmaniasis, *PKDL* post-kala-azar dermal leishmaniasis, *TL* tegumentary leishmaniasis, *TL/HIV* tegumentary leishmaniasis/HIV coinfection
[a]Not TL; it is instead visceral leishmaniasis with cutaneous lesions

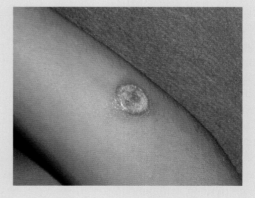

Box 41.9 Clinical Forms of Tegumentary Leishmaniasis

LCL: "classical form"; painless, round-to-oval, craterform ulcer usually on exposed skin area (Fig. 41.42)

LR: a scar with peripheral activity; papules, vesicles, plaques, nodules, in or around previous leishmaniasis healed lesion

Fig. 41.42 Localized cutaneous leishmaniasis, "classical form": painless, round-to-oval, craterform ulcer usually on an exposed skin area (Photograph courtesy of Dr. Ana Lucia França da Costa, Faculdade de Medicina da Universidade Federal do Piauí, Brazil)

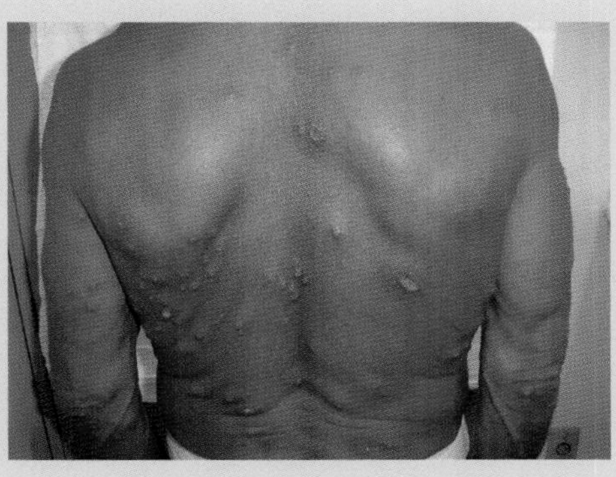

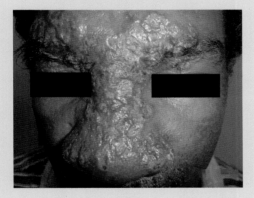

Fig. 41.43 Disseminated cutaneous leishmaniasis: multiple pleomorphic lesions, papules, nodules, and ulcers (Photograph courtesy of Dr. Ana Lucia França da Costa, Faculdade de Medicina da Universidade Federal do Piauí, Brazil)

Fig. 41.44 Mucocutaneous leishmaniasis: extensive infiltrated crusted facial plaque, and involvement of nasal mucosa (Photograph courtesy of Dr. Ana Lucia França da Costa, Faculdade de Medicina da Universidade Federal do Piauí, Brazil)

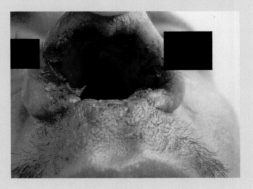

Fig. 41.45 Mucocutaneous leishmaniasis: destructive lesions of mucosal tissues in the upper respiratory tract (Photograph courtesy of Dr. Ana Lucia França da Costa, Faculdade de Medicina da Universidade Federal do Piauí, Brazil)

cutaneous forms can occur in coinfected patients [6, 319]. TL has also been reported to occur during immunologic recovery after ART initiation, as part of the IRIS. Most of these cases occurred 4 months following ART introduction, and the mean baseline (pre-ART) CD4 count was <100 cells/mm³. VL and PKDL were the most commonly reported clinical manifestations, followed by TL and uveitis [16].

Complementary Examinations

Diagnosis of leishmaniasis is based on criteria that consider epidemiologic data, clinical features, and laboratory test results [32, 319]. In endemic areas the typical presentations of leishmaniasis may be suitable to suggest the diagnosis; nevertheless, it is accurate to have the parasitologic and/or immunologic diagnosis confirmed [319]. Table 41.14 lists the diagnostic tools for TL.

Parasitologic Diagnosis

Definitive diagnosis requires demonstration of the parasite by histology, culture, or molecular analysis of tissue samples, which can be obtained by scraping, fine-needle puncture, or biopsy. The edge of a cutaneous lesion is the most appropriate site for skin biopsy [99]. The so-called touch preparation cytology method (imprint; "touch prep") is useful for obtaining rapid interpretations [319]. To perform Giemsa-stained "touch prep" smears, gently grasp the original biopsy sample with forceps and blot the cut surface onto a paper towel or gauze to remove excess blood; gently press the blotted surface onto a clean glass slide using rolling or circular motions while avoiding compressing tissue; air dry the slides, fix in methyl alcohol, and stain with Giemsa [329]. Direct microscopic examination, in vitro culture, and immunohistochemistry are parasitologic diagnostic methods with variable sensitivity that depends on geographic region, *Leishmania* species, and the clinical form of leishmaniasis [100, 115, 319]. In the TL/immunosuppression-associated and in diffuse leishmaniasis the lesions usually present with a high parasite density, whereas

Table 41.14 Diagnostic tests for leishmaniases

Diagnostic tool	Characteristics	Cutaneous leishmaniasis	Mucocutaneous leishmaniasis
Parasitologic diagnosis[a]			
Direct microscopic examination[b]	Detects *Leishmania* parasites in tissues	High specificity	High specificity
	Does not allow species identification	Variable sensitivity[e]	Low sensitivity
		LR and chronic lesions: scarce parasites on samples	Mucosal lesions: scarce parasites due to strong local immune reaction
Immunohistochemistry	Detects *Leishmania* antigens in tissues	CL/HIV: usually numerous parasites on samples	
	Does not allow species identification		
In vitro culture	Allows species identification		
	Reference laboratory required		
	Time consuming		
Molecular diagnosis with PCR-based methods	Detects *Leishmania* DNA	Highly sensitive and specific	
	Allows species identification	Protocols not standardized	
	Reference laboratory required		
Immunologic diagnosis[c]			
Leishmanin intradermal skin test[d] (Montenegro test)	Evaluates anti-*Leishmania* delayed-type hypersensitivity	Variable specificity[f]	
		High sensitivity	
		Positivity increases clinical suspicion	
		Usually positive in DL, LCL and ML	
		Usually negative in DCL, PKDL, and immunosuppressed CL/HIV	
Serologic tests	Anti-*Leishmania* antibody assays (ELISA; IFAT, IIFA)	Variable specificity[f]	Low sensitivity
		Low sensitivity	Positivity increases clinical suspicion
		TL: limited use	
		TL-HIV: usually negative in immunosuppressed	Useful to monitor relapses

Goto and Lindoso [100], Handler et al. [115], WHO [319]

CL/HIV cutaneous leishmaniasis/HIV coinfection, *DCL* diffuse cutaneous leishmaniasis, *DL* disseminated leishmaniasis (cutaneous), *ELISA* enzyme-linked immunosorbent assay, *IIFA* indirect immunofluorescence assay, *LCL* localized cutaneous leishmaniasis, *LR* leishmaniasis recidiva cutis, *ML* mucosal leishmaniasis, *PCR* polymerase chain reaction, *PKDL* post-kala-azar dermal leishmaniasis

[a]Reference standard for tegumentary leishmaniasis diagnosis

[b]Giemsa staining can be useful to highlight parasites

[c]Do not distinguish between past and present infections

[d]Positive test (≥ 5 mm diameter) is indicative of cell-mediated immunity; positive results usually appear within 3 months of infection

[e]Sensitivity depends on geographic location, species, and stage of the lesion; multiple parasitologic diagnostic tests recommended for each patient

[f]Possible cross-reactions with *Trypanosomiasis*, deep mycoses, and mycobacteria infections

chronic lesions such as ML and DL have scarce parasites on samples, and repeat biopsies may be necessary [100]. In vitro culture is the best way to isolate parasites; nevertheless, it may be challenging to perform, because *Leishmania* organisms are fastidious [115]. Molecular approaches using PCR-based methods allow the detection of *Leishmania* DNA as well as the identification of *Leishmania* species. PCR methods can detect *Leishmania* DNA in different biological materials, even with a low parasite load; they are highly sensitive and specific, and provide fast results [99]. PCR is the most sensitive approach to confirm mucosal leishmaniasis [319].

Immunologic Diagnosis

Immunologic tests are used as indirect parameters for the diagnosis, and comprise the leishmanin skin test (Montenegro skin test) and serologic assays. Immunologic tests cannot reliably differentiate between past and present infections. They also show variable specificity, because of possible cross-reactivity between *Leishmania* and other infectious agents, such as *Trypanosoma*, mycobacteria, and some fungi [99, 319]. The leishmanin skin test detects anti-*Leishmania* delayed-type hypersensitivity. It consists of an intradermal injection of killed promastigotes; the response is measured after 48 or 72 h and ≥5 mm induration is considered positive [99]. It is more appropriately used in epidemiologic studies but is of little value in the diagnosis of cutaneous leishmaniasis as an isolated tool. It is usually positive in DL, LCL, and ML, whereas it is negative in DCL, PKDL, and immunosuppressed *Leishmania*/HIV-coinfected patients [100]. The more commonly used serologic assays to detect anti-*Leishmania* antibody are the indirect immunofluorescence assay (IIFA) and ELISA. The sensitivity of serologic tests is variable in *Leishmania*/HIV-coinfected patients depending on the antigen preparation used and the host immune status. Some patients might have *Leishmania*-specific committed memory cells preserved, even in the face of HIV immunosuppression, rendering serologic tests of higher sensitivity [100]. The presence of other OI may complicate the clinical diagnosis in HIV/*Leishmania*-coinfected patients. In endemic areas, patients with unusual presentations of TL should be tested for HIV infection [319].

Therapeutic Approach

Prevention of exposure to leishmanial infection relies on reservoir host control in areas with zoonotic transmission and vector control activities, such as indoor residual spraying and/or use of insecticide-treated bed nets. Personal protective measures include minimizing nocturnal outdoor activities, wearing protective clothing, and applying insect repellent to exposed skin (Panel OI HIV NIH Leishmaniasis 2016).

Few systematic data are available on the efficacy of pharmacologic treatments for tegumentary forms of *Leishmania*/HIV coinfection (Panel OI HIV NIH Leishmaniasis 2016). In the general population the treatment may be either local or systemic, whereas in HIV-infected patients only systemic treatment is recommended [100]. The treatment decision is based firstly on the risk–benefit ratio of the intervention for each patient. Amphotericin B is the first-choice agent for VL and TL; both amphotericin B deoxycholate and lipid formulations can be used for the treatment of TL ([32]; Panel OI HIV NIH Leishmaniasis 2016 [319]). Availability, cost, and side effects should be taken into account when choosing between the two agents. Available guidelines recommend different amphotericin B regimens, as shown in Table 41.15 ([32]; Panel OI HIV NIH Leishmaniasis 2016 [319]). The alternative therapeutic agents include pentamidine isethionate and two pentavalent antimonials: meglumine antimoniate (MG) and sodium stibogluconate (SSG). According to WHO recommendations, amphotericin B should be considered as first choice whereas pentavalent antimonials should be reserved only for areas with no significant *Leishmania*-drug resistance and when amphotericin B lipid formulations are unavailable or unaffordable [319]. Both pentavalent antimonials are chemically similar, and their toxicity and efficacy are related to their pentavalent antimony (Sb^{5+}) content: MG solution contains 8.1% Sb^{5+} (81 mg Sb^{5+}/mL), whereas SSG solution contains 10% Sb^{5+} (100 mg Sb^{5+}/mL) (see Table 41.15) [319]. The treatment efficacy varies according to the geographic region, species of *Leishmania*, and clinical presentation (Goto and Lindoso 2010). Because of drug toxicities the pretreatment assessment of cardiac, hepatic, pancreatic, and renal functions is highly recommended [32].

Clinical parameters are used to assess the response to treatment. If clinical cure is not achieved, it is considered as relapse and new treatment should be provided with the same or an alternative regimen [100]. Long-term follow-up is recommended for *Leishmania*/HIV-coinfection, especially in patients whose CD4 count is <200 cells/mm³ (Panel OI HIV NIH

Table 41.15 Treatment for *Leishmania*-HIV coinfection (tegumentary forms)

Drug	Dose/regimen	Full course of treatment	Contraindications and pregnancy risk	Adverse effects
First choice				
Amphotericin B deoxycholate	Brazil: 1 mg/kg, IV, daily	Total cumulative dose at least 1.5 g	Hypersensitivity to amphotericin	Renal toxicity (lower for liposomal formulation); hypokalemia; hypomagnesaemia; acute infusion reactions (e.g., fever, chills, hypotension)
	CDC and WHO: N/A	Duration of therapy may be variable, depending on patient tolerance	Use with caution in decreased renal and cardiovascular function	
		Daily maximum dose 50 mg	Pregnancy risk category B	
Liposomal amphotericin B[a]	Brazil: 1–4 mg/kg/, IV, daily	LCL and DCL: 1–1.5 g total dose		
		ML: 2.5–3 g total dose		
	CDC: 2–4 mg/kg IV	Daily for 10 days or interrupted schedule up to 20–60 mg/kg (total dose)		
	WHO: 3–5 mg/kg IV	Daily or intermittently[d] for 10 doses, up to 40 mg/kg (total dose)		
Alternatives				
Pentavalent antimonials[b]	Brazil (MG): 15 mg Sb5+/kg, IV[c] or IM, daily	CL: 20 days	Cardiac conduction disorder	Anorexia; arthralgia; cardiac toxicity; hepatic toxicity; myalgia; leukopenia; pancreatitis; skin rash
	CDC (SSG): 20 mg Sb5+/kg, IV[c] or IM, daily	ML: 30 days	Renal and hepatic failure	
	WHO (SSG): 20 mg Sb5+/kg, IV or IM[c], daily	28 days; 10–20 days[e]	Safety in pregnancy not established	
Pentamidine isethionate	Brazil: 4 mg/kg/day, IM or IV, every other day	3– 10 doses for TL[f]	Diabetes mellitus; cardiovascular disease; renal failure; Pregnancy risk category C	Hypoglycemia; hypotension; increased liver enzyme; increased serum creatinine; injection site reaction; leukopenia; renal failure
	CDC: N/A	10 doses for ML caused by *L(V) braziliensis*		
	WHO: 3–4 mg/kg on alternate days	–; 3 to 4 doses		

Brazilian Health Ministry [32], Goto and Lindoso [100], Panel (2016), WHO [319]
CL cutaneous leishmaniasis, *IM* intramuscular, *IV* intravenous, *MG* meglumine antimoniate, *ML* mucosal leishmaniasis, *N/A* not available, *Sb5+* pentavalent antimony, *SSG* sodium stibogluconate
[a]First-choice therapy according USA guidelines; off-label drug in Brazil
[b]Doses are expressed as mg of pentavalent antimony (Sb5+) content; MG has 81 mg Sb5+/mL; SSG has 100 mg Sb5+/mL
[c]Preferred IV route, especially in thrombocytopenic and undernourished patients
[d]Days 1–5, 10, 17, 24, 31, and 38
[e]There is no evidence for the optimal duration
[f]Three doses for *Leishmania* (*V*) guyanensis; ten doses for *L(V)* braziliensis and *L(L)* amazonensis

Leishmaniasis 2016). Although no published data on efficacy are available, maintenance therapy may be indicated for immunocompromised patients with cutaneous leishmaniasis who have multiple relapses after adequate treatment (Panel OI HIV NIH Leishmaniasis 2016).

The impact of ART on tegumentary forms of *Leishmania*/HIV coinfection has not been studied (Alvar et al. 2008). There are no clinical trials demonstrating superiority of any antiretroviral regimens that allow a specific ART recommendation for patients with *Leishmania*/HIV coinfection [32].

Noninfectious Skin Disorders

Xerosis

Xerosis means skin dryness. It is a frequently found dermatologic disorder in approximately 30% of HIV-infected patients, being also a common cause of pruritus [27, 287, 296, 331]. The pathogenesis of HIV-associated xerosis is unknown, and the following factors may be involved: nutritional status; microcirculation, and changes in both skin sweat and sebaceous glands [42]. Rowe et al. reported decreased cutaneous innervation, peptides, and substance P in the skin of HIV patients with xerosis [267]. Xerosis is clinically characterized by diffuse cutaneous dryness with scales, mainly on the extremities. Xerosis is usually more intense in severely immunosuppressed patients, and patients with atopic status and impaired cutaneous barrier. The most severe cases may evolve into eczema craquelé (Fig. 41.46), whereby fissures and cutaneous barrier breakage occurs and favors secondary infection [72]. There are some studies correlating xerosis to low CD4 count, possibly considered a marker of HIV progression [42]. As part of the management it is important to examine the patient's nutritional condition and CD4 count, besides starting ART. Treatment of xerosis includes mild soaps and topical emollients, especially those with urea and lactic acid.

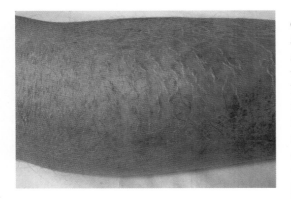

Fig. 41.46 Eczema craquelé: dry scaling and fissures as a result of severe xerosis

Seborrheic Dermatitis

General Epidemiology

Seborrheic dermatitis (SD) is a recurrent chronic inflammatory dermatosis and one of the most common cutaneous manifestations in HIV-infected patients; it may be noticed in up to 40% of seropositive and in up to 80% of AIDS patients, compared with 3% in the general population [91, 181, 191, 225, 263]. SD occurs in any stage of HIV disease, can be the early presentation of HIV infection, worsens as CD4 count decreases, and may also be a cutaneous marker for HIV infection and disease progression, especially when there is an atypical presentation [167, 222].

Etiopathogenesis

Although the exact cause of SD is not completely clear, sebum production, *Malassezia* metabolism, and individual susceptibility play significant roles in triggering inflammatory and hyperproliferative epidermal responses [276]. *Malassezia* is a normal component of the cutaneous flora, although in SD individuals the yeast possibly causes an unspecified immunologic reaction which triggers an inflammatory cascade, resulting in epithelial changes [92, 276]. The severity of SD in HIV patients besides the lesions worsening in parallel with HIV disease progression may also suggest that SD is associated with host immunologic dysfunction facing HIV infection (Chatzikokkinou et al. 2008; [224]).

Clinical Presentation

SD is characterized by erythematous patches and greasy white-yellowish scaling associated with pruritus of variable intensity. It has a predilection for scalp, eyebrows, forehead, paranasal folds (Fig. 41.47), and retroauricular, presternal, interscapular, and pubic areas. The intertriginous folds may also be involved, especially in obese patients. On the scalp the lesions may vary from a slight scaling to adhering crusted patches, possibly resulting in transient alopecia [51, 270]. Eventually there may be an overlapping of SD and psoriasis clinical aspects [72].

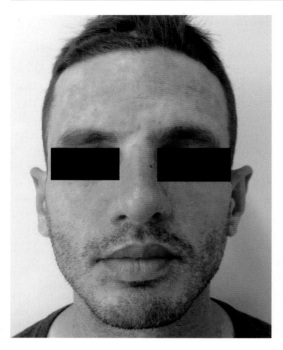

Fig. 41.47 Seborrheic dermatitis: erythema and greasy scales on the face, especially in the nasolabial folds and forehead

On the pigmented skin SD may display hypopigmented annular patches, the so-called petaloid SD, whereby the erythema is less visible and hyperpigmentation is a common finding after resolution of the lesions (Motswaledi et al. 2014). HIV-associated SD may be similar to SD in immunocompetent patients, but is usually more severe or atypical (Chatzikokkinou et al. 2008). In a study by Morar et al., SD caused 12.5% of the erythrodermas in HIV-infected patients [195]. The occurrence of atypical and refractory SD may warn of a possible underlying HIV infection and should prompt HIV testing (Motswaledi et al. 2014).

Complementary Examinations

The diagnosis is usually based on the clinical appearance and topography of the erythematous scaling lesions. A biopsy for histologic study is a resourceful tool on encountering atypical forms of SD.

Therapeutic Approach

SD management aims at reducing the pruritus and the visible signs of disease. Shampoos, topical antifungals, calcineurin inhibitors, and corticosteroids are part of the treatment (Table 41.16). Since SD is a chronic condition, ongoing maintenance therapy is often needed. HIV-associated SD may show itself more extensive resistance to the traditional treat-

Table 41.16 Treatment for seborrheic dermatitis in adults

Scalp seborrheic dermatitis		Facial and body seborrheic dermatitis
Medication	Frequency of use	Frequency of use
Shampoos		
Coal tar shampoo	Twice per week	–
Selenium sulfide shampoo	Twice per week	–
Zinc pyrithione shampoo	Twice per week	–
Topical antifungals		
Ciclopirox 1%	Daily initially, then twice per week	Twice daily for 4 weeks
Ketoconazole 2%	Daily initially, then twice per week	Twice daily for 4 weeks
Topical calcineurin inhibitors	–	
Pimecrolimus 1% cream	–	Twice daily
Tacrolimus 0.1% ointment	–	Twice daily
Topical corticosteroids		
Betamethasone valerate 0.1%	Once daily (lotion)	Once daily (cream)
Fluocinolone 0.01%	Once daily (lotion)	Once daily (cream)
Hydrocortisone 1%		Once daily (cream)
Clobetasol 0.05% shampoo, plus Ketoconazole 2% shampoo	Alternating medications, each twice weekly	

Ang-Tiu et al. [10], Clark [52], Dawson (2007), Dlova and Mosam [72], Firooz et al. [84], Katsambas et al. [135], Moraes et al. [195], Motswaledi et al. (2014), Papp et al. [230], Sampaio et al. [271], WHO [323]

ment, also with more frequent relapses. Symptomatic patients who do not ameliorate under standard treatment should be referred to a dermatologist. For mild scalp SD, the use of shampoos with selenium sulfide, zinc pyrithione, or coal tar may control the symptoms. In case of well-adhered scales emollients can be applied (e.g., mineral oil or petrolatum) at nighttime and removed on the following day [51]. Shampoos must be retained on the scalp for a minimum of 5 min to assure the appropriate scalp exposure to the active ingredient [51]. For long-term control, antifungal shampoos with 2% ketoconazole or 1% ciclopirox can be used on a daily basis, or at least twice or three times a week until remission. The weekly maintenance of these shampoos can prevent recurrences. Depending on the intensity of the scalp inflammation topical corticosteroids may be necessary, although long-term use must be avoided because of adverse effects. For facial and body SD, therapeutic tools include topical antifungals, corticosteroids, and calcineurin inhibitors (pimecrolimus, tacrolimus). Owing to their efficacy, limited adverse effects, and reasonable cost, topical antifungals are the preferred agents for initial SD treatment of the face and body, as well as maintenance therapy [51]. Low- or mid-potency topical corticosteroids alleviate symptoms of the extremely inflammatory SD, showing an efficacy comparable with that of antifungal agents [84, 134]. Because of their safety profile, corticosteroids are regarded as a second-line choice for SD, and their long-term use is contraindicated on account of the risk of cutaneous atrophy and telangiectasias [51]. Topical calcineurin inhibitors have shown similar efficacy to antifungals and topical corticosteroids, but with a lower risk for adverse effects [10, 229]. Facial SD in HIV-infected patients has been successfully managed with topical pimecrolimus regardless of patients' immunologic status, with no changes in CD4, CD8, or viral load counts throughout treatment [194]. Patients undergoing ART may show decreased SD severity and frequency, although there have been reports of aggravation during IRIS [288, 321].

Psoriasis

General Epidemiology

Psoriasis is a chronic papular scaling dermatosis affecting 2–3% of the world's population, and in HIV-patients its prevalence is similar or a little higher [168]. It may be associated with systemic manifestations, corresponding to an autoimmune disorder resulting from keratinocyte proliferation, T-cell mediation, possible genetic susceptibility, and environmental factors [196, 311]. Psoriasis may appear in all phases of HIV infection, although it usually worsens and may become treatment-resistant in the advanced phase. There is a correlation between low CD4 count and psoriasis severity [168]. Moreover, many of these patients are affected with significant psoriatic arthritis [189].

Etiopathogenesis

The pathogenesis of HIV-associated psoriasis seems to be paradoxical, since psoriasis is a T-helper 1 (Th1)-mediated disorder, and there is Th2 immunologic predominance in the HIV-associated advanced disease. Also intriguing is the fact that psoriasis, which is mediated by T-cell activation, becomes more severe with HIV progression, when CD4 count is low [196]. It has been hypothesized that the immunologic deregulation resulting from HIV infection may trigger or exacerbate an existing psoriasis in genetically predisposed individuals [83]. The causal scenario for such a paradox is possibly related to many factors: genetic susceptibility; autoimmunity; destruction of regulatory T CD4 cells by HIV; quantitative increase of memory T CD8 cells and interferon-γ production, especially at the late stage of HIV disease; action of HIV proteins and other pathogens, as the superantigens; and also a direct epidermal proliferative effect of HIV [196, 233].

Clinical Presentation

The typical cutaneous pattern of psoriasis is characterized by circumscribed, erythematous, dry, and scaling plaques of different sizes [311]. Scales are typically silvery and peeling in layers, and when removed tiny bleeding points can be seen (the so-called Auspitz sign). Symmetric lesions are most localized on limbs, abdomen, trunk, scalp, and nails. The lesions may show different patterns: guttata (small drops), follicular, annular, discoid (solid patches) (Fig. 41.48), rupioid (very thick crusts) (Fig. 41.49), and inverse (psoriasis in the flex-

ural areas), among others. The inverse-pattern psoriasis displays erythema and maceration, instead of the typical dry scaling, on the moist flexural areas (Fig. 41.50) and genitals (Fig. 41.51) [196]. Nails are usually affected by distal onycholysis (Fig. 41.51), pitting, oil

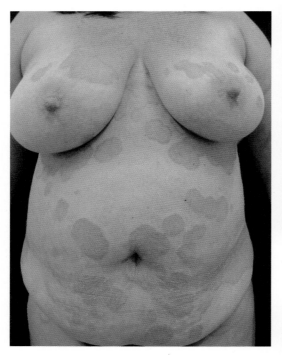

Fig. 41.48 Discoid psoriasis: symmetric erythematous scaling patches and plaques

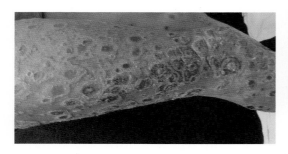

Fig. 41.49 Rupioid psoriasis: large and very thick crusts on limbs

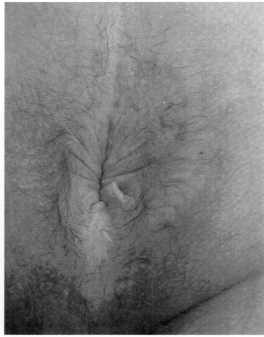

Fig. 41.50 Inverse psoriasis: perianal erythema and maceration

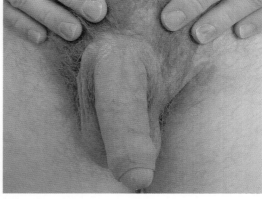

Fig. 41.51 Psoriasis: erythematous annular lesions on the genital area resembling tinea; and onycholysis (Photograph courtesy of Dr. Andre Avelino Costa Beber, Hospital Universitário de Santa Maria, Brazil)

spots, or subungual debris, and hyperkeratosis mimicking onychomycosis. Psoriasis in palms and soles may present as well-circumscribed heavy hyperkeratosis and fissures (Fig. 41.52). Up to 40% of patients with psoriasis may have evidence of arthritis, which presents a variety of different patterns: monoarthritis; oligoarthritis; involvement of the distal interphalangeal joints; and a rheumatoid arthritis-like picture with multiple joints involved or axial disease producing symptoms similar to ankylosing spondylitis [58].

In HIV-associated psoriasis, several morphologic types may coexist in the same patient [217] (Box 41.10). The clinical phenotypes of HIV psoriasis show variable prevalence. In a series in the United States the most common form was patchy psoriasis, whereas in South Africa the erythrodermic variant was prevalent, probably associated with advanced HIV stages [196, 217]. Erythrodermic psoriasis is a severe form that can have a sudden appearance or follow a chronic course (Fig. 41.53). Patients with erythrodermic psoriasis can develop generalized skin failure associated with mortality [196].

Reactive arthritis (Reiter's syndrome) is a seronegative spondyloarthropathy characterized by arthritis, urethritis, and conjunctivitis. Its prevalence is high in HIV patients [196]. Both psoriasis and reactive arthritis can be triggered by infections and might be part of a disease continuum [74]. The most frequently seen presentation is seronegative peripheral arthritis [2]. The classic cutaneous presentation seen in more than half of patients includes palmoplantar psoriasis-like plaques (keratoderma blenorrhagicum) (Fig. 41.54) and circinate balanitis [196]. Studies evaluating HIV-associated reactive arthritis have found human leukocyte antigen (HLA)-B27 in 80–90% of Caucasians while studies of Africans have found nearly all to be HLA-B27 negative [78].

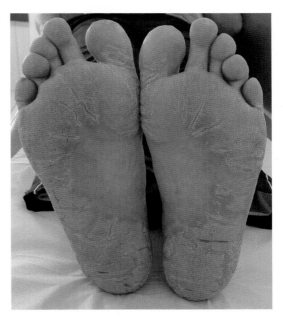

Fig. 41.52 Psoriasis in soles: well-circumscribed heavy hyperkeratosis and fissures (Photograph courtesy of Dr. Andre Avelino Costa Beber, Hospital Universitário de Santa Maria, Brazil)

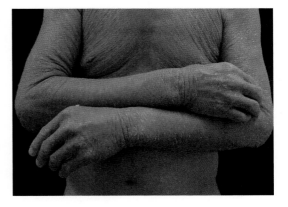

Fig. 41.53 Erythrodermic psoriasis

ing lesions. A biopsy for histologic study is a resourceful tool in face of atypical or erythrodermic psoriasis.

Complementary Examinations

Usually the diagnosis is based on the clinical appearance and topography of the psoriatic scal-

Therapeutic Approach

Given the fact that psoriasis has no cure, the aim of treatment is the provision of a reasonable improvement of the lesions. There are no randomized placebo-controlled trials evaluating the safety and efficacy of treatments for HIV-associated psoriasis. The general principles of management of psoriasis and treating HIV apply [196]. Evidence based therapeutic recommendations for psoriasis management in HIV patients were developed by the Medical Board of the National Psoriasis Foundation, and are summarized in Table 41.17 [189]; Table 41.18 lists pharmacologic options and regimens. The published systematic reviews for topical treatments for psoriasis are not specifically targeted to HIV-infected patients, but could be used for them. For chronic plaque psoriasis, corticosteroids perform at least as well as vitamin D analogs (calcitriol,

Table 41.17 Treatment for HIV-associated psoriasis according severity

	First choice	Second choice
Mild to moderate psoriasis	Topical therapy: calcipotriol, corticosteroids, tazarotene, combined calcipotriol + betamethasone dipropionate	–
Moderate to severe psoriasis	UV-therapy (UVB, PUVA)	Oral retinoids
	Antiretrovirals	
Severe refractory psoriasis	Cyclosporine, methotrexate, TNF-α inhibitors, hydroxyurea	

Menon et al. [189]
PUVA psoralen plus ultraviolet A, *TNF* tumor necrosis factor, *UV* ultraviolet

calcipotriene/calcipotriol), and are associated with a lower incidence of local adverse events. Although topical vitamin D analogs are effective as monotherapy for some patients, a systematic review found that combination therapy with a topical corticosteroid is more effective than either treatment alone [180]. For refractory HIV-associated psoriasis treatment is challenging, and should be tailored to patients based on disease severity and immunologic status. Close monitoring for potential adverse events of systemic therapy is paramount [189]. HIV patients who are adherent to medication regimens and frequent monitoring, and have failed other treatment modalities, could be considered for treatment with tumor necrosis factor α (TNF-α) inhibitors. However, given the limited evidence and the substantial risks associated with their use, TNF-α inhibitors should be reserved for patients with very refractory psoriasis or with debilitating psoriatic arthritis. In addition, these patients should receive optimal ART and close monitoring [94]. Patients with unknown HIV status and with psoriasis unresponsive to therapy should prompt HIV testing.

Papular Pruritic Dermatoses

Among the papular pruritic dermatoses related to HIV infection, two entities are as yet not well differentiated: papular pruritic eruption

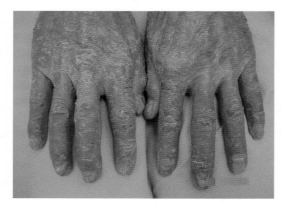

Fig. 41.54 Reactive arthritis with psoriasis-like lesions, severe onychodystrophy; and involvement of the distal interphalangeal joints in in an HIV patient as part of the immune reconstitution inflammatory syndrome (IRIS)

Table 41.18 Pharmacologic treatments for psoriasis and psoriatic arthritis

Drug	Dosage	Monitoring	FDA pregnancy category
Topical therapies	*In affected areas*		
Corticosteroids	Once or twice daily	–	
Tacrolimus; pimecrolimus	Twice daily	–	C
Tazarotene	Once daily	–	X
Vitamin D analogs: calcitriol; calcipotriene (calcipotriol)	Twice daily	–	C
Systemic therapies			
Acitretin	10–50 mg orally per day	Renal function tests, LFTs, lipid panel, and CBC every 1–2 weeks until levels stabilize (typically 4–8 weeks)	X
Cyclosporine[a]	2.5–5.0 mg/kg/day, orally in two divided oral doses	Blood pressure; CBC; LFTs; lipid panel; and magnesium, uric acid, blood urea nitrogen, creatinine, potassium levels every 2 weeks for the first 3 months of therapy, then monthly if stable	C
Methotrexate[a]	7.5–25 mg orally per week	LFTs, renal function tests, CBC, and platelet count every 1–2 months	X

Patel and Weinberg [234], Weigle and McBane [311]
CBC complete blood count, *FDA* US Food and Drug Administration, *LFTs* liver function tests
[a]Useful in patients with psoriatic arthritis

(PPE) and eosinophilic folliculitis (EF). Both are chronic pruritic inflammatory dermatoses usually seen in the advanced phase of HIV infection, although they may also occur as part of IRIS [28, 76, 111, 246, 278, 289]. According to the WHO criteria, the presence of associated PPE defines HIV disease as clinical stage 2, also being a parameter for ART initiation [318]. There are major gaps in the understanding of EF and PPE regarding etiology, natural history, and their role as potential prognostic markers of HIV. PPE mainly affects HIV-infected people living in tropical regions, whereas EF has been described in patients living in developed countries [76, 265]. EF is prevalent in body areas of major concentration of sebaceous glands where the *D. folliculorum* mite is common (Fig. 41.55); PPE, on the other hand, affects mainly the limbs (Fig. 41.56) where insect bites are frequent [278]. The etiopathogenesis hypotheses consider that both diseases may involve deregulated immunologic reactions: in EF a reaction against an unknown antigen, and in PPE a reaction against insect bites, although no specific organism has been identified to date ([80, 253]; Rosatelli et al. 2001; [265]). In a recent study by Chua et al., the presence of PPE in HIV-infected persons undergoing ART was associated with high HIV viral loads at baseline (pre-ART). It has been suggested that the pretreatment of high HIV viremia may have persistent effects even after starting ART and after achieving virologic suppression. The mechanism of this effect on PPE is still unknown. In the same study, PPE in ART-treated HIV-infected persons was not associated with the immune activation markers measured, including CD4 T-cell gains and CD8 T-cell activation [50]. Afonso et al. have suggested that these two entities could possibly be distinguished by histopathologic and immunohistochemical features in addition to clinical characteristics, and that they could both be within the spectrum of the same disease [3]. Since the sole clinical diagnosis is not ideal, a lesion biopsy is important for diagnostic

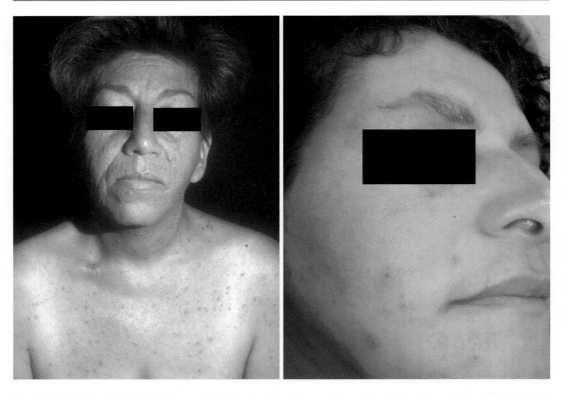

Fig. 41.55 Eosinophilic folliculitis: pruritic follicular edematous papulovesicles with on face and trunk (central body distribution)

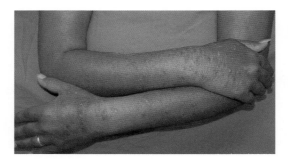

Fig. 41.56 Papular pruritic eruption: skin-colored prurigo-like papules, excoriations, and postinflammatory hyperpigmentation (peripheral location)

confirmation [50]. To date, there have been no randomized clinical trials aimed at therapeutic interventions for EF or PPE. Table 41.19 lists the main characteristics and proposed treatments for EF and PPE.

Antiretroviral Therapy-Associated Manifestations

Cutaneous Toxicities of Antiretroviral Therapy for HIV

The expanded access to ART over the past three decades has led to substantial declines in HIV-related morbidity and mortality. However, multidrug therapy for HIV infected patients is complicated by numerous adverse effects including drug-related toxicities, drug interactions, and IRIS. HIV-infected patients are at higher risk for developing drug-related toxicities than HIV-negative counterparts [121]; and up to 80% of them may experience adverse drug reactions at some point during their therapy, presumably as a result of immune dysregulation, altered drug metabolism, and/or polypharmacy [29, 279]. In addition to the inherent risk

Table 41.19 Summary of characteristics of HIV-associated eosinophilic folliculitis and pruritic papular eruption

	Eosinophilic folliculitis	Pruritic papular eruption
Demographics	Patients most living in developed countries	Populations living in the tropics
Clinical picture	Pruritic follicular edematous papulovesicles, pustules (not predominant)	Pruritic skin-colored papules, pustules rare, prurigo-like nodules, excoriations, postinflammatory hyperpigmentation, scarring
Anatomic pattern	Central distribution: face, neck, postauricular, upper arms, trunk	Peripheral location, or generalized: symmetric, distal extremities, face, trunk, rare on palms and soles
Histologic picture	Folliculocentric lymphocytic and eosinophilic infiltrate; absence of microorganisms, number of mast cells higher than in PPE	Similar to hypersensitivity reaction to insect bites: nonfolliculocentric wedge-shaped dense perivascular and interstitial lymphocytic infiltrates with many eosinophils
Laboratory data	↑ IgE, eosinophilia	↑ IgE, eosinophilia
	CD4 <250/mm³	CD4 <100/mm³
	↑ serum levels of CCL17, CCL26, CCL27	↑ CD8 T cells
		↑ HIV viremia at ART initiation, independent of CD4 count
Improvement under ART	Yes	Yes
Marker for immunosuppression	Yes	Yes; highly predictive of HIV infection in the tropics
Occurrence as part of IRIS	Yes	Yes
Treatment	ART is the primary treatment	ART is the primary treatment
	Potent topical steroids, for the duration of persistent symptoms	Potent topical steroids, for the duration of persistent symptoms
	Topical 1% tacrolimus ointment	Promethazine 25 mg bid
	Topical permethrin 5%	Thalidomide 100 mg daily
	Oral antihistamines	Dapsone 100 mg daily
	Oral metronidazole 250–500 mg bid	Pentoxiphylline 400 mg bid
	Itraconazole 200–400 mg daily	Narrowband ultraviolet B phototherapy
	Oral isotretinoin 20–80 mg/day, 6–8 weeks	
	Dapsone 100 mg daily	
	Ultraviolet B phototherapy	

Afonso et al. [3], Bellavista et al. [22], Chua et al. [50], Eisman [76], Farsani et al. [80], Lakshmi et al. [150], McCalmont et al. [185], Navarini et al. [208], Rajendran et al. [246], Resneck et al. [253], Rosatelli and Roselino [264], Rosenthal et al. [265], Serling et al. [278], Wernham et al. [315], WHO [321], Yokobayashi et al. [328]

ART antiretroviral therapy, *bid*, twice daily, *CCL17* chemokine ligand 17 (thymus and activation regulated chemokine), *CCL26* chemokine ligand (chemotactic for eosinophils and basophils), *CCL27* chemokine ligand 27 (cutaneous T cell-attracting chemokine), *CD4* CD4+ T cell, *CD8* CD8+ T cell, *IgE* immunoglobulin E, *IRIS* immune reconstitution inflammatory syndrome

of cutaneous side effects from the medications themselves, HIV patients are at increased risk for immune-mediated cutaneous reactions to medications of any type, likely because of immune dysregulation [128]. Yang et al. have proposed that HIV infection could represent a predisposition for severe drug reaction by depletion of CD4 T cells and loss of regulatory T cells in the skin, which subsequently leads to an upregulation of cytotoxic CD8 T cells [327]. The adverse reactions may range from life-threatening disorders to cosmetic concerns contributing to increased morbidity and often also leading to discontinuation of ART. Some of these toxicities are family- or even drug-specific (Table 41.20).

ART-associated lipodystrophy syndrome consists of changes in body fat composition usually in association with metabolic abnormalities. These disorders are a side effect of the nucleoside reverse transcriptase inhibitors (NRTI), particularly stavudine and the combination of stavudine and didanosine with or without protease inhibitor (PI) therapy, and the non-nucleoside reverse transcriptase inhibitor (NNRTI) efavirenz [128]. The anatomic characteristics include fat loss in the face (Fig. 41.57), limbs, and buttocks, and the accumulation of dorsocervical ("buffalo hump") and abdominal visceral fat and gynecomastia [104, 310]. The metabolic abnormalities (insulin resistance, hyperinsulinemia, hyperglycemia, and dyslipidemia) can put patients at risk for pan-

Table 41.20 Antiretroviral medications and associated cutaneous reactions

Antiretroviral medications	Cutaneous reactions
Nucleoside reverse transcriptase inhibitors	
Abacavir (ABC)	Skin rash (1–10%), AHR (often described as "maculopapular," but descriptions of urticaria, diffuse erythema, erythema multiforme, or targetoid skin lesions have also been included)
Didanosine (ddI)	Lipodystrophy; pruritus (≤7–9%), skin rash (≤7–9%), xerostomia
Emtricitabine (FTC)	Hyperpigmentation (children: 32%; adults: 2–4); skin rash (17–30%; includes hypersensitivity reaction, maculopapular rash, pruritus, pustular rash, vesiculobullous rash)
Lamivudine (3TC)	Skin rash (5–9%)
Stavudine (d4T)	Skin rash (18–30%), lipodystrophy
Zalcitabine (ddC)[a]	Skin rash (dose-related morbilliform exanthemas, 2%), occasional hypersensitivity syndromes
Zidovudine (AZT, ZDV)	Skin rash (children 12%), nail and mucocutaneous hyperpigmentation
Nucleotide reverse transcriptase inhibitor	
Tenofovir (TDF)	Skin rash (includes maculopapular, pustular, vesiculobullous; pruritus; or urticaria: 5–18%), pruritus (16%)
Non-nucleoside reverse transcriptase inhibitors	
Delavirdine (DLV)	Pruritic rash (18–50%), skin rash (16–32%), desquamation, erythema multiforme, fungal dermatitis, SJS
Efavirenz (EFV)	Skin rash (5–26%), pruritus (≤9%), SJS
Etravirine (ETR)	Skin rash (≥grade 2: 10–15%), hyperhidrosis, gynecomastia, lipohypertrophy, DRESS, SJS, TEN
Nevirapine (NVP)	Skin rash (1–7%; grade 1/2: 13%; grade 3/4: 2%), lipodystrophy, angioedema, DIHS, SJS, TEN, acute generalized exanthematous pustulosis, ulcerative stomatitis
Rilpivirine (RPV)	Skin rash (3–6%)
Protease inhibitors	
Amprenavir (APV)[a]	Self-limited maculopapular rash (20% to 28%), SJS (1%)
Atazanavir (ATV)	Skin rash (adults 3–21%; median onset: 7 weeks; children 14%), asymptomatic jaundice and scleral icterus, DIHS, SJS
Darunavir (DRV)	Skin rash (children: 5–19%; adults: 6–7%)
Fosamprenavir (FPV)	Skin rash (16%), SJS
Indinavir (IDV)	Pruritus (4%), skin rash (1%), lipodystrophy, acute porphyria, SJS
Lopinavir (LPV)	Skin rash (≤28%), pruritus (12%), acne vulgaris (4%), diaphoresis (2–3%), SJS, TEN
Lopinavir/ritonavir boosting (LPV/r) = Kaletra®	Skin rash (children 12%; adults ≤5%), skin infection (3%, including cellulitis, folliculitis, furuncle), SJS, TEN
Nelfinavir (NFV)	Skin rash (1–3%)
Ritonavir (RTV)	Skin rash (≤28%), pruritus (12%)

Table 41.20 (continued)

Antiretroviral medications	Cutaneous reactions
Saquinavir (SQV)	Pruritus (3%), rash (3%), dry lips/skin (2%), eczema (2%), verruca
Tipranavir (TPV)	Rash (children 21%; adults 3–10%)
Fusion inhibitors	
Enfuvirtide (T-20)	Injection site reactions[b] (98%), injection site infection (children: 11%, adults: 2%), folliculitis (2%), generalized rash, hypersensitivity reaction
Integrase inhibitors	
Dolutegravir (DTG)	Pruritus (<2%)
Elvitegravir (EVG)	Skin rash (<2%)
Raltegravir (RAL)	Skin rash with eosinophilia and systemic symptoms (DIHS) <2%
CCR5 antagonists	
Maraviroc	Skin rash (11%), folliculitis (4%), pruritus (4%), acne vulgaris (3%), benign skin neoplasm (3%), alopecia (2%), erythema (2%), tinea (4%)

Bartlett [20], Fletcher [85], Introcaso et al. [128, 129], Phillips and Mallal [238]
AHR abacavir hypersensitivity reactions, *DIHS* drug-induced hypersensitivity syndrome, *DRESS* drug rash with eosinophilia and systemic symptoms, *SJS* Stevens–Johnson syndrome, *TEN* toxic epidermal necrolysis
[a]No longer marketed in most countries
[b]May include at injection site: erythema, induration, ecchymosis, nodule, pruritus, pain

creatitis at any point during therapy and increase their risk of atherosclerotic disease over years of treatment [104, 128]. Morbilliform rashes usually present as a pruritic erythematous maculopapular eruption approximately 2–10 days after starting the medication. NNRTI are the most frequent class of antiretrovirals to cause morbilliform exanthems. Besides the NNRTs, other classes of antiretrovirals and drugs used for treatment of OI can also trigger skin rashes, e.g., sulfonamides, trimethoprim, dapsone, penicillins, cephalosporins, quinolones, ketoconazole, and clindamycin [29, 179]. Most rashes are mild and do not require medication discontinuation, and most resolve quickly during continued administration. However, the implicated drug should be stopped if the rash is associated with fever, blistering, oral mucous membrane involvement, or arthralgias (e.g., suspected hypersensitivity secondary to nevirapine or abacavir). Morbilliform eruptions related to nevirapine may become severe and be associated with systemic hypersensitivity reactions [129]. Abacavir can lead to serious and sometimes fatal hypersensitivity reactions (AHR) with multiple organ involvement. AHR typically presents within the first 6 weeks of treatment (median time of 9 days) with a combination of symptoms, including fever, rash, gastrointestinal disturbances, and

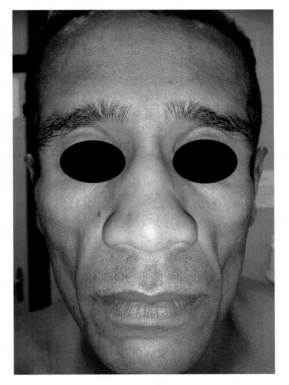

Fig. 41.57 Lipodystrophy: severe fat loss in the face

other constitutional symptoms. [128]. AHR is strongly associated with HLA-B*5701 allele, and genetic screening prior to abacavir exposure has reduced the incidence of hypersensitivity reactions. This association has been present across racial groups in Asia, Europe, Latin America, and the Unites States; nevertheless, pharmacogenetics of drug reactions are drug and population specific [156]. In a large study performed in Uganda, however, HLA-B*5701 was not significantly associated with clinically diagnosed AHR in African patients [204]. It is mandatory to discontinue abacavir if a hypersensitivity reaction is suspected. Reintroduction of abacavir can result in life-threatening or fatal hypersensitivity reactions, even in patients who have no history of hypersensitivity to abacavir therapy [128]. IRIS occurs during the initiation of ART while is not a cutaneous toxicity relating to a specific antiretroviral medication. Given its frequent skin manifestations, IRIS must be distinguished from drug reactions [129, 282].

Immune Reconstitution Inflammatory Syndrome

The use of ART in HIV-infected patients results in reconstitution of the immunologic system and recovery of immunologic response against opportunistic pathogens. However, some patients undergo a worsening of the clinical condition. The restoration of the immunologic reaction against living or dead opportunistic pathogens and many antigens results in immunopathologic damage to the infected tissues, and systemic inflammatory reactions. The term "immune reconstitution inflammatory syndrome," or IRIS, describes a collection of inflammatory disorders associated with paradoxical worsening of pre-existing infectious and noninfectious disorders following the initiation of ART [89, 309]. The syndrome is usually identified during the early months, although it may occur from weeks to years after the start of ART [170]. IRIS incidence is considerably variable among the studies. In controlled studies the reported incidence is up to 25% of patients undergoing ART and varies according to the duration of ART [170]. Skin diseases are very common in HIV-infected patients, and the skin is the organ where IRIS often manifests itself, accounting for 52–78% of all reported events [126, 223, 251]. A great variety of dermatologic

presentations has been described, both infectious and noninfectious. Most authors consider as IRIS any newly dermatologic event occurring after ART initiation, whereas other authors used the term only to describe paradoxical or atypical events [223].

Etiopathogenesis

The immunopathogenesis of IRIS is not clear and involves a combination of factors. IRIS results from a deregulated immunologic reaction to a variety of antigenic stimuli following the initiation of ART [280]. Common immunopathologic characteristics may direct IRIS, although there are specific ways depending on the affected tissue and the involved antigens. In infections the antigenic stimulus can act by means of intact or dead viable organisms and their trace antigens, whereas in noninfectious causes there is involvement of innate autoimmunity against several antigens [170, 176].

Throughout the ART-induced immunologic recovery, chronic activation is a critical factor in the complex interaction between HIV and the immune system. Many components may have a role in the IRIS-exacerbated immune reaction: cell proliferation induced by lymphopenia; quantitative and functional reconstitution of immune cells; redistribution of lymphocytes; impaired T-cell regulatory function; changes in the Th-cell profile; high antigenic exposure; and host genetic susceptibility, all favoring a systemically activated immunologic environment and higher availability of proinflammatory cytokines and circulating chemokines [176, 280]. Such a proinflammatory milieu can be further overwhelmed by OI which activate the innate immune system, allowing recognition of pathogens through molecular patterns released from host cells following tissue injury and necrotic cell death [176]. Chronic systemic immune activation, particularly in severely immunosuppressed patients with OI, affects the immune environment in which immune recovery will emerge. Ongoing research has shed some light on these diverse reaction patterns, but has also engendered new questions.

Risk Factors: IRIS affects mainly HIV patients who initiate ART with a status of

Table 41.21 Risk factors for IRIS associated to HIV

Host-related	Low CD4 count at initiation of ART
	OI or TB prior to ART initiation
	Genetic predisposition: e.g., HLA-A, -B44, -DR4 (associated with herpes virus IRIS);TNFA-308*1, IL6-174*G (associated with mycobacterial IRIS)
	Paucity of immune response at OI diagnosis (in the case of C-IRIS)
Pathogen-related	High pre-ART HIV viral load
	Degree of dissemination of OI/burden of infection (e.g., TB, KS, cryptococcosis)
Treatment-related	Shorter duration of OI treatment prior to starting ART (paradoxical IRIS)
	Rapid suppression of HIV viral load

Walker et al. [309]
ART antiretroviral therapy, *IL6* interleukin-6, *C-IRIS* cryptococcal-associated IRIS, *IRIS* immune reconstitution inflammatory syndrome, *KS* Kaposi's sarcoma, *OI* opportunistic infection, *TB* tuberculosis

advanced immunosuppression, having low CD4 count and high viral load, as well as nondetected microorganisms and other antigens; and resulting in unexpected clinical manifestations. Table 41.21 lists risk factors for HIV-associated IRIS [309].

Clinical Presentation

IRIS is a heterogeneous condition. Clinical and laboratory studies over the two latest decades have defined three categories [44]:

1. Inflammatory disease or cancer resulting from the recovery of an immune reaction against an opportunistic pathogen that causes localized or systemic impairment and can show itself in two ways:
   (a) An IRIS characterized by an exaggerated inflammation and/or atypical inflammation in patients with an already treated OI (paradoxical IRIS), or a subclinical infection (unmasking IRIS).
   (b) A disease of which the presentation cannot be differentiated from the disease typical events over the first 3 months of ART, such as tuberculosis; herpes zoster, and crises of hepatitis caused by the hepatitis B virus (HBV) and the hepatitis C virus (HCV).

2. Autoimmune diseases associated with the immunologic reconstitution, e.g., Graves' disease.
3. Immune-mediated inflammatory diseases and associated with the immunologic reconstitution, e.g., sarcoidosis.

In the paradoxical forms of IRIS, symptoms and signs associated with a known and eventually treated OI recur or severely worsen despite the previous favorable response to therapy, before ART initiation [309]. The unmasked IRIS concept is less defined than the paradoxical IRIS. In paradoxical IRIS a new OI is present with an intensified inflammatory component after the start of ART [309].

Dermatologic IRIS

Dermatologic IRIS represents around half of the IRIS cases in many series, and has been described in association with a wide range of infectious, inflammatory, tumoral, and autoimmune disorders [89, 126, 152, 155, 170, 223]. Usually the condition is associated with mycobacterial, chronic viral, and invasive fungal infections, but the spectrum of the described infections is still expanding (Table 41.22) [152, 153]. Dermatologic manifestations of IRIS comprise genital herpes, herpes zoster, molluscum contagiosum (Fig. 41.58), warts, cutaneous lesions by cytomegalovirus, Kaposi's sarcoma, and fungal infections such as histoplasmosis. The immunologic reconstitution in HIV patients may also be associated with inflammatory and autoimmune diseases, such as sarcoidosis. However, the immunopathogenesis of these diseases seems to be different from the infectious IRIS [89].

Complementary Examinations

IRIS lacks a precise case definition, unequivocal markers and a definitive diagnostic test. Since there are no well-established criteria for the diagnosis of IRIS, a combination of findings is usually necessary to guide clinical suspicion. The clinical diagnosis of IRIS should be considered when inflammatory signs or symptoms occur between 4 and 8 weeks after initiation of ART, reinstatement of an interrupted regimen, or change to a more effective regimen after

Table 41.22 Pathogens and key clinical features of associated IRIS

Condition	Clinical features of IRIS
Pathogen-associated	
Bacteria	
Mycobacterium tuberculosis	Fever, lymphadenitis, cutaneous tuberculosis
Nontuberculous mycobacteria	Fever, lymphadenitis (painful/suppurative), cutaneous lesions: papules, plaques, nodules, abscess
Mycobacterium avium-intracellulare	
Mycobacterium genavense	
Mycobacterium kansasii	
Mycobacterium scrofulaceum	
Mycobacterium xenopi	
BCG	Vaccine associated; local reaction, lymphadenitis
Mycobacterium leprae	Typically tuberculoid or borderline forms, type 1 reactions, neuritis, lepromatous reaction during leprosy and IRIS has similarities
Other	
Chlamydia trachomatis	Reiter's syndrome
Viral	
Herpes viruses	
CMV	Mucocutaneous ulceration
VZV	Dermatologic reactivation (shingles)
HSV-1, HSV-2	Mucocutaneous ulceration
HHV-8	Kaposi's sarcoma (KS)/IRIS; exacerbations of KS can result in tumor enlargement, new lesions, inflammation, and edema
Polyomaviruses	
Molluscum contagiosum virus	Acute new or recurrent cutaneous papules with florid/extensive distribution
HPV	Warts (acute recurrence/relapse or enlargement)
Fungal	
Cryptococcus neoformans	Cutaneous papules, nodules, soft tissue inflammation
Histoplasma spp	Papular/nodular rash
Candida spp	Typically unmasking; mucocutaneous (oral/oesophageal)
Tinea corporis	Inflammatory cutaneous presentation

Table 41.22 (continued)

Condition	Clinical features of IRIS
Malassezia spp	Immune recovery folliculitis
Sporotrichosis	Cutaneous disseminated sporotrichosis; ulcerated lesions
Parasitic	
Leishmania spp	
Leishmania major	Cutaneous, uveitis
Leishmania infantum	Post-kala-azar dermal leishmaniasis, visceral leishmaniasis
Leishmania braziliensis	Cutaneous, mucosal
Nonpathogen-associated	
Autoimmune	
Polymyositis	May occur as a new presentation, or an exacerbation of existing autoimmune condition
SLE	
Cutaneous chronic lupus	
Relapsing polychondritis	
Dermatologic	
Acne	Inflammatory presentation
Demodex folliculitis	
Eosinophilic folliculitis	
Seborrheic dermatitis	
Pruritic papular eruption	
Psoriasis	
Other	
Sarcoidosis	New or recurrent granulomatous inflammation, typically late (around 12 months post-ART initiation) in patients with CD4 counts <200 cells/mm^3; typically pulmonary presentation, but may be cutaneous (erythema nodosum, papular lesions) and/or intra-abdominal
Tattoo and foreign body reaction	Granulomatous reaction

Huiras et al. [126], Manzardo et al. [170], Sharma and Soneja [280], Walker et al. [309]

ART antiretroviral therapy, *BCG* Bacillus Calmette–Guérin, *CMV* cytomegalovirus, *GUD* genital ulcer disease, *HSV* herpes simplex virus, *HHV-8* human herpes virus 8 (Kaposi's sarcoma virus), *HPV* human papilloma virus, *IRIS* immune reconstitution inflammatory syndrome, *NTM* nontuberculous mycobacteria, *OI* opportunistic infection, *SLE* systemic lupus erythematosus, *VZV* Varicella zoster virus

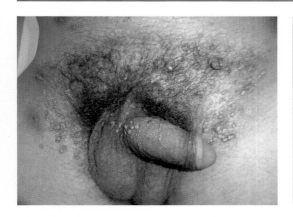

Fig. 41.58 Molluscum contagiosum: sudden appearance of countless lesions as a result of immunologic recovery after antiretroviral therapy initiation

treatment failure [33]. The only reliable predictors of IRIS risk are a low CD4 count and a preexisting OI [89, 281]. The International Network for the Study of HIV-associated IRIS (INSHI) published a consensus to define C-IRIS and TB-IRIS cases [112, 186]. The definitions are appropriate for usage in healthcare centers with limited resources, since CD4 cells and HIV viral load counts are not part of the criteria. Currently there are no consensual case definitions for other forms of IRIS [157]. Shelburne and colleagues have proposed clinical criteria for IRIS, which are displayed in Box 41.11 [281]. In places where resources and laboratory support are limited, IRIS will be an exclusion diagnosis after failure of treatment of other conditions [309].

Therapeutic Approach

Appropriate IRIS management requires acknowledgement of the condition and exclusion of differential diagnoses, especially additional resistant infections and OI. Because of the heterogeneity of IRIS in terms of underlying infection, clinical presentation, and severity, the management should be individualized. When IRIS is suspected the diagnosis must be prioritized and the OI treatment optimized. ART should be interrupted only if IRIS is imminently life-threatening [187]. In most cases, IRIS resolution is spontaneous, only requiring symptomatic treatment such as nonsteroidal anti-inflammatory drugs. Systemic corticosteroid therapy should be used only in severe cases after a careful risk-benefit consideration. Oral prednisone can be prescribed at a 1–2 mg/kg dose, or equivalent, for 1–2 weeks, with subsequent dose tapering. When considering corticosteroid treatment, clinicians should be aware of the side effects of corticosteroids and only use them when the diagnosis of IRIS is certain. In viral forms of IRIS, corticosteroids are generally avoided [187]. According to small series of case reports, thalidomide, which has been shown to inhibit TNF-α production in vitro, could be beneficial for patients who experience IRIS and do not respond favorably and quickly to corticosteroids. Thalidomide may be indicated at a 100–200 mg/day dose [35, 273]. Since the higher risk of IRIS is associated with low CD4 cell count at the time of ART initiation, IRIS events could be preventable with timely initiation of ART, before patients are at risk of OI and advanced immunodeficiency [203]. It is worth pointing out that IRIS has three rules: (1) anything is possible; (2) nothing is as it was in the pre-ART era; (3) IRIS does not mean that ART has failed. In addition, the patients usually have a good prognosis [122].

Neoplastic Disorders

Kaposi's Sarcoma

Described for the first time in 1872 by Moritz Kaposi, a Hungarian dermatologist, Kaposi's sarcoma (KS) is an angioproliferative tumor caused by the human herpesvirus 8 (HHV-8), also known as Kaposi sarcoma herpesvirus (KSHV). Before the AIDS pandemic, KS was considered a rare disease seen mainly in countries around the Mediterranean Sea (classic KS) and in several African countries (endemic KS). In 1981, a disseminated and fulminant form of KS (AIDS-related KS or AIDS-KS) was described in homosexual and bisexual men, and was first reported as part of AIDS [90].

General Epidemiology

In developed countries, the introduction of ART has had a strong influence on the epidemiology of AIDS-KS. The incidence has decreased by up to 80% since its peak in the early AIDS epidemic because of improved control of HIV viremia and preserved CD4 counts and immune function [25]. Before the ART era, HHV-8/HIV-coinfected patients were estimated to be 400–2000 times more likely to develop KS than those with solely HHV-8 infection [25]. Since the introduction of ART, the incidence of KS in HIV-infected persons has diminished in the Western world. It is estimated that AIDS-KS in the United States has decreased by 10% per year from 1990 to 1997; by contrast, the prevalence of KS remains high among Africans, particularly in children [118]. The reasons for this changing epidemiologic trend in different parts of the world remain unclear, although it may be related to incomplete access to ART in resource-limited settings, contrasting with high access to ART in developed countries [118]. Further decreases after 2000 have been more modest, and AIDS-KS remains the second most common tumor arising in HIV-infected persons in the United States [25]. Currently there are four epidemiologic subtypes of KS (Box 41.12).

Box 41.12 Clinical-Epidemiologic Forms of Kaposi Sarcoma

- *Classic KS*: It occurs mainly in elderly men (male/female-ratio 10–15:1) of Mediterranean, Eastern European, or Jewish Ashkenazi origin, with a peak incidence after the 6th decade of life. Usually the lesions are confined to the lower limbs, and it is a slow-progressing disease, patients living 10 or more years after being diagnosed.
- *AIDS-KS*: It is considered an AIDS-defining illness and has a more aggressive behavior compared with the classic form. It usually arises in HIV-infected patients with low CD4 counts. Clinically, AIDS-KS lesions may be more widespread, often involving the face, trunk, lymph nodes, oral mucosa, and visceral organs. It affects mainly MSM and intravenous drug users aged 20–50 years.
- *Endemic (African) KS*: It occurs in people living in all parts of equatorial Africa, particularly in sub-Saharan Africa, mainly middle-aged black adults and children.
- *Iatrogenic or transplant-related KS*: It is described in iatrogenic immunosuppressed organ transplant recipients and patients receiving chronic immunosuppressive therapy (e.g., long-term corticosteroid therapy, cyclosporine, azathioprine, and other biological therapies). This KS form appears about 16 months after transplantation and frequently clears after discontinuation of immunosuppressive therapy. The incidence of KS is 400–500 times higher among organ transplant recipients than in the general population.

Bhutani et al. [25], Curtiss et al. [64], Hengge et al. [118], Radu and Pantanowitz [245]

Etiopathogenesis

HHV-8 is an essential factor in the pathogenesis of any KS type. Like other herpesviruses, HHV-8 establishes a latent infection in KS-spindle cells, eventually undergoing lytic replication, and several latent and lytic viral genes may play a role in its pathogenesis [25, 26, 245]. The lytic gene products seem important for the inflammatory and angiogenic component of KS lesions [119]. According to current knowledge, only individuals with specific conditions of immunodysregulation develop KS. HIV-infected cells produce several inflammatory and growth-promoting cytokines that potentiate HHV-8 activation, leading to increased viral load, antibody titers, and an expanded cell tropism that precedes the clinical appearance of AIDS-KS [119, 295].

Clinical Presentation

KS has a highly variable clinical course ranging from very indolent forms to a rapidly progressive disease. KS lesions typically involve the skin and/or mucosal surfaces (Fig. 41.59), at any location, but are typically concentrated in the lower extremities and the head and neck, in a symmetric linear distribution along tension skin lines [14]. KS presents as purplish, reddish blue, or dark brown/black lesions that evolve from early (patch stage) macules into plaques (plaque stage), which may subsequently develop into larger nodules (tumor stage) (Fig. 41.59). Different stages can coexist in the same individual at the same time. The tumors may easily bleed and ulcerate, may cause pronounced lymphedema (Fig. 41.59), and may invade subjacent tissues [25, 245]. Extracutaneous KS may affect lymph nodes and visceral organs, mainly the gastrointestinal and the respiratory tracts.

Complementary Examinations

The presumptive diagnosis is made based on the clinical history and physical examination, although biopsy is required for definitive diagnosis. Even in resource-limited settings, histologic confirmation is strongly encouraged [8,

321]. The histopathologic aspects are similar for KS subtypes; nevertheless, some studies have documented minor histopathologic differences between AIDS-KS and non-HIV-associated KS cases [245]. The characteristic histologic findings are angiogenesis, inflammation, and proliferation. The lesions usually present two main abnormalities, which are spindle-shaped cells arranged in a snail-like form with leukocyte infiltration and neovascularization [14]. Immunohistochemistry techniques may be useful to confirm the diagnosis and demonstrate endothelial cell markers (CD31, CD34, and factor VIII) as well as markers for lymphatic endothelial cells. Moreover, HHV-8 identification within KS lesion cells by using LNA-1 is the most diagnostically helpful immunostaining technique available to differentiate KS from its mimics [245]. Evaluation of patients with AIDS-KS must include a complete physical examination as well as a detailed checkup of the oral cavity, anogenital region, and lymph nodes, and also a rectal examination. Assessment of visceral involvement is suitable for patients with systemic symptoms, lymphadenopathy, or B-symptoms (unexplained fever, night sweats, >10% involuntary weight loss, or diarrhea persisting more than 2 weeks), occult blood in the stool, or unexplained iron-deficiency anemia [25, 321].

Therapeutic Approach

The treatment decision for AIDS-KS must consider the extent and the rate of tumor growth, patients' symptoms, lesion distribution and evolution pattern, immune status, and concurrent HIV-related complications. Several different therapeutic options are available. Currently there are no standard therapy protocols, the consensus is that all patients should receive ART, regardless of CD4 count [14, 174]. Major treatment goals are symptom palliation, prevention of disease progression, and improved quality of life [14, 25]. ART including protease inhibitors may represent the first treatment step for slowly progressive disease. There are cur-

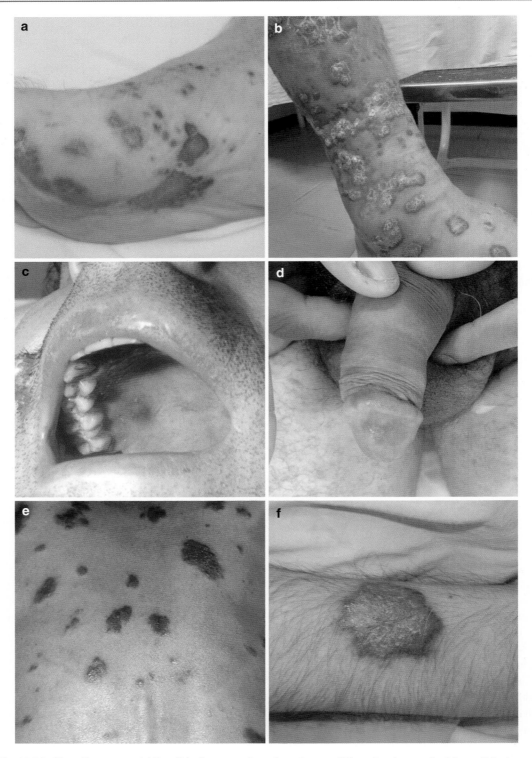

Fig. 41.59 Kaposi's sarcoma. (**a**) Purplish plaques on the feet; (**b**) dark brown nodules, tumors, and marked lymphedema; (**c**) KS lesion on the palate; (**d**) violaceous patches in early-stage KS on the glans penis; (**e**) purplish plaques on the trunk; (**f**) detail of the typical KS lesion at the plaque stage on the forearm

rently no standardized or universally accepted criteria to guide which HIV-infected patients with KS would benefit most from concomitant chemotherapy in addition to receiving ART [321]. Inhibition of HIV replication, amelioration of the immune response against HHV-8, and perhaps some direct antiangiogenic activity of PI are beneficial effects of ART on AIDS-KS. Localized, symptomatic lesions may be treated with local approaches, such as intralesional chemotherapy, liquid nitrogen, laser therapy, localized radiotherapy, or surgical resection. Systemic chemotherapy is applicable for HIV patients not responding to ART and/or with widespread, symptomatic, rapidly progressive, life-threatening AIDS-KS with visceral involvement, and in IRIS-associated flares [25, 146, 174]. Chemotherapy treatment regimens commonly used in high-resource settings are single-agent liposomal anthracyclines (doxorubicin and daunorubicin) and single-agent paclitaxel. Other options, which are more widely used in lower-resource settings, include combination chemotherapy with vincristine, with or without nonliposomal doxorubicin [321].

Glossary

Antigenemia The condition of having an antigen present in the blood.

Cantharidin An odorless, colorless terpenoid secreted by many species of blister beetles, including broadly in genus *Epicauta*, and in species *Lytta vesicatoria* (Spanish fly). Externally, cantharidin is a potent vesicant (blistering agent), exposure to which can cause severe chemical burns.

Dermoscopy A noninvasive method that allows the in vivo evaluation of colors and microstructures of the epidermis, the dermoepidermal junction, and the papillary dermis not visible to the naked eye. These structures are specifically correlated to histologic features.

Dimorphic fungus Fungi that exist either in yeast form or as mold (mycelial form) depending on environmental conditions, physiologic conditions of the fungus, or genetic characteristics.

Gomori methenamine silver Used widely as a screen for fungal organisms and particularly useful in staining carbohydrates. It can be used to identify the yeast-like fungus *Pneumocystis jiroveci*, which causes a form of pneumonia called pneumocystis pneumonia (PCP) or pneumocystosis.

GUD (genital ulcer disease) Located on the genital area, usually caused by a sexually transmitted disease (STD) such as genital herpes, syphilis, chancroid, or chlamydia trachomatis. Genital ulcers are not strictly a sign of an STD.

Immune reconstitution syndrome (IRIS) Some people who start antiretroviral therapy (ART) encounter health problems even though their HIV comes under control. An infection that they previously had might return. In other cases, they develop a new disease. This is linked to improvements in the patients' immune systems. The problems usually occur in the first 2 months after starting HIV therapy. It may occur in about 20% of people starting ART.

LNA-1 (latent nuclear antigen) A Kaposi's sarcoma (KS)-associated herpesvirus (KSHV) latent protein initially found by Moore and colleagues as a speckled nuclear antigen present in primary effusion lymphoma cells that reacts with antibodies from patients with KS. LNA-1 has been suspected of playing a crucial role in modulating viral and cellular gene expression. It is commonly used as an antigen in blood tests to detect antibodies in persons that have been exposed to KSHV.

Majocchi's granuloma Can be defined as a deep folliculitis due to a cutaneous dermatophyte infection.

Meglumine antimoniate (MG) A medication used for treating leishmaniasis. It is manufactured by Aventis and sold as Glucantime in France and Brazil, and Glucantim in Italy. It belongs to a group of compounds known as the pentavalent antimonials. It is administered by intramuscular injection.

p24 antigen test Detects the presence of the p24 protein of HIV (also known as CA), the capsid protein of the virus.

PCR techniques Techniques used in molecular biology to amplify a single copy or a few copies of a piece of DNA across several orders of magnitude, generating thousands to millions of copies of a particular DNA sequence.

Periodic acid-Schiff (PAS) A staining method used to detect polysaccharides such as glycogen, and mucosubstances such as glycoproteins, glycolipids, and mucins in tissues.

Phlebotomine sandflies A subfamily of the family Psychodidae. In several countries, their common name is sand fly. The Phlebotominae include many genera of blood-feeding (hematophagous) flies, including the primary vectors of leishmaniasis and others.

Podophyllotoxin A nonalkaloid toxin lignan extracted from the roots and rhizomes of podophyllum species. it is used on the skin as a topical treatment of external genital warts, caused by some types of the human papillomavirus (HPV), and other warts.

Sodium stibogluconate (SSG) A medication used to treat leishmaniasis, only available for administration by injection. It belongs to the class of drugs known as the pentavalent antimonials, because they contain antimony in its oxidation state of 5. SSG is marketed under the name Pentostam, and is exceedingly phlebotoxic.

Superantigens A class of antigens that cause nonspecific activation of T cells resulting in polyclonal T-cell activation and massive cytokine release. They are produced by some pathogenic viruses and bacteria, most likely as a defense mechanism against the immune system.

Warthin–Starry stain A silver nitrate-based staining method (silver stain) used in histology. Warthin–Starry stains organisms dark brown to black, and the background light golden brown/golden yellow. This technique involves the argyrophilic reaction.

WHO (World Health Organization) A specialized agency of the United Nations concerned with international public health. It was established on 7 April 1948 and is headquartered in Geneva, Switzerland. The WHO is a member of the United Nations Development Group.

References

1. Adenis AA, Aznar C, Couppié P. Histoplasmosis in HIV-infected patients: a review of new developments and remaining gaps. Curr Trop Med Rep. 2014;1:119–28.

2. Adizie T, Moots RJ, Hodkinson B, French N, Adebajo AO. Inflammatory arthritis in HIV positive patients: a practical guide. BMC Infect Dis. 2016;16:100.

3. Afonso JP, Tomimori J, Michalany NS, Nonogaki S, Porro AM. Pruritic papular eruption and eosinophilic folliculitis associated with human immunodeficiency virus (HIV) infection: a histopathological and immunohistochemical comparative study. J Am Acad Dermatol. 2012;67:269–75.

4. Alczuk SSD, Bonfim-Mendonça PS, Rocha-Brischiliari SC, Shinobu-Mesquita CS, Martins HP, Gimenes F, et al. Effect of highly active antiretroviral therapy on vaginal Candida spp. isolation in HIV-infected compared to HIV-uninfected women. Rev Inst Med Trop Sao Paulo. 2015;57(2):169–74.

5. Almeida-Paes R, Oliveira LC, Oliveira MM, Gutierrez-Galhardo MC, Nosanchuk JD, Zancope-Oliveira RM. Phenotypic characteristics associated with virulence of clinical isolates from the Sporothrix complex. Biomed Res Int. 2015;2015:212308. doi:10.1155/2015/212308.

6. Alvar J, Aparicio P, Aseffa A, Den Boer M, Cañavate C, Dedet JP, et al. The relationship between leishmaniasis and AIDS: the second 10 years. Clin Microbiol Rev. 2008;21(2):334–59.

7. Alvar J, Vélez ID, Bern C, Herrero M, Desjeux P, Cano J, Jannin J, den Boer M, WHO Leishmaniasis Control Team. Leishmaniasis worldwide and global estimates of its incidence. PLoS One. 2012;7(5):e35671.

8. Amerson E, Buziba N, Wabinga H, et al. Diagnosing Kaposi's Sarcoma (KS) in East Africa: how accurate are clinicians and pathologists? Infect Agents Cancer. 2012;7(Suppl 1):P6. doi:10.1186/1750-9378-7-S1-P6.

9. Ameen M. The impact of human immunodeficiency virus-related diseases on pigmented skin types. Br J Dermatol. 2013;169(Suppl 3):11–8.

10. Ang-Tiu CU, Meghrajani CF, Maano CC. Pimecrolimus 1% cream for the treatment of seborrheic dermatitis: a systematic review of randomized controlled trials. Expert Rev Clin Pharmacol. 2012;5(1):91–7.

11. Antinori S. New insights into HIV/AIDS-associated cryptococcosis. ISRN AIDS 2013;2013:ID 471363. Accessed on 26 Aug 2016. Retrieved from https://www.hindawi.com/journals/isrn/2013/471363/cta/.

12. Antonelli LR, Mahnke Y, Hodge JN, Porter BO, Barber DL, DerSimonian R, et al. Elevated frequencies of highly activated CD4+ T cells in HIV+ patients developing immune reconstitution inflammatory syndrome. Blood. 2010;116:3818–27.

13. Aquilina C, Viraben R, Sire S. Ivermectin-responsive Demodex infestation during human immunodeficiency virus infection. A case report and literature review. Dermatology. 2002;205(4):394–7.

14. Arruda E, Jacome AA, Toscano AL, Silvestrini AA, Rêgo AS, Wiermann EG, et al. Consensus of the Brazilian Society of Infectious Diseases and Brazilian Society of Clinical Oncology on the management and treatment of Kaposi's sarcoma. Braz J Infect Dis. 2014;18(3):315–26. Erratum in: Braz J Infect Dis. 2014 Jul-Aug;18(4):468.

15. Avelleira JCR, Bottino G. [Sífilis: diagnóstico, tratamento e controle.] [Article in Portuguese]. An Bras Dermatol. 2006;81(2):111–26.

16. Badaró R, Gonçalves LO, Gois LL, Maia ZP, Benson C, Grassi MF. Leishmaniasis as a manifestation of immune reconstitution inflammatory syndrome (IRIS) in HIV-infected patients: a literature review. J Int Assoc Provid AIDS Care. 2015;14(5):402–7.

17. Baddley JW, Sankara IR, Rodriquez JM, Pappas PG, Many WJ Jr. Histoplasmosis in HIV-infected patients in a southern regional medical center: poor prognosis in the era of highly active antiretroviral therapy. Diagn Microbiol Infect Dis. 2008;62(2):151–6.

18. Ballard R, Hook EW III. Syphilis. In: Unemo M, Ballard R, Ison C, Lewis D, Ndowa F, Peeling R, editors. Laboratory diagnosis of sexually transmitted infections, including human immunodeficiency virus. Geneva: World Health Organization (WHO); 2013. p. 93–106. Accessed on 28 Sept 2016. Retrieved from http://www.who.int/reproductivehealth/publications/rtis/9789241505840/en/.

19. Barros MB, de Almeida PR, Schubach AO. Sporothrix schenckii and sporotrichosis. Clin Microbiol Rev. 2011;24:633–54.

20. Bartlett JG. Modifying HIV antiretroviral therapy regimens. In: UpToDate, Hirsch MS (Ed), UpToDate, Mitty J. Accessed on 17 Oct 2016. Retrieved from https://www.uptodate.com/contents/modifying-hiv-antiretroviral-therapy-regimens.

21. Beauman JG. Genital herpes: a review. Am Fam Physician. 2005;72:1527–34. 1541-2.

22. Bellavista S, D'Antuono A, Infusino SD, Trimarco R, Patrizi A. Pruritic papular eruption in HIV: a case successfully treated with NB-UVB. Dermatol Ther. 2013;26(2):173–5.

23. Belum GR, Belum VR, Chaitanya Arudra SK, Reddy BS. The Jarisch-Herxheimer reaction: revisited. Travel Med Infect Dis. 2013;11(4):231–7.

24. Berberi A, Noujeim Z, Aoun G. Epidemiology of oropharyngeal candidiasis in human immunodeficiency virus/acquired immune deficiency syndrome patients and CD4+ counts. J Int Oral Health. 2015;7(3):20–3.

25. Bhutani M, Polizzotto MN, Uldrick TS, Yarchoan R. Kaposi sarcoma-associated herpesvirus-associated malignancies: epidemiology, pathogenesis, and advances in treatment. Semin Oncol. 2015;42(2):223–46.

26. Biberfeld P, Ensoli B, Stürzl M, Schulz TF. Kaposi sarcoma-associated herpesvirus/human herpesvirus 8, cytokines, growth factors and HIV in pathogenesis of Kaposi's sarcoma. Curr Opin Infect Dis. 1998;11(2):97–105.

27. Blanes M, Belinchón I, Merino E, Portilla J, Sánchez-Payá J, Betlloch I. [Current prevalence and characteristics of dermatoses associated with human immunodeficiency virus infection]. [Article in Spanish]. Actas Dermosifiliogr. 2010;101(8):702–9.

28. Boonchai W, Laohasrisakul R, Manonukul J, Kulthanan K. Pruritic papular eruption in HIV seropositive patients: a cutaneous marker for immunosuppression. Int J Dermatol. 1999;38:348–50.

29. Borrás-Blasco J, Navarro-Ruiz A, Borrás C, Casterá E. Adverse cutaneous reactions associated with the newest antiretroviral drugs in patients with human immunodeficiency virus infection. J Antimicrob Chemother. 2008;62:879–88.

30. Brandt AM. How AIDS invented global health. N Engl J Med. 2013;368:2149–52.

31. Braun DL, Kouyos RD, Balmer B, Grube C, Weber R, Gunthard HF. Frequency and spectrum of unexpected clinical manifestations of primary HIV-1 infection. Clin Infect Dis. 2015;61(6):1013–21.

32. Brazilian Ministry of Health. 2015. Secretariat of Health Surveillance, Department of Communicable Disease Surveillance (2015) [Manual of recommendations for diagnosis, treatment and monitoring of patients with Leishmania-HIV co-infection.][Text in Portuguese] Brasília; Ministério da Saúde; 2015. 109 p. Accessed on 18 Oct 2016. Retrieved from http://saudepublica.bvs.br/pesquisa/resource/pt/mis-37506.

33. Brazilian Ministry of Health. Ministério da Saúde. Secretaria de Vigilância em Saúde. Departamento de DST, Aids e Hepatites Virais. Protocolo Clínico e Diretrizes Terapêuticas para Manejo da Infecção pelo HIV em Adultos – PCDT 2015, p 62–63. Brasília: Ministério da Saúde; 2015. Last update: Jul 2015. Accessed on 9th Aug 2016. Retrieved from http://www.aids.gov.br/publicacao/2013/protocolo-clinico-e-diretrizes-terapeuticas-para-manejo-da-infeccao-pelo-hiv-em-adul.

34. Breton G, Adle-Biassette H, Therby A, Ramanoelina J, Choudat L, Bissuel F, et al. Immune reconstitution inflammatory syndrome in HIV-infected patients with disseminated histoplasmosis. AIDS. 2006;20(1):119–21.

35. Brunel AS, Reynes J, Tuaillon E, Rubbo PA, Lortholary O, Montes B, et al. Thalidomide for steroid-dependent immune reconstitution inflammatory syndromes during AIDS. AIDS. 2012;26:2110.

36. Brutti CS, Artus G, Luzzatto L, Bonamigo RR, Balconi SN, Vettorato R. Crusted rosacea-like demodicidosis in an HIV-positive female. J Am Acad Dermatol. 2011;65(4):e131–2.

37. CDC – Centers for Diseases Control. Pneumocystis pneumonia – Los Angeles. Morb Mortal Wkly Rep. 1981;30:250–2.

38. CDC – Centers for Diseases Control. Kaposi's sarcoma and Pneumocystis pneumonia among homosexual men – New York City and California. Morb Mortal Wkly Rep. 1981;30:305–8.

39. CDC – Centers for Disease Control and Prevention. 1993 revised classification system for HIV infection and expanded surveillance case definition for AIDS among adolescents and adults. MMWR Recomm Rep. 1992;41(RR-17):1–19. Accessed on 12 Jul 2016. Retrieved from http://www.cdc.gov/mmwr/preview/mmwrhtml/00018871.htm.

40. CDC – Centers for Diseases Control. Sexually transmitted diseases treatment guidelines. Atlanta: U.S. Department of Health and Human Services; 2015. Accessed on 12 Jul 2016. Retrieved from http://www.cdc.gov/std/tg2015/default.htm.

41. CDC – Centers for Disease Control and Prevention. Sexually transmitted disease surveillance 2015. Division of STD Prevention, National Center for HIV/AIDS, Viral Hepatitis, STD, and TB Prevention. Atlanta: U.S. Department of Health and Human Services; 2016. Accessed on 22 Sept 2016. Retrieved from https://www.cdc.gov/std/stats15/default.htm.

42. Cedeno-Laurent F, Gómez-Flores M, Mendez N, Ancer-Rodríguez J, Bryant JL, Gaspari AA, Trujillo JR. New insights into HIV-1-primary skin disorders. J Int AIDS Soc. 2011;14:5.

43. Chakrabarti A, Bonifaz A, Gutierrez-Galhardo MC, Mochizuki T, Li S. Global epidemiology of sporotrichosis. Med Mycol. 2015;53(1):3–14.

44. Chang CC, Sheikh V, Sereti I, French MA. Immune reconstitution disorders in patients with HIV infection: from pathogenesis to prevention and treatment. Curr HIV/AIDS Rep. 2014;11(3):223–32.

45. Chayakulkeeree M, Perfect JR. Cryptococcosis. In: Hospenthal DR, Rinaldi MG, editors. Diagnosis and treatment of human mycoses. Totowa: Humana Press; 2008. p. 255–76.

46. Chen W, Plewig G. Human demodicosis: revisit and a proposed classification. Br J Dermatol. 2014;170(6):1219–25.

47. Chen CY, Ballard RC, Beck-Sague CM, Dangor Y, Radebe F, Schmid S, et al. Human immunodeficiency virus infection and genital ulcer disease in South Africa: the herpetic connection. Sex Transm Dis. 2000;27:21–9.

48. Chen X, Jiang X, Yang M, González U, Lin X, Hua X, et al. Systemic antifungal therapy for tinea capitis in children. Cochrane Database Syst Rev. 2016;5:CD004685. doi:10.1002/14651858. CD004685.pub3.

49. Chéret A, Bacchus-Souffan C, Avettand-Fenoël V, OPTIPRIM ANRS-147 Study Group, et al. Combined ART started during acute HIV infection protects central memory CD4 T cells and can induce remission. J Antimicrob Chemother. 2015;70(7):2108–20.

50. Chua SL, Amerson EH, Leslie KS, McCalmont TH, Leboit PE, Martin JN, Bangsberg D, Maurer TA. Factors associated with pruritic papular eruption of human immunodeficiency virus infection in the antiretroviral therapy era. Br J Dermatol. 2014;170(4):832–9.

51. Clark GW.Diagnosis and treatment of seborrheic dermatitis. Am Fam Physician 2015 1;91(3):185–190.

52. Clinical Effectiveness Group, British Association for Sexual Health and HIV (BASHH). United Kingdom national guidelines on the management of anogenital warts 2015. Apr 2015. Accessed on 17 Sept 2016. Retrieved from https://www.bashh.org/documents/UK%20national%20guideline%20on%20Warts%202015%20FINAL.pdf.

53. Clyti E, Nacher M, Sainte-Marie D, Pradinaud R, Couppie P. Ivermectin treatment of three cases of demodecidosis during human immunodeficiency virus infection. Int J Dermatol. 2006;45(9):1066–8.

54. Cohen MS, Gay CL, Busch MP, Hecht FM. The detection of acute HIV infection. J Infect Dis. 2010;202(Suppl2):S270–7.

55. Cohen MS, Shaw GM, McMichael AJ, Haynes BF. Acute HIV-1 infection. N Engl J Med. 2011;364(20):1943–54.

56. Coldiron BM, Bergstresser PR. Prevalence and clinical spectrum of skin disease in patients infected with human immunodeficiency virus. Arch Dermatol. 1988;125:357–61.

57. Colombo AL, Guimarães T, Camargo LFA, Richtmann R, Queiroz-Telles F, Salles MJC, et al. Brazilian guidelines for the management of candidiasis – a joint meeting report of three medical societies: Sociedade Brasileira de Infectologia, Sociedade Paulista de Infectologia and Sociedade Brasileira de Medicina Tropical. Braz J Infect Dis. 2013;17(3):283–312.

58. Conaghan PG, Coates LC. Improving recognition of psoriatic arthritis. Practitioner. 2009;253(1724):15–8.

59. Constantine N. HIV viral antigen assays. 2001. HIV InSite knowledge base chapter. Accessed on 25 Aug 2016. Retrieved from http://hivinsite.ucsf.edu/InSite?page=kb-02-02-02-02.

60. Costa JE, Neves RP, Delgado MM, Lima-Neto RG, Morais VM, Coelho MR. Dermatophytosis in patients with human immunodeficiency virus infection: clinical aspects and etiologic agents. Acta Trop. 2015;150:111–5.

61. Costa RO, de Macedo PM, Carvalhal A, Bernardes-Engemann AR. Use of potassium iodide in dermatology: updates on an old drug. An Bras Dermatol. 2013;88(3):396–402.

62. Cunha VS, Zampese MS, Aquino VR, Cestari TF, Goldani LZ. Mucocutaneous manifestations of disseminated histoplasmosis in patients with acquired immunodeficiency syndrome: particular aspects in a Latin-American population. Clin Exp Dermatol. 2007;32(3):250–5.

63. Chatzikokkinou P, Sotiropoulos K, Katoulis A, Luzzati R, Trevisan G. Seborrheic dermatitis - an early and common skin manifestation in HIV patients. Acta Dermatovenerol Croat. 2008;16(4):226–30.

64. Curtiss P, Strazzulla LC, Friedman-Kien AE. An update on Kaposi's sarcoma: epidemiology, pathogenesis and treatment. Dermatol Ther (Heidelb). 2016;6(4):465–470.

65. Daar ES, Pilcher CD, Hecht FM. Clinical presentation and diagnosis of primary HIV-1 infection. Curr Opin HIV AIDS. 2008;3:10–5.

66. Dadabhoy I, Butts JF. Parasitic skin infections for primary care physicians. Prim Care. 2015;42(4):661–75.

67. Darwich E, Darwich L, Cañadas MP, Klaustermeier J, Ercilla G, Alsina-Gibert M, et al. New human papillomavirus (HPV) types involved in epidermodysplasia verruciformis (EV) in 3 HIV-infected patients: response to topical cidofovir. J Am Acad Dermatol. 2011;65(2):e43–5.

68. de Vries HJ. Skin as an indicator for sexually transmitted infections. Clin Dermatol. 2014;32(2):196–208.

69. Delli FS, Mourellou O, Chaidemenos G, Anagnostou E, Amaxopoulos K. Neurosyphilis: a reality again. J Eur Acad Dermatol Venereol. 2007;21:398–9.

70. Dias MF, Quaresma-Santos MV, Bernardes-Filho F, Amorim AG, Schechtman RC, Azulay DR. Update on therapy for superficial mycoses: review article part I. An Bras Dermatol. 2013;88(5):764–74.

71. Dias MF, Bernardes-Filho F, Quaresma-Santos MV, Amorim AG, Schechtman RC, Azulay DR. Treatment of superficial mycoses: review Part II. An Bras Dermatol. 2013;88(6):937–44.

72. Dlova NC, Mosam A. Inflammatory noninfectious dermatoses of HIV. Dermatol Clin. 2006;24(4):439–48. vi.

73. Drali R, Sangaré AK, Boutellis A, Angelakis E, Veracx A, Socolovschi C, et al. Bartonella quintana in body lice from scalp hair of homeless persons, France. Emerg Infect Dis. 2014;20(5):907–8.

74. Duvic M, Johnson TM, Rapini RP, Freese T, Brewton G, Rios A. Acquired immunodeficiency syndrome-associated psoriasis and reactive arthritis. Arch Dermatol. 1987;123:1622–32.

75. Dworkin RH, Johnson RW, Breuer J, Gnann JW, Levin MJ, Backonja M, et al. Recommendations for the management of herpes zoster. Clin Infect Dis. 2007;44(Suppl 1):S1–26.

76. Eisman S. Pruritic papular eruption in HIV. Dermatol Clin. 2006;24:449–57.

77. Elston CA, Elston DM. Demodex mites. Clin Dermatol. 2014;32(6):739–43.

78. Espinoza LR, García-Valladares I. Microbios y articulaciones: la relación entre infección y articulaciones. Reumatol Clin. 2013;9:229–38.

79. Fandiño-Devia E, Rodríguez-Echeverri C, Cardona-Arias J, Gonzalez A. Antigen detection in the diagnosis of histoplasmosis: a meta-analysis of diagnostic performance. Mycopathologia. 2016;181:197–205.

80. Farsani TT, Kore S, Nadol P, Ramam M, Thierman SJ, Leslie K, et al. Etiology and risk factors associated with a pruritic papular eruption in people living with HIV in India. J Int AIDS Soc. 2013;16:1–6.

81. Fatahzadeh M, Schwartz RA. Human herpes simplex virus infections: epidemiology, pathogenesis, symptomatology, diagnosis, and management. J Am Acad Dermatol. 2007;57(5):737–63. quiz 764-6.

82. Fernández-Sánchez M, Saeb-Lima M, Alvarado-de la Barrera C, Reyes-Terán G. Crusted scabies-associated immune reconstitution inflammatory syndrome. BMC Infect Dis. 2012 12:323.

83. Fife DJ, Waller JM, Jeffes EW, Jym K. Unraveling the paradoxes of HIV-associated psoriasis: a review of T-cell subsets and cytokine profiles. Dermatol Online J. 2007;13(2):4. Accessed on 26 Sept 2016. Retrieved from: http://escholarship.org/uc/item/4sf63339.

84. Firooz A, Solhpour A, Gorouhi F, Daneshpazhooh M, Balighi K, Farsinejad K, et al. Pimecrolimus cream, 1%, vs hydrocortisone acetate cream, 1%, in the treatment of facial seborrheic dermatitis: a random-ized, investigator-blind, clinical trial. Arch Dermatol. 2006;142(8):1066–7.

85. Fletcher CV. Overview of antiretroviral agents used to treat HIV. In: UpToDate, Bartlett JG (Ed), UpToDate, Mitty J. Accessed on 17 Oct 2016. Retrieved from https://www.uptodate.com/contents/overview-of-antiretroviral-agents-used-to-treat-hiv.

86. Foucault C, Brouqui P, Raoult D. Bartonella quintana characteristics and clinical management. Emerg Infect Dis. 2006;12(2):217–23.

87. Freitas DF, de Siqueira HB, do Valle AC, Fraga BB, de Barros MB, de Oliveira Schubach A, et al. Sporotrichosis in HIV-infected patients: report of 21 cases of endemic sporotrichosis in Rio de Janeiro, Brazil. Med Mycol. 2012;50(2):170–8.

88. Freitas DF, Valle AC, da Silva MB, Campos DP, Lyra MR, de Souza RV, et al. Sporotrichosis: an emerging neglected opportunistic infection in HIV-infected patients in Rio de Janeiro Brazil. PLoS Negl Trop Dis. 2014;8(8):e3110.

89. French MA. Immune reconstitution inflammatory syndrome: immune restoration disease 20 years on. Med J Aust. 2012;196(5):318–21.

90. Friedman-Kien AE, Laubenstein L, Marmor M, et al. Kaposi's sarcoma and Pneumocystis pneumonia among homosexual men – New York City and California. MMWR Morb Mortal Wkly Rep. 1981;30:305–8.

91. Froschl M, Land HG, Landthaler M. Seborrheic dermatitis and atopic eczema in human immunodeficiency virus infection. Semin Dermatol. 1990;9:230–2.

92. Gaitanis G, Magiatis P, Hantschke M, Bassukas ID, Velegraki A. The Malassezia genus in skin and systemic diseases. Clin Microbiol Rev. 2012;25(1):106–41.

93. Galhardo MC, Silva MT, Lima MA, Nunes EP, Schettini LE, de Freitas RF, et al. Sporothrix schenckii meningitis in AIDS during immune reconstitution syndrome. J Neurol Neurosurg Psychiatry. 2010;81:696–9.

94. Gallitano SM, McDermott L, Brar K, Lowenstein E. Use of tumor necrosis factor (TNF) inhibitors in patients with HIV/AIDS. J Am Acad Dermatol. 2016;74(5):974–80.

95. Gallo RC, Montagnier L. The discovery of HIV as the cause of AIDS. N Engl J Med. 2003;349:2283–5.

96. Garza-Garza R, González-González SE, Ocampo-Candiani J. Cutaneous manifestations of HIV. Gac Med Mex. 2014;150(Suppl 2):194–221. Spanish.

97. Gold JAW, Derado G, Mody RK, Benedict K. Sporotrichosis-associated hospitalizations, United States, 2000–2013. Emerg Infect Dis. 2016. Accessed on 17 Oct 2016. Retrieved from http://dx.doi.org/10.3201/eid2210.160671.

98. Goldani LZ, da Silva LF, Dora JM. Ramsay Hunt syndrome in patients infected with human immunodeficiency virus. Clin Exp Dermatol. 2009;34(8):e552–4. doi:10.1111/j.1365-2230.2009.03228.x. Epub 2009 Jun 1.

99. Gomes CM, Paula NA, Morais OO, Soares KA, Roselino AM, Sampaio RN. Complementary exams in the diagnosis of American tegumentary leishmaniasis. An Bras Dermatol. 2014;89(5):701–9.

100. Goto H, Lindoso JA. Cutaneous and mucocutaneous leishmaniasis. Infect Dis Clin N Am. 2012;26(2):293–307.

101. Greenspan JS, Greenspan D, Webster-Cyriaque J. Hairy leukoplakia; lessons learned: 30-plus years. Oral Dis. 2016;22(Suppl 1):120–7.

102. Gremião ID, Menezes RC, Schubach TM, Figueiredo AB, Cavalcanti MC, Pereira SA. Feline sporotrichosis: epidemiological and clinical aspects. Med Mycol. 2015;53(1):15–21.

103. Griffin JR, Newman CC. Clinical, dermatoscopic, and microscopic findings of infestation with Sarcoptes scabiei var hominis. Mayo Clin Proc. 2011;86(9):e47. doi:10.4065/mcp.2011.0306.

104. Grinspoon S, Carr A. Cardiovascular risk and body-fat abnormalities in HIV-infected adults. N Engl J Med. 2005;352:48–62.

105. Guerra JAO, Coelho LIRC, Pereira FR, Siqueira AM, Ribeiro RL, Almeida TML, et al. American tegumentary leishmaniasis and HIV-AIDS association in a tertiary care center in the Brazilian amazon. AmJTrop Med Hyg. 2011;85(3):524–7.

106. Guerrero-González GA, Herz-Ruelas ME, Gómez-Flores M, Ocampo-Candiani J. Crusted demodicosis in an immunocompetent pediatric patient. Case Rep Dermatol Med. 2014;2014:458046. doi:10.1155/2014/458046. Epub 2014 Oct 12.

107. Gunning K, Pippitt K, Kiraly B, Sayler M. Pediculosis and scabies: treatment update. Am Fam Physician. 2012;86(6):535–41.

108. Günthard HF, Saag MS, Benson CA, del Rio C, Eron JJ, Gallant JE, el al. Antiretroviral drugs for treatment and prevention of HIV infection in adults: 2016 recommendations of the International Antiviral Society-USA Panel. JAMA 2016 12;316(2):191–210.

109. Gupta AK, Cooper EA. Update in antifungal therapy of dermatophytosis. Mycopathologia. 2008;166:353–67.

110. Goto H, Lindoso JA. Current diagnosis and treatment of cutaneous and mucocutaneous leishmaniasis. Expert Rev Anti Infect Ther. 2010 Apr;8(4):419–33.

111. Haddow LJ, Easterbrook PJ, Mosam A, Khanyile NG, Parboosing R, Moodley P, Moosa MY. Defining immune reconstitution inflammatory syndrome: evaluation of expert opinion versus 2 case definitions in a South African cohort. Clin Infect Dis. 2009;49(9):1424–32.

112. Haddow LJ, Colebunders R, Meintjes G, Lawn SD, Elliott JH, Manabe YC, International Network for the Study of HIV-associated IRIS (INSHI), et al. Cryptococcal immune reconstitution inflammatory syndrome in HIV-1-infected individuals: proposed clinical case definitions. Lancet Infect Dis. 2010;10(11):791–802.

113. Hainer BL. Dermatophyte infections. Am Fam Physician. 2003;67(1):101–8.

114. Handler MZ, Patel PA, Kapila R, Al-Qubati Y, Schwartz RA. Cutaneous and mucocutaneous leishmaniasis: clinical perspectives. J Am Acad Dermatol. 2015;73(6):897–908.

115. Handler MZ, Patel PA, Kapila R, Al-Qubati Y, Schwartz RA. Cutaneous and mucocutaneous leishmaniasis: differential diagnosis, diagnosis, histopathology, and management. J Am Acad Dermatol. 2015;73(6):911–26.

116. Harpaz R, Ortega-Sanchez IR, Seward JF, Advisory Committee on Immunization Practices (ACIP) Centers for Disease Control and Prevention (CDC), editors. Prevention of herpes zoster: recommendations of the Advisory Committee on Immunization Practices (ACIP). MMWR Recomm Rep. 2008;57(RR-5):1–30.

117. Havlickova B, Czaika VA, Friedrich M. Epidemiological trends in skin mycoses worldwide. Mycoses. 2008;51(Suppl 4):2–15.

118. Hengge UR, Ruzicka T, Tyring SK, Stuschke M, Roggendorf M, Schwartz RA, Seeber S. Update on Kaposi's sarcoma and other HHV8 associated diseases. Part 1: epidemiology, environmental predispositions, clinical manifestations, and therapy. Lancet Infect Dis. 2002;2(5):281–92.

119. Hengge UR, Ruzicka T, Tyring SK, Stuschke M, Roggendorf M, Schwartz RA, Seeber S. Update on Kaposi's sarcoma and other HHV8 associated diseases. Part 2: pathogenesis, Castleman's disease, and pleural effusion lymphoma. Lancet Infect Dis. 2002;2(6):344–52.

120. Henkle E, Winthrop KL. Nontuberculous mycobacteria infections in immunosuppressed hosts. Clin Chest Med. 2015;36(1):91–9.

121. Hernández-Salazar A, Rosales SP, Rangel-Frausto S, Criollo E, Archer-Dubon C, Orozco-Topete R. Epidemiology of adverse cutaneous drug reactions. A prospective study in hospitalized patients. Arch Med Res. 2006;37:899–902.

122. Hoffmann C. Immune reconstitution inflammatory syndrome (IRIS). In: Hoffmann C, Rockstroh JK, editors. HIV Book 2011.Accessed on 22 Jul 2016. Retrived from https://hivbook.com/tag/hiv-associated-iris/.

123. Hoffmann ER, Daboit TC, Paskulin DD, Monteiro AA, Falci DR, Linhares T, et al. Disseminated histoplasmosis and AIDS: a prospective and multicentre study to evaluate the performance of different diagnostic tests. Mycoses. 2016; doi:10.1111/myc.12536. [Epub ahead of print].

124. Hogan MT. Cutaneous infections associated with HIV/AIDS. Dermatol Clin. 2006;24(4):473–95.

125. Hsu CK, Hsu MM, Lee JY. Demodicosis: a clinicopathological study. J Am Acad Dermatol. 2009;60(3):453–62.

126. Huiras E, Preda V, Maurer T, Whitfeld M. Cutaneous manifestations of immune reconstitution inflammatory syndrome. Curr Opin HIV AIDS. 2008;3(4):453–60.

127. Hung CC, Chang SC. Impact of highly active antiretroviral therapy on incidence and management of human immunodeficiency virus-related opportunistic infections. J Antimicrob Chemother. 2004;54(5):849–53.

128. Introcaso CE, Hines JM, Kovarik CL. Cutaneous toxicities of antirretroviral therapy for HIV: part I. Lipodystrophy syndrome, nucleoside reverse transcriptase inhibitors, and protease inhibitors. J Am Acad Dermatol. 2010;63(4):549–61.

129. Introcaso CE, Hines JM, Kovarik CL. Cutaneous toxicities of antirretroviral therapy for HIV: part II. Nonnucleoside reverse transcriptase inhibitors, entry and fusion inhibitors, integrase inhibitors, and immune reconstitution syndrome. J Am Acad Dermatol. 2010;63(4):563–9.

130. Jackson NA, Herring DB. Primary capsule-deficient cutaneous cryptococcosis in a sporotrichoid pattern in an immunocompetent host. Cutis. 2015;96(1):E26–9.

131. Jacobelli S, Laude H, Carlotti A, Rozenberg F, Deleuze J, Morini JP, et al. Epidermodysplasia verruciformis in human immunodeficiency virus-infected patients: a marker of human papillomavirus-related disorders not affected by antiretroviral therapy. Arch Dermatol. 2011;147:590–6.

132. Johnson RA. Dermatophyte infections in human immune deficiency virus (HIV) disease. J Am Acad Dermatol. 2000;43(5 Suppl):S135–42.

133. Jurevic RJ, Traboulsi RS, Mukherjee PK, Salata RA, Ghannoum MA, Oral HIV/AIDS Research Alliance Mycology Focus group. Identification of gentian violet concentration that does not stain oral mucosa, possesses anti-candidal activity and is well tolerated. Eur J Clin Microbiol Infect Dis. 2011;30(5):629–33.

134. Katsambas A, Antoniou C, Frangouli E, Avgerinou G, Michailidis D, Stratigos J. A double-blind trial of treatment of seborrhoeic dermatitis with 2% ketoconazole cream compared with 1% hydrocortisone cream. Br J Dermatol. 1989;121(3):353–7.

135. Kauffman CA, Bustamante B, Chapman SW, Pappas PG. Clinical practice guidelines for the management of sporotrichosis: 2007 update by the Infectious Diseases Society of America. Clin Infect Dis. 2007;45(10):1255–65.

136. Kauffman CA. Histoplasmosis: a clinical and laboratory update. Clin Microbiol Rev. 2007;20:115–32.

137. Kaushal A, Silver S, Kasper K, Severini A, Hamza S, Keynan Y. Epidermodysplasia verruciformis in an HIV-infected man: a case report and review of the literature. Top Antivir Med. 2012;20(5):173–9.

138. Kaviarasan PK, Jaisankar TJ, Thappa D, Sujatha S. Clinical variations in dermatophytosis in HIV infected patients. Indian J Dermatol Venereol Leprol. 2002;68:2136.

139. Kelly BP. Superficial fungal infections. Pediatr Rev. 2012;33(4):e22–37.

140. Khambaty MM, Hsu SS. Dermatology of the patient with HIV. Emerg Med Clin North Am. 2010;28(2):355–68.

141. Khanna, N. Illustrated synopsis of dermatology and sexually transmitted diseases. 5th ed. India: Elsevier Health Sciences; 2015.

142. Khuraijam R, Lungran P, Yoihenba K, Laishram RS, Pukhrambam P. Pancytopenia and cutaneous cryptococcosis as an indicator disease of acquired immune deficiency syndrome. Indian J Med Microbiol. 2015;33(3):439–42.

143. Kim DK, Bridges CB, Harriman KH, Advisory Committee on Immunization Practices. Advisory committee on immunization practices recommended immunization schedule for adults aged 19 years or older: United States, 2016. Ann Intern Med. 2016;164(3):184–94.

144. Kollipara R, Ekhlassi E, Downing C, Guidry J, Lee M, Tyring SK. Advancements in pharmacotherapy for noncancerous manifestations of HPV. J Clin Med. 2015;4(5):832–46.

145. Kosik-Bogacka DI, Łanocha N, Łanocha A, Czepita D, Grobelny A, Zdziarska B, et al. Demodex folliculorum and Demodex brevis in healthy and immunocompromised patients. Ophthalmic Epidemiol. 2013;20:159–63.

146. La Ferla L, Pinzone MR, Nunnari G, Martellotta F, Lleshi A, Tirelli U, et al. Kaposi' s sarcoma in HIV-positive patients: the state of art in the HAART-era. Eur Rev Med Pharmacol Sci. 2013;17(17):2354–65.

147. Laanani M, Ghosn J, Essat A, Melard A, Seng R, Agence Nationale de Recherche sur le Sida PRIMO Cohort Study Group, et al. Impact of the timing of initiation of antiretroviral therapy during primary HIV-1 infection on the decay of cell-associated HIV-DNA. Clin Infect Dis. 2015;60(11):1715–21.

148. Lacey CJ, Woodhall SC, Wikstrom A, Ross J. 2012 European guideline for the management of anogenital warts. J Eur Acad Dermatol Venereol. 2013;27(3):e263–70.

149. Lacey N, Russell-Hallinan A, Powell FC. Study of demodex mites: challenges and solutions. J Eur Acad Dermatol Venereol. 2016;30(5):764–75.

150. Lakshmi SJ, Rao GR, Ramalakshmi, Satyasree, Rao KA, Prasad PG, Kumar YH. Pruritic papular eruptions of HIV: a clinicopathologic and therapeutic study. Indian J Dermatol Venereol Leprol. 2008;74:501–3.

151. Lama JR, Lucchetti A, Suarez L, Laguna-Torres VA, Guanira JV, Pun M, et al. Association of herpes simplex virus type 2 infection and syphilis with human immunodeficiency virus infection among men who have sex with men in Peru. J Infect Dis. 2006;194:1459–66.

152. Lawn SD, Wilkinson RJ. Immune reconstitution disease associated with parasitic infections following antiretroviral treatment. Parasite Immunol. 2006;28:625–33.

153. Lawn SD, Lipman MC, Easterbrook PJ. Immune reconstitution disease associated with mycobacterial infections. Curr Opin HIV AIDS. 2008;3(4):425–31.

154. LeGoff J, Péré H, Bélec L. Diagnosis of genital herpes simplex virus infection in the clinical laboratory. Virol J. 2014;11:83.

155. Lehloenya R, Meintjes G. Dermatologic manifestations of the immune reconstitution inflammatory syndrome. Dermatol Clin. 2006;24:549–70.

156. Lehloenya RJ, Kgokolo M. Clinical presentations of severe cutaneous drug reactions in HIV-infected Africans. Dermatol Clin. 2014;32(2):227–35.

157. Letang E, Naniche D, Bower M, Miro JM. Kaposi sarcoma-associated immune reconstitution inflammatory syndrome: in need of a specific case definition. Clin Infect Dis. 2012;55(1):157–8.

158. Levin MJ, Weinberg A, Schmid DS. Herpes simplex virus and varicella-zoster virus. Microbiol Spectr. 2016;4(3):1–20.

159. Lindoso JA, Barbosa RN, Posada-Vergara MP, Duarte MI, Oyafuso LK, Amato VS, et al. Unusual manifestations of tegumentary leishmaniasis in AIDS patients from the New World. Br J Dermatol. 2009;160(2):311–8.

160. Lingappa JR, Baeten JM, Wald A, Hughes JP, Thomas KK, Mujugira A, et al. Daily aciclovir for HIV-1 disease progression in people dually infected with HIV-1 and herpes simplex virus type 2: a randomised placebo-controlled trial. Lancet. 2010;375:824–33.

161. Looker KJ, Magaret AS, May MT, Turner KME, Vickerman P, Gottlieb SL, et al. Global and regional estimates of prevalent and incident herpes simplex virus type 1 infections in 2012. PLoS ONE. 2015;10(10):e0140765. Accessed 12 Aug 2016. Retrieved from http://journals.plos.org/plosone/article?id=10.1371/journal.pone.0140765.

162. Looker KJ, Magaret AS, Turner KME, Vickerman P, Gottlieb SL, Newman LN. Global estimates of prevalent and incident herpes simplex virus type 2 infections in 2012. PLoS ONE. 2015;10(1):e114989. Accessed in 2016 Aug 12. Retrieved from http://journals.plos.org/plosone/article?id=10.1371/journal.pone.0114989 Accessed 12 Aug 2016.

163. Lova-Navarro M, Gómez-Moyano E, Pilar LM, Fernandez-Ballesteros MD, Godoy-Díaz DJ, Vera-Casaño A, Crespo-Erchiga V. Tinea capitis in adults in southern Spain. A 17-year epidemiological study. Rev Iberoam Micol. 2016;33(2):110–3.

164. Lowe SM, Katsidzira L, Meys R, Sterling JC, de Koning M, Quint W, et al. Acquired epidermodysplasia verruciformis due to multiple and unusual HPV infection among vertically infected, HIV-positive adolescents in Zimbabwe. Clin Infect Dis. 2012;54:e119–23.

165. MacNeal RJ, Dinulos JG. Acute retroviral syndrome. Dermatol Clin. 2006;24(4):431–8.

166. Maguiña C, Guerra H, Ventosilla P. Bartonellosis. Clin Dermatol. 2009;27(3):271–80.

167. Mahe A, Simon F, Coulibaly S, Tounkara A, Bobin P. Predictive value of seborrheic dermatitis and other common dermatoses for HIV infection in Bamaki Mali. J Am Acad Dermatol. 1996;34(6):1084–6.

168. Mallon E, Bunker CB. HIV-associated psoriasis. AIDS Patient Care STDs. 2000;14:239–46.

169. Manguro GO, Masese LN, Deya RW, Magaret A, Wald A, McClelland RS, Graham SM. Genital HSV Shedding among Kenyan Women Initiating Antiretroviral Therapy. PLoS One. 2016;11(9):e0163541.

170. Manzardo C, Guardo AC, Letang E, Plana M, Gatell JM, Miro JM. Opportunistic infections and immune reconstitution inflammatory syndrome in HIV-1-infected adults in the combined antiretroviral therapy era: a comprehensive review. Expert Rev Anti-Infect Ther. 2015;13(6):751–67.

171. Markowitz LE, Dunne EF, Saraiya M, Chesson HW, Curtis CR, Gee J, et al. Human papillomavirus vaccination: recommendations of the Advisory Committee on Immunization Practices (ACIP). MMWR Recomm Rep. 2014;63(RR-05):1–30.

172. Marques SA, Bastazini I Jr, Martins AL, Barreto JA, Barbieri D'Elia MP, Lastória JC, Marques ME. Primary cutaneous cryptococcosis in Brazil: report of 11 cases in immunocompetent and immunosuppressed patients. Int J Dermatol. 2012;51(7):780–4.

173. Markova A, Kam SA, Miller DD, Lichtman MK. In the clinic. Common cutaneous parasites. Ann Intern Med. 2014;161(5):1–16.

174. Martellotta F, Berretta M, Vaccher E, Schioppa O, Zanet E, Tirelli U. AIDS-related Kaposi's sarcoma: state of the art and therapeutic strategies. Curr HIV Res. 2009;7(6):634–8.

175. Martin P. Interventions for molluscum contagiosum in people infected with human immunodeficiency virus: a systematic review. Int J Dermatol. 2016;55(9):956–66. doi:10.1111/ijd.13267.

176. Martin-Blondel G, Mars LT, Liblau RS. Pathogenesis of the immune reconstitution inflammatory syndrome in HIV-infected patients. Curr Opin Infect Dis. 2012;25(3):312–20.

177. Martin-Iguacel R, Kurtzhals J, Jouvion G, Nielsen SD, Llibre JM. Progressive disseminated histoplasmosis in the HIV population in Europe in the HAART era. Case report and literature review. Infection. 2014;42(4):611–20.

178. Martins AB, Matos ED, Lemos AC. Infection with the *Mycobacterium avium complex* in patients without predisposing conditions: a case report and literature review. Braz J Infect Dis. 2005;9(2):173–9.

179. Martins CR. Cutaneous drug reactions associated with newer antiretroviral agents. J Drugs Dermatol. 2006;5(10):976–82.

180. Mason AR, Mason J, Cork M, Dooley G, Hancock H. Topical treatments for chronic plaque psoriasis. Cochrane Database Syst Rev. 2013;3:CD005028.

181. Mathes BM, Douglass MC. Seborrheic dermatitis in patients with acquired immunodeficiency syndrome. J Am Acad Dermatol. 1985;13:947–51.

182. Maurer TA. Dermatologic manifestations of HIV infection. Top HIV Med. 2005–2006;13(5):149–54.

183. Mayer KH. Sexually transmitted diseases in men who have sex with men. Clin Infect Dis. 2011;53(Suppl 3):S79–83.

184. Maziarz EK, Perfect JR. Cryptococcosis. Infect Dis Clin N Am. 2016;30(1):179–206.

185. McCalmont TH, Altemus D, Maurer T, Berger TG. Eosinophilic folliculitis. The histologic spectrum. Am J Dermatopathol. 1995;17:439–46.

186. Meintjes G, Lawn SD, Scano F, Maartens G, French MA, Worodria W, International Network for the Study of HIV-associated IRIS, et al. Tuberculosis-associated immune reconstitution inflammatory syndrome: case definitions for use in resource-limited settings. Lancet Infect Dis. 2008;8(8):516–23.

187. Meintjes G, Scriven J, Marais S. Management of the immune reconstitution inflammatory syndrome. Curr HIV/AIDS Rep. 2012;9:238–50.

188. Menezes RP, Borges AS, Araujo LB, Pedroso Rdos S, Röder DV. Related factors for colonization by Candida species in the oral cavity of HIV-infected individuals. Rev Inst Med Trop Sao Paulo. 2015;57(5):413–9.

189. Menon K, Van Voorhees AS, Bebo BF Jr, Gladman DD, Hsu S, Kalb RE, et al. Psoriasis in patients with HIV infection: from the medical board of the National Psoriasis Foundation. J Am Acad Dermatol. 2010;62(2):291–9.

190. Meys R, Macedo C, Jones R, Day S, Weir J, Gotch FM, et al. Cutaneous human papillomavirus-related immune reconstitution-associated disease in human immunodeficiency virus: an under-recognized phenomenon. Br J Dermatol. 2011;164(2):458–9.

191. Mirmirani P, Hessol NA, Maurer TA, Berger TG, Nguyen P, Khalsa A, Gurtman A, Micci S, Young M, Holman S, Gange SJ, Greenblatt RM. Prevalence and predictors of skin disease in the Women's Interagency HIV Study (WIHS). J Am Acad Dermatol. 2001;44(5):785–8.

192. Mohle-Boetani JC, Koehler JE, Berger TG, LeBoit PE, Kemper CA, Reingold AL, et al. Bacillary angiomatosis and bacillary peliosis in patients infected with human immunodeficiency virus: clinical characteristics in a case-control study. Clin Infect Dis. 1996;22(5):794–800.

193. Moore RL, de Schaetzen V, Joseph M, Lee IA, Miller-Monthrope Y, Phelps BR, et al. Acquired epidermodysplasia verruciformis syndrome in HIV-infected pediatric patients: prospective treatment trial with topical glycolic acid and human papillomavirus genotype characterization. Arch Dermatol. 2012;148(1):128–30.

194. Moraes AP, Arruda EA, Vitoriano MA, Moraes Filho MO, Bezerra FA, Magalhaes Holanda E, et al. An open-label efficacy pilot study with pimecrolimus cream 1% in adults with facial seborrhoeic dermatitis infected with HIV. Eur Acad Dermatol Venereol. 2007;21:596–601.

195. Morar N, Dlova N, Gupta AK, Naidoo DK, Aboobaker J, Ramdial PK. Erythroderma: a comparison between HIV positive and negative patients. Int J Dermatol. 1999;38:895–900.

196. Morar N, Willis-Owen SA, Maurer T, Bunker CB. HIV associated psoriasis: pathogenesis, clinical features, and management. Lancet Infect Dis. 2010;10:470–8.

197. Moreira JA, Freitas DF, Lamas CC. The impact of sporotrichosis in HIV-infected patients: a systematic review. Infection. 2015;43(3):267–76.

198. Morgan MC, Bartlett BL, Cockerell CJ, Cohen PR. Cutaneous manifestations of HIV infection. In: Motswalw S, Moore AY, Lupi O, editors. Mucocutaneous manifestations of viral diseases: an illustrated guide to diagnosis and management. 2nd ed. London: Informa Healthcare; 2010. p. 263–340.

199. Motswaledi MH, Visser W. The spectrum of HIV-associated infective and inflammatory dermatoses in pigmented skin. Dermatol Clin. 2014;32(2):211–25.

200. Mounsey KE, McCarthy JS. Treatment and control of scabies. Curr Opin Infect Dis. 2013;26(2):133–9.

201. Mukherjee PK, Chen H, Patton LL, Evans S, Lee A, Kumwenda J, et al. Topical gentian violet compared to nystatin oral suspension for the treatment of oropharyngeal candidiasis in HIV-1 Infected participants. AIDS. 2016 Sep 24. Retrieved from http://journals.lww.com/aidsonline/Fulltext/publishahead/Topical_gentian_violet_compared_to_nystatin_oral.97663.aspx.

202. Mulhem E, Pinelis S. Treatment of nongenital cutaneous warts. Am Fam Physician. 2011;84(3):288–93.

203. Muller M, Wandel S, Colebunders R, Attia S, Furrer H, Egger M, IeDEA Southern and Central Africa. Immune reconstitution inflammatory syndrome in patients starting antiretroviral therapy for HIV infection: a systematic review and meta-analysis. Lancet Infect Dis. 2010;10(4):251–61.

204. Munderi P, Snowden WB, Walker AS, Kityo C, Mosteller M, Kabuye G, et al. Distribution of HLA-B alleles in a Ugandan HIV-infected adult population: NORA pharmacogenetic substudy of DART. Tropical Med Int Health. 2011;16:200–4.

205. Murakawa GJ, Kerschmann R, Berger T. Cutaneous cryptococcus infection and AIDS. Report of 12 cases and review of literature. Arch Dermatol. 1996;132:5.

206. Mushi MF, Mtemisika CI, Bader O, Bii C, Mirambo MM, Groß U, Mshana SE. High oral carriage of non-albicans Candida spp. among HIV-infected individuals. Int J Infect Dis. 2016;49:185–8.

207. Narang K, Pahwa M, Ramesh V. Tinea capitis in the form of concentric rings in an HIV positive adult on antiretroviral treatment. Indian J Dermatol. 2012;57(4):288–90.

208. Navarini AA, Stoeckle M, Navarini S, Mossdorf E, Jullu BS, Mchomvu R, Mbata M, Kibatala P, Tanner M, Hatz C, Schmid-Grendelmeier P. Antihistamines are superior to topical steroids in managing human immunodeficiency virus (HIV)-associated papular pruritic eruption. Int J Dermatol. 2010;49:83–6.

209. Navarrete-Dechent C, Ortega R, Fich F, Concha M. [Dermatologic manifestations associated with HIV/AIDS]. [Article in Spanish]. Rev Chil Infectol. 2015;32(Suppl 1):S57–71.

210. Neglected histoplasmosis in Latin America Group. Disseminated histoplasmosis in Central and South America, the invisible elephant: the lethal blind spot of international health organizations. AIDS. 2016;30(2):167–70.

211. Nenoff P, Krüger C, Ginter-Hanselmayer G, Tietz HJ. Mycology – an update. Part 1: dermatomycoses: causative agents, epidemiology and pathogenesis. J Dtsch Dermatol Ges. 2014;12(3):188–209. quiz 210, 188-211; quiz 212.

212. Nenoff P, Krüger C, Schaller J, Ginter-Hanselmayer G, Schulte-Beerbühl R, Tietz HJ. Mycology – an update part 2: dermatomycoses: clinical picture and diagnostics. J Dtsch Dermatol Ges. 2014;12(9):749–77.

213. Neuville S, Dromer F, Morin O, Dupont B, Ronin O, Lortholary O, et al. Primary cutaneous cryptococcosis: a distinct clinical entity. Clin Infect Dis. 2003;36(3):337–47.

214. Noguchi H, Hiruma M, Maruo K, Jono M, Miyata K, Tanaka H, et al. Localized cutaneous cryptococcosis: summary of reported cases in Japan. Med Mycol J. 2016;57(3):E35–9. doi:10.3314/mmj.15-00024.

215. Norman FF, Martín-Dávila P, Fortún J, Dronda F, Quereda C, Sánchez-Sousa A, López-Vélez R. Imported histoplasmosis: two distinct profiles in travelers and immigrants. J Travel Med. 2009;16(4):258–62.

216. Nyitray AG, Iannacone MR. The epidemiology of human papillomaviruses. Curr Probl Dermatol. 2014;45:75–91.

217. Obuch ML, Maurer TA, Becker B, Berger TG. Psoriasis and human immunodeficiency virus infection. J Am Acad Dermatol. 1992;27:667–73.

218. Oliveira PM, Mascarenhas REM, Ferrer SR, Oliveira RPC, Travessa IEM, Gomes MVC, et al. [Vaginal infections in human immunodeficiency virus-infected women] [Article in Portuguese]. Rev Bras Ginecol Obst. 2008;30(30):121–6.

219. Oliveira PM, Mascarenhas RE, Lacroix C, Ferrer SR, Oliveira RP, Cravo EA, et al. Candida species isolated from the vaginal mucosa of HIV-infected women in Salvador, Bahia, Brazil. Braz J Infect Dis. 2011;15(3):239–44.

220. Ollague Sierra JE, Ollague Torres JM. New clinical and histological patterns of acute disseminated histoplasmosis in human immunodeficiency virus-positive patients with acquired immunodeficiency syndrome. Am J Dermatopathol. 2013;35(2):205–12.

221. Olsen JR, Gallacher J, Piguet V, Francis NA. Epidemiology of molluscum contagiosum in children: a systematic review. Fam Pract. 2014;31(2):130–6.

222. Oninla OA. Mucocutaneous manifestations of HIV and the correlation with WHO clinical staging in a tertiary hospital in Nigeria. AIDS Res Treat. 2014;2014:360970.

223. Osei-Sekyere B, Karstaedt AS. Immune reconstitution inflammatory syndrome involving the skin. Clin Exp Dermatol. 2010;35(5):477–81.

224. Ostlere LS, Taylor CR, Harris DW, Rustin MH, Wright S, Johnson M. Skin surface lipids in HIV-positive patients with and without seborrheic dermatitis. Int J Dermatol. 1996;35(4):276–9.

225. Palamaras I, Kyriakis KP, Stavrianeas NG. Seborrhoeic dermatitis: lifetime detection rates. J Eur Acad Dermatol Venereol. 2012;26:524–6.

226. Pan B, Chen M, Pan W, Liao W. Histoplasmosis: a new endemic fungal infection in China? Review and analysis of cases. Mycoses. 2013;56(3):212–21.

227. Panel on Opportunistic Infections in HIV-Infected Adults and Adolescents. Guidelines for the prevention and treatment of opportunistic infections in HIV-infected adults and adolescents: recommendations from the Centers for Disease Control and Prevention, the National Institutes of Health, and the HIV Medicine Association of the Infectious Diseases Society of America. Nov 2016. [Cryptococcosis; M1–11] Accessed 15 Nov 2016. Retrieved from http://aidsinfo.nih.gov/contentfiles/lvguidelines/adult_oi.pdf.

228. Panel on Opportunistic Infections in HIV-Infected Adults and Adolescents. Guidelines for the prevention and treatment of opportunistic infections in HIV-infected adults and adolescents: recommendations from the Centers for Disease Control and Prevention, the National Institutes of Health, and the HIV Medicine Association of the Infectious Diseases Society of America. Nov 2016. [Leishmaniasis; T-15, p 281–91] Accessed 15 Nov 2016. Retrieved from http://aidsinfo.nih.gov/contentfiles/lvguidelines/adult_oi.pdf.

229. Papp KA, Papp A, Dahmer B, Clark CS. Single-blind, randomized controlled trial evaluating the treatment of facial seborrheic dermatitis with hydrocortisone 1% ointment compared with tacrolimus 0.1% ointment in adults. J Am Acad Dermatol. 2012;67(1):e11–5.

230. Pappas PG, Kauffman CA, Andes DR, Clancy CJ, Marr KA, Ostrosky-Zeichner L, et al. Clinical practice guideline for the management of candidiasis: 2016 update by the infectious diseases society of America. Clin Infect Dis. 2016;62(4):e1–50.

231. Park IU, Introcaso C, Dunne EF. Human papillomavirus and genital warts: a review of the evidence for the 2015 centers for disease control and prevention sexually transmitted diseases treatment guidelines. Clin Infect Dis. 2015;61(Suppl 8):S849–55.

232. Patton LL. Oral lesions associated with human immunodeficiency virus disease. Dent Clin N Am. 2013;57(4):673–98.

233. Patel RV, Weinberg JM. Psoriasis in the patient with human immunodeficiency virus, part 1: review of pathogenesis. Cutis. 2008;82(2):117–22.

234. Patel RV, Weinberg JM. Psoriasis in the patient with human immunodeficiency virus, part 2: review of treatment. Cutis. 2008;82(3):202–10.

235. Peeling RW, Hook EW 3rd. The pathogenesis of syphilis: the Great Mimicker, revisited. J Pathol. 2006;208(2):224–32.

236. Perfect JR, Dismukes WE, Dromer F, Goldman DL, Graybill JR, Hamill RJ, et al. Clinical practice guidelines for the management of cryptococcal disease: 2010 update by the infectious diseases society of America. Clin Infect Dis. 2010;50(3):291–322.

237. Pereira GA, Stefani MM, Araújo Filho JA, Souza LC, Stefani GP, Martelli CM. Human immunodeficiency virus type 1 (HIV-1) and mycobacterium leprae

co-infection: HIV-1 subtypes and clinical, immunologic, and histopathologic profiles in a Brazilian cohort. AmJTrop Med Hyg. 2004;71(5):679–84.

238. Phillips EJ, Mallal SA. Abacavir hypersensitivity reaction. In: UpToDate, Bartlett JG (Ed), UpToDate, Mitty J. Accessed on 17 Oct 2016. Retrieved from https://www.uptodate.com/contents/abacavir-hypersensitivity-reaction.

239. Phiske MM. Current trends in congenital syphilis. Indian J Sex Transm Dis. 2014;35(1):12–20.

240. Pialoux G, Vimont S, Moulignier A, Buteux M, Abraham B, Bonnard P. Effect of HIV infection on the course of syphilis. AIDS Rev. 2008;10(2):85–92.

241. Pienaar ED, Young T, Holmes H. Interventions for the prevention and management of oropharyngeal candidiasis associated with HIV infection in adults and children. Cochrane Database Syst Rev. 2010;11:CD003940. doi:10.1002/14651858. CD003940.pub3.

242. Piot P, Quinn TC, Taelman H, Feinsod FM, Minlangu KB, Wobin O, et al. Acquired immunodeficiency syndrome in a heterosexual population in Zaire. Lancet. 1984;2(8394):65–9.

243. Piot P, Quinn TC. The AIDS pandemic – a global health paradigm. N Engl J Med. 2013;368(23):2210–8.

244. Piraccini BM, Alessandrini A. Onychomycosis: a review. J Fungi. 2015;1:30–43.

245. Radu O, Pantanowitz L. Kaposi sarcoma. Arch Pathol Lab Med. 2013;137(2):289–94.

246. Rajendran PM, Dolev JC, Heaphy MR Jr, Maurer T. Eosinophilic folliculitis: before and after the introduction of antiretroviral therapy. Arch Dermatol. 2005;141:1227–31.

247. Ramdial PK, Calonje E, Sing Y, Chotey NA, Aboobaker J. Molluscum-like cutaneous cryptococcosis: a histopathological and pathogenetic appraisal. J Cutan Pathol. 2008;35(11):1007–13.

248. Ramos-e-Silva M, Vasconcelos C, Carneiro S, Cestari T. Sporotrichosis. Clin Dermatol. 2007;25:181–7.

249. Ramos-E-Silva M, Lima CM, Schechtman RC, Trope BM, Carneiro S. Superficial mycoses in immunodepressed patients (AIDS). Clin Dermatol. 2010;28(2):217–25.

250. Ramos-e-Silva M, Lima CM, Schechtman RC, Trope BM, Carneiro S. Systemic mycoses in immunodepressed patients (AIDS). Clin Dermatol. 2012;30(6):616–27.

251. Ratnam I, Chiu C, Kandala NB, Easterbrook PJ. Incidence and risk factors for immune reconstitution inflammatory syndrome in an ethnically diverse HIV type 1-infected cohort. Clin Infect Dis. 2006;42:418–27.

252. Rebbapragada A, Wachihi C, Pettengell C, Sunderji S, Huibner S, Jaoko W, et al. Negative mucosal synergy between herpes simplex type 2 and HIV in the female genital tract. AIDS. 2007;21:589–98.

253. Resneck JS Jr, Van Beek M, Furmanski L, Oyugi J, LeBoit PE, Katabira E, et al. Etiology of pruritic papular eruption with HIV infection in Uganda. JAMA. 2004;292:2614–21.

254. Reusser NM, Downing C, Guidry J, Tyring SK. HPV carcinomas in immunocompromised patients. J Clin Med. 2015;4(2):260–81.

255. Rigopoulos D, Paparizos V, Katsambas A. Cutaneous markers of HIV infection. Clin Dermatol. 2004;22(6):487–98.

256. Rodgers S, Leslie KS. Skin infections in HIV-infected individuals in the era of HAART. Curr Opin Infect Dis. 2011;24(2):124–9.

257. Rodríguez-Cerdeira C, Arenas R, Moreno-Coutiño G, Vásquez E, Fernández R, Chang P. Systemic fungal infections in patients with human inmunodeficiency virus. Actas Dermosifiliogr. 2014;105(1):5–17.

258. Rodwell GE, Bayles CL, Towersey L, Aly R. The prevalence of dermatophyte infection in patients infected with human immunodeficiency virus. Int J Dermatol. 2008;47(4):339–43.

259. Roett MA, Mayor MT, Uduhiri KA. Diagnosis and management of genital ulcers. Am Fam Physician. 2012;85(3):254–62.

260. Rogers HD, Macgregor JL, Nord KM, Tyring S, Rady P, Engler DE, et al. Acquired epidermodysplasia verruciformis. J Am Acad Dermatol. 2009;60(2):315–20.

261. Romani L, Steer AC, Whitfeld MJ, Kaldor JM. Prevalence of scabies and impetigo worldwide: a systematic review. Lancet Infect Dis. 2015;15(8):960–7.

262. Rosamilia LL. Scabies. Semin Cutan Med Surg. 2014;33(3):106–9.

263. Rosatelli JB, Machado AA, Roselino AM. Dermatoses among Brazilian HIV-positive patients: correlation with the evolutionary phases of AIDS. Int J Dermatol. 1997;36(10):729–34.

264. Rosatelli JB, Roselino AM. Hyper-IgE, eosinophilia, and immediate cutaneous hypersensitivity to insect antigens in the pruritic papular eruption of human immunodeficiency virus. Arch Dermatol. 2001;137(5):672–3.

265. Rosenthal D, LeBoit PE, Klumpp L, Berger TG. Human immunodeficiency virus-associated eosinophilic folliculitis. A unique dermatosis associated with advanced human immunodeficiency virus infection. Arch Dermatol. 1991;127:206–9.

266. Rotta I, Ziegelmann PK, Otuki MF, Riveros BS, Bernardo NL, Correr CJ. Efficacy of topical antifungals in the treatment of dermatophytosis: a mixed-treatment comparison meta-analysis involving 14 treatments. JAMA Dermatol. 2013;149(3):341–9.

267. Rowe A, Mallon E, Rosenberger P, Barrett M, Walsh J, Bunker CB. Depletion of cutaneous peptidergic innervation in HIV-associated xerosis. J Invest Dermatol. 1999;112:284–9.

268. Rusiecka-Ziółkowska J, Nokiel M, Fleischer M. Demodex – an old pathogen or a new one? Adv Clin Exp Med. 2014;23(2):295–8.

269. Sahoo AK, Mahajan R. Management of tinea corporis, tinea cruris, and tinea pedis: a comprehensive review. Indian Dermatol Online J. 2016;7(2):77–86.

270. Sampaio AL, Mameri AC, Vargas TJ, Ramos-e-Silva M, Nunes AP, Carneiro SC. Seborrheic dermatitis. [Article in English, Portuguese]. An Bras Dermatol. 2011;86(6):1061–71. quiz 1072-4.

271. Sauerbrei A. Optimal management of genital herpes: current perspectives. Infect Drug Resist. 2016;9:129–41.

272. Sauerbrei A. Diagnosis, antiviral therapy, and prophylaxis of varicella-zoster virus infections. Eur J Clin Microbiol Infect Dis. 2016;35(5):723–34.

273. Sbidian E, Battistella M, Legoff J, Lafaurie M, Bézier M, Agbalika F, et al. Recalcitrant pseudotumoral anogenital herpes simplex virus type 2 in HIV-infected patients: evidence for predominant B-lymphoplasmocytic infiltration and immunomodulators as effective therapeutic strategy. Clin Infect Dis. 2013;57(11):1648–55.

274. Schechtman RC. Sporotrichosis: part I. Skinmed. 2010;8(4):216–20. quiz 221.

275. Schuetz A, Deleage C, Sereti I, Rerknimitr R, Phanuphak N, Phuang-Ngern Y, et al. RV254/SEARCH 010 and RV304/SEARCH 013 Study Groups. Initiation of ART during early acute HIV infection preserves mucosal Th17 function and reverses HIV-related immune activation. PLoS Pathog. 2014;10(12):e1004543. Accessed on 23 Aug 2016. Retrieved from http://journals.plos.org/plospathogens/article?id=10.1371/journal.ppat.1004543.

276. Schwartz JR, Messenger AG, Tosti A, Todd G, Hordinsky M, Hay RJ, et al. A comprehensive pathophysiology of dandruff and seborrheic dermatitis – towards a more precise definition of scalp health. Acta Derm Venereol. 2013;93(2):131–7.

277. Segal E, Frenkel M. Dermatophyte infections in environmental contexts. Res Microbiol. 2015;166(7):564–9.

278. Serling SL, Leslie K, Maurer T. Approach to pruritus in the adult HIV-positive patient. Semin Cutan Med Surg. 2011;30(2):101–6.

279. Sharma A, Vora R, Modi M, Sharma A, Marfatia Y. Adverse effects of antiretroviral treatment. Indian J Dermatol Venereol Leprol. 2008;74:234–7.

280. Sharma SK, Soneja M. HIV & immune reconstitution inflammatory syndrome (IRIS). Indian J Med Res. 2011;134(6):866–77.

281. Shelburne SA, Montes M, Hamill RJ. Immune reconstitution inflammatory syndrome: more answers, more questions. J Antimicrob Chemother. 2006;57:167–70.

282. Shiohara T, Kurata M, Mizukawa Y, Kano Y. Recognition of immune reconstitution syndrome necessary for better management of patients with severe drug eruptions and those under immunosuppressive therapy. Allergol Int. 2010;59(4):333–43.

283. Schofer H, Imhof M, Thoma-Greber E, Brockmeyer NH, Hartmann M, Gerken G, et al. Active syphilis in HIV infection: a multicentre retrospective survey. The German AIDS Study Group (GASG). Genitourin Med. 1996;72:176–81.

284. Silva BC, Paula CR, Auler ME, Ruiz LS, Santos JI, Yoshioka MC, et al. Dermatophytosis and immunovirological status of HIV-infected and AIDS patients from Sao Paulo city, Brazil. Mycoses. 2014;57(6):371–6.

285. Singal A, Khanna D. Onychomycosis: diagnosis and management. Indian J Dermatol Venereol Leprol. 2011;77(6):659–72.

286. Singh A, Preiksaitis J, Ferenczy A, Romanowski B. The laboratory diagnosis of herpes simplex virus infections. Can J Infect Dis Med Microbiol. 2005;16(2):92–8.

287. Singh F, Rudikoff D. HIV-associated pruritus: etiology and management. Am J Clin Dermatol. 2003;4:177–88.

288. Smith K, Kuhn L, Coovadia A, Meyers T, Hu CC, Reitz C, et al. Immune reconstitution inflammatory syndrome among HIV-infected South African infants initiating antiretroviral therapy. AIDS. 2009;23:1097–107.

289. Springinsfeld G, Roth B, Martinot M, Tortel MC, Batard ML. [Immune reconstitution inflammatory syndrome associated with eosinophilic pustular folliculitis in an HIV-infected patient].[Article in French]. Med Mal Infect. 2011;41(1):49–50.

290. Sobel JD. Vulvovaginal candidiasis: a comparison of HIV-positive and -negative women. Int J STD AIDS. 2002;13(6):358–62.

291. Sobel JD. Candidiasis. In: Hospenthal DR, Rinaldi MG, editors. Diagnosis and treatment of human mycoses. Totowa: Humana Press; 2008. p. 137–61.

292. Sobel JD. Recurrent vulvovaginal candidiasis. Am J Obstet Gynecol. 2016;214(1):15–21.

293. Steben M, Garland SM. Genital warts. Best Pract Res Clin Obstet Gynaecol. 2014;28(7):1063–73.

294. Stevenson J, Heath M. Syphilis and HIV infection: an update. Dermatol Clin. 2006;24(4):497–507.

295. Stürzl M, Zietz C, Monini P, Ensoli B. Human herpesvirus-8 and Kaposi's sarcoma: relationship with the multistep concept of tumorigenesis. Adv Cancer Res. 2001;81:125–59.

296. Sud N, Shanker V, Sharma A, Sharma NL, Gupta M. Mucocutaneous manifestations in 150 HIV-infected Indian patients and their relationship with CD4 lymphocyte counts. Int J STD AIDS. 2009;20:771–4.

297. Tan DH, Raboud JM, Kaul R, Walmsley SL. Antiretroviral therapy is not associated with reduced herpes simplex virus shedding in HIV coinfected adults: an observational cohort study. BMJ Open. 2014;4:e004210. Accessed on 19 Sept 2016. Retrieved from http://bmjopen.bmj.com/content/4/1/e004210.full.

298. Tappero JW, Perkins BA, Wenger JD, Berger TG. Cutaneous manifestations of opportunistic infections in patients infected with human immunodeficiency virus. Clin Microbiol Rev. 1995;8(3):440–50.

299. Thurgar E, Barton S, Karner C, Edwards SJ. Clinical effectiveness and cost-effectiveness of interventions for the treatment of anogenital warts: systematic review and economic evaluation. Health Technol Assess. 2016;20(24):v–vi. 1-486.

300. Thurman AR, Doncel GF. Herpes simplex virus and HIV: genital infection synergy and novel approaches to dual prevention. Int J STD AIDS. 2012;23(9):613–9.

301. Tirado-Sánchez A, Bonifaz A, Montes de Oca-Sánchez G, Araiza-Santibañez J, Ponce-Olivera RM. [Crusted scabies in HIV/AIDS infected patients. Report of 15 cases]. [Article in Spanish]. Rev Med Inst Mex Seguro Soc. 2016;54(3):397–400.

302. Towersey L, Cunha MX, Feldman CA, Castro CG, Berger TG. Dermoscopy of Norwegian scabies in a patient with acquired immunodeficiency syndrome. An Bras Dermatol. 2010;85(2):221–3.

303. Tschachler E. The dermatologist and the HIV/AIDS pandemic. Clin Dermatol. 2014;32(2):286–9.

304. UK National Guideline on the Management of Scabies. 2016. Accessed on 23 Sept 2016. Retrieved from [https://www.bashhguidelines.org/media/1099/scabies_guidelines_draft_2016.pdf].

305. Valenti WM. Acute retroviral syndrome: a challenge for primary care. AIDS Read. 2008;18(6):294–6. Accessed on 19 Aug 2016. Retrieved from http://www.theaidsreader.com/articles/acute-retroviral-syndrome-challenge-primary-care.

306. van der Wouden JC, van der Sande R, van Suijlekom-Smit LW, Berger M, Butler CC, Koning S. Interventions for cutaneous molluscum contagiosum. Cochrane Database Syst Rev. 2009;4:CD004767.

307. van Griensven J, Carrillo E, López-Vélez R, Lynen L, Moreno J. Leishmaniasis in immunosuppressed individuals. Clin Microbiol Infect. 2014;20(4):286–99.

308. Vicente A, Pau-Charles I, González-Enseñat MA, Muñoz-Almagro C, Cañadas MP, Noguera-Julian A, et al. High-risk alpha-human papillomavirus types: detection in HIV-infected children with acquired epidermodysplasia verruciformis. J Am Acad Dermatol. 2013;68(2):343–5.

309. Walker NF, Scriven J, Meintjes G, Wilkinson RJ. Immune reconstitution inflammatory syndrome in HIV-infected patients. HIV/AIDS (Auckland, NZ). 2015;7:49–64.

310. Waters L, Nelson M. Long-term complications of antiretroviral therapy: lipoatrophy. Int J Clin Pract. 2007;61:999–1014.

311. Weigle N, McBane S. Psoriasis. Am Fam Physician. 2013;87:626–33.

312. Weis L, Bonamigo RR, Weber MB, Petry V, Luzzatto L. Malignant syphilis and neurolues in an HIV infected patient. Int J Dermatol. 2010;49(5):590–2.

313. Weiss H. Epidemiology of herpes simplex virus type 2 infection in the developing world. Herpes. 2004;11(Suppl. 1):24A–35A.

314. Welsh O, Vera-Cabrera L, Welsh E. Onychomycosis. Clin Dermatol. 2010;28(2):151–9.

315. Wernham AG, Vydianath B, Chua SL. Thalidomide – a novel therapeutic approach for pruritic papular eruption of HIV. JAAD Case Rep. 2015;1(3):109–11.

316. Wheat LJ, Freifeld AG, Kleiman MB, Baddley JW, McKinsey DS, Loyd JE, Infectious Diseases Society of America, et al. Clinical practice guidelines for the management of patients with histoplasmosis: 2007 update by the Infectious Diseases Society of America. Clin Infect Dis. 2007;45(7):807–25.

317. Wheat LJ, Conger NG. Histoplasmosis. In: Hospenthal DR and Rinaldi MG 2008. Diagnosis and treatment of human mycoses. Totowa: Humana Press; p. 317–330.

318. WHO – World Health Organization. Case definitions of HIV for surveillance and revised clinical staging and immunological classification of HIV-related disease in adults and children. Geneva: WHO; 2007. Accessed on 15 Oct 2016. Retrieved from http://www.who.int/hiv/pub/guidelines/hivstaging/en/.

319. WHO – World Health Organization. Control of leishmaniases. Report of a meeting of the WHO Expert Committee, WHO technical report series 949. Geneve: WHO; 2010. p. 1–186. Accessed on 15 Oct 2016. Retrieved from http://apps.who.int/iris/handle/10665/44412.

320. WHO, Rapid Advice. Diagnosis, prevention and management of cryptococcal disease in HIV-infected adults, adolescents and children. Geneva: WHO Press; 2011. Accessed on 22 Oct 2016. Retrieved from http://www.who.int/hiv/pub/cryptococcal_disease2011/en/.

321. WHO – World Health Organization. Guidelines on the treatment of skin and oral HIV-associated conditions in children and adults. Geneva: WHO; 2014. Accessed on 15 Oct 2016. Retrieved from http://www.who.int/maternal_child_adolescent/documents/skin-mucosal-and-hiv/en/.

322. WHO – World Health Organization. Report on global sexually transmitted infection surveillance 2015. Geneva: WHO; 2016. Accessed on 15 Oct 2016. Retrieved frm http://www.who.int/reproductivehealth/publications/rtis/stis-surveillance-2015/en/.

323. WHO – World Health Organization. Guidelines for the treatment of Treponema pallidum (syphilis). Geneva: WHO; 2016. Accessed on 15 Oct 2016. Retrieved from http://www.who.int/reproductivehealth/publications/rtis/syphilis-treatment-guidelines/en/.

324. WHO – World Health Organization. Leishmaniasis in high-burden countries: an epidemiological update based on data reported in 2014. Wkly Epidemiol Rec. 2016;91(22):287–96. Accessed on 15 Oct 2016. Retrieved fromhttp://www.who.int/wer/2016/wer9122/en/.

325. Wiwanitkit S, Wiwanitkit V. Prevalence of eyelash demodex among human immunodeficiency virus infected patients at different CD4+ count status. Int J Trichology. 2013;5(3):166.

326. Yamaoka T, Murota H, Tani M, Katayama I. Severe rosacea with prominent Demodex folliculorum in a patient with HIV. J Dermatol. 2014;41(2):195–6.

327. Yang C, Mosam A, Mankahla A, Dlova N, Saavedra A. HIV infection predisposes skin to toxic epidermal necrolysis via depletion of skin-directed CD4+ T cells. J Am Acad Dermatol. 2014;70(6):1096–102.

328. Yokobayashi H, Sugaya M, Miyagaki T, Kai H, Suga H, Yamada D, et al. Analysis of serum chemokine levels in patients with HIV-associated eosinophilic folliculitis. J Eur Acad Dermatol Venereol. 2013 ;27(2):e212–6. doi: 10.1111/j.1468-3083.2012.04592.x.

329. Zaghi D, Panosian C, Gutierrez MA, Gregson A, Taylor E, Ochoa MT. New World cutaneous leishmaniasis: current challenges in diagnosis and parenteral treatment. J Am Acad Dermatol. 2011;64(3):587–92.

330. Zampetti A, Giurdanella F, Manco S, Linder D, Gnarra M, Guerriero G, et al. Acquired epidermodysplasia verruciformis: a comprehensive review and a proposal for treatment. Dermatol Surg. 2013;39(7):974–80.

331. Zancanaro PC, McGirt LY, Mamelak AJ, Nguyen RH, Martins CR. Cutaneous manifestations of HIV in the era of highly active antiretroviral therapy: an institutional urban clinic experience. J Am Acad Dermatol. 2006;54(4):581–8.

Suggested Reading and Consulting

CDC Sexually Transmitted Diseases Treatment Guidelines 2015. Available at https://www.cdc.gov/std/tg2015/. Although the guidelines emphasize treatment, prevention strategies and diagnostic recommendations also are discussed. This comprehensive document can be the go-to reference for anyone who manages patients at risk for STDs.

Crum-Cianflone NF, Wallace MR. Vaccination in HIV-infected adults. AIDS Patient Care STDs. 2014;28(8):397–410. Available at https://www.ncbi.nlm.nih.gov/pmc/articles/PMC4117268/

Guidelines for the prevention and treatment of opportunistic infections in HIV-infected adults and adolescents: recommendations from the Centers for Disease Control and Prevention, the National Institutes of Health, and the HIV Medicine Association of the Infectious Diseases Society of America. Available at http://aidsinfo.nih.gov/contentfiles/lvguidelines/adult_oi.pdf. A detailed guideline for management of opportunistic infections in HIV-patients also provides useful information on significant pharmacokinetic interactions between antiretroviral agents for HIV and drugs used to treat or prevent opportunistic infections.

Guidelines on the Treatment of Skin and Oral HIV-Associated Conditions in Children and Adults. Geneva: World Health Organization; 2014. Available at http://www.who.int/maternal_child_adolescent/documents/skin-mucosal-and-hiv/en/These guidelines provide a summary of the key evidence and practice recommendations on the diagnosis and treatment of the main skin and oral conditions in HIV-infected adults and children. The primary audience for these guidelines is health professionals who are responsible for providing care to children, adolescents and adults in settings with HIV, primarily where resources are limited.

HIV Book. Hoffmann C, Rockstroh JK, editors. Available at https://hivbook.com. A freely accessible medical information on HIV treatment.

HIV InSite. Available at http://hivinsite.ucsf.edu. Comprehensive, up-to-date information on HIV/AIDS treatment and prevention from the University of California San Francisco, USA.

Liverpool HIV Drug Interactions website. Available at http://www.hiv-druginteractions.org/. A comprehensive, user-friendly, free drug interaction charts. It provides clinically useful, reliable, up-to date, evidence-based information, freely available to healthcare workers, patients and researchers.

Unemo M, Ballard R, Ison C, Lewis D, Ndowa F, Peeling R. Laboratory diagnosis of sexually transmitted infections, including human immunodeficiency virus. Geneva: World Health Organization (WHO); 2013. p. 107–29. Available at http://www.who.int/reproductivehealth/publications/rtis/9789241505840/en/. This manual provides a basic understanding of the principles of laboratory tests in the context of screening and diagnostic approaches, as well as antimicrobial susceptibility testing, as components of STI control. It covers each disease in a separate chapter providing detailed information on specimen collection, transport, and laboratory testing.

Human T-Cell Lymphotropic Virus Type-1 (HTLV-1) Infection in Dermatology

42

Achiléa Lisboa Bittencourt

Key Points

- Brazil is considered the largest endemic area for HTLV-1 and associated diseases. Notwithstanding, the actual prevalence of this infection in Brazil is not yet available
- Nowadays, with the safe sex campaigns to prevent HIV infection and screening of blood donors for HTLV-1/2, breastfeeding constitutes the principal means of HTLV-1 transmission
- ATL and infective dermatitis generally occur in carriers infected vertically. Notwithstanding, in Brazil there is no public health program to prevent transmission through breastfeeding
- HTLV-1 carriers are more susceptible to scabies, strongyloidiasis, superficial mycoses, bacterial skin diseases, and pulmonary tuberculosis than noninfected individuals
- Knowledge of ATL is very important for dermatologists because it affects the skin in a frequency varying from 43% to 72% as a primary or secondary condition.
- The literature on primary cutaneous ATL is very confusing, with different criteria, and for this reason this matter requires standardization
- Most cases of ATL are similar to mycosis fungoides clinically and histologically
- It is mandatory in endemic areas to search for HTLV-1 infection in all cases diagnosed as mature T-cell leukemia/lymphoma even in childhood and puberty.

Human T-Cell Lymphotropic Virus Type (HTLV-1)

Introduction

The human T-cell lymphotropic virus (HTLV-1) is a retrovirus isolated in 1980 from cells of a cutaneous T-cell lymphoma from a patient with adult T-cell leukemia/lymphoma (ATL). Soon after, a second human retrovirus was described, HTLV-2 [1]. Both are retroviruses that infect T lymphocytes and are similar in approximately 70% of their genome sequences; for this reason serologic cross-reactions exist between them [1].

A.L. Bittencourt
Pathology Department, Complexo Hospitalar
Universitario Prof. Edgard Santos,
Salvador Bahia, Brazil
e-mail: achilea@uol.com.br

© Springer International Publishing Switzerland 2018
R.R. Bonamigo, S.I.T. Dornelles (eds.), *Dermatology in Public Health Environments*,
https://doi.org/10.1007/978-3-319-33919-1_42

Although the majority of HTLV-1-infected persons remain asymptomatic carriers, HTLV-1 is associated with many diseases, whereas HTLV-2 is only sporadically associated with neurologic conditions [2]. In 2005 two other related viruses, HTLV-3 and HTLV-4, were described in Central Africa, but to date they have not been linked to human diseases [1].

Epidemiology

Four major geographic subtypes (genotypes) of HTLV-1 have been described: the Cosmopolitan subtype A, the Central African subtype B, the Central African/Pygmies subtype D, and the Australo-Melanesian subtype C. The Cosmopolitan subtype A, which comprises several geographic subgroups, is the most widespread. Until now these subtypes have not been related to the development of diseases [3].

It is estimated that HTLV-1 infects 5–10 million individuals worldwide, with data based on only infected individuals from known endemic areas from available and reliable epidemiologic studies. The actual number of infected people may be much higher because there are regions where epidemiologic data are not yet available. The main HTLV-1 endemic areas are the Southwestern part of Japan, sub-Saharan Africa, South America, the Caribbean area, and foci in Middle East and Australo-Melanesia [3].

Brazil is considered as the largest endemic area for HTLV-1 and associated diseases. Notwithstanding, the real prevalence of this infection in Brazil is not yet available. Most prevalence studies have been performed among pregnant women or blood donors, without discriminating between the viral types 1 and 2, revealing among pregnant women frequencies varying from 0.1% to 0.2% [3]. Among blood donors from 27 Brazilian capitals, from January 1995 to December 2000 prevalence rates were found to range from 0.4/1,000 in Florianopolis to 10.0/1,000 in São Luis [4] (Fig. 42.1).

A study of 6,754 pregnant women with discrimination between HTLV-1 and HTLV-2, in

Salvador, Brazil, found that 0.84% were HTLV-1 carriers [5]. Four years later, in a city near Salvador, a similar frequency (0.98%) was found among 408 HTLV-1-infected pregnant women [6]. More recently, in Southern Bahia, a prevalence of 1.05% of HTLV-1 infection was found among 2,766 pregnant women [7]. A seroprevalence study of HTLV-1 infection among 5,842 blood donors was performed in five state capitals of four regions of Brazil, with results varying from 1.35% to 0.08%. The lowest seroprevalence was found in Florianópolis and Manaus and the highest in Salvador [8]. In this same city, in 2003 a population-based evaluation revealed an overall prevalence of infection of 1.76%. According to this study, infection rates were 2.0% for females and 1.2% for males, and the infection was more prevalent in individuals 51 years of age or older (8.4%) [9].

The transmission of HTLV-1 infection is generally cell associated because this virus is poorly infectious as cell-free particles. It is transmitted in three ways: vertically, from carrier mothers to their children (mainly through breastfeeding); through sexual contact; and parenterally (through blood transfusion or needle sharing among drug users) [10]. Intravenous exposure to contaminated blood is considered the most efficient way of HTLV-1 transmission [1]. Notwithstanding, the screening of blood donors to HTLV-1/2 has been mandatory in Brazil since 1993 [4]. Plasma and industrial blood products (albumin, immunoglobulin, and antihemophilic factors) do not transmit HTLV-1, but transmission occurs through packed red cells and platelets with frequency varying according to the period of storage, being of more risk in the first 14 days [1]. Sexual transmission is considered to occur mainly from males to females. The rate of HTLV-1 transmission from infected males to females is considered to be 60.8%, whereas transmission from infected females to males occurs only rarely (rate of 0.4%) [10].

Serologic surveys of children born to carrier mothers found carrier state rates varying from 15.4% to 25%. The viral transmission rate depends on HTLV-1 proviral load, duration of breastfeeding, and maternal–fetal concordant

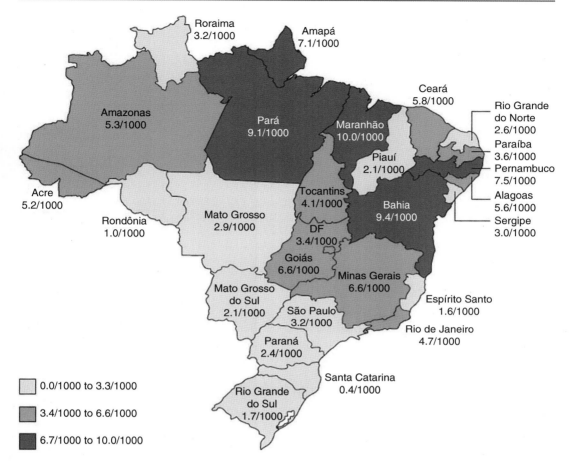

Fig. 42.1 HTLV-1/2 serologic enzyme immunoassay (EIA) screening prevalence rates (per 1,000 donations) in blood donors from the capital cities of 26 states and the Federal District of Brazil (Reprinted from [4] by courtesy of Cadernos de Saúde Pública)

human leukocyte antigen (HLA) class I type [10, 11]. However, bottle-fed children may also become vertically infected. In these children the most probable routes of infection are transplacental or contamination in the birth canal [10]. Transmission via human milk is almost always vertical but may occur by means of breastfeeding by wet-nurses or by cross-nursing (horizontal transmission) [10, 12]. Cross-nursing is a relatively common habit among the poor in Brazil [12].In Brazil there is no public health program to prevent transmission through breastfeeding [13]. Nowadays, with safe-sex campaigns to prevent HIV infection and the screening of blood donors for HTLV-1/2, breastfeeding constitutes the principal means of transmission.

Pathogenicity

HTLV-1 is a complex retrovirus with a single-stranded diploid RNA genome that encodes structural and regulatory proteins and enzymes necessary for the viral replicative cycle [14]. The structural *gag*, *pr*, *pol*, and *env* genes are flanked by 5′ and 3′ long terminal repeats (LTRs). The pX region, situated between *env* and the 3′ LTR, includes regulatory genes encoding Tax, Rex, p21, p12, p13, and p30 proteins as well as the antisense gene encoding the HTLV-1 basic leucine zipper (HBZ) [15, 16] (Fig. 42.2). HTLV-1 protein expression in the infected cells promotes cell cycle progression and survival, and propagation of the proviral DNA by cell division [14].

Fig. 42.2 The HTLV-1 proviral genome. The gag, pr, pol, and env genes are flanked by 5′ and 3′ long terminal repeats (LTRs). In the 3′ portion of the genome is the pX region which includes regulatory genes encoding Tax, Rex, p21, p12, p13, and p30 proteins as well as the antisense gene encoding HTLV-1 basic leucine zipper factor (HBZ) (Modified from Matsuoka and Jeang [15]. Reprinted by courtesy of *Nature Reviews Cancer*)

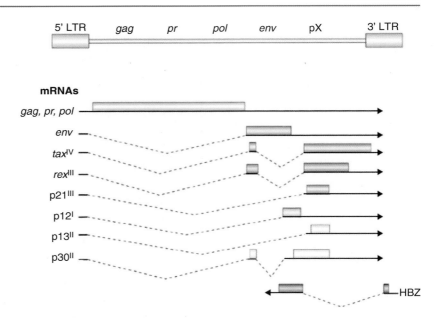

HTLV-1 infect different cells, such as T cells, B cells, fibroblasts, dendritic cells, and macrophages, but the virus persists predominantly in memory CD4+ T cells [14]. The viral propagation occurs through various processes, including the virologic synapse and mitotic clonal proliferation of infected lymphocytes both stimulated by the virus. In the first process the contact between an infected and a target cell induces the formation of a microtubule organizing center through which the viral genome enters the uninfected cell [15] (Fig. 42.3). Within new infected cells, the single-stranded RNA virus is converted to proviral DNA and then integrated into host DNA by viral integrase [11]. Proviral integration in the genome is not random as previously supposed but occurs at different sites, called unique integration sites. In the second mechanism, the HTLV-1 stimulates infected T cells to proliferate by persistent or intermittent expression of Tax and HBZ, resulting in long-lived and abundant clones of infected cells in the circulation, each clone identified by a unique site of integration of the HTLV-1 provirus [16] (Fig. 42.4). As the majority of infected cells harbor only one copy of the provirus, the provirus load indicates the percentage of HTLV-1 infected cells among the circulating host lymphocytes [11].

Clonal proliferation of HTLV-1 infected cells is detected by Southern blot, inverse polymerase chain reaction (PCR), or inverse-long PCR [17]. In Fig. 42.5, a monoclonal pattern of an ATL case detected by inverse-long PCR is shown, determining without doubt the relation between the lymphoma and the virus. Cellular clonality is generally considered qualitatively as polyclonal (Fig. 42.4), oligoclonal, or monoclonal. Clonality of one HTLV-1 infected T-cell population represents the number of distinct clones and the abundance (size) of each clone. Recently, Gillet et al. [18] developed a new method to evaluate clonality which maps and quantifies a great number of HTLV-1 proviral insertion sites. These authors also defined the oligoclonality index to quantify clonality, varying from 0 to 1. The oligoclonality index is low in asymptomatic carriers and patients with HTLV-1-associated myelopathy/tropical spastic paraparesis (HAM/TSP) but this index is significantly greater in ATL patients, in some cases close to 1 (1.0 indicates perfect monoclonality, i.e., all the detected infected cells in an individual presents viral integration at the same point of the genome). Monoclonality equal to 1 is not a real possibility because there are always other small clones. Monoclonality appears when one or two clones became very abundant and predominate over the others, resulting in a sharp rise

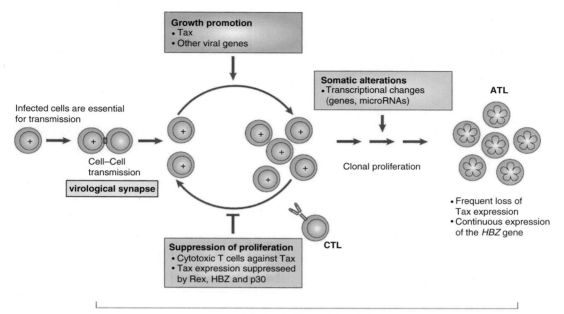

Fig. 42.3 Schematic model of the natural history of HTLV-1 infection to the onset of ATL. An uninfected T cell (empty nucleus) becomes infected (with a + in the nucleus) through a virologic synapse. After infection, HTLV-1 promotes clonal proliferation of infected cells by Tax and HTLV-1 accessory proteins. The proliferation of the infected cells is controlled by the action of the cytotoxic T cells (CTLs). During the latent period of many decades, genetic and epigenetic alterations accumulate in the host genome and ATL may emerge in around 5% of the carriers. Tax expression is suppressed by Rex, HTLV-1 basic leucine zipper factor (HBZ), and p30, in order to escape from CTLs. Tax is needed early to initiate transformation but is not required later to maintain the transformed ATL cells. On the other hand, HBZ is important in all phases (Modified from Matsuoka and Jeang [15]. Reprinted by courtesy of *Nature Reviews Cancer*)

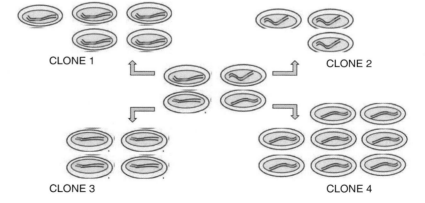

Fig. 42.4 A schematic representation of a polyclonal population. There are four different clones, each one with the same insertion point of the provirus and without great difference in size

in the oligoclonality index and culminating in ATL after a long period of time. An oligoclonality index of 0.48 for an asymptomatic carrier was observed while for ATL cases it varied from 0.79 to 0.85 [18]. This method is important for research, but the demonstration of clonality by Southern blot and inverse or inverse-long PCR (Fig. 42.5) continues to have real importance for

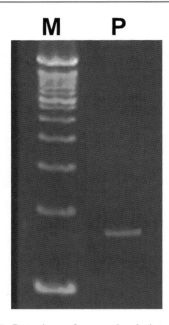

Fig. 42.5 Detection of monoclonal integration of HTLV-1 by inverse and long PCR. The PCR product shown in this figure was sequenced and contains human and virus DNA sequences. *Lane M* DNA molecular weight marker VIII (Roche), *lane P* patient with smoldering ATL (Courtesy of Dr. Lourdes Farré)

the differential diagnosis between ATL and other lymphomas not associated with HTLV-1.

HTLV-1 elicits abundant chronically activated CD8⁺ cytotoxic T lymphocytes (CTLs) [16]. The Tax protein is the main target of these cells, which destroy the host Tax-expressing cells, controlling infection. Notwithstanding, the virus may develop mechanisms to suppress Tax expression because loss of this expression constitutes advantage to the survival of infected cells through the escape from CTLs (Fig. 42.3) [15].

The proviral load depends on the efficiency of the CTL response [16]. It was demonstrated in Southern Japan that the high efficiency of the CTL response in HTLV-1 carriers is related to the host genotype in the HLA Class 1 and killer immunoglobulin-like receptor (KIR) loci, respectively HLA-A*02 and Cw*08, and KIRDL2 [16]. Besides this, there are reports about familial clustering of ATL, HAM/TSP, and infective dermatitis associated with HTLV-1 (IDH), indicating that host genetic background has real influence in the development of HTLV-1 related diseases [15, 19].

The increased number of infected cells in HTLV-1 infection causes an excess of immune reaction, leading to inflammatory diseases such as HAM/TSP, IDH, and HTLV-1-associated uveitis (HAU). HTLV-1-infected individuals with IDH or strongyloidiasis present a significantly increased proviral load and an alteration of HTLV-1 clonality attributable to higher average clone abundance (size) in relation to the asymptomatic carriers. These patients appear to be less capable of reducing clone abundance than HTLV-1 carriers without these associations. Both IDH and strongyloidiasis are considered to increase the risk of development of HTLV-1-associated diseases by the appearance of new clones and an increasing number of infected cells in the pre-existing HTLV-1⁺ clones [20].

The cytokine profile in HTLV-1 infection shows a pattern of a T-helper 1 (Th1) response. A spontaneous cytokine production is seen in asymptomatic carriers and in HAM/TSP and IDH patients with production of higher levels of interleukin (IL)-2, interferon (IFN)-γ, and tumor necrosis factor α (TNF-α) in these patients when compared with asymptomatic carriers. In addition, mononuclear cells from asymptomatic carriers produce high levels of the regulatory cytokines IL-5 and IL-10 when compared with seronegative individuals. The high IL-10 production in asymptomatic carriers downregulates the production of IFN-γ and may explain the asymptomatic status of these carriers, but in vitro such modulation is not seen in HAM/TSP patients [21, 22].

The similarities between the immunologic response in patients with IDH and HAM/TSP (an exaggerated Th1-type immune response) and the high proviral load observed in both diseases would appear to suggest that IDH constitutes a risk factor for the development of HAM/TSP [21]. Moreover, it has been observed that IDH may progress to HAM/TSP, even in childhood and puberty, a severe and disabling form of myelopathy that generally occurs in adulthood [12].

Considering that in ATL patients HTLV-1 infection generally occurs in childhood, a multistep carcinogenesis model has been proposed. Tax is considered to be the main inducer of the early stages of oncogenesis because it stimulates cell proliferation and inhibits apoptosis of the infected cells. The proliferation of the infected cells after a prolonged period may result in the appearance of ATL in approximately 5% of HTLV-1 carriers (Fig. 42.3). There is some evidence that Tax is necessary to initiate transformation but is not required later to maintain the transformed phenotype of ATL cells. However, HBZ is continuously and durably expressed in ATL cells [15].

Host immune competence also plays an important role in controlling the proliferation of infected cells and avoiding leukemogenesis; thus, immunosuppression in HTLV-1-carriers may trigger ATL onset [15].

Diagnosis of Infection

Serology is the most commonly used method for the diagnosis of HTLV-1 infection. The specificity and sensitivity of the tests used to detect HTLV-1 antibodies have improved compared with previous versions. The most commonly used serologic screening test is the enzyme-linked immunosorbent assay (ELISA). Samples that repeatedly test positive in the ELISA must be retested in an immunoblot assay for serologic confirmation to distinguish between HTLV-1 and HTLV-2. For confirmation, the most commonly used method is the highly sensitive western blot 2.4, the specificity of which is 97.5% [17]. Cases that do not meet the criteria for HTLV-1 or HTLV-2 positivity are considered indeterminate. In these cases, molecular testing should be carried out, PCR being the most commonly used method. PCR performed directly on peripheral blood mononuclear cells is able to detect proviral DNA. As a result of its elevated sensitivity and specificity, this method is capable of clarifying indeterminate serologic status and even of detecting the infection in individuals who were defined as seronegative but who had a clinical status suggestive of HTLV-1-associated diseases. PCR is also a confirmatory test for HTLV-1 infection. However, most laboratories are unequipped to perform this method, which is also subject to failure if not performed carefully. PCR is also used to detect the virus in tumor tissue and in other biological specimens [17].

Considering that HTLV/HIV coinfection may have a prevalence of up to 10.9%, it is important to investigate this coinfection in HTLV-1 infected individuals. Besides, there is a suggestion in the literature that the HIV coinfection increases the risk of HAM/TSP [23].

HTLV-1-Related Diseases

HTLV-1 may cause various diseases such as ATL, HAM/TSP, IDH, and HAU, all of which are demonstrably related to the virus [24, 25]. IDH is a childhood disease whereas ATL, HAM/TSP, and HAU are considered adult diseases [26]. HTLV-1 infection has also been linked to polio-myositis, synovitis, thyroiditis, bronchoalveolar pneumonitis, and conjunctivitis sicca [24, 25]. Other conditions significantly more frequently seen among HTLV-1 carriers than in controls are xerostomy, periodontal disease, polyarthralgia, arthritis, erectile dysfunction, and overactive bladder [22]. In some carriers more than one HTLV-1 related disease may occur. In Brazil it has been observed that 14% of the ATL cases are associated with HAM/TSP [27]. Rarely, three HTLV-1-related diseases may appear in some patients simultaneously or sequentially [28, 29].

HTLV-1 acts slowly within the organism, hence the majority of the diseases caused by this virus are considered to be of late onset, emerging in adulthood even when the infection occurred in the early years of life [15]. Notwithstanding, besides IDH, other HTLV-1-related diseases may have a very early onset, occurring even in childhood [26].

HTLV-1 infection causes dysregulation of the immune system, which makes infected individuals more susceptible to other infections such as scabies, strongyloidiasis, superficial mycoses, bacterial skin diseases, and pulmonary tuberculosis in comparison with persons not infected with the virus [1, 17, 30].

In this chapter, only the diseases primarily affecting the skin or those which may cause cutaneous lesions are described.

Infective Dermatitis Associated with HTLV-1 (IDH)

IDH was described in detail as a new disease in 1966, in Jamaica, many years before the discovery of HTLV-1, as a severe form of chronic infected eczema occurring early in childhood [31]. In 1990, it was linked to this virus and in 1998 the criteria for its diagnosis were established [32, 33]. IDH has been reported to be more prevalent in female patients [12, 33].

Cases of IDH have been described, in order of frequency, in Jamaica, Brazil, South Africa, Peru, and Senegal. Isolated cases have been found in French Guyana, Colombia, Dominican Republic, and Chile [26]. In Japan, where the frequency of HTLV-I carriers is high, only three cases of IDH have been reported [34]. In Brazil, 43 reported cases were from Bahia [12, 35], 5 from Rio de Janeiro [36, 37], and 1 from Rio Grande do Sul [38]. It is possible that the majority of Brazilian cases of IDH were found in Bahia, because this is one of the most endemic regions for HTLV-1 in Brazil [4, 9]. In fact in this state there are projects designed to study IDH [12].

Clinical Aspects

This disease appears as a severe chronic eczema associated with a refractory, nonvirulent *Staphylococcus aureus* or β-hemolytic *Streptococcus* infection of skin and nasal vestibules. Its onset is usually under the form of rhinitis at around 18 months of age. IDH begins with an exudative eruption always involving the scalp and usually the external ear, neck, and retro-auricular areas (Figs. 42.6, 42.7, and 42.8). Table 42.1 shows the distribution of the lesions in 42 IDH cases [12]. In addition to the erythematous, scaly, and crusty lesions, pustules, scaly papules, follicular-like papules, and retro-auricular fissures are often found (Table 42.2) [12, 33]. Rhinorrhea and crusting in the nostrils (Fig. 42.9) are a common finding. Patients complain of pruritus, although it is not as intense as in atopic dermatitis. Blepharoconjunctivitis is found in the majority of cases [12].

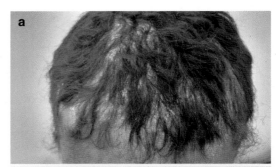
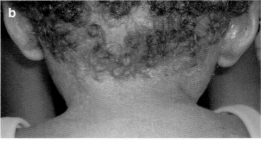

Fig. 42.6 (**a**) Infective dermatitis associated with HTLV-1. Child with severe involvement of scalp with exudative and crusted yellow lesions. (**b**) Adherent yellowish crusts covering the scalp, and scaly and erythematous lesions in the retroauricular areas and neck. Note erosions on scalp

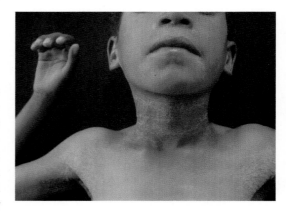

Fig. 42.7 Infective dermatitis associated with HTLV-1. Child with lesions on the neck and axillae. Note crusting of the nostrils

The mean age at onset of IDH is 2.6 ± 2.4 years (range, 2 months to 11 years) and the mean age at complete disappearance of disease is 15 years (range, 10–20 years), but infrequently it may persist until at least 23 years of age [12].

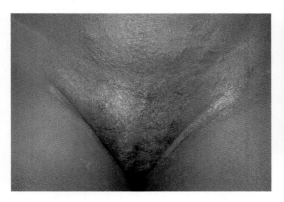

Fig. 42.8 Infective dermatitis associated with HTLV-1. Extensive involvement of genitalia and groins. In the low abdomen there are many follicular papules

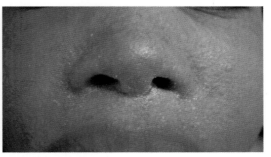

Fig. 42.9 Infective dermatitis associated with HTLV-1. Erythematous-scaly lesions on and around the nose and upper lip. There is crusting on the nostrils covered by yellow crusts

Table 42.1 Distribution of lesions in 42 patients with infective dermatitis associated with the human T-cell lymphotropic virus type 1 [12]

Distribution of lesions	Patients, n (%)
Scalp	42 (100)
Retroauricular regions	42 (100)
Neck	37 (88.0)
Axillae	35 (83.3)
Groin	33 (78.6)
Paranasal skin	30 (71.4)
Ears	30 (71.4)
Thorax	27 (64.3)
Abdomen	26 (62.0)
Antecubital and popliteal fossae	24 (57.1)
Eyelids	24 (57.1)
Forehead	23 (54.8)
Perioral region	21 (50.0)
Umbilicus	17 (40.8)
Limbs	15 (35.7)
External genitalia	14 (33.3)
Buttocks	7 (16.6)

Table 42.2 Frequency of lesions in infective dermatitis associated with the human T-cell lymphotropic virus type 1 [12]

Distribution of lesions	Patients, n (%)
Erythematous-scaly-crusty lesions	42 (100)
Retroauricular fissures	32 (76.2)
Slightly erythematous-scaly papules	32 (76.1)
Crusting of nostrils	27 (64.3)
Fine papular rash	25 (59.5)
Blepharoconjunctivitis	24 (57.1)
Follicular papules	19 (45.2)

Table 42.3 Major criteria for diagnosis of infective dermatitis associated with the human T-cell lymphotropic virus [12, 17]

1. Presence of erythematous-scaly, exudative, and crusted lesions of the scalp, retroauricular areas, neck, axillae, groin, paranasal and perioral skin, ears, thorax, abdomen, and other sites
2. Crusting of nostrils and/or rhinorrhea
3. Chronic relapsing dermatitis with prompt response to appropriate therapy but prompt recurrence on discontinuation of treatment
4. Diagnosis of HTLV-1 infection (by serologic or molecular biological testing)

Modified from La Grenade et al. [33]
Of the four major criteria, three are required for diagnosis, with mandatory inclusion of 1, 3, and 4. To fulfill criterion 1, involvement of ≥3 of the sites is required, including involvement of the scalp and retroauricular areas
HTLV-1 human T-cell lymphotropic virus type 1

Diagnosis

In 2010, Bittencourt and Oliveira [17] proposed a modification in the main criteria established by La Grenade in 1998 [33] for the diagnosis of IDH. The modified criteria are listed in Table 42.3. According to La Grenade et al. [33] the areas affected in IDH are the scalp, axillae and groin, external ear and retro-auricular areas, eyelid margins, paranasal skin, and/or the neck; however, no reference was made to the frequency of the affected areas and which of the involved areas were essential for diagnosis. In 42 cases in Bahia, lesions were present on more areas of the body, being found on ≥3 areas in all cases. Furthermore, the scalp and retro-auricular areas were invariably affected, and the lesions were disseminated in 83% of cases. Thus it was emphasized in the modified criteria that involvement of ≥3 of the sites is required, including involvement of the scalp and retro-auricular regions [12].

Crusting of the nostrils (Fig. 42.9) was absent in some patients, and sometimes appears only during subsequent relapses. Therefore, the presence of crusting of the nostrils cannot be considered an obligatory factor for the diagnosis of IDH, although it represents, when present, an important criterion for diagnosis. Because rhinorrhea is a common symptom in children in several other diseases, it should not constitute a criterion for diagnosis of IDH [17]. However, the relapsing nature of disease, not present in the original main criteria [33], is characteristic of IDH, so this aspect should be considered to be indispensable for diagnosis. On the other hand, the criterion requiring onset in early childhood should be removed, because the disease may begin later in childhood, as late as 11 years of age, or in adulthood [17]. On the other hand, it is important to consider not only the serologic diagnosis, which may fail (albeit infrequently), but also diagnosis of the infection by molecular biology. In seronegative patients with the classic characteristics of IDH, PCR for HTLV-1 must be performed in peripheral blood mononuclear cells to clarify the diagnosis [12].

Differential Diagnosis

The differential diagnosis of IDH should be made mainly with atopic and seborrheic dermatitis. Seropositivity for HTLV-1 is not the only criterion for the diagnosis of IDH; clinical criteria are also very important. In childhood atopic dermatitis occurring after 2 years of age, the lesions partially resemble those of IDH; however, in IDH the lesions are more exudative, infected, and exuberant, and nasal crusting is frequently found. The discovery of lesions in the antecubital and popliteal fossae may sometimes hamper the differential diagnosis with atopic dermatitis [12].

In seborrheic dermatitis, lesions are erythematous and scaling, and less infected than those found in IDH. On the other hand, rhinitis and a papular rash may be present, features that are not found in seborrheic dermatitis. Another very relevant difference is the presence of pruritus in IDH, which is practically nonexistent in seborrheic dermatitis. In seborrheic dermatitis, the squames are oily and *Pityrosporum* is often found. Moreover, IDH responds well to treatment with sulfamethoxazole/ trimethoprim and antibiotics [12].

Infective Dermatitis in Adulthood

The onset of IDH may occur in adult life, characteristics in such cases being similar to those of the infantile-juvenile IDH (Fig. 42.10). In 2006, two cases of late-onset IDH were described in Bahia, Brazil, both in females, one of which was associated with HAM/TSP [39]. Later on, nine more cases were reported, seven of them in females and four associated with HAM/TSP [40–43].

Pathology

IDH cannot be diagnosed by histology. Microscopically, acanthosis, hyperkeratosis, and/ or parakeratosis and crusting are found. Spongiosis is present in only 50% of cases. In some cases, obliteration of the basal layer and epidermotropism of lymphocytes are found, mimicking mycosis fungoides. In the dermis, a slight to moderate infiltration of typical lymphocytes is found, consisting predominantly of CD8+ T lymphocytes with no cytotoxic granulations [44].

According to the literature, CD4+ cells predominate in atopic dermatitis skin lesions; therefore, the finding of CD8+ cells in IDH may represent a distinguishing feature to enable differential diagnosis to be made between these two diseases [44].

Progression to HAM/TSP and ATL

Seventeen of 36 (47.2%) IDH patients followed-up in Bahia progressed to HAM/TSP, a severe

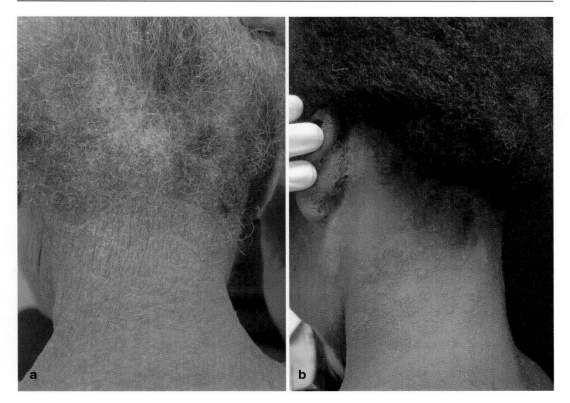

Fig. 42.10 Infective dermatitis associated with HTLV-1 initiated in adulthood. (**a**) Presence of erythematous and scaly lesions on the scalp and neck. (**b**) Another adult patient with retroauricular lesions and many erythematous papules on the posterior aspect of the neck

myelopathy that generally occurs in adulthood [12]. There have also been a few isolated reports on the progression of IDH to ATL [29, 35, 45, 46]. Thirty-seven per cent of ATL cases with skin involvement observed in Bahia reported a history of severe eczema in childhood very suggestive of IDH [47]. On the other hand, abnormal cells, including flower cells, were observed in 17% of a cohort of 30 IDH children and adolescents (Fig. 42.11) [48]. Moreover, proviral monoclonal integration investigated by inverse-long PCR was observed in seven of these IDH patients in whom viral and human DNA sequences were found. In these patients, the percentage of abnormal T cells or flower cells ranged from 2% to 3% and they were not considered as smoldering ATL because they did not have lymphoma or ≥5% of atypical cells in peripheral blood. On the other hand, all of them presented T-cell polyclonality [49]. The pres-

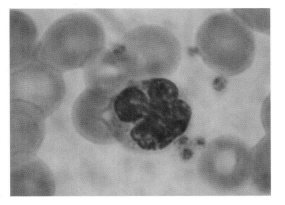

Fig. 42.11 Peripheral blood smear with a flower cell (lymphocyte with condensed chromatin and marked multilobulated nucleus) (Wright stain, ×1,000)

ence of proviral integration without disease is considered a pre-ATL condition [50]. These data may suggest that IDH constitutes a risk factor for the development of ATL.

Treatment

Since IDH is always associated with bacterial infection, it responds well to a combination of trimethoprim/sulfamethoxazole; however, the disease recurs whenever the medication is discontinued. Antihistamine drugs, topical corticosteroids, and emollients are also recommended [12].

Adult T-Cell Leukemia/Lymphoma (ATL)

Knowledge of ATL is very important for dermatologists because it affects the skin in a frequency varying from 43% to 72%, as a primary or secondary condition [17]. In Bahia, Brazil, among cases of primary cutaneous T-cell lymphoma, 26.4% correspond to primary ATL. This result is closer to that found in Lima, Peru, where 19.4% of primary cutaneous T-cell lymphomas were primary cutaneous ATL [51]. These data show that this is a frequent problem in these regions.

ATL is considered as a disease with dismal prognosis and poor response to chemotherapy; however, there are cases with longer survival [52, 53]. ATL is generally reported in adults, the mean age at onset being around 57 years in Japan [54], 49 years in Brazil [27], and 43 years in Jamaica [55]. However, in rare cases onset may be earlier, even in childhood [26].

Classification, Clinical Features, and Diagnosis

ATL has been classified into four types, namely acute, chronic, lymphoma, and smoldering [54]. In 2007, Bittencourt et al. [27] proposed the inclusion in this classification of another clinical type, the primary cutaneous tumoral (PCT). This classification is based on the presence or absence of lymphocytosis and hypercalcemia, percentage of abnormal lymphocytes, levels of lactic dehydrogenase (LDH), sites of involvement, and morphology of skin lesions. These types differ in their presentation, progression, and response to treatment [54, 56]. The characteristics of each type of ATL are summarized in Table 42.4.

The chronic type has been subtyped into favorable and unfavorable, the latter presenting high LDH, high blood urea nitrogen, and/or low albumin levels and a worse prognosis in relation to the favorable subtype [56].

When the patient presents ≥5% of abnormal cells in peripheral blood smoldering, ATL is considered as leukemic [54, 56]. Leukemic smoldering ATL may appear with or without skin or lung involvement (Table 42.4) [57, 58]. When asymptomatic these patients are generally diagnosed by chance during a regular health checkup [58]. Notwithstanding, to recognize these asymptomatic leukemic smoldering

Table 42.4 Clinical classification of adult T-cell leukemia/lymphoma (ATL) modified from the Shimoyama classification [17, 27, 54]

ATL CLINICAL FORMS	Lymphocytosis	Abnormal lymphocytes	LDH levels	Hypercalcemia	Involvement of organs
Smoldering					
1. Primary cutaneous	Absent	<5%	≤1.5 × N	Absent	Only Skin
2. Nonleukemic	Absent	<5%	≤1.5 × N	Absent	Skin and lung or only lung
3. Leukemic	Absent	≥5%	≤1.5 × N	Absent	Skin and/or lung
4. Leukemic	Absent	≥5%	≤1.5 × N	Absent	Without involvement
PCT	Absent	<5	≤1.5 × N	Absent	Skin
Chronic #	Present	Present	≤2 × N	Absent	Any organ except bone, GIT and CNS
Lymphoma	Absent	≤1	Variable	May occur	Lymph node[a] and any other organ
Acute	Usually present	≥5rgg	>1.5 × N	May occur	Any organ

#Subtyped into favorable and unfavorable according to the serum levels of albumin, urea nitrogen, and lactic dehydrogenase (*LDH*). *CNS* central nervous system, *GIT* gastrointestinal tract, *N* normal value, *PCT* Primary cutaneous tumoral
[a]Involvement of lymph node is a mandatory criterion

patients it is necessary to assess systematically abnormal cells in peripheral blood. There are rare references about the outcome of leukemic smoldering ATL in the literature [57, 58]. In one evaluation of 157 smoldering cases, without discrimination between leukemic and nonleukemic cases, 76% had skin lesions and only 2% presented lung involvement, indicating that skin involvement is much more frequent than pulmonary involvement in smoldering ATL [59].

The PCT type is similar to the nonleukemic smoldering type without pulmonary involvement, except for the presence of skin nodules and/or tumors and worse prognosis [47]. In Japan, the smoldering and chronic forms are considered indolent ATL and the PCT type is included within the smoldering ATL [58–62]. The more aggressive forms of ATL are acute, lymphoma, PCT, and unfavorable chronic, survival being longer in patients with the smoldering and favorable chronic types. The diverse forms of ATL may progress to more aggressive types [56].

Similarly to T-cell lymphomas unassociated with HTLV-1, ATL appears on the skin as primary or secondary. Cutaneous lesions appear as patches, plaques, multiple papules, nodules, tumors, diffuse infiltration, and erythroderma (Figs. 42.12 and 42.13a–c) [47]. The lesions are always multiple and are diffuse in 50% of cases [47]. Rarely, purpuric lesions (Fig. 42.13d), vesicles (Fig. 42.14), or bullae are observed [63–65]. Sawada et al. [66], evaluating 119 ATL patients in Japan, observed the following frequency of skin lesions: nodulotumoral (38.7%), plaques (26.9%), multipapular (19.3%), patches (6.7%), erythrodermic (4.2%), and purpuric (4.2%). All of these erythrodermic patients had acute ATL. In Bahia, Brazil, among 80 ATL cases the frequency of the different types of skin lesions were erythroderma (30%), patch/plaque (28.7%), nodulotumoral (22.5%), multipapular (16.25%), and purpuric (2.5%). Erythroderma was observed in all types of ATL, but more frequently in the smoldering and acute types (unpublished data).

The criteria for the diagnosis of ATL are: (1) positive HTLV-1 serology; (2) cytologic or histopathologic finding of leukemia or T-cell lymphoma $CD4^+/CD25^+$; (3) presence of abnormal T

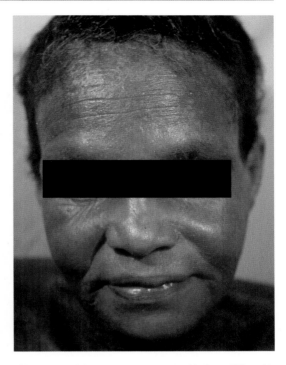

Fig. 42.12 Primary cutaneous smoldering ATL with erythroderma

lymphocytes in blood smears; and (4) demonstration of monoclonal HTLV-1 proviral integration whenever possible [56]. Table 42.5 summarizes the routine for evaluation of ATL patients at diagnosis [56, 67].

The abnormal lymphocytes found in the ATL patients in peripheral blood may consist of several types including flower cells, which are cells with marked polylobulated nuclei containing condensed chromatin [68]. Flower cells, generally found in acute ATL and occasionally in the chronic and smoldering types, are considered to be pathognomonic of ATL [54, 56]. The presence of these cells is important because it represents a fast and simple way of diagnosing ATL using a Giemsa- or Wright-stained blood smear [69].

In cases of doubtful diagnosis, ATL can be differentiated from other T-cell lymphomas unassociated with HTLV-1 but occurring coincidentally in infected individuals through the HTLV-1 proviral integration analysis (Fig. 42.5). However, this analysis is not essential in the diagnosis of most cases [70]. Its importance as scientific evi-

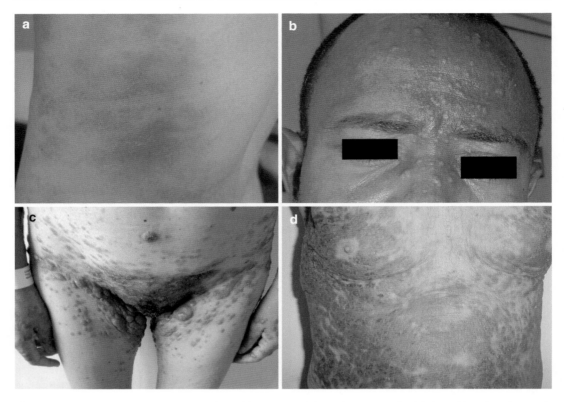

Fig. 42.13 (**a**) Favorable chronic ATL patient with erythematous infiltrated plaques. (**b**) Acute ATL patient with multipapular lesions and few nodules on the face. (**c**) Primary cutaneous tumoral ATL with disseminated nodules and tumors on the skin but without lymphocytosis and systemic involvement. (**d**) Diffuse purpuric lesion with areas of erosion in an acute ATL patient

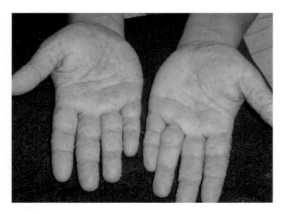

Fig. 42.14 Chronic ATL with vesicles mimicking dyshidrosis on the palms of the hands

dence is higher in patients with atypical features, such as very long evolution or very early appearance [27]. On the other hand, it is known that in endemic areas only rare cases of T-cell lympho-

mas other than ATL have been observed developing in HTLV-1 carriers [56].

Primary Cutaneous Adult T-Cell Leukemia/Lymphoma

It is always important to evaluate whether skin involvement in lymphoma is primary or secondary, since clinical behavior and prognosis are quite different. Among 80 ATL cases with skin involvement, a statistically significant difference was observed between the median survival time of the primary cutaneous ATL in relation to the secondary (58 months versus 10 months for secondary ATL) (Fig. 42.15) (unpublished data).

It has been well established that the principal criterion for considering any type of lymphoma to be primary cutaneous is that it

Table 42.5 Examinations for evaluation of adult T-cell leukemia/lymphoma (ATL) patients at diagnosis [56, 67]

1. *Physical examination*
With full skin inspection and search for adenopathy and hepatosplenomegaly
2. *Laboratory examinations*
Confirmation of HTLV-1 serology (most laboratories in Brazil do not perform confirmation)
Complete blood counts
Blood smears for assessing abnormal lymphocytes including "flower cells"
Determination of serum
LDH (prognostic factor)
Albumin (prognostic factor of chronic ATL)
Urea nitrogen (prognostic factor of chronic ATL)
Calcium (to rule out hypercalcemia)
Soluble IL-2 (prognostic factor), when available
Stool parasitologic examination (Baerman) to rule out strongyloidiasis
Peripheral blood immunophenotyping (necessary to diagnose ATL in patients without histologically proven tumor)
3. *Imaging examinations*
Cervical, thoracic, abdominal, and pelvic CT (when impossible perform at least thoracic X-ray, also to rule out tuberculosis and abdominal and pelvic USG)
CT scan or MRI of the head (in cases with neurologic symptoms unrelated to HAM/TSP)
Skeletal X-ray in patients with hypercalcemia
4. *Cytologic and/or anatomopathologic examinations*
Cutaneous biopsy: histopathology with immunohistochemistry
Puncture or lymph node excision: cytology or histopathology with immunohistochemistry
5. *Useful behaviors in selected cases*
Pregnancy test in women of childbearing age
Endoscopy of the upper digestive tract (patients with digestive symptoms)
Lumbar puncture, in aggressive forms or in patients with neurologic symptoms unrelated to HAM/TSP
Myelogram or bone marrow biopsy (generally not required to make the diagnosis of ATL, but may be useful in the aggressive forms)
PET scan, when indicated and if there is availability
Transplantation evaluation, when indicated

CT computed tomography, *HAM/TSP* HTLV-1-associated myelopathy/tropical spastic paraparesis, *HTLV-1* human T-cell lymphotropic virus type 1, *IL-2* interleukin-2, *MRI* magnetic resonance imaging, *PET* positron emission tomography, *USG* ultrasonography

be confined to the skin. Therefore, the smoldering nonleukemic type with no pulmonary

involvement (primary cutaneous smoldering ATL) and the PCT type represent cases of primary cutaneous ATL (Table 42.4) [17, 47]. In brief, to consider a case of ATL to be primary cutaneous, there should be no lymphocytosis, no hypercalcemia, no extracutaneous involvement, with the LDH levels either slightly elevated or normal and fewer than 5% of abnormal cells found in peripheral blood. Besides, the patient must have a lymphomatous infiltration in the skin [47]. All smoldering ATL patients diagnosed in Bahia, Brazil, to date are nonleukemic smoldering ATL and only present skin involvement [17, 47]. Notwithstanding, the primary cutaneous ATL is not yet universally accepted because it is not included in the classifications of lymphoma defined by the World Health Organization (WHO) and the European Organization for Research and Treatment of Cancer (EORTC) [71, 72].

As the literature regarding primary cutaneous ATL is very confusing with different criteria, this matter requires standardization (Table 42.6) [27, 47, 57, 73–76]. Most authors continue to use the term cutaneous ATL without emphasizing the primary skin condition of this entity.

Amano et al. [74] detected a significantly higher proviral loading in the smoldering form (considered by these authors as leukemic) compared with the cutaneous ATL (nonleukemic smoldering), and considered that this difference could represent a means to distinguish between these two entities. Similarly, Yonekura et al. [57] found a higher proviral load in leukemic smoldering ATL with or without cutaneous lesions than in cutaneous ATL (nonleukemic smoldering). In fact, if cutaneous ATL has a lesser percentage of infected cells in peripheral blood (<5%), the proviral load must be lower than that of the leukemic subtype (≥5%). As already mentioned, the proviral load corresponds to the number of HTLV-1-infected cells in peripheral blood.

Given that the Shimoyama's classification [54] continues to be used and recommended in the literature [56], we believe that the PCT form should be added to this classification and that the

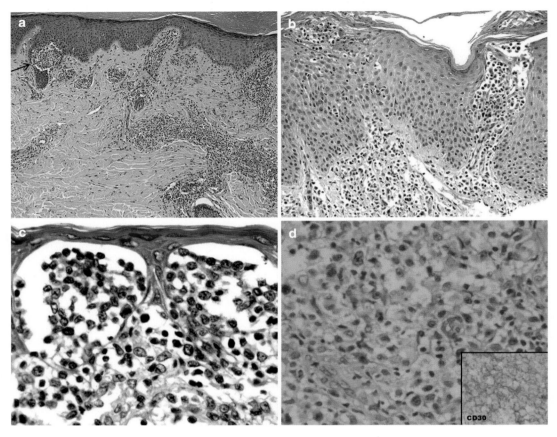

Fig. 42.15 Among 80 ATL cases with skin involvement, a statistically significant difference was observed between the median survival time of the primary cutaneous ATL and that of the secondary atl (58 months versus 10 months for secondary ATL) Oliveira PD, et al, 2016)

variant of the smoldering form that corresponds to primary cutaneous ATL without nodules and tumors should be defined as another type of smoldering ATL (Table 42.4) [17, 27, 47]. Whatever the nomenclature to be adopted in the future, it is important to separate the primary cutaneous tumoral ATL from the nontumoral form (primary cutaneous nonleukemic smoldering) because their prognosis is different and, therefore, the therapeutic approach should be different [17, 47].

One possible means of differentiation between ATL with erythematous papular and nodulotumoral lesions was suggested by Miyata et al. (2010) [75], in Japan, who found distinct genomic profiles in these two subtypes of primary cutaneous ATL. Notwithstanding, this issue should be investigated with a larger number of cases.

Histopathologic and Immunohistochemical Aspects of Skin Lesions

The morphologic appearance of ATL in skin sections is highly variable and often mimics established pathologic types of T-cell lymphomas unassociated with HTLV-1. The diagnosis of ATL can only be made following serologic or molecular evaluation since this T-cell lymphoma has no specific histologic characteristics. Unaware of the serologic findings, the pathologist generally classifies HTLV-1-associated lymphomas as peripheral T-cell lymphoma, unspecified (PTCL-U), mycosis fungoides (MF), or anaplastic large-cell lymphoma (ALCL) [27].

Table 42.6 Different criteria regarding primary cutaneous adult T-cell leukemia/lymphoma (ATL)

Authors	Designation	Subtyping or different cutaneous lesions	Criteria related to Shimoyama classification	Prognosis
Johno et al. (1992) [73][a]	Cutaneous ATL	(a) Erythematopapular (b) Tumoral	The same as for nonleukemic smoldering ATL	Tumoral with worse prognosis
Bittencourt et al. (2007) [27]	Primary cutaneous ATL with two subtypes	1. Smoldering ATL (without nodulotumoral lesions) 2. PCT ATL	1. Smoldering ATL 2. PCT ATL to be added to the Shimoyama classification	PCT with worse prognosis
Amano et al. (2008) [74]	Cutaneous ATL	(a) Erythematopapular	1. The same as for nonleukemic smoldering ATL without lung involvement	–
	Smoldering ATL	(b) Tumoral	2. Leukemic without skin lesions	
Bittencourt et al. (2009, 2010) [17, 47]	Primary cutaneous ATL with two subtypes	1. Primary cutaneous smoldering ATL without nodulotumoral lesions	1. Nonleukemic smoldering ATL without lung lesions and nodulotumoral lesions (<5% of abnormal cells in PB)	PCT with worse prognosis
		2. Primary cutaneous tumoral (PCT) with nodulotumoral lesions	2. PCT: the same but with skin nodulotumoral lesions	
Miyata et al. (2010) [75]	Cutaneous type ATL	(a) Erythema/papule (b) Nodule/tumor	Include leukemic and nonleukemic smoldering and two chronic types	–
Yonekura et al. (2015) [57]	Cutaneous type ATL	–	Include leukemic and nonleukemic smoldering	–
Tsukasaki et al. (2014) [76][b]	Extranodal primary cutaneous variant of lymphoma type ATL	–	Smoldering ATL with primary cutaneous lesions with poor prognosis and histology of high-grade lymphoma	Worse prognosis than smoldering without nodulotumoral lesions

PB peripheral blood, *PCT* primary cutaneous tumoral
[a]Without clearly defining the criteria for differentiation between cutaneous and smoldering adult T-cell leukemia/lymphoma (ATL)
[b]Among eight cases they included seven with nodulotumoral lesions and one with plaques

In cases in which morphology is similar to MF, the infiltrate consists of small, irregular cells frequently associated with epidermotropism of varied intensity, infiltrating the basal layer linearly, forming Pautrier abscesses (Fig. 42.16a) or setting up a pagetoid infiltration (Fig. 42.16b). PTCL-U is characterized by an infiltration of pleomorphic medium-sized to large cells, sometimes infiltrating the subcutaneous tissue. Epidermotropism of lymphocytes and Pautrier abscesses may be present (Fig. 42.16c). Angio- and folliculotropism can be observed less frequently. In ALCL, neoplastic cells are large and cohesive with abundant cytoplasm and anaplastic nuclei (Fig. 42.16d) [47].

In ATL, the immunophenotype most commonly observed is $CD3^+/CD4^+/CD5^+/CD7^-/CD8^-/CD20^-$, $CD79a^-$, $CD25^+$ [72]. However, in 52 cases with skin manifestations, 15 were $CD8^+$ but no statistically significant difference was observed in median survival time between the groups of $CD8^+$ and $CD8^-$ cases. In two cases with ALCL morphology, the phenotype was $CD30^+/ALK^-$ [47]. It is always important to determine the proliferative index of ATL lesions, and this may be performed by immunohistochemistry for which most used marker is Ki-67. This evaluation is important since there is a negative correlation between the rate of the proliferative index and survival in ATL [27].

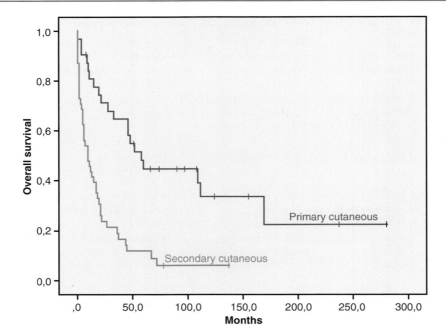

Fig. 42.16 (**a**) Mycosis fungoides pattern in a chronic ATL patient. Presence of small atypical lymphocytes in the upper and mid dermis and one Pautrier microabscess (*arrow*) (H&E, ×200). (**b**) Mycosis fungoides pattern in a primary cutaneous smoldering ATL patient. The atypical lymphocytes present in the dermis infiltrate the epidermis in a pagetoid pattern until the corneous layer (H&E, ×200). (**c**) Peripheral T-cell lymphoma of unspecified pat-tern in a patient with primary cutaneous tumoral ATL. Dermal infiltration of median and large anaplastic lymphocytes with epidermal atrophy and two large Pautrier abscesses (H&E, ×640). (**d**) Anaplastic large cell lymphoma pattern in a patient with primary cutaneous smoldering ATL. Large cells with abundant and eosino-philic cytoplasm and anaplastic nuclei (H&E, ×400). Inset: CD30+ cells (×200)

There was no difference in histopathology between the lesions that were primary and those that were secondary to the skin except for the frequency of histologic types, MF morphology being more common in primary cutaneous ATL while PTCL-U was more frequent in secondary cutaneous ATL [17]. In addition, ATL cases with MF morphology were more frequent in the smoldering and chronic forms and presented a proliferative index <18%, aspects that are indicative of a less aggressive outcome [47]. Most cases of ATL with cutaneous lesions resemble MF clinically and histologically [77, 78].

Histopathologic Differential Diagnosis

In the smoldering primary cutaneous form, the diagnosis of which is frequently based on the finding of a T-cell lymphoma with small and medium-sized cells at skin biopsy, histologic differential diagnosis may be hampered in view of cutaneous lymphoid hyperplasia that mimics lymphoma. In these cases, immunohistochemistry is not usually helpful and analysis of the rearrangement of the genes that codify the T-cell receptors in the skin lesions has to be performed to verify whether there is monoclonal expansion of the T lymphocytes, thus enabling differentiation to be made between these two entities [17]. It should be emphasized that HTLV-I infection in carriers or patients with HAM/TSP may lead to erythematous, inflammatory, noninfectious, and nonlymphomatous skin lesions, often with a histologic suspicion of malignancy [79, 80]. These cases must also be differentiated from cutaneous T-cell lymphomas. On the other hand, patients with HTLV-1 infection often have scabies, even crusted scabies, conditions that may appear histologically as a reactional lymphoid hyperplasia, which often mimics cutaneous T-cell lymphoma [81].

Except for the leukemic types of ATL, which are usually diagnosed by hematopathologists, the diagnosis of ATL is performed by pathologists in tissue biopsy specimens. Thus, it is important that in endemic areas for HTLV-1, these professionals be aware that ATL, besides manifesting histologically as PTCL-U, may also resemble MF or ALCL and that HTLV-I infection should be investigated in these T-cell lymphomas [27].

Prognosis

A study evaluating the type of skin lesions in relation to prognosis indicated that the erythrodermic, followed by the purpuric, nodulotumoral, and multipapular had the poorest prognoses with median survival time of 3.0, 4.4, 17.3, and 17.3 months, respectively. On the contrary, the patch and plaque lesions exhibited much better survival rates (188.4 versus 115.9 months, respectively) [66]. In our experience, the poorer prognosis was also observed in patients with purpuric and nodulotumoral lesions but patients with erythroderma had a median survival time a little better (17 months). However, our cases with erythroderma have also been observed in the smoldering ATL form with the best prognosis in Bahia, Brazil (unpublished data).

The prognosis of smoldering ATL with skin eruptions has been considered poorer than that without skin involvement [62]. Notwithstanding, the smoldering ATL with nodulotumoral lesions presents a worse prognosis [73, 74, 76]. Takasaki et al. [61] in Nagasaki, Japan, evaluating 25 smoldering cases without subtyping and 65 chronic ATL patients, observed that the survival was longer for the chronic (5.3 years) in relation to the smoldering form (2.9 years) and even the 5-year survival was longer for the chronic form (50.2% versus 39.4%). Moreover, in this evaluation the progression rate of smoldering ATL was 60%. Another study in Kyushu, Japan, indicated that among 26 smoldering patients 42% progressed to acute ATL. In Bahia, Brazil, only 18% of the smoldering patients progressed to other ATL types [47]. The poor prognosis of the smoldering ATL with cutaneous involvement in Japan is probably due to the inclusion of the PCT type

within the smoldering primary cutaneous type [57–62].

In Brazil, among 80 cases of ATL with cutaneous involvement, a statistically significant difference was observed between the median survival time of patients with primary cutaneous ATL (58 months) and those with secondary ATL (10 months) (Fig. 42.16). Furthermore, a longer median survival time was found among cases of primary cutaneous smoldering ATL (109 months) compared with the PCT type (20 months), highlighting the importance of making a clear distinction between these two types of primary cutaneous ATL (unpublished data).

The prognosis of the aggressive forms of ATL is considered poor in view of multidrug resistance of malignant cells, a large tumor burden with multiorgan failure, hypercalcemia, and/or frequent infectious complications as a result of a profound T-cell immunodeficiency [56].

Treatment

The treatment decisions should be based on the ATL classification, prognostic factors at diagnosis, and response to initial therapy [56]. The prognostic factors, among others, include age, performance status [82], clinical and histologic types, primary cutaneous versus secondary ATL, levels of LDH, number of involved lesions, hypercalcemia, thrombocytopenia, eosinophilia, bone marrow involvement, and level of Ki-67 expression [47, 56].

In less aggressive forms it is recommended to manage the patients with supportive care and a watchful waiting approach and/or antivirals, the most frequently used being zidovudine (azidothymidine; AZT) and IFN-α and/or skin-direct treatments (topical steroids, ultraviolet B (UVB) phototherapy, psoralen-UVA photochemotherapy, and radiation therapy). In aggressive ATL the patients are generally treated with chemotherapy, antivirals, and/or bone marrow transplantation (Table 42.7). Although some combinations of chemotherapy produce regression in ATL cases, they failed to achieve a significant impact on long-term survival. Other treatment protocols are being tested, such as anti-CCR4 monoclonal

Table 42.7 Strategy for the treatment of adult T-cell leukemia/lymphoma [56]

Smoldering or favorable chronic type

1. Symptomatic patients (skin lesions, opportunistic infections, and so forth): consider AZT/IFN or watch and wait

2. Asymptomatic patients: consider watch and wait

Unfavorable chronic or acute type

If outside clinical trials, check prognostic factors:

1. Good prognostic factors: consider chemotherapy (VCAP-AMP-VECP evaluated by a randomized phase III trial against biweekly CHOP) or AZT/IFN

2. Poor prognostic factors: consider chemotherapy followed by conventional or reduced-intensity allogeneic HSCT

3. Poor response to initial therapy with chemotherapy or AZT/IFN: consider conventional or reduced-intensity allogeneic HSCT

Lymphoma type

If outside clinical trials, consider chemotherapy (VCAP-AMP-VECP)

Check prognostic factors and response to chemotherapy:

   Favorable prognostic profiles and good response to initial therapy: consider chemotherapy

   Unfavorable prognostic profiles or poor response to initial therapy with chemotherapy: consider conventional or reduced-intensity allogeneic HSCT

ATL adult T-cell leukemia/lymphoma, *AZT* zidovudine, *IFN-α* interferon-α, *VCAP-AMP-VECP* vincristine, cyclophosphamide, doxorubicin, and prednisone; doxorubicin, ranimustine, and prednisone; and vindesine, etoposide, carboplatin, and prednisone, *CHOP* cyclophosphamide, doxorubicin, vincristine, and prednisone, *HSCT* hematopoietic stem cell transplantation. Simplified from Table 1 of Tsukasaki et al. [56], originally published by the American Society of Clinical Oncology

antibody [56, 59, 67, 83–85]. Details of treatment options for all types of ATL and response criteria can be found in these references.

Here we emphasize the treatment of primary cutaneous ATL, but it is necessary to take into account that all papers about the treatment of primary cutaneous ATL or cutaneous ATL do not subtype it, and often include the smoldering in general and the favorable chronic forms under the designation of indolent ATL.

The International Consensus Meeting for Definition, Prognostic Factors, Treatment, and Response Criteria of ATL recommended for smoldering ATL the strategy of watchful waiting until disease progression or AZT/IFN-α [56]. In a world meta-analysis study carried out on the use of antiviral therapy versus chemotherapy, analyzing together 23 smoldering and chronic patients, it was observed that those who received first-line antiviral therapy had a better survival (5-year overall survival of 100%) than patients who received first-line chemotherapy (5-year overall survival of 42%) with or without maintenance antiviral therapy [83]. In addition, it has been shown that chemotherapy may result in a poor outcome for indolent ATL [61]. The problem with the treatment using AZT/IFN-α is that continuous therapy is mandatory even after the disappearance of symptoms, because relapse always occurs when treatment is stopped [85].

Katsuya et al. [59], in a retrospective study including 157 smoldering patients, 76% with skin lesions, considered that the standard care for smoldering ATL is watchful waiting with skin-directed therapy (narrow-band UVB therapy or psoralen photochemotherapy), if needed. Kudo et al. [86] obtained good results with UVB phototherapy in a smoldering primary cutaneous ATL patient with localized plaque. The type of phototherapy has to be chosen according to the degree of infiltration of the skin lesions, UVB being used for the less infiltrated lesions.

Employing skin-direct therapies (UVB or radiation therapy) combined or not with etoposide (daily with 25–75 mg combined with 10–20 mg prednisolone, modifying the periods in individual cases) in 62 patients with smoldering ATL, Sawada et al. [84] obtained a better improvement of the overall survival and progression-free survival with the association of etoposide with skin-directed therapy. We emphasize that combination therapy was employed only in patients with nonlocalized lesions and with more than three nodular tumoral lesions in patients with probable poor prognosis. Complete remission was obtained with combined therapies in 68.4% of patients including two with nodules/tumors, with skin-direct therapy alone in 41.4% of patients, all with patch and plaque, and with solely etoposide in only one (7.1%), a patient with plaque. In a recent evaluation of treatment, in Bahia, Brazil, of 29 primary cutaneous smoldering patients with a median survival time of 109 months, good results were obtained with a median survival time of 169 months in the 19 patients submitted to watchful-waiting management, and 11 of them also to phototherapy (unpublished data). Although the watchful-waiting approach for the primary cutaneous smoldering form is the most recommended in the literature [56], combination with phototherapy seems to be the best approach as it leads to a complete or partial remission of the cutaneous lesions (unpublished data). It is important to emphasize the need for regular monitoring of these patients, since they may progress to more aggressive forms. When transformation to acute disease occurs patients, may have the treatments indicated to this form [84].

As the PCT form is generally included in the smoldering type, there is no recommendation in the literature about treatment. Notwithstanding, there are rare cases of PCT type reported with data about therapy and follow-up, one of which was diagnosed as PCT and three others as smoldering ATL and cutaneous-type ATL, respectively [87–90]. All of them had confirmed proviral integration and large cells in histopathology. Three presented complete remission, one with administration of AZT/IFN remaining without lesions during 6 months of follow-up [87], another with intralesional corticosteroids [88], and the third, a rare ATL presentation with only one tumor, with radiotherapy. This last patient had no recurrence during 13 months of follow-up [89]. A fourth patient underwent chemotherapy and bone marrow heterologous transplantation, but failed to achieve a sustained remission [90]. In one report, including five PCT cases, radiotherapy to reduce the size of the tumors combined with chemotherapy and/or IFN-α/AZT were used,

without good results, the median survival time of being only 20 months [47].

Xerosis and Acquired Ichthyosis

Xerosis is dryness of the skin, while acquired ichthyosis is clinically characterized by cutaneous xerosis with the formation of polygonal thin flat squames of varied sizes, principally on the extremities (Fig. 42.17) [91]. Xerosis and acquired ichthyosis have been described in up to 66.7% of cases of HAM/TSP, being more severe in the more advanced cases of the disease [92]. According to Yamaguchi [93], acquired ichthyosis is a consequence of the hypohidrosis found in these patients, which may result from a lesion of the autonomic nerves. However, carriers of this virus may also have acquired ichthyosis [94]. Among 42 cases of infantojuvenile IDH, xerosis was found in 64% and acquired ichthyosis in 10% of the cases [12].

Another theory regarding the cause of acquired ichthyosis is that it may occur following an inflammatory lesion of the eccrine sudoriferous glands. Nested PCR was used to demonstrate the presence of HTLV-1 infection in the epithelial cells of eccrine sudoriferous glands associated with the presence of lymphocyte infiltrate around these glands. It has been suggested that this inflammatory process may lead to sweat disorders, which would be responsible for drying the skin [95].

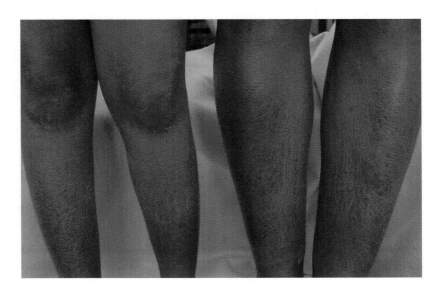

Fig. 42.17 Mother, an HTLV-1 carrier, and daughter with infective dermatitis associated with HTLV-1, both with acquired ichthyosis on the legs

Lenzi et al. [80] evaluated skin biopsies of 32 patients with HAM/TSP and xerosis and found lymphocyte infiltrate in the superficial dermis in seven cases and in the deep dermis in another case, frequently associated with lymphocyte epidermotropism. Atypical lymphocytes were seen in one case. The authors considered these cases to be suggestive of skin lymphoma.

Milagres et al. [91] studied the expression and distribution of keratins K1, K10, K6, K16, involucrin, and the Ki-67 proliferative index of the epidermis in biopsies of HAM/TSP patients with ichthyosis. Taking into consideration the lack of acanthosis and the absence of increased cell kinetics of the epidermis, they concluded that the pattern of acquired ichthyosis related to HTLV-1 is not hyperproliferative but retentive.

An ichthyosis-like pattern may be secondary to diffuse lymphomatous infiltration of the skin (Fig. 42.18); however, clinically, it can be differentiated by the thickness of the skin and by the presence of other lesions. Nevertheless, in cases of doubt biopsy should be performed on the lesion.

Noninfectious Inflammatory Dermatoses

Erythematous patches or plaques may appear in HAM/TSP patients or in HTLV-1 carriers without clinical or laboratory indications of ATL. Histologically a lymphocyte infiltrate with epidermotropism in some cases, albeit with no atypical cells, has been observed [80]. Erythematous lesions of the palms of the hands and the face have already been described as a frequent finding in HAM/TSP, corresponding histologically to perivascular lymphocyte infiltrate [92]. Elevated serum levels of proinflammatory cytokines such as TNF-α have already been reported in HTLV-1 carriers and in patients with HAM/TSP, and this may at least partially explain the occurrence and persistence of these inflammatory skin processes [21].

Seborrheic dermatitis has been reported more frequently among HTLV-1 carriers [94]. Maloney et al. [96] compared 28 HTLV-1 sero-

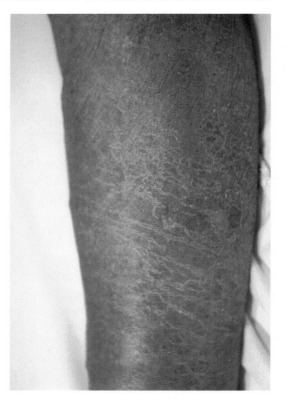

Fig. 42.18 Secondary ichthyosis in a chronic ATL patient associated with lymphomatous infiltration of the skin

positive with 280 seronegative children and observed that seborrheic dermatitis was five times more likely to be present in the infected children compared with the control group. These authors also reported that eczema not referred to as IDH was twice as likely to be found in the infected children compared with the seronegative group.

Infectious and Parasitic Dermatoses

Some infections and parasitic skin diseases such as dermatophytoses and scabies, including crusted scabies, occur more frequently in HTLV-1-infected individuals [94, 97]. In 91 cases of scabies, Brites et al. [97] detected HIV infection in 50%, HTLV-1 infection in 32%, and both infections in 20%. In a cohort of 42 children with IDH,

64% were found to have scabies and two patients had crusted scabies [12]. Less frequently scabies may appear as disseminated nodules (Fig. 42.19) or with diffuse hyperkeratosis and crusts, named crusted or Norwegian scabies (Fig. 42.20) [17].

Protracted *Treponema pallidum* infection has been known to cause syphilitic chancres in HTLV-1-infected rabbits [98]. Figure 42.21 shows a severe form of secondary syphilis, referred to as malignant syphilis, in an HIV-negative HTLV-1 carrier. This may have been the result of a comorbid infection with HTLV-1. The lesions healed completely following antisyphilitic treatment [99].

Salvador et al. [100] found a higher prevalence of HTLV-1 (2.5%) in a cohort of leprosy outpatients in comparison with the prevalence in the general population (1.8%). These authors observed that coinfection with HTLV-1 is associated with a high rate of unfavorable leprosy outcomes such as type 1 and 2 reactions and neuritis.

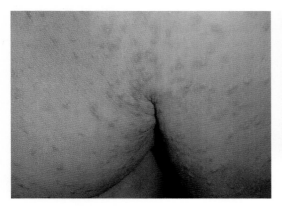

Fig. 42.19 HAM/TSP patient with disseminated nodular scabies. Note numerous papules and nodules

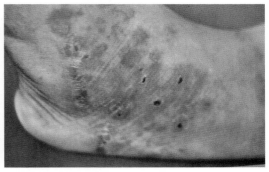

Fig. 42.21 HTLV-1 carrier, HIV negative, with atypical and severe secondary syphilis. Confluent and erythematous papules and plaques on the dorsum of the right foot, some of them with shallow ulcers (Reprinted from Bittencourt and de Oliveira [17])

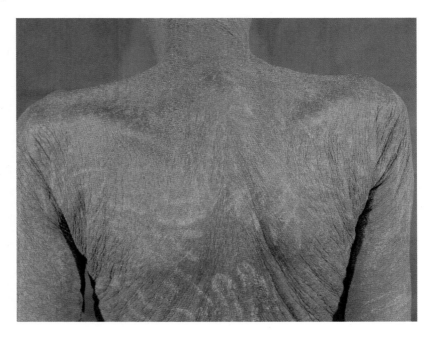

Fig. 42.20 Norwegian scabies in an acute ATL case without skin lymphomatous lesions

Glossary

Acanthosis Epidermal hyperplasia (thickening of the epidermis). It implies increased thickness of the (stratum spinosum).

Anaplastic nuclei Refers to a group of changes in a cell, loss of polarity (cells may not develop connections to one another), pleomorphism (cells vary in size and shape; their nuclei may also vary in size and shape), hyperchromatism (the nuclei of malignant cells often stain darker than normal cells), abnormal mitoses (division of malignant cells often is abnormal, a feature recognized by "abnormal mitotic figures") that point to a possible malignant transformation.

Clonal proliferation In HTLV-1 infection, is the process in which expansion of infected T cells occur by mitosis. When the proliferation is clonal, the generated cells are identical and all of them have the HTLV-1 provirus integrated in the same site in the host genome. The population of identical infected cells constitutes a clone. Thus, each infected clone can be distinguished from other infected clones by the integration site of the provirus in the host human genome. This process is stimulated by HTLV-1 products.

Crusted scabies A rare, highly contagious uncommon form of scabies characterized by presence of huge number of *Sarcoptes scabiei* in the horny layer of the epidermis. As a reaction, the horny layer thickens and forms warty crusts. In most cases it is associated with some underlying diseases and usually affects immunocompromised patients.

Erythroderma Generalized exfoliative dermatitis. It is a disease characterized by erythema and scaling of greater than 90% of the body's surface.

Folliculotropism and angiotropism The invasion of follicular units and vessel walls by lymphocytes. In malignant conditions the lymphocytes show variable degrees of nuclear atypia.

Hyperkeratosis Thickening of the horny layer of the skin.

Ichthyosis It may be inherited (genetic) or acquired during life. The inherited forms are rare, generally present from infancy, and are usually lifelong conditions. Acquired ichthyosis can develop at any age due to a number of medical problems.

Pagetoid infiltration Pagetoid is a term used in dermatology to refer to "upward spreading" of abnormal cells in the epidermis (i.e., from bottom to top). It is a possible indication of a precancerous or cancerous condition.

Parakeratosis A mode of keratinization characterized by the retention of nuclei in the stratum corneum. Parakeratosis is associated with the thinning or loss of the granular layer and is usually seen in diseases of increased cell turnover.

Pautrier's microabscess One of the well-defined collections of mycosis cells located within the epidermis in T-cell lymphomas mainly in mycosis fungoides. They are atypical lymphocytes clusters in the epidermis with little associated spongiosis.

Rhinorrhea A condition whereby the nasal cavity is filled with a significant amount of mucus fluid. The condition, commonly known as a runny nose, occurs relatively frequently.

Spongiosis A microscopic term referring to increased intercellular fluid in the epidermis (intercellular edema) that physically pulls keratinocytes away from each other. If severe, spongiosis will cause intraepidermal vesicles (spongiotic vesicles).

Xerostomy Dryness of mucous membranes of the oral cavity and pharynx. It is a consequence of salivary gland dysfunction. Saliva plays an important role in maintaining the correct condition of the oral cavity mucosa.

References

1. Gonçalves DU, Proietti FA, Ribas JG, Araújo MG, Pinheiro SR, Guedes AC, et al. Epidemiology, treatment, and prevention of human T-cell leukemia virus type 1-associated diseases. Clin Microbiol Rev. 2010 Jul;23(3):577–89.
2. Bertazzoni U. Editorial to the research topic "Comparative studies between HTLV-1 and HTLV-2 function and pathobiology". Front Microbiol. 2015 Jan 14;5:792.
3. Gessain A, Cassar O. Epidemiological aspects and world distribution of HTLV-1 infection. Front Microbiol. 2012;3:388.
4. Catalan-Soares B, Carneiro-Proietti AB, Proietti FA, Interdisciplinary HTLV Research Group. Heterogeneous geographic distribution of human T-cell lymphotropic viruses I and II (HTLV-I/II): serological screening prevalence rates in blood donors from large urban areas in Brazil. Cad Saúde Pública. 2005;21(3):926–31.

5. Bittencourt AL, Dourado I, Filho PB, Santos M, Valadão E, Alcantara LC, et al. Human T-cell lymphotropic virus type 1 infection among pregnant women in northeastern Brazil. J AIDS. 2001;26(5):490–4.

6. Magalhães T, Mota-Miranda AC, Alcantara LC, Olavarria V, Galvão-Castro B, Rios-Grassi MF. Phylogenetic and molecular analysis of HTLV-1 isolates from a medium sized town in northern of Brazil: tracing a common origin of the virus from the most endemic city in the country. J Med Virol. 2008;80(11):2040–5.

7. Mello MA, da Conceição AF, Sousa SM, Alcântara LC, Marin LJ, Regina da Silva Raiol M, et al. HTLV-1 in pregnant women from the Southern Bahia, Brazil: a neglected condition despite the high prevalence. Virol J. 2014;11:28.

8. Galvão-Castro B, Loures L, Rodriques LG, Sereno A, Ferreira Júnior OC, Franco LG, et al. Distribution of human T-lymphotropic virus type I among blood donors: a nationwide Brazilian study. Transfusion. 1997;37(2):242–3.

9. Dourado I, Alcantara LCJ, Barreto ML, Teixeira MG, Galvão-Castro B. HTLV-1 in the general populationof Salvador, Brazil. A city with African ethnic and socio demographic characteristics. JAIDS. 2003;34(5):527–31.

10. Bittencourt AL. Vertical transmission of HTLV-I/II: a review. Rev Inst Med Trop São Paulo. 1998;40(4):245–51.

11. Qayyum S, Choi JK. Adult T-cell leukemia/lymphoma. Arch Pathol Lab Med. 2014;138(2):282–6.

12. Oliveira MFSP, Fatal PL, Primo JR, da Silva JL, Batista ES, Farré L, et al. Infective dermatitis associated with human T-cell lymphotropic virus type 1: evaluation of 42 cases observed in Bahia, Brazil. Clin Infect Dis. 2012;54(12):1714–9.

13. Zihlmann KF, de Alvarenga AT, Casseb J. Living invisible: HTLV-1-infected persons and the lack of care in public health. PLoS Negl Trop Dis. 2012;6(6):e1705.

14. Lairmore MD, Haines R, Anupam R. Mechanisms of human T-lymphotropic virus type 1 transmission and disease. Curr Opin Virol. 2012;2(4):474–81.

15. Matsuoka M, Jeang KT. Human T-cell leukaemia virus type 1 (HTLV-1) infectivity and cellular transformation. Nat Rev Cancer. 2007;7(4):270–80.

16. Bangham CR, Ratner L. How does HTLV-1 cause adult T-cell leukemia/lymphoma (ATL)? Curr Opin Virol. 2015;14:93–100.

17. Bittencourt AL, de Oliveira M. Cutaneous manifestations associated with HTLV-1 infection. Int J Dermatol. 2010;49(10):1099–110.

18. Gillet NA, Malani N, Melamed A, Gormley N, Carter R, Bentley D, et al. The host genomic environment of the provirus determines the abundance of HTLV-1-infected T-cell clones. Blood. 2011;117(11):3113–22.

19. da Silva JL, Primo JR, de Oliveira M, Batista ES, Moreno-Carvalho O, Farré L, et al. Clustering of HTLV-1 associated myelopathy/tropical spastic paraparesis (HAM/TSP) and infective dermatitis associated with HTLV-1 (IDH) in Salvador, Bahia, Brazil. J Clin Virol. 2013;58(2):482–5.

20. Gillet NA, Cook L, Laydon DJ, Hlela C, Verdonck K, Alvarez C, et al. Strongyloidiasis and infective dermatitis alter human T lymphotropic virus-1 clonality in vivo. PLoS Pathog. 2013;9(4):e1003263.

21. Nascimento MCF, Primo JRL, Bittencourt AL, Siqueira I, Oliveira MFSP, Meyer R, et al. Infective dermatitis has similar immunologic features to human T lymphotropic virus-type 1-associated myelopathy/tropical spastic paraparesis. Clin Exp Immunol. 2009;156(3):455–62.

22. Souza A, Tanajura D, Toledo-Cornell C, Santos S, Carvalho EM. Immunopathogenesis and neurological manifestations associated to HTLV-1 infection. Rev Soc Bras Med Trop. 2012;45(5):545–52.

23. Dhasmana D, Taylor GP. Human T-lymphotropic virus/HIV coinfection: a clinical review. Curr Opin Infect Dis. 2014;27(1):16–28.

24. Proietti FA, Carneiro-Proietti AB, Catalan-Soares BC, Murphy EL. Global epidemiology of HTLV-I infection and associated diseases. Oncogene. 2005;24(39):6058–68.

25. Kamoi K, Mochizuki M. HTLV infection and the eye. Curr Opin Ophthalmol. 2012;23(6):557–61.

26. Bittencourt AL. A infecção pelo HTLV-1 na faixa infanto-juvenil. In: HTLV-1. LIVRO HEMOMINAS. vol. XVI, 6ª Ed. Belo Horizonte: Fundação HEMOMINAS; 2015. p. 347–67. Available from: C:/Users/abittencourt/Downloads/livro_htlv-2015.pdf.

27. Bittencourt AL, Vieira MG, Brites C, Farré L, Barbosa HS. Adult T-cell leukemia/lymphoma in Bahia, Brazil: analysis of prognostic factors in a group of 70 patients. Am J Clin Pathol. 2007;128(5): 875–82.

28. Gonçalves DU, Guedes AC, Carneiro-Proietti AB, Pinheiro SR, Catalan-Soares B, Poietti FA, et al. Simultaneous occurrence of HTLV-I associated myelopathy, uveitis and smouldering adult T cell leukaemia. GIPH (Interdisciplinary HTLV-I/II Research Group). Int J STD AIDS. 1999;10(5):336–7.

29. Farré L, de Oliveira MF, Primo J, Vandamme AM, Van Weyenbergh J, Bittencourt AL. Early sequential development of infective dermatitis, human T-cell lymphotropic virus type 1-associated myelopathy, and adult T-cell leukemia/lymphoma. Clin Infect Dis. 2008;46(3):440–2.

30. de Bastos ML, Santos SB, Souza A, Finkmoore B, Bispo O, Barreto T, et al. Influence of HTLV-1 on the clinical, microbiologic and immunologic presentation of tuberculosis. BMC Infect Dis. 2012;12:199.

31. Sweet RD. A pattern of eczema in Jamaica. Br J Dermatol. 1966;78(2):93–100.

32. La Grenade L, Hanchard B, Fletcher V, Cranston B, Blattner W. Infective dermatitis of Jamaican children: a marker for HTLV-1 infection. Lancet. 1990;336(8727):1345–7.

33. La Grenade L, Manns A, Fletcher V, Derm D, Carberry C, Hanchard B, et al. Clinical, pathologic and immunologic features of human T-lymphotrophic virus type I-associated infective dermatitis in children. Arch Dermatol. 1998;134(4):439–44.

34. Tsukasaki K, Yamada Y, Ikeda S, Tomonaga M. Infective dermatitis among patients with ATL in Japan. Int J Cancer. 1994;57(2):293.

35. Oliveira PD, Magalhães M, Argolo JM, Bittencourt AL, Farre L. Double integration band of HTLV-1 in a young patient with infective dermatitis who developed an acute form of adult T-cell leukemia/lymphoma. J Clin Virol. 2013;56(2):163–6.

36. Araujo AP, Fontenelle LM, Padua PA, Maia Filho HS, Araújo AQ. Juvenile human T lymphotropic virus type 1–associated myelopathy. Clin Infect Dis. 2002;35(2):201–4.

37. Lenzi ME, Araujo AQ, Maya TC, Serapião MJ, Leite ACB, Schor D, et al. Dermatite infectiva associada ao HTLV-I: Relato de caso. An Bras Dermatol. 1996;71(2):115–8.

38. Steglich RB, Tonoli RE, Souza PRM, Pinto GM, Riesgo RS. HTLV-1-associated infective dermatitis and probable HTLV-1-associated myelopathy in an adolescent female. An Bras Dermatol. 2015;90(3 Suppl 1):55–8.

39. Bittencourt AL, Oliveira MFSP, Ferraz N, Vieira MG, Muniz A, Brites C. Adult-onset infective dermatitis associated with HTLV-I. Clinical and immunopathologic aspects of two cases. Eur J Dermatol. 2006;16(1):62–6.

40. Nobre V, Guedes AC, Proietti FA, Martins ML, Nassif G, GIPH (HTLV-1/2 Research Interdisciplinary Group), et al. Increased prevalence of human T cell lymphotropic virus type 1 in patients attending a Brazilian dermatology clinic. Intervirology. 2007;50(4):316–8.

41. Maragno L, Casseb J, Fukumori LM, Sotto MN, Duarte AJ, Festa-Neto C, et al. Human T-cell lymphotropic virus type 1 infective dermatitis emerging in adulthood. Int J Dermatol. 2009;48(7):723–30.

42. Okajima R, Casseb J, Sanches JA. Copresentation of human T-cell lymphotropic virus type 1 (HTLV-1)-associated myelopathy/tropical spastic paraparesis and adult-onset infective dermatitis associated with HTLV-1 infection. Int J Dermatol. 2013;52(1):63–8.

43. Di Martino OB, Riveros R, Medina R, Morel M. Infective dermatitis in an adult patient with HTLV-1. Am J Dermatopathol. 2015;37(12):944–8.

44. Bittencourt AL, Oliveira MFSP, Brites C, Van Weyenbergh J, Vieira MG, Araújo I. Histopathologic and immunohistochemical studies of infective dermatitis associated with HTLV-I. Eur J Dermatol. 2005;15(1):26–30.

45. Hanchard B, La Grenade L, Carberry C, Fletcher V, Williams E, Cranston B, et al. Childhood infective dermatitis evolving into adult T-cell leukaemia after 17 years. Lancet. 1991;338(8782–8783):1593–4.

46. Gonçalves DU, Guedes AC, Carneiro-Proietti ABF, Lambertucci JR. HTLV-1 associated infective dermatitis may be an indolent HTLV-1 associated lymphoma. Braz J Infect Dis. 2000;4(2):100–2.

47. Bittencourt AL, Barbosa HS, Vieira MG, Farre L. Adult T-cell leukemia/lymphoma (ATL) presenting in the skin: clinical, histologic and immunohistochemical features of 52 cases. Acta Oncol. 2009;48(4):598–604.

48. Oliveira MFSP, Vieira MG, Primo J, Siqueira IC, Carvalho EM, Farré L, et al. Flower cells in patients with infective dermatitis associated with HTLV-1. J Clin Virol. 2010;48(4):288–90.

49. Bittencourt AL, Argolo JM, Oliveira MFSP, Farre L. Infective dermatitis associated with HTLV-1 represents a pre-adult T-cell leukemia/lymphoma (ATLL) condition. In: Annals of the sixty annual T-cell lymphoma forum. San Francisco; 2014.

50. Imaizumi Y, Iwanaga M, Tsukasaki K, Hata T, Tomonaga M, Ikeda S. Natural course of HTLV-1 carriers with monoclonal proliferation of T lymphocytes ("pre-ATL") in a 20-year follow-up study. Blood. 2005;105(2):903–4.

51. Bittencourt AL, Oliveira PD, Andrade AC, Santos TC, Oliveira RF, Farré L, et al. Analysis of cutaneous lymphomas in a medical center in Bahia, Brazil. Am J Clin Pathol. 2013;140(3):348–54.

52. Bittencourt AL, Barbosa HS, Requião C, Silva AC, Vandamme AM, Van Weyenbergh J, et al. Adult T-cell leukemia/lymphoma with a mixed CD4$^+$ and CD8$^+$ phenotype and a indolent course. J Clin Oncol. 2007;25(17):2480–2.

53. Bittencourt AL, Barbosa HS, Pimenta A, Farré L. A case of adult T-cell leukemia/lymphoma (ATL) with a survival of more than 13 years. Acta Oncol. 2008;47(5):981–3.

54. Shimoyama M. Diagnostic criteria and classification of clinical subtypes of adult T-cell leukaemia-lymphoma. A report from the Lymphoma Study Group (1984–1987). Br J Haematol. 1991;79(3):428–37.

55. Hanchard B. Adult T-cell leukemia/lymphoma in Jamaica: 1986–1995. J Acquir Immune Defic Syndr Hum Retrovirol. 1996;13(Suppl 1):S20–5.

56. Tsukasaki K, Hermine O, Bazarbachi A, Ratner L, Ramos JC, Harrington W Jr, et al. Definition, prognostic factors, treatment, and response criteria of adult T-cell leukemia-lymphoma: a proposal from an international consensus meeting. J Clin Oncol. 2009;27(3):453–9.

57. Yonekura K, Utsunomiya A, Seto M, Takatsuka Y, Takeuchi S, Tokunaga M, et al. Human T-lymphotropic virus type I proviral loads in patients with adult T-cell leukemia-lymphoma: comparison between cutaneous type and other subtypes. J Dermatol. 2015;42(12):1143–8.

58. Ishitsuka K, Ikeda S, Utsunomiya A, Saburi Y, Uozumi K, Tsukasaki K, et al. Smouldering adult T-cell leukaemia/lymphoma: a follow-up study in Kyushu. Br J Haematol. 2008;143(3):442–4.

59. Katsuya H, Ishitsuka K, Utsunomiya A, Hanada S, Eto T, Moriuchi Y, et al., ATL–Prognostic Index Project. Treatment and survival among 1594 patients with ATL. Blood. 2015;126(24):2570–7.

60. Yamaguchi T, Ohshima K, Karube K, Tutiya T, Kawano R, Suefuji H, et al. Clinicopathologic features of cutaneous lesions of adult T-cell leukaemia/lymphoma. Br J Dermatol. 2005;152(1):76–81.

61. Takasaki Y, Iwanaga M, Imaizumi Y, Tawara M, Joh T, Kohno T, et al. Long-term study of indolent

adult T-cell leukemia-lymphoma. Blood. 2010;Jun 3;115(22):4337–43.

62. Setoyama M, Katahira Y, Kanzaki T. Clinicopathologic analysis of 124 cases of adult T-cell leukemia/lymphoma with cutaneous manifestations: The smouldering type with skin manifestations has a poorer prognosis than previously thought. J Dermatol. 1999;26(12):785–90.

63. Oliveira PD, Torres IS, Oliveira RF, Bittencourt AL. Acute adult T-cell leukemia/lymphoma (ATL) presenting with cutaneous purpuric lesions: a rare presentation. Acta Oncol. 2011;50(4):595–7.

64. Bittencourt AL, Mota K, Oliveira RF, Farré L. A dyshidrosis-like variant of adult T-cell leukemia/lymphoma with clinicopathologic aspects of mycosis fungoides. A Case Rep Am J Dermatopathol. 2009;31(8):834–7.

65. Michael EJ, Shaffer JJ, Collins HE, Grossman ME. Bullous adult T-cell lymphoma/leukemia and human T-cell lymphotropic virus-1 associated myelopathy in a 60-year-old man. J Am Acad Dermatol. 2002;46(5 Suppl):S137–41.

66. Sawada Y, Hino R, Hama K, Ohmori S, Fueki H, Yamada S, et al. Type of skin eruption is an independent prognostic indicator for adult T-cell leukemia/lymphoma. Blood. 2011;117(15):3961–7.

67. Yared JA, Kimball AS. Optimizing management of patients with adult T cell leukemia-lymphoma. Cancers (Basel). 2015;7(4):2318–29.

68. Tsukasaki K, Imaizumi Y, Tawara M, Fujimoto T, Fukushima T, Hata T, et al. Diversity of leukaemic cell morphology in ATL correlates with prognostic factors, aberrant immunophenotype and defective HTLV-1 genotype. Br J Haematol. 1999;105(2):369–75.

69. Santos JB, Farré L, Batista Eda S, Santos HH, Vieira MD, Bittencourt AL. The importance of flower cells for the early diagnosis of acute adult T-cell leukemia/lymphoma with skin involvement. Acta Oncol. 2010;49(2):265–7.

70. Foucar K. Mature T-cell leukemias including T-prolymphocytic leukemia, adult T-cell leukemia/lymphoma, and Sézary syndrome. Am J Clin Pathol. 2007;127(4):496–510.

71. Burg G, Kempf W, Cozzio A, Feit J, Willemze R, S Jaffe E, et al. WHO/EORTC classification of cutaneous lymphomas 2005: Histologic and molecular aspects. J Cutan Pathol. 2005;32(10):647–74.

72. Ohshima K, Jaffe ES, Kikuchi M. Adult T-cell leukemia/lymphoma. In: Swerdlow SH, Campo E, Harris NL, et al., editors. WHO classification of tumours of haematopoietic and lymphoid tissues. Lyon: WHO; 2008. p. 281–4.

73. Johno M, Ohishi M, Kojo Y, Yamamoto S, Ono T. Cutaneous manifestations of adult T-cell leukemia/lymphoma. In: Takatsuki K, Hinuma Y, Yoshida M, editors. Advances in adult T-cell leukemia and HTLV-1. Research, Gann monograph on Cancer Research n° 19. Tokyo: Scientific Society Press; 1992. p. 33–42.

74. Amano M, Kurokawa M, Ogata K, Itoh H, Kataoka H, Setoyama M. New entity, definition and diagnos-

tic criteria of cutaneous adult T-cell leukemia/lymphoma: human T-lymphotropic virus type 1 proviral DNA load can distinguish between cutaneous and smoldering types. J Dermatol. 2008;35(5):270–5.

75. Miyata T, Yonekura K, Utsunomiya A, Kanekura T, Nakamura S, Seto M. Cutaneous type adult T-cell leukemia/lymphoma is a characteristic subtype and includes erythema/papule and nodule/tumor subgroups. Int J Cancer. 2010;126(6):1521–8.

76. Tsukasaki K, Imaizumi Y, Tokura Y, Ohshima K, Kawai K, Utsunomiya A, et al. Meeting report on the possible proposal of an extranodal primary cutaneous variant in the lymphoma type of adult T-cell leukemia-lymphoma. J Dermatol. 2014;41(1):26–8.

77. DiCaudo DJ, Perniciaro C, Worrell JT, White JW Jr, Cockerell CJ. Clinical and histologic spectrum of human T-cell lymphotropic virus type I-associated lymphoma involving the skin. J Am Acad Dermatol. 1996;34(1):69–76.

78. Sakamoto FH, Colleoni GW, Teixeira SP, Yamamoto M, Michalany NS, Almeida FA, et al. Cutaneous T-cell lymphoma with HTLV-I infection: clinical overlap with adult T-cell leukemia/lymphoma. Int J Dermatol. 2006;45(4):447–9.

79. Rueda R, Blank A. HTLV-1 associated cutaneous manifestations. In: Zaninovic V, editor. HTLV, truths and questions. Cali: Feriva; 1996. p. 212–22.

80. Lenzi ME, Cuzzi-Maya T, Oliveira AL, Andrada-Serpa MJ, Araújo AQ. dermatologic findings of human T lymphotropic virus type 1 (HTLV-I) associated myelopathy/tropical spastic paraparesis. Clin Infect Dis. 2003;36(4):507–13.

81. Ploysangam T, Breneman DL, Mutasim DF. Cutaneous pseudolymphomas. J Am Acad Dermatol. 1998;38(6 Pt 1):877–95.

82. Oken MM, Creech RH, Tormey DC, Horton J, Davis TE, McFadden ET, et al. Toxicity and response criteria of the Eastern Cooperative Oncology Group. Am J Clin Oncol. 1982;5(6):649–55.

83. Bazarbachi A, Plumelle Y, Ramos JC, Tortevoye P, Otrock Z, Taylor G, et al. Meta-analysis on the use of zidovudine and interferon-alfa in adult T-cell leukemia/lymphoma showing improved survival in the leukemic subtypes. J Clin Oncol. 2010;28(27):4177–83.

84. Sawada Y, Shimauchi T, Yamaguchi T, Okura R, Hama-Yamamoto K, Fueki-Yoshioka H, et al. Combination of skin-directed therapy and oral etoposide for smoldering adult T-cell leukemia/lymphoma with skin involvement. Leuk Lymphoma. 2013;54(3):520–7.

85. Marçais A, Suarez F, Sibon D, Frenzel L, Hermine O, Bazarbachi A. Therapeutic options for adult T-cell leukemia/lymphoma. Curr Oncol Rep. 2013;15(5):457–64.

86. Kudo H, Fukushima S, Masuguchi S, Sakai K, Jinnin M, Ihn H. Cutaneous type adult T-cell leukaemia/lymphoma successfully treated with narrowband ultraviolet B phototherapy. Clin Exp Dermatol. 2012;37(2):183–4.

87. Germain M, Williams J, Skelton HG, Smith KJ. Smoldering HTLV-1-induced T-cell lymphoma localized within the skin; a radiation-resistant tumor. Int J Dermatol. 2000;39(11):815–21.

88. Takahashi K, Tanaka T, Fujita M, Horiguchi Y, Miyachi Y, Imamura S. Cutaneous-type adult T-cell leukemia/lymphoma. A unique clinical feature with monoclonal T-cell proliferation detected by Southern blot analysis. Arch Dermatol. 1988;124(3):399–404.

89. Shimizu S, Yasui C, Koizumi K, Ikeda H, Tsuchiya K. Cutaneous-type adult T-cell leukemia/lymphoma presenting as a solitary large skin nodule: a review of the literature. J Am Acad Dermatol. 2007;57(5 Suppl):S115–7.

90. Lyra-da-Silva JO, de Mello Gonzaga YB, de Melo EO, de Andrada-Serpa MJ, Dib C, et al. Adult T-cell leukemia/lymphoma: a case report of primary cutaneous tumoral type. Dermatol Pract Concepts. 2012;2(2):202–3.

91. Milagres SP, Sanches JA Jr, Milagres AC, Valente NY. Histopathologic and immunohistochemical assessment of acquired ichthyosis in patients with human T-cell lymphotropic virus type I-associated myelopathy. Br J Dermatol. 2003;149(4):776–81.

92. Hashiguchi T, Osame M, Arimura K. Skin manifestations in HTLV-1 associated myelopathy (HAM): xerosis and erythema. In: HTLV-1 and the nervous system. Manhattan: Alan R Liss; 1989. p. 443–8.

93. Yamaguchi K. Human T-cell lymphotropic virus type I in Japan. Lancet. 1994;343(8891):213–6.

94. Gonçalves DU, Guedes AC, Proietti AB, Martins ML, Proietti FA, Lambertucci JR, et al., Interdisciplinary HTLV-1/2 Research Group. Dermatologic lesions in asymptomatic blood donors seropositive for human T cell lymphotropic virus type-1. Am J Trop Med Hyg. 2003;68(5):562–5.

95. Setoyama M, Mizoguchi S, Eizuru Y. Human T-cell lymphotropic virus type I infects eccrine sweat gland epithelia. Int J Cancer. 1999;80(5):652–5.

96. Maloney EM, Wiktor SZ, Palmer P, Cranston B, Pate EJ, Cohn S, et al. A cohort study of health effects of human T-cell lymphotropic virus type I infection in Jamaican children. Pediatrics. 2003;112(2):e136–42.

97. Brites C, Weyll M, Pedroso C, Badaró R. Severe and Norwegian scabies are strongly associated with retroviral (HIV-1/HTLV-1) infection in Bahia, Brazil. AIDS. 2002;16(9):1292–3.

98. Tseng CT, Sell S. Protracted treponema pallidum-induced cutaneous chancres in rabbits infected with human T-cell leukemia virus type I. AIDS Res Hum Retrovir. 1991;7(3):323–31.

99. Carnaúba D Jr, Bittencourt A, Brites C. Atypical presentation of syphilis in an HTLV-I infected patient. Braz J Infect Dis. 2003;7(4):273–7.

100. Machado PR, Machado LM, Shibuya M, Rego J, Johnson WD, Glesby MJ. Viral coinfection and leprosy outcomes: a cohort study. PLoS Negl Trop Dis. 2015;9(8):e0003865.

Suggestions Reading

In Portuguese

HTLV-1. LIVRO HEMOMINAS, vol. XVI, 6ª Ed. Belo Horizonte, Fundação HEMOMINAS, 2015. Available from: C:/Users/abittencourt/Downloads/livro_htlv-2015.pdf.

Oliveira PD, Farre L, Bittencourt AL. Leucemia/linfoma de células T do adulto. Revisão. Rev Ass Méd Bras. Aceito para publicação.

Bittencourt AL, Farré L. Vírus linfotrópico para células T humanas tipo 1 (HTLV-1). Capítulo 32. In: Brasileiro Filho G, editor. Bogliolo, Patologia. 8ª edição ed. Rio de Janeiro: Guanabara Koogan; 2011. p. 1357–68.

Bittencourt AL, Farré L. Leucemia/linfoma de células T do adulto. Adult T-cell leukemia/lymphoma. An Bras Dermatol. 2008;83:351–9.

Bittencourt AL, Oliveira MFSP. Dermatite Infecciosa associada ao HTLV-1- Revisão. An Bras Dermatol. 2001;76:723–32.

In English

Bangham CR, Cook LB, Melamed A. HTLV-1 clonality in adult T-cell leukaemia and nonmalignant HTLV-1 infection. Semin Cancer Biol. 2014;26:89–98.

Cook LB, Melamed A, Niederer H, Valganon M, Laydon D, Foroni L, et al. The role of HTLV-1 clonality, proviral structure, and genomic integration site in adult T-cell leukemia/lymphoma. Blood. 2014;123(25):3925–31.

Ishida T, Joh T, Uike N, Yamamoto K, Utsunomiya A, Yoshida S, et al. Defucosylated anti-CCR4 monoclonal antibody (KW-0761) for relapsed adult T-cell leukemia-lymphoma: a multicenter phase II study. J Clin Oncol. 2012;30(8):837–42.

Tsukasaki K, Utsunomiya A, Fukuda H, Shibata T, Fukushima T, Takatsuka Y, et al. VCAP-AMP-VECP compared with biweekly CHOP for adult T-cell leukemia-lymphoma: Japan Clinical Oncology Group Study JCOG9801. J Clin Oncol. 2007;25(34):5458–64.

Tsukasaki K, Tobinai K. Human T-cell lymphotropic virus type I-associated adult T-cell leukemia-lymphoma: new directions in clinical research. Clin Cancer Res. 2014;20(20):5217–25.

Utsunomiya A, Choi I, Chihara D, Seto M. Recent advances in the treatment of adult T-cell leukemia-lymphomas. Cancer Sci. 2015;106(4):344–51.

Connective Tissue Diseases

43

Jesus Rodriguez Santamaria,
Janyana M.D. Deonizio, and Maira Mitsue Mukai

Cutaneous Lupus Erythematosus

Key Points
- Lupus erythematosus (LE) is a chronic, inflammatory, autoimmune disease. It can affect only the skin (CLE) or also involves internal organs (SLE)
- Several aspects such as genetics, ambient factors, ultraviolet radiation, drugs, infections, inflammatory cells, cytokines, and chemokines participate in the LE pathogenesis

- There are three major forms of CLE: acute (ACLE), subacute (SCLE), and chronic (CCLE)
- Skin biopsy may include findings such as degeneration of the basal cells, dermal mucin deposits, and thickening of the basement membrane
- Treatment includes topical corticosteroids, antimalarials, sun protection, cessation of smoking.

Introduction

Lupus erythematous (LE) is a chronic, inflammatory, autoimmune disease with a wide clinical spectrum and a variable evolution, severity, and prognosis. LE can manifest only as a dermatologic disease, termed cutaneous LE (CLE). Systemic LE (SLE) commonly involves the skin, joints, and several internal organs.

J.R. Santamaria (✉) • J.M.D. Deonizio
M.M. Mukai
Department of Dermatology of Federal, University of Parana - UFPR, Curitiba, Paraná, Brazil
e-mail: jsantamaria@uol.com.br

General Epidemiology

The incidence of LE varies according to the characteristics of the population studied, such as predominant age or sex, race, ethnicity, national origin, or period of time studied, and criteria in diagnostic classification [1–5].

In patients with exclusively cutaneous disease, there is a female-to-male ratio of 3:1. On the other hand, SLE usually affects women during their reproductive years with a female-to-male ratio of 9:1 [6, 7].

Ethnicity is also a major risk factor, the prevalence of SLE being four-fold higher in African American women than in Caucasian American women [6, 7]. African American patients with SLE develop disease at an earlier age and have a higher mortality rate because of organ damage such as nephritis and pneumonitis [6, 7].

© Springer International Publishing Switzerland 2018
R.R. Bonamigo, S.I.T. Dornelles (eds.), *Dermatology in Public Health Environments*,
https://doi.org/10.1007/978-3-319-33919-1_43

Skin Manifestations

In all types of LE, the skin is one of the most frequent sites of involvement. In 1981, James N. Gilliam divided the cutaneous manifestations of LE into those lesions that show histologic changes characteristic of LE (LE-specific skin disease) and those that are not specific for lupus (LE-nonspecific skin disease). CLE refers to LE-specific skin disease and are divided in three major categories: acute CLE (ACLE), subacute CLE (SCLE), and chronic CLE (CCLE) [8]. Moreover, in addition to the classic forms of CLE, uncommon variants often lead to diagnostic difficulties.

Etiopathogenesis

LE is characterized by a mixture of clinical, histologic, immunopathologic, and laboratory findings. The pathogenetic mechanisms responsible for LE-specific skin disease are not fully understood, although recent work has provided many new insights [9–11].

Genetic

Genetics plays an important role in the development of LE. For example, in monozygotic twins with lupus there is a 25% concordance rate compared with a 2% concordance for dizygotic twins [12]. Numerous lupus-associated genes have been identified, and lupus-associated genetic changes have been linked to the clearance of nuclear debris, apoptotic cells, and immune complexes [13].

Some major histocompatibility complex class I and II alleles may confer susceptibility to CLE, such as human leukocyte antigen (HLA) B8, DR3, DQA1, and DRB1 [9]. Rare mutations also contribute to LE pathogenesis [14].

Ultraviolet

Sun exposure can induce the skin lesions of LE or exacerbate the clinical course in a susceptible person [15]. Moreover, cutaneous findings are most frequently found on sun-exposed skin, and lesions can be induced by exposure to arti-ficial sources of ultraviolet (UV) radiation [3, 16–18]. UV light effects include induction of an inflammatory response and generation of apoptotic keratinocytes or "sunburn cells." UV radiation–induced apoptosis causes presentation of autoantigens that can be involved in LE pathogenesis [9].

Infection

Infectious agents can break immunologic tolerance to self-antigens and induce autoimmune disorders [19]. In LE patients, Epstein–Barr virus (EBV), cytomegalovirus, parvovirus B19, and retrovirus (HRES-1, ERV-3, HERV-E 4-1, HERV-K10, and HERV-K18) infections may have an important pathogenetic role [20, 21]. Infections can participate as primers, inducing responses against self-antigens and promoting activation or apoptosis of several immune cells in genetically predisposed individuals [19].

Hormones

LE is a disease with female predilection, suggesting a hormonal influence. High levels of estrogen and progesterone promote humoral autoreactivity, reinforcing the hormonal theory [22]. Oral contraceptives have been thought to produce disease flares [23, 24].

Drugs and Chemicals

Certain medications can induce both CLE and SLE, such as procainamide, isoniazid, quinidine, chlorpromazine, terbinafine, calcium channel blockers, hydrochlorothiazide, and anti–tumor necrosis factor-α (TNF-α) medications, with more than 90 drugs described [25–27]. Clinical and serologic manifestations normally resolve after withdrawal of the suspected medication [25].

Tobacco has been suggested to predispose to the onset or worsening of lupus [28]. Patients who smoke tend to be less responsive to antimalarial treatment in discoid LE.

Apoptosis

Apoptosis is programmed cell death which can be triggered by internal factors, such as DNA mutation, or by external factors, such as infections and UV exposure [10]. Some lupus patients demonstrate increased spontaneous apoptosis or impaired clearance of apoptotic peripheral blood cells [29]. Abnormalities in the clearance of apoptotic cells can generate autoantigens and autoimmune diseases.

Innate Immune System

Dendritic cells (DCs) are important in LE pathogenesis by phagocytosis, B-cell activation, and secretion of cytokine-like interferon (INF)-α, interleukin (IL)-6, and B-lymphocyte stimulator (BLyS) [13]. Patients with LE have impaired phagocytosis of apoptotic cells by the DCs. They also can recognize damage-associated molecular pattern, from microbial and endogenous ligands by pathogen recognition receptors (PRR), mainly Toll-like receptors (TLR). TRL 7, TLR 9, TRL 3, and TRL 8 are important because they can recognize nucleic acids [10]. In addition, several lupus genes encode proteins that mediate or regulate TLR signals and are associated with increased plasma IFN-α [14]. Studies have shown a good correlation between expression of IFN-α-inducible genes and SLE activity, suggesting that the increased IFN activity might contribute to increased immune system activity and tissue damage [10].

Very recently, the role of neutrophils has gained special attention in the lupus pathogenesis [14]. These cells can release chromatin structures called neutrophil extracellular traps (NETs). NETs can trap and kill various bacterial, fungal, and protozoal pathogens, and their release is one of the first lines of defense against pathogens, in a process called NETosis. NETs are able to stimulate DCs to produce IFN-α through, for example, interaction with TLR9 [11]. NETosis has been involved in autoimmune pathogenesis, including LE.

Adaptive Immune System

The combined T- and B-cell abnormalities in SLE result in the production of pathogenic autoantibodies.

B lymphocytes act as antigen-presenting cells and also produce antibodies and cytokines in autoimmune diseases. B-cell tolerance is changed in LE, resulting in autoreactive B cells that induce the production of pathogenic autoantibodies [13]. Several of these autoantibodies are thought to be directly pathogenic, including double-stranded DNA (dsDNA) and Ro/SS-A antibodies, hallmarks of SLE patients. Moreover, B lymphocytes present efficiently autoantigens and activate T cells, amplifying the inflammatory cascade [10].

CD4 T cells are critical players in the pathogenesis of lupus since they regulate B-cell responses and tolerance regulation, and also infiltrate target tissues, leading to tissue damage [10]. In early phase of CLE skin lesions, there is a predominance of CD4 T cells, whereas in the late phase CD8 T cells are more abundant [30]. A T-helper 1 (Th1)-mediated immune response is described in CLE [9, 30].

Th17 cells are responsible for induction of inflammation and autoimmunity through release of IL-17, IL-22, and IL-21. Studies have found these cells in CLE and SLE target tissues [10, 11].

Natural regulatory T cells (Tregs) are important in the prevention of abnormal autoimmune responses. They regulate activities of DCs, monocytes, mast cells, B cells, and CD4 and CD8 T cells. Tregs secrete cytokines as IL-10 and transforming growth factor β (TGF-β), which have inhibitory effects in T cells [9]. In CLE Treg cells are reduced in the lesions but not in the circulation as seen in SLE, suggesting an organ-specific Treg cell defect [9].

Cytokines and Chemokines

Cytokines such as IL-6, IL-10, IL-12, IL-17, and IL-18 have been implicated in the immunopathogenesis of CLE [13]. TNF-α may promote autoreactivity in lupus [30].

Clinical Presentation

In 2012 the revised classification for SLE was proposed. According to the Lupus International Collaborating Clinics (SLICC), patients must meet at least four criteria, including at least one clinical and one immunologic criterion. Alternatively, patients must have biopsy-proven lupus nephritis in the presence of antinuclear and anti-dsDNA.

Cutaneous lesions of LE may be divided into three major forms: acute cutaneous lupus erythematous (ACLE), subacute lupus erythematous (SCLE), and chronic cutaneous lupus erythematous (CCLE). Recently a fourth form has been added to lupus classification, intermittent cutaneous lupus erythematous [31, 32].

Chronic Cutaneous Lupus Erythematous

CCLE can be subclassified into discoid, profundus, and tumidus.

The most common form of cutaneous lesions is the *discoid* form characterized by scaly plaques with dyschromia (usually hyperpigmentation associated with depigmentation) and atrophy (Fig. 43.1). This form of lupus is rarely associated with systemic disease, which occurs in 5–10% of cases. Histologically there is a lymphocytic infiltrate in the dermis–epidermis junction with dermal atrophy. Keratinocyte damage and hyperkeratosis are very characteristic. The dermal–epidermal basement membrane zone is thickened. Hair follicles are involved with damage of keratinocytes and follicular plugging. Dermal mucin deposits may be present.

Lupus profundus is a rare form of CCLE and is characterized by deep nodules involving subcutaneous tissues of proximal extremities, buttocks, face, and trunk, which progress to

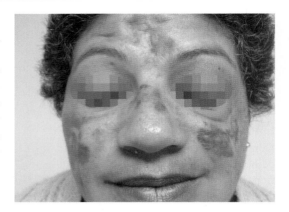

Fig. 43.2 Lupus profundus. Deep nodules on the face. Lipoatrophy and scars

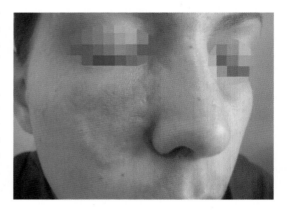

Fig. 43.3 Lupus tumidus. Erythematous plaque on the face

lipoatrophy and scars (Fig. 43.2). Histologically there is a lobular lymphocytic panniculitis.

Lupus tumidus is also a rare manifestation of CCLE and is characterized by erythematous urticarial papules and plaques with annular or centrifugal presentation on the face, proximal upper extremities, and chest (Fig. 43.3). Histologically there is a perivascular and periadnexal lymphocytic infiltrate associated with mucin deposits.

Some authors classify lupus erythematous tumidus as a separate group as intermittent subtype of CLE [32].

SCLE is characterized by annular and papulosquamous lesions with marked photosensitivity (Fig. 43.4). Many times lesions may resemble psoriasis and are often arranged in a reticulated pattern. Usually, arms and torso are involved and the

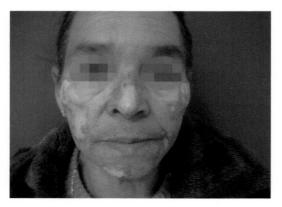

Fig. 43.1 Discoid lupus erythematous. Scarred, dyschromic lesions on the face

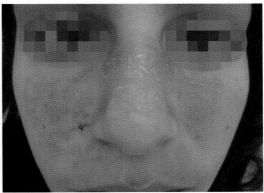

Fig. 43.5 Acute cutaneous lupus erythematosus. Butterfly rash on the center of the face

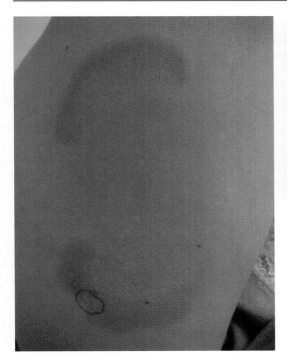

Fig. 43.4 Subacute lupus. Annular lesions on the arms

face is spared. Histologically a common finding is keratinocyte damage and epidermal atrophy. Hydropic degeneration of basal cell layers may be present. Some necrotic keratinocytes may be found in the epidermal layer. The lymphohistiocytic infiltrate is concentrated in the upper dermis with interface and perivascular pattern. The infiltrate tends to be less dense than in discoid cases.

In contrast to CCLE, where there is rarely systemic involvement, half of the patients with SCLE will develop signs and symptoms of SLE.

ACLE is the form most involved with systemic symptoms and is characterized by butterfly rash in the center of the face or a generalized maculopapular exanthema (Fig. 43.5). Histologically the findings are nonspecific and similar to those of dermatitis without significant hyperkeratosis or epidermal atrophy.

The principal characteristics of the three major forms of lupus are summarized in Table 43.1.

Some skin lesions are not specific of LE and are often seen in patients with SLE and other autoimmune diseases. Those include cutaneous vascular disease such as vasculitis and vasculopa-

thies, periungual telangiectasias, livedo reticularis, Raynaud's phenomenon, nonscarring alopecia, rheumatoid nodules, calcinosis cutis, urticaria, leg ulcers, lichen planus, and chilblains [33]. Some specific and nonspecific skin findings in cutaneous lupus erythematous are summarized in Table 43.2.

Cutaneous Lupus Erythematous Variants

Neonatal lupus erythematosus is a rare condition in the neonatal period whereby children have lesions similar to those of SCLE and/or congenital heart block. There is an associated with maternal immunoglobulin G (IgG) antinuclear antibodies. Congenital heart block may require a pacemaker. The children may also have photosensitivity, hepatobiliary disease, hemolytic anemia, thrombocytopenia, and leukopenia [33].

In *bullous lupus erythematosus*, patients have blisters that resemble dermatitis herpetiformis or bullous pemphigoid. Blisters may appear as a result of the intense of the basal cell damage. A second situation is when the blisters are formed by an intense neutrophilic infiltrate in the dermal papillae resembling dermatitis herpetiformis [34].

Hypertrophic lupus is characterized by solitary verrucous and hyperkeratotic lesion [33].

Rowell's syndrome is characterized by skin lesions similar to erythema multiforme and occurs in patients with an established history of LE.

Drug-induced lupus erythematosus is more associated with some drug classes, although

Table 43.1 Principal characteristics of the three major forms of cutaneous lupus erythematous

	Acute	Subacute	Chronic
Clinical	Butterfly rash *OR* generalized maculopapular exanthema	Psoriasiform Annular lesions Marked photosensitivity	Scaly dyschromic plaques Atrophy
Probability of systemic involvement	High	Intermediate	Low
Antibody profile	ANA positive (high titers)	anti-Ro/SS-A and anti-La/SS-B	None *OR* ANA positive (low titers)
Histology	Nonspecific, resembling dermatitis	Similar to discoid with less intense infiltrate	*Discoid*: lymphocytic infiltrate in the dermis–epidermis junction with dermal atrophy. Keratinocyte damage and hyperkeratosis. Follicular involvement *Panniculitis*: lobular lymphocytic panniculitis *Tumidus*: dermal perivascular and periadnexal lymphocytic infiltrate and mucin deposits. Sparse epidermal findings

ANA antinuclear antibody

Table 43.2 Specific and nonspecific skin findings in cutaneous lupus erythematous

Specific lesions	Nonspecific lesions
Acute cutaneous lupus erythematous (ACLE)	Raynaud's phenomenon
Subacute lupus erythematous (SCLE)	Thrombophlebitis
Chronic cutaneous lupus erythematous (CCLE)	Nailfold telangiectasias
	Diffuse nonscarring alopecia
	Calcinosis
	Vasculitis
	Livedo reticularis

more than 40 drugs have been involved. Terbinafine and TNF-α inhibitors are drugs with a high risk of development. Antihypertensives, antipsychotics, anticonvulsants, antihistamines, anti-inflammatories, antimicrobials, and immunosuppressives are all drug classes associated with this form of LE. Patients develop positive antinuclear antibodies (ANA) [35].

Many conditions have to be considered in the differential diagnosis of CLE (Table 43.3).

Complementary Examinations

A skin biopsy may demonstrate some characteristics that corroborate the diagnosis. Each clinical presentation has some specific characteristics in pathology, as discussed previously, and also are related to the stages of the lesions [36]. Degeneration of the basal cells of the epidermis (hydropic degeneration) associated with lymphohistiocytic cellular infiltrate is typical of LE. The hair follicle structure may be involved with keratotic plug. Dermal mucin deposits favor the diagnosis of lupus [34, 35] (Table 43.4).

Direct immunofluorescence of lesional skin may demonstrate granular deposits at the dermal–epidermal junction and around hair follicles. Typically, these are formed by IgG and/or IgM deposits. Complement proteins are also common. Presence of antibody deposits at the dermal–epidermal junction from a normal-appearing skin is called "lupus band" and correlates with systemic disease. Nevertheless, the absence of deposits does not rule out lupus diagnosis [34].

To rule out SLE, ANA profile, urinalysis, complete blood count with differential, platelets count, chemistries, erythrocyte sedimentation rate, and complement levels should be required. Clinically patients with history of diffuse nonscarring alopecia, periungual telangiectasia, Raynaud's phenomenon, livedo reticularis, vasculitis, and lymphadenopathy should be investigated for SLE [34].

Table 43.3 Differential diagnosis of cutaneous lupus erythematosus

Chronic cutaneous lupus erythematosus (CCLE)	Subacute cutaneous lupus erythematosus (SCLE)	Acute cutaneous lupus erythematosus (ACLE)
Actinic keratosis	Plaque psoriasis	Dermatomyositis
Granuloma faciale	Lichen planus	Drug eruptions
Granuloma annulare	Erythema annulare centrifugum	Drug-induced photosensitivity
Keratoacanthoma	Tinea corporis	Seborrheic dermatitis
Lichen planus	Mycosis fungoides	Acne rosacea
Plaque psoriasis	Nummular eczema	
Cutaneous squamous cell carcinoma	Pityriasis rubra pilaris	
Panniculitis	Polymorphous light eruption	
	Sarcoidosis	

Table 43.4 Histologic findings in CLE

Hyperkeratosis with follicular plugging
Epidermal atrophy
Dermal atrophy
Hydropic degeneration of the basal layer
Lymphohistiocytic cellular infiltrate
Apoptotic keratinocytes (Civatte bodies)
Thickening of the basement membrane
Interstitial mucin deposition
Atrophy of pilosebaceous units

Positivity for ANA varies accordingly to the form of lupus. CCLE is rarely associated with systemic disease but low titers of ANA may be present. ACLE is highly associated with systemic involvement and ANA is usually present in high titers. SCLE has an intermediate association with SLE (50% fulfillment criteria for SLE) and usually is associated with positivity for anti-Ro/SSA antibody (70% of cases), ANA (60–70%), and anti-La/SSB (30–50%) [33].

Therapeutic Approach

Treatment includes topical steroids and calcineurin inhibitors such as tacrolimus 0.1% ointment. The latter may be a good alternative because of its fewer side effects, rapid onset, and safety during long-term use [37].

Antimalarials modulate the immune response without increasing the risk of infections. Hydroxychloroquine is associated with skin pigmentation and ocular toxicity. The response with these drugs may be slow and take 2–3 months.

Dapsone and retinoids are used as second-line therapy, especially in patients without response to antimalarials. Thalidomide is also an alternative but is associated with a high risk of relapse and neurotoxicity. Thalidomide analogs such as lenalidomide have less neurotoxicity and may be a good alternative [37]. Other options include immunosuppressors such as mycophenolate mofetil, azathioprine, systemic steroids, sulfasalazine, and cyclophosphamide. For bullous eruption of SLE dapsone may be useful. More recent studies suggest immunobiological drugs such as belimumab as a possible therapeutic alternative [37].

It is believed that UV radiation may induce systemic manifestations and specific skin lesions in LE disease [38]. Skin protection using broad-spectrum sunscreens is recommended in combination with physical protection with clothes and accessories. Although there is an evident association between photosensitivity and LE, light therapies may be an option for recalcitrant cutaneous manifestations [39].

Interestingly, there may be an association between vitamin D deficiency and lupus. Vitamin D has many functions in cellular growth and immune function. In CLE patients, low levels of vitamin D are associated with higher IFN levels and disease activity. Patients with SLE after vitamin D supplementation had lower disease activity scores and decreased anti-DNA antibody level [40]. The levels of vitamin D and calcium should be monitored in these patients.

The definitive role of smoking in lupus is not well established. Current smokers have an increased risk for SLE/CLE, higher disease activ-

Table 43.5 First- and second-line approaches for CLE treatment

First-line therapy	Second-line therapy
Sun protection	Dapsone
Quit smoking	Retinoids
Topical steroids	Thalidomide
Antimalarials	Immunosuppressors

ity scores, and higher frequency of anti-dsDNA compared with ex-smokers or those who never smoked [37]. Smoking is associated with cutaneous manifestations in SLE. Some authors suggest that CLE, but not SLE, is associated with smoking [41]. Smoking is associated with a two-fold decrease in the proportion of patients with CLE achieving cutaneous improvement with antimalarials [42].

First- and second-line approaches for CLE are summarized in Table 43.5.

Dermatomyositis

Key Points
- Dermatomyositis is an autoimmune disease that classically affects skin and muscles
- Vigilance for important associations with lung disease and malignancy can be aided by serology testing
- Distinctive skin findings are readily identifiable and assist in diagnosis
- Dermatomyositis therapy involves the use of corticosteroids, typically with an immunosuppressive agent

Introduction

Dermatomyositis is an idiopathic inflammatory myopathy with characteristic cutaneous findings that occur in children and adults. This systemic disorder most frequently affects the skin and muscles but may also affect the joints, the esophagus, the lungs, and, less commonly, the heart [43, 44]. Dystrophic calcinosis may complicate dermatomyositis and is most often observed in children and adolescents. An association between dermatomyositis and cancer has long been recognized in adult patients.

General Epidemiology

The estimated incidence of dermatomyositis is 9.63 cases per million population. The estimated incidence of amyopathic dermatomyositis is 2.08 cases per million [45].

Dermatomyositis can occur in people of any age. Two peak ages of onset exist: in adults, the peak age of onset is approximately 50 years, whereas in children it is approximately 5–10 years. Dermatomyositis and polymyositis are twice as common in women as in men. Neither condition shows any racial predilection.

Etiopathogenesis

The cause of dermatomyositis is unknown. However, genetic, immunologic, infectious, and environmental factors have been implicated.

A *genetic* component may predispose to dermatomyositis. Dermatomyositis rarely occurs in multiple family members, but a link to certain HLA types (e.g., DR3, DR5, DR7) may exist. Polymorphisms of TNF may be involved; specifically, the presence of the -308A allele is linked to photosensitivity in adults and calcinosis in children [46, 47, 48]. A meta-analysis demonstrated that the TNF-α-308A/G polymorphism might contribute to dermatomyositis susceptibility, especially in a European population [49].

Immunologic abnormalities are common in patients with dermatomyositis. Patients frequently have circulating autoantibodies. Abnormal T-cell activity may be involved in the pathogenesis of both the skin disease and the muscle disease. In addition, family members may manifest other diseases associated with autoimmunity.

ANAs and antibodies to cytoplasmic antigens (i.e., antitransfer RNA synthetases) may be present. Although their presence may help to define subtypes of dermatomyositis and polymyositis, their role in pathogenesis is uncertain.

Infectious agents have been suggested as possible triggers of dermatomyositis. These include the following: viruses (e.g., coxsackievirus, parvovirus, echovirus, human T-cell lymphotropic virus type 1 (HTLV-1), human immunodeficiency virus (HIV)), *Toxoplasma* species, and *Borrelia* species.

Cases of *drug-induced* dermatomyositis have been reported. Dermatomyositis-like skin changes have been reported with hydroxyurea in patients with chronic myelogenous leukemia or essential thrombocytosis [50, 51].Other agents that may trigger the disease include the following: statins, penicillamine, anti-TNF drugs, IFN, cyclophosphamide, bacillus Calmette-Guérin (BCG) vaccine, quinidine, phenylbutazone.

Dermatomyositis may be initiated or exacerbated by silicone breast implants or collagen injections, but the evidence for this is anecdotal and has not been verified in case–control studies. One report detailed HLA differences among women in whom inflammatory myopathy developed after silicone implants [52].

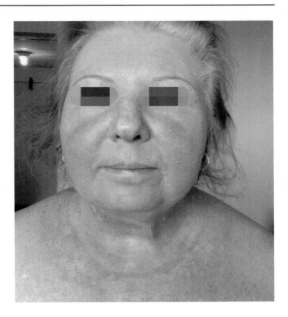

Fig. 43.6 Dermatomyositis. Heliotrope (periorbital erythema and swelling)

Clinical Presentation

The distinctive skin findings of dermatomyositis are periorbital erythema and swelling described as a heliotrope rash (Fig. 43.6). Redness and papules overlying the knuckles are called the papules of dermatomyositis (Gottron papules) and are often seen in conjunction with ragged cuticles, dilated nailfold capillaries, and cuticle hemorrhage (Fig. 43.7).

A less common hand finding is hyperkeratosis along the sides of the fingers and on the palms, sometimes with surrounding erythema known as mechanic's hands.

The finding of erythema, hypopigmentation and hyperpigmentation, and telangiectasia extending over the shoulders, in a V distribution of the neck and lateral thighs, is often described as poikiloderma associated with dermatomyositis (Fig. 43.8). Scale is often present, and the rash is difficult to distinguish from lupus or other papulosquamous disorders. Attention to the characteristic distribution and careful examination of the nailfolds is helpful in these cases. Scalp involvement with erythema, scale,

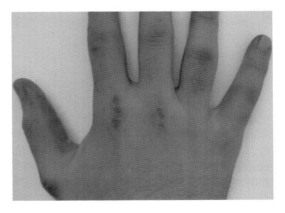

Fig. 43.7 Gottron papules. Erythematous papules overlying the knuckles

and often intense pruritus can persist even when other areas of skin involvement have come under control [53].

Conditions to be considered in the differential diagnosis of dermatomyositis are summarized in Table 43.6.

Complementary Examinations

Skin biopsy is not specific, but can support the diagnosis of dermatomyositis. It shows features

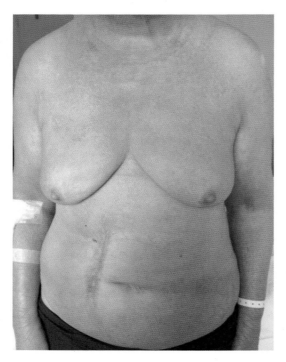

Fig. 43.8 Dermatomyositis. Poikiloderma

Table 43.6 Dermatomyositis: differential diagnosis

Lupus erythematosus
Graft-versus-host disease
Lichen myxedematosus
Lichen planus
Multicentric reticulohistiocytosis
Psoriasis
Parapsoriasis
Polymorphous light eruption
Rosacea
Tinea corporis
Sarcoidosis

similar to those of lupus, with interface dermatitis and perivascular lymphocytic inflammation. Along with strength testing, detection of increased muscle enzyme levels in serum can indicate muscle involvement. Levels of creatine kinase, lactate dehydrogenase, aldolase, aspartate aminotransferase, and alanine aminotransferase are all potentially increased in muscle disease, and checking several is reasonable. Although the complete evaluation of muscle disease is not discussed here, it is important to remember that once dermatomyositis has caused extensive

damage to the muscles and atrophy has occurred, the muscle enzyme levels may return to normal despite significant muscle disease.

A positive ANA test occurs in 80–90% of patients. In addition, multiple myositis autoantibodies can be detected, and increasing relevance and clinical implications are being recognized for these antibodies (Table 43.7) [54]. Clinically important antibodies include Mi-2, MDA5, anti-p155/140, and antisynthetase antibodies. Mi-2 is most specific for dermatomyositis but is not very sensitive. When present, it suggests treatment-responsive disease.

The constellation of rapidly progressive severe interstitial lung disease, myositis, arthritis (often mechanic's hands), and antisynthetase antibodies, sometimes with SSA antibodies, is referred to as the antisynthetase syndrome [55, 56]. Fever and Raynaud's phenomenon may be additional symptoms. There have been eight distinct antisynthetase antibodies detected, and more are likely be to be found in the future. Of these, anti-Jo-1 is the most common. In some cases, lung disease is the initial presenting symptom and other features are less prominent [57].

The presence of MDA5 antibodies is also associated with severe interstitial lung disease [58]. It is found in amyopathic forms of dermatomyositis and may be associated with punched-out-type ulcerations in the skin.

Overlaps exist between dermatomyositis and lupus, as well as systemic sclerosis. In these presentations, a variety of autoantibody patterns can be seen, including positive SSA, anti-RNP, anti-sm, and SCL.

An association between dermatomyositis and malignancy is well recognized. The clinical findings of dermatomyositis may precede, coincide with, or follow the cancer diagnosis. Recent analysis has suggested a five-fold greater occurrence of cancer in these patients than would normally be expected [59]. The malignancies most represented in the setting of dermatomyositis are hematopoietic and lung. A variety of other cancers are also noted to be over-represented, including ovary, colon, bladder, breast, cervix, pancreas, and esophagus [59, 60]. Cancer screening recommendations are not standardized. Consequently, appropriate clinical decision mak-

Table 43.7 Frequency of antibodies in dermatomyositis (DM) and clinical associations

Antibody	Frequency in DM (%)	Clinical association
Mi-2	20–30	Most specific antibody for DM. More responsive disease
MDA5	50	Associated with amyopathic DM. Increased ILD and skin ulcers; levels may decrease in response to therapy
P155/140	20–25 40–75, cancer-associated DM	Cancer-associated myositis, severe skin disease, high negative predictive value for malignancy
Antisynthetase (Jo-1 and others)	5–10	Antisynthetase syndrome high frequency of ILD and arthritis

ILD Interstitial lung disease

ing includes symptom-directed screening and the usual age-appropriate screening. It is reasonable to repeat the screening annually for 3 years, because this is when the risk of cancer-associated dermatomyositis tends to decrease. Because routine screening is not very effective for ovarian cancer, lung cancer, and pancreatic cancer, vaginal ultrasonography and a computed tomography scan of the chest, abdomen, and pelvis is ordered by some experts.

Therapeutic Approach

Although treatment algorithms do not exist for dermatomyositis, a common approach is to start oral prednisone at doses around 1 mg/kg/day for patients with evidence of muscle disease. This dose is tapered slowly, often over months. With long courses of steroids, side effects are a predicted complication. Concurrent addition of a steroid-sparing immunosuppressive drug may shorten the need for high-dose steroids and prevent steroid-associated side effects. Commonly used therapies are methotrexate (10–20 mg per week), mycophenolate (1,000–1,500 mg twice daily), or azathioprine. Often these can be started at the same time as prednisone. In cases resistant to standard therapy, intravenous immunoglobulin or rituximab are reasonable choices. For interstitial lung disease, a more aggressive treatment regimen is usually required.

Once therapy has been initiated it seems that exercise, both resistance and aerobic, may benefit patients with myositis. It is reasonable to recommend an exercise program after about 4 weeks of systemic treatment [61].

Skin disease in patients with dermatomyositis can be resistant, and attention to skin-specific treatments is important.

Photoprotection is recommended, with clothing and broad-spectrum sunscreen. Midpotency topical steroids and topical calcineurin inhibitors are also helpful for the rash and related itching.

Addition of hydroxychloroquine or chloroquine can benefit patients significantly.

In patients with amyopathic forms, escalation of therapy to other systemic agents, including methotrexate and mycophenolate, may be required to control symptoms [44].

Morphea

> **Key Points**
> - Morphea is an idiopathic inflammatory skin disease that causes skin hardening and in some cases loss of function
> - Although understanding of the pathophysiology is incomplete, it seems to share features with systemic sclerosis
> - Despite this common pathophysiology, morphea and systemic sclerosis are readily distinguished clinically and should be thought of separately
> - Morphea is largely confined to the skin and subcutaneous tissues, whereas systemic sclerosis is a multisystem disease

Introduction

Morphea, also known as localized scleroderma, is a disorder characterized by excessive collagen deposition leading to thickening of the dermis, subcutaneous tissues, or both. Morphea is classified into circumscribed, generalized, linear, and pansclerotic subtypes according to the clinical presentation and depth of tissue involvement [62]. Unlike systemic sclerosis, morphea lacks features such as sclerodactyly, Raynaud's phenomenon, nailfold capillary changes, telangiectasias, and progressive internal organ involvement. Morphea can present with extracutaneous manifestations, including fever, lymphadenopathy, arthralgias, fatigue, and central nervous system involvement, as well as laboratory abnormalities, including eosinophilia, polyclonal hypergammaglobulinemia, and positive ANA [62–65].

Although rare, epidemiologic studies suggest that 0.9–5.7% of patients with morphea progress to systemic sclerosis [64]. The transition may be marked by the development of Raynaud's phenomenon and nailfold capillary changes. However, these patients may have been initially misclassified on diagnosis.

General Epidemiology

The incidence of morphea has been estimated as approximately 0.4–2.7 per 100,000 people [66]. The actual incidence is likely higher because many cases may not come to medical attention. Two-thirds of adults with morphea present with plaque superficial circumscribed lesions, with generalized, linear, and deep variants each accounting for approximately 10% of cases. Up to half of all cases of morphea occur in pediatric patients. In this group, linear morphea predominates (two-thirds of cases), followed by the plaque superficial circumscribed (25%) and generalized (5%) subtypes. Of note, as many as half the patients with linear morphea have coexistent plaque-type lesions.

Although morphea occurs in persons of all races, it appears to be more common in whites, who represent 73–82% of patients seen [66].

Women are affected approximately three times as often as men for all forms of morphea except the linear subtype, which only has a slight female predominance.

Linear morphea commonly manifests in children and adolescents, with two-thirds of cases occurring before age 18 years. Other morphea subtypes have a peak incidence in the third and fourth decades of life.

Etiopathogenesis

The cause of morphea is unknown. An autoimmune mechanism is suggested by an increased frequency of autoantibody formation and a higher prevalence of personal and familial autoimmune disease in affected patients [65, 67]. Patients with generalized morphea are more likely to have a concomitant autoimmune disease, positive serology for autoantibodies, particularly ANA, and systemic symptoms [65]. To date, investigations have not described any consistent etiologic factors. Different morphea subtypes often coexist in the same patient, suggesting that the underlying processes are similar. The following are causes and associations.

Radiation therapy Morphea can occur at the site of previous radiation therapy for breast cancer and other malignancies, developing from 1 month to more than 20 years after irradiation [68, 69]. Involvement may extend beyond or distant to the irradiation field [66].

Infections, such as EBV infection, varicella, measles, hepatitis B, and borreliosis, have been reported to precede the onset of morphea and have been proposed as possible triggers [70].

Chimerism Immature chimeric cells have been found in morphea lesions, suggesting that such nonself cells may lead to an autoimmune phenotype [71].

Vaccinations Morphea-like lesions have also been reported to occur following vaccinations, including BCG, tetanus, and mumps-measles-rubella vaccinations. Whether the vaccinations themselves or the trauma from the injections was the inciting event is not clear.

Drug-induced morphea This is only rarely reported (i.e., from bisoprolol, bleomycin, D-penicillamine, L-5-hydroxytryptophan, balicatib) [66, 72].

Trauma Some morphea patients report a history of local trauma directly preceding the onset of disease. Plaques of circumscribed morphea often develop in areas of pressure. Reports of morphea lesions following vitamin B-12 and vitamin K injections suggests that trauma from injections may play a role [66].

Overproduction of collagen, particularly types I and III collagen, by fibroblasts in affected tissues is common to all forms of morphea, although the mechanism by which these fibroblasts are activated is unknown. Proposed factors involved in the pathogenesis of morphea include endothelial cell injury, immunologic (e.g., T-lymphocyte) and inflammatory activation, and dysregulation of collagen production. An autoimmune component is supported by the frequent presence of autoantibodies in affected individuals, as well as the association of morphea with other autoimmune diseases, including SLE, vitiligo, type 1 diabetes, and autoimmune thyroiditis [63, 65].

Endothelial cell injury is currently thought to be the inciting event in the pathogenesis of morphea. This injury results in increased levels of adhesion molecules (circulating intercellular adhesion molecule 1, vascular cell adhesion molecule 1, and E-selectin) and fibrogenic Th2 cytokines such as IL-4, IL-6, and TGF-β. These cytokines recruit eosinophils, CD4+ T cells, and macrophages, which are present in early morphea lesions and in eosinophilic fasciitis. These cytokines and growth factors also increase fibroblast proliferation and induce synthesis of excess collagen and connective-tissue growth factor. TGF-β also decreases production of proteases, inhibiting collagen breakdown [66].

Connective-tissue growth factor is a soluble mediator that enhances and perpetuates the profibrotic effects of TGF-β. The ultimate result of the endothelial injury and inflammatory cascade is increased collagen and extracellular matrix deposition [73–76]. Other proposed pathophysiologic mechanisms in morphea include the formation of anti-matrix metalloproteinase antibodies, as well as increased expression of insulin-like growth factor, which enhances collagen production [77, 78].

Clinical Presentation

The onset of symptoms in morphea may be insidious, and studies have shown a delay in diagnosis of a year or longer [79]. Patients may describe arthralgias, myalgias, and fatigue occurring along with morphea but the systemic symptoms of gastrointestinal reflux, pulmonary symptoms, and cardiac symptoms seen in systemic sclerosis are not characteristic of morphea [80].

In addition to the skin findings, there are some special clinical considerations in patients with morphea. Morphea that involves the scalp or occurs around the eyes can be associated with symptoms of uveitis, headaches, or seizures [81, 82]. Several reports show a strong association between morphea and genital lichen sclerosis. Frank discussion with patients about genital symptoms, including skin changes, itching, or burning, should be included in the history because patients may be reluctant to volunteer these concerns [83].

The course of morphea is one of remission and relapse [84]. Ongoing monitoring is helpful to treat relapses early and avoid additional disability.

Plaque morphea Several distinct patterns of morphea occur on the skin. Plaque-type morphea is the most common. The earliest lesions are often erythematous plaques with little induration; sometimes a lilac border is observed at the periphery of the lesion (Fig. 43.9). This condition progresses to central sclerosis with induration and smooth yellow to white scarring. There is often peripheral erythema or hyperpigmentation. Over time, destruction of the hair and sweat glands occurs in the affected skin. The plaques can increase in size and number. Involvement in the inframammary

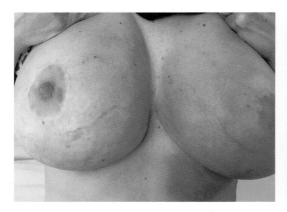

Fig. 43.9 Plaque morphea. Erythematous plaques with induration on mammary area

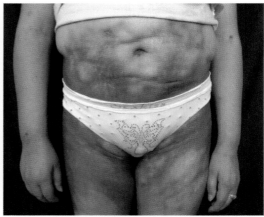

Fig. 43.10 Pansclerotic morphea. Multiple hyperpigmented, atrophic plaques

area, the area around the hips, and on the lower back together as a pattern is common.

Generalized plaque morphea When the plaques are greater than 3 cm in size and there are more than four plaques involving two body areas, it is classified as generalized plaque morphea. Patients can have superficial or deep involvement in the skin.

Pansclerotic morphea In rare patients the course is rapid and progressive with multiple enlarging plaques that eventually result in widespread involvement of almost the entire skin, except for sparing of the hands and feet (Fig. 43.10). This presentation is referred to as pansclerotic and requires aggressive treatment.

Linear morphea The linear subtype of morphea occurs most commonly in children. In this type plaques develop in a linear pattern, eventually coalescing into a single band of scarring that can extend the length of a limb. When it crosses joints it can cause loss of mobility because of scarring. Linear morphea often involves deeper structures, including muscle and bone. When it involves the scalp and forehead it has been referred to as *en coup de sabre* (Fig. 43.11).

Patients often have a mixed presentation with both linear and plaque types. Several less common forms of morphea have been reported,

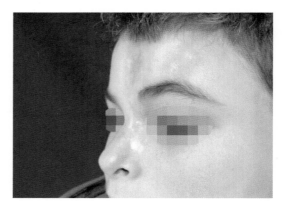

Fig. 43.11 Linear morphea. Band of scarring on the forehead (en coup de sabre)

including superficial morphea [85], guttate morphea, bullous morphea [86], and keloidal morphea [87, 88].

The diagnosis of morphea is made based on history and clinical examination of the skin. Differentiating from systemic sclerosis is an important first consideration. In contrast to systemic sclerosis, which begins with sclerodactyly, morphea usually does not involve the hands. Raynaud's phenomenon is characteristic of systemic sclerosis and is absent in morphea. Nailfold and serologic findings of systemic sclerosis are not present in morphea. Examination of the genital skin is recommended to detect asymptomatic lichen sclerosus and to direct treatment if present.

The most likely clinical differential diagnoses to consider are eosinophilic fasciitis, lipodermatosclerosis, graft-versus-host disease, and nephrogenic systemic fibrosis (Table 43.8).

Complementary Examinations

Skin biopsy shows an inflammatory pattern of lymphocytes and plasma cells in the dermis and subcutis, and in late lesions thickened collagen bundles are present. The histologic findings may be indistinguishable from those of systemic sclerosis.

Table 43.8 Clinical differential diagnosis of morphea

Systemic sclerosis
Eosinophilic fasciitis
Lichen sclerosus
Lipodermatosclerosis
Graft-versus-host-disease
Nephrogenic systemic sclerosis
Panniculitis
Chemical-induced skin hardening (taxane-induced scleroderma, silicone implant/injection complication, toxic oil syndrome)
Scleredema
Scleromyxedema
Myxedema
Dermatofibrosarcoma protuberans
Cutaneous T-cell lymphoma
Radiation-related skin changes
Carcinoma en cuirasse
Porphyria cutanea tarda

There are no specific laboratory tests to confirm the diagnosis of morphea. Patients with morphea, especially the linear and deep subtypes, often have a positive ANA test. The clinical utility of this test is yet to be determined, and routine testing is not clinically useful.

Therapeutic Approach

For patients with early and limited skin involvement, topical therapy with high-potency steroids, topical calcineurin inhibitors, or calcipotriene is recommended. Patients with continued progression or generalized disease should be treated with either phototherapy (narrowband UVB, broadband UVA, or UVA1) or systemic treatment with either methotrexate or methotrexate combined with pulsed-dose steroids (1 g of Solu-Medrol intravenously daily for 3 consecutive days, repeated monthly for 3–6 months). Systemic therapy should be considered for linear morphea, which often is more aggressive and disabling. An alternative to methotrexate is mycophenolate using doses of 1,000–1,500 mg twice daily [89].

Treatment of morphea is summarized in Table 43.9 [90].

Further progression after a period of quiescence is encountered. Treatment should be restarted in these cases. If the clinical findings are not clear and comparison photographs are not available, a skin biopsy may be helpful. The finding of inflamma-

Table 43.9 Treatment algorithm for morphea

Limited plaque morphea	Generalized morphea (without joint contractures)	Linear morphea (involving the face or crossing joints)
▼ Topical steroids (inflammatory phase)	▼ Phototherapy (NB-UVB, UVA, UVA1)	▼ Methotrexate and systemic steroids
▼ If no response after 4–8 weeks	▼ If no response after 4–8 weeks	▼ If no response after 8 weeks
Topical tacrolimus	Methotrexate and systemic steroids	Phototherapy (UVA, UVA1, NB-UVB)
▼ If no response after 4–8 weeks	▼ If no response after 8 weeks	▼ If no response after 8 weeks
Calcipotriol and betamethasone dipropionate or Topical imiquimod or NB-UVB, UVA, UVA1	Change to mycophenolate mofetil	Change to mycophenolate mofetil

NB narrowband

tion on the biopsy suggests clinical activity and may be compelling to restart therapy.

References

1. Ingvarsson RF, Bengtsson AA, Jönsen A. Variations in the epidemiology of systemic lupus erythematosus in southern Sweden. Lupus. 2016;25(7):772–80.
2. Andersen LK, Davis MD. Sex differences in the incidence of skin and skin-related diseases in Olmsted County, Minnesota, United States, and a comparison with other rates published worldwide. Int J Dermatol. 2016;55(9):939–55.
3. Fortuna G, Brennan MT. Systemic lupus erythematosus: epidemiology, pathophysiology, manifestations, and management. Dent Clin N Am. 2013;57(4):631–55.
4. Jarrett P, Thornley S, Scragg R. Ethnic differences in the epidemiology of cutaneous lupus erythematosus in New Zealand. Lupus. 2016;25(13):1497–502.
5. Andersen LK, Davis MD. Prevalence of skin and skin-related diseases in the rochester epidemiology project and a comparison with other published prevalence studies. Dermatology. 2016;232:344–52.
6. Borchers AT, Naguwa SM, Shoenfeld Y, Gershwin ME. The geoepidemiology of systemic lupus erythematosus. Autoimmun Rev. 2010;9(5):A277–87.
7. Pons-Estel GJ, Alarcón GS, Scofield L, Reinlib L, Cooper GS. Understanding the epidemiology and progression of systemic lupus erythematosus. Semin Arthritis Rheum. 2010;39(4):257–68.
8. Gilliam JN, Sontheimer RD. Distinctive cutaneous subsets in the spectrum of lupus erythematosus. J Am Acad Dermatol. 1981;4(4):471–5.
9. Achtman JC, Werth VP. Pathophysiology of cutaneous lupus erythematosus. Arthritis Res Ther. 2015;17:182.
10. Squatrito D, Emmi G, Silvestri E, Ciucciarelli L, D'Elios MM, Prisco D, et al. Pathogenesis and potential therapeutic targets in systemic lupus erythematosus: from bench to bedside. Auto Immun Highlights. 2014;5(2):33–45.
11. Choi J, Kim ST, Craft J. The pathogenesis of systemic lupus erythematosus-an update. Curr Opin Immunol. 2012;24(6):651–7.
12. Sullivan KE. Genetics of systemic lupus erythematosus. Clinical implications. Rheum Dis Clin N Am. 2000;26(2):229–56. v-vi
13. Kirchhof MG, Dutz JP. The immunopathology of cutaneous lupus erythematosus. Rheum Dis Clin N Am. 2014;40(3):455–74. viii
14. Crow MK. Developments in the clinical understanding of lupus. Arthritis Res Ther. 2009;11(5):245.
15. Oke V, Wahren-Herlenius M. Cutaneous lupus erythematosus: clinical aspects and molecular pathogenesis. J Intern Med. 2013;273(6):544–54.
16. Cusack C, Danby C, Fallon JC, Ho WL, Murray B, Brady J, et al. Photoprotective behaviour and sunscreen use: impact on vitamin D levels in cutaneous lupus erythematosus. Photodermatol Photoimmunol Photomed. 2008;24(5):260–7.
17. Orteu CH, Sontheimer RD, Dutz JP. The pathophysiology of photosensitivity in lupus erythematosus. Photodermatol Photoimmunol Photomed. 2001;17(3):95–113.
18. Eyanson S, Greist MC, Brandt KD, Skinner B. Systemic lupus erythematosus: association with psoralen – ultraviolet-A treatment of psoriasis. Arch Dermatol. 1979;115(1):54–6.
19. Rigante D, Esposito S. Infections and systemic lupus erythematosus: binding or sparring partners? Int J Mol Sci. 2015;16(8):17331–43.
20. Esposito S, Bosis S, Semino M, Rigante D. Infections and systemic lupus erythematosus. Eur J Clin Microbiol Infect Dis. 2014;33(9):1467–75.
21. Nelson P, Rylance P, Roden D, Trela M, Tugnet N. Viruses as potential pathogenic agents in systemic lupus erythematosus. Lupus. 2014;23(6):596–605.
22. SongnuanBoonsoongnern P, Faisaikarm T, Sangsuwan P, Weerachatyanukul W, Kitiyanant Y. A role of oestrogen in aggravating SLE-like syndrome in C4-deficient mice. Asian Pac J Allergy Immunol. 2015;33(4):339–48.
23. Lateef A, Petri M. Hormone replacement and contraceptive therapy in autoimmune diseases. J Autoimmun. 2012;38(2–3):J170–6.
24. Guettrot-Imbert G, Morel N, Le Guern V, Plu-Bureau G, Frances C, Costedoat-Chalumeau N. Pregnancy and contraception in systemic and cutaneous lupus erythematosus. Ann Dermatol Venereol. 2016;45:1084–92.
25. Pretel M, Marquès L, España A. Drug-induced lupus erythematosus. Actas Dermosifiliogr. 2014;105(1):18–30.
26. Favalli EG, Sinigaglia L, Varenna M, Arnoldi C. Drug-induced lupus following treatment with infliximab in rheumatoid arthritis. Lupus. 2002;11(11):753–5.
27. Zhang N, Leng XM, Tian XP, Zhao Y, Zeng XF. Clinical analysis of 6 patients with drug-induced lupus. Zhonghua Nei Ke Za Zhi. 2016;55(3):211–5.
28. Privette ED, Werth VP. Update on pathogenesis and treatment of CLE. Curr Opin Rheumatol. 2013;25(5):584–90.
29. Sáenz-Corral CI, Vega-Memíje ME, Martínez-Luna E, Cuevas-González JC, Rodríguez-Carreón AA, de la Rosa JJ, et al. Apoptosis in chronic cutaneous lupus erythematosus, discoid lupus, and lupus profundus. Int J Clin Exp Pathol. 2015;8(6):7260–5.
30. Yu C, Chang C, Zhang J. Immunologic and genetic considerations of cutaneous lupus erythematosus: a comprehensive review. J Autoimmun. 2013;41:34–45.
31. Moura Filho JP, Peixoto RL, Martins LG, Melo SD, Carvalho LL, Pereira AK, et al. Lupus erythematosus: considerations about clinical, cutaneous and therapeutic aspects. An Bras Dermatol. 2014;89(1):118–25.
32. Kuhn A, Bein D, Bonsmann G. The 100th anniversary of lupus erythematosus tumidus. Autoimmun Rev. 2009;8(6):441–8.

33. Grönhagen CM, Nyberg F. Cutaneous lupus erythematosus: an update. Indian Dermatol Online J. 2014;5(1):7–13.

34. Lee L, Werth V. Lupus erythematous. In: Bolognia JL, Jorizzo JL, Schaffer JV, editors. Dermatology. 2, 3 ed. Rio de Janeiro: Elsevier; 2015. p. 615–29.

35. Crowson AN, Magro CM. Cutaneous histopathology of lupus erythematosus. Diag Histopathol. 2009;15(4):157–85.

36. Baltaci M, Fritsch P. Histologic features of cutaneous lupus erythematosus. Autoimmun Rev. 2009;8(6):467–73.

37. Schultz HY, Dutz JP, Furukawa F, Goodfield MJ, Kuhn A, Lee LA, et al. From pathogenesis, epidemiology, and genetics to definitions, diagnosis, and treatments of cutaneous lupus erythematosus and dermatomyositis: a report from the 3rd International Conference on Cutaneous Lupus Erythematosus (ICCLE) 2013. J Invest Dermatol. 2015;135(1):7–12.

38. Kreuter A, Lehmann P. Relevant new insights into the effects of photoprotection in cutaneous lupus erythematosus. Exp Dermatol. 2014;23(10):712–3.

39. Gordon Spratt EA, Gorcey LV, Soter NA, Brauer JA. Phototherapy, photodynamic therapy and photophoresis in the treatment of connective-tissue diseases: a review. Br J Dermatol. 2015;173(1):19–30.

40. Terrier B, Derian N, Schoindre Y, Chaara W, Geri G, Zahr N, et al. Restoration of regulatory and effector T cell balance and B cell homeostasis in systemic lupus erythematosus patients through vitamin D supplementation. Arthritis Res Ther. 2012;14(5):R221.

41. Böckle BC, Sepp NT. Smoking is highly associated with discoid lupus erythematosus and lupus erythematosus tumidus: analysis of 405 patients. Lupus. 2015;24(7):669–74.

42. Chasset F, Francès C, Barete S, Amoura Z, Arnaud L. Influence of smoking on the efficacy of antimalarials in cutaneous lupus: a meta-analysis of the literature. J Am Acad Dermatol. 2015;72(4):634–9.

43. Callen JP. Dermatomyositis Lancet. 2000 Jan 1;355(9197):53–7.

44. Callen JP, Wortmann RL. Dermatomyositis. Clin Dermatol. 2006 Sep-Oct;24(5):363–73.

45. Bendewald MJ, Wetter DA, Li X, Davis MD. Incidence of dermatomyositis and clinically amyopathic dermatomyositis: a population-based study in Olmsted County. Minnesota Arch Dermatol. 2010 Jan;146(1):26–30.

46. Werth VP, Callen JP, Ang G, Sullivan KE. Associations of tumor necrosis factor alpha and HLA polymorphisms with adult dermatomyositis: implications for a unique pathogenesis. J Invest Dermatol. 2002 Sep;119(3):617–20.

47. Pachman LM, Veis A, Stock S, et al. Composition of calcifications in children with juvenile dermatomyositis: association with chronic cutaneous inflammation. Arthritis Rheum. 2006 Oct;54(10):3345–50.

48. Lutz J, Huwiler KG, Fedczyna T, et al. Increased plasma thrombospondin-1 (TSP-1) levels are associated with the TNF alpha-308A allele in children with juvenile dermatomyositis. Clin Immunol. 2002 Jun;103(3 Pt 1):260–3.

49. Chen S, Wang Q, Wu Z, Wu Q, Li P, Li Y, et al. Associations between TNF-a-308A/G polymorphism and susceptibility with dermatomyositis: a meta-analysis. PLoS One. 2014;9(8):e102841.

50. Daoud MS, Gibson LE, Pittelkow MR. Hydroxyurea dermopathy: a unique lichenoid eruption complicating long-term therapy with hydroxyurea. J Am Acad Dermatol. 1997 Feb;36(2 Pt 1):178–82.

51. Noël B. Lupus erythematosus and other autoimmune diseases related to statin therapy: a systematic review. J Eur Acad Dermatol Venereol. 2007 Jan;21(1):17–24.

52. O'Hanlon T, Koneru B, Bayat E, Love L, Targoff I, Malley J, et al. Immunogenetic differences between Caucasian women with and those without silicone implants in whom myositis develops. Arthritis Rheum. 2004 Nov;50(11):3646–50.

53. Kalus A. Rheumatologic skin disease. Med Clin N Am. 2015;99:1287–303.

54. Iaccarino L, Ghirardello A, Bettio S, et al. The clinical features, diagnosis and classification of dermatomyositis. J Autoimmun. 2014;48–49:122–7.

55. Katzap E, Barilla-LaBarca ML, Marder G. Antisynthetase syndrome. Curr Rheumatol Rep. 2011;13(3):175–81.

56. Uribe L, Ronderos DM, Diaz MC, et al. Antisynthetase antibody syndrome: case report and review of the literature. Clin Rheumatol. 2013;32(5):715–9.

57. Hallowell RW, Danoff SK. Interstitial lung disease associated with the idiopathic inflammatory myopathies and the antisynthetase syndrome: recent advances. Curr Opin Rheumatol. 2014;26(6):684–9.

58. Koichi Y, Aya Y, Megumi U, et al. A case of anti-MDA5-positive rapidly progressive interstitial lung disease in a patient with clinically amyopathic dermatomyositis ameliorated by rituximab, in addition to standard immunosuppressive treatment. Mod Rheumatol. 2015;12:1–5.

59. Yang Z, Lin F, Qin B, et al. Polymyositis/dermatomyositis and malignancy risk: a metaanalysis study. J Rheumatol. 2015;42(2):282–91.

60. Olazagasti JM, Baez PJ, Wetter DA, et al. Cancer risk in dermatomyositis: a meta-analysis of cohort studies. Am J Clin Dermatol. 2015;16(2):89–98.

61. Alemo Munters L, Alexanderson H, Crofford LJ, et al. New insights into the benefits of exercise for muscle health in patients with idiopathic inflammatory myositis. Curr Rheumatol Rep. 2014;16(7):429.

62. Laxer RM, Zulian F. Localized scleroderma. Curr Opin Rheumatol. 2006 Nov;18(6):606–13.

63. Zulian F. Systemic manifestations in localized scleroderma. Curr Rheumatol Rep. 2004 Dec;6(6):417–24.

64. Chung L, Lin J, Furst DE, Fiorentino D. Systemic and localized scleroderma. Clin Dermatol. 2006 Sep-Oct;24(5):374–92.

65. Leitenberger JJ, Cayce RL, Haley RW, Adams-Huet B, Bergstresser PR, Jacobe HT. Distinct autoimmune syndromes in morphea: a review of 245 adult and pediatric cases. Arch Dermatol. 2009 May;145(5):545–50.

66. Fett N, Werth VP. Update on morphea: part I. Epidemiology, clinical presentation, and pathogenesis. J Am Acad Dermatol. 2011;64(2):217–28. quiz 229–30.

67. Prinz JC, Kutasi Z, Weisenseel P, Poto L, Battyani Z, Ruzicka T. "Borrelia-associated early-onset morphea": a particular type of scleroderma in childhood and adolescence with high titer antinuclear antibodies? Results of a cohort analysis and presentation of three cases. J Am Acad Dermatol. 2009;60(2):248–55.

68. Kreft B, Wohlrab J, Radant K, Danz B, Marsch WC, Fiedler E. Unrecognized radiation-induced localized scleroderma: a cause of postoperative wound-healing disorder. Clin Exp Dermatol. 2009 Oct;34(7):e383–4.

69. Laetsch B, Hofer T, Lombriser N, Lautenschlager S. Irradiation-induced morphea: x-rays as triggers of autoimmunity. Dermatology. 2011;223(1):9–12.

70. Eisendle K, Grabner T, Zelger B. Morphoea: a manifestation of infection with Borrelia species? Br J Dermatol. 2007 Dec;157(6):1189–98.

71. Zulian F. New developments in localized scleroderma. Curr Opin Rheumatol. 2008 Sep;20(5):601–7.

72. Peroni A, Zini A, Braga V, Colato C, Adami S, Girolomoni G. Drug-induced morphea: report of a case induced by balicatib and review of the literature. J Am Acad Dermatol. 2008 Jul;59(1):125–9.

73. Igarashi A, Nashiro K, Kikuchi K, et al. Connective tissue growth factor gene expression in tissue sections from localized scleroderma, keloid, and other fibrotic skin disorders. J Invest Dermatol. 1996 Apr;106(4):729–33.

74. Kikuchi K, Kadono T, Ihn H, et al. Growth regulation in scleroderma fibroblasts: increased response to transforming growth factor-beta 1. J Invest Dermatol. 1995 Jul;105(1):128–32.

75. Leask A, Denton CP, Abraham DJ. Insights into the molecular mechanism of chronic fibrosis: the role of connective tissue growth factor in scleroderma. J Invest Dermatol. 2004 Jan;122(1):1–6.

76. Yamane K, Ihn H, Kubo M, et al. Increased serum levels of soluble vascular cell adhesion molecule 1 and E-selectin in patients with localized scleroderma. J Am Acad Dermatol. 2000 Jan;42(1 Pt 1):64–9.

77. Fawzi MM, Tawfik SO, Eissa AM, El-Komy MH, Abdel-Halim MR, Shaker OG. Expression of insulin-like growth factor-I in lesional and nonlesional skin of patients with morphoea. Br J Dermatol. 2008 Jul;159(1):86–90.

78. Tomimura S, Ogawa F, Iwata Y, Komura K, Hara T, Muroi E. Autoantibodies against matrix metallo-proteinase-1 in patients with localized scleroderma. J Dermatol Sci. 2008 Oct;52(1):47–54.

79. Johnson W, Jacobe H. Morphea in adults and children cohort II: patients with morphea experience delay in diagnosis and large variation in treatment. J Am Acad Dermatol. 2012;67(5):881–9.

80. Nouri S, Jacobe H. Recent developments in diagnosis and assessment of morphea. Curr Rheumatol Rep. 2013;15(2):308.

81. Chiu YE, Vora S, Kwon EK, et al. A significant proportion of children with morphea en coup de sabre and Parry-Romberg syndrome have neuroimaging findings. Pediatr Dermatol. 2012;29(6):738–48.

82. Polcari I, Moon A, Mathes EF, et al. Headaches as a presenting symptom of linear morphea en coup de sabre. Pediatrics. 2014;134(6):1715–9.

83. Lis-Swiety A, Mierzwinska K, Wodok-Wieczorek K, et al. Coexistence of lichen sclerosus and localized scleroderma in female monozygotic twins. J Pediatr Adolesc Gynecol. 2014;27(6):e133–6.

84. Saxton-Daniels S, Jacobe HT. An evaluation of long-term outcomes in adults with pediatric-onset morphea. Arch Dermatol. 2010;146(9):1044–5.

85. McNiff JM, Glusac EJ, Lazova RZ, et al. Morphea limited to the superficial reticular dermis: an underrecognized histologic phenomenon. Am J Dermatopathol. 1999;21(4):315–9.

86. Fernandez-Flores A, Gatica-Torres M, TinocoFragoso F, et al. Three cases of bullous morphea: histopathologic findings with implications regarding pathogenesis. J Cutan Pathol. 2015;42(2):144–9.

87. Chiu HY, Tsai TF. Images in clinical medicine. Keloidal morphea. N Engl J Med. 2011;364(14):e28.

88. Wriston CC, Rubin AI, Elenitsas R, et al. Nodular scleroderma: a report of 2 cases. Am J Dermatopathol. 2008;30(4):385–8.

89. Fett N, Werth VP. Update on morphea: part II. Outcome measures and treatment. J Am Acad Dermatol. 2011;64(2):231–42. [quiz: 243–4].

90. Careta MF, Romiti R. Esclerodermia localizada: espectro clínico e atualização terapêutica. An Bras Dermatol. 2015;90(1):61–72.

Dermatologic Manifestations in Renal Failure

Lídice Dufrechou Varela, Alejandra Larre Borges, and Andrea Nicola Centanni

Key Points

- The three most common kidney diseases that lead to end-stage of chronic renal failure (CRF) are:
- Vascular nephropathy
- Obstructive nephropathy
- Diabetic nephropathy

  Of note, the latter is the main cause of CRF in American and Spanish populations [1]

- Most skin disorders are seen in patients undergoing HD, probably owing to the fact that it is the most frequently used renal replacement therapy worldwide [2]
- Skin disorders in chronic renal failure are benign, but almost all of them show a significant impact on the quality of life of affected patients [3, 4]
- The prevalence of dermatoses in chronic renal failure is close to 100% [5–7]

L.D. Varela (✉)
Assistant Professor of Dermatology, Hospital de Clínicas "Dr. Manuel Quintela", de Montevideo, Uruguay
e-mail: ldufrechou@gmail.com

A.L. Borges
Adjunct Professor of Dermatology, Hospital de Clínicas "Dr. Manuel Quintela", de Montevideo, Uruguay

A.N. Centanni
Hospital de Clínicas "Dr. Manuel Quintela", Montevideo, Uruguay

Introduction

Chronic renal failure (CRF) is a major public health problem worldwide [3]. (It is defined as an abnormality in renal structure or function, with health implications present for at least 3 months. It is classified according to three variables: glomerular filtration rate (GFR), its etiology, and the amount of albuminuria [8].

Administration of kidney replacement therapy is based on the GFR. Patients with GFR less than 15 mL/min should be admitted to a replacement kidney function plan with any of the existing methods [8]. Replacement of renal function is currently performed by three modalities: hemodialysis (HD), peritoneal dialysis (PD), and renal transplant. Most skin disorders are seen in patients undergoing HD, probably because it is the most frequently used renal replacement therapy worldwide since it has been proved to prolong the life expectancy of patients with CRF [2].

The three most common kidney diseases that lead to end-stage CRF are vascular nephropathy, obstructive nephropathy, and diabetic nephropathy. The latter is the main cause in American and Spanish populations [1].

Of note, this chapter does not discuss dermatologic conditions that are common after transplantation in immunosuppressed patients; this information is available in another chapter.

These patients are considered to have a chronic inflammatory status caused by multiple factors, some of which include the underlying disease, a

© Springer International Publishing Switzerland 2018
R.R. Bonamigo, S.I.T. Dornelles (eds.), *Dermatology in Public Health Environments*,
https://doi.org/10.1007/978-3-319-33919-1_44

permanent fistula or catheter, the membranes used for HD or PD, and the drugs and supplements that they receive [9].

From a dermatologic point of view, there is a high frequency of dermatoses associated with this condition. They can be divided as specific and nonspecific, the latter having the highest prevalence, but all of them showing a significant impact on patients quality of life [3].

Skin changes reported in patients with CRF are diverse [3]. Most skin disorders are benign and do not affect the course of CRF [4]. Sometimes skin disorders can predict the initiation of a renal replacement plan, or may be precipitated by it [3, 4].

Epidemiology

Few worldwide publications describe the prevalence and characteristics of skin alterations observed in patients with CRF and in patients receiving HD. Pico et al. (1992) registered a 100% prevalence of skin lesions in patients with CFR while Bencini et al. (1998) reported 79% prevalence [5–7]. In accordance with these studies, Udayakamur et al. (2006) conducted a study of dermatoses in 100 patients receiving HD, for which the prevalence was 82% [5, 6]. We recently conducted a study in Uruguay about the prevalence of dermatoses in 200 patients in HD, which found a prevalence of 98%.

Multiple factors are described to explain the greatest amount of dermatoses affecting patients with CRF, and these are briefly mentioned in Chart 44.1.

Practically, skin changes in CRF are classified into four groups depending on the relationship with the renal disease or the renal treatment, as described in Chart 44.2.

Cutaneous Manifestations of Chronic Renal Failures

From a dermatologic point of view, a high frequency of dermatoses and skin lesions are associated with this condition. For practical

Chart 44.1 Multiple factors described to explain the greatest amount of dermatoses affecting patients with CRF

Factors described to explain the dermatoses affecting patients with chronic renal failure
Skin dehydration (specially epithelial) with malfunction of the eccrine sweat glands [5, 8]
Dysregulation of calcium and phosphorus metabolism [6]
Chronic systemic proinflammatory condition; for patients receiving hemodialysis, postulating the permanent fistula or catheter as a possible active element [4, 6]
Type of hemodialysis membrane used, which is a questionable concept [9]
Urochrome skin storage [4, 11]
Hypovitaminosis D [5, 8]
Hypervitaminosis A [5, 8]
In hemodialysis patients, higher amount of melanocyte-stimulating hormone β because of poor excretion via hemodialysis [12, 13]
Accelerated erythropoiesis [3, 8]
Altered hemostasis, among other factors mostly by high concentration of urea [10, 11]
Heparin use [10, 11]
Protein malnutrition [5, 10]
Altered cellular immunity [5, 14]
Iron deficiency [3, 8]

Chart 44.2 Classification of skin changes in chronic renal failure according to the relationship with the renal disease or the renal treatment [10]

Causes of skin changes in chronic renal failure
The disease itself that is generating the kidney malfunction
Kidney disease itself
Established treatment
Drugs that the patients receive

purposes, these dermatoses can be grouped into nonspecific (with higher prevalence) and specific. All of them have a significant impact on patients' quality of life [9, 14].

Nonspecific dermatoses are listed in Chart 44.3 and the specific dermatoses are in Chart 44.4.

Besides the aforementioned, there exist iatrogenic dermatoses caused by treatment and adverse drug reactions [6, 10].

Xerosis, bruising, and itching are ubiquitous in this population and are considered multifactorial xerosis, pale skin, and itching were the most prevalent findings according to an Indian study

Chart 44.3 Dermatoses grouped as "nonspecific" in chronic renal failure [8, 9, 14]

Nonspecific dermatoses in chronic renal failure
Xerosis
Pruritus
Dyschromia
Ecchymosis
Gynecomastia
Cutaneous infections
Skin cancer
Mucosal alterations
Faneral disorders

Chart 44.4 Dermatoses grouped as "specific" in chronic renal failures [4, 8–10, 14]

Specific dermatoses in chronic renal failures
Acquired perforating dermatoses (APD)
Bullous dermatoses
Calcification disorders
Nephrogenic systemic fibrosis (NSF)
Specific nail changes
Uremic frost

conducted in 99 patients [4, 10, 14]. This correlates with our findings according to a Uruguayan study, conducted in 2015, of dermatoses in 200 patients receiving HD.

Nonspecific Cutaneous Entities with Higher Prevalence in Patients with Chronic Renal Failure

This grouping mechanism is currently considered controversial since these skin changes could be either coincidental or associated with factors other than CRF, such as the etiologic condition causing renal failure [12].

Xerosis

Xerosis, or dry skin, is a common skin disorder described as the most common skin disorder found among patients with CRF, especially in patients receiving regular HD [4, 9, 10]. It is characterized clinically by rough, scaly, and often itchy skin [2]. A frequency between 50% and 70% in patients undergoing HD is reported [4–6, 8, 10, 11].

Pruritus

Pruritus is one of the most distinctive and troublesome symptoms among patients with CRF, but seems to be absent in patients with acute renal disease [5, 6, 8, 10]. A prevalence rate of 50% has been found in different studies [5, 8–10]. Pruritus has been associated with the degree of renal impairment of the patient and is considered an inflammatory systemic disease rather than a skin disorder per se [5, 9, 15]. It may be accompanied by xerosis but there is no direct correlation between these two entities [15].

The prevalence in patients undergoing HD is between 58% and 90% [5, 11, 15, 16].

Various publications describe that severe pruritus improves after HD, others report no improvement, while some describe patients who report its aggravation after starting HD [5, 9, 10, 16]. Pruritus seems to be more severe in patients with diabetes mellitus (DM) [5, 6].

Dyschromia

Two types of pigmentary changes are described: diffuse hyperpigmentation and citrine yellowish tint [5, 6].

Thomas et al. reported that dyschromia occurs in 32% of HD patients while others refer to prevalence between 25% and 75%, this percentage being higher in patients on maintained HD [10]. In our experience, the prevalence was 31.2% in the 200 patients receiving HD studied.

Diffuse hyperpigmentation is a relatively common early sign and is located in sun-exposed areas [14, 15].

Pallor is observed more frequently in patients receiving sustained HD, with an incidence from 40% to 60% reported. It is difficult to quantify and is defined as an unusual lightness of skin color when compared with normal hue [16], it is attributed to chronic anemia and dysfunctional erythropoiesis [3, 8, 12, 13]. For some authors, pallor is a hallmark in patients with CRF and adds significant morbidity. It correlates with the hemoglobin level, presenting higher incidence in patients with levels lower than 8 g% [6].

Ecchymosis

Ecchymosis prevalence varies from 10% to 60% [5, 10, 11]. It is clinically observed as a subcutaneous lesion characterized by deposits of extravasated blood [16].

Gynecomastia

Gynecomastia has a reported prevalence of 40% in patients undergoing HD [5]. The development of this clinical sign seems to occur 1 or 2 months after starting HD, and spontaneous regression is seen in most cases within a year [17].

Cutaneous Infections

A prospective Indian study of patients undergoing HD reported a prevalence of 26.26% of bacterial, viral, fungal, and parasitic infections, bacterial ones being the most common among diabetic patients [5, 10, 15].

The most common are the fungal infections such as tinea versicolor and onychomycosis; the latter also most prevalent in patients with DM [5, 6]. In Nigeria a high prevalence of tinea versicolor is reported, the predominant location being upper extremities and not in the "classic" areas where sebum production is increased [11].

The most prevalent viral infections reported are warts, herpes simplex, and herpes zoster (VHZ), although in some studies no statistically significant differences were found compared with the general population [5, 7]. Herpes reactivation has been reported more frequently in this population, and supplements with vitamin D and iron have been linked to a lower incidence [18].

Skin Cancer

Immunosuppression in these patients would predispose to higher prevalence of skin cancer, basal cell carcinoma (BCC being) the most frequently reported, although its prevalence has not been compared with that in the general population [5]. In our recent experience the prevalence of BCC and squamous cell carcinoma (SCC) was similar (4% and 4.5%, respectively). One partial possible explanation for the increase in SCC in this study is the fact that we conducted our study in Uruguay, where population is predominantly Caucasian with a high degree of sun exposure as a result of the latitude and social behavior regarding tanning habits. However, in the Uruguayan population BCC is more frequent than SCC. This would favor skin carcinogenesis in susceptible individuals with low phototypes [19]. This study shows that the relationship between the prevalence of BCC and SCC in the HD population would resemble what happens in renal transplant patients in whom the BCC/SCC ratio is reversed [20] (see Box 44.1).

> **Box 44.1 BCC and SCC in the HD Population of Uruguay [19]**
> The authors conducted a study in 2015 about the prevalence of dermatoses in 200 patients receiving hemodialysis. This study allowed the diagnosis of melanoma in two patients, one of them with Breslow thickness of 0.73 mm and the other of 1.3 mm. The reported incidence in Uruguay, where the study was conducted, is 5.2 cases per 100,000 population per year. There are no literature reports on the prevalence of melanoma in hemodialysis patients, this being much higher than that reported in the general population of this country.

Mucosal Alterations

A prevalence of 90% is reported for oral mucous membrane disorders among patients with CRF. Macroglossia ("uremic tongue"), xerostomia, and ulcerative stomatitis are the most frequent findings [5, 10, 21].

Other mucous membrane disorders are angular cheilitis, furred tongue, and uremic breath, the latter being caused by a high concentration of urea in saliva and ammonium degradation [5, 11].

Faneral Disorders

Diffuse hair loss and diffuse alopecia with dull hair are described as distinctive features among patients with CRF [4, 12].

A Brazilian study reported that the prevalence of hair loss and dull hair was between 26% and 33% [11].

Ungular disorders described are koilonychias, subungual hyperkeratosis, onycholysis, Mee's lines (leukonychia transverse bands), Muehrcke's lines (double white cross band), splinter hemorrhage, absence of lunula, and Beau's lines [5, 22]. The prevalence of these entities, plus Lindsay nails (better known as "half and half nails"), is estimated to be 71.4% of patients with CRF [11, 23].

Specific Skin Entities Characteristic of Patients with Chronic Kidney Disease

The prevalence of these entities has been studied in patients receiving HD, but not in patients with CRF. In a case–control study conducted in Egypt a prevalence of 3% was reported among 128 patients receiving HD [12]. These figures do not match with our previously mentioned study, where prevalence was 14%. This difference could be explained in part by the exclusion in the Egypt study of various dermatoses included in our study, such as fistula dermatoses and Lindsay nails.

Acquired Perforating Disorders

Several perforating disorders have been described in patients with CRF. They can be primary or acquired and include perforating folliculitis, Kyrle's disease, reactive perforating collagenosis, and acquired perforating disorder (APD) [5, 8, 10, 13].

The term APD or perforating disorder in kidney disease is used for the description of follicular hyperkeratotic papules in these patients [5, 13]. APD is an acquired skin disease characterized by transepidermal elimination of dermal material with minimal damage to adjacent structures [5, 7, 13, 14, 19].

The reported incidence among patients with CRF varies between 4.5% and 11% [9, 13, 14]. Higher prevalence is described in patients of African descent and patients with DM [7, 9, 13, 19].

Bullous Dermatoses

Bullous dermatoses in renal failures include porphyria cutanea tarda (PCT), pseudoporphyria, and bullous cutaneous drug reactions. The latter is not specific of patients with CRF. The prevalence of these three entities varies from 1.2% to 18% [19].

Porphyria Cutanea Tarda

PCT is a disorder in heme biosynthesis resulting in vesicles and blister rash on sun-exposed areas [14]. It can be divided into inherited or acquired. In acquired PCT the deficient enzyme is located in the liver [8, 13, 14].

The reported incidence of PCT is in the range of 1.8–3%. It was considered a common condition in patients receiving HD in the pre-erythropoietin era, whereby iron overload was common [8, 9, 13, 14].

In PCT the standard HD cannot remove uroporphyrins. These levels in patients with CRF without PCT are similar to the ones found in PCT patients with normal renal function. Currently PCT occurs in anemic HD patients with erythropoietin resistance that requires red blood cell transfusions. In such patients, treatment is based on reducing iron stores and plasma levels of porphyrins [14, 19].

Pseudoporphyria

Pseudoporphyria is a photodistributed vesicobullous disorder with clinical and histologic features similar to those of PCT but without any biochemical porphyrin abnormalities [8, 13, 14, 19, 24].

Calcification Disorders

Disorders of calcification are a heterogeneous group of diseases whose common denominator is the deposit of calcium. Calcium salt deposits in the skin and soft tissues are known as calcinosis cutis [13, 25]. In the context of a patient with chronic kidney disease it is subclassified as benign nodular calcification (BNC) [14]. When intravascular calcium reservoir occurs and is accompanied by initial fibroplasia, vascular occlusion, and soft tissue necrosis, the diagnosis is calciphylaxis, also known as calcifying uremic arteriopathy [7, 9, 14].

Calciphylaxis is a frequently lethal entity because of progressive skin necrosis secondary to calcification of small blood vessels [9, 13, 14]. BNC and calciphylaxis occur more frequently in patients with CRF. While calciphylaxis is more common in patients with CRF, it has also been reported in other entities such as in renal transplant recipients, Crohn's disease, cirrhosis, rheumatoid arthritis, inflammatory bowel disease, neoplasms, systemic lupus erythematosus, human immunodeficiency virus (HIV) infection, and primary hyperparathyroidism [13, 14]. Kidney failure is not a requirement for the development of this phenomenon [8, 25].

The overall incidence of calciphylaxis in HD patients is estimated at between 1% and 4%, women being more commonly affected [8, 13].

Nephrogenic Systemic Fibrosis

Nephrogenic systemic fibrosis (NSF) is a systemic condition with prominent cutaneous manifestations encompassed in fibrosing sclerosis-like disorders, observed in patients with renal disease after exposure to contrast agents based on gadolinium during an imaging procedure [14, 26]. It is a chronic and progressive disease without cure [19, 26, 27].

NSF today is well known by dermatologists and nephrologists, being easily recognized by clinical presentation [14, 27]. While most patients suffering from this condition are undergoing HD, it has also been described in patients receiving peritoneal dialysis and those patients receiving HD because of acute renal failure [7, 14, 19, 27, 28]. The estimated prevalence of NSF among patients with CRF is 0.5–6% [26]. The dominant feature is its presentation during kidney failure, both acute and chronic [14, 28].

Specific Nail Changes

Lindsay nails or "half and half nails" is the most frequent ungual alteration in CRF patients, with an approximate prevalence reported in HD patients from 21% to 40% [4, 5, 8, 10, 22]. In the general population the prevalence is 1.4% [5].

Uremic Frost

Uremic frost is one of the most infrequent skin changes that occurs in patients who suffer an acute episode of severe uremia [5, 8]. It was a common finding in the pre-HD era [5, 6].

Dermatoses on the Arteriovenous Shunt

Udayakumar et al. (2006) reported a prevalence of 8% in patients receiving prolonged HD [5, 6].

The authors found three dermatoses of this topography during the examination of 200 patients on HD.

Kaposi's Pseudosarcoma

Few cases are reported of this entity close to the region of an artificially constructed arteriovenous fistula. They are described as purple nodules or plaques that evolve slowly to lilaceous scaly crusted plaques near the fistula [5].

Adverse Drug Reactions

A higher incidence is described in this population, mainly due to the simultaneous administration of multiple drugs and drugs with prolonged half-life [5].

Recent advances in treatment have improved the quality and life expectancy of these patients, resulting in changes in the frequency and characteristics of skin disease [10].

Etiopathogenic Mechanisms

Xerosis

Cutaneous xerosis may be explained as a dysfunction and reduction in size of eccrine sweat glands, suggesting an alteration in the secretion product that results in epithelial dehydration. The high diuretic regime in these patients could also be involved [4–6, 8, 14, 21]. In the study conducted by Udayakumar et al. (2006), 37% of the patients also had associated pillar-like keratosis lesions on extensor surfaces, xerosis being more severe in patients who also had DM [5]. In our experience, xerosis was found in 79.4% of 200 patients receiving HD. These figures coincide with previous studies in Brazil and in the United States [3, 5]. This Uruguayan study researched the relationship between DM and xerosis with no statistically significant data as reported in the Brazilian study, where 72.5% of patients had DM [3].

Pruritus

The etiopathogenesis and pathophysiology of pruritus is complex, since several uremic and nonuremic factors contribute to its development [5, 10, 25]. In this sense, two hypotheses are described: the immunologic and the opioid hypothesis. The first one is based on considering uremic pruritus as a systemic disease. This idea is based on the proven benefits of the treatment with ultraviolet B (UVB) and thalidomide or calcineurin inhibitor intake such as tacrolimus [9]. UVB radiation attenuates the development of T-helper 1 (Th1) cells for Th2 differentiation, which leads to decreased production of interleukin (IL)-2. In addition, serum levels of proinflammatory markers such as C-reactive protein and IL-6 are increased in CRF patients with pruritus compared with those without pruritus, confirming the inflammatory nature of the condition. Opioid hypothesis proposes that pruritus is part of a change in the endogenous opioid system, overexpressing μ-opioid receptors in dermal skin cells and lymphocytes. This overexpression, with a concomitant decrease of κ-opioid receptors, could cause increased β-endorphin serum in patients with CRF, which would explain the development of pruritus. Use of κ-receptor agonists such as nalfurafine, or naltrexone, a μ-receptor antagonist, improves pruritus in this population [9].

Other possible biological theories proposed to explain pruritus in patients with CRF are urochrome skin reservoir, uremic toxemia, dysregulation of calcium and phosphorus metabolism, proliferation of mast cells with increased levels of histamine, allergy to HD components, and reaction to hypovitaminosis D and hypervitaminosis A [4–6, 8, 10, 11]. Pruritus has been linked to xerosis, although several studies failed to find such a relationship [13]. In HD patients, high plasma histamine levels may be due to allergic sensitization to various components of the HD's membrane and an altered renal excretion of histamine [5, 13]. Parathyroid hormone and divalent ions such as calcium; phosphorus, and magnesium have also been implicated in the pathogenesis of uremic pruritus, since itching is present in severe secondary hyperparathyroidism [5, 7, 10, 19, 29]. The lack of a consistent relationship between levels of parathyroid hormone, calcium, phosphorus, and uremic pruritus indicates that there would be other more important factors

involved in the pathogenesis [9, 10, 13, 29]. A study in Brazil revealed a statistically significant correlation between pruritus and elevated levels of phosphorus and magnesium [11]. A Japanese study 1,773 patients in HD identified male gender, high levels of blood urea/nitrogen, β2-microglobulin, hypercalcemia, and hyperphosphatemia as independent risk factors for the development of severe pruritus, whereas a low level of calcium and intact parathyroid hormone were associated with reduced risk [30].

In our experience, factors described in the literature that could influence the presence of pruritus in this particular population could not be proven statistically, including DM, HD membrane type, calcemia, phosphoremia, C-reactive protein level, and intake of vitamin supplements. On the other hand, we emphasize a significant relationship between vitamin D deficiency (in plasma) and the presence of pruritus. Vitamin D deficiency has been linked to pruritus in HD patients [4, 6].

Dyschromia

Diffuse Hyperpigmentation

Pigmentary alterations are attributed to an increase of melanin pigment in the basal layer of the epidermis and superficial dermis, owing to the greater amount of melanocyte-stimulating hormone because of poor HD excretion [12, 13, 25, 26]. Higher prevalence of this entity has been reported in patients who also had positive serology for hepatitis C virus (HCV) [7].

Sallow Skin

Carotenoid, lipochrome, and urochrome deposits in dermal layer and subcutaneous tissue are thought to be responsible for the yellowish sallow dyschromia so characteristic of these patients [3, 12, 13, 27].

Ecchymosis

Ecchymosis is explained by defects in hemostasis, which generate vascular fragility and platelet dysfunction, to which is added the use of heparin during HD [5, 8, 10, 13]. High concentrations of urea alter platelet aggregation and increase gua-nidinosuccinic acid levels, which inhibits platelet activity induced by adenosine diphosphate [11].

Gynecomastia

Gynecomastia occurs in the early stages of HD and is explained by a "feedback" after starting treatment. Both in CRF and protein malnutrition, pituitary and testicular function remain sup-pressed. When protein supplies increases after starting treatment with HD, a second "pubertal" push generates a transient gynecomastia [5, 10]. It has also been attributed to accumulation of pro-lactin, which inhibits the release of follicle-stimulating hormone and luteinizing hormone, resulting in decreased production of estrogen and progesterone [8].

Cutaneous Infections

HD patients have impaired cellular immunity because of their smaller number of T cells, which could explain the high percentage of infections in this population [9, 14, 15].

Skin Cancer

Patients with CRF receiving HD have been reported have an increased risk of any cancer [31]. Prevalence of skin cancer in CRF patients com-pared with the general population has not been reported [5]. By contrast, kidney transplant recipi-ents with a higher skin cancer prevalence are well studied, with an SCC-versus-BCC incidence ratio of 3.8:1 and an annual incidence calculated at 6.5%, increasing to 10.5% at more than 10 years post transplantation. Duration of immunosuppres-sion, older age at transplantation, presence of actinic keratosis, male sex, and outdoor occupa-tion are significantly associated with both SCC and BCC in kidney transplant recipients [32]. In transplant recipients, immunosuppressive drugs

severely impair the body's immune functions. Among the cell types affected are T lymphocytes, natural killer cells, and dendritic and other anti-gen-presenting cells. The end result is disrupted immune surveillance. Thus, a microenvironment is created that is conducive to unrestricted tumor growth [33]. In our opinion, the same situation is likely to occur in CRF patients as this population is considered as being in a chronic immune-sup-pressed state [5]. As described earlier, this con-cept agrees with the findings of our study wherein the prevalence of SCC was slightly greater than that of BCC in HD patients. In addition, this pop-ulation is at greater risk for developing virus-induced neoplasms.

Nonmelanocytic skin cancer behaves more aggressively in chronically immunosuppressed individuals. The exact mechanism whereby this aggressive phenotype is achieved remains elusive [33].

Faneral Disorders

Dull hair is believed to be due to decreased secre-tion of sebum [5, 10]. On the other hand, all abnormalities in the hair are considered as related to the administration of heparin, hypervitamin-osis A, accumulation of toxins, iron deficiency, and drugs frequently used in HD patients such as β-blockers, methyldopa, cimetidine, allopurinol, and indomethacin [11].

Acquired Perforating Dermatoses

The pathophysiology of APD remains unclear at present, although removal of transepidermal material is thought to be the final pathway. One of the most accepted theories explains the phenom-enon as resulting from diabetic microangiopathy that would prevent proper healing; however researchers have recognized that this theory can-not explain cases of APD in patients without DM [13, 14]. It is suggested that minimal trauma such as scratching triggers tissue necrosis and that the necrotic material is removed by transepidermal elimination [14, 19]. This theory is supported by the fact that lesions exhibit the Koebner phenomenon several times. Saray et al. reported that among 11 patients with coexistent APD and DM, none developed lesions of APD until nephropathy occurred. Other authors propose that the underlying renal disease would be the cause of skin diseases; while other another described that the dermal material is a foreign body reaction to an unknown dermal substance [15].

Bullous Dermatoses

Porphyria Cutanea Tarda

From a pathophysiologic point of view, porphyria is caused by enzyme deficiency related to heme biosynthesis, resulting in blocking heme synthesis and the subsequent accumulation of toxic porphyrins. In PCT the deficient enzyme is uroporphyrinogen decarboxylase, which causes the accumulation of porphyrins, especially water-soluble uroporphyrin, in both liver plasma and skin. The skin porphyrin deposit causes oxygen free radicals when exposed to UV radiation, resulting in photosensitivity, blistering, and scarring. Iron plays an essential role in the development of symptoms of PCT because this metal encourages early enzymatic function for the synthesis of heme and inhibits the already poor decarboxylase uroporphyrinogen. Moreover, iron promotes the oxidation of the porphyrin precursors [14]. In PCT the standard HD cannot remove uroporphyrins [14, 19].

Alcohol, estrogens, HCV, hepatitis B virus (HBV), and HIV are thought to precipitate further uroporphyrinogen decarboxylase dysfunction, possibly through an iron-dependent mechanism [8, 9, 14, 19].

Pseudoporphyria

Pseudoporphyria can develop as a consequence of photosensitizing drugs (including naproxen, furosemide, nalidixic acid, bumetanide, tetracyclines, and amiodarone), excessive exposure to ultraviolet A (UVA) (in the case of tanning beds), or CRF without another precipitant factor. It is more likely to occur when other precipitants are present in a patient receiving HD, such as photosensitization [8, 13]. The mechanism of induction is unknown [14].

Proposed factors that may elicit pseudoporphyria in a patient with CRF and receiving HD include diuretics, aluminum hydroxide, polyvinyl chloride HD tubing, hemosiderosis, silicone particles, erythropoietin, and susceptibility to oxygen free radicals. Keczkes et al. (1976) described five patients with CRF who had bullous dermatoses, all of whom were taking furosemide. The causal role of erythropoietin is discussed because many cases of pseudoporphyria were reported before its use. In addition, through reducing iron stores, it can alleviate pseudoporphyria. Possible aggravating circumstances in some of the case reports of peritoneal dialysis-associated pseudoporphyria include probable HVC infection and the use of nifedipine, a known photosensitizer [34].

Disorders of Calcification

Benign Nodular Calcification

The factors that predispose to such calcification include an increase in calcium and phosphorus products in serum, the degree of secondary hyperparathyroidism, the level of magnesium in plasma, the degree of alkalosis, and the presence of local tissue injury [35].

Calciphylaxis

The pathophysiology of this entity is complex. It is believed that calciphylaxis is the result of an imbalance between inductors and inhibitors of calcification in the vascular wall [8]. The Braun model is practical and divides homeostasis of calcium and phosphorus metabolism into five systems: intestine, kidney, bone, intravascular compartment, and extraosseous calcifications. The only way of removing excess phosphorus in patients with CRF is bone deposition, osseous calcifications, or removal by dialysis. HD removal is insufficient to prevent phosphorus buildup, even with efficient treatment to reduce intestinal absorption. From the aforementioned, extraosseous calcification is a possible consequence [14].

There are increasing reports that support the relationship between bone and vascular calcification. Elevated levels of uremia and phosphatemia cause transdifferentiation of vascular muscle stem cells into osteoblast-like cells [9, 14].

It is concluded that calcium deposit in vascular walls is a dynamic process and not simply due to a passive mineral precipitation secondary to high levels of phosphorus/calcium. There are multiple case reports on patients with calciphylaxis who have normal levels of phosphorus/calcium and normal levels of parathyroid hormone [14, 25].

Calciphylaxis has been linked to acute coronary events. Although calcium deposits generate progressive narrowing of the lumen, the essential event is a thrombotic vascular occlusion [14].

Several risk factors have been linked to the development of calciphylaxis, such as renal failure, female gender, obesity, DM, liver disease, use of systemic corticosteroids, intake of coumarin anticoagulants, serum levels of aluminum higher than 25 ng/mL, hyperparathyroidism, vitamin D exposure, lymphomas, HIV, local trauma, use of calcitriol, salt intake, and production of calcium/phosphorus greater than 70 mg/dL^2 [7, 9, 13, 14, 19]. A series by Dauden Tello et al. (2002) based on 17 patients with cutaneous vascular calcification observed that a large number of patients had hypertension and/or DM and/or atheromatous disease [25].

Nephrogenic Systemic Fibrosis

It is considered that myofibroblasts are involved in this disease, suggesting that certain cytokines, such as TGF-β, could mediate fibroblast proliferation [9, 14, 27].

The etiology is not fully clarified, although exposure to gadolinium (contrast agent) is recognized as an inducing factor of NFS. The lesions appear after approximately 16 days from gadolinium injection [8, 9, 14]. The US Food and Drug Administration (FDA) has created a warning indicating that exposure to gadolinium in patients with renal GFR less than 30 ml/min/1.73 m^2 increases the risk of NSF [9, 14]. This also applies to patients with acute renal failure of any severity associated with hepatorenal syndrome or patients in the perioperative liver transplantation period [14].

Gadolinium is a metal that attracts magnetic forces, making it optimal as magnetic resonance imaging and angioresonance contrast [9, 14]. In its free form it is very toxic to tissues, and combines with chelating agents to create a relatively stable inert compound [14, 26]. After being formed this complex rapidly reaches equilibrium between interstitial and vascular spaces [14].

In patients with normal renal function, 95% of the gadolinium complex is excreted in the first 24 h post administration [9, 14]. In patients with impaired renal function, the removal declines. However, its small molecular weight allows it to be removed via HD up to 95% after three sessions of HD. Current theory suggests that the greater permanence of gadolinium in tissues of patients with CRF allows cytokine signals to activate fibrinogen [14]. The type of gadolinium also appears to be significant [14, 19].

Most cases were exposed to gadodiamide [14, 26]. The challenge is to understand why most patients exposed to gadolinium contrast agents are saved from this entity [14, 19].

Recent surgery, vascular procedures, hypercoagulable states, and thrombotic events have been cited as associated conditions in patients, suggesting that endothelial damage may be a cofactor. High doses of erythropoietin could be a cofactor but without consistent scientific basis [9, 14]. Kidney transplant failure and later onset of HD has also been described as a risk factor [9].

Lindsay Nails

The pathogenesis of this condition is attributed to an increased capillary density in the bed. On the other hand, Lindsay nails are thought to be due to a collapsed venous return in the nail bed [4, 8, 10, 19].

Uremic Frost

Uremic frost due to eccrine deposits of urea crystals on the skin surface in patients with severe uremia [5, 13, 33]. Evaporation of sweat with high urea concentration causes urea to crystallize and deposit onto the skin [36].

Clinical Presentation

Nonspecific Cutaneous Entities with Higher Prevalence in Patients with Chronic Renal Failure

Xerosis

The term xerosis is often used to refer to the concept of dry skin [2]. It is a permanent symptom in CRF patients, with a clinical picture characterized by dry skin appearance, marked scaling and roughness, and poor skin smoothness (Fig. 44.1). Xerosis often affects the entire surface of the body, and may be more intense in some areas. Severe involvement of certain areas, such as the hands and feet, leads to possible functional impairment. As a consequence of an alteration in the cutaneous barrier function, the skin is more easily exposed to external attacks and aggression. As in some other severe xerotic conditions, a greater susceptibility to irritation caused by chemical factors (e.g., soaps and detergents) may be observed [37]. Severe xerosis can lead to fissured and cracked skin [1].

Pruritus

Itching can be localized or generalized, with the back being the most commonly affected site. The intensity and distribution of pruritus may vary significantly over time [16]. It can occur without skin lesions, being a subjective symptom of the patient (better known as pruritus sine materiae), or become clinically present with lesions such as excoriations, lichen simplex, nodular prurigo (see below), or keratotic papules, all resulting from scratching [21]. Variations are described in frequency and severity and often are associated with severe paroxysms that disrupt sleep and impair the quality of life and daily activity [9, 13, 19]. It also contributes to the occurrence of the Koebner phenomenon of APD [13, 19].

As previously stated, prurigo could be a clinical presentation of pruritus. Nodular prurigo is chronic relatively frequent dermatoses among CRF patients. Hyperkeratotic pruritic papular nodules often develop in a symmetric distribution over extensor surfaces of extremities, and may affect the trunk and buttocks. Lesions become hyperpigmented over time and are often excoriated by scratching. The face and palmoplantar region are usually spared [38, 39]. It is the most intense form of lichenification. Itching is the key symptom, being intense and intolerable with nighttime exacerbations. Evolution is chronic and with no tendency to heal [39] (Fig. 44.2).

Dyschromia

Diffuse Hyperpigmentation

Most cases of diffuse hyperpigmentation are reported in sun-exposed areas and in fewer

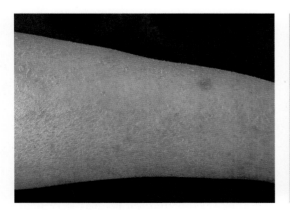

Fig. 44.1 Cracked skin and xerosis of the limb

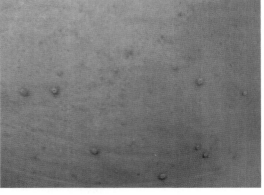

Fig. 44.2 Nodular prurigo

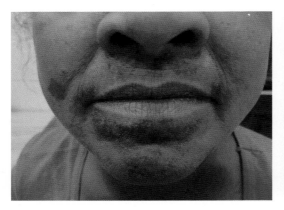

Fig. 44.3 Difuse hyperpigmentation in sun exposed areas

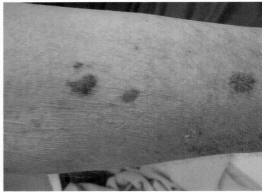

Fig. 44.4 Several ecchymosis of the arm

patients, with hyperpigmented macules on palms and soles [4, 5, 8, 10] (Fig. 44.3).

Sallow Skin

CRF patients may experience sallow complexion or citrine-colored skin, which may present an unhealthy and tired appearance. It occurs mainly as a result of urochrome accumulation in the skin because the impaired kidney cannot function well on its elimination [7, 19, 25].

Ecchymosis

Ecchymosis is characterized by a reddish or bluish macule. The onset of reddish or bluish discoloration of the skin is due to the escape of blood from ruptured blood vessels into the capillaries. It is a subcutaneous nonpalpable purpura. In CRF patients it appears more frequently in regions of trauma, such as arms or legs [13, 14]. It is easily recognized in puncture sites [14, 15] (Fig. 44.4).

Skin-Specific Entities Characteristic of Patients with Chronic Renal Failure

Acquired Perforating Dermatosis

APD is clinically characterized by conical papules with keratotic plugs; the presence of keratotic pits on palms and soles is also described [5, 9, 14]. It predominates in areas of high surface friction or trauma, such as extensor surfaces (most commonly in lower limbs), areas with high density of pilosebaceous follicles,

and the trunk [5, 13, 14, 19] (Fig. 44.5a, b). Etiopathogenically, the constant skin trauma due to pruritus could be the promoting factor [5]. The Koebner phenomenon can be seen [14]. In Caucasians, these papules acquire a pink color while in high phototypes they are brown or hyperpigmented [13, 14]. The most common symptom is severe itching [14]. A minority of patients report pain [13, 14]. The natural evolution is spontaneous resolution of individual lesions with the continuous appearance of new lesions [13].

Porphyria Cutanea Tarda

The clinical presentation does not differ from the one seen in sporadic PCT and is characterized by the development of vesicles and blisters in photo-exposed areas, with a higher prevalence in back of hands and forearms. The presence of scabs and the erosions resulting from trauma are frequently seen, while hyperpigmented scars and milia formation are characteristics in the evolution. It is also common to see subtle face hypertrichosis and hyperpigmentation in sun-exposed areas. Bright, depressed, and slightly infiltrated plaques, known as sclerodermiform plaques, can be observed [8, 9, 13, 14].

Pseudoporphyria

Clinical features are identical to those of PCT but without hypertrichosis, hyperpigmentation, or sclerodermiform plaques [8, 13, 14] (Fig. 44.6).

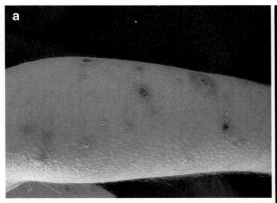

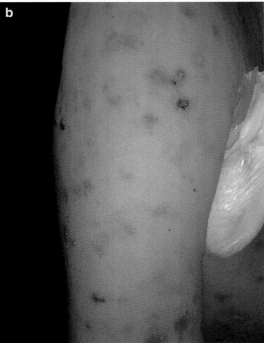

Fig. 44.5 (**a**, **b**) Acquired perforating dermatosis

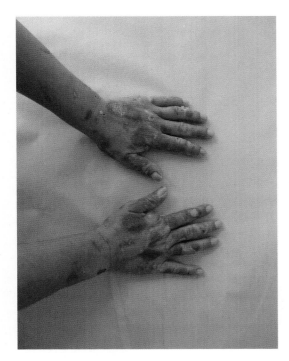

Fig. 44.6 Erosions due to blisters, pseudoporphyria

Benign Nodular Calcification

Also known as calcinosis cutis, this condition presents clinically as papules, plaques, or nodules near joints or fingertips firm to palpation. Most lesions are asymptomatic, although when located in the aforementioned topographies they can compromise joint function and be painful. In some lesions, the output of thick whitish substance can be seen through the skin [8, 14] (Fig. 44.7).

Calciphylaxis

Calciphylaxis is a life-threatening affection that presents acutely by invalidating and severe cutaneous pain. The skin initially shows a small area of erythema or livedo reticularis (retiform purple) that rapidly progresses to shallow or deep stellate ulcerations, with central necrosis or sloughing. In peri-ulcer areas, skin becomes purple with a livedoid pattern on which patients experience exquisite pain [7, 8, 14]. It presents distinctive distribution features that could predict prognosis. Distal acral involvement has a better prognosis than proximal involvement. Peripheral pulses are preserved distal to necrotic areas. When also involved with myopathy, hypotension, fever, dementia, and injury to the central nervous or intestinal system, it is known as systemic calciphylaxis [7, 8, 13]. Ocular ischemic neuropathy commitment has been described [7].

Nephrogenic Systemic Fibrosis

The clinical presentation of NSF is progressive, symmetric, and characterized by skin hardening of extremities and trunk, commonly being described as orange peel or woody induration and reminiscent, in some aspects, of scleromyxedema [5, 8, 14, 19, 26].It firstly shows a clear erythematous papule that may associate with edema of the affected region and then coalesces into brownish indurated plaques at distal areas, generally in the lower limbs, progressing in a cephalic fashion [7, 14, 26]. Sclerosis can generate joint contractures accompanied by numbness, itching, or pain [9, 14, 19, 26]. It tends to spare the head and neck [14]. Latterly, patients develop epidermal atrophy and loss of hair with orange cobblestone peel and hyperkeratosis with pruritus [9, 26]. Some extracutaneous manifestations include yellowish plaques in the sclera, muscle weakness, and deep rib or hip pain [8, 14, 26]. Although progress is slow, a minority of patients may suffer an acute course with immobility lasting several weeks [14].

Lindsay Nails

Lindsay nails are a change on the coloration of the nails characterized by red or chestnut coloration in its distal half (not disappearing with pressure) and white in its proximal half [5, 8, 15, 19]. Both fingernails and toenails are affected [19, 22] (Fig. 44.8a, b).

Uremic Frost

Uremic frost consists of a white-yellowish crystal-like cover, formed by urea in the beard area and other parts of the face, neck, and trunk. In 2 weeks peeling occurs and fissures appear [5].

Complementary Examinations

Most of the aforementioned dermatoses do not require complementary examinations to reach diagnosis. Dermatoses that do require complementary examinations are cited here.

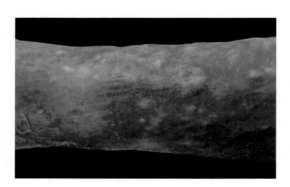

Fig. 44.7 Benign nodular calcification

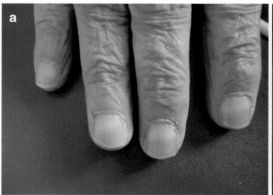
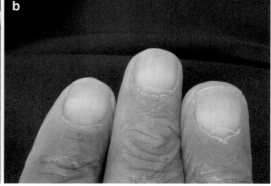

Fig. 44.8 (**a, b**) Lindsay nails

Acquired Perforating Dermatoses

Skin biopsy can help to diagnose this entity in most cases [14]. Differential clinical diagnoses include primary perforating disorders, nodular prurigo, eruptive keratoacanthomas, phrynoderma (vitamin A deficiency), hyperkeratotic lichen, and warts [8, 13, 14].

Histopathology is similar to that of other perforating dermatoses, and overlapping characteristics can be observed in the same skin biopsy sample [8, 13, 14]. An accumulation of keratin is typically observed to fill an epidermal invagination or a dilated hair follicle [8, 14, 19]. The adjacent dermis is characterized by altered and thickened collagen fibers and/or elastic fibers [9, 14]. In evolved lesions, giant foreign body cells due to degenerating inflammatory cells can be seen [8, 13].

Porphyria Cutanea Tarda

Patients with PCT have a large iron reservoir, so high levels of iron and ferritin support this diagnosis. The presence of high levels of urine uroporphyrin I and low urine levels of uroporphyrin III, 8-carboxyl uroporphyrin, and 7-carboxyl uroporphyrin are sufficient for diagnosis. In anuric patients, assessing the stool for high levels of isocoproporphyrin III and plasma for high levels of uroporphyrin may be used to reach diagnosis [14].

Skin biopsy for histopathology and direct immunofluorescence helps to distinguish PCT and pseudoporphyria from other subepidermal bullous dermatoses [14].

Histopathologic findings are subepidermal separation with minimal or no swelling. It is typical to find collections of intraepidermal eosinophilic collagen type IV, called caterpillar bodies, in the basement membrane. Direct immunofluorescence of perilesional skin reveals linear deposits of IgG, complement 3, and fibrinogen along the dermal–epidermal junction and around blood vessels [8, 13, 14].

Serology for HIV, HBV, and HCV should be considered, as well as genetic testing for hemochromatosis in all patients with PCT as they are frequent comorbidities and triggers of this disease [14].

Pseudoporphyria

As already described, porphyrin assays show normal plasma and fecal levels. Biopsy of affected skin reveals subepidermal blisters, lymphocytic perivascular infiltrate, and sclerosis of collagen. In other words, histopathologic features are similar to those of PCT although less thickening of the vessel wall is observed [8, 13, 24]. Direct immunofluorescence may be positive, showing linear IgG deposits in vessel walls and at the basement membrane zone. These results are consistent with a diagnosis of HD-associated pseudoporphyria [24].

Difficulty often arises in establishing a diagnosis of pseudoporphyria in patients undergoing HD because PCT concurrent with CRF may occur. Patients without symptoms undergoing long-term HD have been shown to exhibit higher plasma uroporphyrin levels than normal controls, further complicating the distinction between pseudoporphyria and true PCT. These levels have reached those measured in the plasma of patients with symptomatic PCT. Interestingly, uroporphyrin concentrations are significantly higher in patients undergoing HD in comparison with patients undergoing continuous ambulatory peritoneal dialysis, possibly because of better clearance of larger molecular weight "middle molecules" such as uroporphyrin by continuous ambulatory peritoneal dialysis [34].

Investigation of the dialysis patient poses practical diagnostic difficulties because urinary porphyrin profiles are not available. It is important to investigate anuric patients with fractionation of both fecal and plasma porphyrins [40].

Benign Nodular Calcification

A skin biopsy should be performed to confirm the diagnosis of BNC. Histopathologic calcium reservoir is shown in dermis and subcutaneous tissue. Foreign body giant cells and inflammation can be seen around calcium deposits. Although calcium is clearly distinguishable with hematoxylin and eosin staining, Von Kossa staining (calcium stains black) can highlight deposits [8, 14].

The degree of severity is related to calcium and phosphorus levels in plasma. Normalization of the aforementioned minerals can lead to regression of lesions [8].

Calciphylaxis

Skin biopsy may confirm this entity, although histologic findings are not pathognomonic [8, 13, 14]. Diagnostic features are located in the deeper dermis and subcutaneous tissue, so biopsy should be deep. The distinctive features of intimal hyperplasia and medial calcification are located in dermal small arterioles or subcutaneous arteries and arterioles. Fibrin thrombi in the vascular lumen of dermis and subcutaneous tissue are frequently observed. Overlying dermis and epidermis are necrotic and ulcerated [8, 9, 13, 14]. A few calcium deposits around lipocytes or global calcification of subcutaneous tissue capillaries may be observed [13].

X-ray of the affected area shows the medial calcification as a double reticular fine line in the vessel topography. The commitment of small vessels is radiologically defined as involvement of smaller vessels than 0.5 mm in diameter and is probably the most specific radiologic finding of calciphylaxis. Mammography is more sensitive in many cases, though not routinely performed [13].

The differential diagnosis can be divided into processes of connective tissue such as vasculitides, hypercoagulable states (cryoglobulinemia), deep fungal infection and, on the other hand, embolic events [13, 14]. The crucial point in diagnosis is an adequate sample of tissue for biopsy [14].

Laboratory analysis includes renal function, phosphorus, calcium, parathyroid hormone levels, and urine sediment. Antinuclear antibody (ANA) and antineutrophil cytoplasmic antibody tests may also be necessary. Cryoglobulins and serology for hepatitis are usually requested [13, 14].

Nephrogenic Systemic Fibrosis

Differential diagnosis in these patients includes other fibrosing disorders such as scleromyxedema, sclerederma diabeticorum, and diffuse or limited cutaneous sclerosis [19, 26]. One of the features that differentiate these entities from NSF is the absence of facial involvement in the latter [9, 26]. The absence of Raynaud's phenomenon, periungual capillary dilation, and telangiectasia also excludes other sclerotic disorders [26].

Negativity of antibodies in plasma helps to rule out autoimmune sclerosis, and the absence of circulating paraprotein helps differentiate the NSF from scleromyxedema [26–28].

Gadolinium has been quantified in skin biopsies from patients with NSF. It has been described as 35–100 times higher bone deposits compared with healthy volunteers [14].

The histopathologic features mimic scleromyxedema and depend on the evolutionary stage of the lesion biopsied [5, 14]. The older lesions show CD34, procollagen 1, and CD45Ro in fusiform dermal cells with varied amount of mucin [7, 14]. The expression of CD34 and procollagen 1 suggest that the fusiform dermal cells are circulating fibrocyte infiltrates [14, 19]. The presence of dense fibrous bands that extend into the subcutaneous tissue is related to the clinical presentation of cutaneous induration [14]. Inflammation is absent [9, 14].

Therapeutic Approach

Some of the mentioned dermatoses tend to disappear when the patient is subjected to renal transplant, confirming the role of renal dysfunction in the onset and perpetuation of these disorders [2].

Xerosis

Dry skin affects patients' quality of life, especially when the hands are involved [2]. Treatment is based on skin hydration and treatment of pruritus, if present. Repetitive bathing must be avoided should be short, with warm water avoiding friction with sponges [2, 21]. Once bathing is over, immediate application of emollients preventing transcutaneous water evaporation is mandatory. The application of creams, ointments, or scented lotions is not recommended (especially if they contain alcohol) [2].

The most widely used and effective humectant is glycerol, owing to its excellent hygroscopicity, lipid-modulating, and corneodesmolytic activity. Other humectants include urea and NMF (normal moisturizing factor) components, whereas other corneodesmolytic agents include the hydroxyacids. Topically applied ceramides and other bilayer-forming lipids are, therefore, an option. An equimolar mixture of the three dominant stratum corneum lipids (ceramide, cholesterol, and fatty acids) has been shown to allow normal rates of barrier recovery, whereas adjustment to a 3:1:1 molar ratio accelerates barrier recovery [41].

Pruritus

Despite the almost constant presence of xerosis, classic emollients and keratolytic and antihistamine therapies produce modest benefit in the treatment of pruritus [7, 13]. Antihistamines have limited benefit in uremic pruritus and relies on its side effect to induce drowsiness [9]. Renal transplantation is seen as curative treatment by some authors [13, 19].

In patients undergoing HD, the type of membrane used does not seem to influence the incidence of pruritus, although an uncontrolled study showed a significant reduction when HD was performed with high-flux membrane polymethylmethacrylate [9]. Some authors believe that general measures in the management of pruritus include optimizing the efficiency of HD using biocompatible membranes and improving the nutritional status of the patient [9, 11, 19].

Topical treatments, besides emollients, include capsaicin cream and tacrolimus. Capsaicin is a natural alkaloid found in the hot pepper plant. It acts by reducing levels of substance P in type C sensory cutaneous nerves. The studies carried out show that applications of 0.025% cream significantly relieves itching in

HD patients, with no observed adverse effects. While this is a good choice in localized pruritus, it is impracticable in generalized pruritus [9, 42].

Topical tacrolimus is a calcineurin inhibitor that works by blocking the differentiation of Th1 cells, thereby inhibiting the production of IL-2. There is a single pilot study of 25 patients with uremic pruritus receiving tacrolimus ointment 0.03% for 3 weeks and 0.1% for the next 3 weeks, describing a significant reduction of pruritus without detection of serious toxicity [9]. Since 2006, the FDA has included a warning sign on tacrolimus boxes informing about the risk of cutaneous malignancy after using this agent for long periods. However, to date they have not observed an excessive amount of cutaneous malignancy in 9,800 patients with atopic dermatitis using tacrolimus 0.03% [19].

UVB (280–315 nm) radiation is the most effective treatment for uremic pruritus [8, 13, 19]. The mechanism of action is speculative and is thought to be due to a "photoinactivation" of pruritogenic substances and histamine-releasing factors. UVB also reduces vitamin A levels in the epidermis, which is suggested to contribute to pruritus [5, 13]. Three weekly sessions should be held for several months to obtain benefits. The potential carcinogenic effect of UV radiation requires serious consideration, particularly in patients with Fitzpatrick skin type II or I [9, 19]. Benefits of UVA phototherapy are controversial [7, 13, 19].

Other treatment options include oral cholestyramine, coal, and opioid agonists such as naltrexone or nalfurafine [5, 8]. The latter is successfully used in intractable pruritus in patients receiving HD, based on the hypothesis that endogenous opioids contribute to the development of pruritus. Among various trials the results are controversial [5, 9, 13]. Coal is widely used in England (where phototherapy is a less common treatment modality) as first-line treatment. Six grams daily of activated carbon is used orally and is believed to act by binding pruritogenous substances in the intestinal lumen with absorption preventing action [7, 13]. A limitation of coal is its low tolerance [7]. Cholestyramine, used in other pathologies with high effectiveness, seems not to show similar efficacy in uremic pruritus. The administration of 5 g every 12 h orally is not well tolerated because of gastrointestinal side effects. The risk of acidosis should be considered [19].

Erythropoietin treatment relieves itching in some HD patients by reversibly decreasing plasma histamine levels, according to a small crossover placebo-controlled study that was carried out for 10 weeks in patients receiving HD [5, 9, 19]. Other drugs that have been tested in uremic pruritus are ondansetron orally (a serotonin antagonist receptor and a selective 5-HT$_3$ antagonist) and gabapentin orally, both with good results [5, 7, 19]. Gabapentin at a dose of 100–300 mg is administered after each HD, reducing significantly the severity of pruritus [9, 19]. Neurotoxic side effects such as dizziness, drowsiness, and coma should be considered. In a small uncontrolled study the efficacy of granisetron (another 5-HT$_3$ antagonist) was shown in uremic pruritus [9].

Thalidomide is a suitable drug for uremic pruritus. It is contraindicated in women of reproductive age because of its teratogenic effect, and must be borne in mind as a possible cause of severe polyneuropathy [7, 9].

A controlled double-blind placebo study showed that nitroglycerin, a dopamine receptor and partial α-adrenergic blocker, at doses of 30 mg per day orally plus 5 mg intravenously in HD relieved pruritus in most patients with an effect lasting 24–48 h [19].

Alternative medicine, principally acupuncture, was reported to be useful in several case reports [7].

Pruritus has a substantial effect on the quality of life of this population, causing discomfort, anxiety, depression, and sleep disorders. The latter is associated with chronic fatigue with impaired physical and mental capacity [9, 19].

Dyschromia

Diffuse Hyperpigmentation

Hyperpigmentation, which commonly affects dark-skinned individuals, is often challenging to treat. It has been demonstrated to have a negative impact on quality of life [43].

To date, specific studies on the treatment of diffuse hyperpigmentation in patients with CRF have been lacking. In any event it appears that treatments tend to be ineffective and disappointing. One possible option is tyrosine inhibitors such as hydroquinone, arbutin, aloesin, azelaic acid, kojic acid, licorice extract, proprietary oligopeptide products, phenylethyl resorcinol, mequinol, and free radical scavengers (α-lipoic acid and ascorbic acid) [43, 44].

Hydroquinone is available in strengths up to 4%, with higher concentrations available as a compounded product. Even with diligent application, hydroquinone takes 3 months or more to produce clinical results, and contact dermatitis is often reported. Combining hydroquinone with another product, such as glycolic acid, vitamin C, or vitamin E, may improve efficacy and shorten the time necessary to achieve visible results. A well-known formula is to compound it with a topical retinoid and corticosteroid. Arbutin is a naturally occurring derivative of hydroquinone that also exerts its antimelanogenic activity via tyrosinase inhibition [43].

On the other hand, melanosome transfer inhibitors such as soy-based products, niacinamide, glycolic acid, and cell-turnover inducers are described. The latter are retinoids, commonly used as monotherapy or in combination with other topical medications. Retinoids have a dual mechanism of action; apart from melanosome transfer they stimulate cell turnover, discarding melanized keratinocytes [43, 44].

Currently laser treatment is a reasonable option for the treatment of hyperpigmentation. Among these, good results are described with Q-switched alexandrite laser, Q-switched Nd:YAG 1064/532 nm, and Q-switched ruby laser [45, 46].

Medical makeup, transitory or definite, is an interesting option for the management of hyperpigmentation. Last but not least, external photoprotection is fundamental to the hope of improving hyperpigmentation, whatever its etiology. Sun exposure always plays an aggravating role, considerably reinforcing hyperpigmentation already present and facilitating the appearance of new brown areas [47].

Sallow Skin

To the best of our knowledge there are no published reports to date of cosmetic treatments performed for this type of dyschromia.

Acquired Perforating Disorder

There have been no randomized controlled trials comparing different treatment modalities [13, 14]. There are reported cases of spontaneous resolution [19, 48]. High-potency topical corticosteroids under occlusion and intralesional corticosteroids could collaborate to reduce swelling and itching but do not prevent the appearance of new lesions [7, 8, 14]. Topical and oral retinoids, and oral vitamin A (100,000 U/day) have also been reported as having some therapeutic success, in addition to cryotherapy and topical keratolytic drugs [7, 8, 10, 13, 14, 49]. Kidney transplantation has shown benefits in some cases, although cases of APD after transplantation have been described [9, 14, 19]. A recent report has documented therapeutic success with five patients who were treated with narrowband UVB two or three times per week. Pruritus improved after three to five sessions and smaller lesions began to return after five to seven sessions. A maintenance dose of one or two times per week slowed the development of new lesions for at least 7 months in two of the five patients reported. There are isolated cases mentioning improvement with allopurinol (100 mg/day) and allopurinol combined with psoralen and UVA [3, 28, 48, 49].

Porphyria Cutanea Tarda

As mentioned earlier, standard HD does not remove porphyrins; however, high-flux membranes have led to their reduction, though generally not sufficient to generate clinical remission [8, 9, 13, 14].

Avoidance of sun exposure is a crucial factor in treatment [9]. The mainstay of treatment in patients with normal renal function is based on phlebotomy of 500 mL every 2 weeks, a procedure not feasible in patients with CRF [8, 13, 14]. Chronic kidney disease patients with iron overload and currently not requiring blood transfusion can be treated with small-volume phlebotomy (50–100 mL) once or twice a week. This regime has been reported to induce remission after 8 months of treatment. The normalization of iron and ferritin levels is the ultimate goal of treatment [14].

Chloroquine acts by binding to porphyrins, chelating them and facilitating their excretion. Attempts to remove this complex via HD have been unsatisfactory and may result in an exacerbation of the disease, and for this reason chloroquine is not fully recommended [14, 19].

Deferoxamine has been used as an iron and aluminum chelator in toxicity cases. Several researchers have used this drug in HD patients with PCT, obtaining discordant results depending on the administered dose [8, 14]. More recently another oral-administration iron chelator, deferasirox, is available, with no reported use in patients with PCT [14].

IFN-α treatment has shown to induce remission, suggesting that HCV could play a role in PCT [19].

Benefits of plasma exchange have also been shown, by removing 4 L of plasma twice and separated for 48 h, and reconstruction of erythrocytes with fresh frozen plasma [19].

Complete remission has been reported in patients after receiving a kidney transplant [14].

In every case the withdrawal of precipitating factors such as alcohol, exposure to sunlight, and estrogens is essential [13, 14]. Suspension of iron supplements and vitamin B is highly recommended [9].

Pseudoporphyria

The cornerstone of treatment is based on discontinuation of the suspected photosensitive drug and UVA strict protection [8, 14, 19]. There are increasing numbers of reported cases of pseudoporphyria associated with HD, with complete remission following treatment with *N*-acetylcysteine. The dose ranges from 800 to 1,200 mg per day divided into two doses. It is believed that *N*-acetylcysteine increases production of glutathione, a powerful antioxidant. The improvement mechanism is not clear. However, double-blind controlled studies should be performed to confirm its effectiveness. Even with proper treatment, the symptoms take months to subside [14, 19].

Benign Nodular Calcification

The therapeutic goal is to normalize calcium/phosphorus levels, thereby achieving cure by spontaneous disappearance of lesions [14]. An antacid recently approved (sevelamer), an organic phosphate binder, is recommended as the one of choice [13]. In refractory cases surgery may be considered [13, 14].

Calciphylaxis

Treatment of patients with calciphylaxis is frustrating, with mortality rates of between 60% and 80%. Sepsis remains the leading cause of death [8, 13, 14].

Calciphylaxis prevention is achieved by minimizing risk factors such as obesity, local trauma, calcium/phosphorus intake control, avoidance of excessive vitamin D administration, and secondary hyperparathyroidism [13, 14, 19]. Relieving pain is essential in the therapeutic management of these patients [19]. Most current therapeutic options aim at calcium/phosphorus metabolism disturbances, a diet low in phosphorus (<43 mg/day) being a main therapeutic [7, 9, 13, 14]. Bisphosphonates such as sevelamer have been reported anecdotally as effective, but the overall prognosis is poor. Parathyroidectomy in patients presenting with hyperparathyroidism has shown controversial results, although it has shown some efficacy when autologous transplant of a portion of the parathyroid is made in the forearm [13, 14]. Although all treatments proposed can help in preventing progressive calcification, the ability to restore ischemic tissue perfusion

is questionable, which would explain the low rates of treatment success [14].

Vitamin K is recommended when calciphylaxis is associated with the intake of coumarin [9].

Sodium thiosulfate is gaining support as the agent of choice for calciphylaxis treatment [14]. It likely acts as a chelator by dissolving calcium salts and to inducing an antioxidant effect and, eventually, synthesis of endothelial nitric oxide levels, which improves blood flow and tissue oxygenation [9, 14]. It is well tolerated and considered a safe drug. Adverse effects, especially acidosis and bone resorption by osteoclasts and the activation of intravascular volume overload, are expected [14]. The dose commonly used to treat calciphylaxis is 25 mg administered intravenously three times a week, which can be used for many months to maintain the initial positive response [9, 14]. The biggest limitation is its common side effect, nausea [9].

The use of corticosteroids is controversial, although there is a case report that encourages its use [13].

Meticulous management of ulcers, the generous use of antibiotics, and prevention by debridement are measures universally accepted to increase the survival of these patients. There are studies supporting debridement as part of the treatment and additional use of hydrocolloid patches to guide healing [7, 9, 13, 14, 19]. The hyperbaric chamber has been reported as effective in aggressive debridement of ulcers with consequent greater healing by raising the partial pressure of oxygen in the affected tissues, which improves angiogenesis and phagocytosis, inhibiting bacterial growth and decreasing local tissue edema [7, 13]. The long-term benefit of this therapeutic modality should be validated in larger studies [13, 19].

Sepsis is the leading cause of death [13].

Nephrogenic Systemic Fibrosis

No specific treatment for NSF has universal approval. It seems that the improvement in renal function may be the most beneficial treatment and that transplantation could be the solution, although it does not guarantee symptomatic relief

[5, 7, 9, 14]. There are anecdotal reports of successful trials with thalidomide, pentoxifylline, high doses of intravenous Ig, prednisone, UVA phototherapy, cyclophosphamide, extracorporeal photopheresis, plasmapheresis, sodium thiosulfate, and topical calcipotriol under occlusion [9, 14, 19, 26]. Imatinib mesylate was recently reported to effect a significant improvement in three patients [14, 26]. Enrolling patients into physical treatment sessions such as deep tissue massages seem to be beneficial and do not involve additional risk [7, 14]. There also have been reports of spontaneous remission [19].

While gadolinium plays a major role in the development of NSF, exposure to this agent in patients who present with CRF does not always lead to this condition; it would therefore seem to be a multifactorial process [14].

Glossary

Dyschromia Alteration of the color of the skin.
Gynecomastia Enlargement of the breast in the males, caused by an excess of estrogens.
Macroglossia Excessively large tongue.
Microangiopathy Pathologic processes of the microvessels.
Pruritogenic substances Substances capable of causing pruritus (itching).
Raynaud's phenomenon Abrupt onset of digital paleness followed by cyanosis and erythema in response to cold.
Teratogenic effect Capacity of some substances of generate physical defects in the developing embryo.
Uroporphyrins Porphyrins produced by oxidation of uroporphyrinogen, which can be excreted in excess in the urine in the context of porphyrias.
Xerostomia Decreased salivary flow (dry mouth).

References

1. Registro Uruguayo de Diálisis. www.nefrouruguay.com.
2. Barco D, Giménez-Arnau A. Xerosis: a dysfunction of the epidermal barrier. Actas Dermosifilogr. 2008;99:671–82.
3. Lupi O, Rezende L, Zangrando M, Sessim M, Silveira CB, Sepulcri MAS, et al. Manifestacões cutáneas na doenca renal terminal. An Bras Dermatol. 2011;86(2):319–26.
4. Falodun O, Ogunbiyi A, Salako B, George AK. Skin changes in patients with chronic renal failure. Saudi J Kidney Dis Transpl [serial online]. 2011. Cited 16 Mar 2015.;22:268–72.
5. Udayakumar P, Balasubramanian S, Ramalingam KS, Lakshmi C, Srinivas CR, Mathew AC. Cutaneous manifestations in patients with chronic renal failure on hemodialysis. Indian J Dermatol Venereol Leprol. 2006;72(2):119–25.
6. Leena JA, Noman MU, Islam MMSU, Ahmed AS, Ahmed DS, Rahma MM. Cutaneous manifestations of chronic kidney disease – an observational study in 100 cases. Faridpur Med Coll J. 2012;7:33–6.
7. Brewster UC. Dermatologic disease in patients with CKD. Am J Kidney Dis. 2008;51(2):331–44.
8. Kidney International Supplements. 2013;3:136–50. doi:10.1038/kisup.2012.72.
9. Kuypers D. Skin problems in chronic kidney disease. Nat Clin Pract Nephrol. 2009;5(3):157–70.
10. Thomas EA, Pawar B, Thomas A. A prospective study of cutaneous abnormalities in patients with chronic kidney disease. Indian J Nephrol. 2012;22:116–20.
11. Batista Peres LA, Passarini SR, Ferreira de Barros Tocollini Branco M, Kruger LA. Skin lesions in chronic renal dialysis. J Bras Nefrol. 2014;36(1):1–6.
12. Attia EAS, Hassan SI, Youseef NM. Cutaneous disorders in uremic patients on hemodialysis: an Egyptian case-controlled study. Inter J Dermatol. 2010;49:1024–30.
13. Robinson-Bostom L, DiGiovanna JJ. Cutaneous manifestations of end-stage renal disease. J Am Acad Dermatol. 2000;43(6):987–90.
14. Cordova KB, Oberg TJ, Malik M, Robinson-Bostom L. Dermatologic conditions seen in end-stage renal disease. Semin Dial. 2009;22(1):45–55.
15. Avermaete A, Altmeyer P, Bacharach-Buhles M. Skin changes in dyalisis patients: a review. Nephrol Dial Transplant. 2001;16:2293–6.
16. Fett N, Haynes A, Joy Propert KJ, Margolis DJ. Predictors of malignancy development in patients with chronic pruritus. J Dermatol Sci. 2016;82(2):123–8.
17. Wang A, Elshehadeh R, Rao D, Yap E. Roles of aldosterone receptor antagonists in heart failures, hypertension, and chronic kidney disease. J Nurse Pract. 2016;12(3):201–6.
18. Chao CT, Lai CF, Huang JW. Risk factors for herpes zoster reactivation in maintenance hemodialysis patients. Eur J Intern Med. 2012;23:711–5.
19. Mazen S, Kurban AB, Kibbi A-G. Cutaneous manifestations of chronic kidney disease. Clin Dermatol. 2008;26:255–64.
20. Belloni Fortina A, Piaserico S, Alaibac M. 2009. Squamous cell carcinoma. In: The SCOPE Collaborative Group, editor. Skin cancer after organ

transplantation. Cancer treatment and research 146. Rosen T, Series Editor. Springer, p. 241–61.

21. Chaturvedy M. Dermatologic problems in CKD; ocular manifestations in CKD. Clin Nephrol. 2012;1(4):284–90.

22. Charkhchian M, Beheshti A, Zangivand AA. Nail disorder among patients on maintenance hemodialysis. Dermatol Sin. 2003;31(1):7–10.

23. Saray Y, Seckin D, Gulec AT, Akgun S. Nail disorders in hemodialysis patients and transplant recipients: a case-control study. J Am Acad Dermatol. 2004;50(2):197–202.

24. Green JJ, Manders SM. Pseudoporphyria. J Am Acad Dermatol. 2001;44(1):100–8.

25. Daudén Tello E, Ruiz Genao D, Fraga FJ. Calcificación vascular cutánea. Correlación clínicopatológica y proposición de una nueva clasificación de las calcinosis. Actas Dermosifiliogr. 2002;93(1):23–34.

26. Bernstein EJ, Schmidt-Lauber C, Kay J. Nephrogenic systemic fibrosis: a systemic fibrosing disease resulting from gadolinium exposure. Best Pract Res Clin Rheumatol. 2012;26(4):489–503.

27. Swartz RD, Crofford LJ, Phan SH, Ike RW, Su LD. Nephrogenic fibrosing dermopathy: a novel cutaneous fibrosing disorder in patients with renal failure. Am J Med. 2003;114:563–72.

28. Jimenez SA, Arlett CM, Sandorfi N, Derk C, Latinis K, Sawaya H, et al. Dialysis-associated systemic fibrosis. Study of inflammatory cells and transforming growth factor β1 expression in affected skin. Arthritis Rheum. 2004;50:2660–6.

29. Shavit L, Grenader T, Lifschitz M, Slotki I. Use of pregabalin in the management of chronic uremic pruritus. J Pain Symptom Manage. 2013;45(4):776–81.

30. Narita I, Alchi B, Omori K, Sato F, Ajiro J, Saga D, et al. Etiology and prognostic significance of severe uremic pruritus in chronic hemodialysis patients. Kidney Int. 2006;69:1626–32.

31. Butler AM, Olshan AF, Kshirsagar AV, Edwards JK, Nielsen ME, Wheeler SB, et al. Cancer incidence among US Medicare ESRD patients receiving hemodialysis, 1996–2009. Am J Kidney Dis. 2015;65(5):763–72.

32. Ramsey HM, Fryer AA, Reece S, Smith AG, Harden PN. Clinical risk factors associated with nonmelanoma skin cáncer in renal transplant recipients. Am J Kidney Dis. 2000;36(1):167–76.

33. Athar M, Walsh SB, Kopelvich L, Elmets CA. Pathogenesis of nonmelanoma skin cancers in

organ transplant recipients. Arch Biochem Biophys. 2011;508(2):159–63.

34. Keczkes K, Farr M. Bullous dermatosis of chronic renal failure. Br J Dermatol. 1976;95(5):541–6.

35. Moe SM. Disorders involving calcium, phosphorus, and magnesium. Prim Care. 2008;35(2):251–vi.

36. Mohan D, Railey M. Uremic frost. Kidney Int. 2012;81:1153.

37. Szepietowski JC, Reich A, Schwatrz RA. Uraemic xerosis. Nephrol Dial Transplant. 2004;19(11):2709–12.

38. Winhoven S. Nodular prurigo – a retrospective analysis. Br J Dermatol. 1985;113:431–9.

39. Carrascosa JM, Ferrándiz C. Estrategias terapéuticas en el prurigo nodular. Piel. 2001;16(7):360–4.

40. Glynne P, Deacon A, Goldsmith D, Pusey C, Clutterbuck E. Bullous dermatoses in end-stage renal failure: porphyria or pseudoporphyria? Am J Kidney Dis. 1999;34(1):155–60.

41. Zettersten EM, Ghadially R, Feingold KR, Crumrine D, Elias PM. Optimal ratios of topical stratum corneum lipids improve barrier recovery in chronologically aged skin. J Am Acad Dermatol. 1997;37(3 Pt 1):403–8.

42. Weisshaar E, Dunker N, Gollnick H. Capsaicin therapy in humans with hemodialysis-related pruritus. Neurosci Lett. 2003;345(3):192–4.

43. Molinar VE, Taylor SC, Pandya AG. What's new in objective assessment and treatment facial hyperpigmentation? Dermatol Clin. 2014;32:123–35.

44. Sarkar R, Arora P, Grag KV. Cosmeceuticals for hyperpigmentation: what is available? J Cutan Aesthet Surg. 2013;6(1):4–11.

45. Arora P, Sarkar R, Grag VK, Arya L. Lasers for treatment of melasma and post-inflammatory hyperpigmentation. J Cutan Aesthet Surg. 2012;5(2):93–103.

46. Omi T, Yamashita R, Kawana S, Sato S, Naito Z. Low fluence Q-switched Nd: YAG laser toning and Q-switched ruby laser in the treatment of melasma: a comparative split-face ultrastructural study. Laser Ther. 2012;21(1):15–21.

47. Guerrero D. Dermocosmetic management of hyperpigmentations. Ann Dermatol Venereol. 2012;139(Suppl 3:S1):S115–8.

48. González-Lara L, Gómez-Bernal S, Vázquez-López F, VivancoAllende B. Acquired perforating dermatosis: a report of 8 cases. Actas Dermosifilogr. 2014;105(6):e-39–43.

49. Farrell A. Acquired perforating dermatosis in renal and diabetic patients. 1997;9056(349):895–96.

Dermatologic Manifestations Among Transplant Recipients

45

Lídice Dufrechou and Alejandra Larre Borges

Key Points

- Organ transplant recipients undergo long-term immunosuppressant therapy that leads to reduced immunosurveillance as well as other adverse effects of these drugs
- The high rate of cutaneous complications in this population implies the need for interdisciplinary follow-up care teams with the participation of dermatologists
- Under immunosuppressive treatment, infections can be atypical and unusually disseminated
- Infections caused by rare pathogens must be considered in the differential diagnosis
- A high degree of suspicion and opportune agent isolation are essential
- Skin tumors, particularly squamous cell carcinoma, are of special relevance because of their more aggressive behavior, high risk of metastases, and lethality

- Advanced age at the time of the transplant is one of the most important clinical predictors of squamous cell carcinoma
- A larger ultraviolet radiation accumulation before the transplant also implies an increased risk
- Proactive prevention (i.e.: physical sun protection, use of sunscreens, individually adapted immunosuppressant medication) and the timely treatment of premalignant lesions can lower the risk of squamous cell carcinoma
- In a recent study, melanoma-specific mortality was elevated three-fold compared with nonrecipients, suggesting that melanoma behaves aggressively under transplant-related immunosuppression
- Patients who have had melanoma with lymph node invasion or metastatic disease are not candidates to receive a transplant

L. Dufrechou (✉)
Adjudant Professor, UDELAR, Hospital de Clínicas, Cátedra de Dermatología, Unidad de Lesiones Pigmentadas, Montevideo, Uruguay
e-mail: ldufrechou@gmail.com

A.L. Borges
Assistant Professor, UDELAR, Hospital de Clínicas, Cátedra de Dermatología, Unidad de Lesiones Pigmentadas, Montevideo, Uruguay
e-mail: alarreborges@gmail.com

Epidemiology

Solid organ transplantation constitutes a life-saving intervention for persons with end-stage organ disease. Transplants help increase the survival and quality of life of recipients, lowering treatment costs in most cases. According to the World Transplant Registry, 114,690 solid organ transplants were performed worldwide in 2013,

© Springer International Publishing Switzerland 2018
R.R. Bonamigo, S.I.T. Dornelles (eds.), *Dermatology in Public Health Environments*,
https://doi.org/10.1007/978-3-319-33919-1_45

representing an increase of 1.8% over the previous year; kidney, liver, heart, and lung were the most frequently transplanted organs [1].

Long-term immunosuppression, which aims to downregulate the immune system in order to prevent allograft rejection, is necessary in recipients. New strategies in immunosuppressive therapy are associated with better patient and graft survival rates; however, adverse toxicities and long-term side effects associated with these agents present a number of challenges. Thus, current immunosuppression protocols are individualized and based on combined immunosuppressant therapies aiming to minimize administration of corticosteroids and to achieve a combined and synergic effect [2]. Such protocols vary according to the geographic area and the reference center. Immunosuppressants used with the purpose of maintaining the transplant are corticosteroids, calcineurin inhibitors (cyclosporine, tacrolimus, and tacrolimus MR), antimetabolites (mycophenolate mofetil, sodium mycophenolate, azathioprine), and mammalian target of rapamycin (mTOR) inhibitors (sirolimus and everolimus) [3, 4]. A variety of cutaneous complications and an increase in cutaneous malignancies, having a potentially great impact on patients' quality of life [8, 9], have been reported in this population, particularly among Caucasians [2, 5–7].

Overall, transplant complications can be divided into early and late, the former usually surgical and the latter medical. Infections are a common complication during the immediate postoperative and immediate perioperative periods, up to one month after the surgery. This risk persists as long as the transplant is maintained [10, 11]. Other frequent late complications are neoplasias, probably underreported, the risk of which is increased three to five times compared with in the general population [12].

Skin is a frequently affected organ in solid-organ recipients, affections are reported in 45–100% of patients; the frequency of dermatologic afflictions is 63% in our experience [2, 5]. This is also observed in the pediatric transplant population [13].

Skin Manifestations

Skin complications represent an important burden for transplant recipients for many reasons, such as their frequency, morbidity, and sizable impact on the quality of life of patients. Moreover, there has been increasing awareness of the public health implications of skin cancer in this population.

Most of the literature related to skin manifestations in solid-organ recipients comes from studies of renal and renal-pancreatic recipients. For practical matters we herein classify skin complications from solid organ transplants as infections, neoplasia, and adverse side effects of the immunosuppressant drugs. The aim of this chapter is to describe the most frequent dermatoses in solid-organ recipients regarding their epidemiology, clinical presentation, and therapeutic approach.

Discussion of the etiopathogenesis of the disorders is beyond the scope of this chapter. We focus solely on those etiopathogenic aspects that are distinctive in transplant recipients.

Infections

Skin infections are a relevant cause of death in solid-organ recipients, representing a growing diagnostic and therapeutic challenge [14, 15]. Their frequency varies between 27% and 66% according to different studies, the main causal agents being virus and fungi [2, 6–8, 16, 17]. The type of immunosuppressive drugs and their variable dosage in chronologic sequence after transplantation probably influence the type and appearance of skin infections [15]. The typical chronology of skin infections is wound infections, pyoderma, or the reactivation of herpes viruses in the first month after transplant, followed by opportunistic infections and reactivation of varicella zoster virus between months 2 and 5. After 6 months, as immunosuppression is reduced, the spectrum of causative organisms approaches that of the general population, with mycoses and human papillomavirus (HPV) infections dominating [15] (Fig. 45.1). Vulgar warts caused by different HPV serotypes and the infections caused by the herpesvirus family together with superficial mycoses such as tinea and pityriasis versicolor are the most frequently found in many studies [6–8, 13, 16, 17].

As mentioned, the frequency of these complications is directly proportional to the extent of immunosuppression and exposure to various potential

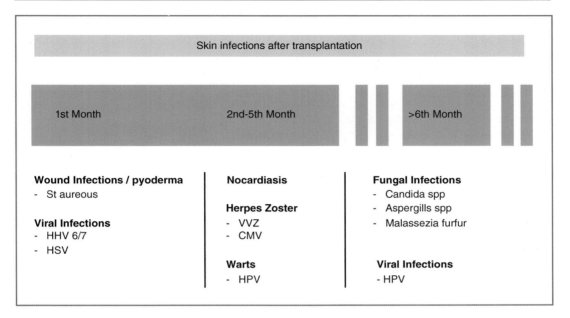

Fig. 45.1 Time frame of typical skin infections in organ transplant recipients. *HHV* human herpesvirus, *HSV* herpes simplex virus, *VZV* varicella zoster virus, *CMV* cytomegalovirus, *HPV* human papillomavirus

pathogens. Moreover, transplant recipients show complex interactions between chronic immuno-suppression and the presence of risk factors such as deficient nutritional status, hyperglycemia, muco-cutaneous barrier integrity loss, and subclinical activity of viral infections [18].

Viral Infections

Cytomegalovirus (CMV) is the most common viral infection following solid organ transplantation [19]. Not only does CMV directly cause morbidity and occasional mortality, but it also affects many short-term and long-term indirect factors that collectively contribute to reduced allograft and patient survival [20].

In light of the aforementioned, we detail cutaneous manifestations of CMV in solid organ recipients, although they are rare [21].

The main cutaneous viral infections among transplant recipients are caused by HPV, herpes simplex virus (HSV), and varicella zoster virus (VZV). The importance of viral infections lies in their morbidity and also in the fact that viral DNA has been found in squamous cell carcinomas (SCCs) as well as in Kaposi sarcoma (KS) of transplant recipients. [2, 22, 23].

Etiopathogenesis

CMV

It has been postulated that the dermis is relatively inhospitable to CMV; therefore, skin disease only occurs in a significantly immunocompromised host. As such, skin infection has generally been associated with disseminated disease, thus reflecting the overall degree of immunosuppression in these patients. The predominant defense against CMV is the major histocompatibility complex-restricted cytotoxic T cells, with growing evidence for the significant contributory role played by CD4+ T cells and humoral immunity. Immunosuppressive therapy suppresses cytotoxic cells in a dose-dependent manner and thus enhances viral replication once stimulated by other factors [24].

Pathogenically, in addition to direct viral effects, the CMV-induced immunomodulatory mechanism probably plays a role. The immuno-suppressive effect of CMV may lead to an increased susceptibility toward opportunistic infection [15].

HPV

Since the advent of improved DNA technology, more than 100 distinct HPV subtypes have been described with probably more to follow. HPV can be classified into two groups: cutaneous and mucosal subtypes. Cutaneous subtypes (cHPV) are predominantly found in cutaneous common and plane warts (mainly subtypes 2 and 4) and mucosal subtypes predominate in anogenital lesions such as condylomata acuminata [12, 22, 25]. Mucosal HPV subtypes can be divided into high-risk (16, 18, 26, 31, 33, 35, 39, 45, 51, 52, 53, 56, 58, 59, 66, 68, 73, and 82) and low-risk (6, 11, 40, 42, 43, 44, 54, 61, 70, 72, 81, and CP6108). Persistent infection with high-risk HPV (hrHPV), especially subtypes 16 and 18, has an essential role in the carcinogenesis of anogenital malignancies. Low-risk HPVs, especially 6 and 11, are responsible for about 90% of condylomata acuminata, which are not considered as precursor lesions of cervical cancer [12]. The HPV types detected in the renal transplant recipient (RTR) population are similar to those described in immunocompetent populations. However, the diversity of HPV types identified and the number of lesions increase in the RTR population [26].

HSV

HSV type 1 and type 2 (HSV-1, HSV-2) belong to the α-herpesvirus family. They are characterized by short replication cycles, rapid growth in culture, lysis of the host cell during replication, and latency in nerve root ganglia [23].

VZV

VZV also belongs to the α-herpesvirus family. Primary infection acquired through direct contact with skin lesions or by the respiratory route usually leads to chickenpox. After initial infection, VZV establishes latency in dorsal root ganglia and cranial nerves, and years or decades later it can reactivate as herpes zoster. The seroprevalence of VZV in adult recipients of solid organ recipients reaches 90%, while rates are lower in pediatric transplant patients. Solid organ transplant-seronegative adult recipients usually acquire infection through exposure in the community. Although very rare, VZV transmission by donor has been described [23]. Recipients with previous VZV disease or who have received vaccination have an increased risk

of herpes zoster. Other predisposing factors are advanced age, being a heart or lung recipient, and the use of mycophenolate mofetil [23].

Clinical Presentation

CMV

Skin infection by CMV has generally been associated with disseminated disease including hepatitis, pneumonitis, pancreatitis, kidney allograft dysfunction, colitis, and meningoencephalitis. As already mentioned, skin involvement is rare [21]. CMV usually presents as generalized maculopapular eruptions, but ulcers, nodules, vesicles, petechiae, and plaques may also be seen and can mimic other skin eruptions and cutaneous viral infections, especially herpetic infections. Cellulitis and ulceration, particularly involving the genital, perineum, and perianal areas, as well as necrosis of the mucosal membranes, can occur in more severe cases (Fig. 45.2)

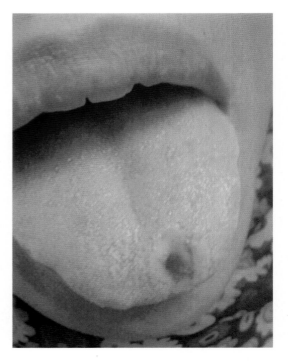

Fig. 45.2 A 31-year-old woman. Renal transplant 2 months ago, taking tacrolimus, mycophenolate mofetil, and prednisone. Oral ulcer due to cytomegalovirus. The patient also presented malaise, asthenia, and weight loss

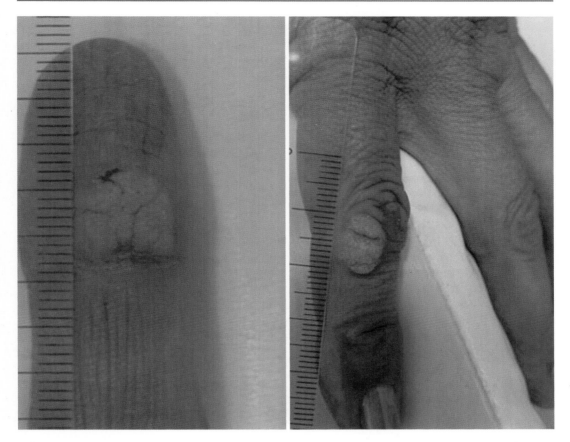

Fig. 45.3 A 52-year-old woman, renal transplant 37 months ago, taking cyclosporine A, mycophenolate mofetil, and prednisone. Recurrent viral warts in fingers

[15, 24]. CMV infection should be considered in a febrile immunosuppressed patient with skin involvement [21].

HPV
Recipients have a 15–50% chance of developing vulgar HPV warts within the first year post transplant, and 77–95% in the first 5 years [18]. These warts appear in multiple forms (hands, feet, and genitalia), predominantly on sun-exposed sites, and display a lesser tendency for spontaneous regression in comparison with the immunocompetent normal population [6, 15, 25] (Figs. 45.3 and 45.4).

HSV
HSV represents another cause of morbidity in these patients. An increased risk of developing HSV reactivations of up to 50% has been described with an incidence of up to 35% within the first 3 weeks following transplantation. In transplant patients HSV has an extensive presentation, together with necrosis, ulceration, prolonged evolution, and a higher risk of dissemination toward noble parenchyma such as the central nervous system, lungs, and liver (Fig. 45.5) [2, 8, 15, 27, 28]. Especially in heart and lung transplant recipients, severe esophagitis, bronchopneumonia, and encephalitis may occur [15]. Primo-infection during the post-transplant period is rare [29].

VZV
VZV is another pathogen that frequently affects transplant recipients [14]. Mustapić et al. (2011) carried out one of the largest trials regarding infection caused by VZV, in a total of 1139

recipients of kidney transplant between 1972 and 2010, showing a frequency of 3.51% and an average time of appearance of 2.13 years. Ninety-five percent of the studied patients presented with herpes zoster, while only 5% presented with chickenpox [30]. The risk of developing herpes zoster seems to increase according to age at the time of the transplant [28, 31]. In this population an increased risk of dissemination, postherpetic

neuralgia, and scars can be seen [28, 32] although in most cases the prognosis is favorable, with minimum morbidity and mortality [14] (Fig. 45.6).

Complementary Examinations

CMV detection using the polymerase chain reaction (PCR) is at present the most specific and sensitive method. The virus can be identified 1–2 weeks earlier than with cell culture or an antigen test [15].

Early skin biopsy is a useful and safe procedure for diagnosis confirmation. It shows cytoplasmic and nuclear inclusions and can be confirmed by immunohistochemistry in endothelial infected cells [33, 34].

Diagnosis of HPV warts, HSV, and VZS is often clinical. Conventional viral detection assays, including serologic assays and growth in cell culture, are not available for the diagnosis and tracking of HPV infection. Several types of HPV DNA tests are now available, including Southern blots, dot blots, in situ hybridization, PCR, and solution hybridization (hybrid capture assay). Of these, the PCR assay is the most sensitive [35].

Cervical Papanicolaou testing to detect and treat cervical intraepithelial neoplasia is one of the most important interventions that can be performed in transplant recipients concerning HPV infections and anal cancer screening [36].

HSV and VZV sometimes may require other diagnostic tools such as viral cultures, cytologic smear/Tzanck preparation of vesicular content, direct fluorescent antibody (DFA) studies, tissue biopsy, viral DNA detection by PCR, and serologic

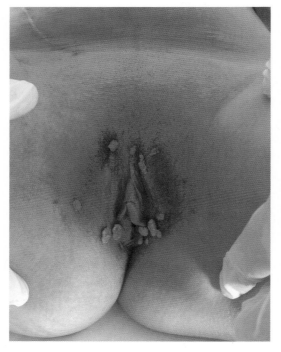

Fig. 45.4 A 23-year-old woman, reno-pancreatic transplant 8 months ago, taking tacrolimus, mycophenolate mofetil, and prednisone. Multiple condylomata acuminata

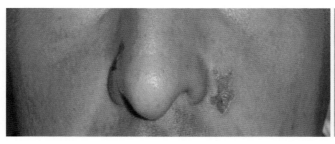
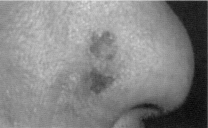

Fig. 45.5 A 43-year-old man, renal transplant 44 months ago, bilateral herpes simplex

Fig. 45.6 Disseminated herpes zoster in a 46-year-old kidney transplant recipient taking tacrolimus, mycophenolate mofetil, and prednisone

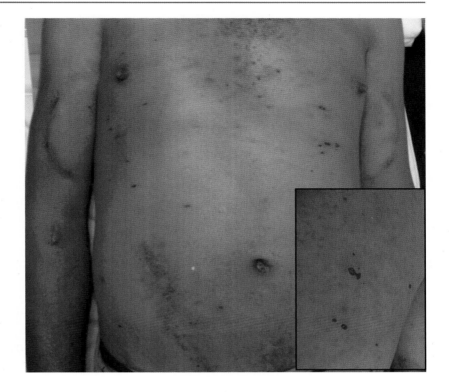

assays. The most rapid, inexpensive, and frequently used diagnostic tool is a cytologic smear (Tzanck smear) taken from the base of a freshly opened vesicle. The collected specimen is typically stained with Giemsa, Wright, or Papanicolaou stain and examined for virally induced cytopathologic features by light microscopy. Although the Tzanck test confirms HSV or VZV infection as the etiology, it cannot differentiate between them. These viral infections share similar cytopathologic features, necessitating immunohistochemical or DFA studies to type the specific virus [37].

Therapeutic Approach

CMV

An increased occurrence of late-onset CMV diseases attributable to prolonged antiviral prophylactic regimens has been seen in solid organ recipients [15].

Prevention of the infection in solid organ recipients includes universal prophylaxis or early therapy considering individual risk factors for the development of CMV infection [38].

Regarding cutaneous manifestations caused by CMV there is no established guideline for treatment, so treatment strategies have been extrapolated from existing successful treatment of solid organ CMV infections and include intravenous ganciclovir and oral valganciclovir [34, 38]. Treatment of the mild or moderate disease consists of oral valganciclovir (900 mg/12 h). Intravenous ganciclovir is reserved for patients with severe disease or in situations where valganciclovir may be inadequately absorbed. The optimal duration of treatment is determined by the clinical and virologic evolution. Weekly determination of viral load or antigenemia should be performed to monitor response to treatment, which must be maintained until viral load decreases or antigenemia is negative. In any case, the minimum duration of treatment should not be less than 14 days [38].

HPV

Treatment strategy for HPV-associated cutaneous and external genital warts depends on the size, location, and grade of the lesion. As cutaneous and external genital warts have very little malignant potential, cosmetics is frequently the main reason for treatment. In immunosuppressed patients, removal of warts may also be necessary because of the development of symptoms such as obstruction (in the case of anogenital warts), itching, and bleeding [36].

Treatment options are categorized as patient or clinician applied. There is no evidence that one modality is superior to the other, and the method chosen should reflect patient and provider preferences [36].

Regarding cutaneous warts, paring down of dead skin using a pumice stone, nail file, emery board, or scalpel is important to maximize the chance of cure. Soaking the affected skin for several minutes prior may help with paring. Products containing salicylic acid, cryotherapy, and imiquimod 5% cream represent the main treatment options. Salicylic acid comes in numerous preparations. It should be used in conjunction with an occlusive dressing such as duct tape that may increase the efficacy of the intervention. Treatment should ideally be continued for 1–2 weeks following the physical removal of the wart so as to minimize the chance of recurrence [36].

Cryotherapy can be performed using liquid nitrogen spray, a liquid nitrogen-soaked swab, or a cryoprobe cooled with nitrous oxide. It can be repeated every 3 weeks and should be a clinician-applied option [36]. Imiquimod 5% cream is a topical immune response modifier that induces cytokines locally without a direct antiviral effect. The usual regimen is to apply it once daily before bedtime, three times a week for up to 16 weeks [36].

For atypically appearing, recalcitrant, and recurrent cases, a biopsy is recommended given the high incidence of skin malignancies in transplant recipients [36].

Patient-applied therapeutic options for condylomata acuminata include imiquimod 5% cream and podofilox 0.5% solution or gel. The usual regimen for imiquimod 5% is to apply it once daily before bedtime, three times a week for up to 16 weeks. Podofilox 0.5% solution or gel arrests the cell cycle in metaphase, leading to cell death.

It should be applied twice daily for 3 days on, 4 days off, with a maximum of four cycles [36].

Dermatologist-applied therapies include cryotherapy, podophyllin resin 25%, and trichloroacetic acid (TCA) 80%. When performing cryotherapy, the freeze margin should extend 2–3 mm beyond the margin of the wart. Cryotherapy can be repeated every 3 weeks. Podophyllin resin 25% in tincture of benzoin is applied to the affected area, left to dry, and washed off after 6 h (maximum 0.5 mL per session). This process can be repeated after 1 week. TCA 80% can be applied to the affected tissue until it appears white or frosted. Multiple cycles of treatment are often needed [36]. Surgical options for the treatment of condyloma acuminata include infrared coagulation, laser surgery, and scissor excision.

The 2009 guidelines issued by the Infectious Diseases Community of Practice of the American Society of Transplantation recommend HPV vaccination before or after transplantation in eligible patients [39].

HSV

Since the cytomegalovirus prophylaxis era began (with drugs such as valganciclovir and ganciclovir), the incidence of HSV reactivation has lowered, nowadays having a 10% frequency [15].

Treatment of disseminated, visceral, or mucosal disease should be conducted with intravenous acyclovir doses of 5–10 mg/kg/8 h. In cases of severe illness the reduction of immunosuppression could also be considered. In limited skin disease, acyclovir, valacyclovir, or famciclovir can be used. In patients who do not respond to acyclovir treatment, resistance to the drug should be suspected, and foscarnet can be used as an alternative. Patients receiving prophylaxis against CMV during the post-transplant period do not require prophylaxis against HSV. When recurrence occurs after the end of treatment, suppressive therapy with antivirals should be considered until the level of immunosuppression can be lowered [37]. Brivudine can also be employed successfully, especially in the setting of renal insufficiency. Adequate clinical experience in organ transplant recipients has not yet been published [15].

VZV

Prevention against CMV used during the early post-transplant period can prevent reactivation of VZV, meaning that no additional prophylaxis is needed during this period. In those patients being evaluated for transplantation who are susceptible to VZV, attenuated Oka virus vaccine should be administered, which has been shown to be safe and effective in patients with advanced kidney disease. This vaccine should be administered at least 2–4 weeks prior to transplantation. Post-transplant vaccination is not recommended for VZV [37]. For children who are to undergo transplantation, prophylactic VZV immunization is strongly recommended [15].

Seronegative recipients who have presented significant exposure to VZV should receive post-exposure prophylaxis. The prophylaxis options for this include passive (VZV immunoglobulin within 96 h after possible exposure) and/or antiviral immunoprophylaxis [15, 37].

Chickenpox treatment is intravenous acyclovir at doses of 10 mg/kg/8 h, which should be initiated as early as possible since earlier initiation leads to greater effectiveness. In cases of serious illness the use of intravenous immunoglobulin can be considered [37].

Herpes zoster can be treated on an outpatient basis with oral acyclovir, valacyclovir, or famciclovir. In cases of ophthalmic or otic involvement, intravenous acyclovir should be used [37]. Especially in patients with renal insufficiency, brivudine has been used successfully as it is metabolized in the liver before renal elimination [15].

Fungal Infections

Despite ongoing refinements in immunosuppressive agents, graft preservation, and surgical techniques, fungal infections remain a significant cause of morbidity and mortality in organ transplant recipients [40]. For practical matters, fungal infections will be classified as systemic, deep cutaneous fungal infections (DCFIs), and superficial.

Systemic fungal infections are associated with very high mortality in recipients [15, 40].

Probably for this reason, in the literature, there are more data on systemic fungal infections than in deep cutaneous and superficial fungal infections, which are mainly of interest to dermatologists.

Etiopathogenesis

Systemic and Deep Cutaneous Fungal Infections

Because of immunosuppression, transplant recipients have a significant risk of invasive fungal disease [41]. The main agents of systemic fungal infections are *Candida* spp., *Aspergillus* spp., and *Cryptococcus neoformans* [11, 15, 40, 41].

Candida species observed in transplant recipients include: *C. albicans*, *C. glabrata*, *C. tropicalis*, *C. parapsilosis*, *C. krusei*, *C. lusitaniae*, *C. rugusa*, *C. kefyr,* and *C. guilliermendii*. *C. albicans* ranks as the most common species with *C. glabrata* and *C. tropicalis* emerging as causative pathogens. *Candida* infections are generally derived from endogenous flora. Conditions that predispose to *Candida* colonization or overgrowth of the hepatobiliary, gastrointestinal, and genitourinary tract can facilitate fungemia and dissemination, especially with mucosal injury or bleeding and surgical manipulation. The frequency of non-*albicans Candida* isolates has increased. Proposed explanations include widespread use of fluconazole in the pre- and post-transplant period, prolonged pretransplant hospitalization and nosocomial acquisition, and the use of broad-spectrum antibiotics [40].

Concerning *Aspergillus*, species of medical importance include *A. fumigatus*, *A. flavus*, *A. niger*, *A. terreus*, *A. nidulans*, *A. glaucus*, *A. ustus*, *A. versicolor*, *A. oryzae*, *A. sydowi*, and *A. chevalieri*. *Aspergillus* infections may include one or more *Aspergillus* species from an individual patient. Lung and liver transplant recipients display the highest risk for invasive *Aspergillus* infection [40].

Aspergillus spores are ubiquitous and are frequently isolated from hospital ventilation systems, especially during periods of construction or renovation; community environmental exposures may also occur. Inhalation of fungal spores is the primary mode of acquiring *Aspergillus*, and the lungs and upper respiratory tract are the most common sites of occurrence. Less commonly, *Aspergillus* from an infected or colonized open wound or surgical drain may pose a risk of airborne transmission to transplant patients housed in an intensive care unit [40].

DCFIs are caused by a variety of mostly tropical organisms, usually when they are implanted into the dermis or the subcutaneous tissue. They are most commonly attributed to traumatic inoculation of the fungi or foreign material containing the fungi into the skin such as thorns, splinters or other soil substrates, vegetation, or animals [42–44]. Agents implicated are *Blastomyces dermatitidis*, *Zygomycetes*, *Alternaria* spp., *Rhizopus* spp., *Fusarium* spp., *Acremonium* spp., and *Pseudoallescheria*, among others [42].

Superficial Fungal Infections

The principal agents involved in superficial fungal infections are *Malassezia* (*Malassezia* spp., *M. furfur*, *M. pachydermatis*) and dermatophytes. *M. furfur* is a dimorphic organism that resides on normal skin and within hair follicles. Dermatophytes include: *Microsporum* (*M. canis*, *M. audouinii*), *Trichophyton* (*T. mentagrophytes*, *T. rubrum*, *T. tonsurans*), and *Epidermophyton* (*E. floccosum*), which represent the etiologic pathogens of dermatophyte infections in recipients. Direct inoculations and traumatic abrasion are the usual routes of entry [40].

Several factors contribute to the high frequency of superficial fungal infections in these patients. This risk depends on factors such as diagnostic criteria, exposure to potentially pathogenic fungi, and geographic, socioeconomic, and hygienic conditions and time of immunosuppression [45]. The failure of cell-mediated immunity and the smaller amount of antigen-presenting Langerhans cells in the epidermis of these patients are essential for the development of infections [46]. Among drugs, corticosteroids in particular cause thickening of the corneal layer and prolong its removal, enabling fungal infections and their chronicity [45, 46].

Clinical Presentation

Systemic and Deep Cutaneous Fungal Infections

Solid organ transplant recipients have a significant risk of invasive fungal diseases (IFD) caused mainly by *Candida* spp. and *Aspergillus* spp., the former being the most frequent agent leading to morbidity and high mortality [11, 15, 41]. The incidence of invasive candidiasis has been estimated at approximately 2% in American adults and pediatric patients. The rate varies according to the organ transplanted: it is particularly high in abdominal solid organ transplants such as intestinal, pancreas, and liver transplantation while it is extremely uncommon after heart transplantation. Most cases of candidiasis occur during the first months after surgery [11, 41]. The main portal of entry is the gastrointestinal tract, followed by endovascular catheters and the urinary tract [41]. By contrast, primary cutaneous fungal infections occur several months after transplantation, have the tendency to progress slowly. and have a benign appearance that leads to a delay in diagnosis [47].

Systemic *Candida* infections can present serious diagnostic problems. In 10–13% of immunosuppressed patients, skin lesions as a result of hematogenous spread were diagnosed and ranged from subcutaneous nodules and pustules up to necrotic plaques [15]. However, the most common clinical forms are mucocutaneous, mainly oropharyngeal, esophageal candidiasis, vulvovaginitis, and wound infections [40, 48].

In general, DCFIs are associated with mortality rates from 4% to 10% in localized infections and can be as high as 83–94% in disseminated disease. Clinical presentation of DCFIs is variable and dependent on host-related factors, the type of fungal organism, and the mode of transmission. Skin lesions are nonspecific and may be misdiagnosed as cutaneous neoplasms or necrotizing lesions caused by coagulation disorders. Pathologic examination and skin tissue cultures are necessary for diagnostic confirmation. In this sense, clinical suspicion is essential [42]. According with González Santiago et al., most common clinical presentations of deep cutaneous fungal infections are encompassed or ulcerated nodules, plaques, ulcers, erythematous macules, and evidence of tissue necrosis [42]. Individual reports exist of cutaneous aspergillosis due to direct inoculation or hematogenous spread. Skin manifestations are often unspecific and present, among others, as hemorrhagic bullae or erythematous plaques [15]. Rarely have cutaneous manifestations of other fungi such as *Cryptococcus neoformans*, *Exophiala jeanselmei*, *Wangiella dermatitidis*, or *Alternaria* species been reported [15].

Phaeohyphomycosis is a rare cutaneous or systemic infection caused by the dematiaceous family of pigmented fungi with several reports in solid organ recipients. Over 100 species have been isolated as etiologic agents, the most common being *Alternaria*, *Curvularia*, *Exserohilum*, and *Bipolaris*. The main route of transmission is traumatic inoculation by thorns, splinters or other soil substrates, vegetation, or animals [43]. Clinical presentation is variable: plaques, nodules, or ulcerative nodules and recurrent cellulitis, commonly in the lower extremities, as well as vegetative or infiltrative lesions. Systemic dissemination with multiple lesions and pulmonary infiltration has also been described [49, 50].

Disseminated histoplasmosis can involve skin and has been described exceptionally as soft-tissue masses and cellulitis [51, 52].

Superficial Fungal Infections

Superficial mycoses are frequently found in transplant recipients [6–8, 16, 17] and can predispose the appearance of deep mycosis [45]. They generally occur 6 months after transplantation[15].

Among the most frequent superficial fungal infections are pityriasis versicolor (*Malassezia* spp.) [8, 17, 29] according to some trials and dermatophytosis according to others [6, 7].

Among 102 organ transplant recipients examined, more than 35% had pityriasis versicolor, followed by mucocutaneous candidiasis (about 25%), onychomycosis (about 13%), and tinea pedis/*Candida* intertrigo (about 12%) [15, 53].

Clinical presentation of cutaneous superficial fungal infection seems to be similar to that in the nonimmunosuppressed host. Non-atypical, more severe, or widespread infections were observed in comparison with controls [5, 46].

Complementary Examinations

Systemic and Deep Cutaneous Fungal Infections

It is essential to develop diagnostic and therapeutic strategies to reduce the mortality attributed to the invasive fungal infections. It is substantial to achieve early accurate diagnosis and elucidate the necessity of establishing prophylactic protocols or not, depending on individual risk factors. To date, blood culture has been the reference procedure for the diagnosis of invasive candidiasis. However, its sensitivity for detecting *Candida* is only 50–75%, and the guidelines for diagnosis and management of *Candida* infections by the European Society of Clinical Microbiology and Infectious Diseases (ESCMID) recommend alternative techniques.

Two serologic diagnostic methods (the combined detection of mannan and antimannan antibodies and the quantification of the 1,3,β-D-glucan) are recommended in the ESCMID guidelines for candidemia detection in adults. PCR-based methods are useful when available [41]. When clinically suspected, an early skin biopsy including direct microscopy and culture of samples should be performed.

For DCFIs, routine histopathologic examination of lesional skin tissue remains the primary confirmatory method. It permits fast, presumptive identification of fungi and can also provide some insight into the diagnostic implication of some culture isolates. Because of the variable and longer turnaround time on tissue culture compared with routine histopathology, the latter is often relied on for the rapid diagnosis of DCFI. However, discrepancies between histopathology and culture results are sometimes seen [42].

Imaging procedures may help in the clinical approach; these include ultrasonography, computed tomography, and magnetic resonance imaging to highlight suspicious lesions for guided biopsies [54].

Superficial Fungal Infections

Although not essential, a laboratory diagnosis is helpful as the clinical diagnosis is not always reliable. The key to diagnosis is the demonstration of the organisms in skin scales, hair, or nails. Scrapings are taken with a scalpel or nail clippers. They are commonly examined in potassium hydroxide and can be cultured on Sabouraud's medium. Skin scales, hair, and nails can be sent to a laboratory folded in a card (transport packs are available). Material from mucosal surfaces is better sent on a moistened swab [55].

Therapeutic Approach

Systemic and Deep Cutaneous Fungal Infections

There are no randomized studies of treatment for invasive or deep fungal infections among solid organ transplant recipients. Treatment should be based on the pathogen recovered as well as on the clinical syndrome and site of involvement, especially taking into account that if the site is accessible, and being possible, surgical removal of the focus is recommended [54].

The drug of choice for the treatment of candidemia is fluconazole (400 mg/day, preceded by initial dose of 800 mg/day). In cases of colonization by *C. glabrata*, prior treatment with azoles or the presence of severe sepsis or septic shock, the initial treatment of choice should be an echinocandin (caspofungin, anidulafungin, and micafungin), which have low toxicity and minor interactions with azoles [38].

Amphotericin B (AmB) deoxycholate has been regarded as the gold standard for therapy, but its administration is often associated with renal toxicity and infusion-related side effects. The lipid-associated amphotericin compounds, mainly the liposomal formulation, have the main advantage of decreasing nephrotoxicity, but there are no data that directly compare these agents with AmB for their efficacy to treat transplant population. The azole antifungal agents have a long-standing role in antifungal therapy. However, their interactions with the cytochrome P450 (CYP) enzyme system produces three- to five-fold increased levels of cyclosporine and tacrolimus in most patients. New antifungal agents currently available require evaluation in solid organ transplant recipients. Drug interactions of a number of antifungal agents with immunosuppressants must be carefully considered when treating these recipients. The triazole agents are potent inhibitors of CYP34A isoenzymes with the potential to increase the levels of calcineurin inhibitors as well as sirolimus and everolimus. Duration of therapy must be individualized according to the fungal pathogen, the resolution of the process, and state of immunosuppression, and be guided by clinical, microbiological, or radiologic means [54].

Superficial Fungal Infections

Topical antifungals (e.g., terbinafine, imidazoles such as clotrimazole) are sufficient in most circumscribed infections including tinea corporis and pityriasis versicolor. The duration of treatment is 1–4 weeks. In the case of widespread lesions of pityriasis versicolor or in patients refractory to topical treatments (ketoconazole ointments and shampoo), oral antifungal therapy may be indicated; in particular fluconazole or itraconazole have been reported to be effective [56]. Nail infections, depending on the implied agent, require systemic treatment with terbinafine, 250 mg daily for 6–12 weeks or itraconazole, 400 mg daily for 1 week every month for at least 3 months [55].

Bacterial Infections

While bacterial extracutaneous infections are of great importance during the immediate posttransplant period [2], pyodermitis are reported with less frequency than the viral and fungal infections, and are mainly folliculitis and, exceptionally, anthrax [6–8, 17, 27].

Ethiopathogenesis

Generally, bacterial infections are the most common ones in tropical and subtropical countries [29].

In the first month after transplantation, perioperative and even nosocomial pathogens predominate. The frequent wound and urinary tract infections of this phase are increasingly being caused by antibiotic-resistant strains (vancomycin-resistant enterococci and methicillin-resistant *Staphylococcus aureus*, MRSA). In a study of 60 liver transplant recipients, 15% demonstrated MRSA on nasal swabs for the first time during inpatient treatment [15, 57].

Clinical Manifestations

Besides observing infections in wounds, the spectrum includes impetigo, folliculitis, abscess, cellulitis, and furuncles [29]. Since the residing bacterial flora is the same in transplant recipient patients as in the general population, causal agents of pyodermitis are the Group A streptococci and *Staphylococcus aureus* [29]. Furthermore, according to Ada et al., screening for nasal *S. aureus* carriage does not seem to assist in preventing staphylococcal bacterial infections in outpatient recipients [58]. The majority of subcutaneous abscesses are caused by staphylococci, and less frequently by Gram-negative bacteria or by a mixed flora. Case reports describe staphylococci following liver transplantation [15, 58].

Complementary Examinations

Isolation of the agent with an antibiogram is essential. Complementary examinations including imaging should be guided by clinical presentation and signs and symptoms of the infection.

Therapeutic Approach

Antibiotic therapy should be oriented on the results of the cultures and antibiogram. For staphylococcal infections, drugs of first choice are sulfonamides such as sulfadiazine and cotrimoxazole or, as an alternative in face of increasing resistance, imipenem/cilastatin combined with amikacin [15]. However, treatment should be individualized according to epidemiology and the bacterial resistance profile of the geographic area.

Other Infections

Numerous nontuberculous *Mycobacterium* (NTM) species can induce cutaneous lesions in solid organ transplant patients. Cutaneous lesions in this patient population characteristically begin as red to violaceous subcutaneous nodules that may be painful or only mildly symptomatic, and may progress to form abscesses or ulcers. Constitutional symptoms are typically absent. Nontuberculous *Mycobacterium* species associated with cutaneous lesions in solid organ transplant patients are *M. kansasii*, *M. marinum*, *M. haemophilum*, *M. fortuitum*, *M. crofulaceum*, *M. chelonae*, *M. avium*, *M. intracellulare*, and *M. abscessus* [59]. Isolation of the agent and directed therapy are essential.

Malignancies and Premalignancies

Skin cancers are more frequently seen in transplanted patients in comparison with the general population, and among them, nonmelanoma skin cancer is the most frequent [60, 61].

Squamous cell carcinomas (SCC) and basal cell carcinomas (BCC) represent over 90% of all the skin cancers in kidney transplant recipients [62].

The risk of developing BCC is proposed to be increased 10–16 times in comparison with the general population. Meanwhile, the risk of developing SCC is about 65–100 times higher in solid organ recipients [6, 60, 61].

Besides its prevalence, SCC in solid organ recipients present themselves more aggressively, with higher morbidity and mortality, and have a risk of metastasis ten times higher than in the general population [60, 63, 64].

Actinic Keratosis and Squamous Cell Carcinoma

Etiopathogenesis

Several risk factors for the development of SCC in transplant recipients can be identified besides those in common with the general population. Advanced age at the time of the transplant is one of the most important clinical predictors of SCC [65, 66]. A larger ultraviolet radiation accumulation before the transplant also implies an increased risk [64–67].

The preferential localization of SCC in photo-exposed areas supports the pathogenic role of ultraviolet radiation, as well as the fact that SCC occurs in areas with extensive actinic damage and epidermal dysplasia known as "field cancerization" [60]. Numerous recent studies that used PCR reported a high prevalence of HPV DNA in skin carcinomas of transplant patients [66]. In fact, immunocompromised patients have 50 times more risk of developing vulvar cancer and 100 times more risk of anal cancer compared with the general population [12]. E6/7 transcripts of HPV 8, 9, and 15 in actinic keratosis (AK) and SCC from these patients have also been found [60].

Having a history of SCC prior to the transplant seems to be one of the strongest predictors of subsequent SCC after transplantation [65, 66].

SCC develops more frequently in patients who have a low Fitzpatrick phototype, blue or light eyes, and male gender, the latter have also been found a factor that does not coincide in all the research studies [10, 64, 65, 68].

With regard to ethnic factors, we must point out the incidence in different populations that live in the same geographic area. In South Africa, SCC was reported only in Caucasian post-transplant patients [69]. The concurrence of factors such as low phototype and living in subtropical areas makes individuals under these conditions particularly susceptible to SCC, as also occurs in Australian non-native residents [64].

However, immunosuppression is the most critical and relevant aspect of transplant recipients in comparison with the general population, which can be explained by a reduction of the anti-tumor surveillance, suggesting that drugs may have an important role in carcinogenesis [70–73].

In addition, duration and level of immunosuppression are well-known risk factors [60].

Several trials suggest that patients who receive therapeutic regimes with three immunosuppressant drugs have more risk of developing skin cancer than patients who receive dual-drug therapy or sirolimus [60].

Azathioprine makes skin more photosensitive to ultraviolet A radiation. Skin DNA of patients with therapeutic doses of azathioprine contains 6-thioguanine, which is capable of accelerating the cutaneous carcinogenesis process [8, 10, 60, 72]. Moreover, maintained immunosuppression with azathioprine has been proved to increase the risk of developing subsequent SCC [74]. In turn, Cyclosporine has been shown to reduce reparation and apoptosis of keratinocytes after ultraviolet B radiation, leading to the accumulation of damaged DNA through inhibition of the mitochondrial permeability transition pore (MPTP) reparation system. The opening of this channel is induced in the presence of oxidative reduction, such as is caused by ultraviolet radiation that leads to cell death. However, in the presence of cyclosporine the damaged cells survive and are capable of initiating the carcinogenesis process [60, 73].

Clinical Presentation

AK is the initial lesion in a disease continuum that progresses to invasive SCC [75] and represents a serious problem in transplant recipients. Among 480 renal transplant recipients, AKs were detected in 54%. However, there have been no studies establishing its true prevalence [61, 62].

The most common clinical presentation of an AK is a red, scaling papule or plaque on a sun-exposed area. It is usually 1–3 mm in diameter, but can be several centimeters in size and numerous or confluent in sun-exposed areas. The surrounding areas may show evidence of sun damage. The scaliness can often be felt before it can be seen, so skin palpation is mandatory [75].

In transplant recipients the AKs clinically appear similarly as they do in the general population, and tend to "gather," which gives way to large areas of "field cancerization" (Fig. 45.7) [61].

The increase in *SCC* frequency among solid organ recipients is well known; its incidence varies

Fig. 45.7 A 66-year-old man, renal transplant 127 months ago, taking cyclosporine A, mycophenolate mofetil, and prednisone. Field of cancerization in the scalp with multiple actinic keratosis. The *arrow* points a basal cell carcinoma

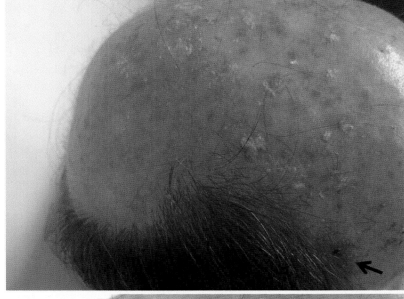

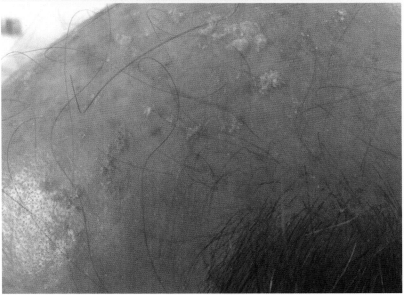

from 1% to 6.5% within the first 5 years after transplant, and from 6% to 35% in the following 10 years [67], reaching between 30% and 70% in kidney transplant recipients depending on the study population [65, 76]. The risk of developing subsequent tumors after the first one has been diagnosed has been less evaluated. A recent trial in New Zealand shows that out of 96 kidney transplant recipients with SCC, practically all developed multiple SCC [77]. Throughout the clinical course, 30% of patients presented a second tumor after the first year, 50% after the second year, 60% after the third year, and 80% after 5 years [77]. Furthermore, a Dutch review confirms this alarming increase in multiple tumor incidence. The authors found a cumulative incidence of a second SCC of 31% after 1 year, 62% after 3 years, and 75% after 5 years [63]. These percentages are clearly high if one takes into account that the cumulative risk of a subsequent SCC is 18% after 3 years in the general population [63, 77, 78].

SCC in solid organ recipients presents more aggressively, with higher morbidity and mortality, and has a risk of metastasis ten times higher than in the general population [60, 63, 64].

Clinically, SCC are characterized by scaling, erythematous skin plaques that initially can be confused with chronic inflammatory dermatitis. Lesions of SCCs are indurated as in immunocompetent patients, and have the characteristic of a slow-growing tumor that is painless, sometimes nodular. This tumor can grow very rapidly in organ transplant recipients, forming exophytic lesions that tend to ulcerate (Fig. 45.8). SCCs are often associated with signs of solar damage, notably elastosis, irregular pigmentation, telangiectasia, and leukokeratosis of the lower lip. However, transplant patients tend to be younger at the time of diagnosis if compared with immunocompetent individuals, and therefore have generally less sun damage [69]. The most common locations for developing SCC in transplant patients are sun-exposed sites, particularly the head and neck, followed by the upper extremity, trunk, and lower extremity. There is an increased incidence of lower trunk and upper extremity SCC compared with immunocompetent patients. The most common sites of SCC in the head and neck region are the scalp and the ear [69].

Contrary to what occurs in the general population where the incidence of BCC surpasses the incidence of SCC, in organ recipients the ratio BCC/SCC is reversed, so that SCC is more frequent than BCC in transplanted patients [10, 60, 67, 69, 79].

The specific mortality attributable to SCC varies between 1.5% and 15% according to different studies, the highest being from Australia. The authors ascribe this increase, among other factors, to the longer follow-up time [63]. Regarding this subject, the most effective measure proposed to decrease SCC morbidity and mortality is exeresis as soon as possible once the tumor is diagnosed [63] (Figs. 45.9 and 45.10).

Complementary Examinations

In general, AKs do not need complementary examinations. When suspected, in areas of field of cancerization, an early biopsy should be performed in order to exclude SCC [74].

Several imaging studies might be needed depending on the size and extension of the tumor. For deep tumors in high-risk areas, consider computed tomography/magnetic resonance imaging scans to evaluate deep extension or nodal involvement [74].

Therapeutic Approach

Treatment of AK and, therefore, the field cancerization is of vital importance, mainly if we take into account that while evolution of AK toward invasive carcinomas among nonimmunosup-

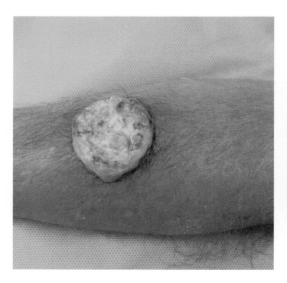

Fig. 45.8 A 78-year-old man, renal transplant 89 months ago, taking cyclosporine A, mycophenolate mofetil, and prednisone. Squamous cell carcinoma in the forearm

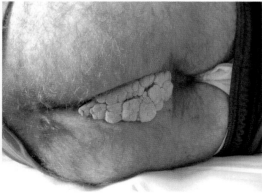

Fig. 45.9 A 35-year-old man, renal transplant 68 months ago, taking cyclosporine A, mycophenolate mofetil, and prednisone. Anal low-grade squamous cell carcinoma (Buschke–Lowenstein tumor)

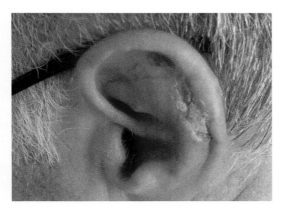

Fig. 45.10 A 65-year-old man, renal transplant 185 months ago, taking cyclosporine A, mycophenolate mofetil, and prednisone. Left helix squamous cell carcinoma

pressed patients is 10%, among transplant recipients this percentage rises to 30% [73].

Among possible treatments of field cancerization, the most tested therapies are photodynamic therapy [59] and systemic retinoids. Patients treated with acitretin at 30 mg/day for 6 months presented a decreased incidence of SCC de novo [80]. Isolated AKs can be treated with classic medical or surgical methods such as cryotherapy. Managing transplant recipients with SCC is a challenge and requires a multidisciplinary approach. The lack of dermatologic control in recipient patients results in a low level of awareness of the problem and incorrect photoprotection, which results in an increased frequency of carcinoma. The appearance of this type of tumoral lesion is an indication for Mohs micrographic surgery if available, and a revision of immunosuppression [74, 81].

Ulrich et al. even proposed to biopsy the sentinel lymph node and to perform systemic therapy with retinoids in patients with clinically or histologically aggressive lesions [82].

Basal Cell Carcinoma

BCC is ten times more frequent in organ transplant recipients than in the general population [83].

Etiopathogenesis

A probable relationship between the occurrence of BCC and HLA DR I allele positivity was explored and confirmed in a Brazilian cohort of transplant recipients by de Carvalho et al. [84].

In addition, PTCH1 haplotypes containing certain alleles were shown to be associated with an increased BCC risk in an Italian population of organ transplant recipients. As in the case of SCC, more research to achieve early identification of individuals at high risk of developing cutaneous cancer after transplantation are needed. This would contribute to the adoption of targeted prevention strategies [83].

Clinical Presentation

In a series of retrospective cases where kidney transplant recipients with BCC were compared with controls, the BCC on the transplant recipients were observed to be more superficial, thinner, and pauci-inflammatory. Lesions were multifocal but without a tendency to metastasize or recur, and the average time for the development of such tumors was 10.5 years [85].

Clinical presentation seems to be similar to that in the general population, but specific studies about the clinical presentation are needed.

The cumulative incidence in renal transplant recipients for a second BCC is lower: 16% 1 year later, 37% after 3 years, and 51% after 5 years [62]. Around 50% of BCC are located on the head and neck, and in those cases where the BCC were multiple and subsequent they were located preferably on the trunk [63].

Complementary Examinations

A biopsy should be performed to confirm diagnosis. Since BBC has a low tendency to metastasize, imaging examinations are not necessary in most cases.

Therapeutic Approach

BCC developing under immunosuppression is generally no more aggressive than in immunocompetent persons, and should be treated surgically if possible [82].

Melanoma

Solid organ recipients have a two- to eight-fold increased risk of developing melanoma compared with the general population, with an average time for its development of 5 years after transplantation [86–89]. However, these data are controversial, since other trials assert that the risk is similar to that for nonrecipient subjects [69].

Hollenbeak et al. published one of the largest trials related to this subject with a total of 89,786 kidney transplant patients between 1988 and 1998. These authors found an increased risk of developing melanoma of 3.6-fold [88].

Etiopathogenesis

Risk factors for melanoma in organ transplant recipients are similar to those in the general population: the presence of multiple nevi (also associated with immunosuppression) and fair complexion, family and personal history of melanoma, and exposure to ultraviolet radiation [90].

The immune system appears to play a role in melanocyte biology, and although the role of immunosuppression in melanoma requires additional study, several studies favor melanocyte proliferation. On a molecular level, a potential role for BRAF gene mutation in both benign nevi and melanoma in organ transplant recipients has been studied, and although preliminary evidence seems to suggest a lower frequency of BRAF mutations in organ transplant recipients, the role of immunosuppression in melanocyte biology remains of interest [60].

Clinical Presentation

There are no studies evaluating clinical characteristics of melanoma in transplant recipients.

The ABCD(E) mnemonic of melanoma has been a cornerstone of public health messaging for the community and physicians to help detect early melanomas. Following this rule, melanomas are characterized by A: *asymmetry*, B: irregular or poorly defined *border*, C: *color* variation from one area to another and different shades of tan, D: *diameter* greater than 6 mm, and E: *evolution* implying changes in size, color, or shape [91].

High-quality evidence suggests that dermoscopy (a noninvasive diagnostic technique for the in vivo observation of pigmented skin lesions performed with a dermoscope) is both more sensitive

and more specific in classifying lesions as melanoma versus nonmelanoma than clinical examination with the naked eye alone [92]. Clinical and dermoscopic characteristics of melanoma are discussed in other chapters and are beyond the scope of this discussion.

Complementary Examinations

The earlier a melanoma is diagnosed and removed, the more likely is a cure for the patient. For this reason, if melanoma is suspected an early excisional biopsy should be performed. The remaining complementary examinations are essential for staging the tumor, and depend mainly on the clinical evaluation and the Breslow thickness in local stages.

Therapeutic Approach

Following a histologic diagnosis, the management of primary cutaneous melanoma is wide local excision with an appropriate clinical margin to minimize the risk of local recurrence and achieve histologic confirmation and accurate local staging while optimizing functional and cosmetic outcomes. The extent of the clinical resection is based on the Breslow thickness of the lesion [93].

In a recent study, melanoma-specific mortality in transplant recipients was elevated three-fold compared with nonrecipients, suggesting that melanoma behaves aggressively under transplant-related immunosuppression [90].

For transplant recipients who develop melanoma, physicians should perform an appropriate staging evaluation, including, if necessary, assessment of lymph node involvement and other distant spread. Along with surgery directed at the primary tumor, treatment should incorporate reduction or revision of immunosuppression, to the extent possible, to facilitate immunologic control of the tumor [90].

Regarding the opportunity for transplant in patients who have presented with melanoma, it is proposed that for patients with a history of melanoma in situ the transplant should not be delayed. In patients with a history of melanoma of Breslow thickness <1 mm and with a negative sentinel lymph node, a 2-year waiting period is recommended in order to control recurrences or metastasis before the transplant. In patients with melanoma of Breslow thickness >2 mm it is advised to wait 5 years before the transplant because of the great risk of recurrence that exists and the uncertain behavior of melanoma against an immunosuppression background. Lastly, patients who have a melanoma with lymph node invasion or metastatic disease are not candidates to receive a transplant [61].

Concerning other malignancies, it is important to point out the larger incidence of KS in solid organ recipients. The risk of developing this neoplasia is thought to be up to 500 times larger in recipient patients than in the general population [2, 61, 93]. The association between human herpesvirus 8 (HHV-8) and KS is evident in transplant patients, although doubt remains over whether this tumor is produced by reactivation of the virus, as a consequence of immunosuppression, or due to a primary infection transmitted by the transplanted organ [94, 95]. The fact that this virus has a larger prevalence in certain geographic areas such as the Mediterranean and Africa implies a larger frequency of KS in recipients coming from these regions. In fact, seven cases of KS were observed in 175 kidney transplant recipients in central and southern Italy, in a 10-year follow-up, with a 14.8% seropositivity for HHV-8 in that population [94].

Contrary to these results, in a total of 3815 solid organ transplants performed over 26 years, only five patients with KS were identified, representing 0.1%, in a central European population where the HHV-8 prevalence is lower [93].

Approximately 23% of seropositive patients at the time of the transplant will develop KS during the following 3 post-transplant years on a standard immunosuppressant regime [96].

KS tends to be more aggressive in kidney transplant recipients. The risk of visceral compromise is related to the transplanted organ and/or the degree of immunosuppression, representing between 25% and 30% among kidney transplant recipients [61].

Since the course of KS depends on the level of immunosuppression, the treatment cornerstone is to taper down immunosuppressive regimens to the lowest possible level associated with lesion regression. Specific local or, less frequently, systemic treatment modalities can be used, such as chemotherapy. Recently, mTOR inhibitors have proved effective in the treatment of KS among kidney recipients. Despite these favorable results, more research on this topic is necessary [97, 98].

Side Effects of Immunosuppressant Drugs

The side effects of immunosuppressant drugs (SEID) comprise dermatoses highly frequent in kidney transplant recipients, and it is estimated that those related to the Cushing syndrome are present in 55–90% of the recipients [17], the latter being specifically related to worse quality of life [7].

Most studies agree that SEID occur more frequently during the first post-transplant stage, and are therefore related to a high immunosuppression charge and tend to reduce as time passes [17, 27].

The most frequently mentioned SEID are acneiform reactions, gingival hyperplasia, striae, skin hyperpigmentation, hirsutism, purpura, and ecchymosis [7, 8, 17, 27].

Glossary

Antibiogram A record of the susceptibility of specific pathogenic bacteria to antibiotics. Antibiograms are often taken into account to define a rational selection of an antimicrobial therapy.

Antimetabolites Drugs that interfere with one or more enzymes or their reactions that are necessary for DNA synthesis. They affect DNA synthesis by acting as a substitute for the actual metabolites that would be used in the normal metabolism.

Calcineurin inhibitors Suppress the immune system by preventing interleukin-2 (IL-2) production in T cells.

Cryotherapy Treatment using low temperature for the removal of some skin lesions by freezing them. The most common product used by doctors is liquid nitrogen.

Mohs micrographic surgery
Microscopically controlled surgery used to treat common types of skin cancer. During the surgery, after each removal of tissue and while the patient waits, the tissue is examined for cancer cells. This examination informs the decision for additional tissue removal. Mohs surgery is one of the many methods of obtaining complete margin control during removal of a skin cancer.

mTOR inhibitors mTOR inhibitors are a class of drugs that inhibit the mTOR, which is a serine/threonine-specific protein kinase belonging to the family of phosphatidylinositol 3-kinase (PI3K)-related kinases (PIKKs). mTOR regulates cellular metabolism, growth, and proliferation.

References

1. Ministerio de sanidad, servicios sociales e igualdad. Gobierno de España [Internet]. Available from: http://www.msssi.gob.es.
2. La Forgia MP. Manifestaciones cutáneas en receptores de órganos sólidos. Dermatol Argent. 2006;11:94–105.
3. Vincent M, Parrott N, Lamerton E. Shared care guideline for immunosuppression after kidney and pancreas transplantation. Central Manchester University Hospitals. Available from: www.nyrdtc.nhs.uk. Consulted: 22nd May 2014.
4. Shahidi S, Moeinzadeh F, Mohammadi M, Gholamrezaei A. Sirolimus-based immunosuppression for treatment of cutaneous warts in kidney transplant recipients. IJKD. 2011;5:351–3.
5. Dufrechou L, Nin M, Curi L, Larre Borges P, Martínez Asuaga M, Noboa O, et al. Clinical spectrum of cutaneous manifestations in renal and renopancreatic recipients in two centers in Uruguay. Transplant Proc. 2014;46:3047–9.
6. Formicone F, Fargnoli MC, Pisani F, Rascente M, Famulari A, Peris K. Cutaneous manifestations in italian kidney transplant recipients. Transplant Proc. 2005;37:2527–8.
7. Sandoval M, Ortiz M, Díaz C, Majerson D, Molgó M. Cutaneous manifestations in renal transplant recipients of Santiago, Chile. Transplant Proc. 2009;41:3752–4.
8. Dufrechou L, Larre Borges A, Nin M, Curi L, González F, Martínez M, et al. Cutaneous manifestations in 100 renal and renopancreatic recipients of Uruguay. Transplant Proc. 2011;43:3377–9.
9. Moloney FJ, Keane D, O'Kelly P, Conlon PJ, Murphy PM. The impact of skin disease following renal transplantation on quality of life. Br J Dermatol. 2005;153:574–8.
10. DePry JL, Reed KB, Cook-Norris RH, Brewer JD. Iatrogenic immunosuppression and cutaneous malignancy. Clin Dermatol. 2011;29:602–13.
11. Quindós G. Candidiasis. Candidiasis, aspergilosis y otras micosis invasoras en receptores de trasplante de órgano sólido. Rev Iberoam Micol. 2011;28(3):110–9.
12. Hinten F, Meeuwis KAP, van Rossum MM, de Hullu JA. HPV-related (pre) malignancies of the female anogenital tract in renal transplant recipients. Crit Rev Oncol/Hematol. 2012;84:161–80.
13. Sitek JC1, Tangeraas T, Bjerre A, Helsing P. The prevalence of skin disorders in Norwegian paediatric renal transplant recipients. Acta Derm Venereol. 2014;94(4):421–4.
14. Netchiporouk E, Tchervenkov J, Paraskevas S, Sasseville D, Billick R. Evaluation of herpes simplex virus infection morbidity and mortality in pancreas and kidney-pancreas transplant recipients. Transplant Proc. 2013;45(9):3343–7.
15. Ulrich C, Hackethal M, Meyer T, Geusau A, Nindl I, Ulrich M, et al. Skin infections in organ transplant recipients. J Dtsch Dermatol Ges. 2008;6(2):98–104.
16. Lugo-Jener G, Sánchez JL, Santiago-Depin E. Prevalence and clinical spectrum of skin diseases in kidney transplant recipients. J Am Acad Dermatol. 1991;24:410–141.
17. Alper S, Kilinc I, Duman S, Toz H, Ceylan C, Unal I, et al. Skin diseases in Turkish renal transplant recipients. Inter J Dermatol. 2005;44:939–41.
18. Valdez-Ortiz R, Sifuentes-Osornio J, Morales-Buenrostro LE, Ayala-Palma H, Dehesa-Lopez E, Alberu J, et al. Risk factors for infections requiring hospitalization in renal transplant recipients: a cohort study. Int J Infect Dis. 2011;15:188–96.
19. Iwami D, Ogawa Y, Fujita H, Morita K, Sasaki H, Oishi Y et al. Successful treatment with foscarnet for ganciclovir-resistant cytomegalovirus infection in a kidney transplant recipient: a case report. Nephrology. 2016;21(Suppl 1):63–66.
20. Eid AJ, Razonable RR. New developments in the management of cytomegalovirus infection after solid organ transplantation. Drugs. 2010;70(8):965–81.
21. Trimarchi H, Casas G, Jordan R, Martinez J, Schropp J, Freixas EA, et al. Cytomegalovirus maculopapular eruption in a kidney transplant patient. Transpl Infect Dis. 2001;3(1):47–50.
22. Gaiser MR, Textor S, Senger T, Schadlich L, Waterboer T, Kaufmann AM, et al. Evaluation of specific humoral and cellular immune responses against the major capsid L1 protein of cutaneous wart-associated alpha-Papillomaviruses in solid organ transplant recipients. J Dermatol Sci. 2015;77:37–45.
23. Carratalà J, Montejo M, Pérez-Romero P. Infections caused by herpes viruses other than cytomegalovirus in solid organ transplant recipients. Enferm Infecc Microbiol Clin. 2012;30(2):63–9.
24. Moscarelli L, Zanazzi M, Rosso G, Farsetti S, Caroti L, Annunziata F, et al. Can skin be the first site of CMV involvement preceding a systematic infection in a renal transplant recipient? NDT Plus. 2011;4:53–5.

25. Schmook T, Nindl I, Ulrich C, Meyer T, Sterry W, Stockfleth E. Viral warts in organ transplant recipients: new aspects in therapy. Br J Dermatol. 2003;149(66):20–4.

26. Martelli-Marzagão F, Santos Junior GF, Ogawa MM, Enokihara MM, Porro AM, Tomimori J. Human papillomavirus detected in viral warts of renal transplant recipients. Transpl Infect Dis. 2016;18(1):37–43.

27. Garay I, Ruiz Lascano A, Ducasse C, Kurpis M, Boccardo G, Massari P. Manifestaciones cutáneas en pacientes receptores de trasplante renal. Dermatol Argent. 2003;9(5):275–83.

28. Tarvade SM, Shahapurkar A, Dedhia NM, Bichu S. Herpes zoster in renal transplant recipient – case report and review of the literature. Indian J Nephrol. 2005;15:245–7.

29. Prakash J, Singh S, Prashant GK, Kar B, Tripathi K, Singh PB. Mucocutaneous lesions in transplant recipient in a tropical country. Transplant Proc. 2004;36:2162–4.

30. Mustapić Ž, Bašić-Jukić N, Kes P, Lovčić V, Bubić-Filipi L, Mokos I, et al. Varicella zoster infection in renal transplant recipients: prevalence, complications and outcome. Kidney Blood Press Res. 2011;34:382–6.

31. Arness T, Pedersen R, Dierkhising R, Kremers W, Patel R. Varicella zoster virus-associated disease in adult kidney transplant recipients: incidence and risk-factor analysis. Transpl Infect Dis. 2008;10(4):260–8.

32. Jantsch J, Schmidt B, Bardutzky J, Bogdan C, Eckardt KU, Raff U. Lethal varicella-zoster virus reactivation without skin lesions following renal transplantation. Nephrol Dial Transplant. 2011;26(1):365–8.

33. Toome BK, Bowers KE, Scott GA. Diagnosis of cutaneous cytomegalovirus infection: a review and report of a case. J Am Acad Dermatol. 1991;24:860–7.

34. Guo RF, Gebreab FH, Hsiang-Ho Tang E, Piao Z, Lee SS, Perez ML. Cutaneous ulcer as leading symptom of systemic cytomegalovirus infection. Case Rep Infect Dis. 2015;2015:723962.

35. Ljubojevic S, Skerlev M. HPV-associated diseases. Clin Dermatol. 2014;32:227–34.

36. Chin-Hong PV, Lough JB, Robles JA. Human papillomavirus in transplant recipients. Infectious disease antimicrobial agents. Available from: http://www.antimicrobe.org/new/t18_dw.html.

37. Fatahzadeh M, Schwartz RA. Human herpes simplex virus infections: epidemiology, pathogenesis, symptomatology, diagnosis, and management. J Am Acad Dermatol. 2007;57:737–63.

38. Castón JJ, López-Oliva MO, Torre-Cisneros J, Del Castillo D, editors. Infecciones en el trasplante renal. [updated 2015, cited 2016 March 10]. Available from: http://nefrologiadigital.revistanefrologia.com/es-monografias-nefrologia-dia-pdf-monografia-64.

39. Danzinger-Isakov L, Kumar D. Guidelines for vaccination of solid organ transplant candidates and recipients. Am J Transplant. 2009;9(Suppl 4):S258–62.

40. Fungal infections. Am J Transplant. 2004;4(Suppl 10):110–34.

41. Gavaldà J, Meije Y, Fortún J, Roilides E, Saliba F, Lortholary O, et al. ESCMID study group for infections in compromised hosts. Invasive fungal infections in solid organ transplant recipients. Clin Microbiol Infect. 2014;20(Suppl 7):27–48.

42. Gonzalez Santiago TM, Pritt B, Gibson LE, Comfere NI. Diagnosis of deep cutaneous fungal infections: correlation between skin tissue culture and histopathology. J Am Acad Dermatol. 2014;71(2):293–301.

43. Salido-Vallejo R, Linares-Sicilia MJ, Garnacho-Saucedo G, Sánchez-Frías M, Solís-Cuesta F, Gené J, et al. Subcutaneous phaeohyphomycosis due to Alternaria infectoria in a renal transplant patient: surgical treatment with no long-term relapse. Rev Iberoam Micol. 2014;31(2):149–51.

44. Pang KR, Wu JJ, Huang DB, Tyring SK. Subcutaneous fungal infections. Dermatol Ther. 2004;17(6):523–31.

45. Vettorato G, Carvalho AVE, Lecompte SM, Trez EG, Garcia VD. Frequency of infectious dermatosis in 208 renal transplant recipients. An Bras Dermatol. 2003;78:283–8.

46. Imko-Walczuka BB, Predotaa A, Okuniewskaa A, Jaskiewiczc J, Zegarskad B, Placeke W, et al. Superficial fungal infections in renal transplant recipients. Transplant Proc. 2014;46:2738–42.

47. Miele PS, Levy CS, Smith MA, Dugan EM, Cooke RH, Light JA, et al. Primary cutaneous fungal infections in solid organ transplantation: a cases series. Am J Transplant. 2002;2:678–83.

48. Fortúna J, Ruiz I, Martín-Dávila P, Cuenca-Estrella M. Fungal infection in solid organ recipients. Enferm Infecc Microbiol Clin. 2012;30(2):49–56.

49. Gilaberte M, Bartralot R, Torres JM, Sánchez Reus F, Rodríguez V, Alomar A, et al. Cutaneous alternariosis in transplant recipients: clinicopathologic review of 9 cases. J Am Acad Dermatol. 2005;52:653–9.

50. Ogawa M, Reis V, Godoy P, Gatti de Menezes F, Enokihara M, Tomimori J. Phaeohyphomycosis caused by Colletotrichum gloeosporioides and Alternaría infectoria in renal transplant recipient. Rev Chil Infectol. 2014;31(4):468–72.

51. Koo HL, Hamill RJ, Gentry LO. Disseminated histoplasmosis manifesting as a soft-tissue chest wall mass in a heart transplant recipient. Transpl Infect Dis. 2008;10:351–3.

52. McGuinn ML, Lawrence ME, Proia L, Segreti J. Progressive disseminated histoplasmosis presenting as cellulitis in a renal transplant recipient. Transplant Proc. 2005;37:4313–4.

53. Gulec AT, Demirbilek M, Seckin D, Can F, Saray Y, Sarifakioglu E, et al. Superficial fungal infections in 102 renal transplant recipients: a case-control study. J Am Acad Dermatol. 2003;49:187–92.

54. Grossi PA, Gasperina DD, Barchiesi F, Biancofiore G, Carafiello G, De Gasperi A, et al. Italian guidelines for diagnosis, prevention, and treatment of invasive fungal infections in solid organ transplant recipients. Transplant Proc. 2011;43(6):2463–71.

55. Hay R. Superficial fungal infections. Medicine (Abingdon 1995, UK ed Print). 2013;41(12):716–8. Available from: 10.1016/j.mpmed.2013.09.011

56. Pedrosa AF, Lisboa C, Gonçalves RA. Malassezia infections: a medical conundrum. J Am Acad Dermatol. 2014;71:170–6.

57. Santoro-Lopes G, de Gouvêa EF, Monteiro RC, Branco RC, Rocco JR, Halpern M, et al. Colonization with methicillin-resistant *Staphylococcus aureus* after liver transplantation. Liver Transpl. 2005;11(2):203–9.

58. Ada S, Seckin D, Azap O, Budakoglu I, Haberal M. Prevalence of cutaneous bacterial infections and nasal carriage of *Staphylococcus aureus* in recipients of renal transplants. Clin Exp Dermatol. 2008;34:156–60.

59. Nathan DL, Singh S, Kestenbaum TM, Casparian JM. Cutaneous mycobacterium chelonae in a liver transplant patient. J Am Acad Dermatol. 2000;43:333–6.

60. Zwald FO, Brown M. Skin cancer in solid organ transplant recipients: advances in therapy and management: part I. Epidemiology of skin cancer in solid organ transplant recipients. J Am Acad Dermatol. 2011;65(2):253–61.

61. Stoff B, Salisbury C, Parkerc D, Zwald FO. Dermato pathology of skin cancer in solid organ transplant recipients. Transplant Rev. 2010;24:172–89.

62. Proby C, Harwood C. Porokeratosis in organ transplantation recipients. In: Otley CC, Stasko T, editors. Skin disease in organ transplantation. New York: Cambridge University Press; 2008. p. 119–21.

63. Wisgerhof HC, Edelbrack JRJ, de Fijter JW, Haasnoot GW, Claas FHJ, Willenze R, et al. Subsequent squamous- and basal-cell carcinomas in kidney transplant recipients after the first skin cancer: cumulative incidence and risk factor. Transplantation. 2010;89:1231–8.

64. Ramsay H, Harden P, Reece S. Polymorphisms in glutathione S-transferases are associated with altered risk of nonmelanoma skin cancer in renal transplant recipients: a preliminary analysis. J Invest Dermatol. 2001;117:251–5.

65. Garg S, Carroll RP, Walker RG, Ramsay HM, Harden PN, Garg S. Skin cancer surveillance in renal transplant recipients: re-evaluation of U.K. practice and comparison with Australian experience. Br J Dermatol. 2009;160:177–9.

66. Ho WL, Murphy GM. Update on the pathogenesis of post-transplant skin cancer in renal transplant recipients. Br J Dermatol. 2008;158:217–24.

67. Queille S, Luron L, Spatz A, Avril MF, Ribrag V, Duvillard P, et al. Analysis of skin cancer risk factors in immunosuppressed renal transplant patients shows high levels of UV specific tandem CC to TT mutations of the p53 gene. Carcinogenesis. 2007;28(3):724–31.

68. Basset-Ségui N, Renaud-Vilmer C, Verola O. Carcinomas Espinocelulares. In: Encilcopedié Medico Chirurgicale. Paris: Editions Scientifiques et Medicales Elservier SAS; 2003. p. 98–625. -A-10.

69. Belloni Fortina A, Piaserico S, Alaibac M, Peserico A. Squamous cell carcinoma. In: Rosen T, editor. Skin cancer after organ transplantation. The SCOPE Collaborative Group (Eds) Springer Science Bussiness Media LLC; 2009, p. 241–61.

70. Martelli-Marzagão F, Yamashiro AS, Ogawa MM, Santos GF Jr, Tomimori J, Porro AM. Clinical and histopathologic characterization and typing of the human papillomavirus in common warts of kidney transplant recipients. An Bras Dermatol. 2010;85(5):743–6.

71. Thoms KM, Kuschal C, Oetjen E, Mori T, Kobayashi N, Laspe P, Boeckmann L, et al. Cyclosporin A, but not everolimus, inhibits DNA repair mediated by calcineurin: implications for tumorigenesis under immunosuppression. Exp Dermatol. 2010;20:232–6.

72. Athar M, Walsh SB, Kopelovich L, Elmets CA. Pathogenesis of nonmelanoma skin cancer in organ transplant recipients. Arch Biochem Biophys. 2011;508:159–63.

73. Norman KG, Canter JA, Shi M, Milne GL, Morrow JD, Sligh JE. Cyclosporine A suppresses keratinocyte cell death through MPTP inhibition in a model for skin cancer in organ transplant recipients. Mitochondrion. 2010;10(2):94–101.

74. Zwald FO, Brown M. Skin cancer in solid organ transplant recipients: advances in therapy and management. Part II: management of skin cancer in solid organ transplant recipients. J Am Acad Dermatol. 2011;65:263–79.

75. Moy RL. Clinical presentation of actinic keratosis and squamous cell carcinoma. J Am Acad Dermatol. 2000;42(1 Pt 2):8–10.

76. Dapprich DC, Weenig RH, Rohlinger AL, Weaver AL, Quan KK, Keeling JH, et al. Outcomes of melanoma in recipients of solid organ transplant. J Am Acad Dermatol. 2008;59:405–17.

77. Mackenzie KA, Wells JE, Lynn KL. First and subsequent nonmelanoma skin cancers: incidence and predictors in a population of New Zealand renal transplant recipients. Nephrol Dial Transplant. 2010;25:300.

78. Marcil I, Stern RS. Risk of developing a subsequent nonmelanoma skin cancer in patients with a history of nonmelanoma skin cancer: a critical review of the literature and meta–analysis. Arch Dermatol. 2000;136:1524.

79. Jensen P, Hansen S, Moller B. Skin cancer in kidney and heart transplant recipients and different long-term immunosuppressive therapy regimens. J Am Acad Dermatol. 2000;40:177–86.

80. Bavinck JN, Tieben LM, Van der Woude F, Tegzess AM, Hermans J, ter Schegget J, et al. Prevention of skin cancer and reduction of keratotic skin lesions during acitretin therapy in renal transplant recipients: a double-blind, placebo-controlled study. J Clin Oncol. 1995;13:1933–8.

81. Stasko T, Brown MD, Carucci JA, Euvrard S, Johnson TM, Sengelmann RD, et al. Guidelines for the management of squamous cell carcinoma in organ transplant recipients. Dermatol Surg. 2004;30:642–50.

82. Ulrich C, Arnold R, Frei U, Hetzer R, Neuhaus P, Stockfleth E. Skin changes following transplantation: an interdisciplinary challenge. Dtsch Arztebl Int. 2014;111(11):188–94.

83. Begnini A, Tessari G, Turco A, Malerba G, Naldi L, Gotti E, et al. PTCH1 gene haplotype association with basal cell carcinoma after transplantation. Br J Dermatol. 2010;163(2):364–70.

84. de Carvalho AVE, Bonamigo RR, da Silva CM, De Zorzi Pinto AC. Positivity for HLA DR1 is

associated with basal cell carcinoma in renal transplant patients in southern Brazil. Int J Dermatol. 2012;51:1448–53.

85. Harwood CA, Proby CM, McGregor JM, Sheaff MT, Leigh IM, Cerio R. Clinicopathologic features of skin cancer in organ transplant recipients: a retrospective case-control series. J Am Acad Dermatol. 2006;54:290–300.

86. Le Mire L, Hollowood K, Gray D, Bordea C, Wojnarowska F. Melanomas in renal transplant recipients. Br J Dermatol. 2006;154(3):472–7.

87. Euvrard S, Kanitakis J, Claudy A. Skin cancers after organ transplantation. N Engl J Med. 2003;348(17):1681–91.

88. Hollenbeak CS, Todd MM, Billingsley EM, Harper G, Dyer AM, Lengerich EJ. Increased incidence of melanoma in renal transplant recipients. Cancer. 2005;104:1962–7.

89. Kasiske BL, Snyder JJ, Gilbertson DT, Wang C. Cancer after kidney transplantation in the United States. Am J Transplant. 2004;4:905–13.

90. Robbins HA, Clarke CA, Arron ST, Tatalovich Z, Kahn AR, Hernandez BR, et al. Melanoma risk and survival among organ transplant recipients. J Investig Dermatol. 2015;135:2657–65.

91. Tsao H, Olazagasti JM, Cordoro KM, Brewer JD, Taylor SC, Bordeaux JS, et al. Early detection of melanoma: reviewing the ABCDEs. J Am Acad Dermatol. 2015;72:717–23.

92. Melanoma: Assessment and Management. National Collaborating Centre for Cancer (UK). London: National Institute for Health and Care Excellence (UK) 2015. National Institute for Health and Care Excellence: Clinical Guidelines. Available from: http://www.ncbi.nlm.nih.gov/.

93. Boeckle E, Boesmueller C, Wiesmayr S, Mark W, Rieger M, Tabarelli D, et al. Kaposi sarcoma in solid organ transplant recipients: a single center report. Transplant Proc. 2005;37:1905–9.

94. Cattani P, Capuano M, Graffeo R, Ricci R, Cerimele F, Cerimele D, et al. Kaposi's sarcoma associated with previous human herpesvirus 8 infection in kidney transplant recipients. J Clin Microbiol. 2001;39(2):506–8.

95. Barozzi P, Luppi M, Facchetti F, Mecucci C, Alù M, Sarid R, et al. Post-transplant Kaposi sarcoma from the seeding of donor derived progenitors. Nat Med. 2003;9:554–61.

96. Frances C, Mouquet C, Marcelin AG, Barete S, Agher R, Charron D, et al. Outcome of kidney transplant recipients with previous human herpesvirus-8 infection. Transplantation. 2000;69(9):1776–9.

97. Campistol JM, Cuervas-Mons V, Manitoc N, Almenar L, Arias M, Casafont F. New concepts and best practices for management of pre– and post-transplantation cancer. Transplant Rev. 2012;26:261–79.

98. Detroyer D, Deraedt K, Schöffski P, Hauben E, Lagrou K, Naesens M, et al. Resolution of diffuse skin and systemic Kaposi's sarcoma in a renal transplant recipient after introduction of everolimus: a case report. Transpl Infect Dis. 2015;17(2):303–7.

Further Information Can Be Found at the Following Internet Addresses

Committee for the Care of Immunosuppressed Patients of the Dermatologic Oncology Working Group: www.ado-homepage.de.

German Transplantation Society (Deutsche Transplantationsgesellschaft e.V., DTG): www.d-t-g-online.de.

German network of dermatologists in private practice specializing in the care of organ-transplant recipients (the ONKODERM e.V. network): www.onkoderm.de.

German Dialysis and Renal Transplantation Board (Kuratorium für Dialyse und Nierentransplantation e.V., KfH): www.kfh-dialyse.de/kfh/index.html.

German Association of Organ-Transplant Recipients (Bundesverband der Organtransplantierten e.V., BDO): www.bdo-ev.de.

German Working Group for Nursing Care in Transplantation (Arbeitskreis AKTX-Pflege e.V.): www.aktxpflege.de.

Skin Care in Organ Transplant Patients Network, Europe: www.SCOPEnetwork.org.

Paraneoplasias

46

Fernanda Razera and Renan Rangel Bonamigo

Key Points
- Paraneoplastic diseases are not directly related to the invasion of the primary tumor or its metastases
- Dermatologic lesions are the second most common form of paraneoplastic syndrome
- They may be the first manifestation of the neoplasia, enabling an earlier diagnosis of the tumor; and may improve the prognosis and help monitor its recurrence
- There is a wide variety of clinical presentation of paraneoplastic dermatoses
- It is important to know the dermatoses with possible association with malignant neoplastic diseases and to conduct appropriate clinical investigation of the patient

F. Razera (✉)
Private office, Rua Regente, 245/504,
Porto Alegre, Brazil
e-mail: ferazera@gmail.com

R.R. Bonamigo, MD, MSc, PhD
Dermatology Service, Hospital de Clínicas de Porto Alegre (HCPA), Federal University of Rio Grande do Sul (UFRGS), Porto Alegre, Brazil

Sanitary Dermatology Service of the Department of Health of Rio Grande do Sul State (ADS-SES), Porto Alegre, Brazil

Graduate Pathology Program of Federal University of Health Sciences of Porto Alegre, Porto Alegre, Brazil

Introduction

Cutaneous manifestations of malignant neoplastic diseases may be classified as metastatic lesions of the skin, genodermatoses associated with neoplasias, dermatoses induced by environmental carcinogens, and paraneoplastic dermatoses [1].

Paraneoplastic diseases are hormonal, neurologic, or hematologic disorders and clinical or biochemical alterations associated with malignant neoplasias that are not, however, directly related to the invasion of the primary tumor or its metastases [2, 3]. Dermatologic lesions are the second most common form of paraneoplastic syndrome, the first being endocrine manifestations [3].

The mechanisms involved in the onset of dermatologic lesions have not yet been recognized for most manifestations. The production or depletion of biologically active mediators such as growth factors, cytokines, or hormones is believed to be involved in the pathogenesis of cutaneous findings [4]. Another possibility is that an immune response induced by the tumor causes skin changes [1].

Although paraneoplastic dermatoses are rare, they are very important in the practice of dermatology because they may be the first manifestation of the neoplasia. Hence, recognizing them enables an earlier diagnosis of the tumor. It may also improve the prognosis and help to monitor its recurrence [1, 4].

© Springer International Publishing Switzerland 2018
R.R. Bonamigo, S.I.T. Dornelles (eds.), *Dermatology in Public Health Environments*,
https://doi.org/10.1007/978-3-319-33919-1_46

In 1976, Helen O. Curth [5] defined six criteria that establish the causal relationship between dermatoses and neoplasia, characterizing the paraneoplastic dermatoses (Box 46.1).

Box 46.1 Curth's Postulates
1. Dermatosis and neoplasia begin almost concurrently
2. Both conditions present a parallel course
3. The condition is not recognized as part of a genetic syndrome
4. A specific tumor occurs with a given dermatosis
5. Dermatosis is not common
6. There is a high percentage of association recognized in the literature

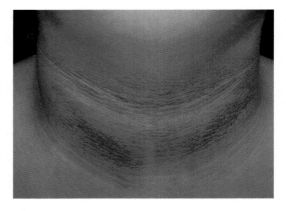

Fig. 46.1 Acanthosis nigricans located in the cervical region

Skin Manifestations

In addition to the clinical presentation, each paraneoplastic dermatosis is discussed regarding its probable etiopathogenesis, complementary examinations for the diagnosis, and the therapeutic approach. All figures in this chapter are provided by the Dermatology Service of UFCSPA (Brazil).

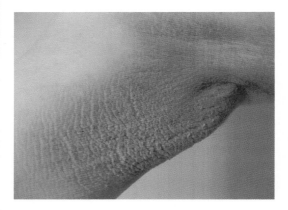

Fig. 46.2 Acanthosis nigricans located in the axilla

Malignant Acanthosis Nigricans

Approximately 80% of cases of acanthosis nigricans are benign and associated with obesity and presentations of insulin resistance. In this situation, onset is usually at an early age. However, patients with abrupt onset and more extensive or severe manifestations in adulthood, above 40 years of age, must be investigated for neoplasias [1, 3].

Malignant acanthosis nigricans (MAN) is clinically characterized by hyperkeratosis, hyperpigmentation, and velvety papillomatosis in body folds (axillae, inguinal region, cervical region, popliteal and cubital fossae) (Figs. 46.1 and 46.2). The lesions can progress to a verru-

cous and thicker appearance. The oral mucosa may be involved, and this presentation is usual in cases of MAN. The palmoplantar regions may also be involved. There may be a complaint of pruritus [1, 4].

The histopathologic findings are in the epidermis and show that it is a proliferative disorder. The main findings are hyperkeratosis, papillomatosis, acanthosis with elongation of the dermal projections, and thickening of the stratum spinosum [1].

The likely mechanism involved in the development of MAN is the production of transforming growth factor α (TGF-α) by the tumor cells that stimulate the proliferation of keratinocytes by the epidermal growth factor [6]. Other growth factors, such as insulin-like growth factor 1, fibroblast growth factor, and α-melanocyte stimulating hormone, may also be involved [7].

There may be an association with other paraneoplastic dermatoses, also with characteristics of dermal proliferation, such as the sign of Leser-Trélat (SLT) and tripe palms, suggesting that these dermatoses share the same pathogenesis [8–11]. This association should increase the suspicion of the presence of neoplasia.

The malignant neoplasias most commonly associated with MAN are adenocarcinomas, especially gastric (73%). Other tumors reported are pulmonary, esophageal, liver, and ovary [11]. The onset of the lesions may occur before, concomitantly with, or after the diagnosis of neoplasias. In a recent series of cases, 22% of lesions preceded the diagnosis of neoplasia and in 57% of the cases they were concomitant [11].

The treatment of the neoplasia generally resolves the skin lesions. The course of MAN is correlated with tumor behavior [1]. The prognosis is poor, and mean survival time is 2 years after the acanthosis is diagnosed [7, 10].

Acquired Pachydermatoglyphy or "Tripe Palms"

This condition is also called palmar acanthosis, palmar acanthosis nigricans, palmar hyperkeratosis, and palmar keratoderma. It presents as palmar thickening with marked palmar ridges and grooves, which exaggerate the dermatoglyph (digital print), giving it a rough, velvety appearance (Figs. 46.3 and 46.4). This clinical aspect recalls the villosities of the intestinal mucosa, thus earning the term tripe palm [3, 12]. There is no predilection for sex, and it occurs more often in elderly patients.

Acanthosis and hyperkeratosis are predominantly observed on histopathology; other findings reported are papillomatosis, dermal mucinosis, and increased mastocytes [1, 13].

As in MAN, there seems to be participation of growth factors and stimulation of epidermal receptors of these factors. High serum levels of TGF-α have already been identified in patients with pachydermatoglyphy [14].

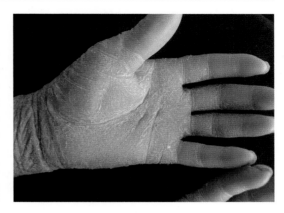

Fig. 46.3 Palmar thickening with marked palmar ridges and grooves, which exaggerate the dermatoglyphs

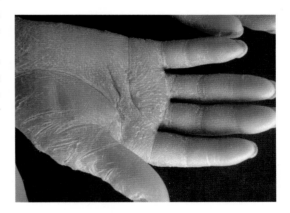

Fig. 46.4 Palmar thickening with marked palmar ridges and grooves, which exaggerate the dermatoglyphs

This dermatosis shares a few epidemiologic, morphologic, and histologic factors with MAN and is present in association with it in 75% of cases [1, 4, 13]. Hence, some authors believe that it may be a palmar manifestation of MAN [1].

About 90% of the cases of dermatoglyphy are associated with malignant neoplasias [1, 13]. The neoplasia most associated is pulmonary, followed by gastric tumors. When there is an association with MAN, the most prevalent neoplasia is gastric [13].

In approximately 60% of cases, the diagnosis of acquired dermatoglyphy occurs before or concomitant with the diagnosis of the tumor [13]. The skin lesions usually run parallel to the course of the neoplasia.

Sign of Leser-Trélat

The SLT presents as a sudden increase in the quantity and rapid growth in the size of seborrheic keratoses. The keratoses are characterized as verrucous papules, with various diameters and colors, located on the trunk, limbs, axillae, neck, and face [3, 4, 15] (Figs. 46.5 and 46.6). There may be inflammatory signs and pruritus. It may be associated with other paraneoplastic manifestations, especially MAN, which increases suspicion regarding the presence of the neoplasia [3].

The SLT primarily affects individuals over 60 years old, without a predilection for sex or race [3].

Its association with malignant neoplasms is still controversial. The age group with the greatest number of seborrheic keratoses is also the one with the most tumors, which makes it difficult to establish a cause–effect relationship [3, 4]. However, it is important to distinguish it from multiple seborrheic keratoses that appear throughout life and whose onset begins in the second or third decade of life [15].

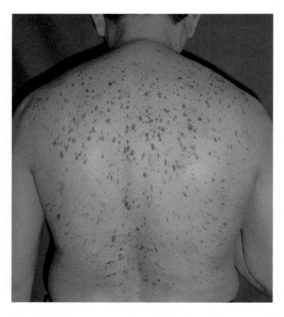

Fig. 46.5 Verrucous papules, with various diameters and colors, located on the trunk

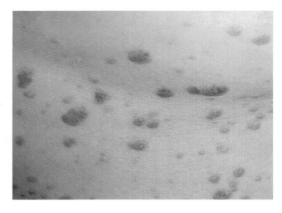

Fig. 46.6 Verrucous papules, with various diameters and colors, located on the trunk

There are reports of cases of an increase in number and size of seborrheic keratoses that are not associated with the onset of neoplasias, even after long periods of observation [16, 17]. Other case–control studies, comparing the number and aspect of seborrheic keratoses in patients with a diagnosis of cancer and paired controls, found that only two patients with tumors presented with SLT as described in the literature, showing that it is a rarer process, which makes it difficult to study [18]. In the other patients studied there was no difference in the number and location of lesions [18].

However, there are hundreds of reports in the literature describing the onset of SLT in many different neoplasias. Most of the tumors are adenocarcinomas, especially in the gastrointestinal tract. There are reports of lymphoproliferative diseases, as well as carcinomas, for instance of the breast, bladder, prostate, kidneys, lungs, ovaries, and melanoma [3, 15].

Skin lesions generally run parallel to the course of the tumor. The neoplasias associated with the SLT are aggressive and may result in an expectation of less than 12 months in most cases [15]. Despite controversy, patients with the SLT must be investigated for the presence of neoplasias by taking a medical history and performing a complete physical examination, biochemical tests, chest X- ray, mammogram, cytopathologic test of the cervix, prostate-specific antigen, endoscopy, and colonoscopy [15].

Acquired Ichthyosis

The clinical aspect of acquired ichthyosis is similar to that of dominant autosomal ichthyosis. However, acquired ichthyosis begins in adulthood, different from the hereditary form which usually begins before the age of 13 years [1]. It is characterized by diffuse, small, white or brownish scales with a rhomboid aspect and high margins. The scales predominate on the trunk and extensor surface of the limbs (Fig. 46.7) [1]. There is no palmoplantar and fold involvement [4].

The histopathologic examination reveals orthokeratosis, a thinner or absent granular layer, and mild acanthosis. There is no dermal inflammation or it is minimal [4].

The great majority of cases of acquired ichthyosis associated with described neoplasias is associated with Hodgkin's lymphoma (70%), but there are reports of an association with non-Hodgkin lymphoma, multiple myeloma, leukemia and, less frequently, solid tumors [4].

Generally the acquired form in adults is associated with various non-neoplastic diseases, such as malnutrition, hypothyroidism, and sarcoidosis, Hansen's disease, the use of medications, and acquired immunodeficiencies, such as human immunodeficiency virus infection, graft-versus-host disease, and disorders post bone marrow transplantation [3].

The pathophysiology involved in the development of acquired ichthyosis is not yet known. Some authors believe that there is malabsorption of vitamin A [19]. Others have published evidence that in patients with Hodgkin's disease there is less synthesis of dermal lipids [20].

Acquired ichthyosis is usually diagnosed weeks or months after the neoplasia is discovered; it is rarely the initial symptom of neoplasia [1, 21]. The course of ichthyosis usually runs parallel to that of the neoplasia. Moreover, ichthyosis can occur in association with other dermatoses such as dermatomyositis (DM), erythema gyratum repens (EGR), and Bazex syndrome [3].

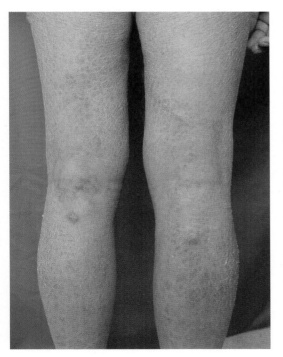

Fig. 46.7 Small, white/brownish scales with a rhomboid aspect and high margins in the extensor surface of the legs

Bazex Syndrome

Also called paraneoplastic acrokeratosis, this condition is associated with malignant neoplasias in the vast majority of cases reported in the literature. It is characterized by erythematous to violaceous colored papulosquamous plaques, located in acral areas such as the nose, auricular pavilion, hands, and feet, besides ungual alterations [1, 22]. The lesions are distributed symmetrically. There may be pruritus [1].

The syndrome is described in three stages: in the first, erythema and psoriasiform scaling is seen on fingers, hands, feet, and margin of the helix, as well as violaceous erythema and pityriasiform scaling on the nasal dorsum. Alterations of the nails often occur, and include fragile nails, subungual hyperkeratosis, and onycholysis (Figs. 46.8 and 46.9). In the second stage the scaling completely covers hands and feet, producing a violaceous keratoderma. The skin becomes edematous and the palms may take on a honeycomb aspect. The scaling may affect the entire auricular

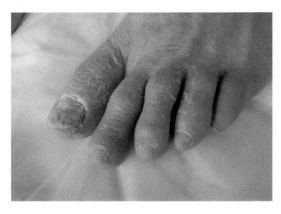

Fig. 46.8 Erythema and psoriasiform scaling on the dorsum of fingers associated with alterations of the nails

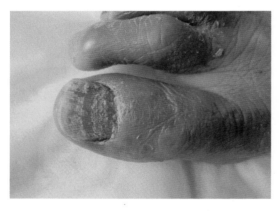

Fig. 46.9 Erythema and psoriasiform scaling on the dorsum of fingers associated with alterations of the nails

pavilion. At this stage the first localized or systemic symptoms of the neoplasia may occur. In the third stage there may be involvement of additional areas, such as knees, arms, and scalp [23].

It predominates in male patients and the age of onset is usually around 60 years [22].

The histologic examination of the papulosquamous lesions shows hyperkeratosis, parakeratosis, acanthosis, dyskeratotic keratinocytes, and a perivascular mononuclear infiltrate [22].

The neoplasias most commonly associated with the Bazex syndrome are squamous cell carcinomas of the head and neck or squamous cell tumors of unknown origin, which present metastases to the cervical lymph nodes [22]. The most frequently described tumors are those of the oro-

pharynx, larynx, esophagus, and lungs. These findings suggest that mechanisms involved in the development of this syndrome are specific to tumors in these locations [22].

In more than 60% of the cases, the onset of skin lesions occurs on average 11 months before the symptoms or tumor diagnosis, and they are one of the earliest signs of neoplasm [22, 24].

The differential diagnosis must be made with psoriasis, eczema resistant to treatment, and superficial fungal infections. In psoriasis generally the entire auricular pavilion is involved and usually affects the palmoplantar area, not the dorsum of the limbs. Furthermore, the involvement of the helix and the bulbous enlargement of the distal phalanx are characteristic of the Bazex syndrome. The Bazex syndrome must always be ruled out in acral dermatoses that do not respond to appropriate treatment [24].

When Bazex syndrome is suspected, the evaluation should begin with a detailed history and physical examination. Initial examinations include complete otorhinolaryngologic evaluation, chest X-ray, complete hemogram, erythrocyte sedimentation rate, biochemistry, iron, tumor markers, and a search for occult blood in the stool. If the otorhinolaryngologic evaluation and chest X-ray are inconclusive, an upper gastrointestinal endoscopy can be indicated. If there is anemia or occult blood in the stool, a colonoscopy is appropriate. Based on findings of the history and physical examination, it may be necessary to perform a computed tomography (CT) evaluation of the chest, abdomen, and pelvis. If the initial evaluation is negative, the patient must be reassessed every 3 months [24].

The lesions are resistant to a variety of topical treatments, but they improve significantly in response to treatment of the neoplasia. Despite the improvement of the skin lesions, the ungual lesions usually do not present a regression [22].

Erythema Gyratum Repens

EGR is a rare and clinically specific pan-neoplastic syndrome associated with a malignant neoplasia in 82% of the cases reported [25]. It is considered mandatory to perform an investigation for neoplasia in patients who have been diagnosed with this syndrome [3, 26].

It is more common in males (2:1) and the mean age of onset of symptoms is 63 years. It predominates in Caucasian patients [26].

EGR is characterized by the presence of polycyclic, serpiginous erythema with scaling on its border and is rapidly progressive (1 cm/day), producing ring-shaped erythematous, concentric figures similar to a wood surface. It is generally located on the trunk and proximal extremities and spares hands, feet, and face. There is usually pruritus [3].

The histologic examination is usually nonspecific with mild to moderate hyperkeratosis, epidermal spongiosis, and perivascular lymphocytic infiltrate [1].

The tumors most commonly associated with EGR are of the lung, esophagus, breast, cervix, and stomach [3, 26, 27]. EGR lesions precede the diagnosis of the neoplasia in 80% of the cases by 4–9 months [3, 4, 26, 27].

The pathophysiology of EGR is still unknown. It is believed that immune mechanisms are involved, since immunosuppression may accompany the resolution of the skin condition [4]. Although it is not a consistent finding, there is evidence of granular deposition of immunoglobulin G (IgG) and protein C3 in the basal membrane of affected areas [28]. Some authors believe that the keratinized cells present proteins that share epitopes with the tumor and its proteins, which would explain a cross-reaction [28].

EGR has already been described in pregnancy and in the presence of non-neoplastic diseases such as tuberculosis, CREST syndrome, and Sjögren syndrome [4].

The lesions usually are completely resolved when the neoplasia is treated and the course of the dermatosis is usually parallel to the course of the neoplasia. In patients with metastatic lesions, the EGR lesions usually persist or recur [4, 27, 28]. The use of antihistamines and topical corticosteroids is not very effective [4].

Necrolytic Migratory Erythema

Necrolytic migratory erythema (NME) is the cutaneous manifestation of the glucagonoma syndrome. This syndrome is characterized by the presence of NME, loss of weight, diabetes mellitus, cheilitis, stomatitis, diarrhea, and anemia [3, 12, 29]. Skin lesions are considered the most specific component of the glucagonoma syndrome and are the first manifestation of the syndrome in 67% of cases, but 100% of the patients with glucagonoma will develop NME lesions at some time during the course of the disease. When the tumor is diagnosed early, there is reasonable potential to cure the neoplasia [29–31].

NME usually appears in the fifth or sixth decade of life, but there are reports of patients aged 19–84 years. There is no predominant gender. The glucagonoma syndrome is an extremely rare disorder with an estimated incidence of 1 in 20 million persons per year, but may be higher. The rate of malignant neoplasia in glucagonoma syndrome is 57–100%. The 5-year survival rate is less than 50% [1, 29–31].

It presents clinically as maculopapular, annular, or arciform erythematous lesions that increase centrifugally, developing blisters that lead to necrosis and erosion. The lesions are confluent and present a crusted periphery. The center of the lesions usually heals with hyperpigmentation, but may take on a lichenified or psoriasiform appearance in intertriginous areas [30]. They predominate in the lower extremities, trunk, face, and inguinal region. The lesions are usually more marked in the perioral and perianal region. Thus, the clinical presentation is similar to that of other dermatoses associated with zinc deficiency and other nutritional deficiencies [4, 12].

Besides the cutaneous findings, the patients present systemic symptoms such as weight loss, glucose intolerance, anemia, thromboembolic disease, hypoaminoacidemia, and psychiatric disorders [1, 3].

Increased glucagon appears responsible for most of the clinical symptoms. However, the deficiency of fatty acids, amino acids, and zinc also contributes to the pathogenesis of skin lesions [4, 30]. The catabolic state produced by the excess of glucagon appears to be responsible for the nutrient depletion [3, 30].

The histologic findings vary according to the phase of evolution of the biopsied lesion. In general the anatomopathologic examination can be characterized by psoriasiform hyperplasia with confluent parakeratosis, epidermal vacuolization, and necrosis with the formation of subcorneal pustules [1, 12].

When associated with tumors, NME is the result of α cell pancreatic tumor [1]. NME is also seen in association with other pancreatic diseases, malabsorption syndromes, liver failure, inflammatory bowel disease, chronic pancreatitis, and celiac disease without the presence of glucagonoma [4, 29]. These conditions are called pseudoglucagonoma syndrome.

The differential diagnosis of NME includes dermatoses such as enteropathic dermatitis, pellagra, psoriasis, seborrheic dermatitis, and pemphigus [29].

Because it is rare the diagnosis is usually late, and therefore it has a worse prognosis. Most of the patients already present metastases at the time of diagnosis and a consequent shorter survival, since the only means of cure is tumor surgery [29].

The treatment of symptoms with the administration of somatostatin/octreotide or chemotherapy is also effective. The effect expected from these treatments is the normalization of glucagon levels, which makes the lesions disappear [32]. In cases of liver metastasis it might be effective to embolize the hepatic artery [30].

Dermatomyositis

DM is a severe inflammatory myopathy associated with cutaneous findings whose cause is unknown. DM has been divided into two groups: (1) idiopathic (not associated with neoplasia) and (2) paraneoplastic (associated with neoplasia) [1]. The clinical findings do not differ between the two groups [3]. The cutaneous findings may occur in the absence of myositis, known as amyo-

pathic DM. Patients with DM appear to have a greater frequency of malignant neoplasia than the general population. Some studies demonstrate a three-fold greater incidence of neoplasia in patients with DM [33]. However, patients with polymyositis appear not to present this association [33, 34].

Patients with DM associated with malignant neoplasia are between the age of 50 and 60 years, a larger age group than that of the patients with the idiopathic form of DM [34]. There is controversy regarding the predilection for sex; in patients without neoplasia DM predominates in women, while DM associated with neoplasia appears to be more frequent among males [1, 33, 34].

The most typical cutaneous lesions in DM are Gottron's papules (erythematous-violaceous papules or plaques, with discrete scaling, located in metacarpophalangeal and interphalangeal joints; Fig. 46.10) and heliotrope (erythematous-violaceous lesions, with or without edema, symmetric, located in the periorbital region). Other cutaneous findings of DM are malar erythema, poikiloderma in photoexposed areas, periungual telangiectasia, cuticular hypertrophy, and cicatricial alopecia. Myositis is characterized primarily by proximal muscular weakness [35].

The anatomopathologic examination that is characteristic of paraneoplastic DM is dermatitis with a vacuolar interface, with irregular lymphocytic inflammation and variable deposition of mucin [1].

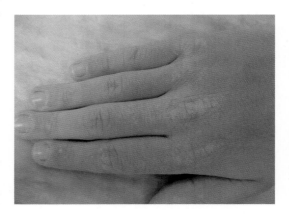

Fig. 46.10 Gottron's papules

Skin lesions generally begin before the diagnosis of neoplasia, and most of the tumors are diagnosed 1 year after the diagnosis of DM [34]. The neoplasias most often associated with DM are ovaries, lung, pancreas, stomach, colorectum, and lymphomas [33].

The factors associated with neoplasia in patients with a diagnosis of DM are the presence of constitutional symptoms, the rapid onset of DM or polymyositis symptoms, the absence of Raynaud's phenomenon, and high levels of erythrocyte sedimentation and creatine phosphokinase [36]. Other factors that also appear to increase the risk of neoplasia in patients with DM are old age, male gender, presence of skin necrosis and dysphagia, while the presence of arthritis and interstitial lung disease appear to be less prevalent in paraneoplastic DM [37].

In patients with DM a careful clinical evaluation, routine laboratory tests, a chest, abdominal, and pelvic CT scan, upper gastrointestinal endoscopy, a mammogram, and a gynecologic assessment should be performed [33, 36]. The risk of a diagnosis of cancer is not diminished even 5 years after DM is diagnosed, indicating the need to remain vigilant for the detection of neoplasia [33]. The 5-year survival rate in patients with DM and neoplasia was reported to be 10% and in patients with idiopathic DM 74% [34].

The treatment of paraneoplastic DM is not different from that for idiopathic disease, and prednisone, azathioprine, and methotrexate can be used, besides topical medication, sunscreen, and hydroxychloroquine [35]. The surgical treatment of the neoplasia appears not to change patients' survival but does diminish progression to myositis [33]. In patients with a prior history of neoplasia and clinical worsening of the DM lesions, it is necessary to investigate the possibility of tumor recurrence [36].

Paraneoplastic Pemphigus

Paraneoplastic pemphigus (PNP) is an autoimmune bullous disease with polymorphic mucocutaneous lesions, associated with benign and malignant lymphoproliferative processes [1, 38].

PNP is associated with a series of autoantibodies that can affect multiple organs such as the kidneys, the smooth and striated muscle system, small bowel, colon, and thyroid. According to some authors PNP is only one of the manifestations of this syndrome, and they therefore propose the term paraneoplastic autoimmune multiorgan syndrome. This term is not yet widely accepted in the literature [39, 40].

In PNP there is no predilection for gender. It may occur at any age from 7 to 80 years, but the mean time of onset is usually around the age of 55 [38].

The typical initial manifestation is progressive and painful stomatitis, which may extend to the pharynx, larynx, esophagus, eyes, nose, and genitals. The oral lesions are located preferentially on the lateral border of the tongue and extend to the vermillion of the lips. It is believed that the pain in stomatitis occurs because of the location of the ulcerated lesions. There are lesions in the palmoplantar region [1, 41, 42].

The cutaneous findings are polymorphic and can occur in a same individual. They can be classified as [40]:

- Pemphigus: superficial, flaccid vesicles and blisters, erosions and crusts, occasionally with some erythema
- Bullous pemphigoid: erythematous papules associated or not with tense blisters
- Multiform erythema: polymorphic lesions, mainly erythematous papules and erosions/ulcers
- Graft versus host: erythematous-squamous papules
- Lichen planus: violaceous, squamous papules, flat, with intense involvement of the mucosae

PNP is the only form of pemphigus that involves tissues not covered only by stratified squamous epithelium. Approximately 40% of the patients develop pulmonary involvement [42]. Bronchiolitis obliterans with progressive ventilatory insufficiency is the main cause of death in PNP [38].

In the histologic examination of PNP, suprabasilar acantholysis, vacuolar degeneration of the interface with necrosis of keratinocytes, and lichenoid inflammatory infiltrate can be observed. The clinical variants present a correlation with the finding of the anatomopathologic examination. This variation represents the different pathogenetic mechanisms involved in the PNP: it may be a disease mediated by B cells, such as pemphigus, or by T cells, as in lichen planus [1, 38, 40]. Direct immunofluorescence shows intercellular deposits of IgG and C3 in the epidermis and/or linearly at the dermoepidermal junction. Indirect immunofluorescence in rat bladders identifies the IgG antibody reaction with simple columnar and transitional epithelium, different from other bullous diseases [1, 4, 38].

The serum autoantibodies are identified by immunoblot analyses of patients' serum samples on human epidermal extracts. The serum autoantibodies identified in PNP are antidesmoglein 1 and 3, as well as members of the family of epithelial proteins plakin (desmoplakin I and II, envoplakin, periplakin), bullous pemphigoid antigen 1 (BPAg1), plectin, and α2-type macroglobulin 1 protein 1 [42] (Table 46.1).

The origin of the disease is not yet clear, but it is believed that the immune response in PNP can originate in two ways: (1) immune response to neoplastic antigens with antibodies that have a cross-reaction to the epithelial antigens or (2) pathogenic autoantibodies synthesized by the tumors that deregulate the immune system by cytokine synthesis [42].

The diagnostic criteria for PNP are shown in Table 46.2:

In two-thirds of the patients with PNP, the neoplasia is diagnosed before the skin lesions. The most commonly associated neoplasias are non-Hodgkin lymphoma, chronic lymphocytic leukemia, and Castleman's disease in children [42]. It has already been described, less frequently, in association with solid tumors such as thymomas and sarcomas [41].

The evaluation of patients with suspected PNP should include a complete physical examination, skin biopsy for histopathology, direct and indirect immunofluorescence, and immunoprecipitation. Evaluation for the presence of neoplasia should include a complete blood count, proteinogram, and a CT scan of the chest, abdomen, and pelvis, besides biopsies directed at lymph nodes, bone marrow, or solid tumors when indicated [45].

The clinical aspects of the disease may mimic those seen in eruptions secondary to drugs, erythema multiforme, Stevens–Johnson syndrome, or toxic epidermal necrolysis [42].

Table 46.1 Paraneoplastic pemphigus: autoantigens in pathogenesis [43]

Antigen	Molecular weight (kDa)	Location
Desmoglein 3	130	Desmosome: extracellular
Desmoglein 1	160	Desmosome: extracellular
Envoplakin	210	Desmosome: intracellular
Periplakin	190	Desmosome: intracellular
Bullous pemphigoid antigen 1	230	Hemidesmosome/lamina lucida
Desmoplakin I	250	Desmosome: intracellular
Desmoplakin II	210	Desmosome: intracellular
Plectin	400	Hemidesmosome: intracellular

Table 46.2 Paraneoplastic pemphigus: diagnostic criteria [44]

1. Clinical	Painful mucosal erosion(s) with a polymorphous skin eruption culminating in vesicles and/or bullae in the context of an occult/confirmed neoplasm
2. Histopathology	Intraepidermal acantholysis, vacuolar interfacial dermatoses, and keratinocyte necrosis
3. Immunofluorescence (direct)	Deposition of complement and IgG in intercellular epidermal spaces and in the epidermal basement zone in linear granular lesions
4. Autoantibodies	Detection in the serum similar to that seen in pemphigus
5. Immune complexes	Characteristic complex of four proteins immunoprecipitated from keratinocytes with serum autoantibodies

The autoimmune disease is difficult to treat and does not improve even when the neoplasia is treated effectively. For autoimmune treatment corticosteroids, immunosuppressive drugs (cyclosporine, cyclophosphamide), plasmapheresis, immunoglobulin, and rituximab may be used [38]. The prognosis for PNP is not favorable; mortality can reach 90% of cases. Most of the patients die of pulmonary complications (bronchiolitis obliterans and pneumonias), infections, or complications resulting from the neoplasia itself [38, 42]. Patents with erythema multiforme-type lesions and the presence of keratinocyte necrosis, especially if associated with extensive lesions at presentation, may have a worse prognosis, with a faster and more severe outcome [44, 46].

Different from the idiopathic form, in the lesions associated with neoplasias there is no history of infection of the upper airways; neutrophilia also may be absent, and the skin lesions are usually more severe and may involve the mucosae [47, 49, 50]. Other common differences in paraneoplastic SS are immature cells in the differential of the blood count, presence of anemia, and thrombocytopenia or thrombocytosis [50]. Anemia and abnormal platelet count appear to be the most readily identified difference between the two groups [47]. Proteinuria is commonly found when there is renal involvement. Therefore the possibility of neoplasia must be considered in all patients with a diagnosis of SS, older age, more severe skin manifestations, and an abnormal differential of leukocytes and/or cytopenias [50,

Sweet Syndrome

Also called acute febrile neutrophilic dermatosis, Sweet syndrome (SS) is characterized by four cardinal aspects: fever, peripheral leukocytosis, painful erythematous plaques on limbs, face, and neck, and dense neutrophilic infiltrate in the dermis. SS has been described in association with different neoplasias, autoimmune diseases, and infections, especially respiratory [47]. Currently it is classified as classic (idiopathic), associated with neoplasias or drug induced [48].

It is believed that 20% of the cases of SS are associated with neoplasias [47, 49, 50]. When associated with neoplasias there is no predilection for the female gender as in idiopathic SS. The median age of the patients with SS and neoplasia is 52 years [1]. Patients with paraneoplastic SS appear to be on average older than patients with the idiopathic and drug-associated subtypes [51].

The lesions usually appear abruptly and evolve within days or weeks. SS is characterized by well-demarcated erythematous-purpuric, painful plaques, with an irregular surface, and because of severe dermal edema they may have the appearance of pseudovesicles. The lesions have annular arrangements and asymmetric distribution, generally on the upper extremities, neck, and face (Figs. 46.11 and 46.12) [1, 47].

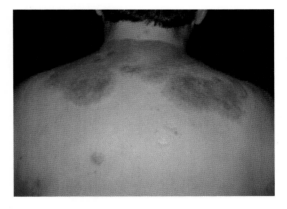

Fig. 46.11 Well-demarcated erythematous-purpuric plaques, irregular surface, annular arrangements, and asymmetric distribution, on the upper trunk

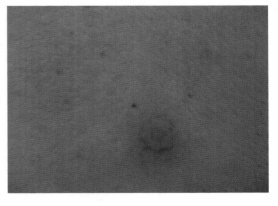

Fig. 46.12 Appearance of pseudovesicles

51]. The characteristics of paraneoplastic SS are described in Box 46.2.

> **Box 46.2 Characteristics of the Paraneoplastic Sweet Syndrome**
> - A history of upper airway infection or other associated conditions is unusual
> - No predominant gender
> - More severe skin lesions
> - Skin lesions precede the diagnosis of neoplasia in most cases
> - Extracutaneous involvement in >50% of the patients
> - Absence of neutrophilia in >50% of the patients
> - Frequent presence of anemia and abnormal platelet count
> - High rate of recurrence generally associated with tumor "relapse"

There may be the presence of hemorrhagic blisters and ulceration, rendering the SS lesions similar to the lesions of atypical gangrenous pyoderma. This led some authors to suggest that it is the same disease with different spectra [47].

There may be symptoms of involvement of other systems in SS. When associated with neoplasias, 50% of the patients will present extracutaneous involvement particularly of the musculoskeletal, renal, and ophthalmic systems, and less commonly of lungs and liver [50].

A dense neutrophilic infiltrate is found in the histopathologic examination, filling the middle and upper dermis. Epidermal alterations are rare. A few patients with SS associated with hematologic neoplasia present leukemia cutis associated with neutrophilia [4, 52]. Histologic aspects of vasculitis are absent, but often endothelial edema and karyorrhexis (nuclear fragmentation of neutrophils) are found [49].

The physiopathogenesis of SS is still unknown. In SS associated with neoplasia, the most accepted pathogenesis mechanism is increased production or inappropriate regulation of inflammatory cytokines such as interleukin (IL)-1, IL-3,

IL-6, IL-8, granulocyte colony-stimulating factor, and granulocyte-macrophage colony-stimulating factor [48].

The tumors most frequently associated with SS (85% of the cases) are the hematologic neoplasias, especially acute myeloid leukemia, lymphoma, myelodysplastic syndrome, and chronic myeloid leukemia. Outstanding among the solid tumors (15% of cases) are those of the genitourinary tract, breast, and gastrointestinal tract [1, 49, 50]. In two-thirds of the patients with paraneoplastic SS, dermatosis is the initial sign either of recurrence/persistence of the tumor or of asymptomatic metastasis [49, 50]. The suggested initial evaluation of patients with suspected paraneoplastic SS is described in Box 46.3.

> **Box 46.3 Initial Evaluation of the Presence of Neoplasias in Patients with Sweet Syndrome [49]**
> - Detailed clinical history
> - Complete physical examination
>   - Evaluation of lymph nodes, thyroid, oral cavity, skin
>   - Digital rectal examination
>   - Gynecologic evaluation in women
>   - Urologic evaluation in men (testicular and prostatic)
> - Laboratory evaluation
>   - Complete blood count
>   - Carcinoembryonic antigen
>   - Biochemical
>   - Qualitative urinalysis
>   - Investigation of occult blood in stool
> - Complementary examinations
>   - Chest X-ray
>   - Endometrial evaluation in menopausal patients, or patients with a history of uterine bleeding, obesity, infertility or hormone treatment
>   - Colonoscopy in patients older than 50 years

Patients with a diagnosis of SS should initially be evaluated for hematologic neoplasia and solid tumors. The hemogram should be repeated every 6–12 months in patients with a diagnosis of SS, since the diagnosis of hematologic neoplasia may be late [49]. A complete blood count must be performed in all patients with a diagnosis of hematologic neoplasia who develop new or recurring SS lesions. It is more unlikely that solid tumors will develop after 12 months' follow-up of these patients, thus there is no indication for an exhaustive investigation. Likewise, the onset of new SS lesions in patients with diagnoses of solid tumors needs evaluation for recurrent or persistent neoplasia [49].

The cutaneous signs and symptoms of SS present a rapid resolution after the administration of corticosteroids, independent of the course of the neoplasia [1, 50].

Pyoderma Gangrenosum

Pyoderma gangrenosum (PG) is an uncommon ulcerative disease whose pathogenesis is still not clear. It is generally associated with other inflammatory diseases such as intestinal inflammatory disease, rheumatoid arthritis, monoclonal gammopathy, systemic lupus erythematosus, and others [53]. Two clinical forms are described [53]:

- Typical form: characterized by painful nodules or pustules that form necrotic ulcers with undermined violaceous borders. It is located preferentially on the abdomen, buttocks, lower extremities and face. Generally associated with intestinal inflammatory disease
- Atypical form; characterized by hemorrhagic blisters and rapidly growing more superficial lesions. Common in the upper extremities, generally associated with hematologic diseases or neoplasias (Fig 46.13)

The age at onset of the lesions is adults on average 45 years old for the typical form and 52 years for the atypical form [53].

The histopathologic findings are not specific, but help rule out other causes of ulcerations and confirm the aspect compatible with PG, and moreover the findings usually vary with the evolution of the lesion and the biopsy site [1, 53]. Earlier PG lesions show a dense neutrophilic

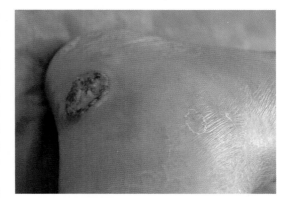

Fig. 46.13 Pyoderma gangrenosum: necrotic ulcers with undermined violaceous borders

infiltrate in the dermis, with a few neutrophils extending to the epidermis. Vasculitis is absent [1, 53, 54].

The clinical and histologic similarity between the hemorrhagic SS and the atypical PG leads some authors to believe that it is the same disease with a different spectrum. The name neutrophilic dermatosis attributable to myeloproliferative diseases has already been suggested [47, 54].

The association of PG with neoplasia is described as 7% [54]. The most common are hematologic neoplasias, especially acute myeloid leukemia [54]. Multiple myeloma is the second neoplasia most frequently described in association with PG [1]. There are reports of an association with solid tumors, but these are rarer, and outstanding among them are colon, prostate, bladder, breast, adrenal glands, and lung [54].

The presence of the bullous variant of PG suggests the need for a careful investigation of the patients for hematologic neoplasias, including bone marrow biopsy. The onset of PG in patients with relatively benign hematologic diseases, such as myelodysplasia and polycythemia rubra vera may indicate the more aggressive progression of the disease, including a malignant transformation, indicating the need for a meticulous evaluation of these patients. In patients with acute myeloid leukemia, the onset of PG indicates a worse prognosis [54].

The treatment of PG is lengthy and based on the use of corticosteroids and immunosuppressors. The lesions of atypical PG usually heal faster than those of the typical PG [53, 54]. The course of PG in association with neoplastic diseases has not yet been well established [1].

Multicentric Reticulohistiocytosis

Multicentric reticulohistiocytosis (MR) is a rare systemic histiocytic disease that preferentially affects skin and synovium. In 40% of the cases the initial symptom is in the joint, and in 30% of cases the initial symptoms are cutaneous [55]. It is a progressive, insidious, and self-limiting disease that disappears within 7 years after onset [1].

The great majority of the cases occur in Caucasian patients, with a slight predominance in females (1.85:1). It may occur at any age, but the mean age of patients at the onset of the symptoms is 50 years [55].

It is characterized by the presence of papules or nodules up to 2 cm in diameter, of pinkish, brownish, or grayish color. Preferential location is the hands, followed by the face, arms, trunk, legs, auricular pavilion, and cervical region [55]. The pathognomonic lesions are the "coral beads," which are papules found along the nail bed. Other characteristic findings are palpebral xanthelasma and vermicular lesions on the nostril rims [4, 55].

Multicentric reticulohistiocytosis is associated with symmetric destructive arthropathy which occurs in any joint, most frequently hands and knees, but it may also affect other joints. The radiologic examination shows well-circumscribed punched erosions and reabsorption of the juxta-articular zone with disproportionate changes compared with the clinical examination [1, 55].

There may be systemic symptoms such as dysphagia, loss of weight, pruritus, weakness, lymphadenopathy, and others [55].

The anatomopathologic examination shows nonencapsulated, well-circumscribed nodular infiltrate of histiocytes and multinucleated giant cells with a "ground-glass" type eosinophilic cytoplasm [1].

In immunohistochemistry the cells are positive for CD68 and CD45, showing that it is an infiltrate originating in monocytes and macro-phages, and it has a variable expression of T-lymphocyte markers (CD3), nonreactivity for B-cell markers (CD10–CD22), Langerhans cells, and dermal dendrocytes (S100 and factor XIIIa) [55, 56].

In laboratory tests there may also be increased erythrocyte sedimentation velocity, anemia, and hypercholesterolemia.

The association of MR with neoplasia varies from 20% to 30% in the literature [55, 56]. There is no predominance of a specific type of tumor associated with MR. MR has already been described in association with cancer of the breast, uterus, ovaries, pleural mesothelioma, lymphomas, melanoma, penis, gastric tract, pancreas, and lung [55, 56]. The clinical course of MR is not predictable or parallel to that of the neoplasia [1, 55]. Although MR does not present all criteria for a paraneoplastic dermatosis, this association appears important. This justifies its investigation for this diagnosis [55].

The use of antiproliferative drugs may alter the course of MR, and outstanding among them are cyclophosphamide, methotrexate, azathioprine, and chlorambucil [55].

Necrobiotic Xanthogranuloma

Necrobiotic xanthogranuloma (NX) is characterized by the presence of plaques and firm, yellowish nodules, which often occur in the periorbital region [57]. NX was distinguished from normo- and hyperlipemic plane periorbital xanthomas by Kossard and Winkelmann in 1980 [58].

The mean age at lesion onset is 52–56 years, but it may appear from the ages of 20 to 80. There is no predilection for gender [59, 60].

NX is characterized by the onset of well-demarcated yellowish-orange plaques (xanthomatosis) or firm subcutaneous nodules, located mainly on the face, more specifically the upper and lower eyelids. Most of the patients also present with lesions on the trunk and extremities [4, 57]. The size may vary from 0.3 to 25 cm in diameter [1]. It may be associated with ulceration, telangiectasias, erythematous-violaceous margins, and atrophy. There may be pruritus [57].

NX is a systemic disease. The most affected extracutaneous sites are the respiratory tract (epiglottis, larynx, pharynx, bronchi, and lungs) and heart [57].

Histopathologically, the epidermis and upper dermis are generally normal. The histopathologic findings extend from the middle dermis to the subcutaneous tissue. Granulomatous inflammation consisting of spumous histiocytes, lymphocytes, foreign body type multinucleated giant cells, and Touton giant cells alternated with foci of collagen necrobiosis is observed [1, 57]. In these necrobiosis foci cholesterol clefts are observed. This characteristic can help distinguish necrobiosis lipoidica from NX [1, 4, 57].

The most frequently found alterations in the laboratory tests in XN patients are leukopenia, C4 deficiency, increased erythrocyte sedimentation velocity and, in the electrophoresis of serum proteins, monoclonal gammopathy of the IgG-κ IgG-λ type [57]. Because of this gammopathy, many patients are submitted to a bone marrow biopsy for investigation. The most often reported findings are plasmocytosis or abnormal plasmocytes, multiple myeloma, and myeloproliferative disease [57].

The association of NX with hematologic disorders has already been clearly established. Benign monoclonal gammopathy is present in the great majority of cases [57, 59–61]. Malignant hematologic diseases associated with NX are multiple myeloma, chronic lymphocytic leukemia, Hodgkin's disease, and non-Hodgkin lymphoma [57, 59–61]. Hematologic alterations may appear before or after the beginning of the skin lesions (8 years before to 11 years after the beginning of the skin lesions) [61]. Hence, patients with NX must be followed for a long time to rule out the development of hematologic diseases [59, 61].

The treatment is usually unsatisfactory, with high rates of recurrence in the options already described. There is a report of the use of alkylating agents (chlorambucil, cyclophosphamide, melphalan), corticosteroids (topical, systemic, and intralesional), laser (CO_2, Nd:YAG), methotrexate, azathioprine, systemic antibiotics, and surgical excision of the lesions [57]. NX is a chronic and progressive process characterized by the onset of new lesions and by the gradual evolution of the oldest lesions [60]. The treatment of the lymphoproliferative disease does not always result in remission of the cutaneous symptoms [57].

Acquired Hypertrichosis Lanuginosa

Acquired hypertrichosis lanuginosa (AHL) is a rare condition with a sudden, late onset, no family history, and strong association with the presence of malignant neoplasias [62].

It occurs predominantly in female patients, and the age of onset of the symptoms usually varies from 40 to 70 years with a mean of 54 years [62, 63].

It is characterized by the development of soft, velvety, nonpigmented hairs, often on the face. It may appear in other regions such as the trunk, axillae, and limbs, but it spares the palmoplantar regions and genitals, since it does not follow a specific distribution according to gender [1, 63]. The progression of the appearance of hairs is craniocaudal. Associated symptoms are glossitis and hypertrophy of the papillae of the tongue. It may be associated with other paraneoplastic manifestations, such as acanthosis nigricans and seborrheic keratoses [1, 63].

In histopathology, the follicle of the lanugo-type hairs is observed, which extend almost parallel to the epidermis surface, different from the normally almost vertical position of the follicles. Besides, many follicles are of the "mantle hair type." The mantle appears to be formed by two buttons or epithelial chords that extend around the follicle, creating a kind of apron at the site where the sebaceous duct would normally be found [62, 64].

The pathogenesis of AHL has not yet been completely elucidated. It is believed that products secreted by the tumors, such as cytokines or growth factors, may stimulate tumor growth, besides promoting the proliferation of other cells such as those of the pilous follicles [63].

In women the neoplasia most associated with AHL is colorectal carcinoma, followed by lung and breast cancer. In men, lung cancer is the most often found neoplasia, followed by colorectal carcinoma [63]. Therefore, patients with AHL without a diagnosis of neoplasia should undergo biochemical tests, chest X ray, colonoscopy, and gynecologic evaluation (in women) [63].

Hair growth may occur 2.5 years before the tumor is diagnosed up to 5 years after the diagnosis. In general, patients with AHL already present advanced metastatic disease at the time of diagnosis; consequently, the prognosis is poor [63].

Successful antitumor therapy is associated with regression of the hairs [63] (Table 46.3).

Pruritus

Paraneoplastic pruritus (PP) is a frequent manifestation in hematologic neoplasias, and may affect 15–50% of the patients with polycythemia vera and lymphomas, but it is quite rare in other forms of neoplasia [65].

PP may be defined as a systemic reaction to the presence of the tumor or of the hematologic neoplasia not produced by the presence of tumor cells or by tumor treatment. PP may precede the diagnosis of a tumor and may also disappear when the tumor is treated. Tumor recurrence leads to the reappearance of the lesions, and the evolution of the tumor disease may also be associated with an increased intensity of the pruritus [65].

The prevalence of pruritus in the population with malignant neoplasias is still unknown. In one study it was demonstrated that generalized pruritus without any other cutaneous manifestation presents a prevalence of 5.9% if we take into account all patients with neoplasias (41/700) evaluated in the study, or 12.97% if we only consider the patients with neoplasias and cutaneous symptoms (41/316) [66].

PP generally appears in skin without any lesions or with lesions secondary to scratching, such as excoriations, nodules, prurigo, lichenification, hyper- or hypopigmentation, and scars [65, 67]. Another clinical form of PP is aquagenic pruritus, characterized by the onset of pruritus within minutes of contact with water at any temperature, without other cutaneous lesions. In more than 30% of the patients, aquagenic pruritus is associated with polycythemia vera or other lymphoproliferative diseases [65, 67]. Pruritus in Hodgkin's disease often begins in the legs and is more severe at night, but soon becomes generalized [68]. Patients with Hodgkin's disease may present a recent onset of eczematous lesions [67].

It has been recognized that the prevalence of pruritus depends on the type of neoplasia [65]. Pruritus is more prevalent in hematologic neoplasias such as Hodgkin's disease, non-Hodgkin lymphoma, leukemia, lymphomas, polycythemia vera, and multiple myeloma [65, 67]. It may occur less frequently in solid tumors such as breast, lung, and gastrointestinal cancer [4, 65, 67].

The type of evaluation to which patients with chronic pruritus of undetermined causes should be submitted is still under discussion. A large 5-year population cohort study with 8,744 patients demonstrated that patients with chronic pruritus had a higher incidence of hematologic (relative risk (RR) 2.02, 95% confidence interval (CI) 1.48–2.75) and bile duct (cholangiocarcinoma) (RR 3.73, 95% CI 1.55–8.97) neoplasias [69]. Despite these relative risks, the incidence of these neoplasias per person per year is extremely low: 0.0003 for cholangiocarcinoma and 0.0016 for malignant neoplasias. Hence, the evaluation for neoplasia in patients with chronic pruritus without skin lesions should be limited to those with signs and symptoms suggesting the presence of a tumor, after clinical evaluation (history and physical examination, with attention to the lymph nodes), initial laboratory tests (complete blood count, lactate dehydrogenase, and liver function) [67, 69]. The initial evaluation will determine the need to complement the evaluation with imaging examinations such as CT [70].

Another large population study [71] showed that patients with pruritus develop 13% more

Table 46.3 Other paraneoplastic dermatoses [1, 4, 78]

Paraneoplastic manifestation	Clinical characteristics	Associated neoplasias	Comments
Scleromyxedema	Papules with a waxy aspect, symmetric on the face, MsSs, and upper chest. Leonine facies due to mucin deposition. Systemic manifestations	IgG-A type monoclonal (meaning not determined) Multiple myeloma, leukemia, non-Hodgkin lymphoma Hodgkin's disease	Are associated neoplasias iatrogenic because melphalan was used?
Scleredema	Indurated edema of the cervical region and upper back. It may progress to disseminated hardened sclerosis	Lymphoma Myeloma	Often associated with diabetes mellitus
Amyloidosis	Purpura in the region of the upper eyelid, face, and neck	Monoclonal gammopathy Multiple myeloma	The amyloid substance is positively stained with Congo red and greenish birefringence is observed under polarized light
	Waxy papules in a region of flexures, eyes, and retroauricular	Multiple endocrine neoplasia (MEN)	
	Macroglossia		
	Carpal tunnel syndrome		
Vasculitis	Palpable purpura on MsIs	Lymphoproliferative diseases (lymphomas, Hodgkin's disease, leukemia)	Rarely associated with malignant neoplasm
Cryoglobulinemia	Purpura	Multiple myeloma	Characterized by the precipitation of immunoglobulins and cryoglobulins in the blood vessels, induced by the cold
	Ischemic ulceration	Waldenstrom's macroglobulinemia	
	Livedo reticularis		
	Acrocyanosis	B-cell neoplasias	
	Raynaud's phenomenon		
	Arterial thrombosis		
Carcinoid syndrome	Episodes of flushing in the face, cervical region, and upper trunk	Carcinoid tumor (endocrine cells of the small bowel) outside the GIT or metastatic to the liver	Diarrhea Bronchospasm Diagnosis: 5-hydroxyindolacetic acid in urine
	Telangiectasias		
	Pellagra type lesions		
Cushing syndrome	Obesity (?)	Anterior pituitary tumor	There may be no presence of obesity
	Hyperpigmentation		
	Acne, striae, telangiectasia, ecchymoses	Carcinoma of the lung Carcinoid tumor	Hyperpigmentation is a common finding in patients with neoplasia
	Proximal muscle weakness	Carcinoma of the thymus, pancreas, thyroid	Late manifestation of the tumor
	Hypertension, hyperglycemia	Pheochromocytoma	
	Hypokalemia	Neoplasias of the male and female reproductive tract	
Pityriasis rotunda	Well-demarcated, circular desquamative plaques of the hypo- or hyperchromic type	Hepatocellular carcinoma, stomach, esophagus, palate, prostate	Rare Associated with non-neoplastic diseases: tuberculosis, Hansen's disease, and pulmonary disease
	Generally on the trunk	Lymphocytic leukemia	
	No pruritus	Multiple myeloma	

MsSs upper limbs, *MsIs* lower limbs, *GIT* gastrointestinal tract malignant neoplasias, hematologic or solid. The greatest risk of cancer diagnosis occurred in the first 3 months of follow-up of the pruritus (RR 2.14, 95% CI 1.67–2.70) dropping to a risk of 1.42 (95% CI 1.19–1.68) in months 4–12 of follow-up. After 12 months of follow-up, the relative risk becomes close to that of the general population. Even so, the authors do not recommend extensive investigations of patients with pruritus [71].

The pathogenesis of paraneoplastic pruritus is still unknown. One of the hypotheses studied is an increase in cytokines (IL-6, IL-8, IL-31) potentiating the T-helper 2 (Th2) response, similarly to what happens in atopy. The tumoral T lymphocytes present a high expression of IL-31 in patients with pruritus who have lymphoma [4, 72].

The treatment of PP is to treat the malignancy when present. Several substances can be used to reduce the symptoms: hydroxyzine, paroxetine, naltrexone, mirtazapine, doxepin, amitriptyline, and others [65].

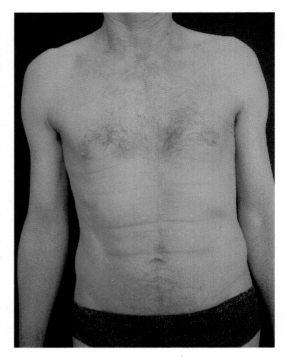

Fig 46.14 Erythroderma: generalized erythema and scaling

Erythroderma

Erythroderma is a condition characterized by generalized erythema and scaling, often associated with pruritus (Figs. 46.14, 46.15, and 46.16) [4]. There may be systemic manifestations such as fever, generalized adenopathies, high-output heart failure, and hypoalbuminemia [4, 73, 74].

It is usually more prevalent in males (2–4:1) and the age of onset of the symptoms is 40–50 years [73–75]. The great majority of cases is associated with the presence of pre-existing dermatoses, such as psoriasis, atopic dermatitis, and pityriasis rubra pilaris, or with the use of medications [73, 74, 76, 77]. Moreover, the reaction can be considered idiopathic in up to 50% of the cases [76, 77].

The prevalence of neoplasia in patients with erythroderma varies from 2% to 11% [73–75]. The most often associated neoplasias are lymphomas and leukemias. In the majority of case

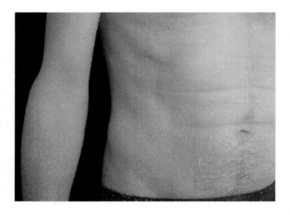

Fig. 46.15 Erythroderma: generalized erythema and scaling. Erythroderma, more closely

series the most frequently associated neoplasia is cutaneous T-cell lymphoma [73, 75]. However, in these patients erythroderma is considered one more direct manifestation of tumor invasion rather than a paraneoplastic dermatosis [76].

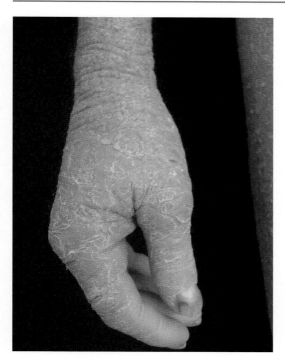

Fig. 46.16 Erythroderma: generalized erythema and scaling. Hands in detail

Among the solid tumors there are reports of the association with cancer of the tongue, liver, lung, stomach, thyroid, and prostate [78].

The histopathologic examination tends to be nonspecific, with acanthosis and hyperkeratosis associated with chronic lymphocytic inflammatory infiltrate, primarily perivascular [76].

The treatment of erythroderma depends on the treatment of the underlying disease when present [76]. Once the neoplasia has been diagnosed it must be treated. Treatment can be aimed at relief of the symptoms with baths, emollients, and topical corticotherapy. In addition, it is necessary to consider the general state of these patients, their hydroelectrolytic balance, and the development of secondary infections [78].

Genetic Syndromes Associated with Malignant Neoplasias and Cutaneous Manifestations (Table 46.4)

These constitute cutaneous manifestations of inherited syndromes that are more susceptible to malignant neoplastic diseases. Since the cutaneous manifestations do not reflect the course of associated neoplasias, they do not fit the definition of paraneoplastic syndromes defined by Curth [77].

Table 46.4 Genetic syndromes associated with neoplasias and skin [79, 80]

Syndrome	Cutaneous manifestations	Associated tumors	Comments
Cowden syndrome (multiple hamartomas)	Brownish papules on the face, neck, tongue, and gingiva (trichilemmomas)	Breast	Autosomal dominant
		Thyroid	Predominates in women
		Endometrium	
	Punctate keratosis	Gastrointestinal polyps	Mutation in the tumor suppressor gene *PTEN/MMAC1* present in chromosome
	Papules on the back of the hands		10q22–23 (codes the tyrosine phosphatase protein that regulates cell proliferation)
	Lipomas		
	Hemangiomas		
Gardner	Epidermoid cysts, fibromas, lipomas, leiomyomas, trichoepitheliomas, neurofibromas	Adenomatous polyps in the gastrointestinal tract (colon and rectum)	Autosomal dominant
	Osteomes (membranous bones of face and head)	Thyroid	Associated with the tumor suppressor gene APC (adenomatous polyposis coli) in chromosome 5q21–q22. Involved in cell migration and cell cycle control
Peutz–Jeghers	Pigmented maculas (ephelide type) on the lips, nose, oral mucosa, subungual	Extensive hamartomatous polyps and carcinomas of the gastrointestinal tract, especially the small bowel	Autosomal dominant
			Extensive hamartomatous polyps and gastrointestinal tract carcinomas, especially of the small bowel
		Appears to have a higher risk of cancer of the pancreas, breast, cervix, ovary, and testicles	Mutation in tumor suppressor gene *STK11/LKB1* In the chromosome
Muir–Torre	Tumors of sebaceous glands, malignant and benign (generally on trunk), keratoacanthomas	GIT neoplasias	Autosomal dominant
		Hematologic cancer	Part of the nonpolyposis syndrome of hereditary colon cancer
		Genitourinary	
		Breast	Mutation of gene MSH-2, located in chromosome 2p22–p21, and MSH-1, located in chromosome 3p21.3
Howel–Evans	Palmoplantar hyperkeratosis	Esophageal cancer	Hyperkeratosis begins in childhood
	Oral leukoplakia		Gene TOC located in chromosome 17q25
Birt–Hogg–Dubé	Skin tags	Renal carcinoma	Mutation of gene17p11.2 codes for folliculin
	Fibrofolliculomas and trichodiscomas on the face and neck		Higher incidence of pulmonary cysts and spontaneous pneumothorax
Hereditary leiomyomatosis/ renal cell cancer syndrome	Cutaneous leiomyomas with segmental or strip distribution (not diffused and symmetric) around 25 years	Papillary renal carcinoma (rapid evolution to lymph nodes and bad prognosis)	Autosomal dominant
			Uterine leiomyomas
			Mutation of gene that codes fumarate hydratase. Mapped in gene 1q42.3–43

Syndrome	Clinical features	Associated tumor	Genetics
Melanoma/pancreatic cancer syndrome (familial atypical multiple mole melanoma-pancreatic cancer syndrome)	Multiple atypical nevi	Pancreatic cancer	Mutation in gene CDKN2A in chromosome 9p21
		Melanoma	
	Increased incidence of melanoma	Breast cancer	
Multiple neuroma syndrome (multiple endocrine neoplasia, MEN type 2B)	Multiple neuromas that appear as whitish nodules on the lips and anterior third of the tongue. They may also appear on the oral mucosa, gingiva, palate, pharynx, conjunctiva, and cornea	Medullary carcinoma of the thyroid	Rare. Autosomal dominant
	Protuberant lips	Pheochromocytoma	Hyperparathyroidism. Mutation in tyrosine kinase receptor (RET) proto-oncogene in chromosome 10
Type I neurofibromatosis	Axillary and inguinal ephelides, café-au-lait macules, cutaneous neurofibromas, plexiform neuromas	Schwann cell tumors. Malignant degeneration of neurofibromas. Pheochromocytomas. Optic glioma	Autosomal dominant. Mutation in gene NF-1 in chromosome 17q11.2 (produces neurofibromin, a tumor-suppressor protein)
Ataxia-telangiectasia syndrome (Louis–Bar syndrome)	Telangiectasias of the conjunctiva, auricular pavilion, palpebrae, malar region, antecubital and popliteal and presternal fossae	Lymphoid tumors (risk 100 times greater than in the general population)	Autosomal recessive. Ataxia (2–3 years of age)
		Leukemia	Immunodeficiency (diminished or absent IgA, IgE, and IgG2). Risk of developing tumors is 37 times greater than in the general population
		Lymphoma	Mutation in gene ATM in chromosome 11q22–23 which signals damage in DNA
Bloom's syndrome	Café-au-lait macules, photosensitivity (center facial erythema), Small stature, thin facies, photosensitivity	Leukemia. Lymphoma. Gastrointestinal adenocarcinoma	Defective gene in DNA helicase (RECQL3) which reduces chromosome stability and the DNA repair capacity
Rothmund–Thomson syndrome (congenital poikiloderma)	Photosensitivity with striated erythema in the first year, telangiectasias, depigmentation and atrophy of the face, extensor extremities, and buttocks (poikiloderma), alopecia	Basocellular and spinocellular carcinomas. Osteosarcoma. Fibrosarcoma, non-Hodgkin lymphoma. Thyroid adenoma	Defective gene in DNA helicase (RECQL4) which reduces chromosome stability and the DNA repair capacity
	Bone abnormalities (frontal protuberance, saddle nose, prognathism)	Gastric carcinoma	
Wiskott–Aldrich syndrome	Petechiae, ecchymoses, eczemas, bacterial infections	Neoplasias, lymphoreticular (Hodgkin lymphoma and B cells)	Gene WAS chromosome Xp11

Glossary

Acanthosis Thickening of the spinous layer. It is a type of epidermal hyperplasia.

Acrokeratosis Clinical condition characterized by erythematous to violaceous papulosquamous plaques arise over accrual areas.

Erythema gyratum repens Disorder characterized by the presence of polycyclic, serpiginous erythema with scaling on its border, rapidly progressive, producing ring-shaped erythematous, concentric figures similar to a wood surface. It is highly associated with neoplasias.

Erythroderma A condition characterized by generalized erythema and scaling, often associated with pruritus and systemic symptoms

Hamartoma A benign tumor-like malformation composed of an abnormal mixture of mature cells and tissues found in areas of the body where growth occurs. It is considered a developmental error and can occur at a number of sites. Example: hemangiomas, melanocytic nevi.

Hypertrichosis Increase in density and length of the hair accepted limits of normal for age, sex, or race.

Ichthyosis Prolonged retention of the stratum corneum, leading to the formation of fishlike scales.

Interleukins Low molecular weight molecules (cytokines), important intercellular messengers, produced by leukocytes, which preferably exert their effect in other white blood cells.

Leiomyomatosis State of having multiple benign tumor of smooth muscle (leiomyomas).

Leser–Trélat sign Sudden increase in the quantity and rapid growth in size of seborrheic keratoses.

Multiple endocrine neoplasias Rare, inherited genetic mutational disorders whereby several endocrine glands develop benign or malignant tumors or grow excessively without forming tumors. A single gene responsible for type 1 disease has been identified. Abnormalities in a different gene have been identified in persons with types 2A and 2B disease.

Necrobiotic xanthogranuloma A disease caused by a granulomatous inflammation that results in the presence of plaques and firm, yellowish nodules, particularly in the face.

Necrolytic Describes processes occurring in cell necrosis and tissue detachment.

Pachydermatoglyphy Palmar thickening with marked palmar ridges and grooves, which exaggerate the dermatoglyphs (digital print) giving it a rough, velvety appearance.

Paraneoplastic disease Clinical or biochemical alterations associated with malignant neoplasias that are not directly related to the invasion of the primary tumor or its metastases.

Poikiloderma Descriptive term that combines atrophy, telangiectasia, and hyper- or hypopigmentation that may occur in different clinical situations.

Reticulohistiocytosis, multicentric
Systemic granulomatous disease of unknown cause. Papulonodular skin lesions containing a proliferation of true histiocytes (macrophages) are associated with arthritis.

References

1. Chung VQ, Moschella SL, Zembowicz A, et al. Clinical and pathologic findings of paraneoplastic dermatoses. J Am Acad Dermatol. 2006; 54(5):745–62.
2. Stedman TL. Dicionário médico. 25th ed. Rio de Janeiro: Guanabara Koogan; 1996. p. 945.
3. Silva JA, Igreja ACDSM, Freitas AF, et al. Paraneoplastic cutaneous manifestations: concepts and updates. An Bras Dermatol. 2013;88(1):9–22.
4. Pipkin CA, Lio PA. Cutaneous manifestations of internal malignancies: an overview. Dermatol Clin. 2008;26:1–15.
5. Curth HO. Skin lesions and internal carcinoma. In: Andrade R, editor. Cancer of the skin: biology, diagnosis, management. Philadelphia: Saunders; 1976.
6. Koyama S, Ikeda K, Sato M, Shibahara K, Yuhara K, et al. Transforming growth factor-alpha (TGFα)-producing gastric carcinoma with acanthosis nigricans: an endocrine effect of TGFα in the pathogenesis of cutaneous paraneoplastic syndrome and epithelial hyperplasia of the esophagus. J Gastroenterol. 1997;32:71–7.
7. Krawczyk M, Mykała-Cieśla J, Kołodziej-Jaskuła A. Acanthosis nigricans as a paraneoplastic syndrome. Case reports and review of literature. Polskie Arch Med Wewn. 2009;119:180–3.
8. Yeh JSM, Munn SE, Plunkett TA, Harper PG, Hopster DJ, et al. Coexistence of acanthosis nigricans and the sign of Leser-Trelat in a patient with gastric

adenocarcinoma: a case report and literature review. J Am Acad Dermatol. 2000;42(3):57–62.

9. Pentenero M, Carrozzo M, Pagano M, Gandolfo S. Oral acanthosis nigricans, tripe palms and sign of Leser-Trélat in a patient with gastric adenocarcinoma. Int J Dermatol. 2004;43:530–2.

10. Brinca A, Cardoso JC, Brites MM, Tellechea O, Figueiredo A. Florid cutaneous papillomatosis and acanthosis nigricans maligna revealing gastric adenocarcinoma. An Bras Dermatol. 2011;86:573–7.

11. Zhang N, Qian Y, Feng AP. Acanthosis nigricans, tripe palms, and sign of Leser-Trélat in a patient with gastric adenocarcinoma: case report and literature review in China. Int J Dermatol. 2015;54:338–42.

12. Lo WL, Wong CK. Tripe palms: a significant cutaneous sign of internal malignancy. Dermatology. 1992;185:151–3.

13. Cohen PR, Grossman ME, Almeida L, Kurzrock R. Tripe palms and malignancy. J Clin Oncol. 1989;7:669–78.

14. Chosidow O, Becherel PA, Piette JC, Arock M, Debre P, Frances C. Tripe palms associated with systemic mastocytosis: the role of transforming growth factor-a and efficacy of interferon-alfa. Br J Dermatol. 1998;138:698–703.

15. Schwartz RA. Sign of Leser-Trélat. J Am Acad Dermatol. 1996;35:88–95.

16. Turan E, Gurel MS, Erdemir AT. Leser-Trélat sign: a paraneoplastic process? Cutis. 2014;94:E14–5.

17. Safa G, Darrieux L. Leser-Trélat sign without internal malignancy. Case Rep Oncol. 2011;4:175–7.

18. Fink AM, Filz D, Krajnik G, Jurecka W, Ludwig H, Steiner A. Seborrhoeic keratoses in patients with internal malignancies: a case-control study with prospective accrual of patients. J Eur Acad Dermatol Venereol. 2009;23:1316–9.

19. Aram H. Acquired ichthyosis and related conditions. Int J Dermatol. 1984;23(7):458–61.

20. Cooper MF, Wilson PD, Hartop PJ, et al. Acquired ichthyosis and impaired dermal lipogenesis in Hodgkin's disease. Br J Dermatol. 1980;102(6):689–93.

21. Moore RL, Devere TS. Epidermal manifestations of internal malignancy. Dermatol Clin. 2008; 26:17–29.

22. Bolognia JL, Brewer YP, Cooper DL. Bazex syndrome (acrokeratosis paraneoplastica). An analytic review. Medicine (Baltimore). 1991;70(4):269–80.

23. Bolognia JL. Bazex syndrome: acrokeratosis paraneoplastica. Semin Dermatol. 1995;14(2):84–9.

24. Valdivielso M, Longo I, Suarez R, et al. Acrokeratosis paraneoplastica: Bazex syndrome. J Eur Acad Dermatol Venereol. 2005;19(3):340–4.

25. Eubanks LE, McBurney E, Reed R. Erythema gyratum repens. Am J Med Sci. 2001;321(5):302–5.

26. Boyd AS, Neldner KH, Menter A. Erythema gyratum repens: a paraneoplastic eruption. J Am Acad Dermatol. 1992;26(5 Pt 1):757–62.

27. Appell ML, Ward WQ, Tyring SK. Erythema gyratum repens. A cutaneous marker of malignancy. Cancer. 1988;62(3):548–50.

28. Bakos N, Krasznai G, Bégány Á. Erythema gyratum repens an immunologic paraneoplastic dermatosis. Pathol Oncol Res. 1997;3:59–61.

29. Kovacs RK, Korom I, Dobozy A, et al. Necrolytic migratory erythema. J Cutan Pathol. 2006;33(3):242–5.

30. Chastain MA. The glucagonoma syndrome: a review of its features and discussion of new perspectives. Am J Med Sci. 2001;321(5):306–20.

31. Wermers RA, Fatourechi V, Wynne AG, et al. The glucagonoma syndrome. Clinical and pathologic features in 21 patients. Medicine. 1996;75:53–63.

32. Beek AP, Haas ERM, Vloten WA, Lips CJM, Roijers JFM, Canninga-van Dijk MR. The glucagonoma syndrome and necrolytic migratory erythema: a clinical review. Eur J Endocrinol. 2004;151:531–7.

33. Hill CL, Zhang Y, Sigurgeirsson B, et al. Frequency of specific cancer types in dermatomyositis and polymyositis: a population-based study. Lancet. 2001;357:96–100.

34. Wakata N, Kurihara T, Saito E, Kinoshita M. Polymyositis and dermatomyositis associated with malignancy: a 30-year retrospective study. Int J Dermatol. 2002;41:729–34.

35. Ramos-E-Silva M, Carvalho JC, Carneiro SC. Cutaneous paraneoplasia. Clin Dermatol. 2011;29:541–7.

36. Sparsa A, Liozon E, Herrmann F, Ly K, Lebrun V, et al. Routine vs extensive malignancy search for adult dermatomyositis and polymyositis: a study of 40 patients. Arch Dermatol. 2002 Jul;138(7):885–90.

37. Wang J, Guo G, Chen G, Wu B, Lu L, Bao L. Meta-analysis of the association of dermatomyositis and polymyositis with cancer. Br J Dermatol. 2013;169:838–47.

38. Ohzono A, Sogame R, Li X, Teye K, Tsuchisaka A, Numata S, Koga H, Kawakami T, Tsuruta D, Ishii N, Hashimoto T. Clinical and immunologic findings in 104 cases of paraneoplastic pemphigus. Br J Dermatol. 2015;173:1447–52.

39. Yong AA, Tey HL. Paraneoplastic pemphigus. Aust J Dermatol. 2013;54:241–50.

40. Nguyen VT, Ndoye A, Bassler KD, et al. Classification, clinical manifestations, and immunopathologic mechanisms of the epithelial variant of paraneoplastic autoimmune multiorgan syndrome: a reappraisal of paraneoplastic pemphigus. Arch Dermatol. 2001;137:193–206.

41. Porro AM, de Caetano L VN, de SN ML, MMS E. Nonclassical forms of pemphigus: pemphigus herpetiformis, IgA pemphigus, paraneoplastic pemphigus and IgG/IgA pemphigus. An Bras Dermatol. 2014;89(1):96–117.

42. Anhalt GJ. Paraneoplastic pemphigus. J Invest Dermatol Symp Proc. 2004;9:29–33.

43. Sehga VN, Srivastava G. Paraneoplastic pemphigus/paraneoplastic autoimmune multiorgan syndrome. Int J Dermatol. 2009;48:162–9.

44. Anhalt GJ, Kim SC, Stanley JR, et al. Paraneoplastic pemphigus. An autoimmune mucocutaneous

disease associated with neoplasia. N Engl J Med. 1990;323:1729–35.

45. Czernik A, Camilleri M, Pittelkow MR, Grando SA. Paraneoplastic autoimmune multiorgan syndrome: 20 years after. Int J Dermatol. 2011;50:905–14.

46. Leger S, Picard D, Ingen-Housz-Oro S, Arnault JP, et al. Prognostic factors of paraneoplastic pemphigus. Arch Dermatol. 2012;148(10):1165–72.

47. Fitzgerald RL, McBurney EI, Nesbitt LT Jr. Sweet's syndrome. Int J Dermatol. 1996;35:9–15.

48. Villarreal-Villarreal CD, et al. Sweet syndrome: a review and update. Actas Dermosifiliogr. 2016. In press. http://dx.doi.org/10.1016/j.ad.2015.12.001.

49. Cohen PR, Kurzrock R. Sweet's syndrome and cancer. Clin Dermatol. 1993;11:149–57.

50. Cohen PR, Talpaz M, Kurzrock R. Malignancy-associated Sweet's syndrome: review of the world literature. J Clin Oncol. 1988;6:1887–97.

51. Rochet NM, Chavan RN, Capel MA, Wada DA, Gibson LE. Sweet syndrome: clinical presentation, associations, and response to treatment in 77 patients. J Am Acad Dermatol. 2013;69:557–64.

52. Cohen PR, Kurzrock R. Sweet's syndrome revisited: a review of disease concepts. Int J Dermatol. 2003;42:761–78.

53. Bennett ML, Jackson JM, Jorizzo JL, Fleischer AB, White WL, Callen JP. Pyoderma gangrenosum. A comparison of typical and atypical forms with an emphasis on time to remission. Case review of 86 patients from 2 institutions. Medicine. 2000;79:37–46.

54. Duguid CM, O'loughlin S, Otridge B, Powell FC. Paraneoplastic pyoderma gangrenosum. Australas J Dermatol. 1993;34:17–22.

55. Luz FB, Gaspar TAP, Kalil-Gaspar N, Ramos-e-Silva M. Multicentric reticulohistiocytosis. J Eur Acad Dermatol Venereol. 2001;15:524–31.

56. Snow JL, Muller AS. Malignancy-associated multicentric reticulohistiocytosis: a clinical, histologic and immunophenotypic study. Br J Dermatol. 1995;133:71–6.

57. Spicknall KE, Mehregan DA. Necrobiotic xanthogranuloma. Int J Dermatol. 2009;48:1–10.

58. Kossard S, Winkelmann RK. Necrobiotic xanthogranuloma with paraproteinemia. J Am Acad Dermatol. 1980;3:257–70.

59. Ugurlu S, Bartley GB, Gibson LE. Necrobiotic xanthogranuloma: long-term outcome of ocular and systemic involvement. Am J Ophthalmol. 2000;129:651–7.

60. Mehregan DA, Winkelmann RK. Necrobiotic xanthogranuloma. Arch Dermatol. 1992;128:94–100.

61. Wood AJ, Wagner MVU, Abbott JJ, Gibson LE. Necrobiotic xanthogranuloma a review of 17 cases with emphasis on clinical and pathologic correlation. Arch Dermatol. 2009;145(3):279–84.

62. Sindhuphak W, Vibhagool A. Acquired hypertrichosis lanuginosa. Int J Dermatol. 1982;21:599–601.

63. Slee PHTJ, Waal RIF, Schagen van Leeuwen JH, Tupker RA, Timmer R, Seldenrijk CA, van Steensel MAM. Paraneoplastic hypertrichosis lanuginosa acquisita: uncommon or overlooked? Br J Dermatol. 2007;157:1087–92.

64. Hegedus SI, Schorr WF. Acquired hypertrichosis lanuginose and malignancy. A clinical review and histopathologic evaluation with special attention to the "mantle" hair of Pinkus. Arch Dermatol. 1972;106:84–8.

65. Weisshaar E, Weiss M, Mettang T, Yosipovitch G, Zylicz Z. Paraneoplastic itch: an expert position statement from the Special Interest Group (SIG) of the International Forum on the Study of Itch (IFSI). Acta Derm Venereol. 2015;95:261–5.

66. Kilic A, Gul U, Soylu S. Skin findings in internal malignant diseases. Int J Dermatol. 2007;46:1055–60.

67. Yosipovitch G. Chronic pruritus: a paraneoplastic sign. Dermatol Ther. 2010;23:590–6.

68. Weisshaar E, Szepietowski JC, Darsow U, Misery L, Wallengren J, et al. European guideline on chronic pruritus. Acta Derm Venereol. 2012;92:563–81.

69. Fett N, Haynes K, Propert KJ, Margolis DJ. Five-year malignancy incidence in patients with chronic pruritus: a population-based cohort study aimed at limiting unnecessary screening practices. J Am Acad Dermatol. 2014;70:651–8.

70. Chiang HC, Huang V, Cornelius LA. Cancer and itch. Semin Cutan Med Surg. 2011;30:107–12.

71. Johannesdottir SA, Farkas DK, Vinding GR, Pedersen L, Lamberg A, Sorensen HT, et al. Cancer incidence among patients with a hospital diagnosis of pruritus: a nationwide Danish cohort study. Br J Dermatol. 2014;171:839–46.

72. Singer EM, Shin DB, Nattkemper LA, Benoit BM, Klein RS, Didigu CA, et al. IL-31 is produced by the malignant T-cell population in cutaneous T-cell lymphoma and correlates with CTCL pruritus. J Invest Dermatol. 2013;133:2783–27.

73. Akhyani M, Ghodsi ZS, Toosi S, Dabbaghian H. Erythroderma: a clinical study of 97 cases. BMC Dermatol. 2005;5:5.

74. Li J, Zheng HY. Erythroderma: a clinical and prognostic study. Dermatology. 2012;225:154–62.

75. Sigurdsson V, Toonstra J, Hezemans-Boer M, Van Vloten WA. Erythroderma. A clinical and follow-up study of 102 patients, with special emphasis on survival. J Am Acad Dermatol. 1996;35:53–7.

76. Kurzrock R, Cohen PR. Mucocutaneous paraneoplastic manifestations of hematologic malignancies. Am J Med. 1995;99(2):207–16.

77. Rothe MJ, Bialy TL, Grant-Kels JM. Erythroderma. Dermatol Clin. 2000;18:405–15.

78. Boyce S, Harper J. Paraneoplastic dermatoses. Dermatol Clin. 2002;20:523–32.

79. Reyes MA, Eisen DB. Inherited syndromes. Dermatol Ther. 2010;23:606–42.

80. Thiers BH, Sahn RE, Callen JP. Cutaneous manifestations of internal malignancy. CA Cancer J Clin. 2009;59:73–9.

Psychiatric Diseases

47

Cecilia Cassal and Ygor Ferrão

Key Points
- Psychodermatology studies the cutaneous manifestations that derive from triggering and aggravating mental factors, and social prejudice and emotional damage resulting from this interaction.
- Skin-related complaints represent 10–58% of primary consultation reasons in general healthcare units in Brazil and North America.
- Self-inflicted dermatosis most prevalent are neurotic excoriation, artifact dermatitis, trichotillomania, delusional parasitosis, and body dysmorphic disorder.
- Lack of control impulse generated by imbalance in serotonergic, noradrenergic, and dopaminergic neurotransmitters and defects in the opioid systems are possible etiologies for psychodermatosis.
- Psychiatric drugs for the treatment of psychodermatosis include selective serotonin reuptake inhibitors, antipsychotics, and mood stabilizers.
- The multifactorial aspects of psychocutaneous diseases require transdisciplinary approach.

C. Cassal (✉)
Sanitary Dermatology Service of the Department of Health of Rio Grande do Sul State, Porto Alegre, Brazil
e-mail: cecilia@cassal.com.br

Y. Ferrão
Federal University of Health Sciences, Porto Alegre, Rio Grande do Sul, Brazil

Anxiety Disorders Outpatient Unit in the Presidente Vargas Maternal and Child Hospital, Porto Alegre, Brazil
e-mail: ygoraf@gmail.com

Epidemiology

The most widely accepted definition of health care refers to a comprehensive approach of individuals in their physical and psychosocial aspects. Embryology explains the common ectodermal origin of the central nervous system and the skin, the largest organ of the human body. With a physiology related to metabolism, thermal and immune modulation, neurosensory perception, and the psyche as a structural border of personality between what is conceived as self and the outer environment, the skin is the first visible aspect of the persona, where it plays a role of social interface, with implications for issues of socialization, self-esteem, and life relationships. The territory of dermatology, psychiatry and psychology, neurology, and endocrinology, the skin

© Springer International Publishing Switzerland 2018
R.R. Bonamigo, S.I.T. Dornelles (eds.), *Dermatology in Public Health Environments*,
https://doi.org/10.1007/978-3-319-33919-1_47

demands a multidisciplinary approach. Psycho-dermatology studies the interaction between skin and psychosocial factors.

Skin-related complaints represent between 10% and 58% of reasons for primary consulta-tion in general healthcare units in Brazil [1] and North America [2]. Among these patients, 4–10% need to be referred to a specialist [3–5], which means, conversely, that 90% of patients not advised to see a referral service will be managed by primary healthcare professionals. The preva-lence of psychological distress/emotional pain in patients with dermatologic disease may reach 25% [6]. A third part of consultations involving the skin as a major complaint corresponds to dis-eases that keep interfaces with dermatology and mental health: psychodermatoses [7]. The chal-lenge to the general practitioner as a first medical contact at the healthcare network, and to the der-matologist, for being referred to as a specialist, is – considering such conceptions and demands – to treat the most prevalent dermatosis properly.

Classification and Diagnosis: Dermatology and Psychiatry Approaches and Systematization of Studies

Dermatology

Psychodermatology has been studied with greater emphasis since the 1950s, and in the 1970s the mechanism by which emotions affect the physical body was unraveled [8]. Several authors, such as Koblenzer [9] and Koo [10], classified the psycho-cutaneous disorders. The different classifications were adapted into six categories in order to sys-tematize the study of psychocutaneous interfaces:

I. Psychophysiologic disorders, whereby a pri-mary cutaneous disease may be exacerbated by emotional factors and stress, such as pso-riasis and atopic dermatitis.

II. Primary psychiatric diseases, whereby the patient does not have skin pathologic sub-strate and all findings are represented by self-induced lesions, as in delusional parasit-osis, artifact dermatosis, neurotic excoria-tion, trichotillomania, and onychophagy.

III. Secondary psychiatric disorders, which occur when the patient develops psycho-logical problems as a consequence of a skin disease that causes physical disfigurement, such as vitiligo and alopecia areata. Difficulties adapting to these disfiguring conditions may be related to depression, anxiety, and the development of social pho-bia [11].

IV. Cutaneous sensory disorders, whereby the patient presents with purely sensory com-plaints, such as itching (pruritus), burning, or tingling, with no evidence of skin disease or other underlying medical condition.

V. Conditions related to the use of psychoac-tive drugs for the treatment of primary dermatologic diseases, such as (a) adminis-tration of doxepin for treatment of chronic urticaria or amitriptyline for postherpetic neuralgia [9, 12]; (b) cutaneous effects due to the use of drugs necessary for the treat-ment of psychiatric disorders, such as acne and psoriasis related to lithium use; and (c) psychological manifestations, such as psy-choses and depression, due to the use of der-matologic drugs, for example, corticoids or interferons.

VI. Multifactorial diseases, such as those whereby psychoneuroimmunologic factors play a synergistic role in triggering or aggravating the cutaneous condition, are exemplified by atopic dermatitis, psoriasis, lichen planus, chronic pruritus, chronic idiopathic urticaria, angioedema, and alo-pecia areata [13]. The role of stress, as well as psychoneuroimmunology, has been widely investigated, as has the genesis of the psychodermatosis (Box 47.1).

Box 47.1 Psychological Problems, Adjusting Process, and the Skin

Dependent on genetic and environmental factors, stress and the presence of associated psychological problems trigger and exacerbate many skin diseases. Producing an inadequate response to stress depends more on the individual's subjective perception about the stressful event than the event itself. By means of a complex interaction of the nervous, endocrine, and immune systems, the biological response to stress varies among individuals: neuropeptides such as vasoactive intestinal peptides and substance P, and chemical mediators such as histamine, are released after stress, inducing inflammation. According to the Stress Model developed by Selye (3-step stress model), dermatologic diseases appear particularly during the adjustment process, which may explain the relationship of stress in the exacerbation of symptoms of many chronic skin diseases such as atopic eczema, psoriasis, alopecia areata, and acne vulgaris [14].

Psychiatry

In the chapter regarding the classification of mental disorders and behavior of the *International Classification of Diseases*, in its 10th edition (ICD-10) [15], Impulse Control Disorders are called Habit and Impulse Disorders [F63] and are inserted in the Section of *Disorders of Adult Personality and Behavior* (F60–F69). It is observed that the disorders are grouped by descriptive similarities and not by the knowledge that they share any other important aspects. The ICD-10 defines disorders as characterized by repetitive actions that do not have any clear rational motivation and that, usually, jeopardize both private and third parties' interests. Such behavior is associated to impulses or actions that cannot be controlled. Importantly, the ICD-10 points out that, for conventional reasons, Habitual Excessive Use of Alcohol or Drugs (F10–F19) and Habit (and Impulse) Disorders involving sexual behavior (F65) or eating behavior (F52) are excluded from this diagnosis group [15].

The ICD-10 describes as major Habit and Impulse Disorders: Pathologic Gambling, Pathologic Incendiary Behavior (pyromania), Pathologic Stealing (kleptomania), and Trichotillomania, inserting Neurotic Excoriation and Intermittent Explosive Disorder into Other Habit and Impulse Disorders.

Until 2013, the *Diagnostic and Statistical Manual of Mental Disorders, Fourth Edition* (DSM-IV) placed Impulse Control Disorders (not classified in other chapters) in one chapter where disorders that are characterized essentially by failure to resist to an impulse or temptation of performing an act that is risky to oneself or to others were included. It pointed out that most patients with these disorders experience either impending tension or excitement before performing the act. Afterward, some patients might feel regret, self-recrimination, or guilt, while others will experience pleasure, gratification, or relief [16].

The main disorders described by the DSM-IV were: Intermittent Explosive Disorder (aggressive impulses that may result in violent assault or destruction of property); Kleptomania (impulse to steal objects that are not necessary for one's personal use or are not worth in terms of financial value); Pyromania (incendiary behavior that results in pleasure, gratification, or tension relief); Pathologic Gambling (maladaptive, recurrent, and persistent behavior related to gambling); Trichotillomania (impulse of pulling and/or plucking one's hair, causing noticeable hair loss); and Impulse Control Disorder with no other specification, where repetitive acts of self-mutilation, onychophagy, oniomania (compulsive shopping), compulsive sexual behavior, and neurotic excoriations could be included.

Besides these disorders, the DSM-IV points out that the occurrence of uncontrolled impulses may occur in other diagnosis categories, such as Substance Related Disorders, Paraphilia, Antisocial and Borderline Personality Disorders, Behavioral Disorders, Schizophrenia and, in some cases, even Mood Disorders, but in the latter the Impulse Control Disorder diagnosis would be secondary [15].

After a series of publications [17–20], some Impulse Control Disorders were moved into other chapters of the DSM-5 [21]. For example, Trichotillomania and Neurotic Excoriation were moved to the group of Obsessive–Compulsive Spectrum Disorders.

Psychodermatosis: Clinical Presentation

Dermatologic

Based on the classification of dermatosis caused primarily by a psychiatric disease, this chapter approaches the skin manifestations of self-inflicted dermatosis, important motivations for either general medical or dermatologic consultation.

Neurotic Excoriation
Artifact dermatitis
Trichotillomania
Delusional parasitosis
Body dysmorphic disorder

The exclusion of other psychiatric or organic diseases, acknowledging or denying the authorship of self-injury, the possibility of impulse control or ritualistic behavior, the intention of anxiety relief or the existence of other secondary gain, and the manifestation of other perceptual issues, such as the presence of delusion, are important factors in determining the diagnosis and the therapeutic approach.

Neurotic Excoriation

Synonyms: skin picking, self-mutilation, dermatotillomania, psychogenic excoriations (Box 47.2).

Box 47.2 General Characteristics of Neurotic Excoriation
- More frequent in middle-aged females
- Affects 2% of all dermatologic patients and up to 10% of those with pruritus complaint
- Scratching, scraping, rubbing, or skin picking urges, acknowledgement of the act, and difficulty in controlling the impulse
- Frequently linear lesions, at various stages, simultaneously
- The middle of the back is typically spared

Epidemiology

Predominantly on females, it has an estimated frequency in 2% of dermatologic patients and in up to 10% of patients with pruritus complaint [22]. Although this condition may occur at any age, more severe and recalcitrant cases have their onset between the third and fifth decades of life [23].

Neurotic excoriations are characterized by repetitive skin scratching because of irritation, sensitivity changes, or benign irregularities on the skin surface, and may adopt obsessive–compulsive ritualistic aspects in some patients. Unlike factitious dermatitis, in neurotic excoriation patients recognize that the lesions are provoked by their self-inflicted acts, although they fail when trying to control such behavior. Gupta [24] describes that the psychiatric disorders most frequently associated with the manifestation of a perfectionist and obsessive personality structure, the obsessive–compulsive disorder, depression, and psychosocial stressors, exacerbate the symptoms in 33–98% of the cases.

Clinical Features

Self-provoked lesions present characteristics of linear trauma, and lesions at several stages may coexist simultaneously, ranging from scars, residual postinflammatory hyper- or hypochromia, erosions, or ulcers. Typically the middle of the back is spared, except when the patient uses tools and not only the nails to reach them. Histopathology is consistent with repetitive local skin trauma [25].

Differential diagnosis should be carried out to exclude other mental disorders, such as borderline personality disorder (frequently associated with suicidal thoughts, dissociation, impulsivity, and aggression) [8], other dermatosis that could cause pruritus, and the use of systemic medication or drugs (Picture 47.1).

Dermatologic compulsions are psychopathologic disorders characterized by a repetitive and uncontrollable impulse to perform certain actions, failed attempts to resist the urge, and increased excitement or tension immediately before the act and pleasure or gratification afterward [26] (Box 47.3).

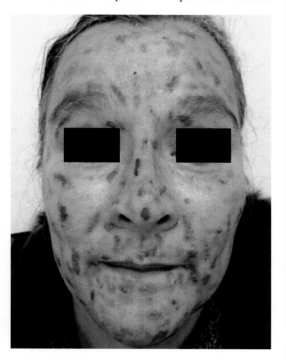

Fig. 47.1 Patient with neurotic excoriations (Photo: personal collection)

> **Box 47.3 Dermatotillomania (Dermatotilexomania)**
> Most psychocutaneous findings reported in children do not fit properly the concepts originally created for the adult population. In this population, the term dermatotillomania is suggested for events whereby the impulse to cause or aggravate one's own skin lesions tends to manifest during times of stress or anxiety. The most frequent clinical forms are erosions on the sides of the nails by tearing, cuticle trauma, nail-fold bleeding, and excoriations in acne lesions. Eventually such behaviors may be associated with dermatophagia, i.e., swallowing of avulsed skin fragments. Onychophagy (titillomania), trichotillomania, and trichophagia have increased frequency, and special events in childhood should draw the attention of the clinician to the possibility of situations of child abuse and family psychopathology, such as Munchausen by Proxy [26, 27] (Table 47.1, Picture 47.2).

Table 47.1 Diagnostic criteria of neurotic excoriation in ICD-10 and DSM-5

ICD-10	DSM-5
Recurrent behavior of harming or excoriating the skin, resulting in noticeable injuries	Recurrent skin picking, resulting in lesions
Sensation of tension increasing, immediately before harming the skin or when the individual tries to resist the behavior	Repetitive attempts to reduce or stop skin picking behavior

Table 47.1 (continued)

ICD-10	DSM-5
Pleasure, satisfaction, or relief when harming the skin	Skin picking behavior causes clinically significant distress or impairment in social, professional, or other important areas of one's life
The disturbance is not better accounted for by another mental disorder and is not caused by a general medical condition (e.g., a dermatologic condition)	Skin picking behavior is not due to physiologic effects of substance use (e.g., cocaine) or to another medical condition (e.g., scabies)
The disturbance causes clinically significant distress or social or occupational impairment as well as impairment in other important areas of one's life. Symptoms may be circumstantial, i.e., appear in childhood or adolescence and disappear with time. The habit of damaging the skin [C1] in a state of increasing anxiety usually does not qualify for a diagnosis of Trichotillomania	Skin picking behavior is not better accounted for symptoms of another mental disorder (e.g., delusions and tactile hallucinations related to a psychotic disorder, attempts to improve a defect or noticeable failure in appearance in body dysmorphic disorder, stereotypes in stereotypic movement disorder, or intent to harm oneself in nonsuicidal self-injury)
Some individuals may present aspects of Neurotic Excoriation, but the resulting skin injury may be difficult to detect when very mild	
In these situations, it is necessary to consider whether the individual experiences or presents more significant psychological, social, or occupational distress. In some cases, after medical consultation with a specialist, the patient undergoes a medical treatment because of the frequency or the damage caused	

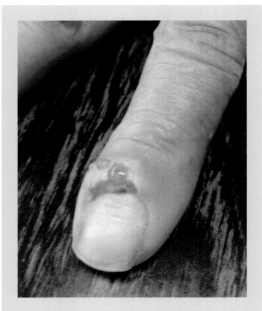

Fig. 47.2 Dermatotilexomania: secondary infections are frequent complications in self-inflicted injury spots (Photo: personal collection)

Artifact Dermatitis

Synonym: factitious dermatitis (Box 47.4)

Box 47.4 General Characteristics of Artifact Dermatitis
- Predominance in females
- Higher incidence in late adolescence and early adulthood, but occurs in elderly patients (loneliness, need for attention)
- Onset after stressor event
- Self-inflicted skin lesions are often induced by objects
- Typically located in areas within easy reach of hands
- Assess substance abuse, other compulsions, and suicide risk

Although patients typically deny, partially or fully, their participation in the origin of injuries, artifact dermatitis is characterized by lesions caused by the use of nails, sharp objects, lit cigarette butts, or chemicals. The disease is associated with personality disorders and occurs predominantly in females [28]. Although described in elderly patients in response to loneliness, losses, and need to obtain attention, the highest incidence is concentrated in late adolescence or early adulthood, as an unconscious response to psychological distress, stress, or as an attempt to a secondary gain [29]. Problems in keeping interpersonal relationships reflect patients' difficulties in controlling self-image and mood control, and self-mutilation behavior develops as a cry for help in response to the stress associated with poorly developed adaptive responses, associated with feelings of emptiness and anger. Sneddon (1975) describes that appearance rate of injuries after situations that cause severe stress such as diseases, accidents, and deprivation was 19–33%, and that lesions disappeared after termination of the stressor event. Besides skin self-mutilation, patients with borderline personality disorder are prone to suicide, substance abuse, or compulsive eating [30].

Clinical Presentation

Lesions typically stand out from normal surrounding skin, with exact geometric edges and bizarre aspect, which may resemble many skin diseases. Obsessive–compulsive disorders, depression, psychosis, mental retardation, and Munchausen syndrome are among the psychiatric disorders that follow artifact dermatitis [31, 32]. Peculiar appearance of lesions, associated with patient's inability to explain how they were formed or evolved, facilitates diagnosis [33] (Picture 47.3).

Trichotillomania

Synonyms: Trichotemnomania, trichoteiromania, scratching-pseudoalopecia, trichocryptomania (Box 47.5).[1]

> **Box 47.5 General Characteristics of Trichotillomania**
> - Most frequent in children and young adults
> - High rate of psychological comorbidities (depression and obsessive–compulsive disorder)

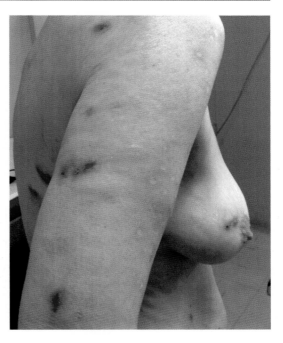

Fig. 47.3 Artifact dermatitis. Several primary lesions and linear ulceration in areas accessible to the hands. Several scarring lesions of previous events are observed (Photo: personal collection)

> - Exclude alopecia areata, fungal infections, and other itchy scalp disorders
> - Dermoscopic and anatomic pathology tests are elucidative
> - Always consider possibility of trichophagia and evaluate risk of trichobezoar

The term "trichotillomania" derives from the combination of the Greek words *trichos* (hair), *tillein* (pull), and *mania* (impulse). Therefore, trichotillomania is defined as the irresistible impulse of pulling the hair, followed by relief [34]. Trichophagia is the act of swallowing hair after avulsion. The most common self-aggressive acts are trichotillomania, trichotemnomania, trichophagia, trichoteironamia, scratching-pseudoalopecia, trichocryptomania, trichorrhexomania, and neuropathic plica, as shown in Table 47.2 [35].

Epidemiology

With an estimated prevalence of 1–2% of the general population, the disease has the highest

---

[1] In this case, synonymia is given by cause-effect approximation – habit control disorder leading to hair behavior.

Table 47.2 Diagnosis features of main compulsive trichosis

Compulsive trichosis	Meaning and clinical features
Trichotillomania	Compulsive act of pulling out the hair, especially from the parietal region and vertex [37], though hair from any part of the body can also be involved in the process. Because of its diffuse characteristics and not being usually the patient's main complaint, hair thinning is often clinically perceived when it affects 30% of a given capillary area [35]
Trichotemnomania	Presence of tonsured areas within a few millimeters of the scalp surface. Hair is cut vertically, with a sharp object. Trichogram, pathology, capillary density within normal limits. Dermatoscopy or common optical microscopy allows observation of cut small and vertical hair. Unlike trichotillomania, trichotemnomania only occurs in older adults, and all cases reported are in psychopathic patients
Trichophagia	Compulsive hair swallowing behavior. Patients with long hair usually put amounts of hair in the mouth and keep chewing them, sometimes swallowing a few. A different form consists of the patient pulling hairs, typical behavior of a trichotillomania, and then taking them to the mouth. Whenever there is a clinical picture of trichotillomania, hair swallowing should be hypothesized. It may result in a trichobezoar
Trichoteiromania Tonsure trichoclasia Scratching-pseudoalopecia	Two-centimeter-long hairs and split, brush-shaped distal extremities. Erythematous and scaly scalp surface is a consequence of scratching. Pathologic anatomy may reveal acanthosis, orthohyperkeratosis, focal parakeratosis, and intraepidermal microvesiculation. Trichoptilosis, trichorrhexis nodosa, incomplete fractures and folds. Trichogram is normal
Tonsure trichotillomania	The terms trichoteiromania, tonsure trichoclasia, tonsure trichotillomania, and scratching-pseudoalopecia represent the same clinical entity. They may all be identified either on the scalp or other region where there is friction, as in the pruritic dermatosis such as lichen planus, atopic dermatitis, or neurodermatitis
Trichokryptomania or trichorrhexomania	The terms trichokryptomania and trichorrhexomania are synonymous and correspond to a compulsive act of cutting the hair with the nails, which can occur either close to the scalp or several centimeters from skin surface. Usually there is no area of alopecia but hairs cut into various sizes, resembling a "bad hair day." The hairs present on their distal end a brush-like appearance. Trichotillomania (pull out) can be concurrent
Neuropathic plica	In psychiatric patients, the presence of too tangled hair, leading to formation of a hardened mass. Differential diagnosis with acute compression of the hair, electrostatic phenomenon that occurs in the hair during washing

Source: Organized by the authors, after a review by Pereira [35]

incidence in children aged 4–10 years, adolescents, and young adults [26], with an incidence of 3.4% in women and 1.5% in men. In the United States, 2–8 million people may have trichotillomania, with 90% being women and 0.6% students; 43% of patients deny the act of pulling the hair [36]. Overall, 40% of cases are not diagnosed and 58% of patients are untreated. In childhood, trichotillomania is seven times more frequent, with an average age of 8 years for boys and 12 for girls [27, 34].

Etiology

Despite variable etiology describing a simple habit reaction to stress and anxiety, the comor-

bidity rate with other diseases is high, the most frequent being obsessive–compulsive disorder and depression. Delusions may be associated with trichotillomania. Other symptoms of anxiety can be evidenced by the presence of onychophagy and onychotillomania, suggesting evaluation for diagnosis of obsessive–compulsive disorder.

Clinical Presentation

Frontotemporal regions of the scalp, eyebrows, eyelashes, beard, and pubic hairs are usually affected; pubic hairs may or may not be sucked and swallowed [36]. Typically, hairs in the affected area have different lengths and the tensile test is negative on peripheral area. Dermatoscopy shows decreased capillary density, hairs broken in different sizes, yanked hairs, vellus, trichoptilosis, and yellow dots with or without black dots [37, 38]. Differential diagnosis should be performed considering alopecia areata, tonsuring tinea, and pruritic dermatosis of the scalp, such as lichens. The lack of typical hair in club (exclamation points) and mycologic test when fungal infection is suspected will exclude these etiologies.

Trichotillomania is one of the rare psychodermatoses is characteristic in hair histopathology, where trichomalacia, characterized by the presence of blackened impregnations (rods remains) in follicular ostia, is only observed in these patients [35, 36]. Pigmentary remains close to follicle isthmus, follicles destroyed by perifollicular hemorrhage, several empty follicle channels, dilated hair follicle infundibulum, and corneal stoppers may also be seen, mostly in the catagen phase or initial anagen without perifollicular inflammatory processes [35]. Trichoptilosis, pili torti, and trichorrhexis nodosa are observed by dermatoscopy. In the semiologic analysis of trichotillomania, other tests described by Pereira [35] are: negative gentle traction test, since most hairs are in anagen phase, not falling off easily. In this test, a breaking damaged hair shaft can produce false positives; the hair pull test, which implies intense hair traction, obtaining fragments, demonstrating hair fragility; and the friction test, which consists of placing a hair pad in the center of the palm of one hand and rubbing it with the finger, obtaining pieces of the hair damage, typical of hair shaft lesion. Trichogram can result in up to 100% of hairs in anagen phase, as telogen hairs are first extracted because they have lower adhesion to the follicle and its extraction is less painful; thus, whole hair restoration is anagen. Analysis of spontaneously eliminated hair, collected by the patient's companion without his knowledge, in places where he has been, and those brought by the patient himself, usually a small sample to justify possible denial and lack of interest in cooperating with the doctor, will reveal the presence of anagen, catagen, or telogen hair with epithelial bag, showing that hairs were extracted by traction. Hair coat study consists of observing small hairs with the aid of a paper card placed perpendicularly to the scalp and removing a sample of them. According to Pereira [35], a hair plucked in the anagen phase results in three possible findings: (a) hair breaks close to the root but will continue to grow soon; (b) hair is fragmented inside the follicular channel and, in this case, may form the trichomalacia; and finally, (c) hair breaks off a few centimeters from scalp surface. Such a test is important for differential diagnosis of androgenetic alopecia, wherein drawn hairs will be predominantly telogen. The fluorescent light test consists of using fluorescent ink (such as text marker pens) close to modified scalp area. Examination of the patient's fingers with a Wood's lamp on the day after will show fluorescence. In the observation window technique, a small area of hair is cut close to the scalp and isolated with scotch tape. This feature will show the patient normal growth of his companion hair (Box 47.6).

> **Box 47.6 Trichobezoar**
>
> *Trichobezoar* occurs in 90% of cases in girls with long hair. Presence of weight loss and imprecise gastrointestinal manifestations should draw attention to the possible diagnosis. Clinically, vomiting and nausea can be observed in 64% of patients, abdominal cramping in 70%, changes in bowel habit in 32%, palpable epigastric mass in 88%, as well as other gastrointestinal disorders. It is often related to the presence of mental retardation. Mortality rate by trichobezoar may reach 50% if there is no early diagnosis with treatment [35] (Pictures 47.4, 47.5, and 47.6).

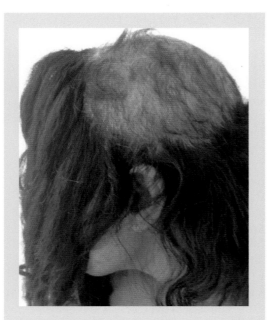

Fig. 47.4 Patient with extensive alopecic area caused by hair pulling (Photo: personal collection)

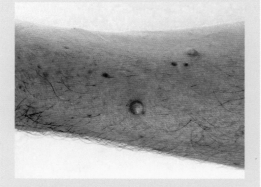

Fig. 47.5 The same patient may pull out hair from more than one site of the body (Photo: Paula Baldissera Tansini collection)

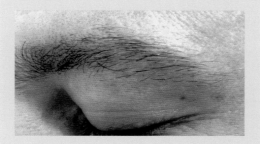

Fig. 47.6 The same patient may pull out hair from more than one site of the body (Photo: Paula Baldissera Tansini collection)

Delusional Parasitosis

Synonyms: *Ekbom syndrome, acarophobia, dermatozoic delirium, psychogenic parasitosis, delirium of internal zoopathy, delusional infestation, Morgellon's disease* [39] (Box 47.7).[2]

Box 47.7 General Characteristics of Delusional Parasitosis

- Starts at the sixth decade, prevalence of one man for every three women over 50 years old
- Irreducible belief of being infested by parasites or other foreign objects
- Exclude psychoses induced by use of substances or drugs, organic causes, cerebrovascular disease, vitamin B12 deficiency
- Can manifest simultaneously in persons in close contact (folie à deux)
- Frequent medical shopping and adhesion issues

Delusional parasitosis (DP) was first reported by Darwin [40], regarding an individual who experienced a wild idea (an itch) so powerfully that it could not be changed suddenly, either by visual sense or reason. In 1894, in relation to other similar cases, Thiberge called it acarophobia, and subsequently Perin published new accounts in 1896. In 1938 the syndrome was defined by Ekbom, who described seven cases and called it *dermatozoenwanh*, dermatozoic delirium. Also known as delusional parasitosis or psychogenic parasitosis, the Ekbom syndrome is infrequent and is characterized by the patient's strong conviction that he is infested with worms that come out of the skin, usually the scalp,

---

[2] *Morgellons disease is a term coined in 2002 by Mary Leitao, founder of the Morgellons Research Foundation (www.morgellons.org). With the advent of the internet, patients go researching for symptoms on the web and self-diagnose, which consists of delusional infestation, when they believe to be infested by inanimate objects, usually multicolored fibers of uncertain origin, but also food, nanotechnology products, fungi, bacteria, etc. The disease is not recognized in the scientific community, but eventually became a mass phenomenon – the first disease "transmitted" via the internet.*

mouth, eyes, or genital area [41, 42]. Dupré described a *délire de zoopathie interne* (delirium of internal zoopathy) and Levy subdivided it into "internal" and "external" types [43]. The main characteristic of these syndromes would be the delusional belief (*délire*) of harboring animals in the body or on the body. The 29 cases described by the author involved rats, birds, worms, snakes, and so forth, but insects were not mentioned. Faure et al. [44], in turn, described two cases in which le *délire zoopathique* involved insects and reiterated the idea that the fundamental problem was "delusional" in its nature. Wilson and Miller [45] suggested the term "delusional parasitosis" and favored their delirious origin. The emergence of other specimens mentioned by patients as responsible for skin symptoms, such as fibers and nanotechnology products, led Freudenmann and Lepping (2009) to advocate the use of the term delusional infestation [39].

With an approximate prevalence of 83.21 affected individuals per million population, the syndrome starts predominantly in the sixth decade, with an average age at onset of 55.6 years [47]. Lyel (1983) describes a male to female ratio of 1:1 in those under 50 years of age and 1:3 in patients over 50. The delirium, with a paranoid character, manifests itself in between 15% and 40% of cases and may develop more often in people with obsessive traits and paranoia. Such descriptions led some authors to consider delusional parasitosis as a picture of monosymptomatic hypochondriacal psychosis [46]. In an extensive discussion on the true nature of delusional parasitosis, Ekbom studies particularly the nature of tactile sensations described by patients, suggesting an organic basis for this syndrome and questioning whether it would be a distortion of real perceptions or a hallucinatory phenomenon [47, 48].

Clinical Presentation

Onset of symptoms can be sudden and slow with complaints of rash, tickling, some feeling of movement inside the skin, tingling, or tactile hallucinations, triggering the feeling of parasitism. Although there is no typical elementary lesion, the skin disorder often found is due to excoriation and scarification, performed to remove parasites

or fibers or other foreign objects that the patient believes are under the skin. Linear or oddly shaped ulcers, erosions, and scars, as well as nodular prurigo, are usually symmetric findings in hand access areas and, for this reason, the center of the back is often spared. Patients retell, obsessively, and in detail, the morphology, life cycle, and habits of these "parasites" as well as the actions taken to avoid and eliminate them. Some patients, in a hallucinatory state, collect pieces of skin, paper, or other specimens, identifying these fragments as parasites. This behavior has been termed the "matchbox sign" [49, 50] in allusion not to the means by which it is presented (matchbox, plastic envelopes, tubes, etc.) but to the agent assigned by the patient as responsible for the infestation. Replacing the classic "matchbox sign," Freudenmann and Lepping (2009) suggest the use of the term "specimen sign," since it is not unusual for patients to submit photographs or videos taken by them to verify the infestation. Sometimes people who live close to the patient (and are influenced by him) share the same feelings and beliefs. This situation is called folie à deux, shared madness [39, 48] (Picture 47.7).

Diagnosis should exclude real skin infestations and other organic, infectious, and metabolic causes, and assess cerebrovascular and psychiatric comorbidities other than monosymptomatic delirium, as well as the use of psychoactive drugs such as opioids, amphetamines, and cocaine.

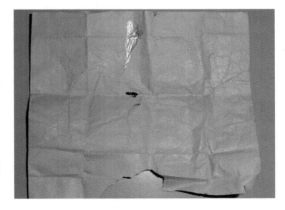

Fig. 47.7 In a variation of the matchbox sign, the patient brought an insect to the medical office, to which he attributed the colonization of his wife, in a folie à deux delusional parasitosis case (Photo: personal collection)

Trichophobia is the belief of the existence of something in the root of the hair, which disappears when it is pulled off, after which normal hair may grow back. Dermatologically it may be expressed as alopecia, and differential diagnosis should pay attention to different forms of trichotillomania. The patient's belief in the presence of parasites or other foreign and non-existent objects provides clues to delusional thinking (Box 47.8).

Box 47.8 Hallucination, Delirium, and Delusion

Conceptual confusion about tactile hallucinations causes the disorder sometimes to be classified from the perspective of perception, sometimes from a cognitive point of view. Regarding a reasonable confusion among the terms hallucination, delirium, and delusion, Berrios (2011) explains that French and German psychiatry have established a less strict line between hallucinations and delusions than English psychiatry, where *"délire"* and *"wahn"* (French and German terms for delirium, respectively) share a less "intellectualist" direction than the English word *"delusion."* *"Délire"* and *"wahn"* assume a personality disorder and a fracture in the "relationship" between the subject and his world, which the English term *"delusion"* lacks, usually defined as a wrong or pathologic "belief" and, thus, a thought disturbance. Hallucinations, therefore, tend to be regarded as a subtype to delusions ("sensory delusions") and, as a consequence, less emphasis is placed on its aspects of "perception" than on those called "cognitive" or "apperception" aspects. Literature on descriptive psychopathology are singularly reticent about tactile hallucination, and the *Traité* by Ey devotes only 16 pages to it, out of a total of 1543 [47, 48].

Body Dysmorphic Disorder

Synonyms: Dysmorphophobia (Box 47.9)

Box 47.9 General characteristics of Hallucination, Delirium and Delusion

- May affect 10–14% of dermatologic patients
- Frequent onset in young adults
- Defined by the concern with minimal or no flaw at all in one's appearance
- Complaints often refer to the nose, mouth, hair, breasts, and genitals
- Typically associated with ritualistic or compulsive behaviors

---

Clinical Presentation

In patients suffering from body dysmorphic disorder (BDD), disturbance in the perception of their own body image, usually a concern with a flaw on the face, nose or mouth, hair, breasts, and genital area, often generates social isolation and adoption of ritualistic behaviors, such as spending a lot of time in front of the mirror and checking it several times, looking for small imperfections. BDD may be manifested as olfactory reference syndrome, whereby the concern relates to an unpleasant odor emitted by the patient, not noticeable by anyone else. These patients often adopt compulsive behaviors to eliminate the perceived odor, such as bathing repeatedly or using products such as deodorants, perfumes, or mouthwashes excessively, as well as arranging multiple medical consultations rationalize their issues. The consequences of ritualistic behaviors can be dermatologic, such as eczemas caused by product contact and, occasionally, erosion in areas burned repeatedly. The spectrum of BDD includes obsessions and delusions – in this case, without the corresponding insight about the problem – which do not meet the criteria for obsessive–compulsive disorder or for the spectrum of psychoses disorders, useful classifications for treatment purposes [23]. It is estimated that BDD affects about 1% of the

United States population and that 10–14% of patients who visit dermatologists have a positive screening for BDD, with an average age around 34 years; it affects both genders equally [23, 51].

Psychiatric/Psychological

Self skin-damaging behavior can occur in response to a delusion (parasitosis), hallucination, or tactile delusion (tingling) as in a psychotic disorder, such as schizophrenia or manic episodes [52, 53]. In such cases, disorder excoriation should be diagnosed as secondary to the main disorder. In general, compulsive or excessive washing in response to contamination fears (which may be the result of any kind of obsessive content) in individuals with obsessive–compulsive disorder can lead to skin lesions [20]. Individuals with BDD may scar or pinch their own skin because of concerns about the appearance of certain body parts (e.g., nose, soles of the feet, jaw, and palms of the hands) [54]. As in psychoses, in such cases the excoriation disorder should also not be considered as a primary diagnosis. Although a stereotypic movement disorder might be characterized as repetitive behavior of self-mutilation, its onset usually occurs in early developmental period. For example, individuals with the neurogenetic condition of Prader–Willi syndrome may have an early-onset behavior of pinching the skin, and its symptoms may meet the criteria for the stereotypic movement disorder [55]. Similarly, although complex motor tics, present in patients with Tourette's disorder, can lead to behaviors of self-mutilation, this is a sudden, automatic, and uncontrollable behavior, which differs considerably from the psychopathologic viewpoint of self-harm behavior in the excoriation disorder [56]. Excoriation disorder should not be diagnosed when skin injury occurs as a consequence of misleading or simulated behavior, such as those occurring in the factitious disorder (or Munchausen syndrome) [57]. Within the heterogeneity of depressive disorders, the excoriation disorder should not be diagnosed if skin pinching is mainly attributed to the intention of hurting oneself in order to reduce psychological distress (anxiety) [58] or to play the role of a cry for help, which occurs in characterological depression, as a result of personality disorders (especially borderline and histrionic personality disorders). [59]. Although the diagnosis of excoriation disorder cannot occur when there is another medical condition present, it may be precipitated or exacerbated by an underlying dermatologic condition. For example, acne can lead to scratching and tearing, which may also be associated with the comorbid excoriation disorder. Differentiation between these two clinical conditions (acne with itching and pinching versus acne with comorbid excoriation disorder) requires an assessment of to what extent skin pinching became independent of the underlying dermatologic condition. Medications of various types (including psychotropic drugs) may also cause itching and, therefore, lead to repetitive abrasions.

Etiopathogenesis of Psychodermatosis

Little is known about which organically based factors are associated with excoriation disorder. If considered as a lack of control impulse, the most accepted hypothesis will be that there is an imbalance in serotonergic, noradrenergic, and dopaminergic neurotransmitters [18]. Modulation of opioid systems is also a possibility, as some patients with neurotic excoriation seem to have a good response to fentanyl, an opioid antagonist, contrary to what was observed in patients with trichotillomania [60], but this study was never replicated and its sample was too small to be conclusive (n = 10).

So far, there is no evidence in neuroimaging studies to substantiate the neurobiology or neurocircuits of excoriation disorder. However, by phenomenological analogy with trichotillomania (both are part of the "grooming behaviors"), it may be speculated that there are changes in the basal ganglia, particularly due to the reduction in volumes of putamen and cerebellar involvement [61].

There seems to be an intersection of the circuits involved in obsessive–compulsive disorder with those potentially involved in neurotic excoriation, but insufficiently so to consider that both are mediated by the same structures or similar neurotransmitters [62].

Psychoanalytic

Historically, individuals with psychogenic excoriation are described by psychoanalytic literature as having an obsessive–compulsive personality configuration; i.e., a rigid, perfectionist, judgmental, controlling, and indecisive personality for fear of making mistakes. These patients would rarely have contact with feelings and struggle with difficulty in dealing with unconscious aggression. This aggression would originate from unresolved feelings toward their parents. Symptoms of psychogenic excoriation are connected to the anxiety generated when aggressive manifestations reach the surface. A broad pathology spectrum is found, ranging from neurotic symptoms that appear only under stress, to the patient who is unable to act because of compulsive behavior that influences many aspects of his or her life.

Social (Family)

In some situations it can be manifested as a reaction to the pressure of psychosocial factors related to family or work, which generates a high level of stress culminating in symptoms, similar to what occurs in trichotillomania.

Treatments: Dermatologic, Psychiatric, and Psychotherapeutic

Dermatologic

Treatment should be conducted with the intention of identifying triggering factors, in association with psychiatric treatment. Lesion occlusion in order to hinder self-harm and identification of best adaptive behaviors as substitutes for self-aggression can help (for example, the use of emollient to replace the act of scarring). Early diagnosis of psychodermatosis can prevent both habit consolidation and chronicity, and severity of skin sequelae caused by injuries. Direct confrontation of the patient is not suggested [63]. Although formal training of dermatologists does not contemplate these therapeutic resources, some authors suggest that hypnosis, biofeedback, and relaxation exercises can be a useful adjunct to the therapy of psychodermatosis, associated or not with psychoactive drugs [9, 23, 64].

Psychiatric

There is no specific pharmacologic treatment for neurotic excoriation, and medicines are used to treat target symptoms or primary conditions such as depression, anxiety, or obsessive–compulsive symptoms. Main drugs used in the treatment of psychodermatosis, their dosages, side effects, and some remarks about their use are listed in Table 47.3. Only drugs that have already been submitted to a clinical trial are listed (open or randomized double-blind trials). Case reports were not considered for this review.

Selective serotonin reuptake inhibitors (SSRIs): only case reports support the use of SSRIs in patients with skin picking, but there is no robust evidence to support their use, except situations of neurotic excoriation secondary to depressive episodes, anxiety scenarios, or obsessive–compulsive disorder [18].

Antipsychotics, especially atypical antipsychotics, which have a serotonergic effect associated with dopaminergic antagonist, seem to be promising in the treatment of excoriation disorder, as well as trichotillomania [18, 65], but there are no studies with adequate methodology and sufficient sample sizes to recommend their use as definitive treatment.

Mood stabilizers (lithium and anticonvulsants): As with SSRIs, mood stabilizers may be promising, but the evidence is based on case reports, especially with the use of lithium carbonate [66].

Table 47.3 Psychiatric drugs with some evidence level used in the treatment of psychodermatosis

Drug (class)	Action	Most common side effects	Dose	Observations
Fluvoxamine (antidepressant)	Selective serotonin reuptake inhibitor (SSRI)	Transient nausea, sexual dysfunction	50–300 mg	Arnold LM et al. J Clin Psychopharmacol. 1999;19(1):15–8. Stanley MA et al. J Clin Psychopharmacol. 1997;17(4): 278–83
Fluoxetine (antidepressant)	SSRI	Transient nausea, decreased appetite, insomnia, anxiety, sexual dysfunction	20–80 mg	Simeon D et al. J Clin Psychiat.1997; 58(8): 341–7. Christenson GA et al., Am J Psychiat. 1991; 148(11): 1566–71. Winchel RM et al. J Clin Psychiat. 1992; 53(9): 304–8. Koran LM et al. Psychopharmacol Bull. 1992; 28(2): 145–9. Streichenwein SM, Thornby JI. Am J Psychiatry. 1995; 152(8): 1192–6(Negative long-term result)
Sertraline (antidepressant)	SSRI	Transient nausea, decreased appetite, insomnia, anxiety, sexual dysfunction	50–250 mg	Dougherty DD et al. J Clin Psychiat. 2006; 67(7): 1086–92
Citalopram (antidepressant)	SSRI	Nausea, headache, sexual dysfunction	20–60 mg	Stein DJ et al. Eur Arch Psychiatry Clin Neurosci. 1997; 247(4): 234–6
Escitalopram (antidepressant)	SSRI	Nausea, headache, sexual dysfunction	10–20 mg	Keuthem NJ et al. Int Clin Psychopharmacol. 2007; 22(5): 268–74. Gadde KM et al. Int Clin Psychopharmacol, 2007; 22(1): 39–42
Clomipramine (antidepressant)	SSRI	Dry mouth, constipation, increased appetite, sexual dysfunction	25–250 mg	McGuire JF et al. J Psychiatr Res. 2014; 58: 76–83. Bloch MH et al. Biol Psychiat. 2007; 62(8): 839–46. Leonard HL et al. Arch Gen Psychiat. 1991; 48(9): 821–7. Swedo SE et al. N Engl J Med. 1989; 321(8): 497–501. Rothbart R et al. Cochrane Database Syst Rev. 2013; 11: CD007662
				Electrocardiogram before starting use is recommended, for possible cardiac conduction problems
Venlafaxine (antidepressant)	Selective serotonin and noradrenaline reuptake inhibitor	Dry mouth, constipation, nausea	37.5–225 mg.	Ninan PT et al. Psychopharmacol Bull. 1998; 34(2): 221–4
Olanzapine (neuroleptic)	Antidopaminergic	Sedation, increased appetite, sexual dysfunction	2.5–15 mg	Rothbart R et al. Cochrane Database Syst Rev. 2013; 11: CD007662. Van Ameringen M et al. J Clin Psychiat. 2010; 71(10): 1336–43. Stewart RS et al. J Clin Psychiat. 2003; 64(1): 49–52
Pimozide (neuroleptic)	Antidopaminergic	Sedation, increased appetite, sexual dysfunction	1–8 mg	Stein DJ et al. J Clin Psychiat. 1992; 53(4): 123–6
				Used to enhance the effect of SSRIs
Risperidone (neuroleptic)	Antidopaminergic	Sedation, increased appetite, sexual dysfunction	0.5–8 mg	Stein DJ et al. J Clin Psychiat. 1997; 58(3): 119–22
				Used to enhance the effect of SSRIs
Aripiprazole (neuroleptic)	Partial dopaminergic and serotonergic agonist	Sedation, increased appetite, sexual dysfunction	10–30 mg	White MP et al. J Clin Psychopharmacol. 2011; 31(4): 503–6

Other medications and therapies: there is no evidence on the use of benzodiazepines or other types of antidepressants in impulsive behavior control related to excoriation disorder. Doxepin, a tricyclic antidepressant with a potent antihistamine effect, has been used by some professionals, especially dermatologists, but there is no strong evidence in the literature to substantiate its use [67, 68]. More recently, N-acetylcysteine, used as mucolytic and as an antidote for acetaminophen overdose, seems to have demonstrated good reduction in symptoms when compared with placebo, especially after 12 weeks of use, in increasing dosages of 1200–3000 mg/day with mild side effects which did not lead to withdrawal of drug use, such as nausea, dry mouth, constipation, and dizziness [69, 70]. Neuromodulation techniques, such as repetitive transcranial magnetic stimulation (rTMS) and transcranial direct current stimulation (tDCS), have not yet been described in cases of excoriation disorder, but as they are treatments with robust evidence for depressive and clinical anxiety settings, they deserve attention in respect of the potential therapeutic arsenal for psychodermatosis.

Psychotherapeutic

Cognitive-behavioral therapy is the psychotherapeutic approach with more evidence of efficacy, especially when behavioral techniques of habit reversal and reinforcement/acceptance are used [71–73]. Habit reversal training (HRT) comprises three basic aspects: behavioral awareness training, competitive behavior training (but healthier), and social support, especially family [74]. Reinforcement/acceptance behavioral techniques consist basically of education on behavioral condition, habit reversal techniques, acceptance techniques, and commitment (especially for avoiding situations) [75].

This combination of techniques also involves the identification of values in one's life and examination of how damaging one's own skin affects the individual's ability to move toward these values.

It also analyzes the attempts to control impulses and other negative personal experiences surrounding the phenomenon of scarring, and how these control strategies worked in the past, providing alternative behaviors and alternative feelings, exercises to undo the merge between feeling/thinking and acting (behavior of automatization), instructing the individual to live through personal emotional experiences as mere thoughts, feelings, or emotions, not as triggers of harmful behavior [73]. These techniques can be performed individually or in groups, but professionals should be well trained to be able to identify situations and correct them properly. There are no reports of family psychotherapeutic approach strategies for neurotic excoriation, but the family should be warned not to be a facilitator of such behaviors and not to allow the patient to become used to self-harm attitudes.

Final Considerations

The body has many languages, and the skin communicates emotions and organ functioning as well as internal systems in a most peculiar way. Frequent medical consultations motivated by skin issues associated with personal, family, and social psychological distress, failure of general and dermatologic medical training particularly regarding a satisfactory approach to the aforementioned issues, as well as the complexity of clinical presentations and their possible comorbidities determine a demand to re-evaluate both health education and care concerning psychodermatology.

More than specific cosmetic issues, innumerable emotional "cries for help" arising from skin manifestations demand teamwork and organized action from primary care medical doctors, dermatologists, psychiatrists, and psychologists, in the same physical setting whenever possible, providing easy access to these specialists for the patient. Valorization of doctor-patient attachment should be shown by attentive listening during a careful account of disease history, including stressor and triggering events, which should be carried out slowly before a physical examination while encouraging the patient to elaborate his concerns and difficulties verbally, instead of showing them through skin injuries.

Usually these patients tend to deny the possibility of underlying psychological conditions and have poor self-esteem: direct confrontation and referral to a psychiatrist may reproduce a sense of latent abandonment and engender suicidal thoughts or other severe psychiatric conditions. Therefore, the inclusion of a mental health professional in the psychodermatosis patient's medical care team should be equally cautious: instead of a routine referral, where the patient – certainly coming from a great deal of medical shopping – would feel worthless or misunderstood in his complaints, issues such as difficult disease control, number of attempts at different sorts of treatment, financial cost, as well as personal investment and frustration (information obtained only by a well-conducted anamnesis) may be discussed with him or her up to the point where the logical consequence would be to consider the benefits of an association of knowledge that the inclusion of psychotherapeutic or drug treatment concomitant with dermatologic follow-up would provide.

Glossary

Anagen phase The growth phase in the hair growth cycle during which a newly formed hair continues to grow. It is generally the longest phase and is followed by catagen.

Borderline personality disorders (BPDs) *BPD* is a pattern of abnormal behavior characterized by extreme fears of abandonment, unstable relationships with other people, sense of self, or emotions, feelings of emptiness, frequent dangerous behavior, and self-harm. Symptoms may be triggered by seemingly normal events. This pattern of behavior typically begins by early adulthood, and occurs across a variety of situations. People with BPD often engage in idealization and devaluation of others, alternating between high positive regard and great disappointment. Substance abuse, depression, and eating disorders commonly coexist with borderline personality disorder. About 6% die by suicide.

Catagen phase The catagen phase is a short transition stage that occurs at the end of the anagen phase. It signals the end of the active growth of a hair. This phase lasts for about 2–3 weeks while the hair converts to a club hair. A club hair is formed during the catagen phase when the part of the hair follicle in contact with the lower portion of the hair becomes attached to the hair shaft. This process cuts the hair off from its blood supply and from the cells that produce new hair. When a club hair is completely formed, about a 2-week process, the hair follicle enters the telogen phase.

Histopathology Refers to the microscopic examination of tissue in order to study the manifestations of disease. Specifically, in clinical medicine histopathology refers to the examination of a biopsy or surgical specimen by a pathologist, after the specimen has been processed and histologic sections have been placed onto glass slides. In contrast, cytopathology examines free cells or tissue fragments.

Intermittent explosive disorder *Intermittent explosive disorder* (sometimes abbreviated as *IED*) is a behavioral disorder characterized by explosive outbursts of anger and violence, often to the point of rage, which are disproportionate to the situation at hand (e.g., impulsive screaming triggered by relatively inconsequential events). Impulsive aggression is unpremeditated, and is defined by a disproportionate reaction to any provocation, real or perceived. Some individuals have reported affective changes prior to an outburst (e.g., tension, mood changes, energy changes).

Munchausen syndrome A psychiatric factitious disorder whereby those affected feign disease, illness, or psychological trauma to draw attention, sympathy, or reassurance to themselves. Casually referred as *hospital addiction syndrome, thick chart syndrome*, or *hospital hopper syndrome*. Munchausen syndrome fits within the subclass of factitious disorder with predominantly physical signs and symptoms, but patients also have a history of recurrent hospitalization, traveling, and dramatic, extremely improbable tales of their past experiences. The condition derives its name from the fictional character Baron Munchausen.

Onychophagy Also known as *nail biting* or *onychophagia*, it is an oral compulsive habit sometimes described as a parafunctional activity, the common use of the mouth for an activity other than speaking, eating, or drinking. Onychophagy is considered an impulse control disorder in the DSM-IV-R, and is classified under obsessive–compulsive and related disorders in the DSM-5. The ICD-10 classifies it as "other specified behavioral and emotional disorders with onset usually occurring in childhood and adolescence."

Paraphilia *Paraphilia* (also known as *sexual perversion* and *sexual deviation*) is the experience of intense sexual arousal to atypical objects, situations, or individuals. No consensus has been found for any precise border between unusual sexual interests and paraphilic ones. The number and taxonomy of paraphilias is under debate. The DSM-5 has specific listings for eight paraphilic disorders. Several subclassifications of the paraphilias have been proposed, and some argue that a fully dimensional, spectrum or complaint-oriented approach would better reflect the evidence.

Prader–Willi syndrome A rare genetic disorder whereby seven genes (or some subset thereof) on chromosome 15 (q 11–13) are deleted or unexpressed (chromosome 15q partial deletion) on the paternal chromosome. It was first described in 1956 by Andrea Prader (1919–2001), Heinrich Willi (1900–1971), Alexis Labhart (1916–1994), Andrew Ziegler, and Guido Fanconi of Switzerland. Characteristic of PWS are "low muscle tone, short stature, incomplete sexual development, cognitive disabilities, behavior problems, and a chronic feeling of hunger that can lead to excessive eating and life-threatening obesity." The incidence of PWS is between 1 in 25,000 and 1 in 10,000 live births.

Psychodermatology The study of skin disorders using psychological and psychiatric techniques, a subspecialty of dermatology. Frequently treated conditions are psoriasis, eczema, hives, genital and oral herpes, acne, warts, skin allergies, pain and burning sensations, hair loss, and compulsive skin picking and hair pulling. Psychological or psychiatric treatments are the primary treatments for some dermatologic disorders, including trichotillomania and skin picking. Techniques include relaxation, meditation, hypnosis and self-hypnosis, psychotropic medications, biofeedback, and focused psychotherapy.

Schizophrenia A mental disorder characterized by abnormal social behavior and failure to understand reality. Common symptoms include false beliefs, unclear or confused thinking, hearing voices, reduced social engagement and emotional expression, and a lack of motivation. People with schizophrenia often have additional mental health problems such as anxiety disorders, major depressive illness, or substance use disorder. Symptoms typically come on gradually, begin in young adulthood, and last a long time.

Social phobia Also known as *social anxiety disorder (SAD)*, it is an anxiety disorder characterized by a significant amount of fear in one or more social situations causing considerable distress and impaired ability to function in at least some parts of daily life. These fears can be triggered by perceived or actual scrutiny from others. It is the most common anxiety disorder and one of the most common psychiatric disorders, with 12% of American adults having experienced it.

Telogen phase The telogen phase is the resting phase of the hair follicle. When the body is subjected to extreme stress, as much as 70% of hair can prematurely enter a phase of rest, called the telogen phase. This hair begins to fall out, causing a noticeable loss of hair. This condition is called telogen effluvium. The club hair is the final product of a hair follicle in the telogen stage, and is a dead, fully keratinized hair. Fifty to 100 club hairs are shed daily from a normal scalp.

Tourette's disorder Tourette's disorder (also called Tourette's syndrome, Gilles de la Tourette syndrome, GTS or, more commonly, simply Tourette's or TS) is an inherited neuropsychiatric disorder with onset in childhood, characterized by multiple physical (motor) tics and at least one vocal (phonic) tic. These tics characteristically wax and wane, can be suppressed temporarily, and are preceded by a premonitory urge. Tourette's is defined as part of a spectrum of tic disorders, which includes provisional, transient, and persistent (chronic) tics.

Trichobezoar Trichobezoars or human hairballs are complications of trichophagia or eating of the hair. Trichophagia occurs when hair that is pulled out is chewed and then swallowed. The hair will eventually collect in a sufferer's stomach and will cause stomach problems such as indigestion and pain. Trichophagia is very commonly associated with trichotillomania.TrichomalaciaA rare genetic condition resulting in patchy hair loss in children. It is an abnormality of the hair shaft and can be due to a compulsive habit of pulling hair on the head or even eyelashes and eyebrows.

Trichotillomania Also known as *trichotillosis* or *hair pulling disorder*, trichotillomania is an obsessive–compulsive disorder characterized by the compulsive urge to pull out one's hair, leading to hair loss and balding, distress, and social or functional impairment. It may be present in infants, but the peak age of onset is 9–13 years. It may be triggered by depression or stress. Owing to social implications, the disorder is often unreported and it is difficult to accurately predict its prevalence. Common areas for hair to be pulled out are the scalp, eyelashes, eyebrows, legs, arms, hands, nose, and the pubic areas.

References

1. Santos Júnior A, Andrade MGGG, Zeferino AB, et al. Prevalência de dermatoses na rede básica de saúde de Campinas, São Paulo-Brasil. An Bras Dermatol. 2007;82(5):419–24.
2. Lowell BA, Froelich CD, Federman DG, et al. Dermatology in primary care: prevalence and patient disposition. J Am Acad Dermatol. 2001;45(2):250–5.
3. Royal College of General Practitioners. Morbidity statistics from general practice: 4th National Study 1991–92. London: HMSO; 1995. p. 54–6.
4. Julian CG. Dermatology in general practice. Br J Dermatol. 1999;141:518–20.
5. Solomon BA, Collins R, Silverberg NB, Glass AT. Quality of care: issue or oversight in health care reform? J Am Acad Dermatol. 1996;34:601–7.
6. Taborda MLV, Weber MB, Freitas ES. Avaliação da prevalência de sofrimento psíquico em pacientes com dermatoses do espectro dos transtornos psicocutâneos. An Bras Dermatol. 2005;80(4):351–4.
7. Savin J, Cotterill J. Psychocutaneous disorders. In: Champion RH, Burton JL, Ebling FJ, editors. Textbook of dermatology. Oxford: Blackwell Scientific; 1992. p. 2479–96.
8. Azambuja RD, Rocha TN, Conrado LA, et al. Psicodermatologia: pele mente e emoções. In: Sociedade Brasileira de Dermatologia. [Org.: Roberto Doglia Azambuja, Tânia Nely Rocha]. 1st. São Paulo: AC Farmacêutica; 2014.
9. Koblenzer CS. Psychocutaneous disease. 1st ed. Orlando: Grune Stratton; 1987.
10. Koo JYM, Pham CT. Psychodermatology: practical guidelines on pharmacotherapy. Arch Dermatol. 1992;126:381–8.
11. Higgins EM, Du Vivier AW. Cutaneous disease and alcohol misuse. Br Med Bull. 1994;50:85–98.
12. Koo J. Psychotropic agents in dermatology. Dermatol Clin. 1993;11:215–24.
13. Gupta MA, Voorhees JJ. Psychosomatic dermatology: is it relevant? Arch Dermatol. 1990;126:90–3.
14. Mercan S, Kivanç Altunay I. Psychodermatology: a collaborative subject of psychiatry and dermatology. Turkish J Psychiat. 2006;17(4):305–13.
15. World Health Organization. The ICD-10 classification of mental and behavioural disorders: clinical descriptions and diagnostic guidelines. Porto Alegre: Artes Médicas; 1992.
16. American Psychiatric Association. Diagnostic and statistical manual of mental disorders. 4th ed. Washington, DC: American Psychiatric Press; 1994.
17. Torres AR, Fontenelle LF, Shavitt RG, Ferrão YA, do Rosário MC, Storch EA, et al. Comorbidity variation in patients with obsessive–compulsive disorder according to symptom dimensions: results from a large multicenter clinical sample. J Affect Disord. 2016;190:508–16.
18. Ferrão YA, Miguel EC, Stein DJ. Tourette's syndrome, trichotillomania, and obsessive–compulsive disorder: how closely are they related? Psychiatry Res. 2009;170:32–42.
19. Phillips K, Stein DJ, Rauch S, Hollander E, Fallon B, Barsky A, et al. Should an obsessive–compulsive spectrum Grouping of disorders be included in dsm-v? Depression Anxiety. 2010;27:528–55.
20. Lovato L, Ferrão YA, Stein DJ, Shavitt RG, Fontenelle LF, Vivan A, et al. Skin picking and trichotillomania in adults with obsessive-compulsive disorder. Compr Psychiatry. 2012;53(5):562–8.
21. American Psychiatric Association. Diagnostic and statistical manual of mental disorders. 5th ed. Washington, DC: American Psychiatric Press; 2013.
22. Dornelles SIT, Dornelles LA. Escoriações Neuróticas. In: Psicodermatologia. [Org.: Weber MB, Fontes Neto PTL]. Yendis Editora: São Caetano do Sul; 2009. p. 71–84.
23. Lee CS, Koo JYM. Psychocutaneous diseases. In: Bologna JL, Jorizzo JL, Schaffer JV, editors.

Dermatology, 3rd ed. St. Louis, Mo: Elsevier Saunders. 2012. p:127–34.

24. Gupta MA, Gupta AK, Haberman HF. The self inflicted dermatoses: a critical review. Gen Hosp Psychiatry. 1987;9:45–52.

25. Van Dijk E, Van Voorst Vader PC. Dermatillomania. Dermatologica. 1979;158:65–71.

26. Silveira VLB. Dermatocompulsões. In: Psicodermatologia. [Org.: Weber MB, Fontes Neto PTL]. Yendis Editora: São Caetano do Sul; 2009. p. 85–93.

27. Manzoni APDS, Grazziotin TC. Psicodermatoses na infância. In: Psicodermatologia. [Org.: Weber MB, Fontes Neto PTL]. Yendis Editora: São Caetano do Sul; 2009. p. 191–202.

28. Koblenzer CS. Dermatitis artefata. Clinical features and approaches to treatment. Am J Clin Dermatol. 2000;1(1):47–55.

29. Gregurek-Novak T, Novak-Bilic G, Vuic M. Dermatitis artefacta: unuasual appearance in an older woman. J Eur A Dermatol Venereol. 2005;19:223–5.

30. Sneddon I, Sneddon J. Self-inflicted injury: a follow-up study of 43 patients. Br J Dermatol. 1975;3:527–30.

31. Gupta MA, Gupta AK. Dermatitis artefacta and sexual abuse. Int J Dermatol. 1993;32:825–6.

32. Stein DJ, Hollander E. Dermatology and conditions related to obsessive compulsive disorder. J Am Acad Dermatol. 1992;26:237–42.

33. Hollander MH, Abraham HS. Dermatitis factitia. South Med J. 1973;66:1279–85.

34. Siddappa K. Trichotillomania. Continuin Med Educ. 2003;69(2):63–8.

35. Pereira JM. Tricoses compulsivas. An Bras Dermatol. 2004;79(5):609–18.

36. Christenson GA, Mackenzie TB, Mitchell JE. Characteristics of 60 adult chronic hair pullers. Am J Psychiatry. 1991;148:365–70.

37. Abraham LS, Torres FN, Azulay-Abulafia L. Pistas dermatoscópicas para diferenciar a tricotilomania da alopecia areata em placa. An Bras Dermatol. 2010;85(5):723–6.

38. Lachapelle JM, Pierard GE. Traumatic alopecia in trichotillomania: a pathogenic interpretation of histologic lesions in the pilosebaceous unit. J Cutan Pathol. 1977;4:51–67.

39. Freudenmann RW, Lepping P. Delusional infestations. Clin Microbiol Rev. 2009;22(4):690–732.

40. Darwin E. Zoonomia. London: J. Johnson; 1796.

41. Alves CJM, Martelli AC, Ceribelli, Prado RBR, Fonseca MS. Variability of psychological diagnosis in patients with psychogenic excoriation. An Bras Dermatol. [Internet]. 2009. [cited 2016 Apr 25];84(5):534–7.

42. Lyell A. Delusions of parasitosis. Br J Dermatol. 1983;108:485–99.

43. Levy H. Les Delires de Zoopathie interne. Paris: These Steinheil; 1906.

44. Faure H, et al. Sur les parasitoses delirantes. L'Evolution Psychiat. 1957;22:357–75.

45. Wilson JW, Miller HE. Delusions of parasitosis. Arch Dermatol Syph. 1946;54:39–56.

46. Alistair M. Monosymptomatic hypochondriacal psychosis manifesting as delusions do parasitosis. A description of four cases successfully treated with pimozide. Arch Dermatol. 1978;114:940–3.

47. Berrios GE. Alucinações táteis: aspectos conceituais e históricos. Rev. latinoam. psicopatol. fundam., São Paulo. 2011;14(3):542–62.

48. Cassal C. Delírio de Parasitose: uma aproximação epistemológica. In: Ensaios filosóficos. [Org.: Guedes W]. Dialógica Editora: São Paulo; 2013. p. 39–48

49. Koo J, Lee CS. Delusions of parasitosis a dermatologist's guide to diagnosis and treatment. Am J Clin Dermatol. 2001;22:85–90.

50. Larsson CE, Otsuka M, Balda AC. Delírio de parasitose (acarofobia): relato de caso em São Paulo(Brasil). An Bras Dermatol. 2000;75:723–8.

51. Phillips KA, Dufresne RG Jr, Wilkel CS, et al. Rate of body dysmorphic disorder in dermatology patients. J Am Acad Dermatol. 2000;42:436–41.

52. Karakus G, Tamam L. Impulse control disorder comorbidity among patients with bipolar I disorder. Compr Psychiatry. 2011;52(4):378–85.

53. Koo JY, Leon A, Levin EC. Psychodermatology. Semin Cutan Med Surg. 2013;32(2):63.

54. Grant JE, Redden SA, Leppink EW, Odlaug BL. Skin picking disorder with co-occurring body dysmorphic disorder. Body Image. 2015;15:44–8.

55. Hustyi KM, Hammond JL, Rezvani AB, Hall SS. An analysis of the topography, severity, potential sources of reinforcement, and treatments utilized for skin picking in Prader-Willi syndrome. Res Dev Disabil. 2013;34(9):2890–9.

56. Gomes de Alvarenga P, de Mathis MA, Dominguez Alves AC, do Rosário MC, Fossaluza V, Hounie AG, et al. Clinical features of tic-related obsessive-compulsive disorder: results from a large multicenter study. CNS Spectr. 2012;17(2):87–93.

57. Boyd AS, Ritchie C, Likhari S. Munchausen syndrome and Munchausen syndrome by proxy in dermatology. J Am Acad Dermatol. 2014;71(2):376–81.

58. Tucker BT, Woods DW, Flessner CA, Franklin SA, Franklin ME. The skin picking impact project: phenomenology, interference, and treatment utilization of pathologic skin picking in a population-based sample. J Anxiety Disord. 2011;25(1):88–95.

59. Harth W, Mayer K, Linse R. The borderline syndrome in psychosomatic dermatology. Overview and case report. J Eur Acad Dermatol Venereol. 2004;18(4):503–7.

60. Frecska E, Arato M. Opiate sensitivity test in patients with stereotypic movement disorder and trichotillomania. Prog Neuro-Psychopharmacol Biol Psychiatry. 2002;26(5):909–12.

61. O'Sullivan RL, Rauch SL, Breiter HC, Grachev ID, Baer L, Kennedy DN, et al. Reduced basal ganglia volumes in trichotillomania measured via morphometric magnetic resonance imaging. Biol Psychiatry. 1997;42:39–45.

62. Stein DJ, van Heerden B, Hugo C, van Kradenburg J, Warwick J, Zungu-Dirwayi N, et al. Functional brain imaging and pharmacotherapy in trichotillomania. Single photon emission computed

tomography before and after treatment with the selective serotonin reuptake inhibitor citalopram. Prog Neuro-Psychopharmacol Biol Psychiatry. 2002;26:885–90.

63. Spraker MK. Cutaneous artifactual disease: an appeal for help. Pediatr Clin N Am. 1983;30:659–68.

64. Azambuja RD, Rocha TN, Conrado LA, et al. Psicodermatologia: pele, mente e emoções. 1st ed. São Paulo: AC Farmacêutica; 2014.

65. Stewart RS, Nejtek VA. An open-label, flexible-dose study of olanzapine in the treatment of trichotillomania. J Clin Psychiat. 2003;64:49–52.

66. Gupta MA. Emotional regulation, dissociation, and the self-induced dermatoses: clinical features and implications for treatment with mood stabilizers. Clin Dermatol. 2013;31(1):110–7.

67. Harris BA, Sherertz EF, Flowers FP. Improvement of chronic neurotic excoriations with oral doxepin therapy. Int J Dermatol. 1987;26(8):541–3.

68. Goldsobel AB, Rohr AS, Siegel SC, Spector SL, Katz RM, Rachelefsky GS, et al. Efficacy of doxepin in the treatment of chronic idiopathic urticaria. J Allergy Clin Immunol. 1986;78(5 Pt 1):867–73.

69. Deepmala, Slattery J, Kumara N, Delheya L, Berkd M, Deand O, et al. Clinical trials of N-acetylcysteine in psychiatry and neurology: a systematic review. Neurosci Biobehav Rev. 2015;55:294–321.

70. Grant JE, Chamberlain SR, Redden SA, Leppink EW, Odlaug BL, Kim SW. N-acetylcysteine in the treatment of excoriation disorder: a randomized clinical trial. JAMA Psychiatry. 2016;73(5):490–6 doi:10.1001/jamapsychiatry.2016.0060.

71. Grant JE, Odlaug BL, Chamberlain SR, Keuthen NJ, Lochner C, Stein DJ. Skin picking disorder. Am J Psychiatry. 2012;169(11):1143–9.

72. Schuck K, Keijsers GP, Rinck M. The effects of brief cognitive-behaviour therapy for pathologic skin picking: a randomized comparison to wait-list control. Behav Res Ther. 2011;49(1):11–7.

73. Flessner CA, Busch AM, Heideman PW, Woods DW. Acceptance-enhanced behavior therapy (AEBT) for trichotillomania and chronic skin picking: exploring the effects of component sequencing. Behav Modif. 2008;32(5):579–94.

74. Azrin NH, Nunn RG. Habit reversal: a method of eliminating nervous habits and tics. Behav Res Ther. 1973;11:619–28.

75. Hayes SC, Strosahl KD, Wilson KG. Acceptance and commitment therapy: an experiential approach to behavior change. New York: Guilford Press; 2003.

Additional Suggested Readings

Azambuja RD, Rocha TN, Conrado LA, et al. Psicodermatologia: pele mente e emoções. Sociedade Brasileira de Dermatologia. 1ª ed. São Paulo: AC Farmacêutica; 2014.

Jafferany M. Psychodermatology: a guide to understanding common psychocutaneous disorders. Prim Care Companion J Clin Psychiat. 2007;9(3):203–13.

Weber MB, Fontes Neto PTL. Psicodermatologia. São Caetano do Sul: Yendis Editora; 2009. p. 71–84.

Part VIII

Emerging Issues of Dermatology in Public Health

Adriano Heemann Pereira Neto, Luiza Metzdorf,
Leandro Linhares Leite, and Renan Rangel Bonamigo

Key Points

- The main polluting agent related to human health problems, according to the WHO, are the particulate materials
- Among the air pollution effects on human health are systemic problems (such as respiratory, cardiac, and rheumatic disorders) and skin disorders
- Early aging, atopic dermatitis, rash, acne, melasma, and skin neoplasias are related to the effects of air pollution
- Global measures and responsibilities of governmental institutions must be demanded to decrease the emission of pollutants noxious to human health
- Individual preventive measures must be stimulated to soothe the impact of air pollution on human health and skin health

A.H.P. Neto, MD, MS (✉) • L. Metzdorf, MD
Federal University of Rio Grande do Sul, Porto Alegre, Brazil
e-mail: adrianohpneto@gmail.com

L.L. Leite, MD
Dermatology Service of Hospital de Clínicas de Porto Alegre, Federal University of Rio Grande do Sul, UFRGS, Porto Alegre, Brazil

R.R. Bonamigo, MD, MSc, PhD
Dermatology Service, Hospital de Clínicas de Porto Alegre (HCPA), Federal University of Rio Grande do Sul (UFRGS), Porto Alegre, Brazil

Sanitary Dermatology Service of the Department of Health of Rio Grande do Sul State (ADS-SES), Porto Alegre, Brazil

Graduate Pathology Program of Federal University of Health Sciences of Porto Alegre, Porto Alegre, Brazil

Introduction

Population increase, propagation of the means of transport accompanied by the burning of fossil fuels, and pursuit of financial gain that triggers an accelerated industrialization process have all increased world pollution [1] by practically immersing the population in particulate residues in the air, garbage, soil chemical products, and waste, as well as contaminated water in the aquatic environment. According to the World Health Organization (WHO), pollution has been defined as the contamination of both the inner and outer environment by any chemical, physical, or biological agent that changes the natural characteristics of the environment [2].

"Pollution" can be classified in different ways Examples include air, land, light, noise, thermal, visual, and water pollution. In this chapter we focus on the impact of external air pollution on the skin, a type of pollution that has concrete relationships with environmental changes, quality of life, and human health [3, 4].

Environmental pollution has its origins in established sources, usually of industrial and mobile origin, such as highways and air traffic.

© Springer International Publishing Switzerland 2018
R.R. Bonamigo, S.I.T. Dornelles (eds.), *Dermatology in Public Health Environments*,
https://doi.org/10.1007/978-3-319-33919-1_48

The multiple types of particles and substances in such emissions are divided into primary and secondary pollutants. According to the Brazilian Environment Ministry (MMA), primary pollutants are substances directly emitted by their sources into the environment, such as particulate materials and gases, whereas secondary pollutants include substances resulting from chemical reactions, or heat reaction, as well as ultraviolet (UV) radiation from primary pollutants with substances present in the lower layer of the atmosphere, for example, ozone and peroxyacetyl nitrate [5].

The main kinds of air pollutants are highly variable depending on the referred author and the literature. According to the Brazilian MMA [5], air pollutants include aldehydes (RCHO), sulfur dioxide (SO_2), nitrogen dioxide (NO_2), hydrocarbons (HCs), particulate matter (PM), carbon monoxide (CO), ozone (O_3), and short-life climate pollutants (PCVC). Furthermore, when the American literature is considered, according to the Environmental Protection Agency, for example, some divergences can be found, since pollutants are divided into six common types [6], so-called criteria, since they are the most common pollutants associated with changes in human health [7].

Among polluting materials, their origins, their significance for pollution, and mainly their relationship with the development of health problems are highly variable. This is important from a physician's perspective because, as will be shown here, it is not merely exposure to a polluted environment that will make an individual more prone to comorbidity, but more importantly the elements to which he or she is exposed. Thus, it is very important that the physician has knowledge of the polluting materials and, moreover, that he knows the environment in which his patients are exposed.

The main polluting agent related to human health problems, according to the WHO, is particulate matter (PM). This form of pollutant is a complex mixture of solid elements of small diameter that comprises different substances (smog, tobacco smoke, pollen, house dust mite allergens, and gaseous contaminants) of different origins, chemical compositions, and physical features [5, 6]. Such substances are divided into three major groups according to their mean diameter: ultrathin particles when their diameter is less than 0.1

μm ($PM_{0.1}$), thin particles when their diameter is less than 2.5 μm ($PM_{2.5}$), and thick particles when their mean diameter is less than 10 μm (PM_{10}).

The variation in diameter is very important for the medical practice, since the smaller the size of the particulate, the greater is its power to penetrate the respiratory tract, possibly reaching the endothelium through cell junctions and gaining access to the interstices and the vascular system, and, of course, the possibility of carrying other toxic substances, bacteria, and viruses. Furthermore, the emission source of those particles is distinct; $PM_{2.5}$ is produced more through combustion, such as in industries, automobiles, and land burning and mainly composed of nitrates, sulfates, and carbon organic compounds, whereas PM_{10} results from mechanical processes that emit bigger particles into the air, such as dust, fog, aerosol, smoke, and soot [8, 9].

The effects of PM on the human health are very diverse. In fact, these particles are the main elements responsible for pollution-related diseases, and therefore are the most commented on in the literature. They encompass systemic assaults, from mainly respiratory ones caused by increased proinflammatory factors and direct cell damage, such as asthma, pulmonary neoplasias, chronic obstructive pulmonary disease (COPD), to exacerbations of cardiac and rheumatic diseases caused by an increased inflammatory reaction, and, as discussed herein, dermatologic diseases [9]. Significant pollutants related to human health are listed in Table 48.1.

According to the WHO report, about 9 out of 10 city dwellers in the world are subject to pollution levels above the acceptable standard levels. In that 2016 report most of the citizens on the planet do not adhere to policies regarding safe levels of air pollution, leaving only 12% of the population in the investigated cities capable of breathing healthy and safe air. Worse is the fact that about half of the investigated urban population is exposed to pollution levels of less than 2.5-fold higher than the recommended levels [11]. In the United States, for example, in 2014 the Environment Protection Agency reported that more than 142 million Americans lived in areas where the air quality did not reach the environmental national standards of quality of the air,

Table 48.1 Primary and secondary compound pollutants related to human health impairment [5, 6, 10]

	What it is	Sources	Effects	Standard levels
$PM_{2.5}$	Composed of particles and organic compounds of <2.5 µm diameter	Car combustion	Respiratory tract diseases (asthma, COPD)	Must not exceed 10 µg/m³ per year, or 25 µg/m³ for 24 h
		Industries	Exacerbation of cardiovascular diseases	
		Natural burning for site clearing	Systemic inflammation	
PM_{10}	Composed of particles and organic compounds with diameter of <10 µm	Combustion processes	Respiratory diseases	Must not exceed 20 µg/m³ (annual mean) and 50 µg/m³ (24-h mean)
		Secondary aerosol		
Nitrogen dioxide (NO_2)	Heavy-smelling gas of chestnut color, highly oxidative	Volcanoes	Photochemical smog	100 ppm, up to 1-h exposure
		Bacterial actions	Acid rain	
		Electrical discharges	Combustion in thermoelectric industries, vehicles, and incinerators	
		Combustion		
Ozone (O_3)	Secondary pollutant resulting from other pollutants. It has a highly oxidative power in the troposphere. It acts in the stratosphere by absorbing solar radiation and refraining part of the UV rays from reaching the Earth's surface	Not directly emitted to the atmosphere, being produced photochemically and by solar radiation over the nitric oxides and volatile organic compounds	Asthma worsening	0.1 ppm
			Respiratory deficiency	
			Emphysemas	
			Bronchites	
			Cardiovascular	
Aldehydes (R-CHO)	Organic compound resulting from the partial oxidation of alcohols, or from photochemical reactions	Fuel burning, mainly ethanol	Mucosal itching	86.5 ppb of formaldehyde over a maximum exposure time of 30 min
		Main examples include formaldehyde and acetaldehyde	Asthmatic crises	
			Carcinogens	
			Cephalea	
Sulfur dioxide (SO_2):	Toxic and highly oxidative colorless gas; a key factor in troposphere ozone development	In nature: volcanoes	Acid rain	0–20 µg/m³
		Burning fossil fuels with sulfur in their composition	Mucosal itching	
		Electric utilities	Burns	
		Industrial processes	Worsening cardiovascular and pulmonary problems	
Methane hydrocarbons (HC)	HC found as gases, thin particles, or drops Methane: colorless and odorless gas, highly explosive	Fossil fuel burning	Ozone development	5000 ppm
		Fuel evaporation	Greenhouse effect	
		Ruminant digestion	Asphyxia	
		Organic waste decomposition	Cardiac arrest	
		Hydroelectric reservoirs	Unconsciousness	
		Extraction of mineral fuels (mainly petroleum);	Damage to the central nervous system	

(continued)

Table 48.1 (continued)

	What it is	Sources	Effects	Standard levels
Carbon monoxide (CO)	Odorless and colorless gas from incomplete burning of carbon-containing fuel	Fuel burning (motor vehicles, fireplaces, heaters)	Headache	9 ppm: maximum levels in closed environments
			Dizziness	10–24 ppm: maximum with no problems for human health
			Weakness	1600 ppm: death after 1 h of exposure
			Nausea and vomiting	
			Quick irregular heartbeat	
			Chest pain	
			Hearing loss	
			Blurry vision	
			Disorientation	
			Death	
Lead	Heavy metal	Combustion of leaded gasoline	Metal refineries	50 $\mu g/m^3$ average over an 8-h workday
			Combustion of leaded gasoline	
			Waste incinerators	
			Battery manufacture	

which represented at that time 44.37% of the nation's population [12].

In underdeveloped and developing countries the situation is even worse. In South America, the rate of urban population growth has increased 1.05% per year resulting in urbanization and, therefore, more problems related to air pollution [13]. In Brazil, air quality standards were settled by the CONAMA n° 3/1990 resolution [14], and estimates are that more than 40% of the population lives in areas where the air quality is less than the ideal one according to the WHO [15].

São Paulo, Brazil's most populated city and one of the major population aggregation areas in the world, is an example of how pollution resulting from motor vehicle emissions has become a critical factor in the development of atmospheric pollution. São Paulo is currently seen as different from all other world megacities since it is the only one with the vehicle fleet working exclusively on biofuel mixtures. Moreover, its air-quality goals are lower than those required of the main Asian and European cities [16]. According to a study presented by the Faculdade de Medicina da Universidade de São Paulo (USP), São Paulo city has a mean $PM_{2.5}$ of 22.17 $\mu g/m^3$, reaching more than 180 depending on the time of the day [17], compared with the WHO reference value for mean $PM_{2.5}$ of 10 $\mu g/m^3$ per year, and of 25 $\mu g/m^3$ as the 24-h mean; in other words, almost two times the rate regarded as safe [18]. These values justify what many research studies already proved: air pollution in São Paulo accounts for more deaths than the combination of car accidents, breast cancer, and AIDS [19]. The same happens in Rio de Janeiro where, according to Reuters, an institution that carries out air quality tests detected $PM_{2.5}$ values of 65 $\mu g/m^3$ in some parts of the city.

However, not only people living in big cities are exposed to risks from air pollution. On the contrary, the ten worst air qualities detected in the world are located in cities where urbanization and industrialization are not actual local concerns. Located in inland Iran, China, India, and Saudi Arabia, although these cities are not areas undergoing an industrialization process, they present incredibly high pollution levels. The three cities occupying the worst position show $PM_{2.5}$ values of 170 $\mu g/m^3$ (Allahabad, India), 176 $\mu g/m^3$ (Gwalior, India), and 217 $\mu g/m^3$ (Zabol, Iran), whose excessive pollution results from climate changes that dry contaminated rivers, therefore elevating the pollutants into the air from coal mines or from extreme drought that produces dust suspension in the air [20].

State of the Art

Skin Damage Mechanisms Induced by Pollution

The skin is the primary interface of the human body and the outer environment, making it an organ directly exposed to environmental pollutants. Nevertheless, most studies on the damaging effects of air pollution are focused on the respiratory and cardiovascular systems. More recently, investigators have shown an increasing interest in skin changes induced by pollution, and there already exists concrete evidence of pollution impact on the health of skin. As reported by Mancebo et al., atmospheric pollution is a known danger to public health and negatively affects many organs, but our knowledge concerning pollution effects on the skin is still limited [6].

Environmental air pollution encompasses many kinds of PM. The increase of such materials in the environment resulting from industrialization and urbanization is highly associated with morbidity and mortality worldwide, and is one of the major concerns related to environmental pollution [9].

The exact mechanisms through which air pollution results in skin-damaging effects are not yet known according to the available literature, and, despite epidemiologic and clinical studies highlighting the noxious effects of pollution in human health, research studies are lacking when the topic involves skin-related effects [8].

Recent epidemiologic studies on the impact of PM on skin show that they affect development and exacerbate skin diseases. Particulate material resulting from pollution induces oxidative stress through the production of reactive oxygen species (ROS), and the secretion of proinflammatory cytokines, such as tumor necrosis factor α, interleukin (IL)-1, and IL-8. Besides, increased ROS production, such as superoxide and radical hydroxyl by exposure to PM, increases matrix metalloproteinases (MMPs), including MMP-1, MMP-2, and MMP-9, resulting in collagen degradation. These processes lead to an increase in inflammatory skin diseases and cutaneous aging. Ultrathin particles (UTPs), including black carbon and polycyclic aromatic hydrocarbons (PAHs), produce a higher incidence of skin cancer [9].

Exogenous Substances Penetrating the Skin

Exogenous substances can cross the cutaneous barrier and reach many different organs, resulting in serious systemic consequences. Agents that penetrate the epidermis include antigens that induce potent hypersensitive late reactions, occupational exposure agents (such as cutting oils to which machine operators are exposed), pesticides (e.g., chlordane insecticide), polychlorinated biphenyls from soil, topical medicines, and cosmetics. Mathematical models that analyze multiple routes and sites of exposure are available.

Some studies show, for example, that among cultivation workers in the Netherlands, there are estimates informing that 75% of the daily dose of pyrene, a substrate of the PAHs, was absorbed through the skin. PAHs are known cancer agents and cytochrome P450 inducers. Road-paving workers are also exposed to significant amounts of PAHs.

Physiology of Skin Absorption

The outer nuclear and dead layer of the stratum corneum is the main barrier to diffusion of exogenous agents. Most penetration occurs through intercellular regions rich in lipids, and highly lipophilic molecules display the highest penetration. Penetration depends on the constant of compound intrinsic diffusion, given that small molecules are often more soluble.

Percutaneous absorption is a process of passive diffusion that follows Fick's first law of diffusion. Often the hydrated stratum corneum shows the highest penetration. Besides this very well defined route, when dermatitis and fissures are present, permeability may be partially increased in comparison with intact normal skin.

The thicker skin is often a more efficient barrier than the thinner stratum corneum, to the extent that the scrotal skin displays higher absorption rates than the body's normal epidermis.

More precise models to determine the importance of percutaneous absorption of many materials are needed, as well as better protective measures for those individuals exposed to such materials [21].

Possible Mechanisms

Modern research studies suggest that each air pollutant on its own has a toxic action specific to the skin. From a theoretical point of view, this may be due to an outside–inside effect, for example, penetration by PM and/or organic compounds connected with a skin PM. Another possibility is an inside–outside mechanism. Therefore, it is well established that PM exposure can cause systemic effects as a consequence of (i) particles which penetrate the lungs and subsequently the circulation, and, eventually, affect the skin, and/or (ii) a resulting inflammatory reaction in the lungs which can then bring about systemic inflammatory reactions that may damage the skin [8].

Vierkötter et al. detected a close association between early skin aging and exposure to soot, a mix of carbon particles covered with PAHs. PAHs are potent binders for the aryl hydrocarbon receptor (AHR), a binder-dependent transcription factor expressed by both keratinocytes and melanocytes. Experimental evidence from cultures of keratinocytes in skin exposed to Asian dust storm particles increased the AHR expression and upregulated proinflammatory mediators.

In addition, in vitro exposure of primary human keratinocytes and melanocytes to the environment containing diesel exhaust particles was recently shown to induce the expression of gene transcription with functional relevance for the development of both wrinkles and hyperpigmented spots.

The regulatory activities of the gene seem to be mediated to a greater extent by AHR activation in both types of cells (Krutmann et al., unpublished data). Moreover, AHR activation

may lead to increased production of ROS, suggesting the possibility that the topical application of antioxidants may be useful to protect the human skin against the harmful effects induced by PMs. These studies do not exclude the possibility that carbon particles on their own, i.e., lacking in PAHs, penetrate the skin, thus resulting in harmful effects as shown in lung epithelial cells [8].

Based on current evidence, there seem to be four active potential physiologic mechanisms that cause harmful skin effects: (1) free radicals, (2) inflammatory cascade and skin barrier, (3) AHRS, and (4) skin microflora.

Free Radicals Development

The ozone in the stratosphere has a protective effect by filtering UV solar radiation; in the troposphere, however, ozone has toxic effects on the skin. Ozone is a highly reactive compound that creates free radicals and depletes the antioxidants present in the epidermis.

Thiele et al. showed that exposure to increasing ozone doses resulted in a dose-dependent depletion of vitamins C and E, and development of malondialdehyde, a marker of lipid peroxidation. Moreover, ongoing low-level exposure to ozone resulted in cumulative oxidative damage to the stratum corneum. Two similar studies conducted by Thiele's group also showed that ozone depletes both the nonenzymatic and the enzymatic antioxidant stores in the skin (i.e., uric acid, vitamin C, tocopherol, glutathione), resulting in lipid peroxidation and protein oxidation, thus suggesting that pollution may induce a dysfunctional barrier [8]. There are two main mechanisms that limit these research studies. Firstly the researchers exposed mice to oxygen levels higher than the levels found in the environment and secondly, the mouse epidermis is significantly thinner than the human epidermis.

McCarthy et al. exposed normal human epidermal keratinocytes (NHEKs) to environmentally relevant ozone levels (e.g., 0.4 and 0.8 ppm) for 30 min. Results showed that exposure to 0.8 ppm of ozone leads to DNA fragmentation and ATP depletion, therefore suggesting that the mitochondrial function can also be impaired.

He et al. tested the effects of environmentally realistic levels of ozone (e.g., 0.8 ppm) in humans. The research assessed the clinical changes occurring in the human skin after short-term in vivo exposure to ozone. There was a 70% decrease in the levels of endogenous vitamin E and a concomitant 230% increase in lipid hydroperoxide in the stratum corneum. By comparison, higher doses of ozone (e.g., 5–10 ppm) were necessary to induce similar increases in the lipid peroxidation markers of mouse skin, thus suggesting that the human stratum corneum may be biochemically more sensitive to the effects of ozone [6].

Other experimental studies with mice showed not only increased levels of oxidative stress markers, but also signs of cell stress modulated by proinflammatory markers (cyclooxygenase-2), heat-shock proteins (HSP32, HSP70, HSP27), nuclear factor κB (NF-κB), and MMPs [8].

Induction of the Inflammatory Cascade and Skin Barrier Disturbances

Many studies have suggested that air pollution instigates inflammation. Cytokines and interleukins are small proteins derived from a great variety of cells involved in cell signaling and inflammatory cascade induction. IL-8 is a proinflammatory mediator of the innate immune system with two primary functions: induction of neutrophil chemotaxis and other granulocytes, and activation of phagocytes. Pollutants, such as diesel exhaust particles (DEPs), have been proved to induce a strong inflammatory reaction in human skin cells, including a significant increase of IL-8 production. Later studies gave more support to these findings by showing that exposure to DEPs in concentrations relevant to humans increases expression of NF-κB, a transitional factor that regulates the expression of proinflammatory cytokines in mouse epidermal cells.

Besides DEPs, dust particles with a complex mixture of heavy metals have been shown to increase the gene expression of proinflammatory cytokines in human epidermal cells. Choi et al. incubated NHEKs over 24 h with sterilized powder from particles derived from three Asian dust storms that happened over the time period 2004 to 2006. The epidermal cells displayed a significant increase in mRNA expression of proinflammatory IL-6 and IL-8 cytokines, and in granulocyte and macrophage colony-stimulating factor. Furthermore, this study showed that epidermal cells significantly expressed caspase-14, a protein found in differentiated keratinocytes and involved in hydration and keratinization of the stratum corneum. The increased caspase-14 suggests that skin cells initiate a compensatory mechanism as a reaction to exposure to dust particles. As a whole, these studies suggest that air pollution induces an epidermal proinflammatory state that probably changes the epidermal differentiation and, consequently, affects the skin's immunologic barrier [6].

Activation of the Aryl Hydrocarbon Receptor

The AHR is a cytosolic transcription factor activated by binders found in many kinds of skin cells which regulate cell proliferation, inflammation, and melanogenesis. AHR activation results in translocation to the nucleus where it becomes a complex with the AHR nuclear translocator, and binds to specific sites of DNA known as a xenobiotic reaction element (XRE). Genes with XREs include the enzymes of cytochrome detoxification P450 (CYP). The AHR activation may have a role as mediator in the toxic effects associated with exposure to xenobiotics, including atmospheric pollutants, such as ozone, dioxins, and PAHs [22]. Many research studies have examined the role of the AHR activation in cutaneous mechanisms, from melanogenesis regulation to the development of skin inflammatory lesions. Tauchi et al. developed a lineage of transgenic mice that expressed the activated AHR in the absence of binder stimulation. In these mice AHR activation led to the development of a severe cutaneous eruption together with pruritus and inflammation similar to atopic dermatitis (AD). The genetic profile analysis of the mouse skin showed a significant positive regulation of genes associated with inflammatory cascade reactions. These results imply that activated AHR and AHR target genes may be involved in the development of skin adverse reactions in reaction to AHR binders [6, 8].

Besides chronic inflammation, AHR has been shown to play a primary role as a melanogenesis regulator. Luecke et al. exposed melanocytes from human donors to 10 nM 2,3,7,8-tetrachlorodibenzo-*p*-dioxin (TCDD) over 5 days, and measured the tyrosinase activity and the melanin content in vitro. After a 3-day exposure to TCDD, the tyrosinase activity was highly increased in the melanocytes, being suppressed by the concomitant treatment with oxy-4′-nitroflovane or β-naphthoflavone, partial antagonists of the AHR. After a 5-day treatment with TCDD, the melanocytes displayed an increased level of tyrosinase activity and a three-fold increase in the total content of intracellular melanin. A similar study carried out in human cells of FM55 melanoma showed that TCDD significantly increases the melanin content, thus verifying that the melanogenic route was positively regulated by AHR activation.

AHR was also identified as an ozone sensor. Afaq et al. exposed NHEKs to 0.3 ppm ozone over 20 min, and collected epidermal cells immediately after, 3 h after, and 6 h after exposure. In this study the ozone induced nuclear translocation of the AHR and increased the expression of mRNA AHR. In addition, the ozone markedly increased the expression of the isoform proteins and mRNA CYP1. CYP1 enzymes are known as compounds that metabolize compounds more toxic than the respective original compounds and activate many xenobiotic procarcinogens [6].

Skin Microflora Alterations

The resident cutaneous microflora is useful to maintain homeostasis and hinder the growth of harmful microorganisms. It was shown that environmental air pollutants change skin microflora.

He et al. showed that in vivo exposure of the human skin to ozone led to a 50% decrease of resident skin microflora, thus suggesting bactericidal effects of ozone.

Sowada et al. investigated the relationship between skin microflora and PAH metabolism. They isolated bacterial species of the human skin that can degrade benzo(a)pyrene (PaB), a PAH prototype. The species of isolated bacteria were able to use PaB as their sole source of carbon and energy. These findings raised the question of whether skin bacteria have a protective or a harmful effect on the skin regarding PAH metabolism, since total metabolism of PAH can protect the skin whereas partial degradation can result in bioactivation and increased skin toxicity [6].

Today our knowledge of the effects of atmospheric pollution on the skin remains limited. Considering the increasing trend of urbanization and increased air pollution in cities around the world, more research studies are necessary to help understand the mechanisms implied in the harmful effects of air pollutants. Prospective research studies must be designed to mimic real-life situations and examine short-term and long-term pollution effects on the skin. Moreover, these studies must deal with the methodological limitations. Lastly, owing to scarce scientific evidence, there are no established guidelines currently available for skin protection against air pollution. Besides decreased exposure, potential protective strategies must focus on rehabilitation of the skin barrier by replenishing antioxidative stores and reducing inflammation caused by air pollutants [6].

Relationship Between Pollution and Systemic Disease

Early studies that analyzed the association of the effects of atmospheric pollution with the human health date back to the twentieth century, and reported significant increases of morbidity and mortality in cities in developed countries [24].

Researchers are increasingly interested in the various effects of pollutants on human health. Recent major epidemiologic research studies identified that exposure to air pollution either in the short or long term, including exposure to PM and ozone, increases respiratory and cardiovascular morbidity. Long-term exposure was also associated with development of some forms of cancer [23].

Cardiopulmonary Morbidity

The impact caused by air pollution particles on morbidity has been a focus of ongoing studies, resulting in a solid scientific consensus on the independent association between air $PM_{2.5}$ and PM_{10} with negative impacts on respiratory and cardiovascular health, both in the short term and in chronic exposures. Furthermore, data strongly suggest that these effects are limitless within the investigated range of environmental concentrations, possibly occurring in PM$_{2.5}$ concentrations, and also that they mostly follow a linear concentration–reaction function. Evidence is well established concerning the reduction in pulmonary function, increase in symptom severity in individuals with asthma, COPD, and ischemic heart disease including heart attacks.

More recently, evidence has linked long-term exposure to PM$_{2.5}$ to atherosclerosis, a condition underlying many cardiovascular diseases. The promotion and the vulnerability of atherosclerotic plaques represent a potential mechanism through which air pollution PM may trigger cardiovascular mortality and morbidity.

Supporting this theory, long-term exposures to PM$_{2.5}$ concentrations, as well as proximity to traffic, are associated with preclinical markers of atherosclerosis (the carotid intima-media thickness and calcification of the coronary artery) [25–28] in addition to pathology progression [27]. Gas and particle atmospheric pollutants also have a close and marked relationship with hospital admissions or mortality resulting from cerebrovascular disorders [33].

Emerging respiratory data link long-term PM exposure to respiratory diseases during childhood. Birth cohort studies have suggested an association between PM exposure during pregnancy and higher respiratory need, airway inflammation, and increased susceptibility to respiratory infections.

The most recent birth meta-analysis of the ESCAPE project also provides solid evidence that postnatal exposure to PM$_{10}$ (but not PM$_{2.5}$) and traffic exposure are associated with an increased risk for childhood pneumonia, as well as evidence of an association with otitis media. In a birth cohort in the Netherlands other associations were reported between long-term exposure to traffic-related air pollution in the place of birth and symptoms of asthma and low-level pulmonary function during childhood [29, 30]. Another interesting epidemiologic observation notes a possible connection between chronic exposure to PM during childhood and COPD vulnerability during adulthood [29].

In regard to nitrogen dioxide, most of the research studies have found an association between NO$_2$ and medical appointments for respiratory diseases. The associations between PM$_{10}$ and nitrogen dioxide on the one hand and respiratory diseases on the other hand were higher among the elderly. Air pollution possibly worsens pre-existing diseases more prone to affect the elderly population. In addition, the aging process is characterized by a decrease in antioxidant defenses, and the elderly constitute a high-risk group for oxidative phenomena induced by air pollution [29].

Long-term exposure to air pollution by thin particles related to exhaust is a significant environmental risk factor for cardiopulmonary and lung cancer mortality. Each 10-µg/m^3 elevation in atmospheric pollution by thin particles was reported to be associated with about 4%, 6%, and 8% more risk for all-cause mortality, cardiopulmonary mortality, and lung cancer mortality, respectively [31].

Some research studies hypothesize that exposure to air traffic pollution, nitrogen dioxide, PM$_{2.5}$, and PM$_{10}$ during pregnancy and the first year of life would be associated with autism. New epidemiologic and toxicologic studies may help determine whether such a causal association exists [32].

Effects of poor-quality air on the population's health are frequently not visible in comparison with other more easily identifiable factors. Epidemiologic studies, however, have shown important correlations between exposure to atmospheric pollutants and effects of morbidity and mortality from respiratory (asthma, bronchitis, pulmonary emphysema, and lung cancer) and cardiovascular problems, even if concentrations of atmospheric pollutants do not exceed the current air quality standards. Children, the elderly, and persons with respiratory diseases are the most vulnerable populations [31].

Cutaneous Diseases Triggered and Aggravated by Pollution

The skin is the primary interface with the external environment and is, therefore, directly exposed to environmental pollution. It is thus reasonable to assume that air pollutants are also involved with the skin disease process. Despite a few persistent doubts, researchers' interest in this topic is increasing, and there already are concrete elements that connect air pollution to dermatologic problems. A discussion of these pathologies follows.

Early Aging

Aging is a natural process that leads to the progressive loss of all tissues' structure and function. The cutaneous aging process is the most perceptible process that brings about functional, social, and psychological impacts.

Skin senescence occurs as a combination of two processes: intrinsic and extrinsic aging. Intrinsic aging is related to the long-term accumulation of cell damage by ROS of the organism itself. Extrinsic aging in its turn is associated with exposure to free radicals created by many environmental factors, such as UV radiation and cigarette smoke. Therefore, the latter process is more easily modifiable from the preventive point of view.

The extrinsic aging process is clinically, histologically, and molecularly different from the intrinsic process. Signs of extrinsic aging include coarse wrinkles, irregular pigment spots, and elastosis [34].

The external cause more associated with extrinsic aging is UV solar radiation exposure, so that for decades words like photoaging and extrinsic aging were almost synonymous. Environmental pollutants, especially PM, are also related to aging [35].

In 2010, an epidemiologic study aimed at assessing the effect of pollution exposure on the skin was published. Letters were sent to 400 women living in rural and urban German areas previously chosen, since these women were exposed to air PM from traffic and steel and coal industries. Follow-up questionnaires were distributed, followed by dermatologic assessment through the SCINEXA (score of intrinsic and extrinsic skin aging), a validated skin-aging score. It was noted that chronic exposure to PM in the air was associated with early aging signs, such as coarse wrinkles and, mainly, the development of pigment spots. An increase in soot and

traffic-driven particles in air concentration was associated with a 20% increase of pigment spots in the forehead and malar region [36]. This study was one of the first to examine the association between environmental pollution and harmful skin effects.

Experimental studies have shown probable mechanisms that associate environmental pollutants with aging. PM can increase the development of oxidative stress through ROS increase, which may speed up the cutaneous aging process by intervening in a series of skin functions, such as prevention of pathogen entry and repair of DNA damage [37, 38]. ROS also inhibits collagen synthesis by activating MMPs [39].

As discussed earlier in the Physiopathology section, exposure to PM can also contribute to the aging process through other mechanisms, such as an increase in the production of proinflammatory cytokines and damage in the repair system of DNA. These added pieces of evidence strengthen the notion of direct involvement of air PM in the cutaneous aging process.

Atopic Dermatitis

AD is a recurrent chronic inflammatory disease that often starts during childhood. It is believed that its development may be related to an environmental trigger in genetically prone individuals. Over its course, the disease usually shows remission and exacerbation periods. Loss of cutaneous barrier integrity is significant for the development of exacerbations, and these may be associated with exposure to environmental allergens. AD incidence is increasing worldwide [40], and environmental pollution has been implicated as a worsening factor in the disease [41].

A research study that assessed the relationship between traffic-driven pollutants and development of allergic diseases showed that long-term exposure to PM in the environment is linked to a greater risk for the development of atopic diseases, such as AD and allergic sensitization [42]. Moreover, it was reported that exposure to NO_2 from vehicle exhaustion was also significantly connected to eczema [42].

Symptom severity also seems to be affected. The intensity of AD symptoms, such as pruritus in children already diagnosed with AD, is higher when high levels of environmental PM_{10}, $PM_{2.5}$, and ultrafine particles (UFP) are detected [43].

The function of the epidermal barrier is fundamental to preventing AD exacerbations. A study assessing the loss of transepidermal water as a parameter of cutaneous barrier integrity showed that short exposure to NO_2, a UFP compound, resulted in damage to the epidermal barrier and exacerbation of AD symptoms [44].

Based on these bibliographic data, we can conclude that exposure to PM is a risk factor for AD development, as well as for exacerbations in children with a previous diagnosis of AD.

Individuals with sensitive skin are also a high-risk population facing the effects of air pollution [8]. It is more a syndrome than necessarily a disease, the concept of which is highly stressed in the specific literature, and its definition deserves some attention in the context of early subjective complaints of discomfort (burning, pruritus, stinging, xerosis, erythema, papules, or scaling) with no immunologic reaction. It is defined as a multifactorial inflammatory syndrome with signs of cutaneous hyperreactivity, while not immune to usually well-tolerated stimuli [45].

It also seems to be associated with the loss of cutaneous barrier integrity and increased permeability of the stratum corneum. Thus, external factors, including environmental pollution, have been associated with complaints by individuals with sensitive skin [45].

Urticaria

Urticaria is an impairment mediated by cutaneous mastocyte degranulation on the surface dermis that affects about 20% of the population. It may be followed by angioedema, a deeper cutaneous edema involving the dermis and the hypodermis. It is clinically characterized by an erythematous and pruriginous plaque. A single reason for the development of urticaria may be found in some patients, mainly those with a recent onset of the presentation. Many cases, nevertheless, do not have an identifiable trigger, a situation more common in cases persisting for weeks or months. The most frequently identified triggers include infections, drugs, food, and insect bites [46].

Although environmental factors can also trigger urticaria, few studies have associated environmental pollutants with its development.

A Canadian research study established a correlation between increased number of visitors to the emergency department because of urticaria with a worsening of the air quality index that used the levels of three known environmental pollutants as parameters: ozone, nitrogen dioxide, and $PM_{2.5}$ [47]. Another Chinese study showed that increased ozone levels led to a statistically significant increase of urticaria (3.84%) and other allergic diseases [48].

Acne

Acne vulgaris is a chronic inflammatory dermatologic disease originating in the pilosebaceous apparatus that leads to clinical changes in the skin, such as open and closed comedones, papules, pustules, and nodules. It has a multifactorial origin, with hormonal, hereditary, and environmental influences.

There is evidence that acne vulgaris can be worsened by increased levels of ROS and IL-8 induced by BaP exposure found in high concentrations in cigarette smoke [49]. BaP is a PAH formed by incomplete combustion of organic matter, present as an air pollutant disseminated through the air, soil, water, and sediments [50, 51]. Therefore, it can be inferred that air pollution can also play a role in acne worsening.

There is, however, one known acne variation closely connected with exposure to environmental pollutants, namely chloracne. Chloracne occurs after the systemic absorption of halogenated aromatic hydrocarbons, and is regarded as one of the most sensitive indicators of intoxication by these compounds. These agents are often called chloracnegens [52].

Chloracne is, thus, more the result of a systemic intoxication than direct contact with the skin. In other words, it is not usually associated with exposure to air pollution. Mostly it results from occupational and non-occupational exposure, the latter being associated with contact with industrial garbage and contaminated food [52].

Table 48.2 Differing characteristics between acne vulgaris and chloracne

	Acne vulgaris	Chloracne
Age group affected	Adolescence and early adulthood	Any age group
Anatomic localization	Face including the nose, upper back, chest	Retroauricular and malar areas, axillae, groin, extremities; nose is spared
Inflammation	Inflammatory lesions are common	Inflammation is very rare (only as a secondary effect after a cyst rupture)
Sebum production	Increased	Decreased; xerosis as a common associated condition
Initial lesion	Limited comedones, papules, pustules, cysts	Myriad comedones
Sebaceous gland	Hypertrophic	Atrophic; gradual replacement with keratinocytes
Sweat gland	Uninvolved	Palmoplantar hyperkeratotic lesions; acrosyringial plugging

Adapted from Panteleyev and Bickers [53]

Dioxins belong to a family of halogenated aromatic hydrocarbons, and are considered the most potent chloracne inducers. They are classified as class 1 carcinogenic [21, 22].

Chloracne is characterized by an acneiform eruption comprising comedones (blackheads and whiteheads), pustules, and cysts. Table 48.2 highlights the main differences between chloracne and acne vulgaris.

The only effective way to prevent chloracne is by avoiding exposure to chloracnegens. The treatment involves moving patients out of contaminated places and allowing the organism itself to eliminate the agent. A synthetic fat substitute, olestra, seems to accelerate the fecal elimination of chloracnegens [54].

Melasma

Melasma is an acquired disorder of multifactorial origin displaying hyperpigmentation on photoexposed areas, mainly the face. It is more common in phototype III and IV women, and causes major aesthetic harm and psychological stress that result in a negative impact on the quality of life [55].

The physiopathology of melasma is not totally understood, although many factors play a role, such as genetic predisposition, UV radiation, hormonal factors (e.g., use of contraceptives and pregnancy), thyroid dysfunction, and use of cosmetics, phototoxic drugs, and anticonvulsants [56–58].

It was recently postulated that environmental pollution might also be a contributing factor in melasma [59]. The author argues that melasma has a higher incidence in Indian and South-East Asian individuals, locations with heavier pollution [60, 61]. By referring to research studies suggesting an association of melasma with factors already linked to pollution, such as extrinsic aging [62], and inflammation [63], the author proposes that air pollution might play a synergistic role with other risk factors for melasma development. Although seeming a plausible hypothesis, there is no evidence as yet that directly correlates melasma with air pollution.

Skin Cancer

Skin cancers are the most common cancer type in the human species. About 40–50% of North Americans up to the age of 65 years will suffer from a basal cellular carcinoma or a spinal cellular carcinoma [64]. Although seen less often, melanoma is the skin cancer displaying the highest potential for fatality, and its incidence is significantly increasing [65].

Air pollution is already acknowledged as an element associated with cancer development. Traditionally lung cancer is the cancer most often associated with air pollution [66], but there are epidemiologic studies showing an association between PM and skin cancers.

In a study conducted among longshoremen in Italy, their occupational exposure to black carbon was investigated and showed an increased incidence of bladder cancer, pleural mesothelioma, and melanoma [67].

Black carbon is classified as a class 1 carcinogen, being a UFP type resulting from diesel exhaustion, so that exposure to it may occur in ways other than the occupational environment. Oddly, an association with other types of skin cancer besides melanoma was not shown [67].

Another epidemiologic study investigated PAHs, also with carcinogen potential, in the occupational environment, and found an association with lung, skin, and bladder cancers [68]. PAHs occur as mixtures within the PM derived from cigarette smoke, coal tar, and diesel exhaust [69]. PAHs may exist in the environment during their particulate and gaseous phases. The gaseous phase is more abundant although it is less carcinogenic than the particulate phase. The particulate-phase PAHs may occur as $PM_{2.5}$ and UFP [9]. PAHs can be absorbed by the skin, and their combination with carcinogenesis takes place through interaction with a specific receptor, the aryl hydrocarbon receptor (AhR) [70].

There are other studies showing the existence of a synergistic effect among environmental pollutants, such as BaP and UVA radiation, in carcinogenesis. If combined, these two agents promote cancer induction in smaller exposure doses than in separate agents [71].

Compounds such as black carbon, PAH, and BaP, are carcinogens present in the environment as compounds of air PM resulting from different human activities, and representing a risk for the whole population beyond the occupational environment. Experimental models have shown that these pollutants induce cellular changes involved with carcinogenesis with consequent skin cancer.

Approach to Pollution-Induced Skin Damage and Preventive Measures

Since it is a recent topic in the literature, there are no established guidelines with recommendations to protect the skin from pollution.

There are, nevertheless, some general measures that can be recommended by dermatologists for skin protection against damage induced by environmental pollutants [9].

- Emollients may be used to preserve and restore the cutaneous barrier, resulting in decreased penetration of pollutants into the skin.
- Daily use of gels and cleaning products may help decrease the particle load of the skin.
- Use of sunscreens may be beneficial against pollution, since there is evidence connecting the synergistic effect of UV radiation with environmental pollutants in carcinogenesis.
- Development of skin barriers with products such as BB foundations and creams may be useful as protection against pollutants, acting as oxidative damage agents through direct contact with the skin.
- Avoidance of excessive skin washing, which may be harmful to the natural cutaneous barrier, is recommended.
- Whenever possible, exposure to environments with high concentrations of pollutants should be avoided.

Experimental studies show that air pollutants, such as ozone, induce skin oxidative damage and deplete its natural antioxidants, such as vitamins C and E [72, 73]. There is also evidence that such effects may be attenuated by the topical application of antioxidants [74]. Therefore, the use of oral or topic antioxidants is an additional strategy to fight cutaneous damage induced by these pollutants.

In closed environments, strategies to control the effects of air pollution on the skin may result in a collective impact. After implementing a program of air quality improvement in nine randomly selected kindergarten in South Korea, the decreased concentrations of indoor PM_{10} brought about a significant reduction in AD symptoms. The eczema area and severity index (EASI) score was significantly decreased from 2.37 to 1.19, and the mean body surface area decreased from 7.06% to 4.22% after the program's implementation [75].

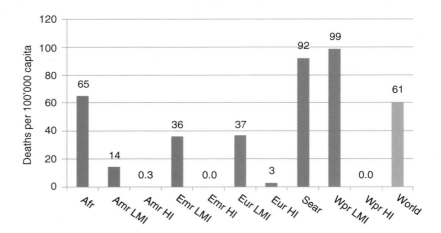

Fig. 48.1 Deaths per capita attributable to PAH in 2012, by region [2]

Future Perspectives

Recent vehicle-controlled clinical studies showed that a new antagonist cosmetic competitive with the AhR was effective in preventing its activation in the human skin [76]. Thus, it may be useful as a promising strategy to prevent skin damage associated with PAHs occurring through a connection to the AhRs expressed in keratinocytes and melanocytes.

A large portion of the research studies that associate environmental pollutants with skin diseases are conducted in occupational environments; therefore, more research studies are necessary at the population level so that we can obtain a more realistic idea of the environmental impact, since in the aforementioned situations exposure can be less intense and pollutants may be in lower concentrations.

Environmental pollution is a public health problem, and its effective management necessarily occurs through a decrease in pollutant exhaust. A concerted effort of companies and governments to implement effective environmental policies that positively affect public health is necessary.

To conclude this chapter, the importance of air pollution related to two indexes is illustrated: deaths attributable by region and by disease (Figs. 48.1 and 48.2, respectively), according to the WHO [2].

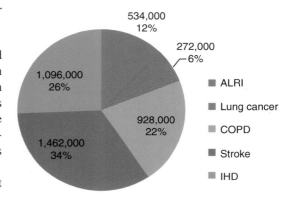

Fig. 48.2 Deaths attributable to PAH in 2012, by disease [2]

Glossary

Aging Natural process that leads to progressive loss of structure and function of all tissues.

Black carbon Environmental pollutant rated ultrafine particulate from diesel exhausts. It is a carcinogen class 1. It is associated with some types of cancer, for example bladder cancer, pleural mesothelioma, and malignant melanoma.

Chloracne Acne variant associated with exposure to environmental pollutants that develops after systemic poisoning by halogenated aromatic hydrocarbons. It is characterized by an acne-iform eruption consisting of comedones (black-heads and whiteheads), pustules, and cysts.

Extrinsic aging Process associated with exposure to free radicals created by numerous environmental factors such as ultraviolet radiation and cigarette smoke. Signs of extrinsic aging are thick wrinkles, irregular pigmentation spots, and elastosis.

Intrinsic aging Process related to the accumulation over time of cell damage by reactive oxygen species from the organism itself.

Sensitive skin Inflammatory multifactorial syndrome with cutaneous hyperreactivity signals not immune to stimuli generally well tolerated, clinically characterized by subjective complaints of discomfort (burning, itching, xerosis, erythema, papules).

References

1. Xinwei L, Xiaolan Z, Loretta YL, Hao C. Assessment of metals pollution and health risk in dust from nursery schools in Xi'an, China. Environ Res. 2014;128:27–34.
2. World Health Organization (WHO). WHO's ambient air pollution database – update 2014. 2014. Available from: www.who.int/phe/health_topics/outdoorair/databases/AAP_database results2014.pdf. Cited 2016 Aug 19.
3. Molina MJ, Molina LT. Megacities and atmospheric pollution. J Air Waste Manage Assoc. 2004;54(6):644–80.
4. Gurjar BR, Butler TM, Lawrence MG, Lelieveld J. Evaluation of emissions and air quality in megacities. Atmos Environ. 2008;42:1593–606.
5. Ministério do Meio Ambiente. Poluentes Atomosféricos [internet]. Brasilia: Ministerio do Meio Ambiente. Cited 2016 Aug 19. Available from: http://www.mma.gov.br/cidades-sustentaveis/qualidade-do-ar/poluentes-atmosf%C3%A9ricos.
6. Mancebo SE, Wang SQ. Recognizing the impact of ambient air pollution on skin health. J Eur Acad Dermatol Venereol. 2015;29(12):2326–32.
7. US Environmental Protection Agency (EPA). Air quality trends [internet]. North Carolina. Updated 2016, Aug. Cited 2016 Aug 09. Available from: https://www.epa.gov/air-trends.
8. Krutmann J, Liu W, Li L, Pan X, Crawford M, Sore G, Seite S. Pollution and skin: from epidemiological and mechanistic studies to clinical implication. J Dermatol Sci. 2014;76:163–8.
9. Kim EK, Cho D, Park HJ. Air pollution and skin diseases: adverse effects of airborne particulate matter on various skin diseases. Life Sci. 2016;152:126–34.
10. DetectCarbonMonoxide. CO Knowledge Center [internet]. Cited 2016 Aug 17. Available from: http://www.detectcarbonmonoxide.com/co-health-risks/.
11. World Health Organization (WHO). Air pollution levels rising in many of the world's poorest cities [internet]. Geneve: WHO [updated 2016 MAY 12; cited 2016 Aug 10]. Available from: http://www.who.int/mediacentre/news/releases/2016/air-pollution-rising/en/.
12. US Environmental Protection Agency. Air quality trends [internet]. [Updated 2014 April 21; Cited 2016 Aug 17]. Available from: http://www.epa.gov/airtrends/aqtrends.html#airquality.
13. Marnitez PJP, Andrade MF, Miranda RM. Traffic-related air quality trends in São Paulo, Brazil. Geophys Res Atmos. 2015;120:6290–304.
14. Ministério do Meio Ambiente. Cidades Sustentáveis: Qualidade do Ar [internet]. Brasilia: Ministerio do Meio Ambiente. Cited 2016 Aug 19. Available in: http://www.mma.gov.br/cidades-sustentaveis/qualidade-do-ar.
15. Copenhagen Consensus Center. Brazil perspectives: air pollution [internet]. Copenhagen. [Cited 2016 Aug 14]. Available from: http://www.copenhagenconsensus.com/publication/brazil-perspectives-air-pollution.
16. Kumar P, de Fatima MA, Ynoue RY, Fornaro A, de Freitas ED, Martins J, et al. New directions: from biofuels to wood stoves: the modern and ancient air quality challenges in the megacity of Sao Paulo. Atmos Environ. 2016;140:364–9.
17. Air Quality Index (AQI). São Paulo air pollution: real-time Air Quality Index (AQI). [Updated 2016 Aug 14. Cited 2016 Aug 14]. Available from http://aqicn.org/city/sao-paulo/.
18. World Health Organization (WHO). Ambient (outdoor) air quality and health [internet]. Geneve: WHO [updated 2014 Mar; cited 2016 Aug 14]. Available from: http://www.who.int/mediacentre/factsheets/fs313/en/.
19. Vormittag EM, Rodrigues CG, Miranda MJ, Cavalcanti JA, da Costa RR, Camargo CA, et al. Avaliação do Impacto da Poluição Atmosférica no Estado de São Paulo sob a Visão da Saúde. Instituto Saúde e Sustentabilidade. 2013. Disponivel em: http://www.saudeesustentabilidade.org.br/site/wp-content/uploads/2013/09/Documentofinaldapesquisapadrao_2409-FINAL-sitev1.pdf. Acesso em 19/08/2016.
20. Lydia Ramsey. About 80% of all cities have worse air quality than what's considered healthy – here are the 15 with the worst air pollution. Business Insider Inc. [updated 2016 May; Cited 2016 Aug 15]. Available from: http://www.businessinsider.com/the-cities-with-the-worlds-worst-air-pollution-who-2016-5/#1-zabol-iran-217-gm3-of-pm-25-15.
21. Goldsmith LA. Skin effects of air pollution. Otolaryngol Head Neck Surg. 1996;114(2):217–9.
22. Suskind RR. Chloracne, "the hallmark of dioxin intoxication". Scand J Work Environ Health. 1985;11:165–71.
23. Beelen R, Raaschou-Nielsen O, Stafoggia M, Andersen ZJ, Weinmayr G. Effects of long term exposure to air pollution on natural cause mor-

tality: an analysis of 22 European cohorts within the multicentre ESCAPE project. Lancet. 2014.; 1;383(9919):785–95.

24. Marcilio I, Gouveia N. Quantifying the impact of air pollution on the urban population of Brazil. Cad Saúde Pública. 2007;23(4):S529.

25. Künzli N, Jerrett M, Mack WJ, Beckerman B, LaBree L, et al. Ambient air pollution and atherosclerosis in Los Angeles. Environ Health Perspect. 2005;113(2):201–6.

26. Bauer M, Moebus S, Möhlenkamp S, Dragano N, Nonnemacher M, et al. Urban particulate matter air pollution is associated with subclinical atherosclerosis. results from the HNR (Heinz Nixdorf Recall) study. J Am Coll Cardiol. 2010;56(22):1803–8.

27. Künzli N, Jerrett M, Garcia-Esteban R, Basagaña X, Beckermann B, et al. Ambient air pollution and the progression of atherosclerosis in adults. PLoS ONE. 2010;5(2):e9096.

28. Hoffmann B, Moebus S, Möhlenkamp S, Stang A, Lehmann N, et al. Residential exposure to traffic is associated with coronary atherosclerosis. Circulation. 2007;116(5):489–96.

29. Kelly FJ, Fussell JC. Air pollution and public health: emerging hazards and improved understanding of risk. Environ Geochem Health. 2015;37(4):631–49.

30. Clark NA, Demers PA, Karr CJ, Koehoorn M, Lencar C, Tamburic L, Brauer M. Effect of early life exposure to air pollution on development of childhood asthma. Environ Health Perspect. 2010;118(2):284–90.

31. Pope CA, Burnett RT, Thun MJ, Calle EE, Krewski D, et al. Lung cancer, cardiopulmonary mortality, and longterm exposure to fine particulate air pollution. JAMA. 2002;287(9):1132–41.

32. Heather E, Volk HE, Lurmann F, Penfold B, Hertz-Picciotto I, McConnell R. Traffic-related air pollution, particulate matter, and autism. JAMA Psychiatry. 2013;70(1):71–7.

33. Anoop SV, Shah ASV, Lee KK, McAllister DA, Hunter A, Nair H, et al. Short term exposure to air pollution and stroke: systematic review and meta-analysis. BMJ. 2015;350:h1295.

34. Yaar M, Eller MS, Gilchrest BA. Fifty years of skin aging. J Invest Dermatol. 2003;120:168–9.

35. Vierkotter A, Krutmann J. Environmental influences on skin aging and ethnic- specific manifestations. Dermatoendocrinology. 2012;4:227–31.

36. Vierkotter A, Schikowski T, Ranft U, Sugiri D, Matsui M, Kramer U, et al. Airborne particle exposure and extrinsic skin aging. J Investig Dermatol. 2010;130:2719–26.

37. Lee JK, Ko SH, Ye SK, Chung MH. 8-Oxo-2′-deoxyguanosine ameliorates UVB-induced skin damage in hairless mice by scavenging reactive oxygen species and inhibiting MMP expression. J Dermatol Sci. 2013;70:49–57.

38. Wolf AM, Nishimaki K, Kamimura N, Ohta S. Real-time monitoring of oxidative stress in live mouse skin. J Investig Dermatol. 2014;134:1701–9.

39. Yun SP, Lee SJ, Oh SY, Jung YH, Ryu JM, Suh HN, et al. Reactive oxygen species induce MMP12-

dependent degradation of collagen 5 and fibronectin to promote the motility of human umbilical cord-derived mesenchymal stem cells. Br J Pharmacol. 2014;171:3283–97.

40. Wolter S, Price HN. Atopic dermatitis. Pediatr Clin N Am. 2014;61:241–60.

41. Kim J, Kim EH, Oh I, Jung K, Han Y, Cheong HK, et al. Symptoms of atopic dermatitis are influenced by outdoor air pollution. J Allergy Clin Immunol. 2013;132:495–8. e491

42. Morgenstern V, Zutavern A, Cyrys J, Brockow I, Koletzko S, Kramer U, et al. Atopic diseases, allergic sensitization, and exposure to traffic-related air pollution in children. Am J Respir Crit Care Med. 2008;177:1331–7.

43. Song S, Lee K, Lee YM, Lee JH, Lee SI, Yu SD, et al. Acute health effects of urban fine and ultrafine particles on children with atopic dermatitis. Environ Res. 2011;111:394–9.

44. Eberlein-Konig B, Przybilla B, Kuhnl P, Pechak J, Gebefugi I, Kleinschmidt J, et al. Influence of airborne nitrogen dioxide or formaldehyde on parameters of skin function and cellular activation in patients with atopic eczema and control subjects. J Allergy Clin Immunol. 1998;101:141–3.

45. Farage M, Maibach HI. Sensitive skin: closing in on a physiological cause. Contact Dermat. 2010;62:137–49.

46. Kaplan AP. Urticaria and angioedema. In: Adkinson NF, Bochner BS, Busse WW, et al., editors. Middleton's allergy: principles and practice, vol. 2. 7th ed. St Louis: Mosby; 2009. p. 1063.

47. Kousha T, Valacchi G. The air quality health index and emergency department visits for urticaria in Windsor. Can J Toxicol Environ Health A. 2015;78(8):524–33. doi:10.1080/15287394.2014.991053.

48. Xu F, Yan S, Wu M, Li F, Xu X, Song W, et al. Ambient ozone as a risk factor for skin disorders. Br J Dermatol. 2011;165:99–228.

49. Tsuji G, Takahara M, Uchi H, Takeuchi S, Mitoma C, Moroi Y, et al. An environmental contaminant, benzo(a)pyrene, induces oxidative stress-mediated interleukin-8 production in human keratinocytes via the aryl hydrocarbon receptor signaling pathway. J Dermatol Sci. 2011;62:42–9.

50. IARC Working Group on the Evaluation of Carcinogenic Risk to Humans. Chemical agents and related occupations. Lyon, International Agency for Research on Cancer; 2012.

51. IARC Monographs on the evaluation of carcinogenic risks to humans, no. 100F. BENZO[a]PYRENE. Available from: http://www.ncbi.nlm.nih.gov/books/NBK304415/.

52. Ju Q, Zouboulis CC, Xia L. Environmental pollution and acne: chloracne. Dermatoendocrinol. 2009;1(3):125–8.

53. Panteleyev AA, Bickers DR. Dioxin-induced chloracne – reconstructing the cellular and molecular mechanisms of a classic environmental disease. Exp Dermatol. 2006;15:705–30.

54. Geusau A, Tschachler E, Meixner M, et al. Olestra increases faecal excretion of 2,3,7,8-tetrachlorodiben zo-p-dioxin. Lancet. 1999;354:1266–7.

55. Balkrishnan R, McMichael AJ, Camacho FT, Saltzberg F, Housman TS, Grummer S, Feldman SR, Chren MM. Development and validation of a health-related quality of life instrument for women with melasma. Br J Dermatol. 2003;149(3):572.

56. Grimes PE. Melasma. Etiologic and therapeutic considerations. Arch Dermatol. 1995;131(12):1453.

57. Lutfi RJ, Fridmanis M, Misiunas AL, Pafume O, Gonzalez EA, Villemur JA, Mazzini MA, Niepomniszcze H. Association of melasma with thyroid autoimmunity and other thyroidal abnormalities and their relationship to the origin of the melasma. J Clin Endocrinol Metab. 1985;61(1):28.

58. Passeron T. Melasma pathogenesis and influencing factors – an overview of the latest research. J Eur Acad Dermatol Venereol. 2013;27(Suppl 1):5–6.

59. Roberts WE. Pollution as a risk factor for the development of melasma and other skin disorders of facial hyperpigmentation – is there a case to be made? J Drugs Dermatol. 2015;14(4):337–41.

60. Shankar D, Somani VK, Kohli M, Sharad J. A cross-sectional, multicentric clinico-epidemiological study of melasma in India. Dermatol Ther (Heidelb). 2014;4:71–81.

61. Sivayathorn A. Melasma in orientals clinical drug investigation. Indian J Dermatol. 2012;10(2 Supplement):34–40.

62. Kang WH, Yoon KH, Lee ES, KIm J, et al. Melasma: histopathological characteristics in 56 Korean patients. Br J Dermatol. 2002;146:228–37.

63. Noh TK, Choi SJ, Chung BY, Kang JS, et al. Inflammatory features of melasma lesions in Asian skin. J Dermatol. 2014;41(9):788–94.

64. UV exposure and sun protective practices. Cancer trends progress report – March 2015 Update. National Cancer Institute. http://progressreport.cancer.gov/prevention/sun_protection. Accessed 18 Aug 2016.

65. Cancer Statistics Review, SEER 1975-2013 (NCI) (2016) http://www.seer.cancer.gov/esr/1975_2013/. Accessed 18 Aug 16.

66. Eftim SE, Samet JM, Janes H, McDermott A, Dominici F. Fine particulate matter and mortality: a comparison of the six cities and American Cancer Society cohorts with a medicare cohort. Epidemiology. 2008;19:209–16.

67. Puntoni R, Ceppi M, Gennaro V, Ugolini D, Puntoni M, La Manna G, et al. Occupational exposure to carbon black and risk of cancer. Cancer Causes Control. 2004;15:511–6.

68. Boffetta N, Jourenkova P, Gustavsson. Cancer risk from occupational and environmental exposure to polycyclic aromatic hydrocarbons. Cancer Causes Control. 1997;8:444–72.

69. Larsen RK 3rd, Baker JE. Source apportionment of polycyclic aromatic hydrocar- bons in the urban atmosphere: a comparison of three methods. Environ Sci Technol. 2003;37:1873–81.

70. Matsumoto Y, Ide F, Kishi R, Akutagawa T, Sakai S, Nakamura M, et al. Aryl hydrocarbon receptor plays a significant role in mediating airborne particulate-induced carcinogenesis in mice. Environ Sci Technol. 2007;41:3775–80.

71. Burke KE, Wei H. Synergistic damage by UVA radiation and pollutants. Toxicol Ind Health. 2009;25:219–24.

72. Thiele JJ, Traber MG, Polefka TG, Cross CE, Packer L. Ozone-exposure depletes vitamin E and induces lipid peroxidation in murine stratum cor- neum. J Invest Dermatol. 1997;108:753–7.

73. Weber SU, Thiele JJ, Cross CE, Packer L. Vitamin C, uric acid and glutathione gradients in murine stratum corneum and their susceptibility to ozone exposure. J Invest Dermatol. 1999;113:1128–32.

74. Thiele JJ, Traber MG, Podda M, Tsang K, Cross CE, Packer L. Ozone depletes tocopherols and tocotrienols topically applied to murine skin. FEBS Lett. 1997;401:167–70.

75. Kim HO, Kim JH, Cho SI, Chung BY, Ahn IS, Lee CH, et al. Improvement of atopic dermatitis severity after reducing indoor air pollutants. Ann Dermatol. 2013;25:292–7.

76. Tigges J, Haarmann-Stemmann T, Vogel CF, Grindel A, Hübenthal U, Brenden H, et al. The new aryl hydrocarbon receptor antagonist E/Z-2-benzylindene-5,6-dimethoxy-3,3-dimethylindan-1-one protects against UVB-induced signal transduction. J Invest Dermatol. 2014;134:556–9.

Photoprotection and the Environment

49

Kátia Sheylla Malta Purim,
Ana Cláudia Kapp Titski, and Neiva Leite

Key Points

- Photoprotection is the primary preventive and therapeutic strategy against sunburn, photoaging, and skin cancer
- Photoprotective resources include broad-spectrum sunscreens, clothing, accessories, an appropriate diet, and the choice of times of lower solar radiation
- The UV index (ultraviolet index) forecast serves to warn of the dangers of excessive sun exposure and the importance of adequate sunscreen application
- Permanent educational measures on photoprotection are required to advise health professionals and the general population from childhood onward

K.S.M. Purim (✉)
Universidade Positivo, Curitiba, Brazil
e-mail: kspurim@gmail.com

A.C.K. Titski
Federal University of Paraná, Curitiba, Brazil

N. Leite
Federal University of Paraná, Curitiba, Brazil

Introduction

Electromagnetic Spectrum

The sunlight that falls on the skin can be absorbed, reflected, or scattered. The electromagnetic spectrum is extremely broad. Medically important wavelength ranges, however, are ultraviolet (UV) rays, visible light, and infrared (IR) radiation [1–5].

Ultraviolet Rays

UV rays have wavelengths of 100–400 nm and are divided into three bands: A (UVA), B (UVB), and C (UVC) (Fig. 49.1).

UVA radiation is subdivided into low UVA (320–340 nm), responsible for the vast majority of physiological effects on the skin, and high UVA (340–400 nm), which causes changes in the dermal structures. UVA has a direct action on the vessels of the dermis, causing vasodilation and gradual erythema. In epidermal cells, it elicits the breakdown of DNA chains that are subsequently repaired by enzymatic mechanisms. Depending on the thickness of the skin and duration of solar exposure, UVA can cause immediate and delayed pigmentation; skin aging; carcinogenesis; and the development of diseases such as lupus erythematosus, polymorphous light eruption, and photoallergies [3, 4, 6].

UVB has a wavelength range of 290–320 nm and is absorbed by ordinary glass. Despite its

© Springer International Publishing Switzerland 2018
R.R. Bonamigo, S.I.T. Dornelles (eds.), *Dermatology in Public Health Environments*,
https://doi.org/10.1007/978-3-319-33919-1_49

Fig. 49.1 Bands of ultraviolet radiation and their wavelengths

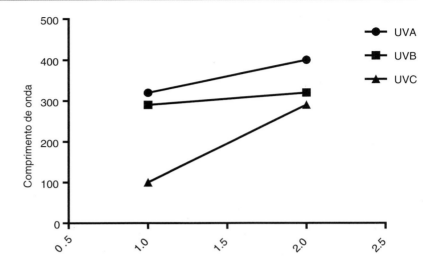

reduced skin penetration, the high energy of UVB is responsible for immediate sun damage and much of the delayed sun damage. UVB causes injury to epithelial cells and induces the formation of vasodilator substances such as prostaglandins. It also takes part in epidermal vitamin D metabolism, although it may cause erythema, burns, delayed pigmentation, epidermal thickening, photoaging, and carcinogenesis [1, 7, 8].

UVC has a wavelength range of 100–290 nm. It is absorbed by the upper layers of the Earth's atmosphere that are rich in ozone. UVC hardly reaches the Earth's surface at all. Recent studies indicate the depletion of the ozone layer. Although the consequences of this are still not fully clear, it is already affecting our lives and the planet [4, 5].

Visible Light

Visible light has a wavelength range between 400 and 780 nm and enables the formation of images by stimulating the retina and helping the brain distinguish between different colors (violet, blue, green, yellow, orange, and red). It may favor the onset of eye and skin diseases [6].

Infrared Radiation

IR radiation corresponds to about 50% of the solar spectrum. It has lower frequencies and generates little power. Because it transports heat

from the sun to the Earth, it is called the "caloric rays band." IR radiation reaches the hypodermis and causes temperature increases, heat, and cutaneous vasodilation. Chronic exposure to heat can lead to the development of erythema ab igne. IR radiation may contribute to pigmentation when combined with visible light [6]. It also contributes to skin aging and carcinogenesis, owing to its additive effects on UV radiation [2, 9].

In addition to the potential for interaction between the different radiation types and wavelength ranges, several environmental factors may influence the intensity of solar radiation that reaches the Earth's surface and the unprotected skin [4].

Personal characteristics, sociocultural aspects, exposure behavior and solar protection, genetic aspects related to skin pigmentation, photosensitive diseases, and immune competence are conditions that affect the health of skin [1].

Radiation Influences on the Environment

The surface levels of UV radiation depend on numerous aspects such as geography (latitude and altitude), weather (ozone levels), time (time of day and season), and sites (weather conditions, environmental pollutants, height, and cloud coverage) [5].

Latitude and Altitude

The intensity of UV rays increases with the increasing altitude of the location. This is because the atmosphere is thinner above it. However, this increase depends on other factors such as the amount of ozone in the lower layers of the atmosphere and the type of surface that reflects the rays and the sun's position [2].

Ozone

Ozone is the main absorber of UV radiation. Its highest concentration (about 80–90%) is located in the layer between 15 and 30 km altitude. This layer is responsible for the intensive absorption of UVB radiation and part of the extinction of UVC radiation [1].

Because of the existing transport mechanisms in the upper atmosphere, much of the ozone produced is transported to higher latitudes. Thus, there are lower ozone levels in the equatorial region of the planet in contrast to the pole and in regions of higher latitudes. Previous research has indicated that a decrease in ozone levels causes an increase in the risk of skin cancer development [4].

Time of Day and Season

UVB radiation is most intense between 10 a.m. and 4 p.m., with peaks recorded near midday. During the summer months, in areas closer to the equator, they increase about 4% every 300 m and can reach us from more than one direction, depending on the reflective surface area [2].

Sites

The intensity of sun radiation varies depending on the surface that it reaches. Snow, ice, white sand, grass, water, glass, and metal reflect radiation. Thus, the intensity of solar radiation striking these objects can be high even in shaded areas. Sand and concrete reflect 17% of UVB radiation while snow reflects 80% of UVB radiation. Pollutants and haze decrease the intensity of radiation, whereas clouds absorb 10–80% of UV radiation and therefore may pose a risk of overexposure [1, 6, 8].

State of Art

Influence of Sun Radiation on the Organism

Primarily due to its psychological and biological effects upon humans, natural light has been linked to positive events, such as lower rates of absenteeism and errors at work, and increased productivity levels. Its psychological effects are considered to be positive attitudes, as well as reduced fatigue and depression in patients with affective disorders. Its biological effects include the production of hormones, body self-regulation, wakefulness, and the sleep cycle [1].

When combined with physical activity, as well as with a proper diet or vitamin supplementation, natural light activates the metabolism of vitamin D [10]. This occurs when the individual receives UVB radiation. Vitamin D regulates bone and mineral physiology, especially the physiology of calcium metabolism, and in addition to having an antioncogenic role, it is also responsible for blood pressure control, the synthesis of natural antibiotics by defense cells, the modulation of autoimmunity, and the synthesis of inflammatory interleukins [11].

The endogenous production of vitamin D is influenced by melanin, and its synthesis begins in the deep layers of the epidermis, where its photochemical precursor 7-dehydrocholesterol is stored [10, 11]. Studies have shown that, regardless of age, ethnicity, geographic location, and sunscreen application, a significant portion of the world's population has low levels of vitamin D [4].

Persons predisposed to possible vitamin D deficiency may require adjustments in diet and oral supplementation with clinical monitoring [6, 7].

The Influence of Sun Radiation on the Skin

Throughout life the human skin, especially the face and back of the hands, is exposed in many ways to the action of UV, visible, and infrared light that can cause acute health problems or chronic health. Solar radiation has significant deleterious effects on the eyes and is the main skin carcinogen [4].

Cumulative sun exposure leads to integumentary system disorders, depending on personal, racial, behavioral, and immunogenetic characteristics. Certain individuals also have a higher risk of sunburn, pigmentation, photoaging, skin injuries, and carcinogenesis than others [6]. Light-skinned people particularly react more intensely to lower doses of UV radiation than dark-skinned people. Pigment sensitivity to UV light indicates ethnic origin and was classified according to phototypes by Fitzpatrick [12] (Table 49.1).

Influence of Sun Radiation on Outdoor Activities

Sports and Recreational Activities

Outdoor physical activities expose not only participants but also the public, organizers, trainers, and the coaching staff to acute and chronic skin changes. The face, the neck, the upper chest area (the "V-neckline" area), and the backs of the hands and arms are usually the most vulnerable sites and are more directly exposed to the environment [1].

The type of sport in which a person participates and the duration of outdoor activities are risk factors for increased exposure to sun radiation. For example, street joggers are exposed to solar radiation at different times of day, which

makes them more vulnerable to the harmful effects of excessive radiation [8, 12]. Physical education teachers who work outdoors are also subject to these effects [13].

Skin lesions must be recognized, treated, and prevented to avoid compromising the participation and performance of athletes in training and competitions [8]. Drug eruptions and dermatoses, such as labial herpes simplex, erythema multiforme, and pemphigus erythematosus, can be activated by sun exposure [4, 12]. The risk of UV radiation-related health effects on the eye and immune system is independent of skin type. Some studies have demonstrated that athletes who stay longer in the sun, such as marathon runners, cyclists, and triathletes, are at greater risk of developing skin cancer [8, 12]. Other athletes who are constantly exposed to sun radiation are surfers, swimmers, boaters, and skiers, as are adventure sports, eco-tourism, mountaineering, and paragliding enthusiasts.

UV radiation exposure tends to be increased on weekends and holidays. Tourists should be informed of UV radiation levels and be encouraged to protect themselves from the sun.

Children and the most vulnerable population groups, who are particularly sensitive to UV radiation, require special protection.

Outdoor Occupational Activities

Professionals such as farmers, gardeners, postmen, public cleaning and street lighting workers, military personnel, lifeguards, sailors, fishermen, and informal trade workers, among others who

Table 49.1 Skin types and response to sun exposure (Fitzpatrick classification) [12]

	I	II	III	IV	V	VI
Skin color	Pale white	White	Cream white to light brown	Moderate brown	Dark brown	Black
Main ethnic representatives	Albinos and redheads	Blondes	Whites	Brunettes and Latinos	Arabs, Mediterraneans, mestizos, Asians Indians	Blacks African people
Response to sun exposure	Always burns, never tans	Always burns, tans minimally	Burns and tans moderately	Burns minimally, always tans well	Rarely burns, always tans well	Never burns, always tans well
Pigment sensitivity to UV radiation	Very sensitive	Very sensitive	Sensitive	Mildly sensitive	Very mildly sensitive	Less sensitive

perform outdoor occupational activities, are continuously and customarily exposed to the sun [4, 5, 14]. Although studies have already demonstrated the relationship between chronic exposure to sunlight and damage to skin health, eyes, and lips, there are still unknown pathologic mechanisms [15]. Nevertheless, the use of protective clothing and measures such as limiting the duration of sun exposure, among others, are preventive, as are therapeutic strategies implemented against the harmful and cumulative effects of radiation on adults who predominantly work outdoors [1, 8, 12]. Health education aims achieve a change in attitudes and behavior [5].

Photoprotective Measures

Effective sun protection is achieved with the use of a set of measures to reduce or mitigate exposure to sun radiation. Photoeducation, as well as the use of sunscreens, clothing, accessories, and shadows, are resources that need to be combined to achieve more effective results [1, 16–21].

Topical Photoprotection

Sunscreens are elements with prophylactic and therapeutic purpose. Its regulation varies between different regions of the world, especially in Europe, the United States, and Australia [22–24].

In Brazil a combination of various physical and chemical filters is used in products to protect against UVA and UVB radiation: namely, SPF (sun protection factor) of 30 or more and UVA protection under international recommendation [4, 6].

Sunscreens should provide broad-spectrum protection, have low cost and good cosmetic acceptance, and be stable, nontoxic, nonirritating, nonsensitizing, easy to use, and water resistant [1, 6, 24]. The active ingredients of sunscreens act through mechanisms that absorb (organic), reflect, or block (inorganic) UV light, according to their chemical nature and physical properties [2].

There is a tendency to add antioxidant factors, DNA repair enzymes, and new compounds to increase the protective efficacy and also mitigate the effects of IR radiation [2, 9, 25, 26]. Research and development of new molecules and technological solutions for photoprotection continues [27].

The sunscreen vehicle should be compatible with the user's specific skin type and with the site of sunscreen application. Shampoos, conditioners, hair sprays, and solutions are indicated for the hair and hairy areas. Creams, lotions, and fluids are particularly suitable for dry skins. Gels are recommended for oily skin, and lipsticks for the mucous membranes. Emulsions and makeups have good cosmetic acceptability and effectiveness [2, 6, 24].

Improper use of sunscreen, however, can create a false feeling of protection. The main problems found are reduced or nonuniform sunscreen application, excessive sunscreen use to prolong the duration of sun exposure, low use of sunscreen, and faulty sunscreen reapplication [6, 20, 28].

In many outdoor work situations, as well as in situations of high sweat secretion, friction, water immersion, and repeated sun exposure, sunscreen has to be applied onto exposed areas every 2–3 h, sometimes even immediately after the first application of the product [1, 4, 13, 15]. Awareness of the dangers of excessive sun exposure should be converted to continuing protection practices and measures.

Photoprotection by Clothing and Accessories

Clothing is simple and practical, and relevant to photoprotection from childhood on [5, 6, 14, 18, 29–31]. Clothing with a sun protection function are subject to international standards and standardized with the term UPF (ultraviolet protection factor) as the category UPF 40–50 (excellent), UPF 25–39 (very good), and UPF 15–24 (good) [4, 32].

Some cotton and viscose fabrics available on the market offer protection against UV radiation. Their protection power, however, decreases as the fabric "ages" after repeated use and washings. Sun protection capacity can be increased according to the design and color of clothing, the fabric weave, the thickness of the threads, additives, and washing conditions [2, 4].

Exposure to sun radiation can be minimized by wearing socks, closed shoes, and accessories such as gloves, helmets, caps, and wide-brim (>7.5 cm) hats. Good-quality sunglasses protect the periorbital region. Clear lenses filter UVB radiation, while dark lenses filter UVA and visible light [6, 30]. The skin coverage provided by clothing and accessories works as a protective barrier against the sun. Moreover, they are easy to use, can be reused, and their cost is diluted over time.

The safety of workers and athletes during outdoor activities can be increased with the use of appropriate clothing and sportswear during work and sports. Increasingly sophisticated, resistant, practical, and easy to maintain products are manufactured to improve performance while protecting the athlete's physical integrity and health [4, 5, 8].

Systemic Photoprotection

More recently, studies have investigated the action of dietary or pharmacologic oral agents and their ability to inhibit or reverse sun damage to healthy or changed skin [6, 26, 33]. Some of the substances studied are β-carotene, green tea, isoflavones, polypodium leucotomos, lycopene, milk thistle, indomethacin, vitamin E, and vitamin C. These agents act by different or synergic mechanisms, and are available in food [34, 35]. Each case must be assessed individually, and caution is advised when prescribing these substances [4, 6, 26, 27].

Photoprotection by Behavioral Strategies

The following strategies should be prioritized as photoprotection behaviors:

Time and Place of Activities

Indoor workers receive 10–20% of outdoor workers' yearly UV exposure [5]. Outdoor activities should be scheduled in the early morning hours or preferably late afternoon, when the incidence of radiation begins to decline [1, 12], causing less damage and injuries.

The place, time of year and day, as well as seasonal and annual climate changes influence the intensity of sun radiation. Sun rays are reflected, dispersed, and absorbed many times on their way to the ground depending on the earth's rotation, tilt, and elliptical orbit around the sun. The intensity of sun rays can also vary depending on the effects caused by the formation of clouds, smog, dust, and mist [2]. The sum of these multiple components results in the overall incidence of solar radiation on a body located on the soil.

On cloudy days with little sunlight, a high percentage of UV rays comes through the clouds, increasing the risk of burns to unprotected body areas [2, 8, 16, 17]. Persons should be encouraged to reduce the occurrence of sunburn and cumulative UV radiation exposure over a lifetime [5].

UV Index

The intensity of UV radiation is wide and variable around the globe. The World Health Organization (WHO) has standardized UV measurement worldwide with the Ultraviolet Index (UV index). This index ranges from 0 to 12 or more in areas of medium altitudes, and is published daily by local meteorological bulletins. The sun protection measures should be triggered with a UV index ≥3. Extra protection is needed with a UV index of ≥7 [4, 5] (Table 49.2).

Shadow Rule

Solar radiation is less damaging the smaller the shadow of persons in relation to their height. Therefore, the larger the size of the lower body shadow, the greater the risk of radiation. This rule is an important and viable resource to identify periods of the day with less solar radiation [32].

Australia and other developed countries invest in intelligent and sustainable ecological solutions in consideration of shade in urban planning. Shade can reduce UV by 50% or more [5]. It is important to promote the modification of public places and educate the population.

Table 49.2 The World Health Organization global solar UV index (UVI)

	UV index				
	0–2	3–5	6–7	8–10	11+
Description	No danger to the average person	Little risk of harm from unprotected sun exposure	High risk of harm from unprotected sun exposure	Very high risk of harm from unprotected sun exposure	Extreme risk of harm from unprotected sun exposure
Recommended protection	Wearing a hat and/or sunglasses is sufficient	Wear a hat and sunglasses. Use SPF 15+ sunscreen	Wear a hat and sunglasses. Use SPF 30+ sunscreen. Cover the body with clothing. Avoid the sun if possible	Wear a hat and sunglasses. Use SPF 30+ sunscreen. Cover the body with clothing. Avoid the sun if possible	Take all precautions possible. It is advised to stay indoors
Sunburn time	1 h+	40 min	30 min	20 min	Less than 15 min

School and all outdoor recreational sites (beaches, sports centers and swimming pools, parks and zoos) provide information about UV radiation levels and sun protection.

The population should be encouraged to use umbrellas, tents, and other coverings especially in the summer months [5].

Eating Habits

A varied diet containing colorful (orange, yellow, and green) and natural food ingredients should be encouraged. Vitamin E, vitamin C, β-carotene, and lycopene are contained in fruits and vegetables and reduce the oxidative effects of UV radiation [33–35]. The intake of minerals (zinc, selenium, iron) and flavonoids and phenolic compounds found in grape, apple, citrus fruits, broccoli, cucumber, soybean, green tea, caffeine, and fish oil also contribute to daily photoprotection because of their antioxidant, anti-inflammatory, and immunomodulatory properties [2, 6, 27, 34].

Self-examination of the Skin

People should be encouraged to regularly check their entire skin surface for changes, including the scalp, armpits, buttocks, genitals, and feet. Self-examination of the skin surface is essential in prevention because it helps in the early detec-

tion of injuries [1]. Patients should seek medical advice if they notice any changes in their skin, or itching or bleeding injuries that do not seem to heal.

Individuals with light-colored skin and eyes, patients with multiple atypical nevi and a personal or family medical history of skin cancer, as well as outdoor athletes and workers are groups who need continuous prevention through extensive sun protection practices, health education, and early diagnosis [4, 20].

Educational Approaches for the Population

The prevention of skin cancer and other sun damage requires the implementation of permanent educational measures and awareness programs to prevent excessive and unprotected exposure to the undesirable effects of radiation [1, 4]. Children and adolescents should be afforded special attention because 50–80% of the estimated individual lifetime sun exposure occurs before 20 years of age. This refers to exposure to radiation resulting from casual exposure to sunlight in cars and other day-to-day routines, or intentional exposure during outdoor recreational and sports activities [6, 29, 31, 32]. Thus, the active participation of the family, schools, communities, businesses, government organizations, and different media is required to disseminate qualified information about the importance of health promotion and the available photoprotective methods.

With regard to sports fans, the characteristics and types of physical activities has changed in recent years, with a special increase in devotion to jogging, sports weekends, and adventure sports [1, 8]. Furthermore, the number of participants in these sports from special populations, such as pregnant women, older people, and disabled athletes, has increased. Both professional physical activities and activities performed to improve the quality of life entail the need for more effective sun protection, which is a cross-cultural challenge [5].

Outdoor workers may be more vulnerable to sun damage because of the amount of radiation accumulated by them over time, as well as episodes of high-intensity exposure [14–16]. Preventive strategies must be contextualized, improved, and constantly updated (Table 49.3).

New sun-protection strategies continue to be developed as several promising substances and products are discovered. However, further studies are still needed in this area. The use of sunscreens, combined with the implementation of a set of photoprotective measures, including photoeducation, is fundamental to achieving effective and lasting results.

Table 49.3 Forms of protection against UV radiation

Photoprotection attitudes	General considerations about the available resources
Healthy interaction with the environment	Observe latitude, altitude, season, reflection and scattering of rays by different surfaces
	Try to stay in the shade of an umbrella, trees, or other shelter
	Avoid sun exposure between 10 a.m. and 3 p.m. (10 a.m. and 4 p.m. in daylight-saving time)
	Be especially careful on cloudy days, because even then
	80–90% of the sun's radiation comes through the clouds
	Pay attention to the UV index of your city
Clothing and accessories	Wear a cap or a hat with an 8 cm wide brim
	Wear sunglasses with good optical quality as well as UVA and UVB lenses for visual comfort
	Wearing gloves protects your hands. The use of gloves should be encouraged, especially during performance of outdoor occupational or sports activities
	Choose fabrics that transmit less UV radiation. Transmission varies according to the texture, color, type, stiffness, and moisture of the fabric
	Avoid wearing wet T-shirts outdoors in the strong sun
Balanced diet	Daily consume colorful (red, orange, and yellow), natural foods rich in β-carotene and lycopene
	Incorporate cucumber, broccoli, and other fruits and vegetables that are sources of polyphenols into your diet, as they help reduce oxidative damage
	Eat natural foods rich in minerals (zinc, selenium, iron) and vitamins E, C, and D
Sunscreens	Confer due value to safety, efficacy, quality, benefits, and cost
	Preferably use products that are specific to your skin type and provide broad UVA and UVB protection
	Choose water- and sweat-resistant sunscreens with SPF 30 or more, and UVB and UVA protection, that do not run into the eyes
	Use sunscreen daily. Apply a generous amount of sunscreen homogeneously onto the skin and make frequent reapplications during the day
	Apply sunscreen liberally and frequently to your face, ears, neck, shoulders, and hands
Permanent education and health promotion	Prevention is the best measure to reduce risks
	Always combine several protection measures
	Perform skin self-examination frequently
	Control sun exposure and see a dermatologist to receive updated information on specific guidelines to follow according to your lifestyle

Future Perspectives

Stratospheric ozone layer depletion, climate changes, increased pollution, and lifestyle changes are factors that expose the individual to sunlight. Unprotected skin exposure to UV radiation can cause burns, photoaging, and skin cancer, in addition to other damage. Studies alert to the need of using appropriate clothing, accessories, and sunscreens for broad-spectrum protection [1–5].

The UV Index, available at public locations of several cities around the world or accessed via mobile electronic devices, has been disseminated as a real-time resource for stimulating photoprotective measures and adequate sunscreen application.

Nevertheless, there are still many controversies with respect to the presence and/or toxicity of certain chemicals used in sunscreen preparations, as well as to whether rigorous photoprotection affects vitamin D3 absorption [4, 7, 10]. There are also concerns and discussions regarding health damage associated with visible light and other currently studied radiations [9, 36].

Given the evidence of global warming, the aging population, and the increased number of cases of skin neoplasms, a systematic and broad photoprotection is recommended as the primary preventive and therapeutic strategy against skin cancer and photoaging, especially for individuals with light skin phototypes, multiple atypical nevi, and previous skin cancer history, outdoor workers, children, and immunologically vulnerable people.

Athletes in particular should be prepared, equipped, and up-to-date on protection practices and the effects of UV radiation on health [1, 12]. Outdoor activities are subject to the dangers, risks, and unpredictable situations associated with natural environments, such as sudden climate variations.

The future of photoprotection in sports will probably include an evolution in the composition and design of sports uniforms and accessories, changes in the times of competitions, the development of photoprotective agents with enzymes to remove or repair DNA damage, and new systemic sunscreens.

Recent research has made possible a better use of renewable energy resources, such as solar power, and has encouraged more conscious use of natural resources. Moreover, there are increased investments in studies of more efficient local and systemic photoprotection methods for the prevention, reduction, or repair of damage caused by sun exposure, with the development and improvement of several photoprotection technologies.

Educational campaigns have been carried out in many countries to promote healthier behaviors and the choice of times of lower solar radiation for the performance of outdoor activities, sports training, work shifts, and school recess, as well as the use of tree shadow, parasols, or covers aimed at habit changing and a more global protection.

Research, innovation, smart technologies, and educational investments point to a promising future in photoprotection. New programs with strong social awareness components will probably be created to educate the population, especially children. In addition, more efficient and objective public health policies should be implemented to reduce skin cancer rates and improve our quality of life.

Conclusion

When used properly and cautiously, sun exposure can bring physical and psychological benefits. Uncontrolled and unprotected exposure to radiation, however, causes damage to the skin, eyes, and health. The conjunctive use of different photoprotective resources and daily preventive measures should be advised and implemented in daily activities from childhood onward to minimize risks and improve the quality of life. The whole society, and particularly physicians, must play an important role in the transmission of knowledge about healthy sun exposure to the population.

Glossary

Malignant skin neoplasm a malignant epithelial neoplasm. The most common types are basal cell carcinoma and squamous cell carcinoma.

Melanoma   A malignant melanocytic neoplasm that can occur on any part of the body. It has a rapid growth rate and high metastasis potential, and may be fatal.

Photoaging   The superimposition of chronic sun damage on the intrinsic skin-aging process.

Photodamage   Skin changes resulting from UV light exposure.

Photoprotection Measures used to avoid or interfere with solar radiation, reducing its deleterious effects.

Phototype   Characterization of the skin according to its color and how it reacts to sun exposure. In brief it has been classified by Fitzpatrick into: (a) fair skin that never tans and is highly susceptible to sunburn (phototypes I and II); (b) white to brown skin with intermediate pigmentation (phototypes III and IV); (c) dark skin with accentuated pigmentation (phototypes V and VI).

Sunburn   The main acute skin reaction to excessive sunlight exposure. It can evolve into erythema, edema, blistering, peeling, and skin pigmentation. The face, neck, and trunk are more sensitive to sunburn than the limbs. The development of erythema is influenced by factors such as duration of exposure, phototype, age, diet, health characteristics, and atmospheric conditions (wind, heat, humidity, clouds).

Sunscreens (or sun filters)   Substances applied to the skin surface in different presentations, which contain in their formulation ingredients capable of absorbing, reflecting, or scattering UV radiation.

Ultraviolet index (UV index)   A scale for measuring the amount of UV radiation reaching the earth's surface and posing a health danger to all humans, not only individuals with certain skin phototypes. The higher the UV index, the greater the potential for damage to the skin. Its aim is to help people prevent excessive sun exposure at their current geographic position.

Ultraviolet radiation   Part of the Sun's light that reaches the earth and the human skin, having both positive and negative health effects.

References

1. Purim KSM, Leite N. Fotoproteção e Exercício Físico. Rev Bras Med Esporte. 2010;16(3):224–9.
2. Balogh TS, Velasco MVR, Pedriali CA, Kaneko TM, Baby AR. Proteção à radiação ultravioleta: recursos disponíveis na atualidade em fotoproteção. An Bras Dermatol. 2011;86(4):732–42.
3. Sklar LR, Almutawa F, Lim HW, Hamzavi I. Lim and Iltefat Hamzavi. Effects of ultraviolet radiation, visible light, and infrared radiation on erythema and pigmentation:a review. Photochem Photobiol Sci. 2013;12:54–64.
4. Consenso Brasileiro de Fotoproteção. Fotoproteção no Brasil. Recomendações da Sociedade Brasileira de Dermatologia. 2014;1:1–23.
5. Unep.org [Internet]. Global solar UV Index: A Practical Guide. A joint recommendation of the World Health Organization, World Meteorological Organization, United Nations Environment Programme, and the International Commission on NonIonizing Radiation Protection. Geneva: WHO; 2002. 28 p. [Cited 2017 20 Jun]. Available from: http://www.unep.org/pdf/solar_Index_Guide.pdf.
6. Gontijo TG, Pugliesi MCC, Araújo FM. Fotoproteção. Surg Cosmet Dermato. 2009;1(4):186–92.
7. Lim HD. Sun exposure and vitamin D level. J Am Acad Dermatol. 2008;58:516.
8. Purim KSM, Titski ACK, Leite N. Hábitos solares, queimadura e fotoproteção em atletas de meia maratona. Rev Bras Ativ Fis e Saúde. 2013;18(5):636–45.
9. Schroeder P, Calles C, Krutmann J. Prevention of infrared-a radiation mediated detrimental effects in human skin. Skin Ther Lett. 2009;14(5):4–5.
10. Kannan S, Lim HW. Photoprotection and vitamin D: a review. Photodermatol Photoimmunol Photomed. 2014;30:137–45.
11. Castro LCG. O sistema endocrinológico vitamina D. Arq Bras Endocrinol Metab. 2011;55(8):566–75.
12. Purim KSM, Leite N. Dermatoses do esporte em praticantes de corrida de rua do sul do Brasil. An Bras Dermatol. 2014;89(4):587–93.
13. Oliveira LMC, Glauss N, Palma A. Hábitos relacionados à exposição solar dos professores de educação física que trabalham com atividades aquáticas. An Bras Dermatol. 2011;86(3):445–50.
14. Reeder AI, Gray A, McCool JP. Occupational sun protection: workplace culture, equipment provision and outdoor workers' characteristics. J Occup Health. 2013;55:84–97.
15. Lucena EES, Costa DCB, Silveira EJD, Lima KC. Prevalência de lesões labiais em trabalhadores de praia e fatores associados. Rev Saúde Pública. 2012;46(6):1051–7.
16. Seité S, Fourtanier AMA. The benefit of daily photoprotection. J Am Acad Dermatol. 2008;58:160–6.

17. Gilaberte Y, González S. Update on Photoprotection. Actas Dermosifiliográficas. 2010;101(8):659–72.
18. Wang SQ, Balagula Y, Osterwalder U. Photoprotection: a review of the current and future technologies. Dermatol Ther. 2010;23(1):31–47.
19. Reyes E, Vitale MA. Avances en fotoprotección. Mecanismos moleculares implicados. Piel. 2012;511:1–13.
20. Purim KSM, Wroblevski FC. Exposição e proteção solar dos estudantes de medicina de Curitiba (PR). Rev Bras Edu Med. 2014;38:477–85.
21. Day AK, Wilson CJ, Hutchinson AD, Roberts RM. The role of skin cancer knowledge in sun-related behaviours: a systematic review. J Health Psychol. 2014;19:1143–62.
22. Loden M, Beitner H, Gonzalez H, Edstrom DW, Akerstrom U, Austad J, et al. Sunscreen use: controversies, challenges and regulatory aspects. Br J Dermatol. 2011;165:255–62.
23. Sambandan DR, Ratner D. Sunscreens: An overview and update. J Am Acad Dermatol. 2011;64(4):748–58.
24. Schalka S, Reis VM. Fator de proteção solar: significado e controvérsias. Anais Bras Dermatol. 2011;86(3):507–15.
25. Allemann B, Baumann L. Antioxidants used in skin care formulations. Skin Ther Lett. 2008;3(7):5–9.
26. Gálvez MV. Antioxidantes en fotoprotección, realmente funcionan? Actas Dermosifiliogr. 2010;101:197–200.
27. Chen L, Hu JY, Wang SQ. The role of antioxidants in photoprotection: a critical review. J Am Acad Dermatol. 2012;67:1013–24.
28. Purim KSM, Avelar MFS. Fotoproteção, melasma e qualidade de vida em gestantes. Rev Bras Ginecologia e Obstetrícia. 2012;34:228–34.
29. Ghazi S, Couteau C, Paparis E, Coiffard LJM. Interest of external photoprotection by means of clothing and sunscreen products in young children. J Eur Acad Dermatol Venereol. 2012;26:1026–30.
30. Almutawa F, Buabbas H. Photoprotection: clothing and glass. Dermatol Clin. 2014;32:439–48.
31. Bonfá R, Martins-Costa GM, Lovato B, Rezende R, Belletini C, Weber MB. Avaliação do conhecimento e hábitos de fotoproteção entre crianças e seus cuidadores na cidade de Porto Alegre. Brasil Surg Cosmet Dermatol. 2014;6(2):148–53.
32. Criado PR, Melo JN, Oliveiras ZNP. Topical photoprotection in childhood and adolescence. J Pediatr. 2012;88(3):203–10.
33. Stahl W, Sies H. Photoprotection by dietary carotenoids: concept, mechanisms, evidence and future development. Mol Nutr Food Res. 2012;56(2):287–95.
34. Nichols JA, Katiyar SK. Skin photoprotection by natural polyphenols: anti-inflammatory, antioxidant and DNA repair mechanisms. Arch Dermatol Res. 2010;302:71–83.
35. Schagen SK, Zampeli VA, Makrantonaki E, Zouboulis CC. Discovering the link between nutrition and skin aging. Dermatoendocrinol. 2012;4:298–307.
36. Skotarczak K, Osmola-Mankowska A, Lodyga M, Polanska A, Mazur M, Adamski Z. Photoprotection: facts and controversies. Eur Rev Med Pharmacol Sci. 2015;19:98–112.

Dermatology and Sports

50

Renato Marchiori Bakos,
Katia Sheylla Malta Purim, Antonio Macedo D'Acri,
and Helena Reich Camasmie

Key Points

- Herpes gladiatorum and tinea gladiatorum are common cutaneous infectious on the face, neck, trunk, and upper limbs that occur more frequently in men performing contact sports.
- Traumatic cutaneous lesions are extremely common among athletes. These reactions may vary in location, distribution, and intensity depending on the sport modality, and history taking is crucial for recognition.
- Sport-induced urticaria is a type of physical urticaria related to angioedema or anaphylactic reactions, which may be food or medication dependent.
- Dermatologic prescriptions may contain substances prohibited by some sports, and dermatologists should contact sports federations whenever necessary.

R.M. Bakos (✉)
Federal University of Rio Grande do Sul,
Porto Alegre, Brazil
e-mail: rbakos@hcpa.edu.br

K.S.M. Purim
Universidade Positivo, Curitiba, Brazil

A.M. D'Acri
Federal University of Rio de Janeiro,
Rio de Janeiro, Brazil

H.R. Camasmie
Hospital Universitário Gaffrée e Guinle,
Rio de Janeiro, Brazil

Introduction

To perform physical activities is nowadays considered an appropriate behavior to achieve good health, leisure, and quality of life. An increasing number of individuals seek sports participation for these reasons and also as a professional career. Nevertheless, because of different personal conditions of the athlete or sports-related and environmental aspects, distinct cutaneous injuries may occur during participation.

Sport-related skin diseases or conditions can be caused by physical, chemical, or biological agents alone or in association. Preexisting medical conditions may also contribute to cutaneous injuries. Most cutaneous reactions are mild and rapid, and easy recovery is expected, although some may be relapsing and have an impact on the athlete's performance. Some cutaneous diseases may also lead to exclusion of athletes from sports events. Consequently, recognizing and controlling sport-associated dermatologic conditions can be also relevant not only to ensure good medical conditions in athletes but also to improve their performance. In this chapter, some of the main sports-related dermatologic diseases and conditions are described.

© Springer International Publishing Switzerland 2018
R.R. Bonamigo, S.I.T. Dornelles (eds.), *Dermatology in Public Health Environments*,
https://doi.org/10.1007/978-3-319-33919-1_50

State of the Art

Lesions Caused by Infectious Agents

In sports, an infectious process has individual and collective impacts as it hinders, limits, or prevents practice. The risk of contagion is greater and more worrying among athletes participating in team and contact sports. It is essential that athletes, coaches, and the multidisciplinary care team have the knowledge to observe skin integrity aimed at preventing injury and providing appropriate action, minimizing transmission within the team [1–4]. Thus, it may be necessary to exclude an athlete from a sports event in order to preserve the health of the others. Immunocompromised players are more vulnerable to infections and, similar to children, pregnant women, and Paralympic athletes, require specific care [3, 4]. Bacterial and fungal infections are common in obesite and diabetic individuals, and have implications for physical activity because they cause pain, discomfort, and difficulty or limitation of movement [5]. Strategies to promote skin health may improve the quality of life of different types of athletes and result in better performance.

Herpes Gladiatorum

This infection is caused by herpes simplex virus in athletes practicing contact sports. It is characterized by grouped vesicles or an erythematous base associated with paresthesia, affecting mainly the cervical and upper thoracic regions of boxers and wrestlers. The main predisposing factors are body contact, chafing caused by uniforms, local trauma, stress, and sun exposure. Clinical diagnosis can be complemented by Tzanck smear, histopathology, and serology. Oral treatment comprises acyclovir (400 mg three times daily or 200 mg five times daily), famciclovir (250 mg three times daily), or valacyclovir (1 g three times daily) for 5 days, on average. In contact sports, when the affected areas are exposed the lesions should be covered or occluded, and there may be a need to exclude the athlete from competition [3].

Common Warts

Warts are seen with some frequency on the hands and feet of athletes of sports whose impact is greater in these areas. In sports such as running, martial arts, and water activities that involve the use of collective dressing rooms, warts are more common in the lower limbs. Pool users, especially if they are atopic individuals, tend to have warts caused by friction, maceration, and microtrauma in the plantar region. Clinical diagnosis is made by localized hyperkeratosis, pinpoint black spots, and disruption of the skin lines in the affected area. There are several therapeutic options with varying success rates, such as chemical cauterization, cryotherapy, electrocoagulation, and use of imiquimod, depending on severity and location. Extensive and exophytic lesions may require surgery and histopathology. In contact sports, when the affected areas are exposed the lesions should be covered or occluded, and there may be a need to exclude the athlete from competition [3].

Tinea Corporis Gladiatorum

This is a dermatophytosis that presents a different clinical pattern, frequently detected in men performing contact sports, mainly wrestlers. The most exposed and affected areas are the face, neck, trunk, and upper limbs. Transmission occurs via skin-to-skin contact or through contaminated objects and surfaces. Clinical diagnosis is based on mycologic examination and culture, usually with identification of *Trichophyton tonsurans*. Lesions are scaly and itchy erythematous plaques, and may assume epidemic proportions in the wrestlers' community. It is treated with topical (ketoconazole, isoconazole, terbinafine, etc.) or systemic (griseofulvin 500 mg/day, itraconazole 100–200 mg/day, fluconazole 150 mg/day, or terbinafine 250 mg/day) antifungals until the lesions heal, along with health measures. If lesions cannot be covered, the athlete will be unable to compete until cured [6].

Tinea Pedis

Tinea pedis, commonly known as athlete's foot (Fig. 50.1), is not exclusive to athletes, although it is common in certain sports. *Trichophyton rubrum* and *Trichophyton mentagrophytes* are mainly responsible for tinea pedis alone or combined with onychomycosis and tinea cruris. This mycosis is favored by individual predisposition, moisture resulting from excessive foot sweating, occlusive shoes, showering in public places, walking barefoot on communal floors, and sharing equipment and towels. Associations with yeasts and bacteria are

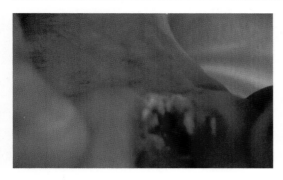

Fig. 50.1 Tinea pedis: athlete's foot (Courtesy of Dr. Renan Bonamigo)

described, and an interdigital attack increases the risk for development of erysipelas or cellulitis of the lower limb. Tinea pedis symptoms are erythema, scaling, fissures and blisters on the feet, associated with itching, discomfort, and social and functional limitation. Clinical diagnosis can be confirmed by direct mycologic examination and culture. Prophylactic measures are essential (wearing sandals in wet environments, changing shoes and socks, drying feet and interdigital areas, not sharing towels or personal items), and treatment can be carried out with topical or systemic antifungals, according to the extent and severity of the clinical picture [7, 8].

Onychomycosis

The highest percentages of nail injuries in athletes are associated with trauma. This condition favors the penetration of fungi and bacteria. The fungal lesions may be restricted or associated with cutaneous lesions. Onychomycosis can evolve to loss of the nail, ingrown toenail, local pain, and limitation of sports movements of the feet [5, 9, 10]. It is necessary to differentiate this from other nail disorders [8, 11].

Swimmer's Ear

Swimmer's ear is caused by bacteria, such as *Pseudomonas aeruginosa* and *Staphylococcus aureus*. Clinical diagnosis is based on symptoms of itching, pain, and redness in the ear canal. Predisposing factors are maceration resulting from long immersion periods in the water leading to ear wax decrease and external ear pH alteration, frequency and quality of activities, pool water treatment, and hygiene. The treatment is based on removing debris from the ear canal and

its acidification using 2% acetic acid in propylene glycol. Relapsing, complicated, or severe cases may cause temporary or permanent limitation on carrying out professional water activities [12].

Sea Bather's Eruption

This dermatitis is caused via contacting marine species of *Cnidaria phylum* (jellyfish, Portuguese man-of-war, sea anemones, corals). It has been described by swimmers and athletes from the Caribbean Sea, Mexico, Australia, and Brazil. Therefore, its importance is growing in recreational and professional water sports activities. Clinical diagnosis is based on body examination for erythematous papules, and pruritic lesions in areas covered or not by the bathing suit after swimming in the sea. Treatment consists in getting out of the sea and applying acetic acid on the affected area. Corticosteroids, antihistamines, and menthol lotions are least effective. Spontaneous regression of the lesions occurs in a few days or up to 2 weeks. Depending on the sea conditions, swimming or competitions should be discontinued [13–15].

Cercarial Dermatitis

People who practice water activities in lakes, streams, rivers, and weirs are subject to skin lesions caused by cercariae of *Schistosoma mansoni* parasites. Diagnosis is made based on epidemiologic history and body examination for erythematous itchy rashes in areas not protected by clothes a few hours after being in contact with water. The symptoms disappear spontaneously or after administering ivermectin orally. Taking into consideration the risks of diseases and accidents involves in this recreational or adventure practice, popular especially in the summer, hygiene orientation should be taught to swimmers and athletes [15].

Other Skin Infections

It should be noted that infectious cutaneous manifestations in athletes vary in their etiology, origin, frequency, and intensity. They include molluscum contagiosum, cutaneous larva migrans, pitted keratolysis, impetigo, folliculitis, scabies, lice infestation, and various mycoses. These diseases may be disguised or worsened by traumatic disorders, inflammatory processes, environmental factors, and pre-existing dermatoses [16].

Most of these conditions are mild and temporary, while others are recurrent and may have an unfavorable outcome. Early recognition and treatment are essential, considering the need for the professional athlete to recover as quickly as possible. One should note the need to exclude the athlete from competition may arise if the condition is contagious [3].

Lesions Caused by Traumatic Conditions

Friction Blisters

The causes of blister development are friction and local skin trauma, commonly on the feet, due to ill-fitting shoes. Other risk factors include various sports equipment (racquets, bats, sticks, bars, etc.) when used in extended and nonideal conditions. The diagnosis is not challenging once the blisters are easily recognized for their discomfort and pain, plus the risk of secondary infection. Treatment consists of hygiene, protection of the affected area, and proper draining if necessary. Prevention of blisters requires comfortable and athlete-adjusted equipment as well as protection on the areas that undergo higher friction [3, 17–19] (Fig. 50.2).

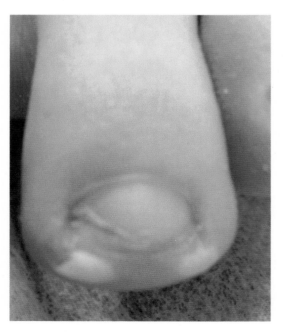

Fig. 50.2 Friction blisters (Courtesy of Dr. Renan Bonamigo)

Calluses and Callosities

These are known as an innate protection mechanism for areas that suffer from constant trauma and friction, sometimes even being the natural evolution of recurrent blisters. Treatment is indicated only if interference of the function is recognized, and includes chemical or physical excision. Prevention with appropriate socks, shoes, and insoles is recommended [5, 10, 20].

Calcaneal Petechiae (Black Heel)

Petechiae are the result of small hemorrhages caused by microtraumatism to the cutaneous capillaries, in areas that suffer from the association of thin fatty tissue, repeated trauma, and bone proximity. They are most common in the calcaneus when practicing sports such as tennis, basketball, and running, caused by rough stop-and-start motions. The lesions may occur on the hands when practicing golf, baseball, weight lifting, or gymnastics. Lentiginous acral melanoma is the differential diagnosis, and dermoscopy may be useful to exclude any suspicion. The lesions disappear if the evolved sport activity is ceased [17, 21, 22].

Jogger's Toe

Subungual or periungual hematoma of the toenails may occur as a result of significant nail trauma (Fig. 50.3), associated with onycholysis and thickening of the nail. The use of poorly adapted or nonideal shoes while practicing sports is the main cause. Painful hematoma can be drained if necessary. Prevention includes the use of appropriate and well-fitting athletic wear, as well as adequate protective silicon insoles to cover the toes [5, 10, 17].

Piezogenic Pedal Papules

These are skin-colored, occasionally painful papules located on the medial or posterolateral side of the heels. Better visualized when standing, their prevalence is found to be up to 10%. Usually symptomatic in long-distance runners, the papules arise from subcutaneous fat herniations through the connective tissue. For painful papules, compression stockings and heel cups are useful [17, 23–25].

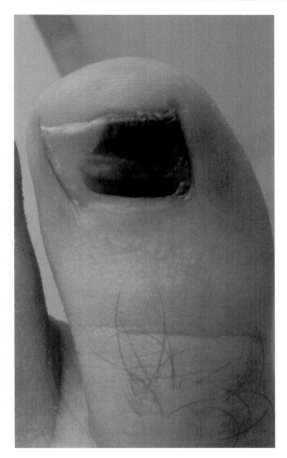

Fig. 50.3 Jogger's toe (subungual hematoma) (Courtesy of Dr. Renan Bonamigo)

Jogger's Nipples

Pain, erosion, and eventual bleeding result from irritation caused by repetitive friction between runners' shirts and their nipples, especially when using coarse-fiber T-shirts. Treatment is easy, for consisting simply of removing the cause. Avoiding such fibers, applying petroleum jelly, or the use of adhesive bandages are good options to prevent this condition. Soft-fiber and well-adapted bras are useful for women [3, 17, 20].

Knuckle Pads

Chronic compression on the knuckles may lead to the development of fibrous skin nodules. Soccer players may present such callosities on the feet, whereas in boxers the nodules occur between the phalanxes of fingers [20, 26].

Environment-Related Cutaneous Conditions

It is common to sports participants to use mandatory equipment, shoe gear, or clothes. This can lead to athletes suffering cutaneous reactions exacerbated from their use or even triggered by them. Some of these conditions might be due to allergic or irritant contact. In addition, weather conditions or even nutritional aspects may aggravate clinical symptoms or diseases. Some of the most relevant conditions are described here.

Contact Dermatitis

Every sport has peculiar aspects as regards its necessary equipment and clothes. Therefore it is common for athletes to present with allergic or irritant contact dermatitis [27]. Allergic contact dermatitis depends on an individual sensitizing predisposition, while irritant contact dermatitis may occur in any athlete depending on time of exposure to a specific substance. Initial clinical suspicion may show after asking the patient appropriate questions about sports participation. Water sports are mostly involved. It is frequent to observe reactions to rubber material such as goggles, underwater masks, and diving suits [28, 29]. Epicutaneous tests might be important in suspicious cases. Allergens such as phenylenediamine and thiourea are good examples of substances involved in the rubber manufacturing process. Topical medications, resins, and inks are other potential causes of dermatitis. Irritant contact dermatitis due to plants might be observed in golfers or hikers. Different sport equipment may also be involved in irritant contact dermatitis, and a careful anamnesis might help to elucidate the scenario. Even the athlete's own body may cause, for example, "swimmer's shoulder" resulting from unshaven hair. The therapeutic approach consists in recognizing the allergenic or irritant agent, and appropriate use of topical steroids and oral antihistamines [27].

Xerosis

Athletes who partake in water sports, especially swimmers, are prone to dry skin. They stay in the water for long periods and lose essential cutaneous oils. Taking hot-water showers after exercise together with soaps worsens the scenario, especially in atopy patients. This is the major cause of pruritus in athletes. Shortening the duration of showers and reducing the water temperature in combination with application of ointments may be a sufficient therapy [3, 27].

Mechanical Acne

This particular acne variant has been described in different sports such as American football, wrestling, and gymnastics. Pre-existing acne is not necessary for its development. It occurs as a result of continuous frictional movements or pressure by sports equipment (helmets, clothes) with occlusion, heat, and humidity [30]. Clinical aspects are very typical, presenting erythematous papules and pustules on body sites associated with equipment-induced pressure or friction. The posterior aspect of the neck and the back are common affected areas. It is important to rule out anabolic steroid use in rapid-onset acne [31]. Recent mild intake has been associated with acne worsening [32]. Moreover, whey protein consumption also precipitated acne development, which was relieved after supplementation suspension [33]. Therefore, nutritional aspects in athletes with acne should always be asked after. Treatment is based on reducing friction or pressure from the equipment and regular acne medications depending on its extent and duration. Total involution of the lesions may occur only at the end of the sport season [27].

Urticaria

Sport-induced urticaria is a type of physical urticaria that, though rarely, can lead to emergency medical situations such as angioedema or anaphylactic reactions [34]. It may be triggered by intense or mild physical exercises. The symptoms may occur just after sport initiation and vary from itching, flushing, burning sensation, and hives to angioedema and cardiovascular collapse [35]. Ninety percent of the athletes refer pruritus as the first symptom. Joggers are particularly affected. Sport-induced urticaria may also be triggered by ingestion of specific foodstuffs (e.g., wheat derivatives) or medications (aspirin or nonsteroidal anti-inflammatory agents) before

exercise [36]. Athletes are also more prone to develop other urticaria variants such as aquagenic, solar, heat, or cold urticaria. Sport-induced urticaria patients should not exercise alone. Use of antihistamines before sport participation may prevent symptoms. If presenting symptoms, patients should suspend exercise immediately. Other measures may be necessary, such as symptomatic medications or subcutaneous epinephrine [3].

Miscellaneous

Striae

Stretch marks are very common in isometric sports participants (70% of female adolescents and 40% of boys), although abrupt striae may also occur in anabolic steroid users. The former situation may be suspected if other androgenic aspects are present, such as acne, oily skin, and androgenetic alopecia. Weightlifting, bodybuilding, gymnastics, and fighting sports are especially associated with striae development caused by skin distension and muscular hypertrophy. Treatment is difficult and should be the same as for other causes. Options include topical tretinoin and laser therapy [3, 37].

Green Hair

Green hair is particularly common among swimmers. The green color is due to copper impregnation and not chlorides as frequently attributed. Increased copper levels in the water may occur because of old pipes or copper-containing algaecides. Showering immediately with shampoos and rinse creams after leaving the swimming pool should be sufficient to avoid the condition [27].

Skin Cancer and Sun Protection

As many sports are performed outdoors, sun protection is always a leading concern among health professionals regarding athletes. Several reports demonstrate that athletes who compete in this scenario receive considerable ultraviolet (UV) doses because of training and competition schedules. UV dosimetric studies have demonstrated that some sports such as skiing, mountaineering, cycling, or triathlon are associated with extreme cumulative UV doses [38]. Moreover, outdoor sports may lead to UV-associated skin lesions even in children. In a cohort it was observed that the nevus count and acquired nevus count were higher in children who practiced outdoor sports [39]. UV radiation is well known as one of the major environmental risk factors for skin cancer. Therefore, some athletes may have an increased risk of developing skin cancer. Indeed in marathon runners it was demonstrated that presence of lentigines correlated with type of sportswear and intense training schedule had an impact on the number of nevi, which are well recognized as melanoma risk factors [40]. In another survey marathon runners presented an increased risk of developing melanoma and other skin cancers in comparison with controls [41]. Fair-skinned athletes competing for the Brazilian national team in the 2003 Pan-American Games stated that they had more sunburn episodes in leisure activities than in sport participation. Therefore, athletes should be educated to adopt sun-protection habits during both periods to prevent UV damage [42]. Prevention strategies to avoid sun exposure include wearing hats, long pants, and long-sleeved shirts, using sunscreens with sun protection factor 30 or higher and avoiding peak UV exposure hours. Unfortunately, the particularities of some sports raise difficulties in dealing with sun protection. It is always important to educate athletes about sun care to improving their sun-care habits. Not only athletes but also the spectators of sporting events should also be very cautious about sun protection, as the duration of events may be sometimes prolonged and occur during peak UV hours [38, 39, 43].

Doping Control and Dermatology

As athletes must regularly undergo doping control tests, dermatologists should be aware of their prescription in this scenario. Some frequently prescribed medications by dermatologists are prohibited in professional sports events. The use of these substances may lead to severe suspensions or even elimination from the sport. The WADA (World Anti-Doping Agency) publishes online (http://www.wada-ama.org) the prohibited substances list every year. Dermatologists should always contact sports federation medical doctors if any substance from the list needs to be used for medical reasons. It may be possible for the athlete to compete using a substance present on the list as long as all the necessary procedures and forms are applied and approved before he/she takes part in sports training or competition ("therapeutic use exemption").

Perspectives: Final Remarks

Sports and dermatology are connected in different ways. Dermatologists should be aware of these scenarios so as to educate athletes about preventive measures against major sport-related skin diseases and to detect and treat them, and finally to avoid harming the athletes through inadequate prescriptions for professional athletes.

Glossary

Flushing Sudden vasodilation by different mechanisms causing skin erythema.

References

1. Diaz JFK, Guillen JR, Carrero JAT. Prevalência de doenças infecciosas no esporte. Rev Bras Med Esporte. 2000;72:343–8.
2. Beck CK. Infectious diseases in sports. Med Sci Sports Exerc. 2000;32(7Suppl):S431–8.
3. Dacri AM., Bakos RM, Purim KSM. Dermatoses do esporte. In: Omar Lupi; Paulo R Criado. Rotinas de Diagnóstico e Tratamento da Sociedade Brasileira de Dermatologia. 2nd. Rio de Janeiro: AC Farmacêutica, 2012, v. 1, p. 165–169.
4. D'Acri AM. Dermatoses excludentes de competições esportivas. J MEx. 2007;51:6–7.
5. Purim KSM, Titski ACK, Leite N. dermatologic aspects influencing the practice of physical activities by obese individuals. Fisioter Mov. 2015;28(4):837–50.
6. Adams BB. Tinea corporis gladiatorum. J Am Acad Dermatol. 2002;47(2):286–90.
7. Purim KSM, de Freitas CF, Leite N. Feet dermatophytosis in soccer players. An Bras Dermatol. 2009;84(5):550–2.

8. Purim KSM, Niehues LP, Queiroz-Telles FF, Leite N. Aspectos epidemiológicos das micoses dos pés em um time chinês de futebol. Rev Bras Med Esporte. 2006;12(1):16–9.

9. Sabadin CS, Benvegnú SA, da Fontoura MM, Saggin LM, Tomimori J, Fischman O. Onychomycosis and tinea pedis in athletes from the State of Rio Grande do Sul (Brazil): a cross-sectional study. Mycopathologia. 2011;171(3):183–9.

10. Purim KSM, Leite N. Sports-related dermatoses among road runners in Southern Brazil. Anais Bras Dermatol. 2014;89(4):587–92.

11. Braswell MA, Daniel CR, Brodell RT. Beau lines, onychomadesis, and retronychia: a unifying hypothesis. JAAD. 2015;73(5):849–55.

12. Adams BB. Dermatologic disorders of the athlete. Sports Med. 2002;32(5):309–21.

13. Haddad V Jr, Cardoso JC, Silveira FL. Seabathers eruption: report of five cases in southeast region of Brazil. Rev Inst Med Trop São Paulo. 2001;43(3):171–2.

14. Rossetto AL, Mora JM, Correa CR, et al. Prurido do traje de banho: relato de seis casos no Sul do Brasil. Rev Soc Bras Med Trop. 2007;40(1):78–81.

15. Haddad V Jr. Dermatologia ambiental: Manifestações dermatológicas de acidentes por animais aquáticos (invertebrados). An Bras Dermatol. 2013;88(4):496–506.

16. Ledoux D, Goffin V, Fumal I, Piérard-Franchimont C, Piérard GE. Cutaneous infections contracted during sports and recreational activities. Rev Med Liege. 2001;56(5):339–42.

17. Mailler-Savage EA, Adams BB. Skin manifestations of running. J Am Acad Dermatol. 2006;55(2):290–301.

18. Burkhart CG. Skin disorders of the foot in active patients. Phys Sportsmed. 1999;27(2):88–101.

19. Brennan FH Jr. Managing blisters in competitive athletes. Curr Sports Med Rep. 2002;1(6):319–22.

20. Tlougan BE, Mancini AJ, Mandell JA, Cohen DE, Sanchez MR. Skin conditions in figure skaters, ice-hockey players and speed skaters: part I – mechanical dermatoses. Sports Med. 2011;41(9):709–19.

21. Urbina F, León L, Sudy E. Black heel, talon noir or calcaneal petechiae? Australas J Dermatol. 2008;49(3):148–51.

22. Basler RS, Hunzeker CM, Garcia MA. Athletic skin injuries: combating pressure and friction. Phys Sportsmed. 2004;32(5):33–40.

23. Rocha BO, Fernandes JD, Prates FV. Piezogenic pedal papules. An Bras Dermatol. 2015;90(6):928–9.

24. Karadag AS, Bilgili SG, Guner S, Yilmaz D. A cases series of Piezogenic pedal papules. Indian Dermatol Online J. 2013;4(4):369–71.

25. Ma DL, Vano-Galvan S. Piezogenic pedal papules. CMAJ. 2013;185(18):E847.

26. Kanerva L. Knuckle pads from boxing. Eur J Dermatol. 1998;8(5):359–61.

27. Adams BB. Sports dermatology. New York: Springer; 2006. p. 180–2.

28. Brooks C, Kujawska A, Patel D. Cutaneous allergic reactions induced by sporting activities. Sports Med. 2003;33(9):699–708.

29. Moritz K, Sesztak-Greinecker G, Wantke F, Götz M, Jarisch R, Hemmer W. Allergic contact dermatitis due to rubber in sports equipment. Contact Dermatitis. 2007;57(2):131–2.

30. Basler RS. Acne mechanica in athletes. Cutis. 1992;50:125–8.

31. Melnik B, Jansen T, Grabbe S. Abuse of anabolic-androgenic steroids and bodybuilding acne: an underestimated health problem. J Dtsch Dermatol Ges. 2007;5(2):110–7.

32. Bronsnick T, Murzaku EC, Rao BK. Diet in dermatology: part I. Atopic dermatitis, acne, and nonmelanoma skin cancer. J Am Acad Dermatol. 2014;71(6):1039. e1-1039.e12

33. Silverberg NB. Whey protein precipitating moderate to severe acne flares in 5 teenaged athletes. Cutis. 2012;90:70–2.

34. Schwartz LB, Delgado L, Craig T, et al. Exercise-induced hypersensitivity syndromes in recreational and competitive athletes: a PRACTALL consensus report (what the general practitioner should know about sports and allergy). Allergy. 2008;63(8):953–61.

35. Jaqua NT, Peterson MR, Davis KL. Exercise-induced anaphylaxis: a case report and review of the diagnosis and treatment of a rare but potentially life-threatening syndrome. Case Rep Med. 2013;2013:610–726.

36. Kim CW, Figueroa A, Park CH, Kwak YS, Kim KB, Seo DY, Lee HR. Combined effects of food and exercise on anaphylaxis. Nutr Res Pract. 2013;7:347–51.

37. Metelitsa A, Barankin B, Lin AN. Diagnosis of sports related dermatoses. Int J Dermatol. 2004;43:113–9.

38. Moehrle M. Outdoor sports and skin cancer. Clin Dermatol. 2008;26(1):12–5.

39. Mahé E, Beauchet A, de Paula CM, Godin-Beekmann S, Haeffelin M, Bruant S, Fay-Chatelard F, et al. Outdoor sports and risk of ultraviolet radiation-related skin lesions in children: evaluation of risks and prevention. Br J Dermatol. 2011;165(2):360–7.

40. Richtig E, Ambros-Rudolph CM, Trapp M, Lackner HK, Hofmann-Wellenhof R, Kerl H, Schwaberger G. Melanoma markers in marathon runners: increase with sun exposure and physical strain. Dermatology. 2008;217(1):38–44.

41. Ambros-Rudolph CM, Hofmann-Wellenhof R, Richtig E, Müller-Fürstner M, Soyer HP, Kerl H. Malignant melanoma in marathon runners. Arch Dermatol. 2006;142(11):1471–4.

42. Bakos RM, Wagner MB, Bakos L, De Rose EH, Granjeiro Neto JA. Queimaduras e hábitos solares em um grupo de atletas brasileiros. Rev Bras Med Esporte. 2006;12(5):275–8.

43. Jinna S, Adams BB. Ultraviolet radiation and the athlete: risk, sun safety, and barriers to implementation of protective strategies. Sports Med. 2013;43(7):531–7.

Dermatosis in Conflict Zones and Disaster Areas

51

Rosana Buffon

Key Points

- The increasing number of natural disasters and armed conflicts in recent decades carries a wide range of clinically relevant dermatoses
- Dermatologic care is presumably required when multiple medical and social problems arise shortly after the onset of an emergency
- About two-thirds of the total deaths in postconflict situations are caused by communicable diseases, some of them skin-related
- Poverty, malnutrition, displacement, poor infrastructure, and inadequate disaster preparedness efforts are the leading causes of communicable skin diseases among refugees
- In response to medical emergencies and disasters, teledermatology has been used to deliver dermatologic care in remote locations

Introduction

At a glance it seems nonsense to include a dermatologist among emergency doctors in a hotspot of a conflict zone or disaster area. It makes sense if in such conditions a dermatologist is called later for elective consultation or intervention. Dermatologic care is presumably required when multiple medical and social problems arise shortly after the onset of an emergency. For instance, a dermatologist's opinion is helpful in complex cases of war burns and outbreaks of measles and cutaneous leishmaniasis, and for specific diagnoses that are not easily detected and managed by emergency doctors (Table 51.1). Apart from a role as a specialist after an emergency, it is opportune to make dermatologists aware of potential risks and imminent skin damage secondary to natural disasters and armed

Table 51.1 Main dermatoses in conflict zones and disaster areas

Main dermatoses in conflict zones and disaster areas
Damage caused by low temperatures
Burns
Wounds
Vitamin deficiencies
Insect bites and other stings
Viral exanthems
Parasite and bacterial infections
Fungal infections
Sexually transmitted diseases
Aggravation of chronic skin diseases

R. Buffon
Dermatologist, Vicenza, Italy
e-mail: rosanabuffon@gmail.com

© Springer International Publishing Switzerland 2018
R.R. Bonamigo, S.I.T. Dornelles (eds.), *Dermatology in Public Health Environments*,
https://doi.org/10.1007/978-3-319-33919-1_51

conflicts, since such conditions are usually unpredictable or unplanned. Understanding the true burden of skin diseases in such situations is difficult as there are many political, logistical, and ethical barriers to conducting programs, surveillance, and research. In fact, the medical literature available for this topic is scarce. Available data are based on reports of nongovernmental organizations or philanthropic foundations, international organizations, volunteering fieldwork, and personal experiences.

By definition, a disaster is a disruption of a society resulting in widespread human, material, or environmental loss that exceeds the affected society's ability to cope by using local resources [1]. Disasters include earthquakes, volcanic eruptions, landslides, tsunamis, floods, and droughts. Populations in developing countries are disproportionately more affected because of poverty, lack of resources, poor infrastructure, and inadequate disaster preparedness efforts [2].

During recent decades, the scale of disasters has expanded owing to increased rates of urbanization, deforestation, and environmental degradation, as well as the intensification of climate variables such as higher temperatures, extreme precipitation, and more violent wind and water storms [3]. The 2004 Indian Ocean tsunami was among the deadliest natural disasters in human history, with at least 230,000 people killed or missing in 14 countries bordering the Indian Ocean [4]. The 2010 earthquake in Haiti killed around 225,000 people in a matter of minutes, destroyed health care facilities, and left many homeless [3]. Deaths associated with natural disasters, particularly rapid-onset disasters, are overwhelmingly due to blunt trauma, crush-related injuries, or drowning. Deaths from communicable diseases after natural disasters are less common [2].

In addition, tens of thousands of other people are dying in armed conflicts around the world, even as the number of conflicts falls, according to an authoritative study that attributes the rising death toll to an inexorable intensification of violence [5]. Sixty-three armed conflicts led to 56,000 fatalities in 2008, whereas 180,000 peo-

ple died in 42 conflicts in 2014. The numbers reflect the extremely violent fighting in Syria and Iraq and the increasing deaths in Afghanistan following the withdrawal of Western combat troops. The Israeli–Palestinian conflict killed 2500 people in 2015, mostly civilians, while fighting in Libya, Yemen, and the Central African Republic also contributed to the rise in overall deaths [5]. In such settings, health systems often collapse or become nonfunctional. Overcrowding, high population density in rudimentary shelters or camps, famine, inadequate safe water and sanitation, and poor vaccination status among victims increase the risk of infectious disease spread [6] and result in higher morbidity and mortality, especially among children.

In 2016, according to Médecins Sans Frontières (also known as Doctors Without Borders), skin diseases and burns are among the main pathologies observed in rescued persons in the Mediterranean Sea, most of them victims of the armed conflicts in Africa and the Middle East [7]. Millions of refugees are detained in reception centers for immigrants and asylum seekers, where physical conditions are extremely poor. In 2013–2014 more than 8% of patients' complaints were related to skin diseases [8]. Again, internal displaced persons (IDPs) who are resident in camps have increased vulnerability to skin infections, environment-associated disorders such as xerosis cutis and eczema, and diseases of psychosomatic origin [9]. Skin infections including scabies, along with acute respiratory tract infections and acute diarrhea, are the leading cause of morbidity [10].

Advances in small-arms technology and struggles over natural resources of international value (oil and rare minerals) make conflict resolution challenging. It is difficult to know whether the nature of conflicts has changed, but recent wars provide evidence of the targeting of health facilities to weaken opposition forces and populations. Refugees cross national borders and are legally entitled to assistance in United Nations (UN)-managed camps but, increasingly since the mid-1980s, people have been unable to cross international frontiers and so remain internally displaced. This population are often at higher risk for malnutrition and disease than residents or refugees [11].

State of the Art

Skin Injuries Related to Chemical Warfare

Blistering or vesicant agents are toxic compounds that produce skin injuries resembling those caused by burns [12]. With its characteristic garlic smell, sulfur mustard (SM) is the vesicant with the highest military significance since its use in World War I. Its last military use was in the Iran–Iraq war. SM injured more than 100,000 Iranians, one-third of whom are still suffering from lingering effects [13]. In modern times it remains a threat on the battlefield as well as a potential terrorist threat because of its simplicity of manufacture and extreme effectiveness [14].

Skin disorders are one of the major complications in SM exposure. The most common signs and symptoms are itching (78%), dry skin (60%), burning sensation (60%), blisters (25%), scarring (18%), dermatitis (13%), and pigmentary changes (hypo- or hyperpigmentation, 11%). Skin injury ranges from sunburn-like erythema to vesicles, which coalesce into blisters. Depending on the level of contamination, SM burns can vary between first- and second-degree burns, although they can also be every bit as severe, disfiguring, and dangerous as third-degree burns. Exposure to SM was lethal in about 1% of cases. Its effectiveness was as an incapacitating agent [13]. Other vesicants of lesser military importance include nitrogen mustard, Lewisite, and phosgene oxime, which are not discussed in detail here.

The use of poison gases, including SM, during warfare is known as chemical warfare, which was prohibited by the Geneva Protocol of 1925 and also by the later Chemical Weapons Convention of 1993. In September 2015 a United States official stated that the rebel militant group ISIS was manufacturing and using SM in Syria and Iraq, which was allegedly confirmed by their group's head of chemical weapons development, Sleiman Daoud al-Afari, who has since been captured [15].

War-Related Burn Injuries

War burns have been described for more than 5000 years of written history, and fire was probably utilized as a weapon long before. Burns and injuries from shrapnel fragments or small arms are the most common wounds to be expected in modern conventional armed conflicts [16]. The overall incidence of burns in current military operations has nearly doubled during the past few years. Unfortunately, civilians are becoming the major targets in modern-day conflicts, accounting for more than 80% of those killed and wounded in present-day conflicts. The provision of military burn care mirrors the civilian standards; however, several aspects of treatment of war-related burn injuries are peculiar to the war situation itself and to the specific conditions of each armed conflict [17].

The critical issue, however, is not the exact number of casualties, but whether the needs of the patients exceed the resources of the healthcare entity at the time they are required. If the facility, materiel, or personnel are hindered or destroyed, there may be insufficient surge capacity to manage the casualties [14]. War-related burn injuries, even among civilians, are unlikely to be the only trauma and are generally more extensive, deeper, more complicated, associated with inhalation injuries, and undertreated in comparison with the accidental burns in our everyday life. Nevertheless, burn injuries that were fatal just a few years ago no longer are, although even with rapid and proper response, burns are still complicated injuries that require lengthy therapy and treatment, particularly when they are complicated by other serious injuries. As the technology of weaponry advances, the number and severity of burn injuries will certainly increase [16].

Dermatology and Bioterrorism

A bioterrorism attack is the deliberate release of viruses, bacteria, or other germs (agents) used to cause illness or death in people, animals, or plants. These agents are typically found in nature, but it is possible that they could be changed to increase their ability to cause disease, make them resistant to current medicines, or increase their ability to be spread into the environment [18]. Biological agents are easy to develop as weapons, are more lethal than chemical weapons, and are less expensive and more difficult to detect than nuclear weapons [19]. The intentional dispersal of anthrax through the United States Postal Service that followed the terrorist attacks of September 11, 2001 brought these issues into clear focus. Five of the 11 victims (45%) of inhalational anthrax succumbed in the Amerithrax mailings of 2001 [20].

Anthrax and smallpox (*Variola* virus) are the most common skin disease agents with the potential of biologic terrorism. A study conducted by the World Health Organization (WHO) showed that Anthrax was somewhat unique in its ability to produce widespread mortality [21]. Smallpox was historically a significant cause of human suffering and death worldwide, responsible for as many as 50 million cases per year in the middle of the last century. The WHO declared smallpox to be eradicated in 1980 after a monumental worldwide vaccination campaign. Significant concern remains that existing laboratory-based *Variola* virus isolates could be reintroduced as a weapon to target an increasingly susceptible population. With an increasing immunologically naive population and the ease of global travel, there is concern that smallpox would spread faster than it has historically [14].

The consequences of using biological weapons are many. They can rapidly produce mass effect that overwhelms services and the healthcare system of communities. Most of the civilian population is susceptible to infections caused by these agents, which are associated with high morbidity and mortality rates. The resulting illness is usually difficult to diagnose and treat early, particularly in areas where the disease is rarely seen.

One kilogram of anthrax powder has the capability to kill up to 100,000 people depending on the mechanism of delivery [22].

Communicable Skin Diseases and Epidemics in Displaced Populations

Disasters and armed conflicts contribute to increased population displacements and densities in camps, creating new conditions for the spread of infectious diseases. In effect, about two-thirds of the total deaths in postconflict situations are caused by communicable diseases because of displacement, malnutrition, and limited access to basic needs [23–25]. In a study published by Salazar, communicable diseases were found to be the predominant syndrome group after three main natural disasters – a flood, an earthquake, and a typhoon – in the Philippines in 2013. Skin communicable diseases were at the top of most common syndromes found [26].

A communicable disease is defined as an illness that arises from transmission of an infectious agent or its toxic product from an infected person, animal, or reservoir to a susceptible host, either directly or indirectly through an intermediate plant or animal host, vector, or environment. An epidemic, or outbreak, occurs when there are more people suffering from a particular illness than would normally be expected. Children younger than 5 years of age (usually about 20% of the displaced population) and the elderly are at the highest risk of morbidity and mortality from infectious diseases, particularly the malnourished [25].

The availability of safe water and sanitation facilities, the degree of crowding, the underlying health status of the population, the size and characteristics of the population displaced, the nutritional status of the displaced population, the level of immunity to vaccine-preventable diseases such as measles, and the availability of healthcare services all interact within the context of the local disease ecology to influence the risk for communicable diseases and death in the affected population [2]. For instance, recurrent scabies outbreaks observed in many detention facilities are indicative of the substandard conditions, as the spread of the disease is directly linked to poor sanitary conditions [8]. Because developing countries may lack resources, infrastructure, and disaster-preparedness systems, they may be disproportionately affected by disasters.

A wide range of skin diseases may be observed according to different phases of a natural disaster. The impact phase occurs from 0 to 4 days, during which extrication of victims and treatment of immediate soft tissue infections takes place. Hypothermia, heat, illness, and dehydration are characteristic of this phase. In the postimpact phase, which takes place from 4 days to 4 weeks after the disaster, airborne, foodborne, waterborne, and vector diseases are seen. Examples of skin diseases in this phase are measles and varicella. The recovery phase begins after 4 weeks, and diseases with long incubation periods, vectorborne, and chronic diseases emerge. Leishmaniasis is an example of skin disease caused by organisms with long incubation periods [27].

Migrants often come from communities affected by war, conflict, or economic crisis and undertake long, exhausting journeys that increase their risks for communicable diseases, particularly measles, and food- and waterborne diseases. This is also true for vectorborne diseases in the Mediterranean area, such as leishmaniasis, with outbreaks recently reported in the Syrian Arab Republic [28].

The length of time that people spend in temporary settlements is an important determinant for the risk of disease transmission. The prolonged mass settlement of refugees in temporary shelters with only minimal provision for essential personal hygiene is typical of a situation that may cause epidemic outbreaks of infectious diseases. Camps established to provide food relief during famine are a special case, as large numbers of people who are already weak and possibly ill are likely to remain in such camps for a long time [29].

Measles Outbreaks

Measles is an important public health concern during disasters involving massive population displacements that end up living in camps.

The WHO recognizes refugees as one of the high-risk groups for measles outbreaks. Several outbreaks have been reported among refugees and in other emergency settings [30–32]. Overcrowding is associated with the transmission of higher infectious doses of measles virus, resulting in more severe cases of clinical disease, which makes measles more often the leading cause of mortality among children in refugee populations. Despite measles control strategies in refugee settings, case-fatality rates (CFR) as high as 34% have been reported. In contrast, measles CFR in stable populations are around 2% [33]. The risk of measles transmission after a natural disaster is also dependent on baseline immunization coverage among the affected population, and in particular among children under 15 years of age [2].

Historically, measles outbreaks have occurred among populations displaced in Africa and Asia where low routine vaccination coverage, even for the general population, has been reported. Almost all measles outbreaks occur in postconflict situations alongside collapse of the health system and disruption of the immunization program [33]. Several conflict-affected countries reportedly have measles coverage below 50%, and widespread outbreaks have been reported in Ethiopia, the Democratic Republic of Congo, and Afghanistan [25].

The highest incidence rate (25.5%) for a measles outbreak was described for Vietnamese children in Hong Kong camps where housing was cramped, consisting of large huts that housed approximately 250 refugees on three-tier bunk beds [34]. The only outbreak that occurred among those with a high coverage of 95% was the outbreak among the tsunami victims. It was suggested that the single-dose vaccination strategy might have been responsible for this outbreak [35].

Measles is an extremely serious disease in severely malnourished children. The age group from 5 to 15 years has been the most affected. Measles impairs the immune system for several months after infection, worsens vitamin A deficiency, and is a precipitating cause of xerophthalmia. In addition, measles often results in rapid and significant weight loss and can trigger cases of kwashiorkor. Severe complications of measles, such as pneumonia, are common in malnourished patients, and the case fatality rate can be as high as 30%. Vitamin A supplements together with measles vaccination have been recommended to minimize mortality [36–38].

Skin and Soft-Tissue Skin Infections

Wound infections are common after disasters. The destruction of the regional health infrastructure, the inability to wash wounds with clean water, and the inability to treat individuals with topical or systemic antimicrobial agents can all lead to severe wound infections, even if the initial trauma was relatively minor [14]. First responders are often not medically trained and, although well intentioned, the treatment they provide is often compromised by a misconception that wounds should be closed to enable them to heal [39]. In addition, damage to the local healthcare infrastructure can compromise the ability to properly treat contaminated wounds, resulting in severe, often polymicrobial, infections [40]. Sepsis with or without necrotizing fasciitis has being frequently seen following flood and tsunami wounds and has been associated with more than doubling of mortality [41]. Among survivors of the tsunami in Thailand in December 2004, traumatic wounds were contaminated with mud, sand, debris, and seawater and had an infection rate of 66.5%. Most wounds (45%) had polymicrobial infection with Gram-negative rods such as *Escherichia coli*, *Klebsiella pneumoniae*, *Proteus*, and *Pseudomonas* species. The risk of wound infection increased with size of the wound and presence of an open fracture [42].

Although considered a common and treatable problem in the Western world, impetigo patients are triaged as urgent in refugee camps and among internally displaced populations, especially if victims are malnourished (Fig. 51.1). Impetigo can progress rapidly from a minor skin infection to septicemia when micronutrient deficiencies and severe malnutrition exist [14]. In 2005, among hurricane Katrina evacuees from the New Orleans area, a cluster of infections with methicillin-resistant *Staphylococcus aureus*

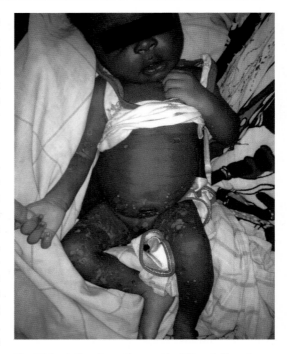

Fig. 51.1 A female newborn with diffuse bullous impetigo admitted to the inpatient department (IPD) of MSF clinic in Doro refugee camp, South Sudan, 2013

(MRSA) was reported in approximately 30 pediatric and adult patients at an evacuee facility in Dallas, Texas [43]. Wounds are at particular risk of becoming infected by MRSA because of conditions that are likely to occur after a natural disaster, such as close skin-to-skin contact with other individuals, use of contaminated items to treat wounds, lack of cleanliness, and crowded living conditions.

The refugee camps are considered the ideal condition for scabies infestation. Patients frequently present with scabies in the outpatient department, and a few "scabies outbreaks" have been reported in refugee populations. Although scabies-related mortality is very low, this is a common health problem among refugees [44].

Disaster-associated fungal infections are uncommon but they are becoming increasingly recognized, and are typically attributable to the impact phase of a disaster because such infections primarily result from inhalation or cutaneous inoculation of fungal spores directly from the environment [45]. Events affecting larger areas, such as earthquakes, tsunamis, and tornadoes, have been linked to the occurrence of fungal infections. Mucormycosis is perhaps the most recognized example of postdisaster fungal soft tissue infection. Necrotizing fasciitis can result, and case-fatality rates of ≈30% are frequently described, although early diagnosis and treatment has been shown to lead to better outcomes [46].

An unusual outbreak of coccidiomycosis occurred following the January 1994 southern California earthquake. The infection is not transmitted from person to person but is caused by the fungus *Coccidioides immitis*, which is found in the soil of certain semi-arid areas of North and South America. This outbreak was associated with exposure to increased levels of airborne dust subsequent to landslides in the aftermath of the earthquake [47].

Plague may become a problem for refugees or returnees in endemic areas because of overcrowding and poor hygienic conditions (if human fleas are playing a role), or when they settle in or enter into contact with areas of wild rodent infection. Cases of plague have been suspected in refugee populations in Malawi and Mozambique [48, 49].

Vector-Mediated Skin Diseases

Natural disasters, particularly meteorological events such as cyclones, hurricanes, and flooding, can affect vector breeding sites and vectorborne disease transmission. While initial flooding may wash away existing mosquito breeding sites, standing water caused by heavy rainfall or overflow of rivers can create new breeding sites. This can result in an increase of the vector population and potential for disease transmission, depending on the local mosquito vector species and its preferred habitat. The crowding of infected and susceptible hosts, a weakened public health infrastructure, and interruptions of ongoing control programs are all risk factors for vectorborne disease transmission [50]. Refugees living in crowded, temporary settings, currently numbering more than 50 million worldwide, are subject to explosive outbreaks of communicable disease of low endemicity, such as cutaneous leishmaniasis (CL) [27].

Leishmaniasis is a neglected tropical disease, endemic in many worldwide foci including the Middle East. Both cutaneous and visceral forms are reported from the region ranging from the Levant to Afghanistan. Several outbreaks have occurred in the Middle East over the past decades, mostly related to war-associated population migration. Refugees, armed forces, and multinational contractors are particularly at risk of acquiring the disease. With the start of the Syrian war, the frequency and magnitude of these outbreaks increased alarmingly [51]. In fact, the recent resurgence of CL in the southern and southeastern Anatolia region in Turkey is a result of the influx of immigrants from neighboring countries where CL incidence is higher. Because of the civil war in Syria, immigrants to this region in the last 3 years have begun to present more frequently with this disease [52].

The sudden increase in leishmaniasis cases in Lebanon in 2013 is also attributed to the increasing numbers and wide distribution of Syrian refugees in Lebanon [51]. There has been an upsurge in leishmaniasis research, especially as new foci are exposed and the need to protect the naive populations moving into endemic areas becomes a public health priority [53].

Malnutrition and Vitamin Deficiencies

Commonly, economic crises and political insecurity (especially war) create and aggravate food insecurity. During these situations, populations try to cope with damaged infrastructure, and looted crops and homes. In conflict situations, individuals or groups may aim to have control over food (of others) in order to manipulate civil populations and feed the militia. This results in a reduction of food availability and accessibility, and an increase in population movements. Armed conflicts can also significantly deteriorate the baseline nutritional status of children and their families; more serious and devastating effects are seen when the conflict persists over time. Natural disasters are rarely the only cause of food insecurity, which can be prompted by a gradual deterioration of food access caused by prolonged or repeated droughts, flooding, large livestock epidemics, and/or economic crisis. As food insecurity progresses to famine there is an increased prevalence of malnutrition, resulting in increased mortality [38]. The analysis of data collected in 42 camps in Asia and Africa indicates a clear association between the prevalence of malnutrition and high mortality rates in refugee camps in the emergency phase [54]. Protein-energy malnutrition (PEM) is known to be a major contributory cause of death in refugee populations, mostly because malnutrition increases vulnerability to diseases and thus its severity, especially in regard to measles [54, 55].

The term PEM applies to a group of related disorders that include marasmus, kwashiorkor, and intermediate states of marasmus-kwashiorkor. The most evident clinical feature in marasmus is severe wasting with loss of muscle and fat mass. Patients are extremely emaciated with thin, flaccid skin and prominent scapulae, spine, and ribs. Loss of facial fat results in the characteristic elderly appearance of affected children. Clinical features in kwashiorkor include bilateral pitting edema of the lower legs and feet; generalized edema in advanced cases (face, hands, arms, trunk); loss of muscle and fat mass (which can be masked by edema); skin lesions (atrophy, patches of erythema, hypo- or hyperpigmentation, desquamation, exudative lesions that resemble burns, fragile skin prone to ulceration and infection); and changes in hair color (lightening or becoming reddish) and texture (dry, thin, brittle, sparse hair that can be pulled out easily and without pain) [56] (Figs. 51.2 and 51.3).

In addition to PEM, micronutrient deficiencies play a key role in nutrition-related morbidity and mortality [54, 55]. Many scurvy outbreaks have occurred in displaced and famine-affected populations, primarily because of inadequate vitamin C in rations. Fortification of foods with vitamin C is problematic because vitamin C cannot be stored in the body. The best solution is to provide vitamin C through a variety of fresh foods, either by including them in the general ration or by promoting access to local markets [44]. Scurvy outbreaks are likely to occur in arid areas, especially during the dry season, when

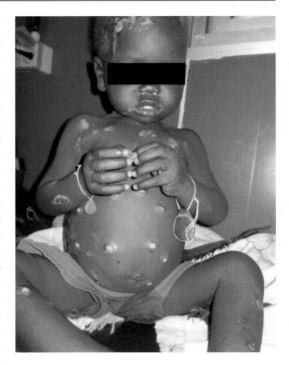

Fig. 51.2 A malnourished boy admitted to the IPD because of exudative skin lesions related to the malnutrition condition. MSF clinic in Doro refugee camp, South Sudan, 2013

refugees have been settled for a few months and have only limited access to fresh fruits, vegetables, or milk on the local market [57, 58].

Pellagra (deficiency in niacin or vitamin B3) is endemic where people eat a maize-based diet with little protein-rich food. Pellagra outbreaks can occur in refugee and displaced populations dependent on food rations based on maize and containing insufficient quantities of groundnuts [59]. A large-scale pellagra outbreak occurred among Mozambican refugees in Malawi (1989 and 1990) [60, 61], and pellagra cases have been reported in several refugee camps (Zimbabwe, Angola, and Nepal in 1993) [62]. Outbreaks of other vitamin B deficiencies have been documented in refugee populations: vitamin B2 in Afghanistan in 1994, and vitamin B5 (nutritional neuropathy) in Afghanistan in 1993 [59]. As these deficiencies are often found in association, the clinical picture may cover a large spectrum of signs: neuropathy with burning feet syndrome, glossitis, conjunctivitis, and angular stomatitis, among others. However, one of these symptoms

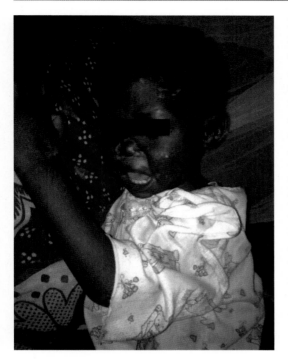

Fig. 51.3 A severely malnourished girl with kwashiorkor admitted to the intensive therapeutic food center for nutritional therapy. Generalized edema and secondary bacterial skin infection are seen. MSF clinic in Doro refugee camp, South Sudan, 2013

will generally be dominant. These outbreaks are probably underreported because the symptoms are nonspecific and may be masked by other deficiencies, or the clinical signs are assumed to be due to other causes. The main recommendation in regard to these deficiencies is to be aware that a sudden increase in the number of cases of stomatitis, conjunctivitis, glossitis, burning feet syndrome, and other signs of neuropathy could be linked to vitamin B deficiencies [59].

Future Perspectives

The front-line field operators in emergency situations are usually volunteers, working for a range of different international nongovernmental organizations, and local health professionals, who frequently have diverse competencies, experience, and background. For instance, at the same emergency operation, European and American doctors share routine tasks with Asian and African ones.

In remote areas, the lack of medical human resources besides the lack of coordination with experts and reference centers make the medical assistance challenging. The nonadoption of standard guidelines and training can aggravate the mishandling of clinical cases. Furthermore, the quality of medical care delivered by international organizations is heterogeneous, even in the same country or population. Humanitarian actors should work closely by using standardized clinical guidelines, mostly focused in nutrition support, public health surveillance, immunization, communicable disease control, epidemic management, and maternal and child healthcare. Such skills are specific to emergencies and are not necessarily acquired in the average medical or nursing school. Once those requirements are achieved, most probably the management of particular conditions such as skin diseases in the field could be ameliorated through specific training and experience sharing. Nevertheless, humanitarian actors need to function effectively in different cultural contexts and, often, in hostile and dangerous environments.

Considering that geographic and political barriers still challenge the access of humanitarian health workers in the field, it is opportune to develop and access alternative tools of communication and technology, such as telemedicine. In response to medical emergencies and disasters, telemedicine has been used to deliver medical care in remote locations. Medical doctors from all over the world can be connected to share knowledge and personal experience, so that an African doctor can contribute by sharing his experiences in managing malnutrition; in turn, a European doctor can provide information on treating severe burns. In areas with no access to dermatologic care because of distance or simple manpower, teledermatology seems like an ideal solution to reach the underserved. However, many factors such as cost, lack of access to modern communication, and underdeveloped infrastructure serve as major obstacles to its widespread use.

The role of teledermatology in emergency care has been sustained by the action of private and nonprofit initiatives that assist poor, sick, and disabled people in the developing world through consultation services, allowing for the provision of access to expert medical advice from consultants around the world to disaster and postconflict areas, including Afghanistan, Iraq, and Nepal. Services are provided in many specialty areas including dermatology, with high-resolution digital cameras and tripods, and training of the local medical staff in the proper use of the equipment, allowing remote hospitals in developing countries to receive assistance free of charge [63]. Natural and man-made disasters both require near-term and long-term interventions to reduce morbidity and mortality among the surviving victims. Information technology and modern portable communication devices should be incorporated in disaster preparedness and recovery training and operations [64]. Future efforts need to focus on expanding the outreach of these existing humanitarian teledermatology networks, and there is a need to invest in inexpensive technology and strategies to sustain programs in developing countries and remote areas that suffer from a high burden of disease with limited resources.

According to the international experience of providing dermatologic services and taking into account that natural disasters and armed conflicts are a global issue, it is reasonable to establish an international coordination center of emergency dermatology, which will unite representatives of national dermatologic societies and other public organizations and nonprofit foundations. The aims are to provide emergency and routine advisory dermatologic care to the affected populations in disaster and conflict areas, to ensure the appropriate care in specialized medical institutions with evacuation of patients when indicated, to encourage interdisciplinary cooperation, and to establish an efficient use of the medical and human resources available.

Glossary

Airborne   Transported by air.
Case-fatality rates (CFR)   A measure of the severity of a disease, defined as the proportion of reported cases of a specified disease or condition which are fatal within a specified time.
Foodborne   (Of a disease) carried by or transmitted through contaminated food.
Glossitis   Inflammation of the tongue. Glossitis is often caused by nutritional deficiencies and may be painless or cause discomfort
Médecins Sans Frontières (MSF) or Doctors Without Borders   An international, independent, medical humanitarian organization that delivers emergency aid to people affected by armed conflict, epidemics, natural disasters, and exclusion from healthcare.
Vectorborne   (Of a disease) transmitted by the bite of infected arthropod species, such as mosquitoes, ticks, triatomine bugs, sandflies, and blackflies.
Waterborne   (Of a disease) transported or transmitted by water.
Xerophthalmia   Abnormal dryness and thickening of the conjunctiva and cornea caused by vitamin A deficiency

References

1. WHO. Definitions: emergencies. WHO.int. Available from: http://who.int/hac/about/definitions/en/index.html. Accessed 25 July 2016.
2. Watson J, Gayer M, Connolly M. Epidemics after natural disasters. Emerg Infect Dis. 2007;13(1):1–5.
3. Leaning J, Guha-Sapir D. Natural disasters, armed conflict, and public health. NEJM. 2013;369(19):1836–42.
4. Wikipedia. 2004 Indian Ocean earthquake and tsunami. Wikipedia 2016. Available from: https://en.wikipedia.org/wiki/2004_Indian_Ocean_earthquake_and_tsunami. Accessed 25 July 2016.
5. Nigel Inkster CMG. Armed conflict survey 2015 Press Statement. IISS.org. Available from: https://www.iiss.org/en/about%20us/press%20room/press%20releases/press%20releases/archive/2015-4fe9/may-6219/armed-conflict-survey-2015-press-statement-a0be. Accessed 20 July 2016.
6. Gayer M, Legros D, Formenty P, Connolly M. Conflict and emerging infectious diseases. Emerg Infect Dis. 2007;13(11):1625–31.
7. Médecins Sans Frontières (MSF). EU migration crisis update. MSF International; June 2016. Available from: http://www.msf.org/en/article/20160617-eu-migration-crisis-update-june-2016. Accessed 25 July 2016.
8. Médecins Sans Frontières (MSF). Invisible suffering: prolonged and systematic detention of migrants and asylum seekers in substandard conditions in Greece. MSF; April 2014. Available from: www.msf.org/sites/msf.org/files/invisible_suffering.pdf. Accessed 25 July 2016.
9. Elfaituri S. Skin diseases among internally displaced Tawerghans living in camps in Benghazi, Libya. Int J Dermatol. 2015;:n/a-n/a.

10. WHO. Iraq (EWARN) Early warning and disease surveillance bulletins. WHO.int. Available from: http://www.who.int/hac/crises/irq/sitreps/erwan/en/. Accessed 25 July 2016.

11. Feikin DR, Adazu K, Obor D, et al. Mortality and health among internally displaced persons in western Kenya following post-election violence, 2008: novel use of demographic surveillance. Bull World Health Organ. 2010;88:601–8.

12. Ganesan K, Raza SK, Vijayaraghavan R. Chemical warfare agents. J Pharm Bioallied Sci. 2010;2(3):166–78.

13. Namazi S, Niknahad H, Razmkhah H. Long-term complications of sulphur mustard poisoning in intoxicated Iranian veterans. J Med Toxicol. 2009;5(4):191–5.

14. Koenig K, Schultz C. Koenig and Schultz's disaster medicine: comprehensive principles and practices. Cambridge: Cambridge University Press; 2010.

15. Wikipedia. Sulfur mustard. Wikipedia 2016. Available from: http://en.wikipedia.org/wiki/Sulfur_mustard. Accessed 25 July 2016.

16. Atiyeh BS, Gunn SWA, Hayek SN. Military and civilian burn injuries during armed conflicts. Ann Burns Fire Disasters. 2007;20(4):203–15.

17. Atiyeh B, Hayek S. Management of war-related burn injuries. J Craniofacial Surg. 2010;21(5):1529–37.

18. CDC. Bioterrorism overview. Emergency.cdc.gov. 2016. Available from: http://emergency.cdc.gov/bioterrorism/overview.asp. Accessed 25 July 2016.

19. Flanagin A, Lederberg J. Biological warfare (themed issue). JAMA. 1997;278:351–72.

20. Wikipedia. 2001 anthrax attacks. Wikipedia. 2016. Available from: https://en.wikipedia.org/wiki/2001_anthrax_attacks. Accessed 25 July 2016.

21. Health aspects of chemical and biological weapons. Geneva: report of a WHO group of consultants; 1970

22. Danzig R, Berkowsky PB. Why should we be concerned about biological weapons. JAMA. 1997;278:431–2.

23. Noji EK, Toole MJ. The historical development of public health response to disasters. Disasters. 1997;21(Suppl 4):366–76.

24. Watson TJ, Gayer M, Connolly AM. Epidemic after natural disasters. Emerg Infect Dis. 2007;13(Suppl 1):1–5.

25. International Federal of Red Cross and Red Crescent Societies. Control of communicable diseases. ICRC. The Johns Hopkins and Red Cross Red Crescent: Public Health Guide in Emergencies. 2nd edition. Geneva: International Federal of Red Cross and Red Crescent Societies; 2008. Available from: http://www.jhsph.edu/research/centers-and-institutes/center-for-refugee-and-disaster-response/publications_tools/publications/_CRDR_ICRC_Public_Health_Guide_Book/Pages_from_Chapter_7_.pdf. Accessed 26 July 2016.

26. Salazar MA, Pesigan A, Law R, Winkler V. Post-disaster health impact of natural hazards in the Philippines in 2013. Glob Health Action. 2016;9:31320. Available from: http://dx.doi.org/10.3402/gha.v9.31320. Accessed 26 July 2016.

27. Lemonick D. Epidemics after natural disasters. Am J Clin Med. Fall. 2011;8(3). Available from: http://www.aapsus.org/wp-content/uploads/ajcmsix.pdf. Accessed 26 July 2016.

28. WHO. Migration and health: key issues. WHO int. Available from: http://www.euro.who.int/en/health-topics/health-determinants/migration-and-health/migrant-health-in-the-european-region/migration-and-health-key-issues#292115. Accessed 26 July 2016.

29. WHO. A field manual – communicable disease control in emergencies. Who.int. Available from: http://www.who.int/diseasecontrol_emergencies/publications/9241546166/en/. Accessed 26 July 2016.

30. Porter JD, Gastellu-Etchegorry M, Navarre I, Lungu G, Moren A. Measles outbreaks in the Mozambican refugee camps in Malawi: the continued need for an effective vaccine. Int J Epidemiol. 1990;19(Suppl 4):1072–7.

31. Taylor WR. Measles in Vietnamese refugee children in Hong Kong. Epidemiol Infect. 1999;122(Suppl 3):441–6.

32. Toole MJ, Waldman RJ. An analysis of mortality trends among refugee population in Somalia, Sudan and Thailand. Bull World Health Organ. 1988;66:237–47.

33. Kouadio IK, Kamigaki T, Oshitani H. Measles outbreaks in displaced populations: a review of transmission, morbidity associated factors. BMC Int Health Hum Rights [Online]. 2010;10:5. Available from: doi: 10.1186/1472-698X-10-5. Accessed 27 July 2016.

34. Feldstein B, Weiss R. Cambodian disaster relief: refugee camp medical care. Am J Public Health. 1982;72(Suppl 6):589–94.

35. Mohan A, Murhekar MV, Wairgkar NS, Hutin YJ, Gupte MD. Measles transmission following the tsunami in a population with high one-dose vaccination coverage, Tamil Nadu, India 2004-2005. BMC Infect Dis. 2006;6:143.

36. Guha-Sapir D, van Panhuis WG, Degomme O, Teran V. Civil conflicts in four African countries: a five-year review of trends in nutrition and mortality. Epidemiol Rev. 2005;27:67–77.

37. Huiming Y, Chaomin W, Meng M. Vitamin A for treating measles in children. Evid-Based Child Health. 2006;1:743–66.

38. Médecins Sans Frontières. Nutritional guidelines. Paris: MSF; 1995. Available from: http://www.unhcr.org/publications/operations/3c4d391a4/nutritional-guidelines-msf.html. Accessed 27 July 2016.

39. Prasartritha T, Tungsiripat R, Warachit P. The revisit of 2004 tsunami in Thailand: characteristics of wounds. Int Wound J. 2008;5:8–19.

40. Ivers LC, Ryan ET. Infectious diseases of severe weather-related and flood-related natural disasters. Curr Opin Infect Dis. 2006;19:408–14.

41. Wuthisuthimethawee P, Lindquist S, Sandler N, Clavisi O, Korin S, Watters D, et al. Wound management in disaster settings. World J Surg. 2015;39(4):842–53.

42. Doung-ngern P, Vatanaprasan T, Chungpaibulpatana J, Sitamanoch W, et al. Infections and treatment of wounds in survivors of the 2004 Tsunami in Thailand. Int Wound J. 2009;6(5):347–54.

43. CDC. Infectious disease and dermatologic conditions in evacuees and rescue workers after Hurricane Katrina – multiple states, August-September, 2005. CDC MMWR. 2005;54(38):961–4.

44. USAID. Field operations guide for disaster assessment and response. Version 4.0 USA: USAID Bureau for Democracy, Conflict, and Humanitarian Assistance Office of U.S. Foreign Disaster Assistance; 2005. Available from: https://www.usaid.gov/sites/default/files/documents/1866/fog_v4_0.pdf. Accessed 27 July 2016.

45. Benedict K, Park BJ. Invasive fungal infections after natural disasters. Emerg Infect Dis. 2014;20(3):349–55.

46. Chamilos G, Lewis RE, Kontoyiannis DP. Delaying amphotericin B-based frontline therapy significantly increases mortality among patients with hematologic malignancy who have zygomycosis. Clin Infect Dis. 2008;47:503–9.

47. WHO. Communicable diseases following natural disasters – risk assessment and priority interventions. Geneva: WHO; 2006. Available from: http://www.who.int/diseasecontrol_emergencies/guidelines/CD_Disasters_26_06.pdf. Accessed 27 July 2016.

48. Bertoletti G. Bubonic plague outbreak in the refugee camp of Mankhokwe, Malawi. Med News. 1995;4(2):21–3.

49. Matthys F. Plague epidemic in Mutarara district, Mozambique. Med News. 1995;4(2):14–20.

50. WHO. Communicable diseases and severe food shortage situations. Geneva: WHO Communicable Diseases Working Group on Emergencies; 2005. Available from: http://www.who.int/diseasecontrol_emergencies/guidelines/CD_Disasters_26_06.pdf. Accessed 27 July 2016.

51. Alawieh A, Musharrafieh U, Jaber A, Berry A, Ghosn N, Bizri A. Revisiting leishmaniasis in the time of war: the Syrian conflict and the Lebanese outbreak. Int J Infect Dis. 2014;29:115–9.

52. Inci R, Ozturk P, Mulayim MK, Ozyurt K, Alatas ET, Inci MF. Effect of the Syrian civil war on prevalence of cutaneous leishmaniasis in Southeastern Anatolia, Turkey. Med Sci Monit: Int Med J Exp Clin Res. 2015;21:2100–4. Available from: doi:10.12659/MSM.893977. Accessed 27 July 2016.

53. Jacobson R. Leishmaniasis in an era of conflict in the Middle East. Vector-Borne Zoonotic Dis. 2011;11(3):247–58.

54. Toole MJ, Nieburg P, Waldman RJ. The association between inadequate rations, undernutrition prevalence, and mortality in refugee camps: case studies of refugee populations in Eastern Thailand, 1979–1980 and Eastern Sudan, 1984–1985. J Trop Pediatr. 1988;24:218–23.

55. CDC. Famine-affected, refugee, and displaced populations: recommendations for public health issues. MMWR Recomm Rep. 1992 Jul 24;41(RR-13):1–76.

56. Médecins Sans Frontières. Nutrition guidelines. 2nd. Paris: MSF; 2006. Available from: https://www.medbox.org/nutrition-guidelines/download.pdf. Accessed 27 July 2016.

57. WHO. Nutrition – scurvy and food aid among refugees in the Horn of Africa. Wkly Epidemiol Rec. 1989;64(12):85–92.

58. Desenclos JC, Berry AM, Padt R, Farah B, Segala C, Nabil AM. Epidemiological patterns of scurvy among Ethiopian refugees. WHO Bull. 1989;67(3):309–16.

59. Médecins Sans Frontières. Refugee health – an approach to emergency situations. London: Macmillan; 1997. Available from: http://refbooks.msf.org/msf_docs/en/refugee_health/rh.pdf. Accessed 27 July 2016.

60. Malfait P, Moren A, Malenga G, Stuckey J, Jonkman A, Etchegorry M. Outbreak of pellagra among Mozambican refugees, Malawi 1990. MMWR. 1991;40(13):209–13.

61. Malfait P, Moren A, Dillon JC, Brodel A, et al. An outbreak of pellagra related to changes in dietary niacin among Mozambican refugees in Malawi. Int J Epidemiol. 1993 Jun;22(3):504–11.

62. Toole MJ. Preventing micronutrient deficiency diseases. Workshop on the improvement of the nutrition of refugees and displaced people in Africa, Machakos, Kenya, Kenya; 1994.

63. The Swinfen Charitable Trust. Available from: http://www.humanitariantelemed.org. Accessed 27 July 2016.

64. Nicogossian AE, Doarn CR. Armenia 1988 earthquake and telemedicine: lessons learned and forgotten. Telemed J E Health. 2011;17:741–5.

Suggested Literature

CDC. Centers for Disease Control and Prevention. Emergency preparedness and response. Available from: https://emergency.cdc.gov/.

Council on Foreign Relations. Global conflict tracker. Available from: www.cfr.org/globalconflicttracker.

EM-DAT. The international disaster database. Centre for Research on the Epidemiology of Disasters – CRED. Available from:http://www.emdat.be/database.

ICRC. The International Red Cross and Red Crescent Movement. Available from: https://www.icrc.org/.

IISS. International Institute for Strategic Studies. Available from: https://www.iiss.org/.

MSF. Médecins Sans Frontières. Available from: http://www.msf.org/.

WHO. World Health Organization. Refugees. Available from: http://www.who.int/topics/refugees/en/.

WHO. World Health Organization. Maternal, newborn, child and adolescent health. Available from: http://www.who.int/maternal_child_adolescent/topics/child/malnutrition/en/.

Vaccines and the Prevention of Dermatologic Diseases

52

Giancarlo Bessa

Key Points

- The impact of vaccines in the control of various infectious diseases is a very relevant topic in public health
- The HPV vaccines are most effective when administered before the onset of sexual activity
- A major obstacle to widespread use of zoster vaccine is the high cost
- Despite its variable protective efficacy, BCG is the best available vaccine for the prevention of leprosy

Introduction

Immunization is the process of inducing immunity through the administration of antigens or antibodies. Active immunization is the situation whereby a person is stimulated to produce antibodies by antigen administration. Sometimes the protection achieved is permanent and occasionally is partial, requiring reinforcements. Passive immunization corresponds to the administration of exogenously produced antibodies for temporary protection [1]. Classification of vaccines according to their composition is provided in Table 52.1.

Table 52.1 Classification of vaccines according to their composition [1]

Toxoid vaccine	Composed by a bacterial toxin modified to become nontoxic while retaining the ability to stimulate antibody formation
Attenuated vaccine	Vaccine that includes live bacteria or viruses that have lost virulence after growing under adverse conditions, but retain the ability to replicate and produce immunity without causing disease
Inactivated vaccine	Vaccine that contains killed bacteria or viruses, which are inactivated by chemical or physical procedures. This type of vaccine generally requires multiple doses for primary immunization and posterior booster doses to maintain adequate serum concentrations of antibodies
Subunit vaccines	The infectious organism is processed to purify those components to be included in the vaccine. These vaccines are categorized in three groups: protein-based, polysaccharide, and conjugate vaccines
Combined vaccines	Vaccines that comprise different antigens from several infectious agents in the same presentation, applied in a single administration. The necessary condition for combined vaccines is the preservation of the efficacy of the various components without increasing adverse reactions

Vaccination is considered the most efficient and cost-effective strategy to prevent infectious

G. Bessa
University Hospital, Luteran University of Brazil, ULBRA, Canoas, Brazil
e-mail: giancarlobessa@gmail.com

© Springer International Publishing Switzerland 2018
R.R. Bonamigo, S.I.T. Dornelles (eds.), *Dermatology in Public Health Environments*,
https://doi.org/10.1007/978-3-319-33919-1_52

diseases [2]. The impact of vaccines in the control of various infectious diseases is a very relevant topic in public health. Mass vaccination campaigns promoted in the past century led to drastic reductions in the incidence or even eradication of major childhood infectious diseases including smallpox, polio, tetanus, diphtheria, pertussis, measles, rubella, mumps, and *Haemophilus influenzae* type b–related diseases [3]. Although they are fundamental in childhood, specific vaccination schedules also exist for adolescents, adults, the elderly, and select groups such as immunocompromised persons, health professionals, and travelers.

Available vaccines are generally well tolerated. Some precautions are necessary in conditions that can increase the risk of adverse reactions or compromise the ability of the vaccine to produce immunity. Common precautions are moderate to severe acute illness, mild or moderate allergies to vaccine components, pregnancy, anticoagulation, and immunosuppression. Previous anaphylactic reaction to a vaccine is a contraindication for application of subsequent doses of the product [4]. Vaccines with live components generally should not be given to pregnant women and immunocompromised individuals. The use of immunosuppressants, corticosteroids at high doses, immunoglobulins, and blood products is a temporary contraindication to the application of certain live attenuated vaccines. Anticoagulated individuals should avoid intramuscular administration. Subcutaneous or intradermal routes may be used if previously authorized by the manufacturer [1, 4]. Antipyretics such as acetaminophen reduce the incidence of vaccine-related febrile reactions, although they should not be routinely used because they can reduce the antigenic response [5].

State of the Art

Routine vaccination schedules can protect the population from infectious diseases both individually and through induction of herd immunity. Herd immunity refers to indirect immunity, when the vaccination of a portion of the population

(the "herd") provides protection to unvaccinated individuals, through the theory that the chain of infection is interrupted when large numbers of the population are immune. Herd immunity requires vaccination rates to be high [3].

The World Health Organization (WHO) periodically reviews the medical literature on immunizations and publishes Position Papers providing global vaccine and immunization recommendations for diseases that have an international public health impact [6]. These recommendations are designed for immunization managers worldwide and are summarized in tables (Table 52.2). The WHO emphasizes that the recommendations are not intended for direct use by health workers; rather, their purpose is to aid technical decisions with respect to national vaccination schedules.

Vaccines are available for prevention of various infectious diseases. This chapter focuses on discussing the vaccines of dermatologic interest.

Vaccines Against HPV

The family of human papillomavirus (HPV) comprises more than 200 genotypes, approximately 40 of which can induce infections in the anogenital area [57]. Visible anogenital warts (condylomata acuminata) are commonly induced by HPV-6, -11, -42, -44, -51, -55, and -69 strains. Subtypes HPV-16, -18, -31, -33, -35, -39, -45, -51, -52, -56, -58, -59, -66, and -68 are known for the potential of inducing malignant lesions, notably invasive cervical carcinomas in women. Mixed infections (presence of more than one oncogenic HPV genotype within a lesion), are not uncommon [57, 58].

Most HPV infections are asymptomatic and clear up within a few years [59]. Persistence of infection by an oncogenic HPV subtype in female genital tract was associated with higher risk of invasive cervical cancer [60].

The reason for failure of the immune system in otherwise healthy individuals to clear HPV infections for months or years remains incompletely understood. Some possible mechanisms are poor antigen presentation and effector

Table 52.2 WHO recommended routine immunizations for all immunization programs [7]

Vaccine	Children	Adolescents	Adults
BCG	One dose		
Hepatitis B	Three to four doses	Three doses (for high-risk groups if not previously immunized)	
Polio	Three to four doses (at least one dose of IPV) with DTP		
DTP	Three doses		
	Booster (DTP) 1–6 years of age	Booster (Td)	Booster (Td) in early adulthood or pregnancy
Haemophilus influenzae type b	Three doses, with DTP		
	OR		
	Two or three doses, with booster at least 6 months after last dose		
Pneumococcal (conjugate)	Three doses, with DTP		
	OR		
	Two doses before 6 months of age, plus booster dose at 9–15 months of age		
Rotavirus	Rotarix: two doses with DTP		
	RotaTeq: three doses with DTP		
Measles	Two doses		
Rubella	One dose	One dose (adolescent girls and/or child bearing aged women if not previously vaccinated)	
HPV		Two doses (females)	

Adapted from: WHO recommendations for routine immunization – summary tables. Available from: http://www.who.int/immunization/policy/immunization_tables/en

response, or virally induced local immunosuppression resulting in the development of tolerance [61].

The HPV vaccination rationale is to avoid genital infections and its associated morbidity. HPV is implicated in virtually all invasive cervical cancers (and precancerous lesions) and genital warts [62]. Although screening programs have significantly reduced the incidence of cervical cancer, it remains a considerable public health burden [59]. HPV infection is also the cause of a proportion of cancers of the anus, the oropharynx, the vulva and vagina, and of the penis, although the incidence rates for these cancers are much lower than for cervical cancer [64]. The prevalence of HPV infection is higher among teenagers and in the early twenties, decreasing with advancing age [63].

The WHO position paper [10] recommends that HPV vaccines should be included in national immunization programs if prevention of cervical cancer and other HPV-related diseases constitutes a local public health priority and vaccine introduction is feasible, considering sustained financing and cost-effectiveness. The priority target group for HPV vaccination is girls aged 9–13 years, prior to becoming sexually active, because HPV vaccines are most efficacious in those who have not previously been exposed to the virus. There is no specific recommendation for any formulation of the vaccine. The document also highlights the need for a comprehensive strategy that should include education about reducing risky sexual behaviors, training of health workers, and maintenance or improvement of programs of screening, diagnosis, and treatment of precancerous lesions and cancer.

Formulations

Three prophylactic vaccines are currently available: a bivalent vaccine that targets HPV types 16 and 18; a quadrivalent vaccine that targets HPV types 6, 11, 16, and 18; and more recently a 9-valent vaccine that targets HPV types 6, 11, 16, 18, 31, 33, 45, 52, and 58. The three vaccines were developed using recombinant technology and are prepared from purified L1 structural proteins. Neither of these vaccines contains live biological products or viral DNA, and are therefore noninfectious. They are administered as an intramuscular injection [65].

Schedules

The HPV vaccines are most effective when administered before the onset of sexual activity, i.e., before first exposure to HPV infection. However, sexually active individuals can be vaccinated according to recommendations based on age. The USA Advisory Committee on Immunization Practices (ACIP) recommends routine HPV vaccination (bivalent, quadrivalent, or 9-valent) for women at 11 or 12 years old, and for those aged 13–26 years who have not been previously vaccinated [2]. ACIP also recommends routine use of quadrivalent or 9-valent HPV vaccine for men at 11 or 12 years old and those aged 13–21 years if they have not yet been vaccinated. Men who have sex with men (MSM) and those immunocompromised, in particular, could benefit from vaccination to prevent condyloma and anal cancer [66, 67]. This is why ACIP recommends routine vaccination for this group through age 26 (if not previously vaccinated). Other men aged 22–26 years can be vaccinated but are not considered to be a priority for inclusion in routine vaccination schedules [20].

The WHO suggests that vaccination strategies should initially prioritize high coverage in the WHO-recommended primary target population of young females of 9 through 13 years of age. Vaccination of other populations is recommended only if this is feasible, affordable, and cost effective, and does not divert resources from vaccinating the primary target population or from cervical cancer screening programs [10].

HPV vaccines were originally licensed and marketed using a three-dose immunization schedule. The second dose can be administered in 1–2 months after the first, and the third dose is administered 6 months after the first (at least 24 weeks after first dose) [20]. A systematic review of quadrivalent and bivalent vaccines indicated that a two-dose (0 and 6 months) schedule in girls aged 9–14 years were noninferior to the three-dose schedule in terms of immunogenicity [29]. Based on this the WHO recommends administration of quadrivalent HPV vaccine for girls and boys aged 9–13 years according to the two-dose schedule, and the same for bivalent HPV vaccine for girls aged 9–14 years. The nonavalent (9-valent) vaccine was not considered in the current WHO position paper (2014) because it was under regulatory assessment at that time [10].

Pre- or postvaccination serology or HPV DNA testing are not recommended because prevaccinal serostatus is not a criterion for HPV vaccine candidacy, and there is no evidence that the measurement of postvaccination antibody titers is useful for determining immunity [73].

Clinical Evidence

Quadrivalent vaccine efficacy was assessed in two large randomized trials that enrolled more than 17,000 young women [68, 69]. In the major study, the efficacy of the vaccine for preventing the composite outcome of cervical intraepithelial neoplasia grade 2 or 3, adenocarcinoma in situ, and invasive carcinoma of the cervix due to HPV types included in the vaccine, among HPV-naive women, was 97–100%. In the overall population of study participants (intention-to-treat analysis), the efficacy of the vaccine was significantly lower (approximately 44%), which was associated with the fact that the most of subjects were sexually active and many had previous contact with vaccine HPV types [68]. In the other study, the efficacy for preventing external anogenital and vaginal lesions due to vaccine-type HPV, among HPV-naive women, was 100%. In the intention-to-treat analysis, the efficacy was 73% for HPV types included in the vaccine and 34% for lesions associated with any HPV type [69].

Quadrivalent vaccine efficacy was also evaluated in a trial of 4065 men aged 16–26 years (3463 heterosexual and 602 MSM with ≤5 sexual partners) [66]. Among HPV-naive males, the efficacy for preventing incidence of external genital lesions (primary endpoint) due to HPV types included in the vaccine was 90%. Efficacy against persistence of HPV infection (secondary endpoint) was 86%. In the overall population of study participants (intention-to-treat analysis), the efficacy was 66% for preventing external genital lesions and 48% for preventing persistent HPV infection. The efficacy of the HPV quadrivalent vaccine in preventing anal intraepithelial neoplasia secondary to vaccine-types HPV was assessed in the subpopulation of 602 MSM of the study [67]. The vaccine efficacy for this group was 78% among HPV-naive men and 50% in the overall MSM population.

Bivalent vaccine efficacy was assessed in two large randomized trials [70, 76]. The major study enrolled more than 18,000 women aged 15–25 years [70]. The efficacy of the vaccine for preventing the composite outcome of cervical intraepithelial neoplasia grade 2 or 3, adenocarcinoma in situ, and invasive carcinoma of the cervix due to HPV types included in the vaccine, among HPV-naive women, was 93%. In intention-to-treat analysis (overall population of study), the efficacy was 53%. Bivalent vaccine efficacy in older women was evaluated in a trial of 5752 women ≥25 years [71]. Among HPV-naive females, the efficacy for preventing the composite outcome (persistent cervical infection for 6 months or cervical intraepithelial neoplasia grade 1 or more severe disease, both associated with vaccine-type HPV) was 81%. For the overall participants in the study, the efficacy was 44%.

The nonavalent HPV vaccine efficacy was assessed in a large trial of 14,215 women aged 16–26 years who were randomized to receive the 9-valent or the quadrivalent HPV vaccine [72]. The composite outcome included cervical intraepithelial neoplasia grade 2 or more severe disease, vulvar intraepithelial neoplasia grade 2 or 3, and vaginal intraepithelial neoplasia grade 2 or 3, associated with HPV types 31, 33, 45, 52, and 58. The efficacy of the vaccine among HPV-naive women was 97%. For the overall participants the rate of high-grade cervical, vulvar, or vaginal disease irrespective of HPV type was the same in both vaccine groups (14.0 per 1000 person-years).

Long-term data about bivalent and quadrivalent vaccines reported persistent serum antibody levels and protection against HPV infection up to 9 years after vaccination [79, 80].

Special Populations

Cases of pregnant women inadvertently enrolled in phase III clinical trials were reported in the HPV vaccine groups, and abnormal pregnancy outcomes following administration do not appear to be associated with vaccination [68]. However, vaccination during pregnancy is not recommended because of limited data on safety. Lactating mothers may be vaccinated [73].

The HPV vaccine can also be administered to subjects with a history of genital warts or abnormal Papanicolaou test or positive HPV DNA test result, because immunization can still prevent infection by vaccine-type HPV that was not already acquired [73].

HPV vaccines do not have live virus particles and can be administered to individuals with immunosuppression due to infections (including human immunodeficiency virus (HIV) infection), illness, or medications. The vaccine is recommended for immunocompromised patients through age 26 years [73]. There is evidence of immunogenicity and safety of quadrivalent vaccine in HIV-infected patients [74, 75]. However, data on effectiveness are not yet available.

Safety

HPV vaccines appear to have satisfactory safety profile in the context of clinical trials [66, 68, 72]. Local reactions, particularly pain, occur at relatively high rates, having been reported in up to 80% of immunized individuals for both bivalent and quadrivalent vaccines, but this is usually of short duration and resolves spontaneously. Systemic reactions have generally been mild and self-limited [77]. Fever occurred about 2% more frequently in vaccine groups. Other minor systemic adverse events such as headache, dizziness, myalgia, arthralgia, and gastrointestinal symptoms were reported, but with <0.5% difference in the vaccinated group [10]. Postvaccination syncope has occurred, but can be avoided with appropriate care [77]. Serious vaccine-attributable adverse events, such as anaphylaxis, are rare (0.1 per 100,000 doses of quadrivalent vaccine in the United States) [78].

Vaccines Against Varicella Zoster

The causal agent of both varicella (chickenpox) and herpes zoster (shingles) is the varicella zoster virus (VZV), a highly prevalent virus affecting the human race. Only one serotype is known, and in nature VZV infects only humans [15]. The majority of primary infections occur as varicella in early childhood, which is generally a benign, self-limiting disease in immunocompetent children. Varicella infection usually confers immunity for life. Second attacks of varicella are rare in immunocompetent persons but have been documented. After resolution of varicella VZV remains latent, with occasional reactivation as the herpes zoster (HZ) disease [8].

Varicella
Vaccines against both varicella and HZ are based on live attenuated VZV (Oka strain) but at different virus titers. Although Oka strain is clinically attenuated, it can cause mild varicella, establish latency, and, theoretically, reactivate to cause HZ [14]. The United States introduced universal varicella vaccination in 1996, and Australia in 2000. Both countries have subsequently experienced a substantial decrease in disease burden [17, 18].

The varicella vaccination rationale is to avoid associated morbidity (which may be mediated either by VZV or secondary bacterial infection) such as encephalitis, cerebellar ataxia, pneumonia, sepsis, and the congenital varicella syndrome [9]. Although complications are more frequent at the extremes of age and in individuals with underlying chronic disease, most cases of complications arise in previously healthy individuals [16]. Rarely these complications may result in

death, especially among neonates and immunocompromised persons [13]. The WHO position paper [9] considers that varicella vaccination is of value for public health by lowering morbidity and mortality arising from VZV, particularly in vulnerable population groups. It suggests that authorities should consider introducing varicella vaccination in the routine childhood immunization programs in countries where varicella is a relatively important public health problem and where the resources are sufficient to ensure high (85–90%) and sustained vaccine coverage. Additionally the vaccine may be offered in any country to individual adolescents and adults without a history of varicella, mainly with a high average age (≥15 years) of acquisition of infection, indicating a high proportion of susceptible persons in the population.

Formulations
The varicella vaccine is available either as a monovalent (varicella only) or in combination with measles, mumps, and rubella (MMR) vaccine, and is administered subcutaneously [19]. All vaccines are licensed for use in persons aged ≥12 months; one monovalent and two combined vaccines are licensed for use from 9 months of age in some countries. There is an acceptable variability in the virus concentrations among different varicella vaccines, and currently licensed vaccine content varies from 1000 to 17,000 plaque-forming units [9].

Schedules
The WHO suggests that the first dose be administered at age 12–18 months. Each country should decide on the number of doses of the schedule, depending on the goal of the vaccination program. One dose can reduce mortality and severe morbidity from varicella but does not prevent limited virus circulation and outbreaks. Two doses have higher effectiveness and are recommended for countries where the programmatic goal includes the reduction of the number of cases and outbreaks. The second dose (for countries with a two-dose schedule) should be administered as recommended by the manufacturer, ranging from 4 weeks to 3 months after the first

dose [9]. The ACIP recommends routine two-dose varicella vaccination for children, with the first dose administered at 12–15 months of age and the second dose at age 4–6 years [19]. It is also recommended for adolescents ≥13 years and adults without evidence of immunity, which requires a two-dose schedule separated by 4–8 weeks [20]. Some European countries, such as the United Kingdom and France, do not recommend universal immunization [41]. It is particularly important to immunize susceptible individuals who have close contact with immunocompromised patients at high risk of severe disease, such as healthcare workers and household contacts [9, 19, 20].

Since the routine schedule for varicella vaccine generally is the same as that for MMR vaccine, either monovalent or combination MMRV vaccines can be used, taking into consideration the safety and effectiveness profiles, including a higher risk for febrile seizures after the first dose (when administered at 12–18 months) but not after the second dose [9]. Based on this the ACIP and the American Academy of Pediatrics suggest that the first doses of varicella and MMR vaccines should be administered at different sites for children 12 through 47 months of age (even if given at the same visit). The first doses for children 48 months through 12 years of age and the second doses for children 15 months through 12 years of age can be administered as MMRV vaccine. Adolescents and adults should receive single-antigen varicella vaccine [21, 22].

Pre- or postvaccination serology is not recommended because available commercial tests do not detect low levels of antibody and cannot reliably exclude immunity in exposed or vaccinated individuals [31].

Clinical Evidence

Pre- and Postlicensure studies have demonstrated that the vaccine against VZV is effective in preventing varicella, decreases disease severity in breakthrough cases, minimizes the risk of transmission, and reduces varicella-associated health care utilization [23–27]. Indirect protection of persons outside the vaccinated cohorts was also documented [28].

A systematic review [29], provided by the WHO Strategic Advisory Group of Experts (SAGE), of 40 studies about varicella vaccine effectiveness, showed that a single dose of varicella vaccine had an approximate effectiveness in preventing 80% of varicella cases of any severity; 95% of moderate disease; and 99% of severe cases. Two doses were demonstrated to be more effective, yielding a mean effectiveness of 93% against varicella of any severity.

The strategy of including the vaccine in routine immunization at 15–18 months of age seems to be better than vaccinating susceptible adolescents [42].

Contraindications and Special Populations

Varicella vaccine is contraindicated in pregnant women (pregnancy should be delayed for 4 weeks after vaccination) and in persons with a history of severe allergic reactions to a previous dose of varicella vaccine or a component of it [9, 19]. Breastfeeding is not a contraindication to administration. Varicella vaccine is usually contraindicated in the context of congenital or acquired immune deficiencies [32]. However, varicella vaccination (two doses) may be considered in these groups:

- Clinically stable HIV-infected children or adults without severe immunosuppression (CD4+ T-cell levels ≥15% or ≥200 cells/µL), including those receiving highly active antiretroviral therapy (HAART), may receive single-antigen varicella vaccine [9, 20, 30].
- Children with leukemia in remission and patients with certain solid tumors who have successfully completed chemotherapy and are unlikely to relapse (administered at least 3 months after all chemotherapy has been completed) [9, 33]
- Isolated B-lymphocyte (humoral) deficiencies are not a contraindication to single-antigen varicella vaccine [9]
- Low-dose systemic glucocorticoid therapy (prednisone ≤20 mg per day or ≤2 mg/kg per day in children who weigh <10 kg, or equivalent) is not a contraindication to varicella vaccine. However, the vaccine should not be

administered in persons receiving higher doses of prednisone; immunosuppressive agents, such as those given to patients who have undergone solid organ or hematopoietic stem cell transplant; and during treatment with tumor necrosis factor α inhibitors and other biological agents for autoimmune conditions [32].

Postexposure Prophylaxis

Small trials suggest that vaccination of children within 3 days after an exposure to VZV decreases the risk of infection (23% versus 78%) and the severity of disease. The efficacy of postexposure prophylaxis in adolescents or adults remains uncertain [35].

Safety

It is advisable to delay vaccination in persons who have recently received immune globulin, blood products, or antiviral therapy, because of the potential inhibition of the immune response. The vaccine manufacturer also recommends that salicylates be avoided for at least 6 weeks after VZV vaccine [19].

Evidence on the safety of varicella vaccines concludes that monovalent varicella vaccine is generally well tolerated [36]. Local reactions (tenderness and redness at the injection site and localized varicella-like rash) are the most common adverse event (up to 25% of children which received combined or monovalent varicella vaccine) [34]. Fever was reported in 15% of children [9]. The risk of a febrile seizure after separate injections of varicella vaccine and MMR is approximately 1 in 2500 [21]. Urticaria was rarely reported, mainly after receipt of varicella vaccine in combination with other vaccine (2.2/100,000 doses). Postlicensure data from the United States showed the incidence of serious adverse events to be 2.6/100,000 doses [36]. Review of evidence for severe adverse events associated with varicella vaccines supports causality for rare occurrences: disseminated cutaneous infection by vaccine strain virus; disseminated vaccine strain virus infection with internal organ involvement in individuals with immunodeficiencies; vaccine strain reactivation (HZ) with or without organ involvement; and anaphylaxis [9].

Varicella vaccination raised concerns about its impact on the incidence of HZ, either by a risk of vaccine-associated HZ in immunized individuals or by an increase in general population incidence of HZ due to a reduction of exogenous boosting of immunity by naturally circulating VZV [39]. None of these concerns were supported by evidence. The incidence of HZ in vaccinated children is approximately 14 cases per 100,000 person-years [40]. Long-term follow-up of a group of individuals who received varicella vaccine as healthy young adults found that the incidence of HZ was similar to historical data in the prevaccine era in the United States [37]. Also, if given in childhood the vaccine does not appear to affect the incidence of HZ in individuals older than 65 years in general population [38].

It should be noted that varicella vaccine is licensed only to protect against varicella disease; it is not indicated for protection against HZ disease.

Herpes Zoster

About 10–30% of people infected by VZV will develop an episode of HZ during their lifetime. HZ incidence is related to waning specific cell-mediated immunity and is particularly high in elderly and immunocompromised subjects [43]. The most frequent complication of HZ is postherpetic neuralgia (PHN), defined as a pain along the affected sensory nerves lasting more than 90 days after the healing of the rash, which has a high impact on patients' quality of life [44].

Zoster immunization rationale is to boost VZV-specific T-cell immune responses, preventing or attenuating HZ disease [45]. The first developed HZ vaccine contains the same VZV Oka strain used in varicella vaccine, but at a much higher dose [29]. Zoster vaccination can help to reduce the occurrence and severity of HZ or the risk of PHN [46]. Therefore, it might be an interesting option for introduction into national immunization programs. The WHO position paper [10] does not offer any specific recommendation concerning the routine use of HZ vaccine in public health. The reason is due to the unknown burden of HZ in most countries and insufficient data concerning the use and duration of protection of HZ vaccine. However, countries with high demographic shift toward older ages may consider introducing routine HZ vaccination if they have an important burden of disease.

Formulations

HZ vaccine composed by a live attenuated virus is administered as a single 0.65-mL subcutaneous injection [29]. Recently an inactivated zoster vaccine composed by VZV glycoprotein E in combination with an adjuvant has been developed. This vaccine requires two doses for protection [47].

Schedule

Despite the US Food and Drug Administration (FDA) having licensed zoster vaccine for use in persons over 50 years of age, the ACIP recommends beginning vaccination at age 60 years [48], independently of patient's previous history of varicella or HZ disease. There are no studies about vaccination of patients who have received the varicella vaccine. The ACIP does not recommend zoster vaccination in such patients.

The manufacturer of the pneumococcal vaccine, indicated for a similar age group, recommends that the zoster vaccine should be administered separately by at least 4 weeks, because coadministration would reduce the immunogenicity of the zoster vaccine [49]. Despite this, to reduce the probability of low adherence to both vaccines the ACIP has recommended the administration of pneumococcal and HZ vaccine at same visit [48], based on findings of an observational study that did not find differences in incidence of HZ between both situations [49].

Clinical Evidence

A large placebo-controlled primary prevention clinical trial of the live attenuated zoster vaccine, including 38,546 immunocompetent adults aged 60 years and older, has demonstrated a significant reduction in the burden of illness due to both clinical HZ and PHN. Immunization reduced the incidence of HZ by 51% compared with placebo (1.6% versus 3.3%, respectively) and of PHN by 67% (0.1% versus 0.4%, respectively) [46].

The HZ vaccine reduces disability related to pain by two-thirds and the impact on quality of life by half [53]. Most of this reduction was attributed to the prevention of HZ infection.

A meta-analysis of eight randomized trials that included 52,269 individuals 60 years of age or older showed results similar to those of the original study [50].

The efficacy of the vaccine in the age group from 50 to 59 years of age was tested in another placebo-controlled trial which showed significant reduction in the incidence of HZ (2 per 1000 person-years versus 6.6 per 1000 person-year in the placebo group) [52].

A major obstacle to widespread use of zoster vaccine is the high cost. Multiple cost-effectiveness analyses have been performed. A systematic review of 14 cost-effectiveness studies of HZ vaccination [54] showed that duration of vaccine-induced protection affected the ratio considerably. In general, HZ immunization is cost-effective when the vaccine is administered between the age of 60 and 75 years and the duration of vaccine-induced protection is longer than 10 years. However, long-term follow-up of individuals from the major trial suggest that the efficacy of the zoster vaccine is somewhat reduced approximately 8 years after vaccination [51]. It is not known whether a second dose can preserve immunity conferred by the HZ vaccine.

The efficacy of two doses of the new inactivated zoster vaccine was evaluated in a placebo-controlled clinical trial including 15,411 individuals aged 50 years and older. The overall vaccine efficacy to prevent HZ disease was 97.2% without significant adverse effects reported [47]. This vaccine may be particularly helpful in immunocompromised individuals.

Contraindications and Special Populations

As varicella vaccine, the live attenuated zoster vaccine is contraindicated in pregnant women. Also, it should not be administered to persons with history of an anaphylactic reaction to gelatin or neomycin [48]. Zoster vaccine should be avoided the context of congenital or acquired immune deficiencies [9]. However, low-level immunosuppressive therapy, such as prednisone

≤20 mg per day or methotrexate ≤0.4 mg/kg/week, is not a contraindication for vaccination [32]. The indications of zoster vaccine in HIV-infected individuals are not yet established. It can be considered in those with CD4 counts >200 cells/μL who are aged 60 years or older [55]. Healthcare providers can consider vaccination of candidates for solid organ transplants prior to transplantation, although its efficacy in preventing HZ disease during immunosuppression therapy following transplantation is unknown [56].

Zoster vaccine is not indicated for the treatment of HZ disease or PHN.

Safety

Clinical trials as well as postlicensure studies of the live attenuated zoster vaccine demonstrated a good tolerability and safety profile [9]. In a large study the incidence of serious adverse events was <0.1% [52]. Immunized subjects reported more frequent (26–35%) reactions involving the site of injection (erythema, pain, tenderness, swelling, and pruritus). An HZ-like rash (usually mild) has been registered in 0.1% of immunized individuals [9]. Transmission of the vaccine virus has not been reported. One patient had an anaphylactic reaction on the day of vaccination [52].

Vaccines Against Herpes Simplex

There are no vaccines currently available for protection against infection with either HSV-1 or HSV-2. Clinical studies of herpes simplex virus type 2 (HSV-2) subunit vaccines containing glycoproteins showed that, overall, the vaccine was not efficacious [81–83].

BCG Vaccination Against Tuberculosis and Leprosy (Hanseniasis)

The Bacillus Calmette–Guérin (BCG) vaccine was produced by in vitro attenuation of a strain of *Mycobacterium bovis* in the early twentieth century and is one of the most widely used vaccines. The objective of vaccinating neonates and infants is for prevention of severe tuberculosis (TB) [84]. BCG vaccine has a documented protective effect against meningitis and disseminated TB in children [85]. Evidence about the protection of BCG vaccine against *Mycobacterium tuberculosis* primary infection has been scarce. Recently, the development of modern techniques allowed discrimination of recent *M. tuberculosis* infection from previous BCG vaccination or contact with most nontuberculous mycobacterial infections, which was not possible with the tuberculin skin test [86]. Based on this, a meta-analysis of 14 studies demonstrated that BCG protects against *M. tuberculosis* infection (overall efficacy of 19% among vaccinated children after exposure) as well as progression from infection to disease (efficacy of 58% among those infected) [87].

By blocking the progression of *M. tuberculosis* infection, BCG could, theoretically, confer protection over some forms of cutaneous TB. However, the role of BCG as a preventive measure against cutaneous TB is controversial. In some reports, BCG vaccination appeared to protect against disseminated disease [88] and also to be effective in adults against cutaneous TB (efficacy of 60.9%) [89]. Nevertheless, other studies did not find any difference between the vaccinated and the unvaccinated groups in preventing cutaneous TB [90, 91].

The cross-reactivity between BCG and *Mycobacterium leprae* has been exploited in attempts to induce immunity against leprosy (also known as hanseniasis). BCG started to be used for the prophylaxis of leprosy in the 1940s [92] and the presence of a BCG scar has been recognized as a protective factor for the disease [95]. However, the efficacy of BCG in preventing leprosy has varied widely in studies. Meta-analyses demonstrated an overall efficacy of 26–41% in experimental studies and 61% in observational studies [93, 94]. BCG is mostly known as a vaccine for prevention of TB but, curiously, studies that tested the efficacy of the same BCG vaccine for TB and leprosy in the same populations have shown BCG to be more effective against leprosy than against TB [103].

Because of BCG's efficacy against leprosy, Brazil has officially recommended two doses of

BCG to be administered to household contacts of leprosy cases, as a boost to routine BCG vaccination in newborns, when it is applied as a TB prophylactic vaccine [104]. This approach was evaluated in a cohort study of 5376 contacts of 1161 leprosy patients in Brazil [105], showing that the efficacy of BCG was 56% and was not substantially affected by previous BCG vaccination (50% with and 59% without a scar). Interestingly, the risk of tuberculoid leprosy was high during the initial months among those vaccinated with no scar [105]. Another study in Bangladesh also identified a high proportion of healthy contacts of leprosy patients who presented with paucibacillary leprosy within 12 weeks after receiving BCG vaccination (all 21 contacts who developed leprosy in this period) [106]. This can be attributed to the boosted cell-mediated immunity due to antigens in BCG, which may accelerate and modulate clinical manifestations in subjects infected with *M. leprae* before or immediately after BCG vaccination [105].

In addition to BCG, the vaccine potential of killed *M. leprae* has also been assessed in clinical trials, but in most studies, BCG plus *M. leprae* vaccine did not offer better protection against leprosy than BCG alone [96, 97].

Protective efficacy of BCG has been reported to decrease with time and is generally thought to last no more than 10–15 years [11]. In contrast to what occurs with vaccination for TB, for which studies indicate no substantial benefit of BCG revaccination, the evidence suggests that multiple BCG doses enhance protective efficacy against leprosy [97], although this has been questioned by some studies [98].

Formulations

All BCG vaccine used nowadays contains descendant strains from the original *M. bovis* isolate obtained by Calmette and Guérin. The manufactured vaccine is a lyophilized compound which, after reconstitution, contains both living and dead bacilli. The number of cultivable bacilli per dose and the biochemical composition of the vaccine vary considerably depending upon the strain and production method [11].

Schedule

The WHO recommends that a single dose of BCG vaccine should be given to all infants as soon as possible after birth in countries with a high burden of TB and also to infants and children at particular risk of TB exposure in otherwise low-endemic areas. BCG revaccination for TB is not supported [11]. BCG is also administered at birth in most countries with high rates of leprosy, a fact that generally coincides with the WHO recommendation for TB because both diseases are common in low-income countries.

To date, despite its variable protective efficacy, BCG is the best available vaccine for the prevention of leprosy [94]. Besides the dose administered at birth, the Brazilian Ministry of Health recommends two doses of BCG to be administered to household contacts of leprosy patients [104].

BCG vaccine application should be intradermal, preferably on the deltoid region of the arm. Newborns normally receive half the dose given to older children, because they have a higher risk of vaccine-induced suppurative lymphadenitis. BCG vaccine can be given simultaneously with other childhood vaccines [11].

BCG vaccination of adults is not normally recommended but may be considered for tuberculin-negative persons in close contact with cases of multidrug-resistant *M. tuberculosis* [11].

Contraindications and Special Populations

BCG vaccination is contraindicated for persons with impaired immunity (symptomatic HIV infection, known or suspected congenital immunodeficiency, leukemia, lymphoma or generalized malignant disease); for patients under immunosuppressive treatment (corticosteroids, alkylating agents, antimetabolites, radiation); and in pregnancy [11].

Neonates of known HIV-positive mothers are at risk of disseminated BCG disease if they have rapid development of immunodeficiency. Based on this, the WHO recommends that [12]:

- In infants born to women of unknown HIV status, benefits outweigh risks for BCG vaccination and they should be immunized
- In infants whose HIV infection status is unknown and do not demonstrate signs or symptoms suggestive of HIV infection, but who are born to known HIV-infected women, the benefits usually outweigh risks for BCG vaccination and they should be immunized after consideration of local factors (prevalence and potential exposure to TB; capacity to conduct follow-up of immunized children; capacity to perform early virologic infant diagnosis)
- In infants who are known to be infected with HIV, risks outweigh benefits for BCG vaccination and they should not be immunized
- In infants whose HIV infection status is unknown but who have signs or symptoms suggestive of HIV infection and who are born to HIV-infected mothers, risks usually outweigh benefits for BCG vaccination and they should not be immunized.

Safety

After 2–6 weeks of BCG vaccination a variable local reaction usually occurs (erythema, induration, tenderness, and ulceration), often followed by a small scar at the site of the injection.

Complications following BCG vaccination are rare. Fatal dissemination of BCG occurs almost exclusively in inadvertently immunized persons with severely compromised cellular immunity. Extensive ulceration and regional lymphadenitis sometimes occurs, but is also much more common in immunodeficient persons [11].

Specific complications caused by the BCG organism include lupus vulgaris at the vaccination site [99]. Case reports have also documented occurrence of scrofuloderma [100], papular tuberculids [101], and erythema induratum of Bazin [102] following vaccination. Antituberculous therapy is not necessary for these hypersensitivity reactions to *M. bovis* in immunocompetent patients.

Future Perspectives

Despite major advances in the field of vaccinology over the last decades, there are still possibilities for improvement. Vaccines are being developed both to prevent and to aid in the treatment of HSV-2 infection [107]. Multiple molecules are under study for the development of new vaccines against varicella and HZ. Complete prevention of both varicella and HZ is the only path that will lead to eradication of VZV, and future research should consider the reduction of VZV infection in the general population as a primary outcome [108].

Regarding HPV vaccines, it is important to generate more data on longer-term clinical efficiency and to define the duration of protection and cost-effectiveness after two-dose and three-dose schedules. Additional studies in low-income countries among healthy young females and among special populations (e.g., HIV-infected, malnourished, endemic malaria) would provide evidence of the impact of the vaccine in those populations [10].

Despite the positive impact of the WHO treatment campaign on the global prevalence of leprosy, there is still a need for further efforts toward eradication of the disease. These efforts should include an effective vaccine with potential for both prophylactic and therapeutic use. The development of an improved BCG vaccine, BCG booster, or alternative vaccine strain that could benefit control of both TB and leprosy is currently an important global research goal [109]. The most favored research strategies include recombinant modified BCG vaccines, attenuated strains of *Mycobacterium*, subunit vaccines, and DNA vaccines [11].

Glossary

Anaphylaxis A severe, potentially life-threatening allergic reaction. It can occur within seconds or minutes of exposure to an allergen. The flood of chemicals released by the immune system during anaphylaxis can lead the body into shock; the blood pressure drops suddenly and the airways narrow, blocking normal breathing. Signs and symptoms of anaphylaxis include a rapid, weak pulse, a rash, and nausea and vomiting.

Genotypes   The genotype of an organism is the inherited map it carries within its genetic code. It is the part (DNA sequence) of the genetic makeup of a cell, and therefore of an organism or individual, which determines a specific characteristic (phenotype) of that cell/organism/individual.

Revaccination   The vaccination administered some time after an initial vaccination, especially to strengthen or renew immunity.

References

1. American Academy of Pediatrics. Red book: 2015 report of the committee on infectious diseases. In: Kimberlin DW, Brady MT, Jackson MA, Long SS, editors. 30th ed. Elk Grove Village; 2015.
2. Del Giudice G, Weinberger B, Grubeck-Loebenstein B. Vaccines for the elderly. Gerontology. 2015;61(3):203–10.
3. Scully IL, Swanson K, Green L, Jansen KU, Anderson AS. Anti-infective vaccination in the 21st century – new horizons for personal and public health. Curr Opin Microbiol. 2015;27:96–102.
4. Centers for Disease Control and Prevention. General recommendation on immunization: recommendation of the Advisory Committee on Immunization Practices. MMWR Morb Mortal Wkly Rep. 2011;60(02):1–64.
5. Prymula R, Siegrist C-A, Chlibek R, Zemlickova H, Vackova M, Smetana J, et al. Effect of prophylactic paracetamol administration at time of vaccination on febrile reactions and antibody responses in children: two open-label, randomised controlled trials. Lancet. 2009;374(9698):1339–50.
6. Position papers [internet]. Geneva: World Health Organization [cited 2016 Feb 26]. Available from: http://www.who.int/immunization/policy/position_papers/en/.
7. WHO recommendations for routine immunization – summary tables [internet]. Geneva: World Health Organization [cited 2016 Feb 26]. Available from: http://www.who.int/immunization/policy/immunization_tables/en/.
8. Duncan CJ, Hambleton S. Varicella zoster virus immunity: a primer. J Infect. 2015;71(Suppl 1):S47–53.
9. Varicella and herpes zoster vaccines: WHO position paper, June 2014. Wkly Epidemiol Rec. 2014; 89:265.
10. Human papillomavirus vaccines: WHO position paper, October 2014. Wkly Epidemiol Rec. 2014; 89:465.
11. BCG vaccine: WHO position paper, January 2004. Wkly Epidemiol Rec. 2004; 79:27.
12. Revised BCG vaccination guidelines for infants at risk for HIV infection: WHO position paper, May 2007. Wkly Epidemiol Rec. 2007; 21:193.
13. Meyer PA, et al. Varicella mortality: trends before vaccine licensure in the United States, 1970–1994. J Infect Dis. 2000;182(2):383–90.
14. Quinlivan M, Breuer J. Clinical and molecular aspects of the live attenuated Oka varicella vaccine. Rev Med Virol. 2014;24(4):254–73. doi:10.1002/rmv.1789. Epub 2014 Mar 29.
15. Gershon AA1, Gershon MD. Pathogenesis and current approaches to control of varicella-zoster virus infections. Clin Microbiol Rev. 2013;26(4):728–43. doi:10.1128/CMR.00052-13.
16. Helmuth IG, Poulsen A, Suppli CH, Mølbak K. Varicella in Europe – a review of the epidemiology and experience with vaccination. Vaccine. 2015;33(21):2406–13. doi:10.1016/j.vaccine.2015.03.055. Epub 2015 Apr 1. Review.
17. Marin M, Meissner HC, Seward JF. Varicella prevention in the United States: a review of successes and challenges. Pediatrics. 2008;122:e744–51. http://dx.doi.org/10.1542/peds.2008-0567.
18. Heywood AE, Wang H, Macartney KK, McIntyre P. Varicella and herpes zoster hospitalizations before and after implementation of one-dose varicella vaccination in Australia: an ecological study. Bull World Health Organ. 2014;92:593–604. http://dx.doi.org/10.2471/BLT.13.132142
19. Marin M, Güris D, Chaves SS, et al. Prevention of varicella: recommendations of the Advisory Committee on Immunization Practices (ACIP). MMWR Recomm Rep. 2007;56:1–40.
20. Kim DK, Bridges CB, Harriman KH. Advisory Committee on Immunization Practices. Advisory committee on immunization practices recommended immunization schedule for adults aged 19 years or older: United States. Ann Intern Med. 2016;164:184.
21. Centers for Disease Control and Prevention (CDC). Advisory Committee on Immunization Practices (ACIP). Update: recommendations from the Advisory Committee on Immunization Practices (ACIP) regarding administration of combination MMRV vaccine. MMWR Morb Mortal Wkly Rep. 2008;57:258.
22. Committee on Infectious Diseases. Policy statement – Prevention of varicella: update of recommendations for use of quadrivalent and monovalent varicella vaccines in children. Pediatrics. 2011;128:630.
23. Weibel RE, Neff BJ, Kuter BJ, et al. Live attenuated varicella virus vaccine. Efficacy trial in healthy children. N Engl J Med. 1984;310:1409–15.
24. Seward JF, Marin M, Vázquez M. Varicella vaccine effectiveness in the US vaccination program: a review. J Infect Dis. 2008;197(Suppl 2):S82.
25. Vázquez M, PS LR, Gershon AA, et al. The effectiveness of the varicella vaccine in clinical practice. N Engl J Med. 2001;344:955.

26. Centers for Disease Control and Prevention (CDC). Evolution of varicella surveillance – selected states, 2000–2010. MMWR Morb Mortal Wkly Rep. 2012;61:609.

27. Zhou F, Harpaz R, Jumaan AO, et al. Impact of varicella vaccination on health care utilization. JAMA. 2005;294:797.

28. Waye A, Jacobs P, Tan B. The impact of the universal infant varicella immunization strategy on Canadian varicella-related hospitalization rates. Vaccine. 2013;31:4744.

29. World Health Organization. Background documents for the meeting of the Strategic Advisory Group of Experts (SAGE). 2014. http://www.who.int/immunization/sage/meetings/2014/april/presentations_background_docs/en/. Accessed on 26 Feb 2016.

30. Levin MJ, Gershon AA, Weinberg A, et al. Administration of live varicella vaccine to HIV-infected children with current or past significant depression of CD4(+) T cells. J Infect Dis. 2006;194:247–55.

31. Schmid DS, Jumaan AO. Impact of varicella vaccine on varicella-zoster virus dynamics. Clin Microbiol Rev. 2010;23(1):202–17.

32. Rubin LG, Levin MJ, Ljungman P, et al. 2013 IDSA clinical practice guideline for vaccination of the immunocompromised host. Clin Infect Dis. 2014;58:e44.

33. Gershon AA, Steinberg SP. Persistence of immunity to varicella in children with leukemia immunized with live attenuated varicella vaccine. N Engl J Med. 1989;320:892–7.

34. Prymula R, Bergsaker MR, Esposito S, Gothefors L, Man S, Snegova N, Stefkovičova M, Usonis V, Wysocki J, Douha M, Vassilev V, Nicholson O, Innis BL, Willems P. Protection against varicella with two doses of combined measles-mumps-rubella-varicella vaccine versus one dose of monovalent varicella vaccine: a multicentre, observer-blind, randomised, controlled trial. Lancet. 2014;383(9925):1313–24. doi:10.1016/S0140-6736(12)61461-5. Epub 2014 Jan 29.

35. Macartney K1, Heywood A, McIntyre P. Vaccines for post-exposure prophylaxis against varicella (chickenpox) in children and adults. Cochrane Database Syst Rev. 2014;6:CD001833. doi:10.1002/14651858. CD001833.pub3.

36. Chaves SS, Haber P, Walton K, et al. Safety of varicella vaccine after licensure in the United States: experience from reports to the vaccine adverse event reporting system, 1995–2005. J Infect Dis. 2008;197(Suppl 2):S170.

37. Hambleton S, Steinberg SP, Larussa PS, et al. Risk of herpes zoster in adults immunized with varicella vaccine. J Infect Dis. 2008;197(Suppl 2):S196–9.

38. Hales CM, Harpaz R, Joesoef MR, Bialek SR. Examination of links between herpes zoster incidence and childhood varicella vaccination. Ann Intern Med. 2013;159:739.

39. Ogunjimi B, van Damme P, Beutels P. Herpes zoster risk reduction through exposure to chickenpox patients: a systematic multidisciplinary review. PLoS One. 2013;8(6):e66485.

40. Uebe B, Sauerbrei A, Burdach S, Horneff G. Herpes zoster by reactivated vaccine varicella zoster virus in a healthy child. Eur J Pediatr. 2002;161:442–4.

41. Carrillo-Santisteve P1, Lopalco PL. Varicella vaccination: a laboured take-off. Clin Microbiol Infect. 2014;20(Suppl 5):86–91. doi:10.1111/1469-0691.12580.

42. Gil-Prieto R, Walter S, Gonzalez-Escalada A, Garcia-Garcia L, Marín-García P, Gil-de-Miguel A. Different vaccination strategies in Spain and its impact on severe varicella and zoster. Vaccine. 2014;32(2):277–83.

43. Volpi A, Gross G, Hercogova J, et al. Current management of herpes zoster. The European view. Am J Clin Dermatol. 2005;6:317–25.

44. Kawai K, Gebremeskei BG, Acosta CJ. Systematic review of incidence and complications of herpes zoster: towards a global perspective. BMJ Open. 2014;4:e004833.

45. Weinberg A, Zhang JH, Oxman MN, et al. Varicella-zoster virus-specific immune responses to herpes zoster in elderly participants in a trial of a clinically effective zoster vaccine. J Infect Dis. 2009;200:1068.

46. Oxman MN, Levin MJ, Johnson GR, et al. A vaccine to prevent herpes zoster and postherpetic neuralgia in older adults. N Engl J Med. 2005;352:2271–84.

47. Lal H, Cunningham AL, Godeaux O, et al. Efficacy of an adjuvanted herpes zoster subunit vaccine in older adults. N Engl J Med. 2015;372:2087.

48. Hales CM, Harpaz R, Ortega-Sanchez I, et al. Update on recommendations for use of herpes zoster vaccine. MMWR Morb Mortal Wkly Rep. 2014;63:729.

49. Tseng HF, Smith N, Sy LS, Jacobsen SJ. Evaluation of the incidence of herpes zoster after concomitant administration of zoster vaccine and polysaccharide pneumococcal vaccine. Vaccine. 2011;29:3628.

50. Gagliardi AM, Gomes Silva BN, Torloni MR, Soares BG. Vaccines for preventing herpes zoster in older adults. Cochrane Database Syst Rev. 2012;10:CD008858.

51. Morrison VA, Johnson GR, Schmader KE, et al. Long-term persistence of zoster vaccine efficacy. Clin Infect Dis. 2015;60:900.

52. Schmader KE, Levin MJ, Gnann JW Jr, et al. Efficacy, safety, and tolerability of herpes zoster vaccine in persons aged 50–59 years. Clin Infect Dis. 2012;54:922.

53. Schmader KE, Johnson GR, Saddier P, Ciarleglio M, Wang WW, Zhang JH et al.; for the Shingles Prevention Study Group. Effect of a zoster vaccine on herpes zoster-related interference with functional status and health-related quality-of-life measures in older adults. J Am Geriatr Soc. 2010; 58(9):1634–41.

54. de Boer PT, Wilschut JC, Postma MJ. Cost-effectiveness of vaccination against herpes zoster.

Hum Vaccin Immunother. 2014;10(7):2048–61. doi:10.4161/hv.28670.

55. Aberg JA, Gallant JE, Ghanem KG, et al. Primary care guidelines for the management of persons infected with HIV: 2013 update by the HIV medicine association of the Infectious Diseases Society of America. Clin Infect Dis. 2014;58:e1.

56. Pergam SA, Limaye AP, AST Infectious Diseases Community of Practice. Varicella zoster virus in solid organ transplantation. Am J Transplant. 2013;13(Suppl 4):138.

57. Choi YJ, Park JS. Clinical significance of human papillomavirus genotyping. J Gynecol Oncol. 2016 Mar;27(2):e21.

58. Gross G. Condylomata acuminata und andere HPV – assoziierte Krankheitsbilder des Genitale und der Harnröhre. Hautarzt. 2001;52:405–10.

59. Sycuro LK, Xi LF, Hughes JP, Feng Q, Winer RL, Lee SK, O'Reilly S, Kiviat NB, Koutsky LA. Persistence of genital human papillomavirus infection in a long-term follow-up study of female university students. J Infect Dis. 2008;198(7):971–8.

60. Wallin KL, Wiklund F, Angstrom T, et al. Type-specific persistence of human papillomavirus DNA before the development of invasive cervical cancer. N Engl J Med. 1999;341:1633–8.

61. Frazer IH. Interaction of human papillomaviruses with the host immune system: a well evolved relationship. Virology. 2009;384:410–4.

62. Bosch FX, Lorincz A, Munoz N, Meijer CJ, Shah KV. The causal relation between human papillomavirus and cervical cancer. J Clin Pathol. 2002;55:244–65.

63. Datta SD, Koutsky LA, Ratelle S, et al. Human papillomavirus infection and cervical cytology in women screened for cervical cancer in the United States, 2003–2005. Ann Intern Med. 2008;148:493–500.

64. de Martel C, Ferlay J, Franceschi S, et al. Global burden of cancers attributable to infections in 2008: a review and synthetic analysis. Lancet Oncol. 2012;13:607–15.

65. Dochez C, Bogers JJ, Verhelst R, Rees H. HPV vaccines to prevent cervical cancer and genital warts: an update. Vaccine. 2014;32:1595–601.

66. Giuliano AR, Palefsky JM, Goldstone S, et al. Efficacy of quadrivalent HPV vaccine against HPV Infection and disease in males. N Engl J Med. 2011;364:401.

67. Palefsky JM, Giuliano AR, Goldstone S, et al. HPV vaccine against anal HPV infection and anal intraepithelial neoplasia. N Engl J Med. 2011;365:1576.

68. FUTURE II Study Group. Quadrivalent vaccine against human papillomavirus to prevent high-grade cervical lesions. N Engl J Med. 2007;356:1915.

69. Garland SM, Hernandez-Avila M, Wheeler CM, et al. Quadrivalent vaccine against human papillomavirus to prevent anogenital diseases. N Engl J Med. 2007;356:1928.

70. Paavonen J, Naud P, Salmerón J, et al. Efficacy of human papillomavirus (HPV)-16/18 AS04-adjuvanted vaccine against cervical infection and precancer caused by oncogenic HPV types (PATRICIA): final analysis of a double-blind, randomised study in young women. Lancet. 2009;374:301.

71. Skinner SR, Szarewski A, Romanowski B, et al. Efficacy, safety, and immunogenicity of the human papillomavirus 16/18 AS04-adjuvanted vaccine in women older than 25 years: 4-year interim follow-up of the phase 3, double-blind, randomised controlled VIVIANE study. Lancet. 2014;384:2213.

72. Joura EA, Giuliano AR, Iversen OE, et al. A 9-valent HPV vaccine against infection and intraepithelial neoplasia in women. N Engl J Med. 2015;372:711.

73. Markowitz LE, Dunne EF, Saraiya M, et al. Human papillomavirus vaccination: recommendations of the Advisory Committee on Immunization Practices (ACIP). MMWR Recomm Rep. 2014;63:1.

74. Wilkin T, Lee JY, Lensing SY, et al. Safety and immunogenicity of the quadrivalent human papillomavirus vaccine in HIV-1-infected men. J Infect Dis. 2010;202:1246.

75. Kojic EM, Kang M, Cespedes MS, et al. Immunogenicity and safety of the quadrivalent human papillomavirus vaccine in HIV-1-infected women. Clin Infect Dis. 2014;59:127.

76. Hildesheim A, Wacholder S, Catteau G, Struyf F, Dubin G, Herrero R, CVT Group. Efficacy of the HPV-16/18 vaccine: Final according to protocol results from the blinded phase of the randomized Costa Rica HPV-16/18 vaccine trial. Vaccine. 2014;32(39):5087–97. doi:10.1016/j.vaccine.2014.06.038.

77. Macartney KK, Chiu C, Georgousakis M, Brotherton JM. Safety of human papillomavirus vaccines: a review. Drug Saf. 2013;36(6):393–412.

78. Slade BA, Leidel L, Vellozzi C, et al. Postlicensure safety surveillance for quadrivalent human papillomavirus recombinant vaccine. JAMA. 2009;302:750.

79. Naud PS, Roteli-Martins CM, De Carvalho NS, et al. Sustained efficacy, immunogenicity, and safety of the HPV-16/18 AS04-adjuvanted vaccine: final analysis of a long-term follow-up study up to 9.4 years post-vaccination. Hum Vaccin Immunother. 2014;10:2147.

80. Ferris D, Samakoses R, Block SL, et al. Long-term study of a quadrivalent human papillomavirus vaccine. Pediatrics. 2014;134:e657.

81. Corey L, Langenberg AG, Ashley R, et al. Recombinant glycoprotein vaccine for the prevention of genital HSV-2 infection: two randomized controlled trials. Chiron HSV Vaccine Study Group. JAMA. 1999;282:331.

82. Stanberry LR, Spruance SL, Cunningham AL, et al. Glycoprotein-D-adjuvant vaccine to prevent genital herpes. N Engl J Med. 2002;347:1652–61.

83. Belshe RB, Leone PA, Bernstein DI, Wald A, Levin MJ, Stapleton JT, et al. Efficacy results of a trial of a herpes simplex vaccine. N Engl J Med. 2012;366(1):34–43.

84. Springett VH, Sutherland I. A re-examination of the variations in efficacy of BCG vaccination against tuberculosis in clinical trials. Tuber Lung Dis. 1994;75:227–33.

85. Trunz BB, Fine P, Dye C. Effect of BCG vaccination on childhood tuberculous meningitis and miliary tuberculosis worldwide: a meta-analysis and assessment of cost-effectiveness. Lancet. 2006;367:1173–80.

86. Lalvani A, Millington KA. T cell-based diagnosis of childhood tuberculosis infection. Curr Opin Infect Dis. 2007;20:264–71.

87. Roy A, Eisenhut M, Harris RJ, Rodrigues LC, Sridhar S, Habermann S, Snell L, Mangtani P, Adetifa I, Lalvani A, Abubakar I. Effect of BCG vaccination against *Mycobacterium tuberculosis* infection in children: systematic review and meta-analysis. BMJ. 2014;349:g4643.

88. Kumar B, Rai R, Kaur I, Sahoo B, Muralidhar S, Radotra BD. Childhood cutaneous tuberculosis: a study over 25 years from northern India. Int J Dermatol. 2001;40:26–32.

89. Zodpey SP, Shrikhande SN, Maldhure BR, Kulkarni SW. Effectiveness of Bacillus Calmette Guerin (BCG) vaccination in the prevention of tuberculosis of skin: a case control study. Indian J Dermatol. 1998;43:4–6.

90. Singal A, Sonthalia S. Cutaneous tuberculosis in children: the Indian perspective. Indian J Dermatol Venereol Leprol. 2010;76(5):494–503.

91. Ramesh V, Misra RS, Beena KR, Mukherjee A. A study of cutaneous tuberculosis in children. Pediatr Dermatol. 1999;16:264–9.

92. Azulay RD. Antileprosy vaccinations. An Bras Dermatol. 2002;77(4):489–94.

93. Setia MS, Steinmaus C, Ho CS, Rutherford GW. The role of BCG in prevention of leprosy: a meta-analysis. Lancet Infect Dis. 2006;6:162–70.

94. Merle CS, Cunha SS, Rodrigues LC. BCG vaccination and leprosy protection: review of current evidence and status of BCG in leprosy control. Expert Rev Vaccines. 2010;9:209–22.

95. Goulart IM, Bernardes Souza DO, Marques CR, Pimenta VL, Goncalves MA, Goulart LR. Risk and protective factors for leprosy development determined by epidemiological surveillance of household contacts. Clin Vaccine Immunol. 2008;15:101–5.

96. Convit J, Sampson C, Zuniga M, Smith PG, Plata J, Silva J, et al. Immunoprophylactic trial with combined *Mycobacterium leprae*/BCG vaccine against leprosy: preliminary results. Lancet. 1992;339:446–50.

97. Karonga Prevention Trial Group. Randomised controlled trial of single BCG, repeated BCG, or combined BCG and killed *Mycobacterium leprae* vaccine for prevention of leprosy and tuberculosis in Malawi. Lancet. 1996;348:17–24.

98. Cunha SS, Alexander N, Barreto ML, Pereira ES, Dourado I, de Fatima Maroja M, et al. BCG revaccination does not protect against leprosy in the Brazilian Amazon: a cluster randomised trial. PLoS Negl Trop Dis. 2008;2:e167.

99. Handjani F, Delir S, Sodafi M, et al. Lupus vulgaris following bacille Calmette–Guérin vaccination. Br J Dermatol. 2001;144:444–5.

100. Atasoy M, Aliagaoglu C, Erdem T, et al. Scrofuloderma following BCG vaccinatiosn. Pediatr Dermatol. 2005;22:179–80.

101. Muto J, Kuroda K, Tajima S. Papular tuberculides post-BCG vaccination: case report and review of the literature in Japan. Clin Exp Dermatol. 2006;31:611–2.

102. Inque T, Fukumoto T, Ansai S, et al. Erythema induratum of Bazin in an infant after bacille Calmette–Guerin vaccination. J Dermatol. 2006;33:268–72.

103. Zodpey SP. Deciphering the story of Bacillus Calmette Guerin (BCG) vaccine in prevention of leprosy. Indian J Public Health. 2006;50(2):67–9.

104. Brazilian Ministry of Health. Guia para o Controle da hanseníase. Brasília; 2002.

105. Duppre NC, Camacho LA, da Cunha SS, Struchiner CJ, Sales AM, Nery JA, et al. Effectiveness of BCG vaccination among leprosy contacts: a cohort study. Trans R Soc Trop Med Hyg. 2008;102(7):631–8.

106. Richardus RA, Butlin CR, Alam K, Kundu K, Geluk A, Richardus JH. Clinical manifestations of leprosy after BCG vaccination: an observational study in Bangladesh. Vaccine. 2015;33(13):1562–7.

107. Status of vaccine research and development of vaccines for herpes simplex virus [internet]. Geneva: World Health Organization [cited 2016]. Available from: http://www.who.int/immunization/research/meetings_workshops/HSV_vaccineRD_Sept2014.pdf.

108. Silver B, Zhu H. Varicella zoster virus vaccines: potential complications and possible improvements. Virol Sin. 2014;29(5):265–73.

109. Duthie MS, Gillis TP, Reed SG. Advances and hurdles on the way toward a leprosy vaccine. Hum Vaccin. 2011;7(11):1172–83.

Suggested Literature

World Health Organization. Information about available and "in development" vaccines in world. Available at: http://www.who.int/immunization/diseases/en/.

American Academy of Pediatrics. Red book: 2015. Report of the Committee on Infectious Diseases. In: Kimberlin DW, Brady MT, Jackson MA, Long SS (editors). 30th ed. Elk Grove Village; 2015. Available for subscribers at: http://redbook.solutions.aap.org/redbook.aspx.

Centers for Disease Control and Prevention. Advisory Committee on Immunization Practice (ACIP). General recommendations on use of vaccines in USA. Available at: http://www.cdc.gov/vaccines/acip/.

Human Skin Bank

Eduardo Mainieri Chem, Luana Pretto,
Aline Francielle Damo Souza,
and Angelo Syrillo Pretto Neto

Introduction

The skin bank has as its main functions the harvesting, processing, preservation, and supply of fine human skin allografts for burn treatment and polytrauma centers. Allograft skin acts as a temporary biological dressing to cover superficial and deep skin wounds. Its main clinical indication is for cases in which an extensive body surface area is compromised, impeding autograft transplantation [1].

Skin Harvesting

Skin can be donated from individuals who have died from brain death or cardiac arrest. As occurs for other organs and tissues regarding the possibility of donation, the donor's family is interviewed regarding the desire to donate organs and tissues, signing a consent form for donation.

Skin harvesting involves removing, with the aid of a dermatome or graft knife, thin slices of skin with thicknesses ranging from 0.8 to 1.0 mm [1].

In this process, slices are removed from the epidermis and a small part of the dermis, which are the most superficial layers of the skin [1].

The skin is removed from sites that can be "hidden" during the donor's funeral, such as thighs, legs, and back (Fig. 53.1) [1]. After removing the skin, the donor sites have a lighter color compared with the donor's skin tone; however, skin harvesting does not cause bleeding or harm to the donor's body (Fig. 53.2). Furthermore, the sites where the skin was removed are reconstituted with wound dressings, bandages, and plasters—the end of the skin-harvesting process. This minimizes possible loss of liquid following the removal of the body tissue barrier [1].

The whole process of skin harvesting must necessarily be performed in an operating room. To preserve tissue conditions and minimize potential microbial contamination, the skin-harvesting protocol is very similar to that of in vivo surgery. Clean rooms, antisepsis of hands and forearms, surgical scrubs, and use of sterile materials are part of the routines of skin harvesting [2].

Chronologically, the stages of skin harvesting are: (i) The Center of Notification, Procurement and Distribution of Organs informs the skin bank team about the donation process (donor data, such as clinical history and serology, cause of death, age, and place and time of skin harvesting). (ii) The skin bank team (plastic surgeon and biomedical) moves to the

E.M. Chem • L. Pretto (✉)
A.F.D. Souza • A.S.P. Neto
Irmandade Santa Casa de Misericórdia de Porto
Alegre, Porto Alegre, RS, Brazil
e-mail: luana.pretto@santacasa.tche.br

© Springer International Publishing Switzerland 2018
R.R. Bonamigo, S.I.T. Dornelles (eds.), *Dermatology in Public Health Environments*,
https://doi.org/10.1007/978-3-319-33919-1_53

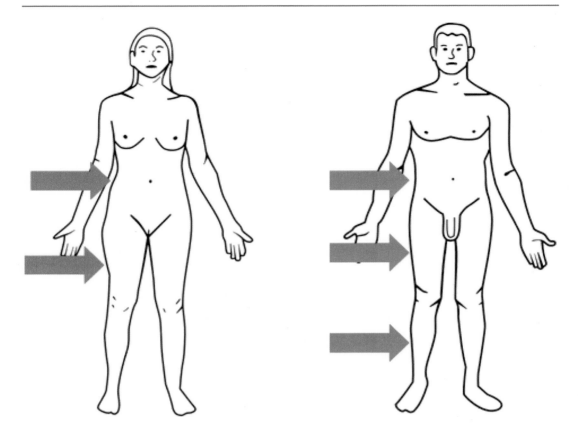

Fig. 53.1 Skin harvesting body sites

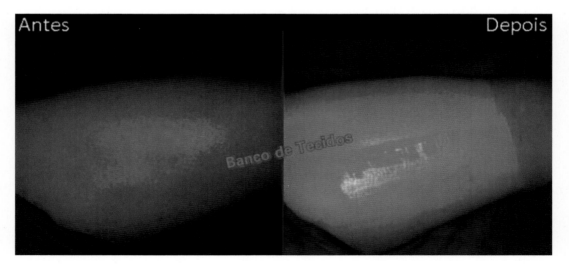

Fig. 53.2 Donor skin site before (*left*) and after (*right*) harvesting

hospital where the skin harvesting is to takes place and starts organizing the process. (iii) In the surgery center, the plastic surgeon responsible for the skin harvesting performs the physical examination of the donor body (evaluation of the skin quality). (iv) If the skin is viable for harvest, skin preparation is initiated: trichotomy and antisepsis of the donor sites. (v) The work area is prepared (placement of sterile fields) for the skin-harvesting process.

While in the operating room, the skin-harvesting process is initiated. The responsible biomedical technician performs a double wash of the skin slices with sterile saline solution. Soon after, microbiological screening of the tissue is performed by passing rayon swabs on the surface of each skin slice and small fragments are collected for subsequent placement in culture media (tryptone soya broth and thioglycolate). The skin is then packaged in bottles containing sterile 50% glycerol and transferred to a coolbox with periodic temperature control. The skin is taken to the tissue bank and kept under refrigeration (2–6 °C).

Skin Processing

Skin processing can be divided into three phases (Fig. 53.3). The first step is to wash the skin again with sterile saline and place it in more concentrated glycerol (85%). The second phase aims to "massage" the skin so that the free edges of the slice does not stick, as well as changing it over to a new 85% glycerol solution. The third and final stage consists in trimming the edges of the skin slices, packaging, and measurement of tissue in cm^2. In the case of skin contamination in the processing period, it is subjected to a specific antibiotic treatment in an attempt to eliminate the microorganisms, repeating as necessary after the three stages of processing.

Tissue Quality Control

After each stage of processing, collection of skin fragments is performed for microbiological analysis. The fragments are placed in culture media

that favor the growth and recovery of aerobic bacteria, anaerobic bacteria, and fungi that may be present in the tissue.

The tissue bank follows international guidelines [1], whereby the tissue acceptability criteria take into account the degree of pathogenicity of the organism and its potential to produce toxins. Thus, the presence of Gram-negative bacteria, *Staphylococcus aureus*, and fungi in tissue lead to its summary disposal. However, if the skin is colonized by bacteria of microbiota (coagulase-negative staphylococci) or environmental contaminants (such as those belonging to the genus *Bacillus*), it can be treated with antibiotics or physical methods such as irradiation, in order to leave sterile tissue [1].

Preservation Methods and Tissue Storage

Storage of the skin can be accomplished in two distinct forms, each of which has a direct relationship with the type of processing performed: glycerol under refrigeration at 2–6 °C or cryopreservation [3, 4].

The method using glycerol is cheaper and involves exposing the tissue to high concentrations of glycerol. Glycerol is a polyol which has as one of its properties the "sequestration" of water molecules, being characterized as a preserving solution. Accordingly, the tissue can be stored under refrigeration (4 ± 2 °C) for up to 2 years from the skin-harvesting date. On the other hand, in cryopreservation the skin associated with a cryopreservant is subjected to a slow and progressive decrease in temperature with subsequent storage at − 80 to −196 °C (in liquid nitrogen). The main advantage of this method is the longer storage time of 5 years [3, 4].

Tissue Release and Distribution

The release and distribution of allogeneic skin for clinical use only occurs after certification of tissue sterility.

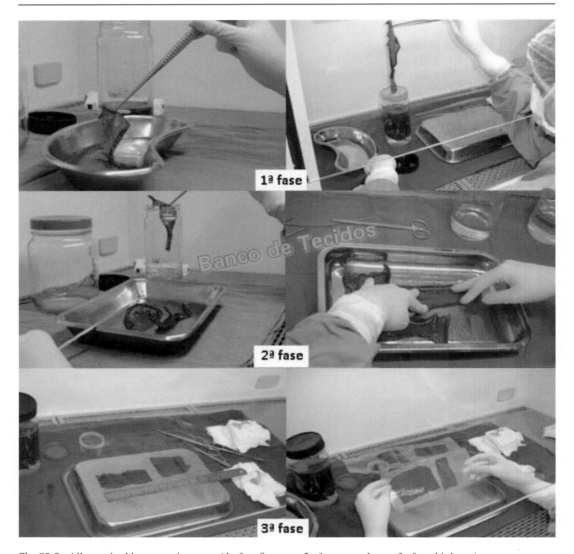

Fig. 53.3 Allogeneic skin processing steps (*1a fase* first step, *2a fase* second step, *3a fase* third step)

Tissue Release

The tissue is released after completing the three aforementioned processing steps in the absence of any microbial contaminant. Each pack of tissue is identified by a standard label which states: contact information of the tissue bank (address and telephone), the donor code, the type of processing (glycerol 85%), the expiration date (from the date of harvesting), the tissue area contained in each package (in cm²), if there was contact with antibiotics during processing, the indication:

"Product Released for Use in Human," and the temperature of the tissue storage (4 ± 2 °C) [2].

Distribution of Tissue for Clinical Use

Tissue distribution is made to all burn treatment units of the country, being governed by the National Center of Transplants and Regional Center. The function of these regulators is to assess the skin request content, verify that both the doctor and the transplantation hospital are properly registered in the National Center of Transplants, and issue an authorization for sending and carrying out the transplant.

The tissue bank separates from the stock of released tissue the amount of skin required and organizes its delivery to the center of transplantation. Shipping can be done by land or air according to the distance from the burns unit.

Sent along with the tissue are instructions for handling and use of allogeneic skin, as well as documents containing the record about the tissue, a "Consent Form" to perform the transplant, which must be signed by a person responsible for the recipient patient previously to transplant, a "Notification of Performed Transplant," and a "Notification of Side Effects." All documents duly completed by the transplant physician must be returned to the tissue bank for traceability control of the procedure and subsequent archiving [2].

Clinical Use of Allogeneic Skin

The main clinical indications for the use of allogeneic skin are deep and extensive burns and large skin defects caused by trauma. One of the most critical factors in handling and repairing lesions in patients with major skin loss is adequate coverage of the damaged area to prevent further blood loss and opportunistic bacterial infections [5].

The gold standard in surgical treatment in these cases is autologous skin grafting. However, this approach is somewhat limited when large extensions of skin are affected or large areas are injured by physical trauma, because of the restriction of skin donor sites in the affected patient. In these cases, utilization of allografts is a providential treatment and can mean the difference between life and death for these patients, with a reduction in mortality from extensive burns when this alternative is provided [5]. Observations of the clinical course of patients with full-thickness burns has shown that the earlier the removal of necrotic tissue and healthy tissue grafting is performed, the better can the recovery outcome [6, 7].

Burns

Skin defects may occur for many reasons, including skin diseases, acute trauma, chronic wounds, or even surgical interventions. However, the most common cause for their occurrence is thermal injury whereby large areas of skin may be damaged, often without the possibility of regeneration [8]. These defects compromise the functional integrity of the skin because they break the electrolyte homeostasis and alter the internal temperature control resulting from an immediate loss of physical barrier. This loss causes body fluids to directly come into contact with the environment and are lost through evaporation that causes severe dehydration in the individual [7, 9].

Classification of Burns and the Use of Allogeneic Skin

First-Degree Burns

First-degree burns affect the topmost layer of skin, the epidermis. The injured area presents hyperemia and painful erythema. Important electrolyte or clinical changes do not occur. Allogeneic skin grafting is not indicated for this type of burn [9, 10].

Second-Degree Burns

A second-degree burn reaches beyond the epidermis into the dermis layer and may be superficial or deep. Its main characteristic is the formation of blisters (bubbles containing liquid formed beneath the epidermis) which can rupture easily, leading to exposure of the dermal layer. Re-epithelialization results from the migration of cells in the basal layer of the annexes (sebaceous and sweat glands, and hair follicles) to the surface, with resolution of the lesion within 15–20 days after trauma [9, 10].

As a result of capillary stasis in the bed of burning during the first 48 h, there is the chance of bed drying, making the burn deeper. This can be prevented by an allogeneic skin graft within the first 6 h after the occurrence of the burn. A significant reduction in pain is immediately apparent after the application of the graft. At first, the donor skin is sticky and remains in place as a flexible graft. In general, rapid epithelialization follows and the graft begins to dry and detach [9, 10].

Third-Degree Burns

In third-degree lesions there is necrosis of the epidermis and dermis, with destruction of all dermal attachments as well as the nerve endings, with consequent anesthesia of the damaged areas. The healing process in these cases is time consuming and delicate, requiring appropriate management of the patient. After surgical removal of necrotic tissue, the wound can be covered with autograft depending on the availability of healthy donor regions and the clinical condition of the patient. This graft can be covered with an allogeneic skin graft, known as "sandwich" or mesh graft, which provides cover for the exposed areas. In cases where there is no possibility of autografting or when the patient has a more delicate clinical condition, the exclusive use of allogeneic skin is possible. The time to permanence grafted tissue at the injury site ranges from 3 to 5 weeks [9, 10].

Skin Defects Caused by Trauma

The allogeneic skin can also be used to cover skin defects caused by trauma, such as scalping and amputations [9, 10].

Chronic Wounds

The allogeneic skin preserved in glycerol can be useful as a first surgical step prior to conducting autologous grafts in cases of chronic wounds.

This tissue has a stimulating effect by cleaning and granulating the wound bed. An important effect is the reduction of pain [9, 10].

Glossary

Allogeneic skin Skin from an individual of the same species, but genetically distinct.

Autograft transplantation A skin graft transplantation from a donor area of the same patient.

Cryopreservation Preservation method of cells and tissues consisting in a progressive and slow decrease of temperature which, when combined with the use of cryoprotectants and buffered saline solutions, maintains cell viability.

References

1. Euro Skin Bank. [citado 31 de agosto de 2015]. Disponível em: http://www.euroskinbank.nl/.
2. Agência Nacional de Vigilância Sanitária - ANVISA. Resolução da Diretoria Colegiada – RDC n° 55, de 11 de dezembro de 2015.
3. Kearney JN. Guidelines on processing and clinical use of skin allografts. Clin Dermatol. 2005;23:357–64.
4. Blondet R, Gibert-Thevenin MA, Pierre C, et al. Skin preservation by programmed freezing. Br J Plast Surg. 1982;35:530–6.
5. Kagan RJ, Robb EC, Plessinger RT. Human skin banking. Clin Lab Med. 2005;25(3):587–605.
6. Papini R. Management of burn injuries of various depths. BMJ. 2004;329(7458):158–60.
7. Wood FM, Kolybaba ML, Allen P. The use of cultured epithelial autograft in the treatment of major burn injuries: a critical review of the literature. Burns. 2006;32(4):395–401.
8. Shevchenko RV, James SL, James SE. A review of tissue-engineered skin bioconstructs available for skin reconstruction. J R Soc Interface. 2010;7(43):229–58.
9. Rocha C. Histofisiologia e classificação das queimaduras: consequências locais e sistêmicas das perdas teciduais em pacientes queimados. Rev Interdiscip de Estudos Experimentais. 2009;1:140–7.
10. Carreirão S, Cardim V, Goldenberg D. Cirurgia Plástica. 1st ed. São Paulo: Editora Atheneu; 2005.

Marketing Influence on Body Image Perception: A Bioethical Perspective

54

João Batista Blessmann Weber

Key Points

- There has been a steady increase in the search for aesthetic-related procedures in the medical field
- The controversy about plastic surgery is based on the analysis of the patients' reasons for requesting surgical treatment
- Patients who undergo aesthetic surgery are members of a group of particularly vulnerable people
- Mass media plays a huge role in spreading stereotypes related to the aesthetics of body image
- Concerns about body image are often influenced by the media and social networks, leading to unhealthy behaviors

Introduction

Modern society has encountered countless ethical dilemmas in recent decades, mostly attributable to technological progress in biomedical sciences. These dilemmas may be related to the need to establish limits to the use of new technologies in order to ensure the integrity of people and all components of the environment [1].

Revolutionary advancements have occurred in the understanding, development, marketing, and dissemination of medical knowledge. There have recently been significant changes in the methods of research and practicing medicine, as well as in the variety of services that are considered relevant to healthcare. Linked to industrial progress, advances in medical technology have been remarkable. Sophisticated technologies have expanded the limits of diagnosis on one hand, and of intervention efficacy on the other [2].

This new scientific and technological reality, whose impact on the global economy is substantial, began about half a century ago. Undoubtedly, its capacity of transforming and intervening in the environment and in the human species has caused scientific and ethical perplexities for some time. Among the several healthcare technological innovations with immediate repercussions on people's lives, the production of highly potent antibiotics, assisted reproduction, gene therapy, and the use of new materials and medications in the field of aesthetics are worthy of mention. Furthermore, consumerism has led the world to a market economy, contributing to a situation whereby wealthy nations maintain other peoples under their economic, ideological, and, in some cases, religious domination [3].

A recurrent issue in today's society is how to establish limits between normal and abnormal,

J.B.B. Weber
Pontifical Catholic University of Rio Grande do Sul,
Porto Alegre, Brazil
e-mail: jbweber@pucrs.b

natural and artificial. Are people willing to break the rules of anatomic and physiologic normality they have created? Will they be dissatisfied with merely adapting their biological structure for the preservation of the species [3]?

Health sciences have seen a constant increase in the demand for aesthetic procedures. New techniques and products with this purpose have appeared on the market, and countless aesthetic clinics have opened across the world.

In the field of aesthetic surgery, bioethicists have focused on the discussion regarding freedom and autonomy of individuals requesting a procedure. However, aspects such as social pressure and the fact that the human body has been converted into a depository of contemporary society's imaginary ideals should be considered. This situation leads to the analysis of a patient's vulnerability and medical responsibility, which is much higher in aesthetic surgery than in cases with clear clinical indications or in medical emergencies [4].

Thus, a question arises: What would be the reason for patients to be increasingly seeking procedures aimed at improving or changing their appearance? Evidently, every human being is concerned with personal aesthetics. Everyone wants to have a pleasant appearance and good health. However, is this search for aesthetic procedures always aimed at improving the patient's health? What is the limit between health and sickness in the pursuit of an often unreachable perfection? All such aspects are inserted in a new form of reflection, so-called bioethics, which seeks to establish a dialogue between health sciences and morality. This reflection is an attempt to understand the consequences of the application of human knowledge for life and for the future of our planet [3].

Aesthetics

The word "aesthetics" derives from the Greek *aisthetiké* and means to perceive, to feel. It is a branch of philosophy concerned with the nature of beauty. Yet, how can we define what makes something beautiful? What are the traits and features that make a person beautiful? Are such standards constant over time [5]?

Throughout history, great philosophers have tried to define what makes something beautiful. For Plato (428–347 BC) and René Descartes (1596–1650), beauty would be inherent to the object, not depending, therefore, on the subject that perceives it. For Aristotle (384–22 BC), people are responsible for seeking the ideal of beauty, by means of order, proportion, and symmetry. For Hegel (1770–1831), beauty would be inherent to each individual's spiritual activity. In the Middle Ages, the concept of beauty was directly related to identification with God, and Thomas Aquinas (1225–1274) was the most important representative of that time. Finally, for David Hume (1711–1776), the taste for the beautiful would come from each individual, not being directly linked to the object itself [5].

As we can see, not even great philosophers have been able to determine what makes something beautiful, what is universally pleasing with no clear explanation. Then why do beauty standards change so frequently? How can aesthetic standards present, for instance, in Renoir's works, in which female bathers exhibit curvy, voluptuous bodies, have completely changed into today's anorexic standards? We need, therefore, to reflect on the relentless quest for bodily perfection through medical and dental procedures, which often offer great risks to the patient's health and are sometimes unnecessary or even futile.

Naini, Moss, and Gill have questioned whether human notions of facial beauty depend on each person's sense of perception or whether this sense is common to all persons. Is facial beauty a quality of the face observed, or does the sensitivity of the observer also depend on his or her own ideas, feelings, and judgments? The authors quote the philosopher David Hume (1741), who said "Beauty in things exists in the mind that contemplates them," and the writer Margaret Wolfe Hungerford (1878), famous for the sentence "Beauty is in the eye of the beholder." Both quotations, and their philosophical ideologies, assume that sensitivity is subjective to each person. However, if a specific face is universally pleasing, some part of our sensitivity must be common to all human beings [6].

Aesthetic Surgery and Bioethics

The popularity achieved by aesthetic surgery, the development of technological resources, and the proliferation of aesthetic clinics and cosmetic methods indicate the social pressure that currently exists, as a result of intolerance toward old age and the need to conform to universal and cultural standards of beauty. The strategies to confront this need or social desire have challenged the field of bioethics in an almost unprecedented way. Based on bioethics, we should ask ourselves: "For what purpose or reason should I analyze the case of a patient requesting an aesthetic treatment, if their decision is founded on the ultimate expression of freedom and autonomy of being or looking the way they like, and also if the satisfaction of this desire reflects directly on their project and quality of life?" So far, both plastic surgeons and general surgeons have been governed by the same morality and similar codes of ethics.

The term "aesthetic" is broad, since it includes all body interventions, with no necessity of experiencing psychological suffering. Such interventions are part of a satisfaction, a vanity, and a submission to a society that has placed a commercial aesthetic value on bodily beauty, through which it often profits [4].

The controversy over plastic surgery arises from the questioning of psychologists, anthropologists, sociologists, feminists, physicians, and even the general population about the motivation of those requesting an intervention. Assessing the patient's mental health is essential. Excessive concern is expressed by those undergoing aesthetic surgery when they do not adapt to social and cultural standards of beauty, according to the dictates of fashion. Body dissatisfaction, often imperceptible to others, may cause great psychological suffering, resulting in pain, shame, rejection, and emotional and mental instability, reducing the level of personal satisfaction. Since these are all subjective factors, adopting a common standard to all individuals is impossible. This suffering is rooted in the desire and the imagination of beauty. Thus, physical and mental well-being should guide us for meeting the patient's needs [4].

Patients undergoing aesthetic surgeries are part of a particularly vulnerable group. Therefore, they should receive special attention and care in order to prevent physical and mental issues derived from both interventions and results that do not meet their often unrealistic expectations [4].

In aesthetic surgery practice, there are two types of ethical issues. The primary issues arise when decision-making about a surgical procedure involves few ethical issues, because these individuals evidently suffer from a body malformation, such as congenital malformations and injuries caused by burns or serious accidents. The secondary issues, however, are seen with distrust and some ethical objection, because they are superficial or vanity-driven interventions that may unnecessarily place a healthy body at risk in order to improve its image, such as liposuction, rhinoplasty, facelift, and abdominoplasty [7], which often do not have medical indications or are even contraindicated in some cases.

The World Medical Association (WMA) Declaration on aesthetic treatments adopted at the 65th General Assembly, which took place in October of 2014 in Durban, South Africa, establishes ethical principles to be observed in aesthetic treatments (Box 54.1). According to the WMA, aesthetic treatment is defined as an intervention performed not to treat a lesion, disease, or deformity, but for nontherapeutic reasons, with the sole purpose of improving or changing the patient's physical appearance [8].

Box 54.1 Ethical Principles to Be Observed in Aesthetic Treatments Defined by the World Medical Association [8]

Ethical principles on aesthetic treatment

1. The patient's dignity, integrity, and confidentiality must always be respected
2. Physicians have a role in helping to identify unhealthy body images and to address and treat disorders when these exist
3. Aesthetic treatments must only be performed by practitioners with sufficient knowledge, skills, and experience of the interventions performed

4. All practitioners providing aesthetic treatments must be registered with and/or licensed by the appropriate regulatory authority. Ideally, the practitioner should also be authorized by this authority to provide these specific aesthetic treatments

5. All aesthetic treatments must be preceded by a thorough examination of the patient. The practitioner should consider all circumstances, physical and psychological, that may cause an increased risk of harm for the individual patient and should refuse to perform the treatment if the risk is unacceptable. This is especially true in the case of minors. Practitioners should always choose the most appropriate treatment option, rather than the most lucrative one

6. Minors may need or benefit from plastic medical treatments, but pure aesthetic procedures should not be performed on minors. If, in exceptional cases, aesthetic treatment is performed on a minor, it should only be done with special care and consideration and only if the aim of the treatment is to avoid negative attention rather than gain positive attention. All relevant medical factors, such as whether the minor is still growing or whether the treatment will need to be repeated at a later date, must be considered

7. The patient must consent explicitly to any aesthetic treatment, preferably in writing. Before seeking consent, the practitioner should inform the patient of all relevant aspects of the treatment, including how the procedure is performed, possible risks, and the fact that many of these treatments may be irreversible. The patient should be given sufficient time to consider the information before the treatment starts. When the patient requesting the treatment is a minor, the informed consent of his or her parents or legally authorized representative should be obtained

8. All aesthetic treatments performed should be carefully documented by the practitioner. The documentation should include a detailed description of the treatment performed, information on medications used, if any, and all other relevant aspects of the treatment

9. Aesthetic treatments must only be performed under strictly hygienic and medically safe conditions on premises that are adequately staffed and equipped. This must include equipment for treating life-threatening allergic reactions and other potential complications

10. Advertising and marketing of aesthetic treatments should be responsible and should not foster unrealistic expectations of treatment results. Unrealistic or altered photographs showing patients before and after treatments must not be used in advertising

11. Advertising and marketing of aesthetic treatments should never be targeted to minors

12. Practitioners should never offer or promote financial loans as a means of paying for aesthetic treatment

Next, we discuss some basic concepts of bioethics that are very important to lay the foundations for a reflection about this pursuit of body perfection through medical procedures, which is increasingly influenced by a globalized media and standardized ethical patterns.

Principles of Bioethics

The term bioethics emerged in 1971 with the publication of the book *Bioethics: A Bridge to the Future* by American oncologist Van Rensselaer Potter. The author suggested that there was need for a balanced relationship between human beings and the ecosystem in order to preserve life on Earth [1].

The scope of bioethics has become more comprehensive, especially in terms of biomedical sciences. There is concern about ethics in the care of human beings, whether they are patients seeking health care at public healthcare facilities, private healthcare clinics, and teaching hospitals, or individuals who participate in scientific research.

According to Nunes and Nunes, bioethics consists of a continuous search for wisdom, criticism, and use of information and knowledge to improve living conditions and preserve life. Bioethics involves a combination of humility, responsibility, and rationality aimed both at individual and collective welfare [9].

The purpose of clinical bioethics is to analyze and discuss the application of new values resulting from scientific development within a society that respects pluralism and accepts the differences. The conflicts that may arise in the patient–healthcare professional relationship must be analyzed according to ethical values; that is, a science of the foundations or principles of actions and moral values that constitute a set of cultural rules that regulate human actions [10].

The book by Beauchamp and Childress, *Principles of Biomedical Ethics*, written in 1979, led bioethics toward a line of thought known as "Principlism," a system of ethics used in the analysis of the problems related to biomedicine based on four basic moral principles to guide decision-making, both in clinical practice and in biomedical research with humans [11].

The four principles are nonmaleficence, beneficence, respect for autonomy, and justice. These are basic principles but are not absolute. Beauchamp and Childress did not establish a lexicographic order between these four fundamental principles. Only the context and the consequences of a specific ethical conflict will be able to establish the criteria to order them [11].

The application of these four basic principles is not an easy task, let alone a conclusive task. However, these principles can help people involved in a conflict seek the most ethical way to act, thus supporting the role of principlism [1].

The Principle of Respect for Autonomy

The word *autonomy* derives from the Greek terms *autos* (self) and *nomos* (rule or law) [11]. The principle of respect for autonomy accepts people's self-determination and their ability to make the best decisions based on what they believe [1]. In the context of clinical bioethics, this basic concept of principlism is the basis of informed consent as an active process in the health professional/patient relationship.

The concept of respect for autonomy is widely used to refer to a decision taken in terms of health care and research, both by patients and research subjects [11]. People must be able to decide on a course of action and implement this plan to practice autonomy [12]. Autonomous individuals act

freely according to their own will. By contrast, people who have reduced autonomy are controlled by others because they are unable to decide or act according to their desires and values. For instance, a person with severe mental disorder is not able to decide on what is best for her/him. Some people may also have reduced freedom, such as prisoners or other institutionalized individuals [11], therefore constituting a vulnerable population.

Hence, two fundamental conditions are necessary for an individual to be able to practice autonomy: freedom (to be free from controlling influences) and ability to act intentionally. However, the principle of autonomy can sometimes be overlapped by another moral principle. Therefore, the individual's autonomy is restricted when, for example, a personal choice is harmful to public health or to another person [11], or even during emergency medical care when the patient is not able to make a decision.

Children and adolescents may not have maturity and ability to make autonomous decisions; nevertheless, this does not mean that they do not deserve moral respect. Their legal guardians are responsible for protecting them and making the decisions. Clinical studies involving children and adolescents require the participants to sign an informed consent form in order to show their willingness to participate in the study. However, an informed consent form must also be signed by the participant's legal guardian, and must be written in a clear manner so that the child or adolescent is able to understand it.

The Principle of Nonmaleficence

The principle of nonmaleficence consists of a moral obligation not to create harm to the patient intentionally [12]. This obligation is often stricter than the obligation to help the patient. In any particular case health care may cause little harm to the patient, such as bleeding caused by needle puncture, but, at the same time, may confer greater associated benefit, such as the cure of a disease. Therefore, the obligation of beneficence takes priority over the obligation of nonmaleficence [11].

The Principle of Beneficence

The principle of beneficence is aimed at assuring the patient's well-being and interests according to the criteria of beneficence provided by the healthcare facility where people are seen. In practice, this principle involves using all skills and technical knowledge available to provide health care to patients to increase benefits and reduce risks [1].

Common morality requires us to contribute to other people's well-being. Based on the ethical principles, moral is responsible for determining what is "good" in a scenario or situation and measuring the weight of "good" against the risks in specific actions [12].

Morally, people must be treated not only with respect for their autonomy and without associated harm, but the treatment must also contribute to their well-being. The principle of beneficence is potentially more demanding than the principle of nonmaleficence, because the actions should be positive in helping others and not merely avoiding harmful acts [11]. Medical procedures that neither cause direct benefit to the patient nor produce harm can be described as futile treatments.

The Principle of Justice

The principle of justice is associated with equity issues related to the distribution of healthcare services, respect for people's rights, and respect for the laws morally accepted by the population [12]. The term "justice" cannot be confused with the term "moral." Justice is a moral principle, whereas the law enforces this principle within social life. According to Beauchamp and Childress, the principle of justice is a distributive expression of justice, that is, a fair, equitable, and appropriate distribution in society, according to rules that establish the terms of social cooperation [11].

The Patient–Health Professional Relationship and Decision-Making

Health interventions are focused on diagnosis and preventive or therapeutic treatment to achieve the maximum benefit for each patient. In addition, in clinical practice, risks are justified by the potential benefits associated with the procedure for each patient [11].

The medical visit is a factor that has an impact on autonomy and vulnerability. During these visits, patients deliberately express their willingness to change their bodies, talking about their reasons, desires, or fantasies, and trusting the physician to make their desires come true. After considering the type of treatment requested by the patient, the surgeon often lists the procedures that could improve the patient's appearance [4].

All procedures and techniques aimed at changing the body at the expense of health, putting the patient at risk, should be deeply analyzed considering their ethical aspects. No clinical or surgical intervention in the human body is totally safe. Biomedical or biotechnological interventions should be carried out according to ethical conducts consistent with the physical and moral integrity of the person [3].

However, there has been considerable discussion about the patient's role in decision-making in clinical situations that often involve conflict between respect for the patient's autonomy and care for his/her health, and between the patient's values and the health professional's values [13].

Unlike the old Hippocratic model, patients' needs, values, and moral principles must be taken into consideration. Patients can actively participate in decision-making in unique situations in their lives [14]. Health professionals keep their authority because they hold the technical knowledge on indications and contraindications of a specific treatment, always taking into account the needs and wishes of the patient. However, health professionals cannot transfer the full responsibility for these choices to patients, thus becoming mere service providers [11].

Hence, in an optimal model of the patient–health professional relationship, the professional is not the only one responsible for making the decisions. Instead, the decision-making process must be based on mutual and respectful participation. The role of health professionals is to help patients understand their situation and their illness, evaluating possible courses of action and expressing their desires and values. In this relationship, health professionals provide their scientific knowledge, including knowledge on different options available for the diagnosis and treatment of the patient's condition. At the same time, patients express their goals and values, according to which the risks and benefits of various treatment options can be evaluated. Based on this approach, choosing the best treatment for each specific patient includes the participation of both the patient and the health professional [13]. The decision is made with both agents sharing the responsibility. The patient expresses his or her will, and the health professional holds the scientific knowledge and is responsible for determining the most recommended actions for each case.

Informed Consent

As already mentioned, the principle of respect for the patient's autonomy is essential to understanding the informed consent as an active process in the patient–health professional relationship.

The code of ethics of health professionals and the standards for research involving human beings require the signatures of an informed consent form. Informed consents are required to make it possible for persons who undergo medical treatment or participate in studies to make independent choices, thus protecting patients and research subjects from harm. Such consents are also aimed at encouraging health professionals and researchers to take responsible actions when dealing with other people's life and health [11].

The objective of requiring patients and research subjects to provide informed consent is neither to protect health professionals against possible negligence claims nor even to produce evidence of good clinical practice. The main objective is to provide patients with all the information they need to make an autonomous decision in accordance with their interests. Therefore, providing informed consent is an active process of mutual decision-making to reduce the risk of alleged illegal actions. Communication between patients and health professionals is the beginning of a trust-based relationship [15].

Thus, the informed consent form should not be a document solely aimed at providing legal protection for health professionals. Instead, it should be an active process of mutual decision-making between patients and health professionals, considering technical issues (of professional responsibility) as well as the patients' values [16].

It is worth noting that judging values is a complex task because each individual has his or her own peculiarities. Therefore, it is essential that health professionals are aware of all the facts related to specific cases and that patients receive clear information on all possible outcomes of a specific treatment, as well as the risks and consequences that may arise. Only then will patients be able to decide on what they believe to be the best for them in an autonomous and informed manner.

Every patient must be respected, especially regarding the privacy and confidentiality of their data. Also, whenever there is associated conflicts of interest, this should be made clear to patients.

Aesthetic Medicine and the Media

Aesthetic medicine covers all types of medical procedures aimed at improving patients' physical appearance and psychological satisfaction by means of noninvasive or minimally invasive techniques for cosmetic procedures [17]. In a systematic review assessing the effect of experimental presentation of thin media images on body satisfaction, Groesz et al. [18] concluded that, from a sociocultural perspective, mass media disseminates a slender ideal that can lead to body dissatisfaction [18].

In a meta-analysis on the role of the media in the concepts of body image among young women, Grabe et al. [19] found that the body image shown in the media is directly related to women's widespread dissatisfaction with their own bodies, higher expenses to change their body appearance, and increased number of eating disorders. These effects are present in several outcomes in both experimental and correlational studies. Therefore, exposure in the media seems to be negatively related to women's body image regardless of assessment method, differences in individual variables, media type, age, or other characteristics of the studies. In addition, based on the result of this meta-analysis, the authors emphasized the importance of prevention and intervention, particularly in education and advertising. In terms of education, the media can be used to teach girls and women to become more active and more critical consumers of products related to body appearance to prevent the development of body dissatisfaction and disturbed eating behaviors. The use of models with medium-sized bodies in advertisements could help protect some women from developing body dissatisfaction or at least prevent the exacerbation of strict concepts about body image [19].

The current sociocultural theory provides a robust theoretical basis for understanding body dissatisfaction, claiming that the slender ideal is enhanced by various social influences [20]. The media is the most powerful and widespread type of influence [18].

Women who see skinny models in media images tend to have negative feelings about their bodies; and this is particularly truer for overweight women, because there is a larger discrepancy between the size of their bodies and those typically thin images shown in the media today [21].

Bergstrom, Neighbors, and Malheim conducted a study evaluating the effect of the media on body image disorder in 197 university students. The objective of the study was to investigate whether women who were overweight would care more about their appearance after seeing thin women in media images. The authors found that women with low self-esteem related to their body mass index cared more about their appearance after seeing images of thin women in comparison with women with high self-esteem or those who did not see the images. They also reported that the magnitude of the threat to the perception of their own body image depends, among other factors, on the discrepancy between their bodies and the comparison target [21]. Prieler and Choi stressed that the concern with body image dissatisfaction should go beyond the slender ideal as it may be related to various body parts, such as breast size, skin color, and shape of the eyes [22].

Mass media plays a huge role in spreading stereotypes related to the aesthetics of body image. The media can also establish and reinforce the standards for a perfect male body, emphasizing leanness and muscularity. Taking part in conversations on social networks about physical appearance may increase perceptions that the ideal male body is slim, tall, and muscular. Social media can also have a significant impact on body image in some men when they compare themselves with real or computer-manipulated muscular figures [23].

The interactive format and content of social media, such as the strong presence and exchange of multiple images, suggest that social media can significantly influence body image concepts through negative social comparisons [23]. Social media and contemporary digital technologies represent the arena where lessons are learned, attitudes are adopted, and body image concepts are created, disseminated, and transformed into strong beliefs [23]. Unlike conventional media, the Internet and social networks enable users to create and share messages in a streamlined manner. In addition, instant communication with other users on mobile devices is also made possible [23].

Body Image Disorders

As mentioned earlier, concerns with body image, often influenced by the media and social networks, exceeds a healthy limit when disorders related to body image are developed both in women and men. Diseases such as body dysmorphic disorder (BDD) and dysmorphophobia are increasingly common, affecting both men and women at different ages and from different sociocultural groups.

BDD has been included in the International Statistical Classification of Diseases and Related Health Problems (ICD-10 Version: 2016) of the World Health Organization, in Chapter V of the Mental and Behavioral Disorders within Somatoform disorders (F45), being classified as a hypochondriacal disorder (F45.2) [24]. Its essential feature is a persistent preoccupation with the possibility of having one or more serious and progressive physical disorders. Patients manifest persistent somatic complaints or a persistent preoccupation with their physical appearance. Normal or commonplace sensations and appearances are often interpreted by patients as abnormal and distressing, and attention is usually focused upon only one or two organs or systems of the body. Marked depression and anxiety are often present, and may justify additional diagnoses. The following conditions are classified as hypochondriacal disorder: body dysmorphic disorder, dysmorphophobia (nondelusional), hypochondriacal neuroses, hypochondriasis, and nosophobia; as well as delusional dysmorphophobia and fixed delusions about bodily functions or shape, which are classified as schizophrenia, schizotypal, and delusional disorders [24].

Dysmorphophobia is a psychiatric condition that is often diagnosed in doctor's offices. This disorder is problematic for patients and can be confusing for health professionals. A commonly undiagnosed condition, it can be detected by a few simple steps. Referral to a psychiatrist can be beneficial for most patients suffering from this disease [25].

When body dysmorphophobia is a possible diagnosis, any medical treatments with aesthetic purposes should be avoided and patients should be referred to a mental health center. This is very important for the patient's mental health but also because it is unlikely that the patient will be satisfied with the results of any aesthetic interventions [26].

Individuals with BDD may develop a variety of compulsive behaviors related to the body part of interest [27]. These behaviors are called compulsive because they occur repeatedly. Some examples include checking a specific part of the body in the mirror, comparing their body with other people's bodies, repeatedly using makeup, or camouflaging a body part with clothes [27].

BDD is a condition associated with dissatisfaction with physical appearance in combination with repetitive behaviors associated with these defects. BDD affects both men and women with approximately the same intensity, but a variant called muscle dysmorphia develops more often in men [28]. Muscle dysmorphia is a pathologic concern that the body is not muscular enough. It occurs as a relatively new form of body image disorder in men. Men with this disorder believe that they are small, when they actually are of normal size or even very muscular. Men with any type of BDD should be carefully evaluated for the presence of muscle dysmorphia, because men with concerns about other parts of their bodies may also have muscle dysmorphia, which appears to be associated with a major psychopathology [29].

Pope et al. [29] evaluated men with BDD and compared those with a history of muscle dysmorphia with those with BDD who did not have muscle dysmorphia. Men with muscle dysmorphia were similar to other men in terms of demographic factors, severity of BDD, delusion, and number of body parts with related muscular dissatisfaction [29].

Future Perspectives

As we can see, marketing has a negative influence on body image perception in both men and women from different sociocultural groups, bringing many severe diseases. Ethical dilemmas, such as respect for autonomy, can arise when an increasing number of patients seek perfection in their bodies through aesthetic procedures.

We must reflect on this incessant search for perfection of the body through medical and dental procedures, which can bring risks to patient health and often be unnecessary or futile.

It is therefore essential that prevention of such body image disorders becomes a major priority in the care of human health. This can be achieved by using the media to spread concepts of health and to prevent the development of body dissatisfaction and disturbed eating behaviors.

References

1. Clotet J, Feijó AGS. Bioética: uma visão panorâmica. In: Clotet J, Feijó AGS, Oliveira MG, editors. Bioética: uma visão panorâmica. Porto Alegre: EDIPUCRS; 2011. Cap. 1. 280p.

2. Kalekin-Fishman D. The impact of globalization on the determination and management of ethical choices in the health arena. Soc Sci Med. 1996;43(5):809–22.

3. Drumond JGF. Ética, Bioética y los desafios del siglo XXI. Rev Fac Derecho. 2012;69:65–79.

4. Viesca MRR. La Vulnerabilidad humana frente a la cirugía estética. Rev Med Ins Mex Seguro Soc. 2012;50(1):81–6.

5. Weber JBB. Estética e Bioética. Rev AMRIGS. 2011;55(3):302–5.

6. Naini FB, Moss JP, Gill DS. The enigma of facial beauty: esthetics, proportions, deformity and controversy. Am J Orthod Dentofac Orthop. 2006;130:277–82.

7. Hans T. Aspectos éticos de la cirurgia plástica y reconstructiva. Cuadernos de Bioética. 1989;XIX(1):131–45.

8. World Medical Association. WMA statement on aesthetic treatment. Available at: http://www.wma.net/en/30publications/10policies/a13/. Accessed on 25 Jan 2016.

9. Nunes CRR, Nunes AP. Bioética Rev Bras Enferm. 2004;57(5):615–6.

10. Oliveira RA, Jorge FI. Bioética Clínica: como praticá-la? Rev Col Bras Cir. 2010;37(3):245–6.

11. Beauchamp TL, Childress JF. Principles of biomedical ethics. New York: Oxford University Press; 2013.

12. Lawrence DJ. The four principles of biomedical ethics: a foundation for current bioethical debate. J Chiropr Humanit. 2007;14:34–40.

13. Emanuel EJ, Emanuel L. The physician-patient relationship. JAMA. 1992;267(16):2221–6.

14. Francesconi CF, Goldim JR. Bioética clínica. In: Clotet J, Feijó AGS, Oliveira MG, editors. Bioética: uma visão panorâmica. Porto Alegre: EDIPUCRS; 2011. Cap. 4. 280p.

15. Petruzzi MNMR, Pithan LH, Figueiredo MAZ, Weber JBB. Informed consent in dentistry: a standard of good clinical practice. Rev Odonto Cienc. 2013;28(1):23–7.

16. Pithan LH. O consentimento informado como exigência ética e jurídica. In: Clotet J, Feijó AGS, Oliveira MG, editors. Bioética: uma visão panorâmica. Porto Alegre: EDIPUCRS; 2011. Cap. 10. 280p.

17. American Academy of Aesthetic Medicine. What is aesthetic medicine? Available at: https://www.aaamed.org/aesthetic_med.php. Accessed on 19 Jan 2016.

18. Groesz LM, Levine MP, Murnen SK. The effect of experimental presentation of thin media images on body satisfaction: a meta-analytic review. Int J Eat Disord, Int J Eat Disord. 2002;31(1):1–16.

19. Grabe S, Hyde JS, Ward LM. The role of the media in body image concerns among women: a meta-analysis of experimental and correlational studies. Psychol Bull. 2008;134(8):460–76.

20. Thompson JK, Heinberg LJ, Altabe M, Tantleff-Dunn S. Exacting beauty: theory, assessment, and treatment of body image disturbance. Washington, DC: American Psychological Association; 1999. 396p.

21. Bergstrom RL, Neighbors C, Malheim JE. Media comparisons and threats to body image: seeking evidence of self-affirmation. J Soc Clin Psychol. 2009;28(2):264–80.

22. Prieler M, Choi J. Broadening the scope of social media effect research on body image concerns. Sex Roles. 2014;71:378–88.

23. Perloff RM. Social media effects on Young women's body image concerns: theoretical perspectives and agenda for research. Sex Roles. 2014;71:363–77.

24. World Health Organization. International statistical classification of diseases and related health problems 10th Revision (ICD-10)-WHO Version for:2016. Available at: http://apps.who.int/classifications/icd10/browse/2016/en. Accessed on 26 Jan 2016.

25. Varma A, Rastogi R. Recognizing body dysmorphic disorder (dysmorphophobia). J Cutan Aesthet Surg. 2015; Jul-Sep;8(3):165–8.

26. Newton JT, Cunningham SJ. Great expectations: what do patients expect and how can expectations be managed? J Orthod. 2013;40:112–7.

27. Phillips KA, Menard W, Fay C, Pagano ME. Psychosocial functioning and quality of life in body dysmorphic disorder. Comp Psychiat. 2005;46:254–60.

28. Phillipou A, Castle D. Body dysmorphic disorder in mem. Aust Fam Physician. 2015;44(11):798–801.

29. Pope CG, Pope HG, Menard W, Roberto O, Phillips KA. Clinical features of muscle dysmorphia among males with body dysmorphic disorder. Body Imag. 2005;2(4):395–400.

Recommended Reading

Ethics in Medicine. University of Washington School of Medicine. https://depts.washington.edu/bioethx/topics/consent.html.

Potter VR. Bioethics: bridge to the future. Prentice-Hall; 1971. 205p.

Quality of Life in Dermatology

Magda Blessmann Weber, Mariele Bevilaqua, and Rebeca Kollar Vieira da Silva

Key Points Summary

- This chapter presents the importance of quality of life evaluation in dermatology, and the clinician's role in this new treatment approach
- Reviews and describes quality of life scales used in dermatology in general
- Sets scales used in pediatric dermatology and their importance in treatment compliance
- Provides, in addition, information about specific scales made for particular dermatoses and family members

Introduction

Quality of life (QoL) is an expression that suggests considerable interpretation and involves important issues such as social welfare, health, family, prosperity, emotional condition, and others [1, 2]. This expression was clearly defined by the Quality Group of Life from the World Health Organization (WHO) as "the individuals'

perception of their role in life, in the context of culture and value systems in which they are supported to, and in related to their goals, expectations, standard of living and concerns" [3].

Dermatologic diseases frequently have an unpleasant effect on patients' emotional conditions, social life, and daily activities because of the stigmas resulting from the lesions' appearance [4, 5]. It is estimated that one-third of dermatologic patients have emotional aspects associated with their dermatosis [6]. Because of the common trajectory between ectoderm, skin, and the central nervous system, they present a close connection. This connection leads to the assumption that the skin and central nervous system can influence each other, which has been shown in several studies of skin diseases, such as systemic lupus erythematosus, psoriasis, acne, and alopecia areata. In these specific dermatoses it is clear that an unbalanced psychic condition can be triggered and negatively exacerbated by the underlying skin disease [7–9].

Moreover, the context of psychological distress related to acne does not affect only the patient. Considering health as a multifactorial concept, family members are also affected by the consequences of acne, and they too could develop emotional disorders. According to a dermatologic study in 2013, conducted by researchers from southern Brazil, this connection between psychological factors and dermatosis is substantive. The authors pointed out that 42% of

M.B. Weber (✉) • M. Bevilaqua • R.K.V. da Silva
Dermatology Service of Federal University of Health Sciences of Porto Alegre, Porto Alegre, Brazil
e-mail: mbw@terra.com.br

© Springer International Publishing Switzerland 2018
R.R. Bonamigo, S.I.T. Dornelles (eds.), *Dermatology in Public Health Environments*,
https://doi.org/10.1007/978-3-319-33919-1_55

caregivers of pediatric patients suffering vitiligo had anxiety symptoms and 26% had depressive symptoms [10].

The importance of having standard tools that consider QoL is based on the appreciation of the patient's subjective experience of living with the disease. This subjective aspect is a measure of the relationship between the patient's living conditions and psychosocial state. Monitoring the report from the patient's point of view on the feelings regarding the disease is the best way to conduct an assessment of QoL [11].

The analysis of the responses in QoL questionnaires allows clinics to accurately set this connection [12]. In arbitrary clinical trials, the estimation of QoL was recently added as the third dimension to be studied in addition to the efficiency and safety of the medications [4]. Tools that assess QoL should not be limited to the reporting of symptoms but should also include the way the patient faces the disease and its improvement [13].

Table 58.1 Main scales measuring quality of life in a global evaluation of the patient

Name of scale	First time mentioned in	Version in Portuguese
WHOQOL-100 (World Health Organization Quality of Life Assessment)	The WHOQOL Group [3]	WHOQOL-100 Fleck et al. [14]
WHOQOL-Bref	The WHOQOL Group [15]	WHOQOL – Bref Fleck et al. [16]
SF-36 (36-Item Short Form Health Survey)	Ware et al. [18]	Brasil SF-36 Ciconelli et al. [20]
NHP (Nottingham Health Profile)	Lindholm et al. [21]	Perfil de Saúde de Nottingham Teixeira-Salmela et al. [22]
SIP (Sickness Impact Profile)	Gilson et al. [23]	PSIP Feio et al. [26] (Portuguese version for Portugal)
PGI (Patient-Generated Index)	Ruta et al. [30]	–

State of Art

The assessment of QoL in dermatology as measured by scales began with the Dermatology Quality of Life Index (DLQI) designed by Finlay and his team [1]. Since then, the use of similar instruments has become increasingly common. Moreover, it is confirmed as valid and effective, a fact that indicates QoL as one of the pillars of medical care in dermatology and a standard part of routine clinical dermatology [13].

The use of QoL questionnaires, associated with both detailed study of subdivisions covering the different areas that constitute the concept of QoL to be evaluated, and the use of more than one scale for the same analysis, constitutes an effective tool.

Quality of Life Scales in General

Questionnaires for QoL assessment can be applied in three forms: by personal interview or phone, by mail, or by self-application. The first requires more resources, but ensures compliance and reduces errors and losses; the second is

cheaper, but increases the number of losses because of lower reliability of the data; while the third reduces errors and losses, but is limited by its simple structure. Besides these there is a form of administration by Internet, which is not very practical [2]. The most widely used tools for global patient consideration nowadays are listed in Table 58.1.

World Health Organization Quality of Life Assessment (WHOQOL-100)

Given the importance of the concept of QoL and after several discussions about questionnaires that assess QoL, the WHO developed, in 1994 [16], a tool whose intention is general in nature [3]. The WHOQOL-100 consists of 100 items that assess QoL in six areas: physical, psychological, level of independence, personal relationships, environment, and spiritual aspects/religion and beliefs [18]. This instrument, also valid for Brazilian practice [14], although rather comprehensive and complete, requires a long time for its completion, making it difficult its use in routine care.

WHOQOL-Bref

Because of the time taken for completion of WHOQOL-100, in 1998 the same WHO group developed the WHOQOL-Bref, a shorter tool with similar internal validity. It consists of 26 questions, two of which are related general issues of QoL; the other questions are divided into four areas: physical, psychological, personal relationships, and environment [16].

The 36-Item Short-Form Health Survey (SF-36)

This instrument evaluates both the health condition and the QoL generally, and is used in research and clinical practice [17–19]. It can be implemented by phone or interviewer, or be self-administered. It consists of 36 items, divided into eight areas: functional capacity, physical aspects, pain, general health, mental health, emotional aspects, social functioning, and vitality. It also contains a question of comparative assessment between current mental health conditions and the same conditions 1 year previously [18]. Despite being relatively short, it is a comprehensive questionnaire with broad coverage of all areas related to the concept of health, enabling the detection of small to moderate differences among groups [18, 19]. It can be used by different populations to allow comparison between several diseases [20].

Nottingham Health Profile (NHP)

The NHP was developed in England and was also validated in Switzerland. It considers questions about the patient's discomfort related to pain, physical mobility, sleep, energy, emotional reactions, and social isolation, items presented in the first part of the instrument, and has been used to check the impact on QoL of chronic leg ulcer patients [21, 22].

Sickness Impact Profile (SIP)

This tool is not connected to the disease diagnosis but considers the patient's conduct, and is considered widely applicable among different diseases and cultural groups [23, 24]. It is a validated, estimated, and effective instrument to assess the health conditions of a specific population and the changing nature of these conditions over time, or also to compare different population groups [23, 25]. It covers appropriate healthcare effects and can be used for assessment, planning, and formulation of health policy, aiming not only at improving mortality/morbidity rates but also reducing the impact of diseases on daily activities [23, 24]. The SIP is composed of 136 statements about health related to disorders in 12 areas of activity, and can be self-administered; it has a Portuguese version fulfilled in Portugal [23–26]. The respondent points out only those statements that seem to be true at that time [23]. There is an English version of the SIP, the UKSIP (United Kingdom Sickness Profile), in a similar format to the previous one, but with particular percentage results. It has high internal consistency and reproducibility and has been used for psoriasis [27], acne [28], and atopic dermatitis (AD) [29].

Patient-Generated Index (PGI)

The PGI is a three-step assessment instrument developed in 1994. As a first step, the patient sets the five most affected areas by disease; in the second step, the patient grades the less important to more important areas that affect life quality between 0 and 100; and finally the patient shares "60 points" among the listed items according to his/her concept of necessity of improvement in those areas. The index ranges from 0 to 100: the higher the score, the lower the QoL. The purpose of this questionnaire is to calculate the effect of the disease on QoL according to relevance in the context of daily life as estimated by the patient [30].

Quality of Life Scales in Dermatology

The development and the confirmation of specific QoL questionnaires for Dermatology is a new tool of assessment [31]. General questionnaires, used for all types of dermatoses, allow comparisons

Table 58.2 Main scales measuring quality of life in a dermatologic evaluation of the patient

Name of scale	First time mentioned in	Version in Portuguese
DLQI (Dermatology Life Quality Index)	Finlay et al. [5]	DLQI Ferraz et al. [48]
Skindex	Chren et al. [38]	Skindex-29 Paula et al. [52]
DSQL (Dermatology-Specific Quality of Life)	Anderson et al. [37]	–

between them and also an overview of their involvement in the patient's QoL. These questionnaires can be applied to patients in different clinical categories and can also be applied to groups under control [19]. There is also a trend toward the combination of two questionnaires, a general and a dermatologic one, with combined evaluation of each measurement [32]. In addition, there are questionnaires for childhood dermatosis, some of them containing images [33–35].

The most validated and currently used questionnaires are the DLQI (Dermatology Life Quality Index) – QoL Index for Dermatology, Skindex (with its simplified version, Skindex-29) m and DSQL (Dermatology-Specific Quality of Life) – Specific QoL for Dermatology. These instruments are self-applicable, reproducible, with shelf life and acceptable confidence [36–38]; some of these tools can even be sent by mail [19, 35, 39], as described below and summarized in Table 58.2.

Dermatology Life Quality Index (DLQI)

In 1995, Finlay et al. [5] created and validated this instrument in order to allow simple, minor, and regular assessment of skin diseases in general, such as psoriasis [40–43], AD [41, 44], other eczemas [40, 43], and vitiligo [45]. The questions refer to facts from a week before the administration of the questionnaire, which can be completed in about 3–5 min, and are relevant to outpatients aged between 15 and 75 years [5, 36].

The instrument consists of ten items divided into six groups: symptoms and feelings, daily activities, recreation, job, school, personal relationships, and treatment. Responses set scores of 0–3, and the final calculation is a simple sum of these scores, with the highest rates indicating the worst QoL associated with the disease [5].

This tool is easily used in many contexts, such as clinical or research situations, for inpatients, outpatients, or control patients [19, 36, 46, 47]. By the end of 2003, the DLQI was translated and validated in Brazil in 2006 [48], allowing the assessment of the impact of diseases such as alopecia areata, Darier's disease, lichen planus, and viral warts [49, 50].

Skindex-29

The Skindex-29 is a simplified version of the self-administered questionnaire Skindex. This version, widely used at present, was designed in 1997 and contains 61 items divided into eight levels: cognitive effects, social effects, depression, fear, embarrassment, anger, physical discomfort, and physical limits [38].

The Skindex-29 version contains 29 items and an additional one related to adverse effects of treatment, divided into three different parts: symptoms, functionality, and emotions [51]. The probable answers are: never, rarely, sometimes, often, and always, given in a scale from 1 to 5 points, with the final score calculated either by the average of obtained points from the 29 questions (total score) or by the average from the items of each domain (domain score). In Brazil the validation and adoption of this tool is recent, being conceived in 2014 [52].

Dermatology-Specific Quality of Life (DSQL)

The DSQL was developed as an easy to use comprehensive tool for use in dermatologic clinical trials and observational studies [37, 53]. It is more elaborate and takes longer in its application (15 min) than previous versions. It contains 52 items, 43 of them specific and nine related to emotional well-being, in general, taken from the SF-36 questionnaire. It includes seven different levels: physical symptoms, day-to-day activities, social functioning, general mental health, vitality, job functionality, and school [37].

Quality of Life Scales Specific for the Evaluation of Pediatric Patients in Dermatology

At present, the estimation of the QoL in pediatric patients is relevant in medical practice. Because of this, in randomized clinical trials it has been added as a third particular aspect to be studied besides the safety and efficacy of the medication [54].

Dermatoses are taken as a relevant subject, given the aspects of negative psychological impact the disease confers, such as problems in the cognitive process, and difficulties in school learning and in the social and family environment. In addition, the disease could cause mild to severe mood disorders and personality disorder. Moreover, even interest in sports activities can be adversely affected by skin disease because of its strong relationship with low infant self-esteem [55].

In an extensive study of skin disease in the United Kingdom including a group of 64 pediatric patients with pruritus, AD, or psoriasis, a relationship between clinical worsening and an adverse event in patients' life was observed. As a result, a clinical improvement occurred 5 years later, after these stress factors were removed [56].

Over recent years further studies evaluating the QoL in children with specific dermatoses such as AD [57], vitiligo [58] and epidermolysis bullosa [59] have been conducted worldwide, reflecting the increasing importance of this aspect of treatment, demonstrating a shift in the relevant position of improving the effectiveness of health care for such conditions.

A study conducted in São Paulo in 2008 compared pediatric patients with chronic diseases with apparently healthy patients and observed a lower QoL in patients with chronic diseases using the Quality Index Pediatric Life (PedsQL) questionnaire. The study distributed the questionnaire separately, with the same queries, among pediatric patients and the relative who was accompanying them to consultations, whereby a correlation between the information in the physical and educational aspects was observed, but there was disagreement with their views on the psychological aspects [60]. Another study has successfully applied the PedsQL, translated to Portuguese, in pediatric patients with neoplasms [61].

The family impact that acne causes is extremely important in the treatment and needs to be addressed during patient care, since the child's environment is greatly affected by conditions caused by the disease, in addition to the stigma suffered. The need to evaluate the QoL of the family heralds the development and improvement of this type of analysis in order to effectively evaluate how the disease can change the functioning of the group [57–59].

This section describes the most widely used scales for the assessment of QoL in pediatric patients (Table 58.3).

Table 58.3 Main scales measuring quality of life in a dermatologic evaluation of the pediatric patient

Name of scale	First time mentioned in	Version in Portuguese
PedsQL (Pediatric Quality of Life Inventory)	Varni et al. [62]	BR-PedsQL Scarpelli et al. [61]
DFI (Family Dermatosis Family Impact)	Lawson et al. [94]	O Impacto da Dermatite Atópica Infantil na Família Weber et al. [66]
CDLQI (Children's Dermatology Life Quality Index)	Lewis-Jones et al. [33]	BR-CDLQI Prati et al.[63]
IDQoL (Infants' Dermatitis Quality of Life Index)	Lewis-Jones et al. [35]	Índice de Qualidade de Vida da Dermatite Atópica em Crianças Alvarenga et al. [109]
AUQEI (Quality of Life Scale for Children)	Manificat and Dazord [64]	AUQEI Assumpção et al. [65]

Pediatric Quality of Life Inventory (PedsQL 4.0)

The general questionnaire PedsQL assesses items in physical, emotional, social, and educational dimensions. The PedsQL (Pediatric Quality of Life Inventory™) version 4 [61] has 23 issues in: (1) physical dimension (eight items); (2) emotional dimension (five items); (3) social dimension (five items); and educational dimension (five items). These dimensions were developed by discussion groups, cognitive interviews, pretests, and protocols of mensuration development. Completion of the tool takes 5 min [62]. It is compose by parallel forms of self-evaluation of children's and parents' questionnaires. The child self-evaluation includes children aged 5–7, 8–12, and 13–18 years. The parents' questionnaire includes ages 2–4 (preschool), 5–7 (toddler), 8–12 (child), and 13–18 years (teenager), and assesses the parental perception of QoL in the child. Besides the PedsQL, other questionnaires have been developed to evaluate relatives' QoL.

Children's Dermatology Life Quality Index (CDLQI)

This questionnaire was made to assess the QoL of patients aged 4–16 years, presenting a structure similar to that of the DLQI and FDI [33], and a scale that assesses pediatric patients' welfare in dermatologic-specific fashion, with the goal of allowing a simple, compact, and uniform assessment in several contexts for patients presenting general dermatologic disease such as psoriasis, AD, other eczemas, vitiligo, and nevus.

The CDLQI tool in its nonillustrated form was previously translated and validated in Brazil by Prati et al. as *Escore da Qualidade de Vida na Dermatologia Infantil*. Besides giving a general index of QoL related to the patient's skin disease, it helps to assess how each patient's life aspect is affected [63].

This tool consists of ten questions subdivided into six categories: symptoms and feelings, daily activities, recreation, school, personal relation-ships, and treatment. The answers score between 0 and 3 and the final count is a simple sum of these scores. The highest score indicates the worst QoL related to the evaluated disease.

In 2003, a more appealing illustrated version of the CDLQI emerged [34]. Colorful and friendly dog drawings were added to questions, keeping the original text. The comparison among the versions shows that they produce similar results, suggesting that they may be equivalents. However, the illustration was quickly adopted as it was considered easier by children and parents.

The Infants' Dermatitis Quality of Life Index (IDQoL)

The IDQOL was developed as a method to assess impairment of QoL in infants with AD in a clinical setting and in conjunction with an instrument for assessing clinical severity, such as the SCORAD [14] or SASSAD [15].

The IDQOL was derived from parental views of the impairment of QoL caused by their children's eczema. It was produced and validated in 2001, with the goal of assessing children under 4 years old. It is quick and simple to complete, containing ten questions about symptoms and difficulties of mood, sleep (two questions), play time, family activities, mealtime, treatments, dressing, and bathing. The highest score for each question is 3, leading to a maximum total possible score of 30. There is an additional question scored separately, asking for the parents' assessment of current dermatitis severity, giving four options, from none to extremely severe (0–4).

It is sensitive to treatment changes but presents a weak correlation with severity of the clinical condition [35]. It is estimated that some of the parameters used by parents may show some impairment in "normal" infants. The authors demonstrated that the IDQOL is simple to use in an outpatient setting or by postal survey. It is not based on clinicians' views and has been characterized from the test–retest results to have good reproducibility.

The Quality of Life Scale for Children (AUQEI)

The AUQEI was developed by Manificat and Dazord [64], and assessed and translated by Assumpção et al. [65]. This questionnaire gives a profile of the child's satisfaction and welfare degree in different situations, based on four images that represent the answers: very happy, happy, discontented, and very discontented, associated with several QoL domains.

In studies conducted in 2012 in a dermatology referral center in southern Brazil [66], it was observed that the results taken from AUQEI and CDLQI indicate that the general QoL of the child is less affected than the QoL domains specifically related to dermatosis.

Quality of Life Scales in Specific Dermatoses

The QoL assessment in dermatologic patients is affected by the stigma and the disease's presentation characteristics, and for this reason some scales are applied in a specific way, according to the patient's dermatosis, as shown in Table 58.4.

Psoriasis

Psoriasis can initiate deep effects in patients' functionality and welfare [32, 67]. The dermatologic treatments are sometimes only temporary, with a large impact on QoL of these patients. There are several tools for the assessment of QoL in psoriasis, with the correct choice of instrument depending on the study subject, the patient's characteristics, and the psychometric measures of the chosen questionnaire [32, 42]. Among the available tools, the following are worthy of mention.

Psoriasis Disability Index (PDI)
Inability caused by psoriasis is defined by the PDI as practical aspects of a patient's life changed by the disease appearance that can be confirmed by an observer.

Table 58.4 Main scales measuring quality of life in specific dermatoses

Name of scale	First time mentioned in	Name in Portuguese
Psoriasis		
PDI (Psoriasis Disability Index)	Finlay et al. [68]	–
PLSI (Psoriasis Life Stress Inventory)	Gupta et al. [70]	–
PSORIQoL (Psoriasis Index of Quality of Life)	McKenna et al. [71]	–
Acne		
ADI (Acne Disability Index – Índice de Incapacidade para a Acne	Motley and Finlay [76]	–
CADI (Cardiff Acne Disability Index)	Motley and Finlay [77]	–
APSEA (Assessment of the Psychological and Social Effects of Acne)	Oakley [74]	–
Acne-QoL	Martin et al. [79]	–
UKSIP (United Kingdom Sickness Profile)	Salek et al. [28]	–
Vitiligo		
VLQI (Vitiligo Life Quality Index)	Senol et al. [110]	–
VitiQol (Vitiligo Specific Health Related Quality of Life Instrument)	Lilly et al. [111]	VitiQoL-PB Boza et al. [108]
VIS-22 (Vitiligo Impact Scale-22)	Gupta et al. [112]	–
Melasma		
MelasQoL (Melasma Quality of Life Scale)	Lieu et al. [85]	MelasQol-PORT Cestari et al. [86]
Dermatitis of the scalp		
Scalpdex	Chen et al. [97]	–
Atopic dermatitis		
QoLIAD (Quality of Life Index for Atopic Dermatitis)	Whalley et al. [100]	–
ADDI (Atopic Dermatitis Disability)	Eun et al. [101]	–
Itch		
ItchyQo	Poindexter et al. [95]	–
Latex allergy		
QoLLA-C e QoLLA-P (Quality of Life in Latex Allergy – Children and Parents)	Lewis-Jones et al. [107]	–

This scale, translated to Brazilian Portuguese as *Índice de Incapacidade Causada Pela Psoríase*, includes 44 variables distributed as: 28 questions related to loss on daily activities, professional activities, personal relationship, recreation, and treatment, all of them during the last 4 weeks; and nine additional questions that refers to the patient's symptoms and feelings related to the disease. In addition, the involved area is analyzed [68].

Finlay et al., comparing the use of the PDI questionnaire in a compact version (15 questions) with the questionnaire to assess the general SIP QoL, showed a good correlation between these two methods, demonstrating a good applicability of PDI because of the short time necessary for completion [25]. A second study suggests the use of 10 questions from the compact questionnaire (15 questions) proposed by Finlay. The author advocates that three of these questions would not distinguish patients with psoriasis from those with dermatologic conditions, while the other two must be punctuated negatively (the opposite of the proposed, whereby a low assessment would result in a high score) [69].

Psoriasis Life Stress Inventory (PLSI)

The PLSI assesses the resulting stress from the impact of the disease on QoL, involving 15 situations associated with psoriasis and the degree of stress associated with these events. With an average completion time of between 10 and 15 min, it must be used in subgroups of patients with a high psychological impact level associated with the disease [70].

Psoriasis Index of Quality of Life (PSORIQoL)

This is the newest tool to evaluate QoL in psoriasis. McKenna et al. [71] developed 25 dichotomous items, which inform about, among others, issues such as socialization, self-esteem, limitations in personal freedom, emotional stability, and sleep disturbance. The authors claim that the questions do not access direct injuries or deficits, as in the other questionnaires, but highlight the impact of these and other influences in the QoL. The applicability of PSORIQoL in clinical studies has yet to be demonstrated [71].

Acne

Acne causes emotional, social, and psychological changes severe enough to justify specific tools to assess the QoL of these patients [72]. Tools made for acne have been more specific than the general questionnaire [73]. The most widely uses nowadays include the following.

Acne Disability Index (ADI)

Consisting of 48 questions, the ADI has eight dimensions: psychological, physical, recreational, professional, self-image, social reaction, skin care, and financial care [74, 75]. It associates the patient's social and psychological prejudice with the severity of the acne on different parts of the body [76].

Cardiff Acne Disability Index (CADI)

The CADI consists of a form with five questions derived from the ADI [77] and presents good internal consistency in comparison with ADI and UKSIP [17, 31]. It correlates the acne severity on the face and midsection, and is useful to identify patients with low self-esteem who are seeking less invasive treatment, and to assess the treatment effect [77, 78]. Scores, however, do not correlate well with the severity of the clinical condition [74].

Assessment of the Psychological and Social Effects of Acne (APSEA)

This scale was developed by the use of a psychological and social approach in different questionnaires about disability related to acne beyond ADI [79].

Overall, 15 items comprise the APSEA, nine of which are scored on a linear visual analog scale from 0 to 10, and the remaining six by response selection with score allocation of 0, 3, 6, and 9. The maximum achievable score of 144 represents the greatest disability. Although none of the questions are specific for facial acne, the APSEA correlates with facial acne grade but not the total acne grade [80].

Acne Quality of Life Scale (Acne-QoL)

This tool estimates the effect of facial acne in QoL and the impact of treatment in clinical trials.

The 19 questions explore four dimensions: personal perceptions, social life, emotional condition, and symptoms related to acne [81]. The Acne-QoL presents good applicability, shelf life, and internal consistency [82], and the scales of QoL strongly correlate with the severity reported by patients in comparison with that reported by the clinician, suggesting that the patient's perceptions of the disease may be more important than the obtained results [32].

United Kingdom Sickness Profile (UKSIP)

This is the UK version of the SIP, developed by Salek in 1986. It is a self-administered questionnaire containing 136 health-related statements covering 12 areas of daily activity, seven of them aggregated into physical and psychosocial dimensions. The final score is expressed as a percentage. The questions in the UKSIP relate to the situations on the day of completion based on the respondent's usual activity. In addition to the detailed statement questions, patients are also asked to rate their "overall health" on a 5-point scale ranging from "very good" to "very poor" [28].

Vitiligo

Parsad et al., in 2003, evaluated the impact of social and psychological difficulties in treatment response of patients suffering vitiligo, using the DLQI for the assessment. According to the results, a worse index of QoL would be related to responses less favorable to treatments, suggesting that a psychological approach could be more valuable, attesting the importance of measurement not only of lesion severity but also the leverage on patients' day-to-day activity [47]. The QoL assessment of patients suffering vitiligo by the DLQI in a nonclinical scenario also appeared to be effective, but with a weak correlation with sex and age [83].

Vitiligo Life Quality Index (VLQI)

In 2012, Asl Şenol et al., in Turkey, created the VLQI in English, evaluating specifically the QoL in patients suffering vitiligo. The scale is com-

posed of 25 questions that assess emotions, personal relationships, anxiety, work/school life, leisure, and symptoms. The answer for each question can be evaluated as: "never" = 1; "sometimes" = 2; "often" = 3; "all the time" = 4. The total score varies between 25 and 100. Higher scores mean worse QoL.

Vitiligo-Specific Health-Related Quality of Life Instrument (VitiQoL)

In the United States the Vitiligo Specific Health Related Quality of Life Instrument (VitiQoL) has been validated by Lilly et al. It is a questionnaire to specifically evaluate the QoL in individuals suffering vitiligo. The VitiQoL has 15 items, scoring from 0 ("not at all") to 6 ("all the time") for each question, and therefore achieves a total score between 0 and 90. It assesses the domains of participation limitation, stigma, and behavior. Moreover, it presents a personal assessment of vitiligo severity via a scale ranging from 0 (without skin involvement) to 6 (most severe), which leads to the 16th question in the questionnaire. This questionnaire is promising as a study tool, both epidemiological and clinical, presenting very good discriminatory power [17]. In 2014, Boza et al. translated and validated this questionnaire for use in Brazil (the VitiQoL-PB) [108].

Vitiligo Impact Scale-22 (VIS-22)

More recently, in 2014, Gupta et al. validated the VIS-22 questionnaire, which can be used as a guide for therapeutic decisions including psychological interventions in patients suffering vitiligo. It has 22 questions, covering domains of self-confidence, anxiety, depression, marriage, family worries, social interactions, school/college-related, occupation-related, treatment-related, and attitude. Each question is scored as "not at all" = 0; "a little" = 1; "a lot" = 2; "very much" = 3.

Melasma

The Melasma Quality of Life Scale (MelasQoL) is a questionnaire developed and assessed by Balkrishnan in 2003. This new instrument was made for an English-speaking population and focuses on the effect of melasma on emotional aspects such as attractiveness, productivity, and vitality. It is composed of ten questions, scored from 1 to 7, whereby higher indices indicate a worse QoL.

MelasQoL has a high internal consistency, validity, and a good discriminatory power, meaning that the questionnaire can also be used for other dermatosis. The original MelasQoL study evaluated 102 female patients, aged between 18 and 65 years, most of them being high school graduates (87%) and free of any other disease (64%). The results established that the personal areas most affected by melasma were social life, recreation, leisure, and welfare.

The Melasma Area and Severity Index (MASI) is a tool to evaluate the extent and severity of melasma, however, MelasQoL values bear only a slight correlation with this scale demonstrating that, for patients, the impact of the disease is typified by criteria other than its clinical severity as assessed by clinicians. This difference clearly illustrates the need to broaden the evaluation of therapeutic results and possibly how dermatologic consultations are conducted. MelasQoL has been translated and adapted culturally for Spanish and Brazilian Portuguese-speaking populations in accordance with WHO guidance and other published recommendations [6, 17].

Recently, Balkrishnan et al. developed the MELASQOL (Melasma Quality of Life Scale), which collects valuable information about the impact of this dyschromia. It has high internal consistency, shelf life, and good discriminatory power in comparison with other questionnaires [84–86].

Contact Dermatitis

The recurrent characteristic of this disease confers an important social and occupational impairment, mainly if there is hand involvement. There is no specific questionnaire for QoL measurement in contact dermatitis, so clinicians usually resort to a general questionnaire in combination with a more specific one [19, 51, 87].

Dermatitis of the Scalp

The Scalpdex was developed in 2002 for the assessment of QoL in patients with psoriasis and seborrheic dermatitis on the scalp, and consists of 23 questions divided into three tables [88]. When compared with Skindex, this questionnaire showed better capacity of response detention over time [89].

Atopic Dermatitis

AD is a characteristically recurrent disease whose symptoms usually appear during childhood, and in which one-third of patients retain the disease in adult life [35]. Psychological aspects and emotional stress have a role in its pathogenesis [90, 91]. The difference between clinical severity and the socio-psychological impact of the disease illustrates a need to expand the assessment of therapeutic results and the integral attendance of patients.

Quality of Life Index for Atopic Dermatitis (QoLIAD)

This is the most specific tool to analyze QoL in patients with AD. It was developed and initially validated in 1994, with the intention being applied to literate adult patients without other conditions that could influence the QoL. It is composed of 25 items, each with a simple and dichotomous response system, making its use simple and rapid. It is available in English, German, French, Spanish, Italian, and Dutch languages. Among the tools compared in the initial study, it presented the closest correlation with the DLQI [92].

Atopic Dermatitis Disability Index (ADDI)

The ADDI was developed in 1989, with 11 questions referring what happened in the previous 12 months [93]. Because of its evaluation format it is considered a long-term perception of the patient's QoL and has not been used frequently in practice, since the evolution of QoL during treatment is not easily accessed by this method.

Pruritus

Pruritus is a common symptom that is present in several dermatoses. Recently the measurement of its impact on QoL has been made possible by a specific tool, the ItchyQoL, which contains 27 questions and was validated in English [95]. Initial studies demonstrated it to be a questionnaire with sufficient sensibility to detect the emotional, functional, and symptomatic impact between different levels of severity and frequency of pruritus [96, 97].

Quality of Life Assessment in Family Members

It is known that diseases have a significant impact not only on patients' lives but also that of their relatives and partners. Thus, questionnaires to assess QoL in relatives are of major importance. It is well known that when the relatives' QoL is affected they find it more difficult to give support to the sick patient. The following describes the noteworthy questionnaires that assess this aspect (Table 58.5).

Pediatric Quality of Life Inventory: Family Impact Module (The PedsQL Family Impact Module)

The PedsQL™ measures parent self-reported physical, emotional, social, and cognitive functioning, communication, and worry [98]. It presents 36 items and was designed to measure the impact of pediatric chronic health conditions on relatives, similar to the DFI scale, which measures parent-reported family daily activities and family relationships. The Brazilian version was validated by Scarpelli et al. in 2008 [99].

Family Dermatology Life Quality Index (FDLQI)

The FDLQI is a questionnaire designed for adult relatives or partners of patients with any skin

Table 58.5 Scales measuring quality of life in family members

Name of scale	First time mentioned in	Version in Portuguese
The PedsQL family impact module	Varni et al. [62]	The Brazilian version of the PedsQL™ family impact module
		Scarpelli et al. [61]
DFI (Family Dermatosis Family Impact)	Lawson et al. [67]	Weber et al. [113]
FDLQI (Family Dermatology Life Quality Index)	Basra et al. [100]	–
PIQoL-AD (Parents' Index of Quality of Life in Atopic Dermatitis)	McKenna et al. [103]	–
CADIS (Childhood Atopic Dermatitis Impact Scale)	Chamlin et al. [104]	–
PFI-15 (Psoriasis Family Index)	Eghlileb et al. [105]	Boza et al. [106]

disease. As it is self-explanatory, the FDLQI is an easily administered questionnaire. Its scoring is calculated by summing the score of each question, resulting in a maximum of 30 and a minimum of 0 [100]. As in the DLQI, the higher the score, the more the QoL is impaired. There is as yet no validated version of this instrument for the Brazilian setting.

Dermatitis Family Impact (DFI)

In the adapted Brazilian version, the DFI examines the consequences of AD involvement in pediatric patients in daily life [66, 101, 113]. Consisting of ten questions, it analyzes the impact of dermatosis in the child's and relatives, lives in the week before the appointment, including several daily domains common to a family, such as sleep, recreation, feeding, and house cleaning. Considering that the disease affects an individual's QoL and its role in triggering and worsening of some dermatoses, the search for more data about this relationship is needed to help improve therapeutic evaluations and behavior in the pediatric patient population [94, 102].

Parents' Index of Quality of Life in Atopic Dermatitis (PIQoL-AD)

The PIQoL-AD instrument was developed for the UK, Netherlands, Italy, France, Germany, USA and Spain. It has 28 dichotomous items, making it short and practical to use, and is designed to be completed by the parents of children aged 8 or younger. It is a valuable instrument for inclusion in clinical trials and routine clinical practice. The PIQoL-AD provides distinct and complementary information to existing dermatology-specific measures and has been shown to be responsive to changes in QoL in clinical trials.

The PIQoL-AD assesses the QoL of parents of young children who have AD. It is not intended to measure the direct impact of the condition on the children, although it is likely that this will be related to the impact on the main caregiver. The PIQoL-AD will serve as an invaluable addition to the outcome measures already available for use in dermatology, most notably those assessing functional limitations: the IDQOL for children under 4 years old and the CDLQI for older children [103].

Childhood Atopic Dermatitis Impact Scale (CADIS)

The CADIS is self-administered by the patient's parents. Standardized answers consist of five category choices relating to frequency ("never," "rarely," "sometimes," "often," and "all the time"). The CADIS looks at the parent's perceptions during the last 4 weeks and evaluates the conceptual framework to consist of two dimensions with five domains: child dimensions (symptoms and activity limitation/behavior) and parent dimensions (family/social function, sleep, and emotions). It is a measurement of the effects of AD on young children and their parents [104].

The Psoriasis Family Index (PFI-15)

Several psoriasis-specific QoL instruments are available to measure the impact of psoriasis on patients. However, the impact caused by many skin diseases is not limited to the patient but may extend to the rest of the family.

To this end, Eghlileb and coworkers [105] developed and validated a new tool to assess family members and partners of patients suffering psoriasis, the PFI-15. The questionnaire consists of questions applied to relatives, which evaluate psychological aspects of the disease, collateral effects of treatment, sleep, daily activities such as reading, travel, shopping, and others, with answers chosen from one of four alternatives ranging from "not applicable" to "a lot." It is a questionnaire validated for Portuguese and easy to apply, direct, and complete. The preliminary results are promising [106].

Conclusion

From the clinical point of view, the importance of measurement of QoL is obvious when patients arrive at the clinic with a serious complaint about the effect on daily life that symptoms cause and their perception of welfare, while the assessment of relatives is also essential [103, 107]. Some individuals are more affected than others by the disease, even when the disease severity and length are similar [94]. Several factors affect the degree of impact the disease could have on QoL: the individual characteristics of patients, the disease's natural history, the affected body location, and disease time before diagnosis [51]. To date, QoL questionnaires have been used frequently in clinical studies, showing good correlation with other analyzed characteristics [107]. The assessment of QoL in general patient evaluation is fundamental in deciding the therapeutic strategy and its course. The development of tools in dermatology that assess this aspect must be increasingly stimulated, not only in respect of translation and validation but also the elaboration of new instruments for different cultures or social groups, following the inevitable evolution of integral care of individuals.

It is clearly important that these instruments are adapted to both the language and culture of each population; as the use of

QoL measures become more commonplace the need for validated, adapted instruments becomes more apparent.

The health of individuals depends on the harmony between the physical, psychological, and social dimensions and correlates directly with QoL, being understood as a multifactorial entity. Thus, the individual's appreciation as a whole and an interdisciplinary intervention are imperative for any therapy to be effective in improving patients' QoL.

References

1. Gill TM, Feinstein AR. A critical appraisal of the quality of quality-of-life measurements. JAMA. 1994;272(8):619–26.
2. Guyatt GH, Feeny DH, Patrick DL. Measuring health-related quality of life. Ann Intern Med. 1993; 118(8):622–9.
3. The WHOQOL Group. The World Health Organization quality of life assessment (WHOQOL): position paper from the World Health Organization. Soc Sci Med. 1995;10:1403–9.
4. Weber MB, Mazzotti NG, Prati C, Cestari TF. Quality of life assessment in the overall evaluation of dermatology patients. HCPA. 2006;26(2):35–44.
5. Finlay AY, Khan GK. Dermatology life quality index (DLQI) – a simple practical measure for routine clinical use. Clin Exp Dermatol. 1994;19:210–6.
6. Madhulika A, Aditya K. Psychodermatology: an update. J Am Acad Adermatol. 1996;34:1030–46.
7. Folks DG, Warnock JK. Psycocutaneous disorders. Curr Psychiatry Rep. 2001;3:219–25.
8. Walker C, Papadopoulos L. Psychodermatology: the psychological impact of skin disorders. New York, Cambridge University Press, 2005. JAMA. 2007; 297:97–8.
9. Tucker P, et al. The psychosocial impact of alopecia areata. J Health Psychol. 2009;14(1):142–51.
10. Manzoni APDS, Weber MB, Nagatomi ARS, Pereira RL, Townsend RZ, Cestari TF. Assessing depression and anxiety in the caregivers of pediatric patients with chronic skin disorders. An Bras Dermatol. 2013;88:894.
11. Gaspar, Tania et al. Qualidade de vida e bem-estar em crianças e adolescentes. Rev Bras Ter Cogn Dez. 2006;2(2):47–60. ISSN 1808-5687.
12. Chren MM. Measurement of vital signs for skin diseases. J Invest Dermatol. 2005;125(4):viii–x.
13. Finlay AY. Quality of life in dermatology: after 125 years, time for more rigorous reporting. Br J Dermatol. 2014;170:4–6. doi:10.1111/bjd.12737.
14. Fleck MPA, Leal OF, Louzada S, et al. Desenvolvimento da versão em português do instrumento de avaliação de qualidade de vida da OMS (WHOQOL-100). Rev Bras Psiquiatr. 1999;21(1):19–28.
15. Development of the World Health Organization WHOQOL-Bref quality of life assessment. The WHOQOL Group. Psychol Med. 1998;28(3):551–8.
16. Fleck MPA, Louzada S, Xavier M, et al. Aplicação da versão em português do instrumento abreviado de avaliação da qualidade de vida "WHOQOLbref". Rev Saude Publica. 2000;34(2):178–83.
17. Finlay AY. Quality of life measurement in dermatology: a practical guide. Br J Dermatol. 1997;136(3):305–14.
18. Ware JE Jr, Sherbourne CD. The MOS 36-item short-form health survey (SF-36). I. Conceptual framework and item selection. Med Care. 1992;30(6):473–83.
19. Skoet R, Zachariae R, Agner T. Contact dermatitis and quality of life: a structured review of the literature. Br J Dermatol. 2003;149(3):452–6.
20. Ciconelli RM, Ferraz MB, Santos W, Meinão I, Quaresma MR. Brazilian-Portuguese version of the SF-36. A reliable and valid quality of life outcome measure. Rev Bras Reumatol. 1999;39(3):143–150., maio-jun.
21. Lindholm C, Bjellerup M, Christensen OB, Zederfeldt B. Quality of life in chronic leg ulcer patients. An assessment according to the Nottingham health profile. Acta Derm Venereol. 1993;73(6):440–3.
22. Teixeira-Salmela LF, Magalhães LC, Souza AC, Lima MC, Lima RCM, Goulart F. Adaptação do Perfil de Saúde de Nottingham: um instrumento simples de avaliação da qualidade de vida. Cad Saude Publica. 2004;20(4):905–14.
23. Gilson BS, Gilson JS, Bergner M, et al. The sickness impact profile. Development of an outcome measure of health care. Am J Public Health. 1975;65(12):1304–10.
24. Bergner M, Bobbitt RA, Carter WB, Gilson BS. The sickness impact profile: development and final revision of a health status measure. Med Care. 1981;19(8):787–805.
25. Bergner M, Bobbitt RA, Kressel S, Pollard WE, Gilson BS, Morris JR. The sickness impact profile: conceptual formulation and methodology for the development of a health status measure. Int J Health Serv. 1976;6(3):393–415.
26. Feio ALJ, Batel Marques FJ, Alexandrino BM, Salek MS. Portuguese cultural adaptation and linguistic validation of Sickness Impact Profile (PSIP). Qual Life Res. 1995;4:424–5.
27. Finlay AY, Khan GK, Luscombe DK, Salek MS. Validation of sickness impact profile and psoriasis disability index in psoriasis. Br J Dermatol. 1990;123(6):751–6.
28. Salek MS, Khan GK, Finlay AY. Questionnaire techniques in assessing acne handicap: reliability and validity study. Qual Life Res. 1996;5(1):131–8.
29. Salek MS, Finlay AY, Luscombe DK, et al. Cyclosporin greatly improves the quality of life of adults with severe atopic dermatitis. A randomized, double-blind, placebo-controlled trial. Br J Dermatol. 1993;129(4):422–30.

30. Ruta DA, Garratt AM, Leng M, Russell IT, MacDonald LM. A new approach to the measurement of quality of life. The patient- generated index. Med Care. 1994;32(11):1109–26.

31. Halioua B, Beumont MG, Lunel F. Quality of life in dermatology. Int J Dermatol. 2000;39(11):801–6.

32. De Korte J, Mombers FM, Sprangers MA, Bos JD. The suitability of quality-of-life questionnaires for psoriasis research: a systematic literature review. Arch Dermatol. 2002;138(9):1221–7.

33. Lewis-Jones MS, Finlay AY. The Children's Dermatology Life Quality Index (CDLQI): initial validation and practical use. Br J Dermatol. 1995;132(6):942–9.

34. Holme SA, Man I, Sharpe JL, Dykes PJ, Lewis-Jones MS, Finlay AY. The children's dermatology life quality index: validation of the cartoon version. Br J Dermatol. 2003;148(2):285–90.

35. Lewis-Jones MS, Finlay AY, Dykes PJ. The infants' dermatitis quality of life index. Br J Dermatol. 2001;144(1):104–10.

36. Hahn HB, Melfi CA, Chuang TY, et al. Use of the Dermatology Life Quality Index (DLQI) in a midwestern US urban clinic. J Am Acad Dermatol. 2001;45(1):44–8.

37. Anderson RT, Rajagopalan R. Development and validation of a quality of life instrument for cutaneous diseases. J Am Acad Dermatol. 1997;37(1):41–50.

38. Chren MM, Lasek RJ, Quinn LM, Mostow EN, Zyzanski SJ. Skindex, a quality-of-life measure for patients with skin disease: reliability, validity, and responsiveness. J Invest Dermatol. 1996;107(5):707–13.

39. Kadyk DL, McCarter K, Achen F, Belsito DV. Quality of life in patients with allergic contact dermatitis. J Am Acad Dermatol. 2003;49(6):1037–48.

40. Kurwa HA, Finlay AY. Dermatology in-patient management greatly improves life quality. Br J Dermatol. 1995;133(4):575–8.

41. Lundberg L, Johannesson M, Silverdahl M, Hermansson C, Lindberg M. Health-related quality of life in patients with psoriasis and atopic dermatitis measured with SF-36, DLQI and a subjective measure of disease activity. Acta Derm Venereol. 2000;80(6):430–4.

42. Mazzotti E, Picardi A, Sampogna F, Sera F, Pasquini P, Abeni D, IDI Multipurpose Psoriasis Research on Vital Experiences Study Group. Sensitivity of the dermatology life quality index to clinical change in patients with psoriasis. Br J Dermatol. 2003;149(2):318–22.

43. Badia X, Mascaro JM, Lozano R. Measuring health-related quality of life in patients with mild to moderate eczema and psoriasis: clinical validity, reliability and sensitivity to change of the DLQI. The Cavide Research Group. Br J Dermatol. 1999;141(4):698–702.

44. Kiebert G, Sorensen SV, Revicki D, et al. Atopic dermatitis is associated with a decrement in health related quality of life. Int J Dermatol. 2002;41(3):151–8.

45. Parsad D, Pandhi R, Dogra S, Kanwar AJ, Kumar B. Dermatology life quality index score in vitiligo and its impact on the treatment outcome. Br J Dermatol. 2003;148(2):373–4.

46. Zachariae R, Zachariae C, Ibsen H, Mortensen JT, Wulf HC. Dermatology life quality index: data from Danish inpatients and outpatients. Acta Derm Venereol. 2000;80(4):272–6.

47. Harlow D, Poyner T, Finlay AY, Dykes PJ. Impaired quality of life of adults with skin disease in primary care. Br J Dermatol. 2000;143(5):979–82.

48. Ferraz LB, Almeida FA, Vasconcellos MR, Facina AS, Ciconelli RM, Ferraz MB. The impact of lupus erythematosus cutaneous on the quality of life: the Brazilian-Portuguese version of DLQI. Qual Life Res. 2006;15:565–70.

49. Lewis V, Finlay AY. 10 years experience of the Dermatology Life Quality Index (DLQI). J Investig Dermatol Symp Proc. 2004;9(2):169–80.

50. Loo WJ, Diba V, Chawla M, Finlay AY. Dermatology life quality index: influence of an illustrated version. Br J Dermatol. 2003;148(2):279–84.

51. Chren MM, Lasek RJ, Flocke SA, Zyzanski SJ. Improved discriminative and evaluative capability of a refined version of Skindex, a quality-of-life instrument for patients with skin diseases. Arch Dermatol. 1997;133(11):1433–40.

52. Paula HR, Haddad A, Weiss MA, Dini GM, Ferreira LM. Translation, cultural adaptation, and validation of the American Skindex-29 quality of life index. An Bras Dermatol. 2014;89(4):600–7.

53. Anderson R, Rajagopalan R. Responsiveness of the Dermatology-specific Quality of Life (DSQL) instrument to treatment for acne vulgaris in a placebo-controlled clinical trial. Qual Life Res. 1998;7(8):723–34.

54. Bech P. Quality of life measurement in the medical setting. Eur Psychiatry. 1995;10:83–5.

55. Loney T. Psychosocial effects of dermatological-related social anxiety in a sample of acne patients. J Health Psychol. 2008;13(1):47–54.

56. Capoore HS, et al. Does psychological intervention help chronic skin conditions? Postgrad Med J. 1998;74:662–4.

57. Lifschitz C. The impact of atopic dermatitis on quality of life. Ann Nutr Metab. 2015;66(Suppl 1):34–40.

58. Silverberg JI, Silverberg NB. Quality of life impairment in children and adolescents with vitiligo. Pediatr Dermatol. 2014;31(3):309–18.

59. Eismann EA, Lucky AW, Cornwall R. Hand function and quality of life in children with epidermolysis bullosa. Pediatr Dermatol. 2014;31(2):176–82.

60. Klatchoian DA, et al. Qualidade de vida de crianças e adolescentes de São Paulo: confiabilidade e validade da versão brasileira do questionário genérico Pediatric quality of life inventory TM versão 4.0. J Pediatr. 2008;84(04):308–25.

61. Scarpelli, Ana C et al. The Pediatric Quality of life inventory™ (PedsQL™) family impact module:

reliability and validity of the Brazilian version. Health and Quality of Life Outcomes. 2008;6:35–42.

62. Varni JW, Seid M, Rode CA. The PedsQL: measurement model for the pediatric quality of life inventory. Med Care. 1999;37:126–39.

63. Prati C, Comparin C, Boza JC, Cestari TF. Validação para o português falado no Brasil do instrumento Escore da Qualidade de Vida na Dermatologia Infantil (CDLQI). Med Cutan Iber Lat Am. 2010;38:229–33.

64. Manificat S, Dazord A. Évaluation de la qualité de vie de l'enfant: validation d'un questionnaire, premiers résultats. Neuropsychiatr Enfance Adolesc. 1997;45:106–14.

65. Assumpção Jr, Francisco B, Kuczynski E, Sprovieri MH, Aranha EMG. Escala de avaliação de qualidade de vida: (AUQEI – Autoquestionnaire Qualité de Vie Enfant Imagé) validade e confiabilidade de uma escala para qualidade de vida em crianças de 4 a 12 anos. Arq Neuro-Psiquiatr. 2000;58(1):119–27.

66. Weber MB, Lorenzini D, Reinehr CPH, Lovato B. Assessment of the quality of life of pediatric patients at a center of excellence in dermatology in southern Brazil. An Bras Dermatol. 2012 Oct;87(5):697–702.

67. Shikiar R, Bresnahan BW, Stone SP, Thompson C, Koo J, Revicki DA. Validity and reliability of patient reported outcomes used in psoriasis: results from two randomized clinical trials. Health Qual Life Outcomes. 2003;1(1):53.

68. Finlay AY, Kelly SE. Psoriasis – an index of disability. Clin Exp Dermatol. 1987;12(1):8–11.

69. Kent G, al Abadie M. The psoriasis disability index – further analyses. Clin Exp Dermatol. 1993;18(5):414–6.

70. Gupta MA, Gupta AK. The psoriasis life stress inventory: a preliminary index of psoriasis-related stress. Acta Derm Venereol. 1995;75(3):240–3.

71. McKenna SP, Cook SA, Whalley D, et al. Development of the PSORIQoL, a psoriasis specific measure of quality of life designed for use in clinical practice and trials. Br J Dermatol. 2003;149(2):323–31.

72. Mallon E, Newton JN, Klassen A, Stewart-Brown SL, Ryan TJ, Finlay AY. The quality of life in acne: a comparison with general medical conditions using generic questionnaires. Br J Dermatol. 1999;140(4):672–6.

73. Klassen AF, Newton JN, Mallon E. Measuring quality of life in people referred for specialist care of acne: comparing generic and disease-specific measures. J Am Acad Dermatol. 2000;43(2 Pt1):229–33.

74. Oakley AM. The acne disability index: usefulness confirmed. Australas J Dermatol. 1996;37(1):37–9.

75. Zaraa I, Belghith I, Ben Alaya N, Trojjet S, Mokni M, Ben OA. Severity of acne and its impact on quality of life. Skinmed. 2013;11(3):148–53.

76. Motley RJ, Finlay AY. How much disability is caused by acne? Clin Exp Dermatol. 1989;14(3):194–8.

77. Motley RJ, Finlay AY. Practical use of a disability index in the routine management of acne. Clin Exp Dermatol. 1992;17(1):1–3.

78. Gupta A, Sharma YK, Dash KN, Chaudhari ND, Jethani S. Quality of life in acne vulgaris: relation-ship to clinical severity and demographic data. Indian J Dermatol Venereol Leprol. 2016;82(3):292–7.

79. Martin AR, Lookingbill DP, Botek A, Light J, Thiboutot D, Girman CJ. Health-related quality of life among patients with facial acne – assessment of a new acne-specific questionnaire. Clin Exp Dermatol. 2001;26(5):380–5.

80. McLeod LD, Fehnel SE, Brandman J, Symonds T. Evaluating minimal clinically important differences for the acne-specific quality of life questionnaire. PharmacoEconomics. 2003;21(15):1069–79.

81. Ladbrooke S, Finch C, Fryatt E, Allgar V, Eady A, Layton A. Twenty years on APSEA still hits the spot: validation of the Assessment of the Psychological and Social Effects of Acne (APSEA) questionnaire in a large cohort of patients with acne. Br J Dermatol. 2015;173(Suppl. S1):21–76.

82. Fehnel SE, McLeod LD, Brandman J, et al. Responsiveness of the Acne-Specific Quality of Life Questionnaire (Acne-QoL) to treatment for acne vulgaris in placebo-controlled clinical trials. Qual Life Res. 2002;11(8):809–16.

83. Kent G, al-Abadie M. Factors affecting responses on dermatology life quality index items among vitiligo sufferers. Clin Exp Dermatol. 1996;21(5):330–3.

84. Balkrishnan R, McMichael AJ, Camacho FT, et al. Development and validation of a health-related quality of life instrument for women with melasma. Br J Dermatol. 2003;149(3):572–7.

85. Lieu TJ, Pandya AG. Melasma quality of life measures. Dermatol Clin. 2012;30(2):269–280., viii. doi:10.1016/j.det.2011.11.009.

86. Cestari TF, Hexsel D, Viegas ML, Azulay L, Hassun K, Almeida ART, Rêgo VRPA, Mendes AMD, Filho JWA, Junqueira H. Validation of a melasma quality of life questionnaire for Brazilian Portuguese language: the MelasQoL-BP study and improvement of QoL of melasma patients after triple combination therapy. Br J Dermatol. 2006;156:13–20.

87. Wallenhammar LM, Nyfjall M, Lindberg M, Meding B. Health-related quality of life and hand eczema – a comparison of two instruments, including factor analysis. J Invest Dermatol. 2004;122(6):1381–9.

88. Zampieron A, Buja A, Fusco M, Linder D, Bortune M, Piaserico S, Baldo V. Quality of life in patients with scalp psoriasis. G Ital Dermatol Venereol. 2015;150(3):309–16. Epub 2014 Sep 18

89. Chen SC, Yeung J, Chren MM. Scalpdex: a quality of life instrument for scalp dermatitis. Arch Dermatol. 2002;138(6):803–7.

90. Buske-Kirschbaum A, Geiben A, Hellhammer D. Psychobiological aspects of atopic dermatitis: an overview. Psychother Psychosom. 2001;70(1):6–16.

91. Rajka G, Langeland T. Grading of the severity of atopic dermatitis. Acta Derm Venereol Suppl (Stockh). 1989;144:13–4.

92. Whalley D, McKenna SP, Dewar AL, et al. A new instrument for assessing quality of life in atopic dermatitis: international development of the Quality of Life Index for Atopic Dermatitis (QoLIAD). Br J Dermatol. 2004;150(2):274–83.

93. Eun H, Finlay AY. Measurement of atopic dermatitis disability. Ann Dermatol. 1990;2:9–12.
94. Lawson V, Lewis-Jones MS, Finlay AY, Reid P, Owens RG. The family impact of childhood atopic dermatitis: the dermatitis family impact questionnaire. Br J Dermatol. 1998;138:107–13.
95. Poindexter G, Monthrope Y, Shah N, Chen S. Pruritus quality of life instrument. J Am Acad Dermatol. 2005;52(3 Suppl 1):P106.
96. Shah N, Palubin K, Lucero M, Chen S. Measuring quality of life impact in patients with pruritus. J Am Acad Dermatol. 2005;52(3 Suppl 1):P105.
97. Love EM, Marrazzo GA, Kini S, Veledar E, Chen SC. ItchyQoL bands: pilot clinical interpretation of scores. Acta Derm Venereol. 2015;95(1):114–5.
98. Varni JW, Sherman SA, Burwinkle TM, Dickinson PE, Dixon P. The PedsQLTM family impact module: preliminary reliability and validity. Health Qual Life Outcomes. 2004;2:55. doi:10.1186/1477-7525-2-55.
99. Scarpelli AC, Paiva SM, Pordeus IA, Varni JW, Viegas CM, Allison PJ. The Pediatric Quality of Life InventoryTM (PedsQLTM) family impact module: reliability and validity of the Brazilian version. Health Qual Life Outcomes. 2008;6:35. doi:10.1186/1477-7525-6-35.
100. Basra MKA, Sue-Ho R, Finlay AY. Family dermatology life quality index: measuring the secondary impact of skin disease. Br J Dermatol. 2007;156:528–38. Erratum: Br J Dermatol. 2007;156:791.
101. Weber MB, Fontes Neto PT, Prati C, Soirefman M, Mazzotti NG, Barzenski B, et al. Improvement of pruritus and quality of life of children with atopic dermatitis and their families after joining support groups. JEADV. 2008;22:992–9.
102. Dodington SR, Basra MK, Finlay AY, Salek MS. The dermatitis family impact questionnaire: a review of its measurement properties and clinical application. Br J Dermatol. 2013;169(1):31–46.
103. McKenna SP, Whalley D, Dewar AL, Erdman RA, Kohlmann T, Niero M, Baró E, Cook SA, Crickx B, Frech F, van Assche D. International development of the Parents' Index of Quality of Life in Atopic Dermatitis (PIQoL-AD). Qual Life Res. 2005;14(1):231–41.
104. Chamlin SL, Cella D, Frieden IJ, Williams ML, Mancini AJ, Lai JS, Chren MM. Development of the childhood atopic dermatitis impact scale: initial validation of a quality-of-life measure for young children with atopic dermatitis and their families. J Invest Dermatol. 2005;125:1106–11.
105. Eghlileb AM, Basra MKA, Finlay AY. The psoriasis family index: preliminary results of validation of a quality of life instrument for family members of patients with psoriasis. Dermatology. 2009;219:63–70.
106. Catucci BJ, Basra Mohammad KA, Caminha VR, Rosa CR, Blessmann WM, Ferreira CT. Traducao e validacao do instrumento indice de qualidade de vida para familiares de pacientes com psoriase para o portugues falado no Brasil. An Bras Dermatol. 2013;88(3):488–9.
107. Lewis-Jones MS, Dawe RS, Lowe JG. Quality of life in children with type 1 latex allergy and their parents: use and primary validation of the QoLLAC and QoLLA-P questionnaires. Br J Dermatol. 2005;153(Suppl 1):83–4.
108. Boza JC, Kundu RV, Fabbrin A, Horn R, Giongo N, Cestari TF. Tradução, adaptação cultural e validação do instrumento de avaliação da qualidade de vida de pacientes com vitiligo (VitiQol) para o Português falado no Brasil. An Bras Dermatol. 2015;90(3):355–60.
109. Alvarenga Tassiana MM, Caldeira Antônio P. Qualidade de vida em pacientes pediátricos com dermatite atópica. J Pediatr. 2009;85(5):415–20.
110. Şenol A, Yücelten AD, Ay P. Development of a quality of life scale for vitiligo. Dermatology. 2013;226(2):185–90. doi:10.1159/000348466. Epub 2013 May 28
111. Lilly E, Lu PD, Borovicka JH, Victorson D, Kwasny MJ, West DP, Kundu RV. Development and validation of a vitiligo-specific quality-of-life instrument (VitiQoL). J Am Acad Dermatol. 2013;69(1):e11–8. doi:10.1016/j.jaad.2012.01.038. Epub 2012 Feb 25
112. Gupta V, Sreenivas V, Mehta M, Khaitan BK, Ramam M. Measurement properties of the vitiligo impact scale-22 (VIS-22), a vitiligo-specific quality-of-life instrument. Br J Dermatol. 2014;171:1084–90.
113. Cardiff's Department of Dermatology [homepage]. Quality of life questionnaires. Available in: http://sites.cardiff.ac.uk/dermatology/quality-of-life/.

Dermatoscopy in the Public Health Environment

56

Alejandra Larre Borges, Sofía Nicoletti, Lídice Dufrechou, and Andrea Nicola Centanni

Key Points

- Dermoscopy has been shown to improve diagnostic accuracy, sensitivity, and specificity of skin cancer diagnosis
- If you don't have a dermoscope … You can always perform tape dermoscopy!
  - Use immersion fluid (i.e., water, olive oil, disinfectant spray) to place it on the flat or slightly elevated lesion;
  - Cover the lesion with transparent adhesive tape with lateral tension;
  - Use ambient indoor or outdoor lighting for illumination (rather than flash photography);
  - Position your photographic device at an angle of approximately 45° from the side of the lesion to avoid light reflection;
  - Record a focused image with your mobile phone or digital camera at a distance of approximately 25–30 cm from the lesion; and
  - Enlarge the image on the screen of the device.

  Done! Even though you have better have your own dermoscope!
- Interpretation of colors and structures is essential for dermoscopic diagnosis since both have a histopathologic correlate. Recognition of specific structures permits the classification of a lesion as a melanocytic or nonmelanocytic tumor
- Through dermoscopy four main morphologic groups of benign nevi can be identified: globular, reticular, starburst, and structureless blue nevi. There are some special nevi due to their specific body site (facial, acral, nails, mucosal).
- The atypical nevus is not a precursor of melanoma but a risk marker. Atypical nevus has a higher chance of being a melanoma but not a higher chance of becoming a melanoma. Most melanomas start de novo and not in a pre-existing nevus of any type, and if they start in a pre-existing nevus it is often a completely "benign" nevus and not a large dysplastic one

A. Larre Borges (✉) • S. Nicoletti
L. Dufrechou • A. Nicola Centanni
Hospital de Clínicas "Dr. Manuel Quintela",
Montevideo, Uruguay
e-mail: alarreborges@gmail.com

© Springer International Publishing Switzerland 2018
R.R. Bonamigo, S.I.T. Dornelles (eds.), *Dermatology in Public Health Environments*,
https://doi.org/10.1007/978-3-319-33919-1_56

- Once the patient is examined clinically and by dermoscopy:
  - Patient who has a single lesion or few lesions: if a lesion seems benign it may be left; but if it is suspicious, it should be removed or monitored, depending on the degree suspicion of malignancy
  - Patient with multiple nevi: start monitoring program with an analytic dermoscopic approach for early diagnosis of melanoma
  - Low-risk patient with a single or a few slightly atypical melanocytic lesions: long term monitoring versus excision

Introduction

Much effort has been made in developing non-invasive in vivo imaging techniques to improve dermatologic diagnostics. Dermoscopy, also known as dermatoscopy, epiluminescence microscopy, incident light microscopy, and skin surface microscopy, is performed using a handheld instrument called a dermatoscope or dermoscope, which has a transilluminating light source and standard magnifying optics (usually 10×). A dermatoscope can diminish the refraction and reflection of light at the skin and facilitates the recognition of colors and structures of subsurface skin located within the epidermis, dermoepidermal junction, and papillary dermis, which are otherwise not visible to the naked eye [1, 2].

Dermatoscopes illuminate the skin by use of light-emitting diode bulbs, with or without the use of polarizing filters. Dermatoscopes using nonpolarized light require direct contact between the skin and the scope, and require a liquid interface, such as ultrasound gel or alcohol, to be placed between the skin and the glass plate of the dermatoscope to overpass refraction and reflection. Thus dermoscopy can be contact nonpolarized, contact polarized, or noncontact polarized,

each of which provides complementary information. A cross-polarized dermatoscope allows visualization of deeper skin structures (60–100 μm), and accordingly may have higher sensitivity for detecting skin cancer based on its ability to enhance the visualization of vascular and crystalline structures, both of which are commonly seen in skin cancer. On the other hand, nonpolarized dermoscopy improves specificity as it permits easier visualization of other superficial structures commonly seen in benign lesions, such as milia-like cysts in seborrheic keratosis [2–4].

This diagnostic technique represents a link between the macroscopy (clinical dermatology) and microscopy (dermatopathology). Besides its relevance for evaluating pigmented structures, dermoscopy enables the recognition of vascular structures and other subtle features that usually are less visible to the naked eye [5]. Dermoscopy has mainly been developed to diagnose skin tumors, especially pigmented tumors, and reduce the number of benign lesion excisions. It has also recently played a relevant role in other diseases including inflammatory and infectious disorders.

Dermoscopy has been shown to improve diagnostic accuracy, sensitivity, and specificity for skin cancer diagnosis by dermatologists [2, 6]. Its accuracy is enhanced if physicians are trained in its use. A nontrained individual has a worse result using dermoscopy than with visual examination [7]. A short training course in dermoscopy increases the diagnostic performance of both inexperienced and experienced dermatologists [6]. The main use of dermoscopy is to aid in the decision of whether to perform a biopsy [2]. It is also helpful in the evaluation of amelanotic lesions and inflammatory and infectious diseases. Furthermore, it helps in the evaluation of treatment for different dermatoses.

Two strategies for the approach to dermatoscopic diagnosis of pigmented skin tumors have been described: the verbal-based *analytic* and the more visual-global *heuristic* method [8]. The analytic method implies the application of a catalog of semantic criteria and thereby the detailed analysis of individual features of a given lesion to reach a logical deductive diagnostic conclusion. The heuristic method evaluates the overall pattern of a given lesion and relies on a so-called gut feeling or some form of intuition. The diagnostic conclusion is drawn from unconscious insight into given relationships without rational or causal deduction. While being taught an explicit analytic method, a student may develop intuitive heuristic mechanisms independently, so in this chapter we focus on the former approach while the other strategy develops. Both strategies are essential in the diagnostic process as applied by a clinician. On one hand, a clinician needs to learn analytically the "alphabet" of a morphologic medical discipline and, on the other, he or she also needs experience to correctly interpret the many variations that a morphologic structure can show in real life. Tschandl et al. [8], in 2015, described a tendency toward sex-related differences in the improvement of diagnoses depending on the approach used, proposing that women would probably be more likely to learn using the heuristic method.

Lower-Cost "Instruments"

As many medical doctors do not have access to a dermoscope, a simple and cost-effective technique that can be easily used is "tape dermoscopy." One of its disadvantages is that dermoscopic features that are only visible under polarized light, such as crystalline structures, cannot be detected [9]. The technique involves:

1. Placing immersion fluid (i.e., water, olive oil, disinfectant spray) on the flat or slightly elevated lesion
2. Covering the lesion with transparent adhesive tape with lateral tension
3. Using ambient indoor or outdoor lighting for illumination (rather than flash photography)
4. Positioning a photographic device at an angle of approximately 45° from the side of the lesion to avoid light reflection
5. Recording a focused image with a mobile phone or digital camera at a distance of approximately 25–30 cm from the lesion
6. Enlarging the image on the screen of the device

This technique has many other disadvantages and so should be used only in "emergency" cases [9].

Colors and Structures

The principal dermoscopic features for making a diagnosis are the interpretation of colors and structure distribution. Colors and structures have a specific histologic correlation [3, 4, 10].

The number of colors is relevant mainly in melanocytic lesions; most benign ones are monochrome. Polychromy is associated with more advanced malignant tumors [11]. Colors depend on the location of keratin, blood, collagen, and melanin. Accordingly, colors visualized include yellow, red, and white for keratin, blood, and collagen, respectively [2].

Colors for keratin show a yellowish-brown pigmentation, depending on its oxidation process, and the presence of melanin. It is yellow to whitish in cystic lesions, and darker in keratin plugs. Colors for hemoglobin are red, blue, purple, or black depending on its location and on its oxidation and presence or absence of thrombosis. The easiest way to visualize blood vessels is to use a noncontact polarized dermatoscope. If a contact dermatoscope is used, it is beneficial to use ultrasound gel as the liquid interface because it minimizes the pressure applied to the vessels. The analysis of morphology and organization of vessels is a very helpful tool, especially in the recognition of amelanotic lesions as exist in some melanomas. A review of vascular structures is beyond the scope of this chapter [12, 13]. Colors for melanin, because of the Tyndall effect, depend on the depth in the corneous stratum, the epidermis, dermoepidermic union, or papillary dermis; this pigment will range from black to dark brown, light brown, gray, and blue [11] (Fig. 56.1).

At times, the presence of colors seems to incorrectly trump the presence of structures and patterns when making a diagnosis. In 2016 Bajaj et al. proposed that color and color variegation can distract dermoscopy users from recognizing or placing appropriate emphasis on morphologic structures and patterns present in skin lesions, leading to the possibility of misdiagnosis and incorrect prognosis. They concluded that there is no statistically significant difference in the ability of novices to correctly diagnose common cutaneous neoplasms in grayscale versus color

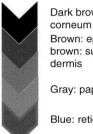

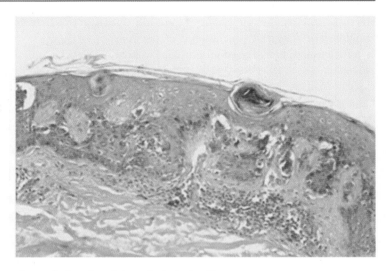

Dark brown: stratum corneum

Brown: epidermis -Light brown: superior dermis

Gray: papillary dermis

Blue: reticular dermis

Fig. 56.1 Colors in dermoscopy according to the location of the melanin in the skin

dermoscopic images. Participants were thus able to render a diagnosis based on morphologic characteristics alone (i.e., structure and pattern) without any appreciable loss in their diagnostic confidence level when evaluating grayscale images. These results conclude that dermoscopic diagnosis based on structures and patterns may prove to be more objective and accurate compared with diagnosis based on color [14]. In fact structures have a histopathologic correlate, which is the reason why they help diagnosis. Their recognition is basic for differentiating between melanocytic and nonmelanocytic lesions. The presence of specific structures permits the classification of a lesion as a melanocytic or a nonmelanocytic tumor. An analytic method to classify them is the two-step dermoscopy algorithm [2].

Two Step Dermoscopy Algorithm

The two-step dermoscopy algorithm (Fig. 56.2) guides the observer toward the most likely diagnosis and helps in the decision-making process. This algorithm was introduced in 2001 by a panel of the virtual Consensus Net Meeting on Dermoscopy [15]. Its primary aim is to help clinicians to avoid missing the diagnosis of melanoma, and its secondary aim is to segregate

lesions into melanocytic and nonmelanocytic categories and provide the observer with the most probable diagnosis [2].

The two-step dermoscopy algorithm has high sensitivity, specificity, and accuracy, and can be relied on to provide an accurate and specific pre-biopsy diagnosis and to help guide management decisions. In 2015 Chen et al. reported that there are some lesions that have a higher chance of being misclassified, intradermal nevi being the most common. The authors proposed that other imaging methods such as confocal microscopy may aid in the further evaluation of these lesions. In addition, they arrived at the conclusion that this algorithm helps in maximizing the detection of skin cancer to ensure that malignant lesions are not missed, and aims at making more precise clinical diagnoses [16].

A major critique of the two-step algorithm is that initial errors in the classification of melanocytic status will render the second step irrelevant [16].

First Step: Melanocytic versus Nonmelanocytic Lesions

The first step is to define whether a lesion is melanocytic or nonmelanocytic. The former

Fig. 56.2 Two-step dermoscopy algorithm

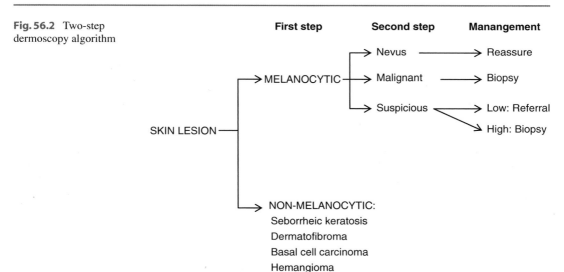

Table 56.1 Melanocytic lesion criteria

Pigment network
Negative pigment network
Aggregated globules
Streaks (pseudopods and radial streaming)
Homogeneous blue pigmentation
Pseudonetwork (facial skin)
Parallel pigment pattern (acral lesions of palms and soles)

should have one of the following criteria (Table 56.1): pigment network, negative pigment network, aggregated globules, streaks (pseudopods and radial streaming), homogeneous blue pigmentation, pseudonetwork (facial skin), and parallel pigment pattern (acral lesions on palms and soles). Lesions classified as non-melanocytic are further subclassified as benign (i.e., dermatofibroma, seborrheic keratosis (SK), hemangioma, and angiokeratoma) and malignant (basal cell carcinoma (BCC) and squamous cell carcinoma (SCC)) in the first step [16]. Lesions that are classified as melanocytic are further evaluated in the second step, which is intended to differentiate benign melanocytic neoplasms from melanoma [2].

If it cannot be defined that a lesion is melanocytic or not it should be classified as suspicious to ensure that cutaneous malignancies will not be missed [17].

Second Step: Benign Versus Malignant Melanocytic Lesions

The second step is to distinguish benign nevi, i.e., melanocytic nevi, blue nevi, Spitz nevi, and atypical nevi, from melanoma [2].

There are multiple methods that can be used to differentiate nevi from melanoma, including pattern analysis, the three-point checklist, the seven-point checklist, the ABCD rule, the Menzies method, the chaos and clues, and CASH (color, architecture, symmetry, and homogeneity) [18]. The first one is preferred by experts, while the others were developed to facilitate a novice's ability to distinguish skin cancer (especially melanomas and BCC) from nevi with high diagnostic accuracy [2, 16, 18].

Here we explain two methods: the three-point checklist and pattern analysis. The three-point checklist is considered the simplest method for novices to learn and use while pattern analysis is the more holistic and complete, and is the most chosen by experts.

The three-point checklist has the highest sensitivity for identifying melanoma [2]. It is intended as a screening algorithm for detecting skin cancer (melanoma and pigmented BCC) and applies only to pigmented skin lesions. One point is assigned to each of the following criteria present in the lesion [19]:

- Asymmetry in distribution of dermoscopic colors and/or structures in one or two perpendicular axes. The contour or silhouette of the lesion does not factor into whether the lesion is symmetric or not.
- Irregular or atypical pigment network consisting of thick lines and irregular holes.
- Blue-white veil and/or white scar-like depigmentation and/or blue pepper-like granules.

A total score of 2 or 3 is considered positive, in which case the lesion should be biopsied or the patient referred for further evaluation [19]. Given its simplicity and high sensitivity for detecting pigmented skin cancer, the three-point checklist may be ideally suited for clinicians with little experience in dermoscopy and for use as a screening tool in the primary care setting [2].

Pattern analysis is a qualitative method that evaluates dermoscopic structures and their distribution [20].

State of the Art

Benign Melanocytic Nevi

Dermoscopy requires the ability to recognize, and experience in recognizing, benign patterns. It also requires the ability to recognize the ten melanoma-specific structures defined by Marghoob et al. in 2013. Any melanocytic lesion that deviates from one of these benign patterns, while also revealing at least one of the ten melanoma-specific structures, should be biopsied to rule out melanoma [2] (Table 56.2).

Through dermoscopy, four main morphologic groups can be identified: globular, reticular, starburst, and structureless blue nevi. There are some structural combinations of the precedent morphologic groups: diffuse reticular, peripheral reticular with central hypopigmentation, patchy reticular, peripheral reticular with central hyperpigmentation, peripheral globules/starburst, peripheral reticular with central globules, and two components symmetric in structure [2] (Figs. 56.3, 56.4, 56.5, 56.6, and 56.7).

Table 56.2 Ten suspicious structures for melanoma adapted from Marghoob et al. [2]

Irregular or atypical pigment network
Negative pigment network
Streaks
Off-centered blotch
Atypical dots or globules
Regression structures
Blue-white veil overlying raised areas
Atypical vascular structures
Crystalline structures
Peripheral brown structureless areas and shape of the holes

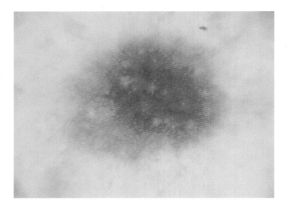

Fig. 56.3 Diffuse reticular pattern in a melanocytic nevus

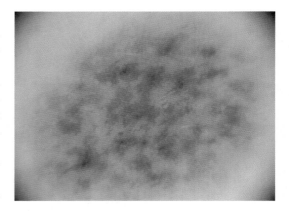

Fig. 56.4 Patchy reticular pattern in a melanocytic nevus

Some nevi are specific according to their special body site: face, acral (palms and soles), and nails. Another group, called special nevi, consists of nevi typified by peculiar clinical–histopathologic findings. These can be subdivided into "melanoma

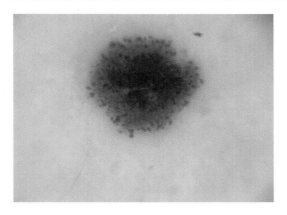

Fig. 56.5 Peripheral globules in a melanocytic nevus

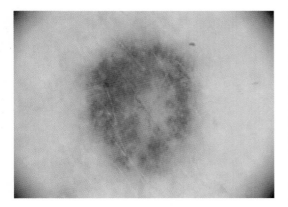

Fig. 56.6 Peripheral reticular with central hypopigmentation in a melanocytic nevus

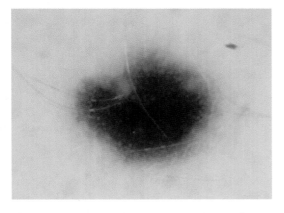

Fig. 56.7 Peripheral reticular with central hyperpigmentation in a melanocytic nevus

simulators" including combined nevi, recurrent nevi, and sclerosing nevi with pseudomelanomatous features, "targetoid" nevi (i.e., halo, cockade, irritated targetoid hemosiderotic, and eczematous nevi) and uncommon histopathologic variants such as desmoplastic, white dysplastic, or balloon cell nevus. The description of special nevi is beyond the scope of this chapter [21].

Atypical Nevi or Clark Nevus

The term "dysplastic nevus" (DN) is derived from Greek *dys-* (bad or malfunction) and *-plasia* (growth development or change). The name implies that this nevus exists as a different defined entity of potential detriment to its host. Indeed, we prefer to keep this term for histology and preserve the word atypical for clinical and dermatoscopic use. From our point of view, the atypical nevus is not a precursor of melanoma but a risk marker. Atypical nevus has a higher chance of being a melanoma but not a higher chance of becoming a melanoma. Most melanomas start de novo and not in a pre-existing nevus of any type, and if they start in a pre-existing nevus it is often a completely "benign" nevus and not a large dysplastic one [22].

Atypical nevi share some clinical and dermatoscopic features with melanoma so it is often difficult to distinguish one from the other. Atypical nevi are diagnosed with at least three of the following characteristics: (1) diameter more than 5 mm; (2) ill-defined borders; (3) irregular margin. (4) varying shades in the lesion; (5) simultaneous presence of papular and macular components. Dermoscopically they can have three main dermoscopic patterns: reticular, globular, and homogeneous. They have also two descriptors of pigmentation: uniformly and central hypo- or hyperpigmented, eccentric peripheral hypo- or hyperpigmented, and multifocal hypo- or hyperpigmented. Most patients have one type of atypical nevus [23] (Figs. 56.8, 56.9, 56.10, 56.11, and 56.12).

The recently described criteria with strong discriminatory power and moderate levels of interobserver agreement to dermoscopically distinguish nevi from melanoma. Regarding melanoma: architectural disorder, pattern asymmetry, contour asymmetry; and regarding nevi: comma vessels, and absence of vessels [18].

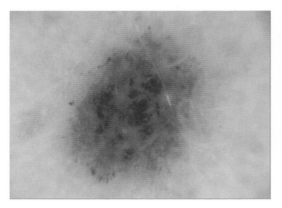

Fig. 56.8 Atypical nevus showing asymmetrical network, irregular margin, irregular size, and distribution of globules

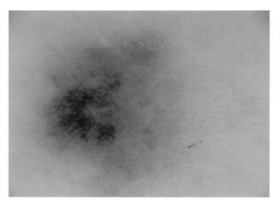

Fig. 56.9 Atypical nevus showing asymmetry and eccentric peripheral hyperpigmented network

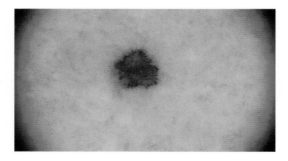

Fig. 56.10 Atypical nevus showing asymmetry and peripheral projections and irregular borders

Atypical Mole Syndrome

Some patients have many atypical moles (>5), and there are two options for managing these

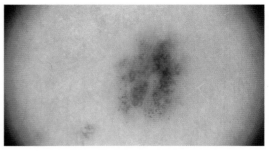

Fig. 56.11 Atypical nevus showing ill-defined borders, eccentric hyperpigmented area, irregularly distributed globules, and variegated shades

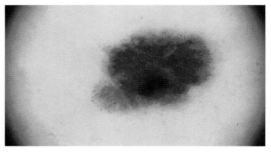

Fig. 56.12 Atypical nevus showing three main dermatoscopic patterns – globular, reticular, and homogeneous – irregularly distributed in the lesion

patients: removing all atypical lesions, with a high number of unnecessary excisions of benign melanocytic nevi, or dermoscopic follow-up and excision of only those lesions that change over time, considering that probably they were the initial melanomas [24].

Total Nevi, Atypical Nevi, and Melanoma Thickness

A case study from Geller et al. in 2016 of 566 patients in the United States having recently been diagnosed with melanoma demonstrated that most patients had 0–20 total nevi and absence of atypical nevi, this finding being most pronounced among older patients, for whom both total nevi and atypical nevi were uncommon. Therefore, physicians and patients should not rely on the total nevus count as a sole reason to perform skin examinations or to determine a risk status patient. Younger should be educated on their incresed risk of thicker melanomas, which is associated with having more atypical nevi [25].

Nevi in Specific Body Sites

The anatomic structure of specific body sites results in unique dermoscopic features.

Facial Nevi

On the face, differential diagnoses of pigmented skin lesions are lentigo maligna (LM), LM melanoma, seborrheic keratosis, actinic lentigo, pigmented actinic keratosis (AK), and lichen planus-like keratosis.

Stratum corneum of facial skin is thinner than that of the trunk and limbs, while pilosebaceous units and sweat glands are densely present in the facial skin. The thin epidermis allows blood vessels or melanophages to be observed more easily on facial skin than elsewhere on the extrafacial skin. In addition, the pseudonetwork and sundamaged elastosis are often present (Fig. 56.13). Facial nevi are usually characterized by unpigmented or poorly pigmented elevated lesions, which correspond histopathologically to dermal nevi [26].

Acral Volar

Saida et al. first performed dermoscopic studies of nevi and melanomas located on the palms and soles in 2002 [27].

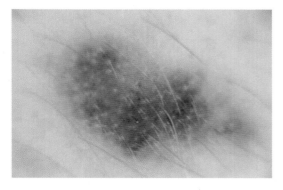

Fig. 56.13 Facial nevi showing a pseudonetwork

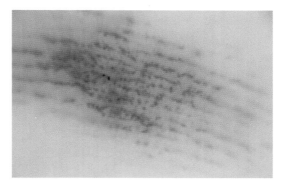

Fig. 56.14 Acral melanocytic nevus showing a parallel furrow pattern

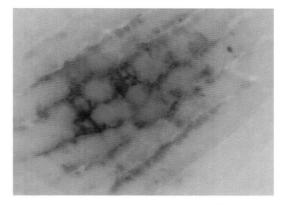

Fig. 56.15 Acral melanocytic nevus showing a lattice-like pattern

Specific dermoscopic major benign patterns are [28–30]:

1. The parallel furrow pattern with its variants, whereby pigmentation is seen in the parallel sulci of the skin (Fig. 56.14)
2. The lattice-like pattern, characterized by pigmented lines that follow and cross the skin margins (Fig. 56.15)
3. The fibrillar pattern, consisting of pigmented lines that cross the skin markings diagonally (Fig. 56.16)

Other patterns are: the nontypical (showing neither malignant features nor the benign patterns described above), the globular pattern (brown globules regularly distributed within the lesion, Fig. 56.17), the homogeneous pat-

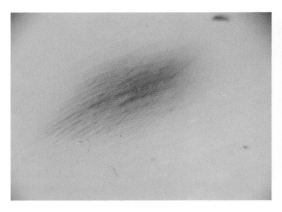

Fig. 56.16 Acral melanocytic nevus showing a fibrillar pattern

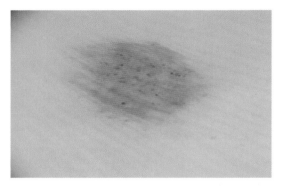

Fig. 56.17 Globular acral pattern

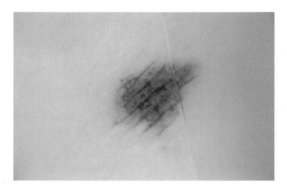

Fig. 56.18 Reticular acral pattern

tern (diffuse light brown or blue pigmentation), the reticular pattern (black or brown network similar to that seen in nonglabrous skin, Fig. 56.18), the transition pattern (combination of specific dermoscopic features characteristic of volar and nonglabrous skin, Fig. 56.19) and

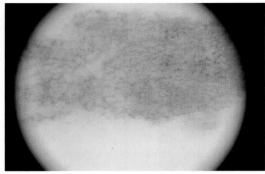

Fig. 56.19 Acral melanocytic nevus showing a transition pattern

globulostreak-like pattern (dark brown globules and brown linear or curvilinear streak-like structures) [28, 29, 31, 32].

All of these patterns are similar among populations worldwide. In our study, performed in the Latin American population, the parallel furrow pattern, followed by the lattice-like and homogeneous patterns, were the most prevalent acral melanocytic nevi [33].

The fibrillar pattern is exclusively found on the soles of feet, since high-pressure points and shearing forces contribute to its dermoscopic features [32, 34].

Mucosal

Pigmented lesions on the mucocutaneous junction and mucous membrane include mucosal melanotic macule (mucosal melanosis), melanocytic nevus, malignant melanoma, and nonmelanocytic lesions, such as bowenoid papulosis. Nevi of the mucosal membrane tend to be associated with younger age compared with melanoma or melanosis. Clinically they present as single 5-mm to 9-mm flat, slightly elevated, or nodular brown to gray lesions. Common melanocytic nevi on the mucosal membranes are brown to gray symmetric lesions with a globular or homogeneous pattern [35].

Benign vulvar lesions including nevi and melanosis have the following patterns: globular, cobblestone, ring-like, reticular-like, homogeneous, parallel, or mixed [36] (Figs. 56.20 and 56.21).

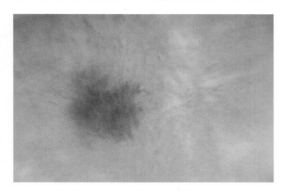

Fig. 56.20 Globular mucosal pattern

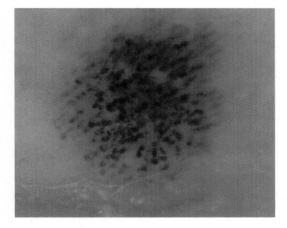

Fig. 56.21 Vulvar globular nevus

Melanoma

Unlike other life-threatening internal cancers, cutaneous melanoma allows diagnosis through noninvasive approaches [37]. The ABCD acronym for melanoma screening was described in 1985 by Riger et al. to provide the lay public and primary healthcare professionals with a useful and memorable mnemonic to aid in the early recognition of potentially curable cutaneous malignant melanoma. It consists of Asymmetry, Border irregularity, Color variegation, and Diameter greater than 6 mm. The E was latterly included for emphasizing change over time as an important additional criterion in differentiating melanoma from benign pigmented lesions [38, 39]. It should be noted that many melanomas do not have all four ABCD features [37]. Besides the

ABCD that helps to recognize an individual lesion, the examination of the rest of the patient's melanocytic lesions is relevant. Another clinical and or dermoscopically important concept is the "ugly duckling" sign, which is a pigmented lesion that "looks different from all of its neighbors," thus arousing suspicion of melanoma [40].

Early diagnosis of melanoma is crucial because its prognosis is directly proportionate to the depth of the neoplasm. The earlier the tumor is detected the thinner it is, so early diagnosis is of central importance in saving lives [37]. In this sense, clinical ABCD seems not enough, as melanoma is already melanoma when it is smaller than 6 mm, and shape, border, and color might be relatively regular at this stage. The advantage of dermoscopy is that equivocal features are often present in very small melanomas, thus increasing our index of suspicion even in the context of small and clinically banal-looking melanomas [24]. The diagnosis of skin cancer, however, is complex, and individual clinicians place varying degrees of emphasis on patient history, clinical evaluation, dermoscopic examination, and heuristic method [8, 41].

Traditional melanoma classification is based on clinical and pathologic characteristics and includes four melanoma subtypes: superficial spreading melanoma, LM, nodular melanoma, and acral lentiginous melanoma [42]. However, today there are other melanomas related to particular genetic status, anatomic location, and degree of sun exposure [43]. Besides the classical melanoma subtypes, here we review the main dermoscopic features of *specific* melanomas: lentiginous nonfacial melanomas in chronically damaged skin, hypomelanotic melanoma, and mucous melanoma. Relevant meta-analysis demonstrated that the use of dermoscopy, for trained users but not novices, improves diagnostic accuracy for melanoma [44, 45].

Regarding the ABCDE rule in melanoma, it should be pointed out that symmetry or asymmetry in dermoscopy does not factor in the contour or shape, but rather the distribution of colors and structures within the lesion, so a lesion could be symmetric for the clinical ABCDE and asymmetric for the dermatoscopic one. Therefore there are

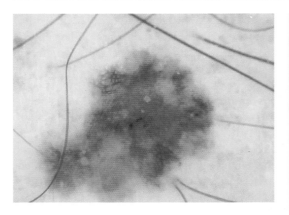

Fig. 56.22 Atypical pigment network, increased variability in the thickness and color of the lines of the network, melanoma in situ

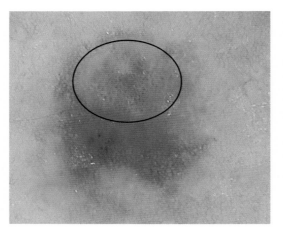

Fig. 56.23 Negative pigment network. The *circle* marks an area with interconnecting hypopigmented lines resembling a "white network"

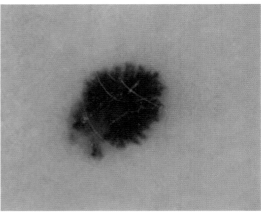

Fig. 56.24 Streaks asymmetrically distributed, melanoma in situ

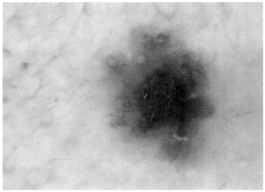

Fig. 56.25 Off-centered blotch

ten melanoma-specific dermoscopic structures as mentioned earlier (Table 56.2) [2]:

1. Irregular or atypical pigment network: Network with increased variability in the thickness and color of the lines of the network, and increased variability in the size (Fig. 56.22)
2. Negative pigment network: Serpiginous interconnecting hypopigmented lines that surround irregularly shaped pigmented structures resembling elongated curvilinear globules [46] (Fig. 56.23)
3. Streaks (pseudopods and radial streaming): Radial projections at the periphery of the lesion that are focally and asymmetrically distributed (Fig. 56.24)
4. Off-centered blotch: Asymmetrically or focally located at the periphery of the lesion. Irregular blotch will often reveal differing hues (Fig. 56.25)
5. Atypical dots or globules: Multiple dots or globules of different size, shape, and color. Asymmetrically or focally distributed within the lesion (Fig. 56.26)
6. Regression structures: Include scar-like depigmentation and peppering, which, when combined, give the appearance of a blue-white veil (Fig. 56.27)

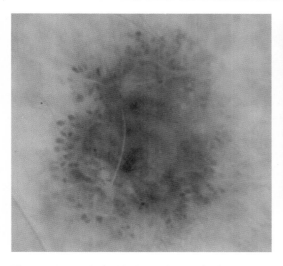

Fig. 56.26 Atypical globules, melanoma in situ

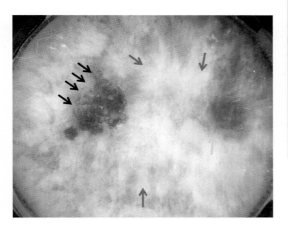

Fig. 56.27 Scar-like depigmentation (*black arrows*) and peppering (*red arrows*) as regression structures. *Yellow arrow*: blue-white veil

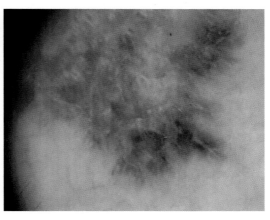

Fig. 56.28 Atypical vascular structures, melanoma

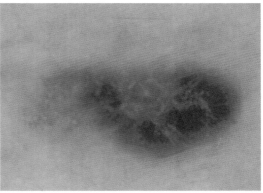

Fig. 56.29 White shiny structures, crystalline structures

7. Blue-white veil overlying raised areas: Tends to be asymmetrically located or diffuse throughout the lesion with differing hues (Fig. 56.27)
8. Atypical vascular structures: Dotted vessels over milky-red backgrounds. Serpentine irregular linear vessels. Polymorphous vessels (Fig. 56.28)
9. White shiny structures, including three groups: (a) crystalline structures: white shiny streaks or lines organized orthogonally or parallel; (b) rosettes: four shiny points; (c) white shiny areas: larger structureless shiny areas (Fig. 56.29) [47]
10. Peripheral brown structureless areas and shape of the holes: Tan areas located at the periphery of the lesion that encompass greater than 10% of the lesion (Fig. 56.30)

Nodular Melanoma

Nodular melanoma apparently does not have the initial radial growth phase, beginning with a vertical phase. Nodular melanoma often exhibits features associated with deep tumor extension and less commonly displays the classic dermoscopic features of superficial spreading melanoma [48].

The ABCD warning signs for melanoma were made to identify superficial spreading

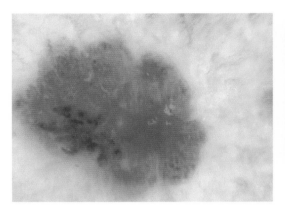

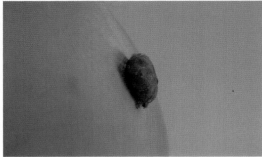

Figs. 56.32 Nodular melanoma following the EGF rule (elevated, firm on palpation, continuous growth over 1 month)

Fig. 56.30 Peripheral brown structureless areas

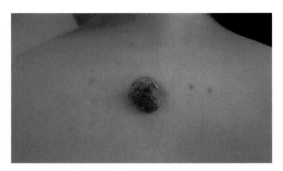

Figs. 56.31 Nodular melanoma following the EGF rule (elevated, firm on palpation, continuous growth over 1 month)

melanoma rather than nodular melanoma, as the latter is often small in diameter, symmetric, with regular borders and less color variegation, and is frequently amelanotic [48]. For this reason, the "EFG" rule (Elevated, Firm on palpation, continuous Growth over 1 month) summarizes the classical characteristics of nodular melanoma [49] (Figs. 56.31 and 56.32). The presence of ulceration, a homogeneous disorganized pattern, and homogeneous blue pigmented, structureless areas are significant independent prognostic factors for nodular versus superficial spreading melanoma. Nodular melanoma is frequently symmetric, with regular borders and less color variegation, and is frequently amelanotic. In nodular melanoma the colors are distributed in a disorganized and asymmetric fashion, characterizing the overall disorganized homogeneous pattern [48].

Peripheral light-brown structureless areas are absent in nodular melanoma as they are associated with thin melanoma [48]. The main clues for the diagnosis of pigmented nodular melanoma and its differentiation from other pigmented nodular lesions (nonmelanocytic and benign melanocytic nevi) are asymmetric pigmentation, blue-black pigmented areas, homogeneous disorganized pattern, the combination of polymorphous vessels and milky-red globules/areas, and polymorphic vessels associated with homogeneous red areas [48].

The thicker the lesion, the more vascular polymorphism is seen. Blue-black pigmented areas may be the only clue for the correct diagnosis of pigmented nodular melanoma in examining asymmetrically pigmented lesions with a homogeneous disorganized pattern [48, 50].

Acral Melanoma

Four patterns are suggestive of melanoma in acral volar skin: the parallel ridge pattern, irregular diffuse pigmentation, the serrated pattern, and the multicomponent pattern (Fig. 56.33).

Melanoma in Facial Chronically Damaged Skin: Lentigo Maligna

LM has many differential diagnoses in facial skin: actinic lentigo, seborrheic keratosis, pigmented AK, and lichen planus-like keratosis. These are all

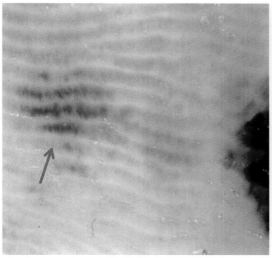
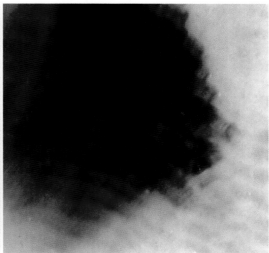

Fig. 56.33 Different images in an acral melanoma of the sole. *Red arrow*: parallel ridge pattern of incipient stages. On the right, multicomponent pattern: parallel ridge pattern, fibrillar pattern, irregular diffuse pigmentation, and black eccentric blotch

common facial lesions that typically develop after the fourth decade of life [51]. The lesions have a similar clinical appearance of a flat, pigmented macule of different size and color. Typically solitary lesions appear to be more suggestive of LM, but this difference is not very trustworthy. Accordingly, neither age nor clinical criteria appear useful for differentiating these entities [51].

Throughout this section we describe the dermatoscopic features that differentiate the aforementioned lesions.

Schiffner et al., Stolz et al., and Pralong et al. have identified specific, dermoscopic criteria for facial LM [52–54].

The paradigmatic progression model consists of four subsequent steps of malignancy. The first step consists in regular/irregular, hyperpigmented follicular openings corresponding to the earliest invasion of the hair shaft histopathologically. Subsequently, the signet-ring-shaped structures (thickening of the hyperpigmented follicular openings) and annular–granular pattern (multiple, gray dots and globules round the pilosebaceous units) appear with further invasion. The third step is composed of pigmented, rhomboidal structures that are created in the perifollicular area while progressing. Finally, the follicular opening is completely covered with uniformly

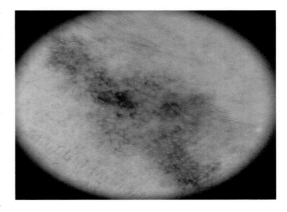

Fig. 56.34 Lentigo malignant melanoma of the face. Hyperpigmented follicular openings. In the center of the lesion, follicular openings completely covered with uniformly pigmented area

pigmented areas. Structureless blue areas, white scar-like areas, and milky-red areas can be also seen [51, 53, 54] (Figs. 56.34 and 56.35).

As characterized by Paralong et al. in 2012, the newly identified dermoscopic patterns include increased density of the vascular network, red rhomboidal structures, target-like patterns, and darkening at dermoscopic examination (when compared with naked-eye examination) [54]. It is very important to never perform ablative treatment of equivocal lesions [51].

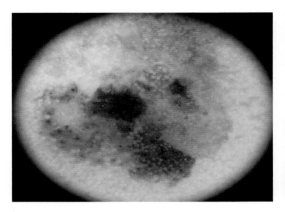

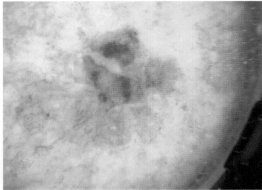

Fig. 56.35 Lentigo malignant melanoma: structureless blue areas and white scar-like areas

Fig. 56.37 Extrafacial lentigo malingnant melanoma

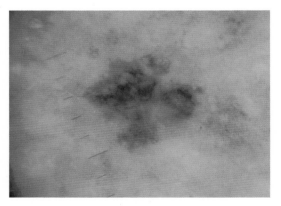

Fig. 56.36 Extrafacial lentigo malingnant melanoma

Melanoma with Special Characteristics

Melanoma in nonfacial chronically damaged skin: extrafacial LM.

Dermoscopic patterns seen in melanomas on nonfacial chronically sun-damaged skin are patchy peripheral pigmented island, angulated line pattern, structureless tan, and granularity pattern [55, 56] (Figs. 56.36 and 56.37).

Mucosal Melanoma

Early mucosal melanomas present brown-black macules with shades of gray. The diameter is larger than 1 cm and multifocal growth is possible. Advanced mucosal melanomas present as black or dark brown nodules com-bined frequently with the macular part at the base of a tumor [35].

Mucosal melanoma has the following patterns: gray, white, or blue color plus structureless zones, irregular dots or globules, and atypical vessels [36].

Non-nodular Hypomelanotic Melanoma

These represent 2–8% of all melanomas and are an important diagnostic pitfall for clinicians. Any of the four subtypes of melanoma (superficial spreading, nodular, acrolentiginous, and LM) can occur as an amelanotic melanoma. To avoid missing it, a high index of suspicion is needed when evaluating isolated and persistent pink outlier lesions. From a dermoscopic perspective pure amelanotic melanomas reveal no pigment while hypomelanotic ones have subtle pigment, which is often present only focally. They present as symmetric erythematous macules and plaques with well-defined borders in 80% of the cases. Light-brown structureless areas have been associated with thin melanomas with a 93.8% positive predictive value. Melanomas with decreased or absent skin markings are significantly thicker than those with increased or normal skin markings [57].

It is important to consider amelanotic melanoma in the differential diagnosis of isolated and persistent erythematous outlier lesions, even if the lesion does not manifest any of the melanoma ABCD criteria [57].

How Reliable Is Dermoscopy and How Much Time is Needed to Perform it?

Our main objective is not to miss any skin cancer. The risk of missing a skin cancer in patients who are seen by a dermatologist for a localized problem (which does not involve examination of the whole cutaneous surface) is on the order of 1 in 50 patients, whereas the risk of missing a melanoma is about 1 in 400 patients [58]. With regard to dermatologists, a total body skin examination to all patients is recommended. Zalaudek et al. estimated that the time required to complete a total body skin examination with manual dermatoscopy was on the order of only 2–3 min [59].

Once examined clinically and by dermoscopy, patients will follow two distinct management paths, depending on their risk profile: (1) patients who have a single lesion or few lesions and (2) patients with multiple nevi. In the first group, if a lesion seems benign it may be left, but if it is suspicious it should be removed or monitored depending on the degree of suspicion. Monitoring is a specific procedure that helps reduce the number of unnecessary excisions in higher-risk patients, particularly those with multiple nevi. On the other hand, in low-risk patients with a single or a few slightly atypical melanocytic lesions, long term monitoring versus excision can be implemented. An alternative method to manage indeterminate or equivocal melanocytic lesions is short-term clinical and dermoscopic follow-up (2–4 months) [60].

Patients with multiple nevi should be on a monitoring program to ensure a comparative and analytic dermoscopic approach for early diagnosis of melanoma [60]. By this means the reduction in the number of unnecessary removals of benign lesions is around 75% [61]. The patient with multiple nevi should be included in a long-term clinical and dermoscopic monitoring program for the detection of subsequent melanoma [62, 63].

It is noteworthy that patient compliance is typically significantly higher for short-term (2–4 month) than longer-term (6–12 month) reviews [64].

Nonmelanocytic Lesions

As discussed earlier, the two-step dermoscopy algorithm allows the differentiation between melanocytic and nonmelanocytic lesions. Absence of melanocytic lesion criteria should lead us to think that we are facing a nonmelanocytic lesion and evaluate the presence of distinctive criteria of nonmelanocytic lesions.

Nonmelanocytic lesion criteria were described for SK, BCC, dermatofibroma, and vascular lesions (hemangioma and angiokeratoma). In this section, we revise these criteria with a brief description of clinical aspects.

Seborrheic Keratosis

SK is the most common benign epidermal tumor. Its importance lies in its high frequency and its similarity, in some cases, to malignant tumors such as BCC, SCC, and melanoma. SKs are more common in middle-aged individuals but they may also arise in adolescence. Its etiology is unknown. Genetic factors, sun exposure, and infections have been implicated as possible risk factors. Many patients with SK have a family history. Most lesions are asymptomatic, but itch and discomfort in friction areas are not uncommon. SK can appear in any topography except mucous membranes, palms, and soles [65].

The clinical presentation of SKs is polymorphous. They can present as macular, papular, polypoid, or cerebriform lesions, generally multiple and varied in size, usually between 2 to 20 mm in diameter. They have generally well-defined limits, as "stuck" on the skin surface, and may be warty, rough, or velvety. The color is very variable between beige, brown, brown-black, gray, and black with or without keratin cysts on the surface. SKs tend to persist and grow slowly over the years with no malignant potential [65] (Fig. 56.38).

Clinical polymorphism correlates with histologic subtype: acanthotic, hyperkeratotic, webbed, clonal, irritated, and melanoacanthoma. Some of these varieties can be melanoma simulators [65].

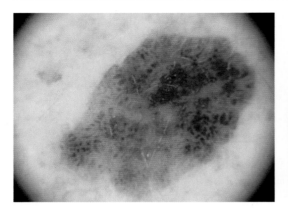

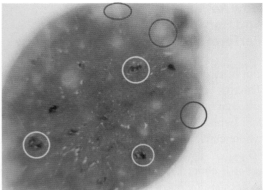

Fig. 56.38 Seborrheic keratosis: abrupt edges on the skin

Fig. 56.39 Seborrheic keratosis. *Red*: milia-like cysts. *Yellow*: comedo-like openings. *Blue*: abrupt edges

Table 56.3 Dermoscopic criteria of seborrheic keratosis

Dermoscopic structures
Abrupt edge
Milia-like cysts
Comedo-like openings
Cracks and ridges
Hairpin vessels
Fingerprint-like structures

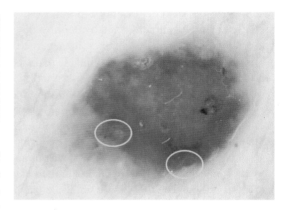

Fig. 56.40 Seborrheic keratosis. *Yellow*: comedo-like openings

The first described dermoscopic features of SK were comedo-like openings and milia-like cysts. In 2001, the Dermoscopy Consensus NetMeeting defined more criteria for the diagnosis such as multiple milia, comedo-like openings, cracks and ridges (cerebriform aspect), and light-brown fingerprint structures [66]. In 2002, Braun et al. evaluated dermoscopic features of 203 pigmented SKs and added additional criteria such as cracks, hairpin vessels, demarcated borders, and moth-eaten edge. In addition, crypts, exophytic papillary structures, and the jelly sign were described, improving diagnostic sensitivity [66].

Dermatoscopic criteria of SK are listed in Table 56.3.

- Milia-like cysts: Yellowish white circular structures of 0.1–1 mm of diameter, present in 14–66% of SK [67]. Because milia-like cysts and comedo- like openings are less conspicuous with polarized dermoscopy, they blink when the observer toggles between light sources (nonpolarized and polarized), which are useful for identifying them [67–69]. SK

can be also observed in melanocytic lesions, congenital melanocytic nevi, and in some melanomas [67, 68] (Fig. 56.39).

- Comedo-like openings: Circular structures similar to a comedo, light or dark brown, yellowish, or black in color. They are observed in 71–80% of SKs and can be also present in papillomatous nevi [67, 69–71] (Figs. 56.39 and 56.40).

- Cracks and ridges: These have the same meaning. The former are described as linear depressions that resemble brain surface. The latter are hypo- or hyperpigmented and resemble "fat fingers" [69, 70] (Fig. 56.41).

- Hairpin vessels: Elongated looped vessels at the periphery of the lesion, regularly distributed, with monomorphic appearance and usu-

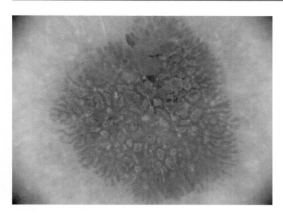

Fig. 56.41 Seborrheic keratosis: cracks (*blue*) and ridges (*red*)

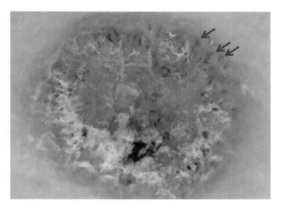

Fig. 56.42 Irritated seborrheic keratosis. *Red*: hairpin vessels with *white* halo

ally surrounded by a whitish halo, which is a keratinization sign. They are usually present in head and neck lesions [67, 69–71]. In irritated SK, hairpin vessels are irregular, polymorphous, elongated, twisted, or double-stranded and different in size, simulating melanomas. They are present in 63% of SKs and in 94% of irritated SKs [67] (Fig. 56.42).

- Fingerprint-like structures: Dark-brown, fine parallel cord-like structures characteristically seen in the periphery of SK and solar lentigo [69–71]. These structures are present in 55–100% of plane SKs [67].
- Treatment of SK is not necessary. They are usually treated for cosmetic purposes or when symptoms appear. Among therapeutic options

there are different destructive methods such as cryotherapy, electrodesiccation with curettage, or laser ablation, which are very effective. Most common complications include depigmentation, scarring, and recurrence as a consequence of incomplete excision [65].

Basal Cell Carcinoma

BCC is a primary malignant epithelial skin tumor derived from immature stem cells of the basal layer of the epidermis and its annexes. BCC grows slowly, in close relationship with the surrounding stroma, with minimal metastatic potential [72].

BCC is the most common cancer in humans. Its incidence has been increasing at a rate of 4–8% annually since 1960 [73].

It produces considerable morbidity although its death rate is low [74].

Clinically, nodular BCC is the most common variant. Its presents in the head and neck, posing as a nodule or smooth papule, solitary, erythematous, translucent, shiny, and pearlescent, showing telangiectasia on its surface [72, 74, 75]. Ulceration of the lesion is common as well as pigmentation (named pigmented BCC) [76].

Superficial BCC presents as a flat erythematous scaly patch or papule, well defined in shape, with slow centrifugal growth, most often located in the trunk [72, 74, 77]. Dermoscopy has been extensively described for nodular and superficial BCC.

Dermoscopic criteria for BCC are as follows [78] (Table 56.4).

- Leaf-like areas: Gray, brown or blue, shiny, discrete bulbous structures that resemble a maple leaf. They are seen on the edges of pigmented BCC [69]. Leaf-like areas show a 100% specificity and 20% sensitivity for the diagnosis of pigmented BCC [71] (Fig. 56.43).
- Spoke wheel structures: Radially arranged [69, 71, 79] projections with a more pigmented brown, blue, or gray center. They are seen in 10% of cases and have a specificity of 100% [70, 80] (Fig. 56.43).

Table 56.4 Dermoscopic criteria of basal cell carcinoma

Classic criteria	New criteria
Leaf-like areas	Concentric structures
Spoke wheel structures	Multiple blue-gray focused points
Multiple blue-gray globules	Crystalline structures
Large blue-gray ovoid nests or blotches	Thin and short superficial telangiectasia
Linear and arborizing (branch-like) telangiectasia	Multiple small erosions
Single or multiple ulceration	

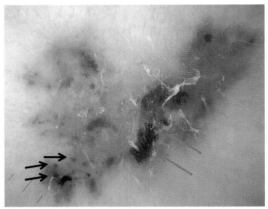

Fig. 56.44 *Black arrows*: multiple blue-gray globules. *Red arrows*: ulceration

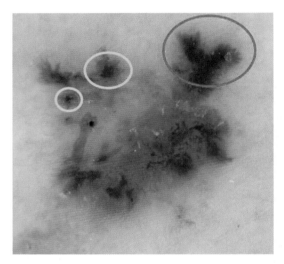

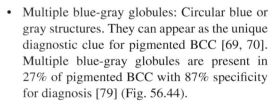

Fig. 56.43 Basal cell carcinoma. *Red*: leaf-like areas. *Yellow*: spoke wheel structures

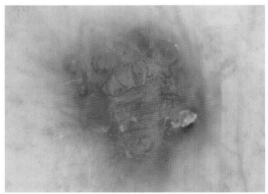

Fig. 56.45 Basal cell carcinoma: linear and arborizing (branch-like) telangiectasia

- Multiple blue-gray globules: Circular blue or gray structures. They can appear as the unique diagnostic clue for pigmented BCC [69, 70]. Multiple blue-gray globules are present in 27% of pigmented BCC with 87% specificity for diagnosis [79] (Fig. 56.44).
- Large blue-gray ovoid nests or blotches: Round or ovoid formations larger than globules, homogeneously bluish [69–71]. They are present in more than half of the cases of pigmented BCC, with 97% specificity [79].
- Linear and arborizing (branch-like) telangiectasia: Thick- and thin-branched vessels. This may be the unique criterion of unpigmented BCC [69, 70, 79]. These vessels are present in more than half of the cases and in 90% of

superficial BCCs. Its specificity is 77% [79] (Figs. 56.45 and 56.46).
- Single or multiple ulceration: Areas with interruption of the epidermis that show a sero-hematic orange or yellow crust in its surface. Ulceration of a BCC may occur early, unlike melanoma where this is usually a late event [71] (Fig. 56.44).

Nonclassical criteria of BCC were latterly described. These are present in 26% of cases and include the following structures [78]:

- Concentric structures: Similar to globules, irregularly shaped, blue, gray, or brown with a darker central area. They may represent the

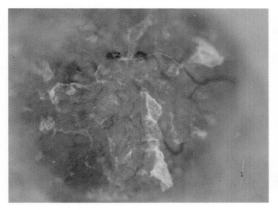

Fig. 56.46 Basal cell carcinoma: linear and arborizing (branch-like) telangiectasia

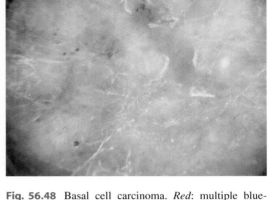

Fig. 56.48 Basal cell carcinoma. *Red*: multiple blue-gray focused points

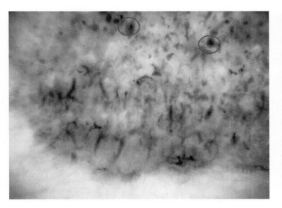

Fig. 56.47 Basal cell carcinoma. *Red*: concentric structures

Fig. 56.49 Basal cell carcinoma: thin and short superficial telangiectasia

early stage of spoke wheel structures. They are present in 7.6% of BCCs [78, 81] (Fig. 56.47).

- Multiple blue-gray focused points: It is postulated that they would be the initial form of the blue-gray globules; they are present in 5% of BCCs [78, 81] (Fig. 56.48).
- Bright white-red areas: Areas without structures, pink or pearly, present in 100% of the superficial BCCs [78].
- Crystalline structures: Short, thick and shiny, pearly whitish lines due to the presence of collagen bundles in thickened dermis. These structures are only visible with polarized light dermoscopy. They can also be seen in dermatofibromas, scars, Spitz nevi, and melanomas [47, 78, 80, 82].
- Thin and short superficial telangiectasia: Also known as microarborizing vessels. They are

telangiectasias with a smaller caliber than 1 mm with little or no ramifications. They are present in more of the 91% of superficial BCCs and are considered the initial form of branched vessels [78] (Fig. 56.49).

- Multiple small erosions: Erosions of less than 1 mm in diameter, reddish-brown in color. They adopt a peripheral distribution in the lesion with a frequency of 8.5–70% in superficial BCCs [78] (Fig. 56.50).

Treatment options for BCC are beyond the scope of this chapter and are discussed in Chap. 15.

Dermatofibroma

Dermatofibroma, or superficial benign fibrous histiocytoma, is a common benign tumor, more

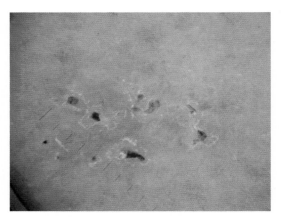

Fig. 56.50 Superficial basal cell carcinoma: multiple small erosions

Table 56.5 Dermoscopic criteria of dermatofibroma [83]

Pattern 1: Total delicate pigment network
Pattern 2: Peripheral delicate pigment network and central white scar-like patch
Pattern 3: Peripheral delicate pigment network and central white network
Pattern 4: Peripheral delicate pigment network and central homogeneous area
Pattern 5: Total white network
Pattern 6: Total homogeneous area
Pattern 7: Total white scar-like patch/multiple white scar-like patches
Pattern 8: Peripheral homogeneous area and central white scar-like patch
Pattern 9: Peripheral homogeneous area and central white network
Pattern 10: Atypical pattern

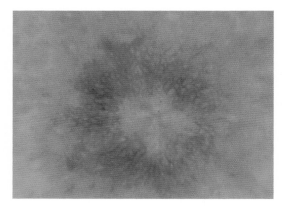

Fig. 56.51 Dermatofibroma: peripheral delicate pigmented network and central white scar-like patch (pattern 2)

frequently located in the lower extremities of young females, but not exclusively. Clinically it presents as a papule or firm nodule with smooth surface in shades of brown. It can be unique or multiple. The pinch test is helpful and easy for diagnosis, and consists of squeezing the lesion from the sides, resulting in dimpling of overlying skin [83].

The most frequent dermoscopic feature is the presence of a fine peripheral pigmented network and a white central scar-like patch (Fig. 56.51) [69, 70]. In 2008 Zaballos et al. described ten different dermoscopic patterns for dermatofibroma [83] (Table 56.5, Figs. 56.51, 56.52, and 56.53).

Atypical patterns can often be difficult to differentiate from melanocytic lesions including melanoma (Fig. 56.54) [84]. Many histopathologic variants have been described. Surgical excision should be performed in high-risk patients who present with changes in the lesion [85].

In 2013 Ferrari et al. described a group of dermatofibromas showing a pattern of atypical lesions as "nondermatofibroma-like patterns", including melanoma-like, vascular tumor-like, BCC-like, tumor-like collision, and psoriasis-like [85].

A significant association between the pattern of melanoma-like dermatofibroma and the histopathologic variant hemosiderotic/aneurysmal was found. This shows in dermoscopy a multicomponent pattern with a homogeneous bluish-red central area. The histologic correlation in these central structures is the presence of intra- and extracellular spaces filled with blood and hemosiderin deposits [84].

Vascular Lesions: Hemangioma and Angiokeratoma

Capillary hemangiomas are common skin tumors that can appear as single or multiple lesions. Clinically they present as macules or papules that vary in size, characterized by bright red or purple color. The diagnosis is usually clinical, but often

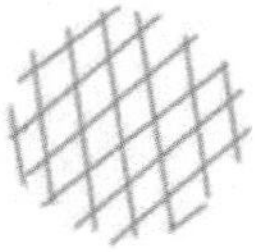 Pattern 1	Total delicate pigment network
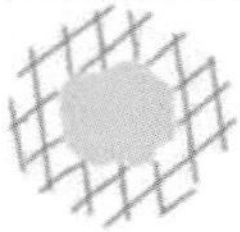 Pattern 2	Peripheral delicate pigment network and central white scarlike patch
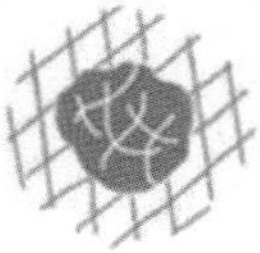 Pattern 3	Peripheral delicate pigment network and central white network
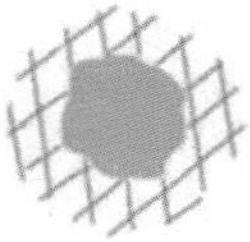 Pattern 4	Peripheral delicate pigment network and central homogeneous area
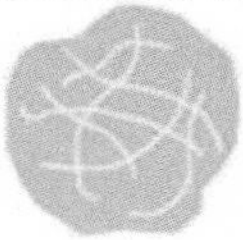 Pattern 5	Total white network
Pattern 6	Total homogeneous area
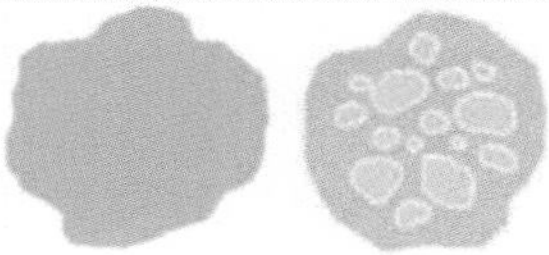 Pattern 7	Total white scarlike patch/multiple white scarlike patches
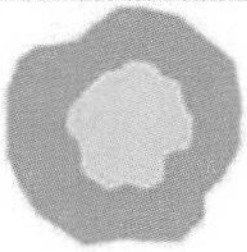 Pattern 8	Peripheral homogeneous area and central white scarlike patch
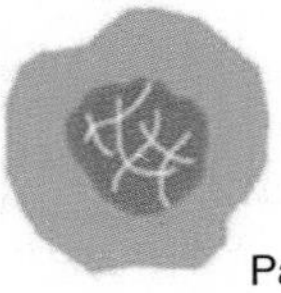 Pattern 9	Peripheral homogeneous area and central white network
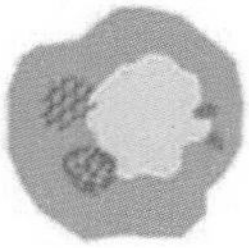 Pattern 10	Atypical pattern

Fig. 56.52 Dermoscopic patterns of dermatofibroma (Modified from Zaballos et al. [83])

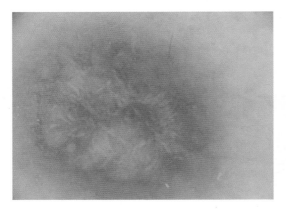

Fig. 56.53 Dermatofibroma: total white network (pattern 5)

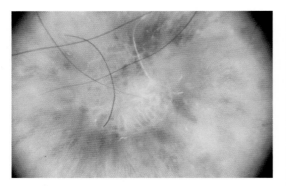

Fig. 56.54 Dermatofibroma: atypical pattern (pattern 10)

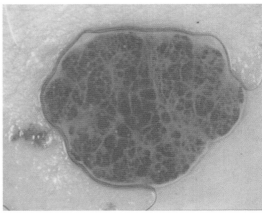

Fig. 56.55 Hemangioma: red lagoons

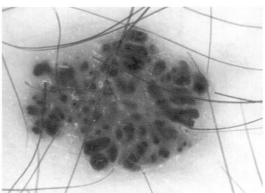

Fig. 56.56 Angiokeratoma: vascular lagoons and hyperkeratosis covering the lesion like a veil

can simulate a nodular melanoma or metastatic melanoma, and it is in these cases is where dermoscopy is useful [69].

Dermoscopic features are the presence of red lagoons which could show bluish-red or black color, posing as well-defined structures, circular or ovoid, which vary in size and color within the same lesion [70–72]. These criteria have a sensitivity of 83.9% and specificity of 99.1% for the diagnosis [86] (Fig. 56.55).

Angiokeratomas are vascular malformations that clinically appear as dark-red to blue-black lesions, single or multiple, and circumscribed [24]. They consist in the combination of vascular ectasia with hyperkeratosis [69].

Angiokeratomas have five clinical presentations: single or multiple lesions, circumscribed, Fordyce angiokeratomas, angiokeratomas of Mibelli, and diffusum corporis [87].

Dermoscopy shows the presence of dark red-blue lagoons and white veil with peripheral erythema that may have a bleeding scab [87] (Fig. 56.56).

Lagoons in angiokeratomas tend to be less defined than that those of hemangiomas. Hyperkeratosis covering the lesion with yellowish white coloring is observed. In early lesions the differentiation between hemangioma and angiokeratoma may be difficult [70].

Often angiokeratomas pose differential diagnosis with other pigmented lesions such as melanocytic nevi, Spitz nevi, melanoma, BCC, SK, and other benign vascular lesions such as pyogenic granuloma. Dermoscopy is useful to define the diagnosis when it shows characteristic red-bluish lagoons with white veil covering the lesion [87].

Actinic Keratosis

AK is considered to be an in situ epidermal dysplasia that frequently develops on chronic sun-damaged skin [88–90]. Its main clinical and management aspects are discussed in Chap. 14.

The diagnosis of AK is usually simple, with no need of histologic evaluation, and is based on its typical clinical appearance of nonpigmented, circumscribed, rough and scaly reddish papule or plaque located in a photodamaged site such as the face, lower neck, and back of hands [89, 91]. Less frequently it can be pigmented, making the differential diagnosis with melanoma difficult (or even impossible) [89]. Most AKs are asymptomatic and rarely develop as solitary tumors [91, 92].

The diagnostic sensitivity and specificity of dermoscopy for classical AK has been reported to reach 98% and 95%, respectively, with a high level of concordance between this technique and histopathology [88, 93]. Four dermoscopic criteria have been established, and a similar pattern is seen in each individual for different AKs [88, 92].

Classical Nonpigmented Actinic Keratosis

According to Zalaudek et al., three different grades are described [93].

- Grade 1: When the AK is a slightly palpable lesion (better felt than seen) and exhibits a pink to red pseudonetwork pattern surrounding hair follicles and discrete white to yellow scale upon dermoscopy [88, 93] (Fig. 56.57).
- Grade 2: Refers to a moderately thick lesion that is easily felt and seen. This lesion is dermoscopically typified by an erythematous

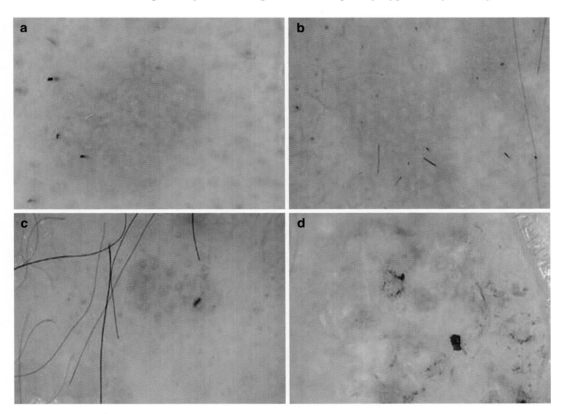

Fig. 56.57 Nonpigmented actinic keratosis (**a**) grade 1: red pseudonetwork; (**b**) grade 2: "strawberry pattern"; (**c**, **d**) grade 3: hyperkeratosis and enlarged follicular openings filled with keratotic plugs over a scaly and white to yellow appearing background or a structureless area

pseudonetwork that is intermingled with white to yellow, hyperkeratotic, partially confluent, and enlarged follicular openings surrounded by white halo (targetoid appearance). It is called a "strawberry pattern" and is seen in 95% of AKs [12, 88, 92, 93]. Of note, the term "strawberry pattern" is a metaphorical term that sticks in the memory and represents a useful diagnostic clue [94] Fig. 56.57.

• Grade 3: When the AK is very thick, hyperkeratotic, and can exhibit by dermoscopy either enlarged follicular openings filled with keratotic plugs over a scaly and white to yellow appearing background, or a structureless area [93] (Fig. 56.57).

Last but not least, bowenoid AK is an infrequent type of AK that exhibits a vascular pattern shown by regularly distributed glomerular vessels with no clustering arrangement as seen in classic Bowen disease [12, 95].

Pigmented Actinic Keratosis

Owing to the overlapping of clinical and dermoscopy patterns with LM, the diagnostic sensitivity and specificity for pigmented AK is much lower than that for nonpigmented AK.

Classically, pigmented AK shows a superficial, broken pseudonetwork consisting of brown, curved double lines that surround enlarged, partially confluent, hyperkeratotic follicles of various sizes. Scales can be associated [89, 92, 93]. A feature typically described for solar lentigo and seborrheic keratosis, such as the moth-eaten border, has been reported for pigmented AK [92].

In addition, pigmented AK may sometimes reveal pigmented structures that overlap with those of LM. These structures include annular granular pattern (multiple grayish-brown dots and globules which coalesce around hair follicles), rhomboidal structures around the follicular openings, and asymmetric, pigmented follicular openings. In such cases, a biopsy is mandatory to rule out LM [89, 92, 93] (Fig. 56.58).

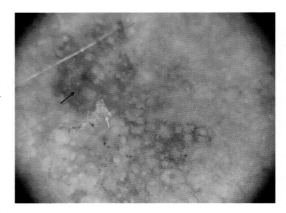

Fig. 56.58 Pigmented actinic keratosis: hyperkeratosis, scale (*yellow arrow*), rhomboidal structures (*black arrow*), and pigmented follicular openings

Other Frequent Uses of Dermoscopy

Common Daily Uses for Infections

Four parameters should be assessed when applying dermoscopy in the realm of inflammatory and infectious diseases: (i) morphologic vascular patterns; (ii) arrangement of vascular structures; (iii) colors; and (iv) follicular abnormalities. The presence of other specific features should also be evaluated [96].

Molluscum Contagiosum

The diagnosis of molluscum contagiosum, a common skin viral infection of the epidermal keratinocytes caused by a poxvirus, is generally easy because of its characteristic cutaneous feature of umbilicated translucent papules [97–99]. Lesions are generally numerous, characteristically of 2–4 mm diameter, with glossy appearance [99].

In adults it may raise diagnostic doubts when it presents as a single lesion or when the lesion is inflamed. In locations such as the face, molluscum can be mistaken for BCC, sebaceous hyperplasia, or other adnexal tumor [100]. Dermoscopy may facilitate the clinical diagnosis [99].

Molluscum contagiosum shows a characteristic dermoscopy pattern consisting of a central polylobular white to yellow amorphous structure

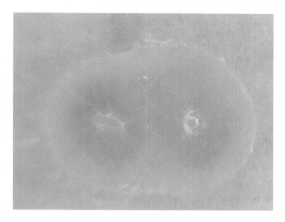

Fig. 56.59 Molluscum contagiosum showing a skin-colored surface with a central white to yellow amorphous structure

(Fig. 56.59) [95]. The hallmark dermoscopic pattern is crown vessels at the periphery of the lesion with a radial distribution (not crossing the center of the lesion) that resembles a red crown [95, 98, 99]. These crown vessels are also described for sebaceous hyperplasia. Other frequent dermoscopy findings are a whitish peripheral halo and hyperkeratosis [95].

In 2011 a study conducted on dermoscopy of 211 lesions of molluscum contagiosum led to a further vascular pattern being described: the punctiform vascular pattern. This consists of small reddish dots inside the lesion (also described in melanoma, clear cell acanthoma, lichen planus, and eccrine poroma, among others). The punctiform pattern prevails in inflamed and/or excoriated lesions and in lesions with perilesional eczema [98].

Warts

Cutaneous and mucosal viral infections due to human papillomavirus are extremely common in clinical practice. The diagnosis is generally easy in all its clinical forms: common warts, flat warts, filiform warts, plantar warts, and genital warts. However, in some cases the diagnosis may be challenging, as it occurs in traumatized and irritated lesions or those previously treated [100].

Dermoscopy has been demonstrated to be a valuable tool in these infections, both for diagnosis and monitoring treatment [95, 98].

Common warts display a whitish halo that corresponds to dense papillomatosis, each containing a central red dot [95, 98, 100]. The halo may not be visible if there is significant vascular occlusion. This vascular pattern is described as multiple homogeneous but with nonspecific distribution of dots, ranging in color from red to black [100]. Black dots indicate thrombosed vessels [95]. Plantar warts show more prominent hemorrhages and black lines corresponding to thrombosed capillaries and microbleeds caused by trauma from ambulation. The identification of the aforementioned structures in hyperkeratotic plantar lesions helps to distinguish warts from common conditions such as calluses and corns [95, 98].

Flat warts exhibit small dotted vessels with regular distribution on a yellowish brown background [98, 100] (Fig. 56.60).

Genital warts, also known as condylomas, show a mosaic pattern consisting of a white reticular network surrounding central small islands of unaffected mucosal skin [98]. Higher magnification demonstrates that those islands correspond to a vascular pattern, given by many punctate (dotted vessels) and/or red globules (bigger vessels) [100, 101]. Dermoscopy in genital warts can be useful to differentiate them from vestibular papillae and pearly penile papules, normal features of female and male external genitalia, respectively [98].

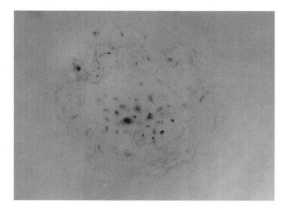

Fig. 56.60 Vulgar wart showing homogeneously distributed dots, from red to violet, and hemorrhages. Whitish peripheral halo

Squamous Cell Carcinoma

In the field of SCC a progression model has been described, and alongside it specific dermoscopic patterns associated with different stages of progression have been identified. Dermoscopy findings allow the differentiation between AK, intraepidermal carcinoma (IEC) also commonly named Bowen's disease or SCC in situ, and invasive SCC [93, 102].

Intraepidermal Squamous Cell Carcinoma or In Situ Squamous Cell Carcinoma

Dermoscopy exhibits classically dotted/glomerular vessels arranged in small clusters and discrete yellowish or white opaque scales, representing hyperkeratosis [13, 102]. Both dotted and glomerular vessels are frequently seen in the same lesion [13].

Invasive Squamous Cell Carcinoma

SCC shows highly polymorphous vascular structures [13, 95]. The prevailing ones are elongated, linear vessels and/or hairpin vessels of varying shape and distribution, without grouping into clusters. In addition to vascular patterns, signs of keratinization (representing further important clues for diagnosis) are usually seen as white structureless amorphous areas, a central mass of keratin, or, less frequently, targetoid appearance follicular openings consisting of an opaque, yellow center surrounded by a white halo (white circles). Variable areas of ulceration are often seen [13, 93, 95, 102].

Keratoacanthoma

Keratoacanthoma is actually regarded as a variant of SCC due to its resemblance to the histopathology of SCC [13].

The most stereotypical dermoscopic pattern is typified by a central amorphous, structureless whitish mass of keratin, which is surrounded by elongated telangiectasias of large caliber and few branches [13, 93, 102]. These large-caliber vessels may be sometimes mistaken for the arborizing vessels of BCC; however, they are less focused, with fewer branches, and are frequently associated with signs of keratinization [93, 102].

Future Perspectives

Future perspectives for dermoscopy are enormous.

It now has an increasing role in the recognition of several inflammatory and infectious diseases, as well as their discrimination from skin tumors [96].

Moreover, recent data indicate that it might also be worthwhile for the assessment of the outcome and adverse effects of various treatments [103].

Dermoscopy is also a promising bridge connecting clinical with basic molecular research in dermato-oncology [104]. A correlation between an individual genetic status and dermoscopy patterns of nevi and melanoma can be made. For example, melanomas with BRAF V600E mutation or NRAS mutations reveal dermoscopic signs of regression at higher frequency compared with melanoma, which are wild-type for these mutations [105, 106].

Dermoscopy will also be a link between new technologies and clinical practice. Likewise, dermoscopy and reflectance confocal microscopy represent complementary/synergistic methods for the evaluation of skin tumors [107].

References

1. Pehamberger H, Binder M, Steiner A, et al. In vivo epiluminiscence microscopy: improvement of early diagnosis of melanoma. J Invest Dermatol. 1993;100:356S–62S.
2. Marghoob AA, Usatine RP, Jaimes N. Dermoscopy for the family physician. Am Fam Physician. 2013;88(7):441–50.
3. Ochaita P, Avilés JA. Dermatoscopia digital. Análisis de los diferentes sistemas. Piel. 2004;19(7):395–401.
4. Marghoob AA, Swindle LD, Moricz CZ, et al. Instruments and new technologies for the in vivo diagnosis of melanoma. J Am Acad Dermatol. 2003;49:777–97.

5. Zalaudek I, Argenziano G, Di Stefani A, Ferrara G, Marghoob AA, Hofmann-Wellenhof R, et al. Dermatology. 2006;212:7–18.

6. Chevolet I, Hoorens I, Janssens A, Speeckaert R, Van Geel N, Van Maele G, et al. Short dermoscopy training increases diagnostic performance in both inexperienced and experienced dermatologists. Australas J Dermatol. 2015;56(1):52–5.

7. Vestergaard ME, Macaskill P, Holt PE, Menzies SW. Dermoscopy compared with naked eye examination for the diagnosis of primary melanoma: a meta-analysis of studies performed in a clinical setting. Br J Dermatol. 2008;159(3):669–76.

8. Tschandl P, Kittler H, Schmid K, Zalaudek I, Argenziano G. Teaching dermatoscopy of pigmented skin tumours to novices: comparison of analytic vs. heuristic approach. J Eur Acad Dermatol Venereol. 2015;29(6):1198–204.

9. Blum A, Giacomel J. "Tape dermoscopy" consists in six steps: "Tape dermatoscopy": constructing a low-cost dermatoscope using a mobile phone, immersion fluid and transparent adhesive tape. Dermatol Pract Concept. 2015;5(2):17.

10. Longo I, Chaeta P. Novedades en dispositivos y software en dermatoscopia digital. Piel. 2007;22(3):107–8.

11. Malvhey J, Puig S. Parámetros dermatoscópicos: definición e histopatología. En Principles of dermoscopy. 2009 Ed 2011. www.cege.es. 37–38.

12. Zalaudek I, Kreusch J, Giacomel J, Ferrara G, Catricalà C, Argenziano G. How to diagnose non-pigmented skin tumors: a review of vascular structures seen with dermoscopy: part I. Melanocytic skin tumors. J Am Acad Dermatol. 2010;63(3):361–74.

13. Zalaudek I, Kreusch J, Giacomel J, Ferrara G, Catricalà C, Argenziano G. How to diagnose nonpigmented skin tumors: a review of vascular structures seen with dermoscopy: part II. Nonmelanocytic skin tumors. J Am Acad Dermatol. 2010;63(3):377–86.

14. Bajaj S, Marchetti MA, Navarrete-Dechent C, Dusza SW, Kose K, Marghoob AA. The role of color and morphologic characteristics in dermoscopic diagnosis. JAMA Dermatol. 2016;152(6):676–82.

15. Argenziano G, Soyer HP, Chimenti S, Talamini R, Corona R, Sera F, et al. Dermoscopy of pigmented skin lesions: results of a consensus meeting via the internet. J Am Acad Dermatol. 2003;48(5):679–93.

16. Chen LL, Dusza SW, Jaimes N, Marghoob AA. Performance of the first step of the 2-step dermoscopy algorithm. JAMA Dermatol. 2015;151(7):715–21.

17. Marghoob AA, Braun R. Proposal for a revised 2-step algorithm for the classification of lesions of the skin using dermoscopy. Arch Dermatol. 2010;146(4):426–8.

18. Carrera C, Marchetti MA, Dusza SW, Argenziano G, Braun RP, Halpern AC, et al. Validity and reliability of dermoscopic criteria used to differentiate nevi from melanoma: a web-based International Dermoscopy Society study. JAMA Dermatol. 2016;152(7):798–806.

19. Soyer HP, Argenziano G, Zalaudek I, Corona R, Sera F, Talamini R, et al. Three-point checklist of dermoscopy. A new screening method for early detection of melanoma. Dermatology. 2004;208(1):27–31.

20. Nachbar F, Stolz W, Merkle T, Congetta AB, Vogt T, Landthaler M, et al. The ABCD rule of dermatoscopy: high prospective value in the diagnosis of doubtful melanocytic skin lesions. J Am Acad Dermatol. 1994;30(4):551–9.

21. Larre Borges A, Zalaudek I, Longo C, Dufrechou L, Argenziano G, Lallas A, et al. Melanocytic nevi with special features: clinical-dermoscopic and reflectance confocal microscopic-findings. J Eur Acad Dermatol Venereol. 2014;28(7):833–45.

22. Kittler H, Tschandl P. Dysplastic nevus: why this term should be abandoned in dermatoscopy. Dermatol Clin. 2013;31(4):579–88.

23. Hofman-Wellenhof R, Carrera C. Dermoscopic classification of Clark Nevi. In Malvhey J, Puig S. Principles of dermoscopy. 2009 Ed. www.cege.es www.dermoscop.com. Chap 8.3 377–84.

24. Argenziano G, Albertini G, Castagnetti F, De Pace B, Di Lernia V, Longo C, et al. Early diagnosis of melanoma: what is the impact of dermoscopy? Dermatol Ther. 2012;25(5):403–9.

25. Geller AC, Mayer JE, Sober AJ, Miller DR, Argenziano G, Johnson TM, et al. Total nevi, atypical nevi, and melanoma thickness: an analysis of 566 patients at 2 US centers. JAMA Dermatol. 2016;152(4):413–8.

26. Cengiz FP, Cengiz AB, Emiroglu N, Comert E, Wellenhof RH. Dermoscopic and clinical features of head and neck melanoma. An Bras Dermatol. 2015;90(4):488–93.

27. Saida T, Oguchi S, Miayazaki A. Dermoscopy for acral pigmented skin lesions. Clin Dermatol. 2002;20:279–85.

28. Zaballos P, Llambrich A, Puig S, Malvehy J. Criterios Dermatoscópicos de las lesiones melanocíticas palmplantares. Piel. 2006;21:31–6.

29. Saida T, Koga H. Dermoscopic patterns of acral melanocytic nevi. Their variations, changes and significance. Arch Dermatol. 2007;143:1423–6.

30. Miyazaki A, Saida T, Koga H, Oguchi S, Suzuki T, Tsuchida T. Anatomical and histopathologic correlates of the dermoscopic patterns seen in melanocytic nevi on the sole: a retrospective study. J Am Acad Dermatol. 2005;53:230–6.

31. Malvehy J, Puig S. Dermoscopic patterns of benign volar melanocytic lesions in patients with atypical mole syndrome. Arch Dermatol. 2004;140:538–44.

32. Altamura D, Altobelli E, Micantonio T, Piccolo D, Fargnoli MC, Peris K. Dermoscopic patterns of acral melanocytic nevi and melanomas in a white population in central Italy. Arch Dermatol. 2006;142:1123–8.

33. Barquet V, Dufrechou L, Nicoletti S, Acosta MA, Magliano J, Martínez M, et al. Dermoscopic patterns of 158 acral melanocytic nevi in a Latin American population. Actas Dermosifiliogr. 2013;104(7):586–92.

34. Bowling J. Fibrillar pattern of an acquired plantar acral melanocytic naevus: correspondence between

epiluminiscence light microscopy and transverse section histology. Clin Exp Dermatol. 2006;31:449–51.

35. Hofmann-Wellenhof R. Special criteria for special locations 2: scalp, mucosal, and milk line. Dermatol Clin. 2013;31(4):625–36.

36. Murzaku EC, Penn LA, Hale CS, Pomeranz MK, Polsky D. Vulvar nevi, melanosis, and melanoma: an epidemiologic, clinical, and histopathologic review. J Am Acad Dermatol. 2014;71(6):1241–9.

37. Rigel DS, Russak J, Friedman R. The evolution of melanoma diagnosis: 25 years beyond the ABCDs. CA Cancer J Clin. 2010;60(5):301–16.

38. Friedman RJ, Rigel DS, Kopf AW. Early detection of malignant melanoma: the role of physician examination and self-examination of the skin. CA Cancer J Clin. 1985;35:130–51.

39. Abbasi NR, Shaw HM, Rigel DS, Friedman RJ, McCarthy WH, Osman I, et al. Early diagnosis of cutaneous melanoma: revisiting the ABCD criteria. JAMA. 2004;292(22):2771–6.

40. Grob JJ, Bonerandi JJ. The "ugly duckling" sign: identification of the common characteristics of nevi in an individual as a basis for melanoma screening. Arch Dermatol. 1998;134:103–4.

41. Marghoob AA, Scope A. The complexity of diagnosing melanoma. J Invest Dermatol. 2009;129(1):11–3.

42. McGovern VJ, Mihm MC Jr, Bailly C, Booth C, Clark WH Jr, Cochran AJ, et al. The classification of malignant melanoma and its histologic reporting. Cancer. 1973;32:1446–57.

43. Curtin JA, Fridlyand J, Kageshita T, Patel HN, Busman KJ, Kutzner H, et al. Distinct sets of genetic alterations in melanoma. N Engl J Med. 2005;353:2135–47.

44. Kittler H, Pehamberger H, Wolff K, Binder M. Diagnostic accuracy of dermoscopy. Lancet Oncol. 2002;3(3):159–65.

45. Bafounta ML, Beauchet A, Aegerter P, Saiag P. Is dermoscopy (epiluminescence microscopy) useful for the diagnosis of melanoma? Results of a meta-analysis using techniques adapted to the evaluation of diagnostic tests. Arch Dermatol. 2001;137(10):1343–50.

46. Pizzichetta MA, Talamini R, Marghoob AA, Soyer HP, Argenziano G, Bono R, et al. Negative pigment network: an additional dermoscopic feature for the diagnosis of melanoma. J Am Acad Dermatol. 2013;68(4):552–9.

47. Balagula Y, Braun RP, Rabinovitz HS, Dusza SW, Scope A, Liebman TN, et al. The significance of crystalline/chrysalis structures in the diagnosis of melanocytic and nonmelanocytic lesions. J Am Acad Dermatol. 2012;67(2):194.e1–8.

48. Pizzichetta MA, Kittler H, Stanganelli I, Bono R, Cavicchini S, De Giorgi V, et al. Italian Melanoma Intergroup. Pigmented nodular melanoma: the predictive value of dermoscopic features using multivariate analysis. Br J Dermatol. 2015;173(1):10614.

49. Kalkhoran S, Milne O, Zalaudek I, et al. Historical, clinical, and dermoscopic characteristics of thin nodular melanoma. Arch Dermatol. 2010;146:311–8.

50. Argenziano G, Longo C, Cameron A, Cavicchini S, Gourhant JY, Lallas A, et al. Blue-black rule: a simple dermoscopic clue to recognize pigmented nodular melanoma. Br J Dermatol. 2011;165:1251–5.

51. Lallas A, Argenziano G, Moscarella E, Longo C, Simonetti V, Zalaudek I. Diagnosis and management of facial pigmented macules. Clin Dermatol. 2014;32(1):94–100.

52. Schiffner R, Schiffner-Rohe J, Vogt T, Landthaler M, Wlotzke U, Cognetta AB, et al. Improvement of early recognition of lentigo maligna using dermatoscopy. J Am Acad Dermatol. 2000;42:25–32.

53. Stolz W, Schiffner R, Burgdorf WH. Dermatoscopy for facial pigmented skin lesions. Clin Dermatol. 2002;20:276–8.

54. Pralong P, Bathelier E, Dalle S, Poulalhon N, Debarbieux S, Thomas L. Dermoscopy of lentigo malignant melanoma: report of 125 cases. Br J Dermatol. 2012;167:280–7.

55. Jaimes N, Marghoob AA, Rabinovitz H, Braun RP, Cameron A, Rosendahl C, et al. Clinical and dermoscopic characteristics of melanomas on nonfacial chronically sun-damaged skin. J Am Acad Dermatol. 2015;72(6):1027–35.

56. Vanden Daelen A, Ferreira I, Marot L, Tromme I. A digital dermoscopy follow-up illustration and a histopathologic correlation for angulated lines in extrafacial lentigo maligna. JAMA Dermatol. 2016;152(2):200–3.

57. Jaimes N, Braun RP, Thomas L, Marghoob AA. Clinical and dermoscopic characteristics of amelanotic melanomas that are not of the nodular subtype. J Eur Acad Dermatol Venereol. 2012;26(5):591–6.

58. Argenziano G, Zalaudek I, Hofmann-Wellenhof R, Bakos RM, Bergman W, Blum A, et al. Total body skin examination for skin cancer screening in patients with focused symptoms. J Am Acad Dermatol. 2012;66:212–9.

59. Zalaudek I, Kittler H, Marghoob AA, Balato A, Blum A, Dalle S, et al. Time required for a complete skin examination with and without dermoscopy: a prospective, randomized multicenter study. Arch Dermatol. 2008;144:509–13.

60. Argenziano G, Giacomel J, Zalaudek I, Blum A, Braun RP, Cabo H, et al. A clinicodermoscopic approach for skin cancer screening: recommendations involving a survey of the International Dermoscopy Society. Dermatol Clin. 2013;31(4):525–34.

61. Argenziano G, Catricala C, Ardigo M, Buccini P, De Simone P, Eibenschutz L, et al. Dermoscopy of patients with multiple nevi: improved management recommendations using a comparative diagnostic approach. Arch Dermatol. 2011;147:46–9.

62. Salerni G, Carrera C, Lovatto L, Puig-Butille JA, Badenas C, Plana E, et al. Benefits of total body photography and digital dermatoscopy ("twostep method of digital follow-up") in the early diagnosis of melanoma in patients at high risk for melanoma. J Am Acad Dermatol. 2011;67(1):e17–27.

63. Salerni G, Lovatto L, Carrera C, Puig S, Malvehy J. Melanomas detected in a follow-up program compared with melanomas referred to a melanoma unit. Arch Dermatol. 2011;147:549–55.

64. Argenziano G, Mordente I, Ferrara G, Sgambato A, Annese P, Zalaudek I. Dermoscopic monitoring of melanocytic skin lesions: clinical outcome and patient compliance vary according to follow-up protocols. Br J Dermatol. 2008;159:331–6.

65. Valencia D, Neil A, Ken K. Benign epithelial tumors, hamartomas, and hyperplasias. In: Fitzpatrick. Dermatología en medicina general. Madrid: Panamericana. 2008; p. 1054–76.

66. Lin J, Han S, Cui L, Song Z, Gao M, Yang G, et al. Evaluation of dermoscopic algorithm for seborrheic keratosis: a prospective study in 412 patients. J Eur Acad Dermatol Venereol. 2014;28:957–62.

67. Ruiz AB, Quiñones R, Domínguez AE. Dermatoscopía de las queratosis seborreicas y sus diferentes caras. Dermatol Rev Mex. 2012;56(3):193–200.

68. Braun RP, Scope A, Marghoob AA. The "blink sign" in dermoscopy. Arch Dermatol. 2011;147(4):520.

69. Malvehy J, Puig S, Braun R, Marghoob A, Kopf A. Manual de Dermatoscopía. Barcelona: Editorial BCN Art Directe; 2006. p. 1–20.

70. Cabo H, Argenziano G, Sabban C, et al. Lesiones no melanocíticas en Dermatoscopía. 2nd ed. Argentina: Ediciones Journal; 2008. p. 83–117.

71. Carrera C, Zaballos P, Puig S, Malvehy J, Mascaró-Galy JM, Palou J. Correlación histológica en dermatoscopía; lesiones melanocíticas y no melanocíticas. Criterios dermatoscópicos de nevus melanocíticos. Med Cut Iber Lat Am. 2004;32(2):47–60.

72. Basset-Séguin N, Chaussade V, Vilmer C. Carcinomas basocelulares. EMC. Dermatología. Paris: Elsevier Masson SAS; 2011.

73. Nelson SA, Scope A, Rishpon A, Rabinovitz HS, Oliviero MC, Laman SD, et al. Accuracy and confidence in the clinical diagnosis of basal cell cancer using dermoscopy and reflex confocal microscopy. Int J Dermatol. 2016; doi:10.1111/ijd.13361.

74. Wong CSM, Strange RC, Lear JT. Basal cell carcinoma. BMJ. 2003;327(7418):794–8.

75. Mackiewicz-Wysocka M, Bowszyc-Dmochowska M, Strzelecka-Węklar D, Dańczak-Pazdrowska A, Adamski Z. Basal cell carcinoma – diagnosis. Contemp Oncol (Pozn). 2013;17(4):337–42.

76. Chinem PV, Miot HA. Epidemiologia do carcinoma basocelular. An Bras Dermatol. 2011;86(2):292–305.

77. Lallas A, Tzellos T, Kyrgidis A, Apalla Z, Zalaudek I, Karatolias A, et al. Accuracy of dermoscopic criteria for discriminating superficial from other subtypes of basal cell carcinoma. J Am Acad Dermatol. 2014;70(2):303–11.

78. González V, Gramajo M, Escobar C, Romero Costas L, Ruzzi I, Picardi N, et al. Dermatoscopía del carcinoma basocelular: criterios clásicos y actuales. Arch Argent Dermatol. 2012;62:87–91.

79. Menzies SW, Westerhoff K, Rabinovitz H, Kopf AW, McCarthy WH, Katz B. Surface microscopy of pigmented basal cell carcinoma. Arch Dermatol. 2000;136(8):1012–6.

80. Puspok-Schwarz M, Steiner A, Binder M, Partsch B, Wolff K, Pehamberger H. Statistical evaluation of epiluminiscence microscopy criteria in the differential diagnosis of malignant melanoma and pigmented basal cell carcinoma. Melanoma Res. 1997;7:307–11.

81. Altamura D, Menzies S, Argenziano G, Zalaudek I, Soyer P, Sera F, et al. Dermatoscopy of basal cell carcinoma: morphologic variability of global and local features and accuracy of diagnosis. J Am Acad Dermatol. 2010;62:67–75.

82. Quiñones R, Verduzco AP, Guevara E. Hallazgos dermatoscópicos del carcinoma basocelular en relación con su tamaño. Dermatol Rev Mex. 2012;56(3):172–6.

83. Zaballos P, Puig S, Llambrich A, Malvehy J. Dermoscopy of dermatofibromas: a prospective morphological study of 412 cases. Arch Dermatol. 2008;144(1):75–83.

84. Laureano A, Fernandes C, Cardoso J. Hemosiderotic dermatofibroma: clinical and dermoscopic presentation mimicking melanoma. J Dermatol Case Rep. 2015;9(2):39–41.

85. Ferrari A, Argenziano G, Buccini P, Cota C, Sperduti I, De Simone P, et al. Typical and atypical dermoscopic presentations of dermatofibroma. JEADV. 2013;27(11):1375–80.

86. Zaballos P, Daufí C, Puig S, Argenziano G, Moreno-Ramirez D, Cabo H, et al. Dermoscopy of solitary angiokeratomas. A morphological study. Arch Dermatol. 2007;143(3):318–25.

87. Kim JH, Kim MR, Lee S-H, Lee SE, Lee SH. Dermoscopy: a useful tool for the diagnosis of angiokeratoma. Ann Dermatol. 2012;24(4):468–71.

88. Malvehy J. A new vision of actinic keratosis beyond visible clinical lesions. JEADV. 2015;29(Suppl. 1):3–8.

89. Zalaudek I, Ferrara G, Leinweber B, Mercogliano A, D' Ambrosio A, Argenziano G. Pitfalls in the clinical and dermoscopic diagnosis of pigmented actinic keratosis. J Am Acad Dermatol. 2005;53:1071–4.

90. Aviles JA, Suárez R, Lázaro P. Diagnostic utility of dermoscopy in pigmented actinic keratosis. Actas Dermosifiliogr. 2011;102(8):623–6.

91. Rigel DS, Stein Gold LF. The importance of early diagnosis and treatment of actinic keratosis. J Am Acad Dermatol. 2013;68:S20–7.

92. Giacomel J, Lallas A, Argenziano G, Bombonato C, Zalaudek I. Dermoscopic "signature" pattern of pigmented and nonpigmented facial actinic keratoses. Am Acad Dermatol. 2015;72:e57–9.

93. Zalaudek I, Argenziano G. Dermoscopy of actinic keratosis, intraepidermal carcinoma and squamous cell carcinoma. Curr Probl Dermatol. Basel, Karger. 2015;46:70–6.

94. Kittler H, Marghoob AA, Argenziano G, Carrera C, Curiel-Lewandrowski C, Hofmann-Wellnhof R, et al. Standardization of terminology in dermoscopy/dermatoscopy: results of the third consensus conference of the International Society of Dermoscopy. J Am Acad Dermatol. 2016;74:1093–106.

95. Martín JM, Bella-Navarro R, Jordaa E. Vascular patterns in dermoscopy. Actas Dermosifiliogr. 2012;103(5):357–75.

96. Lallas A, Giacomel J, Argenziano G, García-García B, González-Fernández D, Zalaudek I, et al. Dermoscopy in general dermatology: practical tips for the clinician. Br J Dermatol. 2014;170(3):514–26.

97. Mun J, Ko H, Kim B, Kim MB. Dermoscopy of giant molluscum contagiosum. J Am Acad Dermatol. 2013;69:e287–8.

98. Mical G, Lacarruba F, Massimino D, Schwartz RA. Dermatoscopy: alternative uses in daily clinical practice. J Am Acad Dermatol. 2011;64(6):1136–46.

99. Ianhez M, da Costa P. Cestari S, Yoshiaki Enokihara M, Bandeira de Paiva Melo Seize M. Dermoscopic patterns of molluscum contagiosum: a study of 211 lesions confirmed by histopathology. An Bras Dermatol. 2011;86(1):79–4.

100. Segura Tigell S. Dermatoscopia en el diagnóstico de las infecciones cutáneas. Dermoscopy in the diagnosis of skin infections. Piel (barc). 2014;29(1):20–8.

101. Michajłowski I, Michajłowski J, Sobjanek M, Włodarkiewicz A, Matuszewski M, Krajk K. Usefulness of dermoscopy for differentiation of pearly penile papules and genital warts. Eur Urol Supl. 2008;8:567–605.

102. Zalaudek I, Giacomel J, Schmid K, Bondino S, Rosendahl S, Cavicchini S. Dermatoscopy of facial actinic keratosis, intraepidermal carcinoma, and invasive squamous cell carcinoma: a progression model. J Am Acad Dermatol. 2012;66:589–97.

103. Rhee DY, Won KH, Lee YJ, Won CH, Chang SE, Lee MW. Successful treatment of multiple vemurafenib-induced keratoacanthomas by topical application of imiquimod cream: confirmation of clinical clearance by dermoscopy. J Dermatolog Treat. 2016;19:1–2.

104. Woltsche N, Schwab C, Deinlein T, Hofmann-Wellenhof R, Zalaudek I. Dermoscopy in the era of

dermato-oncology: from bed to bench side and retour. Expert Rev Anticancer Ther. 2016;16(5):531–41.

105. Pozzobon FC, Puig-Butille JA, Gonzalez-Alvarez T, Carrera C, Aguilera P, Alos L, et al. Dermoscopic criteria associated with BRAF and NRAS mutation status in primary cutaneous melanoma. Br J Dermatol. 2014;171(4):754–9.

106. De Giorgi V, Savarese I, D'Errico A, Gori A, Papi F, Colombino M, et al. CDKN2A mutations could influence the dermoscopic pattern of presentation of multiple primary melanoma: a clinical dermoscopic genetic study. J Eur Acad Dermatol Venereol. 2015;29(3):574–80.

107. Guitera P, Menzies SW, Argenziano G, Longo C, Losi A, Drummond M, et al. Dermoscopy and in vivo confocal microscopy are complimentary techniques for the diagnosis of difficult amelanotic and light colored skin lesions. Br J Dermatol. doi:10.1111/bjd.14749.

Recommended Reading

108. Malvhey J, Puig S. Handbook of dermoscopy. 1st ed. Barcelona: Taylor and Francis Group, CRC Press; 2006.

109. Malvehy J, Puig S. Principios de dermatoscopia. 1st ed. Barcelona; 2011.

110. Kittler H, Rosendahl C, Cameron A, Tschandl P. Dermatoscopía. Un método algorítimico basado en el análisis de patrones. 1st ed. Gdansk; 2015.

111. Cabo H. Dermatoscopía. 2ª ed. Buenos Aires: Ediciones Journal; 2012.

112. Rezze G., Paschoal, FM., Hirata, S. Atlas de Dermatoscopia aplicada. 1era Edición. San Pablo: Lemar Livraria e editora Marina; 2014.

113. Larre Borges A, Nicoletti S, Salerni G. Dermatoscopía elemental: lesiones pigmentadas. Primera Edición. Montevideo; 2013.

Teledermatology

57

Daniel Holthausen Nunes

Key Points
- Teledermatology is a new tool that bridges the distance between the dermatologist and remote areas
- Teledermatology aims to screen severe cases and support to general physicians
- The effectiveness of teledermatology is greater if the photos obtained are systematic and follow specific protocols.
- There is a considerable reduction in costs of referral flow with the implementation of teledermatology, especially in countries where the health system is public or distribution of specialists is uneven.

Introduction

Dermatology is one of the most visual specialties in medicine and is also suited for modern telemedicine techniques. It is not difficult to see the potential for telemedicine to be widely disseminated. Since dermatology is the field of medicine responsible for the care of the skin and its appendages, it is often possible to make a diagnosis, with due respect to the patient's medical history, through images/pictures and visualization of the lesions [1].

Teledermatology refers to the delivery of dermatologic care via information and communication technology [2]. Thus, it can be said that teledermatology represents the field of telemedicine that aims to apply new communication and information technologies to dermatologic practices in order to reduce the need for the patient and the specialist to meet face to face, with a view toward ensuring effective health planning, research, education, clinical discussion, second opinion, and expert dermatologic care. Given the strong visual component of dermatology as a specialty it has a significant benefit for the use of telemedicine, whose basic function is remote diagnostics—in other words, health care at a distance [1, 3–6].

In teledermatology, dermatologists use telemedicine techniques to diagnose and treat patients from a distance, which involves the clinical evaluation of skin lesions and the review of laboratory findings. The primary aim is to ensure that patients from remote areas receive specialized dermatologic care. Other aims are to decrease the number of hospital visits and increase diagnostic efficiency. One objective of teledermatology is to deliver

D.H. Nunes
Federal University of Santa Catarina – HU-UFSC, Florianópolis, Brazil
e-mail: daniel.holthausen@ufsc.br; danieldermato@gmail.com

© Springer International Publishing Switzerland 2018
R.R. Bonamigo, S.I.T. Dornelles (eds.), *Dermatology in Public Health Environments*,
https://doi.org/10.1007/978-3-319-33919-1_57

1189

high-quality healthcare more efficiently by moving a patient's information rather than moving the actual patient [7, 8].

The merit of teledermatology was aptly described as follows: "teledermatology makes three promises: better, cheaper, and faster dermatologic care." "Better" quality is achieved by reliance on sophisticated devices for remote diagnosis and by extending the reach of dermatologists to serve patients in need of a specialist. "Cheaper and faster" are achieved by improved efficiency from increased volumes of patients, as well as "avoiding unnecessary and time-consuming face-to-face appointments" [9].

Thus, we have as a means, through telemedicine and teledermatology, to gain a second formative opinion that can be defined as the search for and delivery of medical information from a trained professional when distance no longer constitutes a barrier. Moreover, the second formative opinion has as one of its greatest benefits assisting the applicant in identifying the professional health problem and the therapeutic strategy [10, 11].

Two modalities of exchange of information in telediagnostics can be used in gaining the second formative opinion: synchronous mode (real-time), whereby the third party and the applicant, with the patient, participate in a real-time query; and asynchronous mode (store and forward), whereby the question is transported to a database and subjected to further consultation [12].

State of the Art

Nowadays telediagnosis, specifically in dermatology, lacks clear regulation, unlike other specialties that already have such specific protocols contemplated as an established procedure. In dermatology, perhaps because of easy access to the patient's own skin lesions and technology (digital photography, computers, and smartphones), the boundaries between the ideal and the actual are cloudy, besides being ethically prohibited [13].

The possibility of having a remote diagnostics service can ultimately end "consultations" by emails/social networks, including formalizing fees. It is important to clarify that this interaction should always be "medical doctor–specialist–medical doctor" and not directly between the specialist and the patient. However, this point is subject to an extensive discussion of responsibility around the medical act itself. In this case, the specialist accepts unlimited liability for any risks he/she undertakes [14].

We should bear in mind that face-to-face consultation remains the gold standard for diagnosis; and while the aim of teledermatology is to achieve the quality of this reference standard, the conventional service should be maintained as long as the resources and conditions for offering it are available. It is impossible to properly manage a disease without a precise diagnosis [15].

Some models of teleconsulting, such as second formative opinion and tele-education, often occur between peers, with clarification of intent on specific questions, theoretical basis or continuing education, respectively. In this regard, the sooner we define and establish rules, the lower will be the risk of incurring serious ethical shortcomings by omission or negligence. The use of social networks, such as Facebook or WhatsApp, which are excellent in function for homogeneous groups, are not ideal discussion forums because of, for example, patient exposure.

Some patients themselves search the Internet to seek further information or advice regarding their illness. Patients are connecting to databases or emailing their physicians for more advice. However, patients obtaining advice by using the Internet may increase their level of anxiety or reach false conclusions, which may lead to poor outcome [16].

Telediagnosis thus aims to include the mandatory requirement of (1) a specialist who is responsible for providing a report (diagnosis), based on relevant clinical information provided by the physician, and (2) good-quality images. Owing to the large number of dermatologic diseases and their clinical and chronologic variability and difficulty in standardizing photos, the creation of specific protocols and tools is essential for enabling remote diagnostics in dermatology [10, 12, 17]. The method, as employed for example in the second formative opinion, should be asynchronous; however, the program can be developed via the technology to enable a dialogue between professionals simultaneously and synchronously in specific and selected cases [18, 19].

Teledermatology relies on the use of electronic devices to capture, transfer, and process information gathered by remote providers, typically general practitioners (GPs). It can be conducted in either synchronous fashion (with patient and provider interacting in real time) or asynchronously. The latter, also referred to as "store-and-forward" (S&F) modality, is often preferred by providers for convenience, better workflow, and greater efficiency. Because skin disorders all manifest on the surface of the body, digital photography is the most common tool for capturing diagnostic information, as a substitute for visualization and touch. Other devices include dermoscopes (surface contact microscopes that provide high-resolution images) and ex vivo confocal laser microscopy (an optical imaging technique for increasing optical resolution and contrast to eliminate out-of-focus light). Clinical notes and observations also constitute important sources of information.

The teledermatology process is based on photography, dermoscopy, or newer technologies (confocal microscopy), and consists of three basic models: (1) primary teledermatology, or direct service for patients for initial diagnosis and referral; (2) secondary teledermatology, or service for primary care providers for consults and triage; and (3) tertiary teledermatology, or specialist-to-specialist consults [9].

Currently it is difficult not to notice that one of the impediments to the achievement of a comprehensive and effective health system is the collision with economic restrictions. In this sense, the second formative opinion and remote diagnostics introduce alternatives to overcome this barrier, since these are procedures that are inexpensive in relation to their concrete results [20–27].

Another notable fact is the geographic maldistribution of physicians [23, 28]. Most specialists, for several reasons, prefer the large urban centers and tend to stay on the outskirts of urban centers, leaving outlying areas under the responsibility of often less skilled professionals. Remote diagnostics in dermatology enables the assessment of patients by a medical expert distant from the home, preventing the possibility of delay in simple treatments because of the distance between patient and expert. In addition, this new technique of exchanging information enables appropriate treatment for residents of remote regions [1, 3, 13, 20, 27].

It is true that an accurate diagnosis is the precursor of a successful therapeutic intervention; however, the dynamics of medicine as well as the various ways in which a dermatologic disease can manifest interferes in the skill of clinical judgment. Given this reality, coupled with the aforementioned economic and geographic factors, the remote diagnostics teledermatology looms large as an innovative method of assistance to professionals and a facilitator of proper access to healthcare.

Four factors that may account for a successful teledermatology program have been identified : (1) preselection of patients, (2) image quality, (3) dermoscopy for pigmented lesions, and (4) an effective culture and infrastructure. Three of these four critical factors for teledermatology programs should be implemented in any teledermatology system: first, preselection of patients; second, quality clinical photographs; and third, quality dermoscopic photographs of potentially malignant lesions. Any system planning to start a teledermatology service must anticipate that there can be a steep learning curve for the referring providers and imagers. It is crucial to establish training and standardized guidelines for referring providers and teleimagers and to facilitate continuous feedback among referrers, imagers, and readers [9].

The development of specific protocols and guidelines should be used to familiarize the GPs about the methods and procedures, such as for skin cancers (melanoma and nonmelanoma), psoriasis (severe), and leprosy, facilitating access of the patients to specialized clinics, creating the culture and the need for teledermatology for other skin diseases. In this way, a generic protocol can be used for remote diagnostics in dermatology with risk classification, making an appointment for a face-to-face consultation with a specialist easier and faster [29].

The fourth identified factor, culture and infrastructure, directly affects teledermatology success but is not as easy to implement in all programs. The capacity of primary doctors to participate effectively in teledermatology, either because of attitude or resources, plays a crucial role in the success of teledermatology programs. This issue must be addressed particularly when planning expansion of a successful teledermatology pilot program, as the larger pool of primary care providers may not have the enthusiasm of the pilot participants, for a variety of reasons, e.g., already feeling overburdened, lack of interest in technology, or other competing demands.

Some procedures can increase the effectiveness of teledermatology.

During conventional face-to-face consultation with the GP in a primary health unit the relevant patient data is entered on a virtual platform, which allows referral to the specialist when needed. Indications of all patients who show signs or symptoms of skin disease for whom the treating physician deems referral to the specialist necessary are forwarded.

The patient selected for consultation with dermatologist is then requested to undergo the examination, where agreement to the collection and holding of data is granted by signing the free and informed consent form.

The photographic record for the investigation of suspected cases is carried out following a protocol consisting of three steps: a panoramic photo, a close-up photo with scale, and a photo contact/dermatoscopy in cases of suspicion of skin cancer [30] (Fig. 57.1).

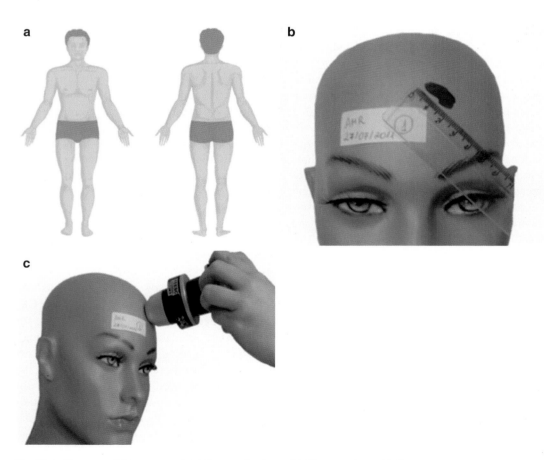

Fig. 57.1 Photo acquisition protocol. (**a**) Panoramic photo. (**b**) Close-up photo. (**c**) Dermoscopy

Regarding the panoramic photo, the technician is advised to identify each injury, using a label with date, initials of the patient, and lesion number, in order to create a panoramic image of the body region (head, torso, arms and legs, may be front or back) affected by one or more lesions. At this stage, the technician is advised not to use the zoom mode [30].

At the second stage, the close-up photo with scale, the technician is instructed to shoot at a distance of about 30 cm from the injury without the use of a zoom function, and to place a scale parallel to the injury to serve as reference to the actual size of the lesion.

Finally, the third photo is taken using dermoscopy. The dermatoscope is connected to the digital camera. The technician applies gel on the lens of the camera and photographs each lesion by using the dermatoscope placed against the patient's skin and maximizing the zoom level.

After collection, the data are transmitted through an internet environment developed exclusively for sending data corresponding to each patient. Whenever a new case is loaded into the portal, the examinations are available for an evaluation report by the dermatologist and can be accessed through a restricted site.

All reports are published in a structured and standardized way, obligatorily consisting of the description of the study, primary elementary lesion, secondary lesion, color, morphology, size, location, and distribution. The report concludes with the compatibility of diagnosis (medical assistant) with the remote diagnostics (dermatologist), whereby another hypothesis may be suggested according to the interpretation of clinical data and photographs provided for each case. According to the diagnosis, a risk classification is added in the report, making the GP's decision for each specific case easier [31].

This structure is necessary and essential to providing standardization and reproducibility of these reports. In specific situations there is an open field so that the specialist can make comments relevant to the case or suggestions for diagnostic elucidation to the doctor. In short, it is a diagnostic test, in terms of a pathology, whereby the expert is responsible for the generated diagnosis and its consequences.

With the information for making the report inserted at the end, the report is published automatically and a protocol number is generated to access the doctor or the patient. This report can then be accessed through the portal and printed if necessary.

It is true that the correlation between the initial diagnosis and teledermatology diagnosis when obtained by dermatologists varies between 80.5% and 91.6% [4, 32]. However, with structuring of the acquisition of images through a fixed protocol, it is possible to increase the accuracy of a report by accessing appropriate specialists up to 40 times [6].

For example, with full service installation, during the first year 5,158 reports were issued. Of these 40.4% were suspected by the attending physician to be skin cancer in patients who would be scheduled for referral for consultation with the specialist. Through teledermatology, we were able to screen more than two-thirds of the patients who had benign lesions (seborrheic keratoses, nevi) without referrals [33] (Fig. 57.2).

Future Perspectives

This model, with the acquisition protocol photos and the structured reports, demonstrates the importance of using teledermatology as a modern health access tool. This diagnostic method enables the early detection of skin cancer and other skin diseases and reduces the number of unnecessary referrals to dermatologists, and therefore can reduce the waiting time for face-to-face consultations, as well as the costs associated with this process.

High rates of accuracy can be obtained with teledermatology both for adults and children, with affordable technical requirements. Furthermore, high rates of agreement are found for most common dermatologic lesion referrals.

Teledermatology can be used as a complementary tool in daily consultations at primary care centers and as an effective means to filter dermatology referrals. Nevertheless, integration with the health system (whether private or public) is essential to reduce the teleconsulta-

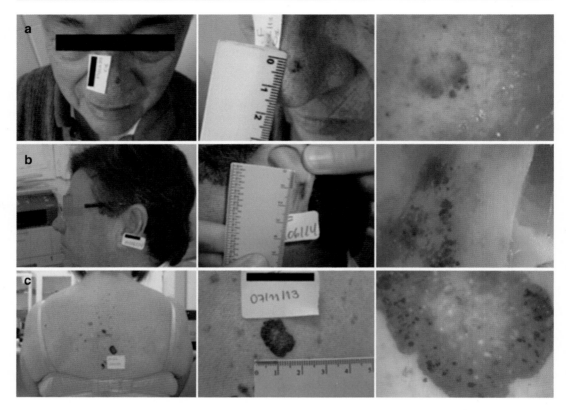

Fig. 57.2 Teledermatology cases. (**a**) Pigmented basal cell carcinoma. (**b**) Malignant melanoma. (**c**) Seborrheic keratosis

tion time, and training is needed to improve the quality of images [34].

Glossary

Second formative opinion Systematic response, based on literature review of the best scientific and clinical evidence and the directive role of primary health care. The questions originate from teleconsultation and are selected from criteria of relevance.

Tele-education Lectures, classes, and courses provided through the use of information and communication technologies.

Teleconsulting Registered consultation conducted among workers, professionals, and managers of health through bidirectional telecommunication instruments in order to answer questions about clinical procedures, health

actions, and issues related to the work process. They can be of two types: (a) Synchronous – teleconsulting performed in real time, usually by chat, web, or video conferencing; or (b) asynchronous – teleconsulting performed by off-line messages.

Telediagnostics Autonomous service that uses information technology and communication to perform diagnostic support services through distance and time; e.g., Teleradiology, Teledermatology, Tele-electrocardiography.

References

1. Miot HA, Paixão MP, Wen CL. Teledermatologia: passado, presente e futuro. An Bras Dermatol. 2005;80:523–32.
2. Perednia DA, Brown NA. Teledermatology: one application of telemedicine. Bull Med Libr Assoc. 1995;83(1):42–7.

3. Heffner VA, Lyon VB, Brousseau DC, Holland KE, Yen K. Store-and-forward teledermatology versus in-person visits: a comparison in pediatric teledermatology clinic. J Am Acad Dermatol. 2009;60(6):956–61.

4. Ribas J, Cunha MDGS, Schettini APM, Ribas CBDR. Concordância entre diagnósticos dermatológicos obtidos por consulta presencial e por análise de imagens digitais. An Bras Dermatol. 2010;85:441–7.

5. Armstrong AW, Wu J, Kovarik CL, Goldyne ME, Oh DH, McKoy KC, et al. State of teledermatology programs in the United States. J Am Acad Dermatol. 2012;67(5):939–44.

6. Piccoli MF, Amorim BD, Wagner HM, Nunes DH. Teledermatology protocol for screening of skin cancer. An Bras Dermatol. 2015;90(2):202–10.

7. Burdick AE, Berman B. Teledermatology. Adv Dermatol. 1997;12:19–45; discussion 6.

8. Pak HS. Teledermatology and teledermatopathology. Semin Cutan Med Surg. 2002;21(3):179–89.

9. Landow SM, Mateus A, Korgavkar K, Nightingale D, Weinstock MA. Teledermatology: key factors associated with reducing face-to-face dermatology visits. J Am Acad Dermatol. 2014;71(3):570–6.

10. Miot HA, Paixão MP, Paschoal FM. Fundamentos da fotografia digital em Dermatologia. An Bras Dermatol. 2006;81:174–80.

11. Neira RAQ, Puchnick A, Cohrs FM, Lopes PRDL, Lederman HM, Pisa IT. Avaliação de um sistema de segunda opinião em radiologia. Radiol Bras. 2010;43:179–83.

12. Wen C. Telemedicina e Telessaúde – Um panorama no Brasil. Inf Pública. 2008;10(2):7–15.

13. CFM. Resolução 1974/2011. Brasília: Conselho Federal de Medicina; 2011.

14. CFM. Resolução 1643/2002. Brasília: Conselho Federal de Medicina; 2002.

15. de Argila D. Reflections on the future and usefulness of teledermatology. Actas Dermosifiliogr. 2008;99(7):503–5.

16. Huntley AC. The need to know: patients, e-mail, and the internet. Arch Dermatol. 1999;135(2):198–9.

17. Eedy DJ, Wootton R. Teledermatology: a review. Br J Dermatol. 2001;144(4):696–707.

18. Warshaw EM, Hillman YJ, Greer NL, Hagel EM, MacDonald R, Rutks IR, et al. Teledermatology for diagnosis and management of skin conditions: a systematic review. J Am Acad Dermatol. 2011;64(4):759–72.

19. Whited JD, Warshaw EM, Kapur K, Edison KE, Thottapurathu L, Raju S, et al. Clinical course outcomes for store and forward teledermatology versus conventional consultation: a randomized trial. J Telemed Telecare. 2013;19(4):197–204.

20. Loane MA, Bloomer SE, Corbett R, Eedy DJ, Gore HE, Hicks N, et al. Patient cost-benefit analysis of teledermatology measured in a randomized control trial. J Telemed Telecare. 1999;5(Suppl 1):S1–3.

21. High WA, Houston MS, Calobrisi SD, Drage LA, McEvoy MT. Assessment of the accuracy of low-cost store-and-forward teledermatology consultation. J Am Acad Dermatol. 2000;42(5 Pt 1):776–83.

22. Loane MA, Bloomer SE, Corbett R, Eedy DJ, Hicks N, Lotery HE, et al. A comparison of real-time and store-and-forward teledermatology: a cost-benefit study. Br J Dermatol. 2000;143(6):1241–7.

23. Loane MA, Oakley A, Rademaker M, Bradford N, Fleischl P, Kerr P, et al. A cost-minimization analysis of the societal costs of realtime teledermatology compared with conventional care: results from a randomized controlled trial in New Zealand. J Telemed Telecare. 2001;7(4):233–8.

24. Hockey AD, Wootton R, Casey T. Trial of low-cost teledermatology in primary care. J Telemed Telecare. 2004;10(Suppl 1):44–7.

25. Bonnardot L, Rainis R. Store-and-forward telemedicine for doctors working in remote areas. J Telemed Telecare. 2009;15(1):1–6.

26. Eminovic N, Dijkgraaf MG, Berghout RM, Prins AH, Bindels PJ, de Keizer NF. A cost minimisation analysis in teledermatology: model-based approach. BMC Health Serv Res. 2010;10:251.

27. Parsi K, Chambers CJ, Armstrong AW. Cost-effectiveness analysis of a patient-centered care model for management of psoriasis. J Am Acad Dermatol. 2012;66(4):563–70.

28. CFM. In: Scheffer M, Cassenote A, Biancarelli A, editors. Demografia Médica no Brasil. São Paulo: Conselho Regional de Medicina do Estado de São Paulo: Conselho Federal de Medicina; 2013. p. 256.

29. SES-SC SES. DELIBERAÇÃO 366/CIB/13 (disponível em: in: http://portalses.saude.sc.gov.br/index.php?option=com_docman&task=doc_download&gid=7285&Itemid=128). Florianópolis: Comissão Intergestores Bipartite – Governo de Santa Catarina; 2013.

30. Wangenheim AV, Wagner HM, Santos MIAD. Novo Manual de Realização de Exames Dermatológicos – Relatórios Técnicos do INCoD. Florianópolis: Sistema Catarinense de Telemedicina e Telessaúde. Laboratório de Telemedicina Lab|Med Universidade Federal de Santa Catarina – UFSC; 2014.

31. Wangenheim Av, Wagner HM, Santos MIAD. Manual – Laudador de Exames Dermatológicos – Relatórios Técnicos do INCoD. Florianópolis: Sistema Catarinense de Telemedicina e Telessaúde. Laboratório de Telemedicina Lab|Med Universidade Federal de Santa Catarina – UFSC; 2014.

32. Miot HA. Desenvolvimento e sistematização da interconsulta dermatológica à distância. São Paulo: Universidade de São Paulo; 2005.

33. Nunes DH, Inacio ADS, Wagner HM, Wangenheim AV. Banco de dados da Telemedicina da SES-SC (disponível em: https://telemedicina.saude.sc.gov.br/rctm/). Florianópolis: Sistema Catarinense de Telemedicina e Telessaúde. Laboratório de Telemedicina Lab|Med Universidade Federal de Santa Catarina – UFSC; 2014.

34. Lasierra N, Alesanco A, Gilaberte Y, Magallon R, Garcia J. Lessons learned after a three-year store and forward teledermatology experience using internet: strengths and limitations. Int J Med Inform. 2012;81(5):332–43.

Part IX

Signs and Symptoms of Skin Diseases in Public Health: A Practical Guide to Management

Stains

58

Roberta Castilhos da Silva, Mariele Bevilaqua, and Jenifer de Morais Silva

Key Points
- Stains configure an elementary dermatologic lesion of several common skin diseases in public health
- Pigmentary changes can be described as hyperchromic, hypochromic, and achromic stains
- Stains can be caused by vascular injuries or even be related to blood pigment
- This chapter provides an overview of the most prevalent skin diseases in public health that manifest as stains
- It is very important for the general physician to have a strategic flowchart to reach the etiologic diagnosis of each dermatosis that presents with stains

Introduction

The most important pigments that primarily determine the normal color of the skin are melanin, oxygenated reduced hemoglobin, and carotene [1].

R.C. da Silva (✉) • J. de Morais Silva
Dermatology, University of Caxias do Sul, School of Medicine, Caxias do Sul, Brazil
e-mail: betacs@gmail.com

M. Bevilaqua
Dermatology Service of Federal University of Health Sciences of Porto Alegre, Porto Alegre, Brazil

Other factors such as vascular supply, including number, caliber, and reactivity of blood vessels in the dermis, and epidermal thickness also influence the appearance of skin [2].

Melanocytes are located in the basal layer of the epidermis and contain specialized organelles that synthesize melanin released by dendrites as mature melanosomes. They arise from the neural crest during embryonic development. Three different types of melanin exist in human skin: eumelanin (brown or black), pheomelanin (red or yellow), and trichromes (present in various chemically well-defined variants). The gene for the melanocortin receptor 1 determines the level of melanin production. It is present in melanocytes and controls sensitivity to light exposure and sunburn, influences skin and hair color, and partly determines the individual risk of melanoma. The number and size of melanosomes cause variations in individual skin color and between persons of various ethnicities. Melanin synthesis is influenced by genetic factors and varies greatly among individuals, families, and ethnicities. Other factors include exposure to ultraviolet (UV) light, hormonal influences, and biochemical substances [3].

The term "stain" is used to describe an elementary dermatologic lesion that is flat and not palpable. It considers the term "spot" for a stain with a diameter less than 5 mm. The color of the lesion, which often is the first visual assessment, is an important additional feature and is repeatable in certain pathologies such as the destruction of melanocytes, dilation of blood vessels in the dermis, or inflammation of the vascular wall with extravasation of red blood cells. Pigmentary changes can be described as hyperchromic, hypochromic, and depigmented or achromic [4].

Hyperpigmentation or hyperchromia results from increased melanin production caused by tyrosinase activity, increased melanocytes, and delayed breakdown and removal of melanin. On the other hand, hypopigmentation or hypochromia results from a reduction in the number of mature melanosomes and/or melanocytes or the abnormal transfer of mature melanosomes to neighboring keratinocytes [3].

From the point of view of semiology, we can divide the injuries of vascular stains into three main groups:

Transient or functional: always flat (stains), generally represented by erythema, which consists of reddish stain caused by cutaneous vasodilation; thus the digital pressure disappears

Cyanosis: characterized by a bluish spot on the skin due to lower local blood supply

Permanent: related to vascular proliferation (angiomas, hemangiomas), vascular dilatation (telangiectasia), and functional vascular constriction (nevus anemicus)

Furthermore, stains are also related to the blood pigment, when they are named purpura or hemorrhagic suffusion [5].

State of the Art and Future Perspectives

Skin disease is a common medical problem, becoming one of the most frequent reasons for consulting a general physician [6]. It represents 8.4% of primary care cases and can be a challenge to general physicians because of their general lack of knowledge and training in this area [7].

A study from the United Kingdom showed that, in primary care, the top three diagnoses were eczema (22.5%), infection and infestation (20.3%), and benign tumors (11.4%) [7], whereas

in secondary care the top three diagnoses were benign tumors (23.8%), malignant tumors (16.4%), and eczema (16.3%). The Brazilian Society of Dermatology conducted a study of the reasons for seeking a medical specialist in dermatology. Skin diseases with stains were common, with eczema, vitiligo, and leprosy being major reasons for visits [8].

As with other semiologic signs studied in dermatology, stains configure elementary lesions of several common skin diseases in public health. Recognizing and knowing how to characterize this sign makes performing a correct clinical diagnosis more simple and contributes to the solving capacity at the primary level of public health, whereby most of the problems presented by the population can be answered without the need to refer the patient to a specialist.

Hypochromic Stains

Leukoderma and hypopigmentation are general terms used to describe disorders characterized by whitening of the skin, which results from the decrease in epidermal melanin content (related to melanin) or cutaneous blood supply (related to hemoglobin).

Hypomelanosis is a specific term that expresses a level of deficiency or reduction of melanin, whereas melanosis is defined as total deficiency of skin color caused by lack of melanin pigments initially existent, as occurs in vitiligo. "Pigment breaking" is a term used to describe general reduction of skin color and hair color, as occurs in oculocutaneous albinism.

A summary of hypochromic stains is provided in Flowcharts 58.1 and 58.2.

Acquired Hypomelanosis

Vitiligo

Vitiligo is an acquired hypomelanosis of unknown etiology that is characterized by achromic stains, the result of a selective breakdown of functional epidermal melanocytes causing depigmentation

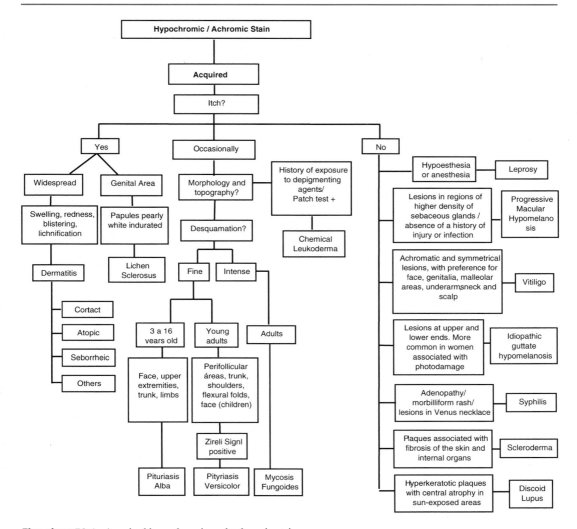

Flowchart 58.1 Acquired hypochromic and achromic stains

of the skin [8]. It is apparent in 0.1–2% of the world population, regardless of gender, age, or race [5]. Heredity is attributed to 30% of the cases [9–12]. Dermatologic lesions can also occur after trauma (Koebner's phenomenon), emotional stress, and sunburn [13, 14]. It is important to note that the evolution of the disease is unpredictable, and the lesions, likewise, can be extant or even slowly increase over the years.

Vitiligo clinically consists of the appearance of achromic stains that can initially be hypochromic, with clear limits and no associated symptoms; they generally have centrifugal growth [14]. The

pattern shown by the disease is symmetric and predominantly focuses on malleolus, wrists, legs anterolaterally, back of hands, underarms, neck, scalp, and genitals (Fig. 58.1) [15]. Diagnosis is clinical and can be complemented using Wood's lamp or, rarely, a skin biopsy.

However, a fully effective treatment against vitiligo is not yet available. The main goal is the repigmentation of the skin and stability of the disease [15]. Among the factors to be considered in treatment strategies are the degree of the disease (stable or in progress), the psychological impact, and the age of the patient. Therefore, pho-

Flowchart 58.2
Congenital hypochromic
and achromic stains

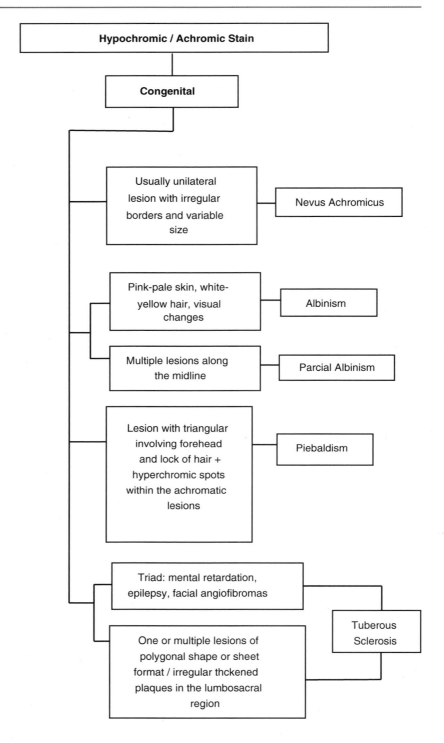

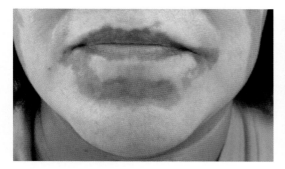

Fig. 58.1 Vitiligo: achromic stains on the face (Image courtesy of dermatology service of Federal University of Health Sciences of Porto Alegre – UFCSPA)

toprotection, topical and systemic corticosteroids, calcineurin inhibitors, analogs of vitamin D3, phototherapy, excimer laser, surgery, depigmentation, and covering are the therapeutic tools currently available [15, 16].

Guttate Leukoderma (Idiopathic Guttate Hypomelanosis)

Guttate leukoderma is an acquired and very common benign and asymptomatic dermatosis [17]. It is characterized by hypopigmented stains of about 0.5 mm diameter and has a smooth surface [18]. Guttate leukoderma affects mainly older people and women from all races [18, 19]. However, it is more common in dark skin pigmentation. It refers to a multifactorial disease that comprises repeated small traumas, genetic influence, and sun exposure as casual factors [20].

Lesion coverage includes mainly exposed areas of upper and lower extremities of the body, but other regions are, in the same way, commonly affected, except the facial area (Fig. 58.2) [21]. The lesions continuously change their dimensional aspect but increase in number. For this reason, aesthetic concerns become the main motivation for a dermatologic appointment.

The diagnosis is clinical [18]. A biopsy only is necessary when there is the need to differentiate from other diseases, such as vitiligo. Cryotherapy, superficial dermabrasion, topical retinoids, and topical tacrolimus 0.1% are some of the available therapeutic options [22, 23].

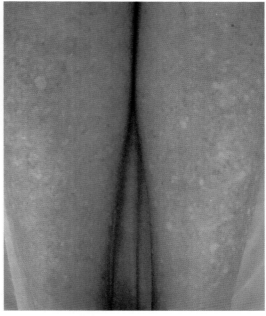

Fig. 58.2 Guttate leukoderma or idiopathic guttate hypomelanosis: hypopigmented stains on the lower limbs (Image courtesy of dermatology service of Federal University of Health Sciences of Porto Alegre – UFCSPA)

Progressive Macular Hypomelanosis

Progressive macular hypomelanosis is a disease that affects mainly adults and young people [24]; the recommended pathogenesis consists in the use of *Propionibacterium acnes* as an element for the skin-lightening factor production that takes part in melanogenesis and causes hypopigmentation stains [5, 25, 26].

It is clinically defined as multiple nummular and confluent hypochromic macules, symmetric and asymptomatic [27]. The lesions mainly appear in areas of higher density of sebaceous glands, as in the midsection and they tend to converge in the midline, although they also can move to the neck and the upper extremities [28, 29] (Fig. 58.3). Progressive macular hypomelanosis has clearly been shown to be a persistent disease that develops over several years and then becomes stabilizing; in some cases it can regress.

The diagnosis is clinical and is completed by use of the Wood's lamp method, which shows red follicular fluorescence restricted to the injured area [30].

The treatment is off-label. However, the likely implication of *P. acnes* in the pathogenesis has prompted the use of drugs with activity against the bacteria. The use of topical benzoyl peroxide 5%, or clindamycin 1%, or systemic use of lymecycline 300 mg/day or minocycline 100 mg, for 3 months, are some of the recommended drugs [5, 31]. Phototherapy has been proved to be effective, but it does not prevent recurrence of the disease [32]. In some patients, there is transient pigmentation after sun exposure.

Postinflammatory Hypomelanosis

Pityriasis Alba

Pityriasis alba is a benign dermatosis that affects mainly children between the ages of 3 and 16 years old. Although no definitive cause has yet been found, it has been associated with atopy and sun exposure [33–35].

The disease affects the patient's face and upper extremities and, occasionally, the midsection and the lower extremities. Its development follows three steps: erythematous plaques that can cause itching come first; after a few weeks, the rash disappears and fine scale stains appear; in the final stage of disease development, hypopigmentation macules [34, 36] round or oval from 0.5 to 5 cm diameter, with defined edges, and usually asymptomatic, are observed [36, 37]. These hypopigmentation macules can remain for years or regress in some months.

The main differential diagnosis is pityriasis versicolor, and mycologic examination is often essential in order to confirm the differential [38]. For treatment, low-dose topical glucocorticoids, calcineurin inhibitors, and emollients are preferable to moisturize the skin and speed up the pigmentation [35].

Hypopigmented Mycosis Fungoides

Hypopigmented mycosis fungoides is a variation of the first phase of mycosis fungoides, and is much more common in individuals with intensive

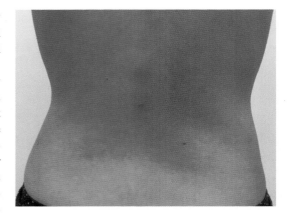

Fig. 58.3 Progressive macular hypomelanosis: confluent hypopigmented macules involving the torso (Image courtesy of dermatology service of Federal University of Health Sciences of Porto Alegre – UFCSPA)

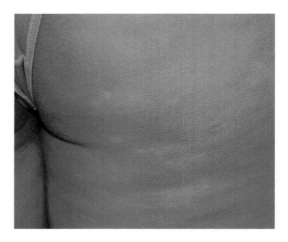

Fig. 58.4 Hypopigmented mycosis fungoides: hypopigmented lesions in the proximal lower limbs (Image courtesy of dermatology service of Federal University of Health Sciences of Porto Alegre – UFCSPA)

sun exposure and evidence of lesions. The hypopigmented lesions occur in the midsection or the extremities of the body (Fig. 58.4), possibly accompanied by uncomfortable itching and erythema. The appropriate treatment consists in the use of nitrogen gas or phototherapy [18].

Scleroderma

Scleroderma is a connective tissue disease of unknown origin and slow evolution that leads to fibrosis of skin, blood vessels, and internal organs

[39]. The disease presents two types: restricted scleroderma (morphea) and systemic [40]. The morphea also presents in other forms: cutaneous hypochromic stain (Fig. 58.5), consisting of a clear erythematous plaque of ivory and yellow center, smooth and shiny blue and violet shades; hypochromic atrophic plaque, with central depression, papule, or skin-colored plaque that resembles keloids; and injury to the frontal or frontoparietal region that causes grooves [40, 41]. It can be progressive and can affect the entire hemiface (morphea "en coup de sabre"). The systemic scleroderma can develop either in a hyperchromic or hypochromic way [42]. It is characterized by retaining segments at the level of the hair follicles, causing an appearance that resembles salt and pepper. Systemic scleroderma appears commonly in the upper midsection and on the patient's face [43]. The options for treatment are scarce; in general, therapy attempts to control the characteristics of the affected organ [43, 44].

Lichen Sclerosus

Lichen sclerosus is a disease of unknown origin, but is multifactorial disease [45]. Although lichen sclerosus seems to be a skin disorder, it predomi-

nantly affects the external genitalia and anal region; in males, the disease affects most frequently the area of the glans [45–47]. Genital and extragenital lesions of lichen sclerosus are often hypopigmented (Fig. 58.6). Other characteristics of the disease are pearly white, polygonal, and flattened papules, atrophy, and corneal pimples [46, 48]. The main purpose of treatment is to gain control over the symptoms, and to detect and treat early overlying neoplasms [9].

Discoid Lupus

Lupus is an autoimmune and multisystemic disease whose appearance is much more common in women; it clinically appears in all skin areas [49]. Lupus can have only a cutaneous appearance and can be associated with systemic disorders, although it is rarely a systemic injury.

The appearance of chronic cutaneous lupus, such as discoid injury, is less likely to develop into systemic involvement [50]. The injuries are initially apparent as well-limited erythematous hyperkeratotic plaques, with adherent scaling and

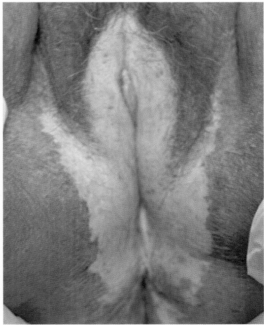

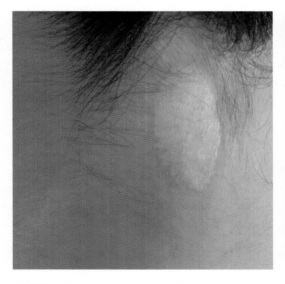

Fig. 58.5 Scleroderma: hypochromic and atrophic stain (morphea) on the neck (Image courtesy of dermatology service of Federal University of Health Sciences of Porto Alegre – UFCSPA)

Fig. 58.6 Lichen sclerosus: hypopigmented stain in the genital area (Image courtesy of dermatology service of Federal University of Health Sciences of Porto Alegre – UFCSPA)

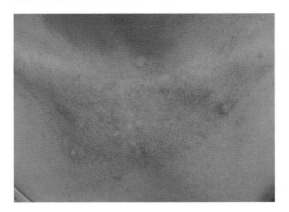

Fig. 58.7 Discoid lupus: erythematous lesions with achromic (vitiligoid) and hypochromic areas associated with atrophy (Image courtesy of dermatology service of Federal University of Health Sciences of Porto Alegre – UFCSPA)

Table 58.1 Vitiligo × chemical leukoderma

1. Acquired vitiligo-like depigmented lesion(s)
2. History of repeated exposure to specific chemical compounds
3. Patterned vitiligo-like macules conforming to site of exposure
4. Confetti macules

gradual development to central atrophy [49]. The achromia, which refers to a vitiligoid or hypochromic feature on the lesion, is frequently associated with skin atrophy (Fig. 58.7) [51]. The most affected areas are those exposed to sunlight.

The diagnosis is reached by clinical examination and confirmed by histopathologic examination [52]. Glucocorticoid and calcineurin inhibitors are used for topical treatment. For systemic treatment, antimalarials, retinoids, and thalidomide are suggested drugs, according to the degree of injury [49, 53].

Leukoderma by Chemical Substance

Chemical leukoderma is an acquired dermatosis caused by repeated exposure to certain chemical or pharmacologic compounds, which carry consequences of burning, destruction of melanocytes, and achromatic scars. The main depigmentation groups are phenols/catechol, sulfhydryl, and miscellaneous, harmful only to genetically susceptible persons [5, 18]. The effect caused by the use of these compounds can be: (a) selective destruction of melanocytes; (b) inhibiting the function or structure of the melanosome; (c) inhibition of tyrosinase biosynthesis; (d) inhibiting the nature of melanin; (e) involvement in the transfer from melanosomes to keratinocytes; (f) the effect of chemicals compound on melanin or damage to melanin [54].

For treatment, the most widely recommended phenolic compound is monobenzyl ether of hydroquinone, often used in the rubber industry (gloves, shoes, glasses, condoms, etc.) [5]. This compound can cause achromatic stains with morphotopography of the object it contacts. For cosmetic treatment against the melasma, the depigmentation caused by use of the compound is supposed to be definitive, and appears as a confetti pattern [54, 55]. Other phenol compounds and catechols (bultifenol and aminophenol) exist in germicides, insecticides, resins, deodorants, and detergents, and can cause hypochromia or achromia of the skin, even in areas where close contact, by inhalation, does not occur [5, 12].

However, it is noteworthy that clinical differentiation between chemical leukoderma and vitiligo is not easy [56] (Table 58.1).

In some cases, chemical leukoderma can also cause pruritus. Patch tests are a useful tool for this diagnosis. Repeated examinations are important for it to be effective (e.g., in 2 weeks, repeated at 4 weeks and 6 weeks) [18]. Biopsy is only necessary in controversial cases [57]. In some situations, after removal of the causative agent, monitoring of the skin pigmentation is advisable.

Infectious/Parasitic Hypomelanosis

Pityriasis Versicolor

Pityriasis versicolor is a chronic fungal infection of the skin caused by *Malassezia furfur* [58]. These fungi normally settle in sebum areas (scalp, face, back, midsection) and clinical development occurs in certain circumstances whereby the equilibrium of the skin changes, such as age, sex, race, genetic capacity, high level of hydration, and oily substances in skin, allowing the pseudofilaments of yeast to grow [9, 58]. Pityriasis versicolor can appear as outbreaks or becomes recurrent or chronic.

The diagnosis is clinical and easily noticed by multiple round or oval stains or thin plaques with desquamation (noticeable by Zireli's sign) which shows glossy or matt smooth surface, usually asymptomatic (Fig. 58.8) [59]. The stains can vary in color from white to brown and, more rarely, erythema [9, 60]. For this reason the name, versicolor, is one of the disease features. The hypopigmentation lesions occur by the action of inhibitory effects on the melanocytes, through the production of dicarboxylic acids by the yeast [61]. Initially, the filaments present a perifollicular feature, but after time grow and merge to form irregular stains of larger extent.

The final diagnosis is by direct mycologic examination and Wood's lamp, which confirm a yellow or silver fluorescent characteristic in the stains [62].

Treatment comprises the use of topical agents alone or in combination with systemic therapy [9, 62]. The prophylaxis is acceptable for recurrent cases. The hypopigmentation may persist for several months even after conclusion of the treatment.

Leprosy

Leprosy is a chronic, contagious, and infectious disease of potentially disabling outcome, caused by *Mycobacterium leprae*, which mainly affects the skin and the peripheral nerves [5, 63]. The patient who carries the infected bacillus is the main source of infection, and transmission occurs through the upper airway or by direct contact with the injury [5, 63–65]. Leprosy can be divided into two groups: tuberculoid (paucibacillary) and virchowian (multibacillary); and into two unstable types: indeterminate (which can develop into any form of leprosy) and dimorphic or borderline [12]. The World Health Organization has proposed a simple classification for operational purposes: paucibacillary (indeterminate and tuberculoid) and multibacillary (virchowian and borderline) [9].

Paucibacillary forms of the disease present with hypochromic stains, and for this reason they are included in the differential diagnosis for other dermatoses showing similarly appearing lesions. Indeterminate leprosy is the first manifestation of the disease and presents as hypochromic macules or slight erythema with hypoesthesia (Fig. 58.9) [66, 67]. There are usually few injuries with no specific area of affection, and the edges of lesions can be a clear or strongly outlined. Generally in the injured area there is some nerve fiber loss. In this case, the largest diameter of nerves is not impaired and, therefore, there is no resulting disability [9].

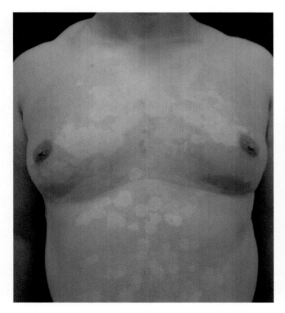

Fig. 58.8 Pityriasis versicolor: multiple round and oval stains with desquamation on the trunk (Image courtesy of dermatology service of Federal University of Health Sciences of Porto Alegre – UFCSPA)

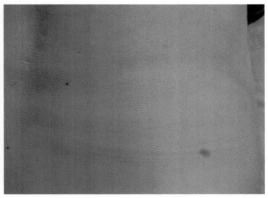

Fig. 58.9 Indeterminate leprosy: hypochromic stain with hypoesthesia on the back (Image courtesy of dermatology service of Federal University of Health Sciences of Porto Alegre – UFCSPA)

In other cases, different from paucibacillary forms in tuberculoid leprosy, lesions are macules and erythematous plaques of varying sizes, with strong outline and regular papular rash [67]. They appear in classical form, being circular and asymmetric lesions, usually single or in a cluster. The sensorial disturbances are severe, and important asymmetric and neural involvement, with thickening of peripheral nerves, can occur; the reduction or absence of nerve fibers in the affected area can occur [5, 67].

The diagnosis is clinical and the treatment has been effective. The first-line drugs are dapsone, rifampicin, and clofazimine [65, 66]. The differential diagnosis of paucibacillary leprosy includes achromic nevi, pityriasis alba, tinea versicolor, discoid lupus erythematosus, secondary and tertiary syphilis, circular granuloma, multiform granuloma, lichen planus, leishmaniasis, sarcoidosis, and vitiligo, among other diseases [63, 68, 69]. As a rule, no hypochromic lesion with preserved thermal and pain sensitivity is leprosy.

Syphilis

Syphilis is a contagious and infectious disease caused by the bacterium *Treponema pallidum* and is mainly transmitted through sexual intercourse [70, 71]. It follows a systematic pattern and if left untreated, and progresses to chronically alternating periods of activity and remission. Acquired syphilis comprises two types: recent (1 year or less of evolution; it encompasses the primary form, secondary and latent) and late (more than 1 year of evolution; it encompasses the tertiary form) [9].

In secondary syphilis the rash appears in different forms and structures and frequently similar to injuries of other diseases; for this reason secondary syphilis is named "the great imitator," a factor that has always been included in differential diagnosis of hypochromic macules [5].

In secondary disease a nonpruritic morbilliform rash comes first, exhibiting round or oval erythematous macules and papules, named syphilitic rose stains [70, 72]. These progress symmetrically through the midsection and continue throughout the body, including the palm and the sole regions [73]. Peripheral desquamation, in some lesions, is known as Biett's collarette. Residual hypochromic lesions form a lens shape around the neck, known as "necklace of Venus," and can be present after secondary degree syphilis [12].

The diagnosis of syphilis is by direct search of *T. pallidum* in a dark-field and serum area examination. The treatment comprises penicillin G benzathine in varying dosages according to the degree of the disease [74].

Hereditary and Congenital Hypomelanosis

Albinism

Albinism is a group of genetic diseases, of autosomal recessive pattern, characterized by a defect in melanin synthesis, but with the structure and complement of ordinary melanocytes [5]. The oculocutaneous albinism segment, which comprises four different diseases, constitutes hypopigmentation of the skin, hair, and eyes. It becomes ocular albinism when it focuses on the retinal epithelium [5, 18]. Skin involvement can occur by itself, but this is less common.

Albinism can be categorized in two branches: complete (universal) or incomplete (partial) [75]. Incomplete albinism is a variant of the disease whereby the skin tends to have slight pigmentation, the hairs are clear, and the ophthalmologic changes are less frequent. It is identified by hypopigmented lesions that are usually multiple and have been present along the midline of the body since the patient's birth [18]. The main difference, related to the diagnosis, in this case, is the vitiligo.

The primary treatment against the disease is strong photoprotection of the skin and the eyes, beginning at the patient's birth, as well as no exposure to UV radiation [5, 18, 75]. Cryosurgery, curettage, electrocoagulation, and early ablation of keratosis and malignant neoplasms are normally the methods used as therapy in cases of photoinjuries to the skin [75].

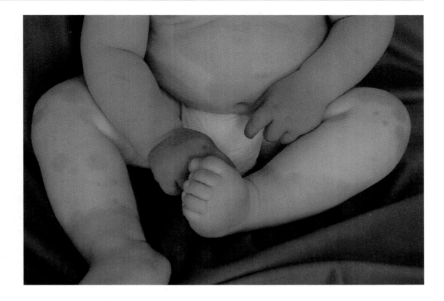

Fig. 58.10 Piebaldism: symmetric achromic stains on the abdomen and extremities (Image courtesy of dermatology service of Federal University of Health Sciences of Porto Alegre – UFCSPA)

Piebaldism

Piebaldism is a rare congenital autosomal dominant leukoderma, caused by a mutation in the involved gene, in the development of melanoblast (C-KIT gene) [5].

Clinically the disease initially presents at the patient's birth, and consists of achromic and triangular-shaped stains specifically placed on the forehead with a lock of hair (poliosis) next to it, including the eyelashes; the skin discolorations, strictly symmetric, can also affect the chest, abdomen, and extremities, although the back is spared (Fig. 58.10) [5, 12].

The leukoderma is, generally, a stable disease that follows the growth of the patient. An interesting characteristic of this disease is the presence of pigmented stains or hyperchromic macules in the achromic injury, which aids the differential diagnosis of vitiligo [5]. Photoprotection is essential, and the recommended treatment involves transplantation of melanocytes, assuming the lesions do not respond to topical treatment and phototherapy [12, 76].

Tuberous Sclerosis

Tuberous sclerosis is a complex, autosomal dominant neurocutaneous syndrome characterized by hamartomas in many organs, especially the skin.

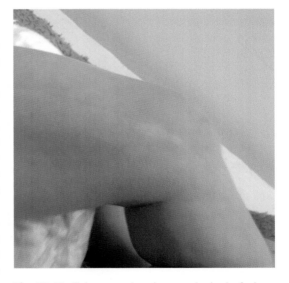

Fig. 58.11 Tuberous sclerosis: macule in leaf shape located on the leg (Image courtesy of dermatology service of Federal University of Health Sciences of Porto Alegre – UFCSPA)

The classic triad consists of mental retardation, epilepsy, and facial angiofibromas [77].

Cutaneous lesions of many types occur. The hypochromic macules (usually present at birth) vary in number from one to tens and are mostly small, polygonal, or in a fingerprint shape [78]. Another version of the hypochromic lesion is macules in leaf shape (Fig. 58.11), which is less common but characteristic. Also part of the syndrome's cutaneous manifestations are thick irregular plaques that occur in the midsection, commonly in the lumbosacral region (Shagreen patches) [79].

The treatment is complex. For skin lesions, electrosurgery, dermabrasion, and laser therapy are more common [78, 80].

Nevus Achromicus

Nevus achromicus (also known as nevus depigmentosus) is a achromic congenital stain with irregular border and variable size and stability [81, 82] (Fig. 58.12). It manifests segmentally or, less commonly, is widespread. Usually it is a single lesion diagnosed at birth or in childhood. In most patients, it appears in midsection or proximal portion ends and does not cross the midline [81]. It can affect both men and women

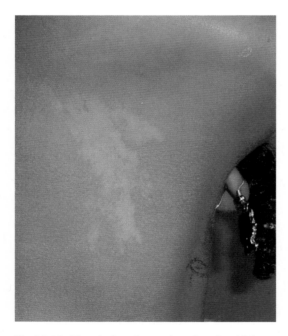

Fig. 58.12 Nevus achromicus: achromic stain with irregular border on the neck (Image courtesy of dermatology service of Federal University of Health Sciences of Porto Alegre – UFCSPA)

Table 58.2 Diagnostic criteria for nevus achromicus

1. Leukoderma presents at birth or early childhood
2. Leukorderma distribution unchanged for the entire life
3. No texture or sense change in the affected area
4. Absence of hyperpigmentation border around the achromic area

equally, and its physiopathology is likely associated with a defective development of fetal melanocytes. The diagnosis is clinical [83] (Table 58.2). The biopsy typically displays a hypomelanotic, but not melanocytic, lesion, rendering the term "nevus achromicus" inappropriate [84].

The main differential diagnoses are vitiligo and nevus anemicus for strict shape and Ito hypomelanosis for target and systematic shapes. The Wood's lamp examination indicates hypochromia, but without the whitish-pink color from vitiligo [81]. The appearance and frequency of the lesions are also important criteria in determining vitiligo. The treatment available for repigmentation are phototherapy, excimer laser and surgical grafting [85, 86]. However, the results of these therapies are inconsistent and recurrence is possible.

Hyperchromic Stains

Hyperpigmentation is due to an increased melanin production caused by increased melanocyte and tyrosinase activity, as well as delayed breakdown and removal of melanin [18]. Hyperchromic stain appears as brown shades over the skin. It can be single, isolated, or multiple and widespread, in many geometric patterns. Many hyperpigmentation disorders are acquired or idiopathic, although some may be influenced by genetic, systemic, or environmental factors [18].

A summary of hyperchromic stains is provided in Flowchart 58.3.

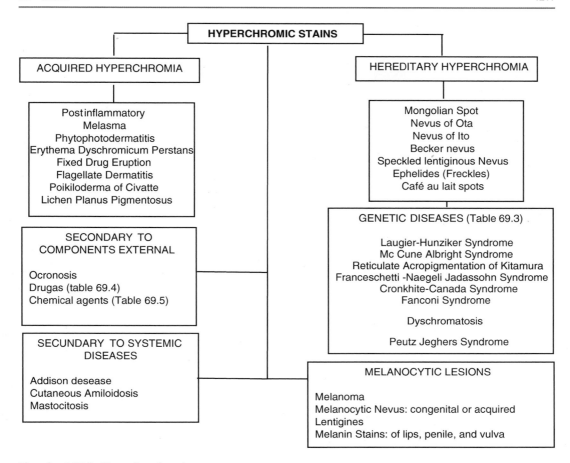

Flowchart 58.3 Hyperchromic stains

Acquired Hyperchromic Stains

Postinflammatory Hyperpigmentation

Postinflammatory hyperpigmentation represents an excess of melanin acquired after inflammation or skin lesion. It is extremely common and it can occur on any part of the skin surface, including mucous membrane and nails. It affects individuals of any age, regardless of gender preference. People with high phototypes tend to be affected more frequently and severely. Lesions can become worse after uninterrupted inflammation, trauma, or sun exposure [18].

The stains are asymptomatic, their color varying from brass color to dark brown or from bluish gray to greyish brown. The primary lesions of underlying inflammatory disorder may or may not be evident when mixed with hyperpigmentation. When there is no primary lesion the size, shape, and pattern of hyperpigmentation lesion distribution suggest the underlying etiology (Fig. 58.13) [18].

Disorders that cause postinflammatory hyperpigmentation include acne, insect bites, pyoderma, atopic dermatitis, psoriasis, pityriasis rosea, lichenoid drug reactions, systemic lupus erythematosus, and fixed drug eruptions.

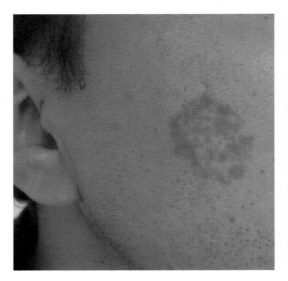

Fig. 58.13 Postinflammatory hyperpigmentation: hyperchromic stain caused after using trichloroacetic acid (Image courtesy of dermatology service of Federal University of Health Sciences of Porto Alegre – UFCSPA)

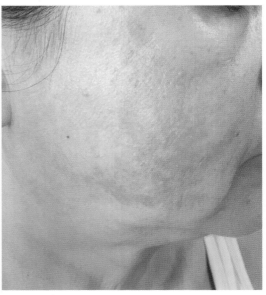

Fig. 58.14 Melasma: hyperchromic stains on the malar and mandibular regions (Image courtesy of dermatology service of Federal University of Health Sciences of Porto Alegre – UFCSPA)

Treatment focuses on treating the underlying cause, even with lesion regression that ceases over time; treatment can take months or years in patients with darker skin [18].

Melasma

Melasma is an acquired disorder characterized by symmetric and hyperpigmented stains of irregular shape that occurs more often on the face. It is most prevalent in young and middle-aged women. Exacerbating factors include pregnancy, use of oral contraceptives, sun exposure and, rarely, use of phenytoin on human immunodeficiency virus (HIV) patients. Although the exact pathogenesis of melasma is unknown, there is no evidence that after sun exposure (or another inductor) the hyperfunctional melanocytes in exposed skin cause an increased production of melanin [18].

The most common clinical pattern according to region of the lesion is the centrofacial (malar region, supralabial, nose, and mentum). Other patterns are malar (cheeks and nose) and mandibular (mandible branches) (Fig. 58.14).

The disease can be epidermal (resulting from increase of melanin in the basal and suprabasal layer of epidermis) or dermal (melanin in perivascular macrophage clusters). The diagnosis is essentially clinical, and a combination of hydroquinone (2–4%), tretinoin (0.05–0.1%), and a corticosteroid is the most common treatment [87].

Phytophotodermatitis

Phytophotodermatitis is a common disease characterized by a rash that occurs after contact with photosensitizing compounds in plants and sun exposure. It does not need previous exposure to furocoumarins. The acute form of the disease may be asymptomatic or can cause itching and burning, with erythema and vesiculation depending on the amount of skin contact, the skin color, and intensity of sun exposure. After resolution of the inflammation, the affected area has marked hyperpigmentation (Fig. 58.15). Many plants have been identified that contain furocoumarins,

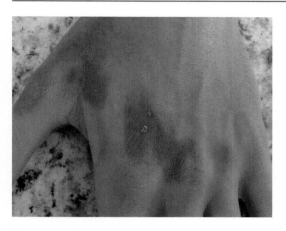

Fig. 58.15 Phytophotodermatitis: hyperpigmentation on the hand due to contact with plant and subsequent sun exposure (Image courtesy of dermatology service of Federal University of Health Sciences of Porto Alegre – UFCSPA)

including limes, lemons, and celery. The extract of this plant makes use in chemical components of some perfumes and colognes, inducing "Berloque dermatitis" or "au-de-cologne dermatitis" [88].

The diagnosis is clinical, and treatment for acute inflammatory lesions includes the use of a topical steroid and cold compress. After the reduction of inflammation, it is advisable to discontinue the topical steroids. To prevent more hyperpigmentation, the use of sunscreen is fundamental. The hyperpigmentation areas usually fade with time, but a bleaching agent is an option if skin discoloration persists [89].

Erythema Dyschromicum Perstans

Erythema dyschromicum perstans is an uncommon disease of unknown etiology and it well known for its chronic appearance, also known as "gray dermatosis." It is more common in people with high phototypes and can be associated with endocrinopathies, ingestion of ammonia nitrate, radiologic contrast, vitiligo, HIV, and chronic hepatitis C infection. Most of the cases do not have an identifiable triggering factor. Some studies point to an immune-mediated dermatosis, likely with a genetic predisposition, as initiating the disease. The lesions described are asymptomatic and symmetric stains colored

gray-brown, located on the midsection, face, and extremities, except the palms, sole, scalp, and hands.

Diagnosis focuses on clinical presentation and histopathologic findings. Differential diagnosis includes lichen planus pigmentosus, idiopathic eruptive macular pigmentation, postinflammatory hyperpigmentation, fixed pigmented erythema, Addison's disease, and hemochromatosis. Treatment is based on the topical use of hydroquinone, topical corticosteroids, and tretinoin, although the results may be not so good because of the dermal deposits of melanin. Clofazimine and dapsone can be used in adult patients because of their anti-inflammatory and immunomodulatory activity [87].

Fixed Pigmented Erythema

Fixed pigmented erythema is a type of pharmacodermia characterized by lesions that occur for 1–2 weeks after the first exposure to certain medicines, with resurgence within 24 h in the same place via a new exposure.

Clinically it is visible as erythematous and edematous rounded stains or plaques, sharply demarcated, and sometimes with gray and violet hue (Figs. 58.16 and 58.17), in addition to the central blister. It can be found anywhere on the body but prevails in the lips, face, hands, feet, and genitalia. The lesions gradually disappear in several days, leaving a postinflammatory

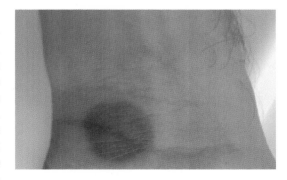

Fig. 58.16 Fixed pigmented erythema: erythematous and edematous rounded stain on the wrist (Image courtesy of dermatology service of Federal University of Health Sciences of Porto Alegre – UFCSPA)

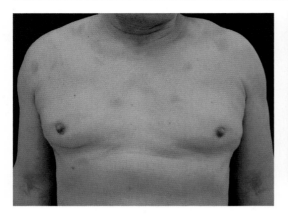

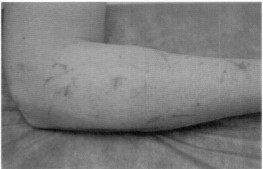

Fig. 58.18 Flagellate dermatitis: erythematous and hyperchromic linear stains on the upper limbs (Image courtesy of dermatology service of Federal University of Health Sciences of Porto Alegre – UFCSPA)

Fig. 58.17 Fixed pigmented erythema: multiple stains with *violet* hue on the trunk (Image courtesy of dermatology service of Federal University of Health Sciences of Porto Alegre – UFCSPA)

hyperpigmentation residue. The most common medications used for treatment are sulfonamides, anti-inflammatories, barbiturates, tetracycline, acetaminophen, and tetryzoline. It is a clinical and sometimes histopathologic diagnosis. The treatment consists of removing the triggering agent [18].

Flagellate Dermatitis

Flagellate dermatitis, or flagellate erythema, is a cutaneous toxic effect unleashed by bleomycin, with a rate of incidence of 8–20% regardless of the path of administration or the types of malignant disease to be treated. The reaction usually occurs after accumulative doses of 100–300 mg. The time between drug administration and the appearance of lesions varies and can last up to 6 months. Clinically it presents as linear stains with adjacent pruritic erythematous papules that may show occasional bleeding or pustules. It appears on the upper chest and back, but also on the limbs and flanks (Fig. 58.18) [87].

As the rashes become less erythematous, the affected areas become hyperpigmented. Most cases can be reverted after discontinuation of the offending agent. Antihistamines and the use of topical and oral corticosteroids can reduce pruritus [18].

Poikiloderma de Riehl-Civatte

Poikiloderma of Civatte is an acquired and commonly benign dermatosis that affects fair-skinned, middle-aged, and elderly people. The etiology is multifactorial and includes chronic sun exposure, menopause-related hormonal changes, contact hypersensitivity, and genetic predisposition. Clinically it consists of telangiectasia, cutaneous atrophy, and macular hypo- and hyperpigmentation that appears symmetrically on the sides, as a V-shaped area on the neck, and on the lateral parts of the face with sparing of anatomically shaded areas (Fig. 58.19) [90, 91].

Because of the variations in clinical appearance, a classification proposes to categorize the disease into erythematotelangiectatic type, pigmented type, and mixed type, which also assists in determining the most appropriate treatment [92]. Treatment consists mainly of educating patients to avoid sun exposure and regular use of sunscreen. Laser treatment can be used, but with varying results.

Lichen Planus Pigmentosus

Lichen planus pigmentosus is an uncommon variation of lichen planus that affects mostly middle-aged adults with high cutaneous phototypes. Its etiology is still unknown, but sun exposure may be involved because of the

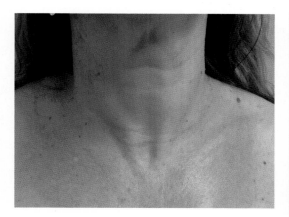

Fig. 58.19 Poikiloderma of Civatte: symmetric telangiectasias and hyperpigmentation on the V-shaped area on the neck (Image courtesy of dermatology service of Federal University of Health Sciences of Porto Alegre – UFCSPA)

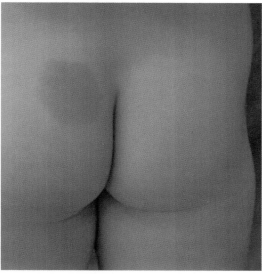

Fig. 58.20 Mongolian spot: stain with *blue-black* pigmentation located on the gluteal area (Image courtesy of dermatology service of Federal University of Health Sciences of Porto Alegre – UFCSPA)

photodistribution. It appears as stains and plaques with irregular oval shape, usually symmetric and with coloration ranging from brown to grayish-brown in sun-exposed or scarred areas. The early lesions differ from erythema dyschromicum perstans by not presenting an erythematous border. It is usually asymptomatic, although some patients describe a light itch or burning sensation. The clinical diagnosis is obtained by histopathology; as yet there is no effective treatment [18].

Hereditary Hyperchromic Stains

Mongolian Spot

Mongolian spot is a congenital stain with blue-black pigmentation, unique or multiple, located on lumbosacral and gluteal areas and lower portion of the scapula with varying size and shape (Fig. 58.20). It is frequent in yellow and black races. It is present at birth and tends to disappear between 3 and 5 years old, but can remain during childhood or adulthood. The diagnosis is clinical and there is no need for treatment, since it usually regresses spontaneously and presents benign features [18].

Nevus of Ota

Nevus of Ota derives from melanocytes located on the innervation of the ophthalmic and maxillary branches of the nerve trigeminal areas. It appears at birth or in adolescence, mostly in women. Clinically it is an irregular stain, edge set, and grayish blue in color, unilaterally located in the periorbital, malar, or nasal region (Fig. 58.21). It usually affects the sclera of the ipsilateral eye. As it can be associated with increased intraocular pressure, it is important to request an ophthalmologic examination and careful follow-up [18].

Nevus of Ito

This nevus presents the same characteristics as nevus of Ota, but differs in location. It occurs in innervated areas of the tracheocutaneous lateral and anterior supratrochlear nerves (shoulders, supraclavicular, and neck regions). The indicated therapy is similar to that for nevus of Ota [18].

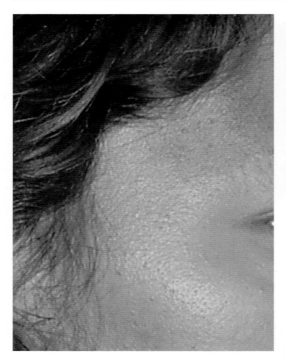

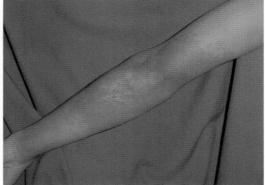

Fig. 58.22 Nevus of Becker: irregular pigmented stain on the upper limb (Image courtesy of dermatology service of Federal University of Health Sciences of Porto Alegre – UFCSPA)

Fig. 58.21 Nevus of Ota: irregular stain, with *grayish blue* color, unilaterally located on the periorbital region (Image courtesy of dermatology service of Federal University of Health Sciences of Porto Alegre – UFCSPA)

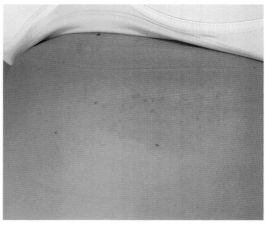

Fig. 58.23 Speckled lentiginous nevus: an irregular *brownish* stain (similar to café-au-lait) with darker pigmentary punctate lesions on the inframammary region (Image courtesy of dermatology service of Federal University of Health Sciences of Porto Alegre – UFCSPA)

Becker Nevus

Becker nevus is a hamartoma that affects mostly young men. It appears as an irregular pigmented stain located on the shoulder, upper chest, or scapular region (Fig. 58.22). During puberty, dark and thick hair appears in the lesion, and does not always affect the pigmentation area [18].

Speckled Lentiginous Nevus

Speckled lentiginous nevus appears as an irregular brownish stain (similar to coffee with milk) with darker pigmentary punctate lesions and histological features of simple lentiginous or compound nerves (Fig. 58.23). It begins usually at pre-school age, and the data regarding malignant potential are insufficient [18].

Ephelides (Freckles)

Freckles are caused by an increase of melanin pigment in the melanocytes. They are macules of brownish color that are prevalent in sun-exposed areas of the skin. Freckles occur on the nose and

malar area, forehead, and dorsum of the hands, as a sign of photoaging, but may also appear in younger age groups, especially in those with fair skin. The diagnosis is clinical and the treatment is purely for cosmetic reasons, including the use of chemicals such as α-hydroxy acids, trichloroacetic acid, phenol, and Jessner's solution. Electrosurgery, cryotherapy, and lasers are also treatment options. These treatments have not proved to be completely satisfactory and have a common risk of postinflammatory hyperpigmentation [93, 94].

Café-au-Lait Spots

Café-au-lait spots may be present at birth or develop during the first years of life. They have a uniform pigmentation and a sharp border, and range in size from 0.2 to 30 cm in diameter. They are also indicators for various genodermatoses, especially neurofibromatosis. More than five café-au-lait lesions are suggestive of neurofibromatosis. Examinations of axillary freckling (Crowe sign) and iris hamartomas (Lisch nodules) are advisable. Other rare genetic syndromes such as Albright syndrome and Cowden syndrome are also associated with café-au-lait stains [3].

Other Genetic Hyperpigmentations

Other genetic diseases that can cause hyperpigmentation are listed in Table 58.3.

Hyperchromia Secondary to Systemic Diseases

Addison Disease

Addison's disease is a primary adrenal insufficiency that results in glucocorticoid and mineralocorticoid deficiency. Acute adrenal crisis results from orthostatic hypotension, fever, and hypoglycemia. Chronic primary adrenal insufficiency is characterized by a more frequent history of malaria, anorexia, diarrhea, weight loss, and joint and back pain [95].

The cutaneous manifestations include darkening of the skin, especially in sun-exposed areas, and hyperpigmentation of the palmar creases, frictional surfaces, vermilion border, recent scars, genital skin, and oral mucosa. Measurement of basal plasma cortisol is an

Table 58.3 Other genetic diseases associated with hyperpigmentation

Peutz–Jeghers syndrome
Laugier–Hunziker syndrome
McCune–Albright syndrome
Reticulate acropigmentation of Kitamura
Franceschetti–Naegeli–Jadassohn syndrome
Cronkhite-Canada syndrome
Fanconi syndrome
Dyschromatosis
Incontinentia pigmenti

insensitive screening test. Synthetic adrenocorticotropin 1–24 at a dose of 250 µg is an effective dynamic test. Elevated plasma levels of adrenocorticotropin and renin confirm the diagnosis. Treatment involves hormonal replacement therapy [96].

Cutaneous Amyloidosis

Cutaneous amyloidosis is a deposit of amyloid substance in the skin and internal organs. It can be classified in primary and secondary, systemic or localized, and hereditary or acquired. The primary and secondary forms can be systemic or localized. The form most associated with neoplasms is the primary systemic, which appears at a rate of 10–20% in individuals with multiple myeloma. The dermatologic clinical condition usually adopts a general systemic appearance and begins with hemorrhagic lesions caused by a deposit of amyloid in the vessels walls, causing vascular fragility. Features around the eyes may appear as ecchymotic lesions, known as raccoon sign. Alopecia and cutis verticis gyrata in the scalp could appear. Linear hemorrhagic lesions in the midsection (Koebner's phenomenon) may be present. Macroglossia presents in 40% of cases. The clinical diagnosis by histopathology is definitive. Systemic change occurs throughout the affected organ. There is no effective treatment. Some studies showed good response to melphalan in conjunction with prednisone. The progression of the disease most commonly leads to death within 2 years [18].

Mastocytosis

Cutaneous mastocytosis is a spectrum of disorders characterized by accumulation of normal mast cells in the skin and sometimes other organs. Systemic signs and symptoms include flushing, blistering, pruritus, and diarrhea, due to histamine degranulation and by release of physical and dermatologic impulse. Systemic disease may involve the gastrointestinal tract, the bone marrow, or other organs. In children, the disease is typically limited to the skin; however, painless systemic mastocytosis is also common. The classic form related to hyperpigmentation is urticaria pigmentosa, when patients develop stains and brown to reddish-brown papules, presenting as a

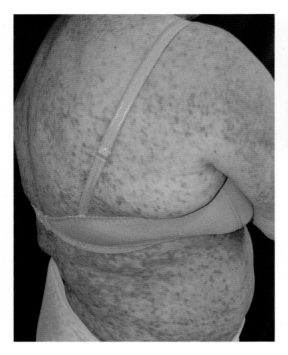

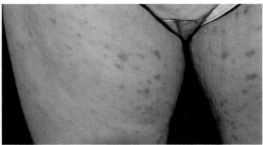

Fig. 58.25 Darier's sign: the cutaneous mastocytosis lesions usually become irritated after suffering friction (Image courtesy of dermatology service of Federal University of Health Sciences of Porto Alegre – UFCSPA)

Hyperchromia Secondary to External Components

The affinity of melanin biopolymers for metal ions, drugs, and other organic compounds is an important factor in the etiology of some hyper-pigmentation disorders [98].

Ocronosis

Exogenous ochronosis is an unintended side effect for patients who already being treated with hydroquinone for long-term hyperpig-mentation disorders in sun-exposed areas. Early diagnosis is the key in ensuring that the offending agent is suspended. The diagnosis is clinical, the presence of dark stains in areas previously treated with hydroquinone being important (Fig. 58.26). Dermatoscopy can be useful and may negate the need for a biopsy. It is necessary to identify this disorder at the earliest stage and discontinue hydroquinone immediately [99].

Miscellaneous Hyperchromia

Acquired hyperpigmentation of the skin is sometimes interpreted as an adverse effect of drugs (Table 58.4) or secondary to chemical agents (Table 58.5).

Melanocytic lesions are also part of the differential diagnosis of hyperchromic lesions such as melanoma, a subject already discussed in Chap. 17; others are mentioned in Table 58.6.

Fig. 58.24 Urticarial pigmentosa: stains and *brown* to *reddish-brown* papules, as a prickly rash mostly in mid-section spreading symmetrically (Image courtesy of dermatology service of Federal University of Health Sciences of Porto Alegre – UFCSPA)

prickly rash mostly in the midsection, spreading symmetrically (Fig. 58.24).

The cutaneous mastocytosis lesions usually become irritated after suffering friction (Darier's sign, Fig. 58.25). Skin lesions may or may not accompany systemic mastocytosis. Even when the physician considers mastocytosis as a possible diagnosis, it can be difficult to identify because of special technical requirements necessary for a biopsy and because of problems with biochemical testing. The level of serum tryptase is useful to examine the possibility of systemic disease and is mainly used during the initial diagnostic evaluation. Drug therapy stabilizes mast cell membranes to reduce the severity of the attacks and block the action of inflammatory mediators. The primary therapy is histamine H1 and H2 blockers, and the avoidance of triggering factors. While the prognosis for urticaria pigmentosa in early childhood is excellent, with spontaneous resolution in months or years, the disease in adulthood is often persistent [97].

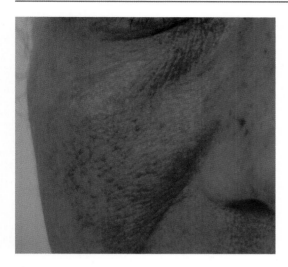

Fig. 58.26 Exogenous ochronosis due to long-term use of hydroquinone to treat dark circles (Image courtesy of dermatology service of Federal University of Health Sciences of Porto Alegre – UFCSPA)

Table 58.4 Other medicines that cause hyperpigmentation

Clofazimine
Amiodarone
Antimalarials
Chemotherapeutics: carmustine, bleomycin, busulfan, cyclophosphamide, dactinomycin, hydroxyurea, methotrexate
Azidothymidine
Diltiazem
Minocycline
Psoralen
Psychotropic drugs
Hormones: oral contraceptives, melanotropic and adrenocorticotropic hormones

Table 58.5 Hyperpigmentation due to metals

Arsenic
Bismuth
Gold
Steel
Lead
Mercury
Silver (argyria)

Table 58.6 Melanocytic hyperchromic lesions

Melanoma
Melanocytic nevus: congenital or acquired
Lentigines
Melanin stains: of lips, penis, and vulva

Vascular and Blood Stains

Purpura

Purpura is mucocutaneous bleeding from blood vessel leakage in the dermis, which measures at least 5–10 mm in diameter, is palpable or nonpalpable, and does not disappear with added pressure. It may have different causes to be investigated, firstly by history and physical examination. Clinical manifestations differ according to the cause, including petechiae (purpura with a diameter less than or equal to 4 mm), contusion, ecchymosis (with generally diameter larger than 1 cm), linear petechiae, and hematoma (shows slight rise, unlike ecchymosis). The color helps determine the etiology, being typically red (hemoglobin saturated with flow and adequate skin perfusion), bright red (superficial bleeding), and blue (restricted blood flow). If there is more hemorrhaging and therefore more swelling and inflammation of the skin resulting from purpura, it is more likely that the lesion is palpable. The retiform purpura is a branched purple complex that indicates microvascular occlusion.

Nonpalpable Purpura

Idiopathic thrombocytopenic purpura is a hematologic disorder characterized by isolated thrombocytopenia without a clinically apparent cause. The major causes of accelerated platelet absorption include immune thrombocytopenia, decreased bone marrow production, and increased splenic sequestration. Its clinical manifestation may be acute, with severe bleeding, mild, or asymptomatic. Treatment should be restricted to those patients with moderate or severe thrombocytopenia who are bleeding or at risk of bleeding [100].

Thrombotic thrombocytopenic purpura is more common in adults, while the hemolytic-uremic syndrome is more common in children. Associated factors are pregnancy, cancer, medications, bone marrow transplantation, and autoimmune diseases. Clinical signs include fever, renal disorders, and changes to the central nervous system. Hemolytic uremic syndrome due to *Escherichia coli* infection is common. The available treatment consists of fresh frozen plasma [101].

Purpura fulminans is a hematologic emergency with skin necrosis and scattered intravascular coagulation. It may progress rapidly and complicate severe sepsis, or may occur as an autoimmune response to otherwise benign childhood infections. The initial appearance of these lesions is well-demarcated erythematous macules that progress rapidly to develop irregular central areas of blue-black hemorrhagic necrosis [102].

A summary of nonpalpable purpuras is provided in Flowchart 58.4.

Palpable Purpura

Any process that occludes or damages the cutaneous vessels results in purpura. When palpable, it may be due to vasculitis or vascular occlusion.

Henoch-Schönlein Purpura

Henoch-Schönlein purpura (HSP) is an acute immunoglobulin A-mediated disorder characterized by a generalized vasculitis involving small vessels of the skin and other organs. It is the most common vasculitis in children, with an incidence of 10–20 cases per 100,000 children per year.

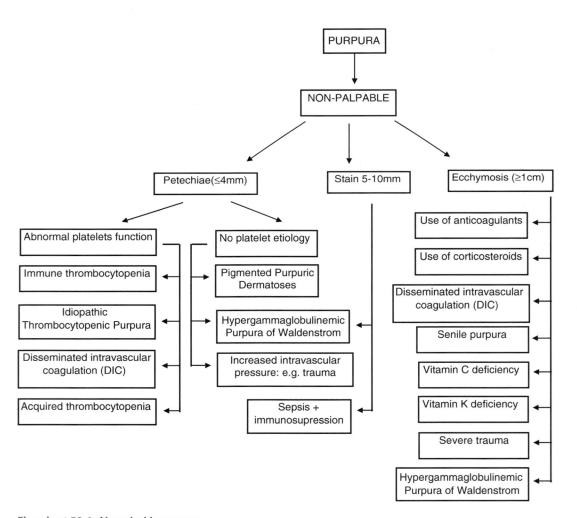

Flowchart 58.4 Nonpalpable purpuras

The etiology of the disease is still not clear and is probably multifactorial. Up to 50% of patients develop the disease after a respiratory infection. Several bacterial and viral infectious agents have been associated with the development of HSP, and some cases have been reported after the ingestion of drugs or vaccines [103].

Generally there are prodromic symptoms such as headache, anorexia, and fever. Subsequently, other developing symptoms may include the following.

Rash (95–100% of cases) is the characteristic feature of the disease, which appears in nearly all patients and usually lasts an average of 3 weeks. Lesions occur on the buttocks and upper thighs in younger children and on the feet, ankles, and lower legs in older children and adults. The primary difference between children and adults is the chronicity and severity of the eruption in adults. The eruption is commonly symmetric and begins as erythematous stains or urticarial lesions, progressing to blanching papules and later to palpable purpura. Usually the face, palms, soles, and mucous membranes are spared. In general, the lesion regresses spontaneously.

The gastrointestinal tract can be involved, with abdominal pain, vomiting, and bloody stools. Other symptoms included arthritis, especially involving the knees and ankles, glomerulonephritis, pulmonary involvement, subcutaneous edema, and scrotal edema [104].

The diagnosis of HSP is clinical. Laboratory tests are usually normal, but sometimes help in the exclusion of other diagnoses and evaluation of renal and hematologic function. Diagnosis is by evidence of immunoglobulin A in the skin or kidney documented by immunofluorescence. The prognosis is generally good, with full recovery and, less commonly, recurrent episodes or persistent disease. This disease does not require specific therapy in the majority of symptomatic cases, except in severe ones that require specific treatments [105].

Pigmented Purpuric Dermatoses

Pigmented purpuric dermatosis is a term used to describe a group of asymptomatic benign eruptions with periods of clinical remission. The lesions present petechiae and pigmentary stains of the skin primarily localized to the lower limbs

in the absence of venous insufficiency or hematologic disorders. Their cause is unknown, but several underlying diseases and drugs can be related to the disorder [106].

Pigmented purpuric dermatosis shares common histopathologic features including capillaritis, extravasation of erythrocytes, and hemosiderin deposits. Clinical variations between eruptions lead to subclassification as shown in Table 58.7 [107] (Fig. 58.27).

There is no fully effective treatment. There are several therapies reported, including topical steroids, oral antihistamines, pentoxifylline, and treatment based on UV light [108].

Table 58.7 Pigmented purpuric dermatoses

Schamberg's disease	Usually in women about 50 years
	Insidious onset, in one or both legs
	Irregular reddish-brown stains and asymptomatic
Purpura annularis telangiectodes (Majocchi's disease)	Usually in young women
	Asymptomatic annular spots, telangiectasias and purpura, symmetric, in the lower extremities
Lichen aureus	Usually in young men
	The dermal dense inflammatory infiltrate type band distinguishes golden lichen other pigmented purpuric dermatoses
	Circumscribed areas of papules or yellowish, reddish, or violet stains
	Usually asymptomatic and unilateral (lower extremities)
Itching purpura	Usually middle-aged men
	Abrupt onset, in the lower extremities (can become widespread)
	Reddish-brown stains with intense itching
Gougerot-Blum	Usually in males approximately 40 years
	Primary lesion consists of papule lichenoides polygonal or round, red-brown, in combination with purpura or telangiectasia, in lower extremities
Eczematid-like purpura of Doucas-Kapetanakis	Usually women about 40 years
	Seasonal: spring and summer
	Light peeling on the reddish-brown spots on the lower limbs
	Abrupt onset

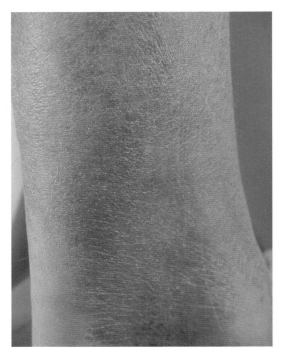

Fig. 58.27 Schamberg's disease: irregular *reddish-brown* stains on both legs (Image courtesy of dermatology service of Federal University of Health Sciences of Porto Alegre – UFCSPA)

Raynaud's Phenomenon

Raynaud's phenomenon presents a bilateral cold hypersensitivity and episodic digital color changes in the absence of vascular pathology or digital trophic changes. It affects about 10% of the population, predominantly young women. This condition can be classified as primary (idiopathic) and secondary (known occurrences or because of disease). Vasospasm occurs with exposure to cold, leading to white coloration and severe cyanosis to the fingers, which extends from the fingertips in proximal direction to varying degrees. The distal finger to the line of ischemia is cold, while the proximal portion is warm and rosy. During reheating, the whitish fingers may become cyanotic and then brilliant-red, via reactive hyperemia. Persistent discoloration suggests the secondary cause of disease. Not all patients with Raynaud's present these three color changes [109]. Connective tissue diseases, particularly systemic sclerosis, are most commonly associated with the secondary phenomenon. Current treatment options include general

care, keeping the hands and feet warm, quitting smoking, and avoiding caffeine and stress. In severe cases, the most commonly prescribed class of medications is calcium channel blockers such as nifedipine. If a secondary cause appears, a specific treatment must be applied [110].

Livedo Reticularis

Livedo reticularis is a well-known, relatively common physical dermatologic finding that consists of macular, violaceous, connecting rings that form a net-like pattern, characterized by a cyanotic discoloration or erythematous-cyanotic aspect (Fig. 58.28). It is defined as livedo reticularis when the crosslinked pattern is fully formed with a clear interconnection, with certain areas of the skin within having a normal appearance, even pallor. In livedo racemosa, the crosslinked pattern is not made up of lines that converge and close, and in general is followed by pathologic states. Livedo reticularis is divided into congenital or acquired:

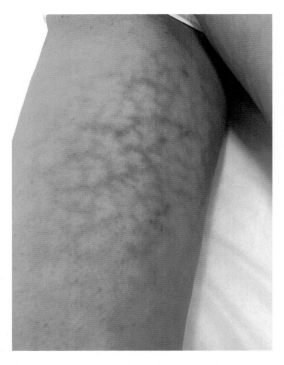

Fig. 58.28 Livedo reticularis: violaceous stains, connecting rings that form a net-like pattern, characterized by a cyanotic discoloration or erythematous-cyanotic aspect (Image courtesy of dermatology service of Federal University of Health Sciences of Porto Alegre – UFCSPA)

Congenital (cutis marmorata telangiectatica congenita): congenital form of livedo reticularis typically presenting at birth, confined to the lower extremities

Acquired: physiologic livedo reticularis or cutis marmorata are synonymous and refer to a normal livedo pattern that occurs in response to cold. It occurs more frequently in neonates, children, and young adults, and can appear in up to 50% of children.

Idiopathic or primary livedo reticularis occurs predominantly in young adults and middle-aged women. Generally it is most widespread, particularly in the lower extremities and sometimes in the upper extremities. Although varying with temperature fluctuations, it continues upon heating. It can manifest with stains, sores, swelling, and numbness. It is a diagnosis of exclusion; it is important to rule out secondary causes, especially in disseminated cases [111].

Livedo reticularis by vasospasm is the most common cause of reticular livedo. It is usually associated with connective tissue diseases and reflects a vasospastic trend, occurring most commonly in patients with Raynaud's phenomenon.

Livedo reticularis racemosa is associated with systemic diseases and is caused by intravascular disorders, disease of the vessel walls, or clogging of vessels (see Table 58.8).

Treatment of livedo reticularis is based on the etiology. The aim of treatment of primary livedo is to limit exposure to cold, and sometimes it may be necessary to use vasodilators. Livedo racemosa treatment also focuses on the causative disorder [112].

Table 58.8 Some conditions associated with livedo racemosa

Vasculitis (vasculitis in systemic lupus erythematosus, polyarteritis nodosa, microscopic polyangiitis, Wegener granulomatosis, Churg–Strauss syndrome, vasculitis due to drugs, and others)
Antiphospholipid antibody syndrome
Sneddon syndrome
Thrombophilias
Sickle cell anemia
Myeloproliferative syndromes
Vasculopathy livedoid
Cryoglobulinemia
Calciphylaxis
Hyperoxaluria
Medicines
Infections
Necrosis by coumarin

Glossary

Cryotherapy A technique that uses an extremely cold liquid or instruments to freeze and destroy abnormal skin cells that require removal. It can be used to destroy a variety of benign skin growths, such as warts, actinic keratoses, and some malignant lesions (such as superficial basal cell and squamous cell cancers).

Cutis verticis gyrata A condition of the skin of the forehead with hypertrophy and deep vertical folds so as to resemble the surface of the brain. It is a feature of acromegaly, local inflammation, and acute myeloid leukemia. A rare primary form, which affects males only, is associated with neurologic problems.

Darier's sign Skin change produced when the skin lesion in urticaria pigmentosa is rubbed briskly. The area usually begins to itch and becomes raised and surrounded by erythema.

Dermabrasion A technique whereby a dermatome or abrading device is used to remove the epidermis and superficial dermis, allowing regeneration of the epithelium to occur from underlying adnexal structure.

Excimer laser A powerful form of laser which is nearly always operated in the ultraviolet spectral region and generates nanosecond pulses.

Furocoumarins A class of organic chemical compounds produced by a variety of plants. They sensitize the skin to the effects of the sun, thus leading to irregular pigmentation and increasing the risk of sunburn and phototoxicity.

Koebner's phenomenon (isomorphic response) The appearance of new skin lesions on areas of cutaneous injury in otherwise healthy skin, with the same clinical and histologic features as lesions of the patient's original skin disease.

Phototherapy A technique used for the treatment of some skin diseases by exposure to light, including ultraviolet and infrared radiation. It is defined as either medium-wave light energy (ultraviolet-B light [UVB]) or long-wave light (ultraviolet-A [UVA]). UVB is available as narrowband or broadband.

Wood's lamp   Created by Robert Williams Wood, this lamp used especially to detect some skin conditions by the fluorescence induced in the affected areas by ultraviolet radiation.

Zireli's sign   Scaling of macules made prominent by stretching the affected skin. It is present in pityriasis versicolor.

References

1. Barsh GS. What controls variation in human skin color? PLoS Biol. 2003;1:19–22.
2. Nordlund JJ, Boissy RE, Hearing VJ, King R, Oetting W, Ortonne JP. The pigmentary system: physiology and pathophysiology. 2nd ed. Oxford: Wiley-Blackwell; 2006.
3. Fistarol SK, Itin PH. Disorders of pigmentation. JDDG. 2010;8:187–202.
4. Wolff K, Goldsmith LA, Katz SI, Gilchrest BA, Paller AS, Leffell DJ, editors. Fitzpatrick Tratado de Dermatologia. 7a edição, Rio de Janeiro: Revinter; 2010.
5. Azulay RD, Azulay DR, Abulafia LA. Azulay Dermatologia. 6th ed. Rio de Janeiro: Guanabara Koogan; 2015.
6. Rübsam ML, Esch M, Baum E, Bösner S. Diagnosing skin disease in primary care: a qualitative study of GP's. Fam Pract. 2015;32(5):591–5.
7. Kerr OA, Tidman MJ, Walker JJ, Aldridge RD, Benton EC. The profile of dermatologic problems in primary care. Clin Exp Dermatol. 2010;35(4):380–3.
8. Sociedade Brasileira De Dermatologia. Perfil nosológico das consultas dermatológicas no Brasil. An Bras Dermatol. 2006;81(6):549–58.
9. Lupi O, Cunha PR. Rotinas de Diagnóstico e Tratamento da Sociedade Brasileira de Dermatologia. 2nd ed. Itapevi: AC Farmacêutica; 2012.
10. Majumder PP, Nordlund JJ, Nath SK. Pattern of familial aggregation of vitiligo. Arch Dermatol. 1993;129:994.
11. Handa S, Kaur I. Vitiligo: clinical findings in 1436 patients. J Dermatol. 1999;26:653.
12. Rivitti E. Manual de dermatologia clínica de Sampaio e Rivitti. São Paulo: Artes Médicas; 2014.
13. Jin Y, Birlea SA, Fain PR, Gowan K, Sheri L, Riccardi BS, et al. Variant of TYR and autoimmunity susceptibility loci in generalized vitiligo. N Engl J Med. 2010;362(18):1686–97.
14. Taïeb A, Picardo M. Vitiligo. N Engl J Med. 2009;360:160–9.
15. Taïeb A, Alomar A, Böhm M, Dell'Anna ML, Pase De A, Eleftheriadou V, et al. Guidelines for the management of vitiligo: the European Forum consensus. Br J Dermatol. 2013;168:5–19.
16. Grimes PE. New insights and new therapies in vitiligo. JAMA. 2005;293:730.
17. Falabella R, Escobar C, Giraldo N, Rovetto P, Gil J, Barona MI, et al. On the pathogenesis of idiopathic guttate hypomelanosis. J Am Acad Dermatol. 1987;16(1):1.
18. Bolognia JL, Jorizzo JL, Schaffer JV; Kalil CLPV (organization); Corrêa ADC (translation), et al. Dermatologia. 3rd ed. Rio de Janeiro: Elsevier; 2015.
19. Kakepis M, Havaki S, Katoulis A, Katsambas A, Stavrianeas N, Troupis TG. Idiopathic guttate hypomelanosis: an electron microscopy study. JEADV. 2015;29:1435–8.
20. Kaya TI, Yazici AC, Tursen U, Ikizoglu G. Idiopathic guttate hypomelanosis: idiopathic or ultraviolet induced? Photodermatol Photoimmunol Photomed. 2005;21:270–1.
21. Shin MK, Jeong KH, Oh IH, Choe BK, Lee MH. Clinical features of idiopathic guttate hypomelanosis in 646 subjects and association with other aspects of photoaging. Int J Dermatol. 2011;50:798–805.
22. Friedland R, David M, Feinmesser M, Fenig-Nakar S, Hodak E. Idiopathic guttate hypomelanosis-like lesions in patients with mycosis fungoides: a new adverse effect of phototherapy. JEADV. 2010;24:1026–30.
23. Rerknimitr P, Disphanurat W, Achariyakul M. Topical tacrolimus significantly promotes repigmentation in idiopathic guttate hypomelanosis: a double-blind, randomized, placebo-controlled study. JEADV. 2013;27:460–4.
24. Tey HL. Approach to hypopigmentation disorders in adults. Clin Exp Dermatol. 2009;35:829–34.
25. Ayres EL, Magrin PF, Bentivoglio F, Costa A. Progressive macular hypomelanosis: an epidemiological study of 103 cases in Southeast Brazil. Surg Cosmet Dermatol. 2015;7(1):56–60.
26. Hwang SW, Hong SK, Kim SH, Hoon Park JH, Seo JK, Sung HS, et al. Progressive macular hypomelanosis in Korean patients: a clinicopathologic study. Ann Dermatol. 2009;21(3):261–7.
27. Almeida ART, Bedani TP, Debs EAF, Ferreira JAD. Estudo piloto para avaliar a eficácia da minociclina no tratamento da hipomelanose macular progressiva (HMP). Surg Cosmet Dermatol. 2009;1(1):25–8.
28. Relyveld GN, Menke HE, Westerhof W. Progressive macular hypomelanosis: an overview. Am J Clin Dermatol. 2007;8(1):13–9.
29. Rodríguez-Lojo R, Verea MM, Velasco D, Barjaa JM. Hipomelanosis macular progresiva y confluente. Actas Dermosifiliogr. 2010;101(3):268–83.
30. Tey HL. A practical classification of childhood hypopigmentation disorders. Acta Derm Venereol. 2010;90:6–11.

31. Cavalcanti SMM, Magalhães V, Magalhães M, Querino MCD, França ERD, Alencar E. Uso da limeciclina associada com o peróxido de benzoíla no tratamento da hipomelanose macular progressiva: um estudo prospectivo. An Bras Dermatol. 2011;86(4):813–4.

32. Duarte I, Della Nina BI, Gordiano MC, Buense R, Lazzarini R. Hipomelanose macular progressiva: estudo epidemiológico e resposta terapêutica à fototerapia. An Bras Dermatol. 2010;85(5):621–4.

33. In SI, YI SW, Kang HY, Lee ES, Sohn S, Kim YC. Clinical and histopathologic characteristics of pityriasis alba. Clin Exp Dermatol. 2008;34:591–7.

34. Malik TG, Khalil M, Bhatti MM. Pityriasis alba with poliosis. J Coll Phys Surg Pak. 2014;24(2):138–40.

35. Weber MB, Ávila LGS, Albaneze R, Oliveira OLM, Sudhaus BD, Cestari TF. Pityriasis alba: a study of pathogenic factors. JEADV. 2002;16:463–8.

36. Cruz BM, Cázares JPC, Álvarez BT, Gonzáles BM. Pitiriasis alba. Dermatol Rev Mex. 2010;54(2):67–71.

37. Du Toit MJ, Jordaan HF. Pigmenting pityriasis alba. Pediatr Dermatol. 1993;10(1):1–5.

38. Sandhu K, Handa S, Kanwar J. Extensive pityriasis alba in a child with atopic dermatitis. Pediatr Dermatol. 2004;21(3):275–6.

39. Pla VF, Aznar CPS. Esclerodermia. Med Clin (Barc). 2004;122(11):418–9.

40. Nieves AT, Holguera RM, Atrio AS. Esclerodermia. Medicine. 2013;11(32):1981–90.

41. Zancanaro PCQ, Garcia LT, Isaac AR, Costa IMC. Esclerodermia localizada na criança: aspectos clínicos, diagnósticos e terapêuticos. An Bras Dermatol. 2009;84(2):161–72.

42. Macedo PA, Shinjo SK, Goldenstein-Schainberg C. Esclerodermia juvenil. Acta Reumatol Port. 2008;33:289–97.

43. Garza-Rodríguez V, Villarreal-Alarcón MA, Ocampo-Candiani J. Etiopatogenia y tratamiento de la esclerodermia: conceptos actuales. Rev Med Inst Mex Seguro Soc. 2013;51(5):50–7.

44. Bossini-Castillo L, Martín JE, Días-Gallo LM, Rueda B, Javier M. Genética de la esclerodermia. Reumatol Clin. 2010;6(S2):12–5.

45. McPherson T, Cooper S. Vulval lichen sclerosus and lichen planus. Dermatol Ther. 2010;23:523.

46. Powell JJ, Wojnarowska F. Lichen sclerosus. Lancet. 1999;353:1777.

47. Higgins CA, Cruickshank ME. A population-based case-control study of etiological factors associated with vulval lichen sclerosus. J Obstet Gynaecol. 2012;32:271.

48. Neill SM, Lewis FM, Tatnall FM, Cox NH. British Association of Dermatologists' guidelines for the management of lichen sclerosus. Br J Dermatol. 2010;163:672.

49. Rothfield N, Sontheimer RD, Bernstein M. Lupus erythematosus: systemic and cutaneous manifestations. Clin Dermatol. 2006;24:348.

50. Kuhn A, Sonntag M, Richter-Hintz D, et al. Phototesting in lupus erythematosus: a 15-year experience. J Am Acad Dermatol. 2001;45:86.

51. Kuhn A, Ruland V, Bonsmann G. Photosensitivity, phototesting, and photoprotection in cutaneous lupus erythematosus. Lupus. 2010;19:1036.

52. Kuhn A, Gensch K, Haust M, et al. Photoprotective effects of a broad-spectrum sunscreen in ultraviolet-induced cutaneous lupus erythematosus: a randomized, vehicle-controlled, double-blind study. J Am Acad Dermatol. 2011;64:37.

53. Wahie S, Daly AK, Cordell HJ, et al. Clinical and pharmacogenetic influences on response to hydroxychloroquine in discoid lupus erythematosus: a retrospective cohort study. J Invest Dermatol. 2011;131:1981.

54. Boyle J, Kennedy CTC. Leucoderma induced by monomethyl ether of hydroquinone. Clin Exp Dermatol. 1985;10:154–8.

55. Williams H. Skin lightening creams containing hydroquinone. Br J Dermatol. 1992;305:903–4.

56. Ghosh S, Mukhopadhyay S. Chemical leucoderma: a clinicoetiological study of 864 cases in the perspective of a developing country. Br J Dermatol. 2009;160:40–7.

57. Petit A. Prise en charge des complications de la dépigmentation volontaire en France. Ann Dermatol Venereol. 2006;133:907–16.

58. Fernández-Vozmediano JM, Armario-Hita JC. Etiopatogenia y tratamiento de la pitiriasis versicolor. Med Clin (Barc). 2006;126(1):7–13.

59. Schwartz RA. Superficial fungal infections. Lancet. 2004;364:1173.

60. Centeno LBZ, Pacheco AML, Murillo EE, Huerta EA, Calvo AMG. Pitiriasis versicolor. SEMERGEN. 2001;27:48–50.

61. Hu SW, Bigby M. Pityriasis versicolor: a systematic review of interventions. Arch Dermatol. 2010;146:1132.

62. Drake LA, Dinehart SM, Farmer ER, et al. Guidelines of care for superficial mycotic infections of the skin: pityriasis (tinea) versicolor. Guidelines/Outcomes Committee. American Academy of Dermatology. J Am Acad Dermatol. 1996;34:287.

63. Britton WJ, Lockwood DNJ. Leprosy. Lancet. 2004;363(10):1209–19.

64. Ministério da Saúde do Brasil. Guia para o Controle da Hanseníase. 3rd ed. Brasília: Ministério da Saúde, 2002.

65. Ministério da Saúde do Brasil. Protocolo de Atendimento em Hanseníase. 1st ed. Brasília; Subsecretaria de Vigilância à Saúde, 2007.

66. Faye O, Hay RJ, Ryan TJ, Keita S, Traore AK, Mahe A. A public health approach for leprosy detection based on a very short term-training of primary health care workers in basic dermatology. Lepr Ver. 2007;78:11–6.

67. Walker SL, Lockwood DNJ. Leprosy. Clin Dermatol. 2007;25:165–72.

68. Ustianowski AP, Lockwood DNJ. Leprosy: current diagnostic and treatment approaches. Curr Opin Infect Dis. 2003;16:421–7.

69. Moschella SL. An update on the diagnosis and treatment of leprosy. J Am Acad Dermatol. 2004;51:417–26.

70. Peterman TA, Kahn RH, Ciesielski CA, et al. Misclassification of the stages of syphilis: implications for surveillance. Sex Transm Dis. 2005;32:144.

71. Patton ME, Su JR, Nelson R, et al. Primary and secondary syphilis – United States, 2005–2013. MMWR Morb Mortal Wkly Rep. 2014;63:402.

72. Calonge N, U.S. Preventive Services Task Force. Screening for syphilis infection: recommendation statement. Ann Fam Med. 2004;2:362.

73. Hook EW, Peeling RW. Syphilis control – a continuing challenge. N Engl J Med. 2004;351:122.

74. Douglas JM Jr. Penicillin treatment of syphilis: clearing away the shadow on the land. JAMA. 2009;301:769.

75. Summers CG. Albinism: classification, clinical characteristics, and recent findings. Optom Vis Sci. 2009;86:659.

76. Hartmann A, Brocker EB, Becker JC. Hypopigmentary skin disorders: current treatment options and future directions. Drugs. 2004;64(1):89.

77. Crino PB, Nathanson KL, Henske EP. The tuberous sclerosis complex. N Engl J Med. 2006;355:1345.

78. Curatolo P, Bombardieri R, Jozwiak S. Tuberous sclerosis. Lancet. 2008;372:657.

79. Schwartz RA, Fernández G, Kotulska K, Józwiak S. Tuberous sclerosis complex: advances in diagnosis, genetics, and management. J Am Acad Dermatol. 2007;57:189.

80. Kwiatkowski DJ, Manning BD. Molecular basis of giant cells in tuberous sclerosis complex. N Engl J Med. 2014;371:778.

81. Bolognia JL, Lazova R, Watsky K. The development of lentigines within segmental achromic nevi. J Am Acad Dermatol. 1998;39:330–3.

82. Hewedy ESS, Hassan AM, Salah EF, Sallam FA, Dawood NM, Al-Bakary RH, Al-Sharnoby HA. Clinical and ultrastructural study of nevus depigmentosus. J Microsc Ultrastruct. 2013;1:22–9.

83. Lee HS, Chun YS, Hann SK. Nevus depigmentosus: clinical features and histopathologic characteristics in 67 patients. J Am Acad Dermatol. 1999;40:21–6.

84. Kim SK, Kang HY, Lee ES, Kim C. Clinical and histopathologic characteristics of nevus depigmentosus. J Am Acad Dermatol. 2006;55:423–8.

85. Sanjeev M, Ahmed AI, Abdullah AE. Nevus depigmentosus treated by melanocyte-keratinocyte transplantation. J Cutan Aesth Surg. 2011;4(1):29.

86. Shim JH, Seo SJ, Song KY, Hong CK. Development of multiple pigmented nevi within segmental nevus depigmentosus. J Korean Med Sci. 2002;17:133–6.

87. Cestari TF, Dantas LP, Boza JC. Acquired hyperpigmentations. An Bras Dermatol. 2014;89(1):11–25.

88. Pathak MA. Phytophotodermatitis. Clin Dermatol. 1986;4(2):102–21.

89. Weber IC, Davis CP, Greeson DM. Phytophotodermatitis: the other "lime" disease. J Emerg Med. 1999;17(2):235–7.

90. Katoulis AC, Stavrianeas NG, Katsarou A, Antoniou C, Georgala S, Rigopoulos D, Koumantaki E, Avgerinou G, Katsambas AD. Evaluation of the role of contact sensitization and photosensitivity in the pathogenesis of poikiloderma of Civatte. Br J Dermatol. 2002;147:493–7.

91. Katoulis AC, Stavrianeas NG, Georgala S, Katsarou-Katsari A, Koumantaki-Mathioudaki E, Antoniou C, Stratigos JD. Familial cases of poikiloderma of Civatte: genetic implications in its pathogenesis? Clin Exp Dermatol. 1999;24:385–7.

92. Nofal A, Salah E. Acquired poikiloderma: proposed classification and diagnostic approach. J Am Acad Dermatol. 2013;69:e29–140.

93. Dummer R, Graf P, Grief C, Burg G. Treatment of vascular lesions using the versapulse variable pulse width frequency doubled neodymium:YAG laser. Dermatology. 1998;197:158–61.

94. Adrian RM. Treatment of leg telangiectasias using a long-pulse frequency-doubled neodymium:YAG laser at 532 nm. Dermatol Surg. 1998;24:19–23.

95. Addison T. On the constitutional and local effects of diseases of the supra-renal capsules. London: Warren and Son; 1855.

96. Nieman LK, Chanco Turner ML. Addison's disease. Clin Dermatol. 2006;24:276–80.

97. Alto WA, Clarcq L. Cutaneous and systemic manifestations of mastocytosis. Am Fam Physician. 1999;59(11):3047–54.

98. Buszman E, Betlej B, Wrześniok D, Radwańska-Wala B. Effect of metal ions on melanin–local anaesthetic drug complexes. Bioinorg Chem Appl. 2003;1(2):113–22.

99. Martins VM, Sousa AR, Portela Nde C, Tigre CA, Gonçalves LM, Castro Filho RJ. Exogenous ochronosis: case report and literature review. An Bras Dermatol. 2012;87(4):633–6.

100. Kayal L, Jayachandran S, Singh K. Idiopathic thrombocytopenic purpura. Contemp Clin Dent. 2014;5(3):410–4.

101. Wolff K, Goldsmith LA, Katz SI, Gilchrest BA, Paller AS, Leffell DJ, editors. Fitzpatrick Tratado de Dermatologia. 7th ed. Rio de Janeiro: Revinter; 2010.

102. Chalmers E, Cooper P, Forman K, Grimley C, Khair K, Minford A, Morgan M, Mumford AD. Purpura fulminans: recognition, diagnosis and management. Arch Dis Child. 2011;96(11):1066–71.

103. Gardner-Medwin JM, Dolezalova P, Cummins C, Southwood TR. Incidence of Henoch-Schönlein purpura, Kawasaki disease, and rare vasculitides in children of different ethnic origins. Lancet. 2002;360:1197–202.

104. Gonzalez-Gay MA, Calvino MC, Vazquez-Lopez ME, Garcia-Porrua C, Fernandez-Iglesias JL, Dierssen T, et al. Implications of upper respiratory tract infections and drugs in the clinical spectrum of Henoch-Schönlein purpura in children. Clin Exp Rheumatol. 2004;22:781–4.

105. Saulsbury FT. Henoch-Schönlein purpura. Curr Opin Rheumatol. 2001;13:35–40.

106. Magro CM, Schaefer JT, Crowson AN, Li J, Morrison C. Pigmented purpuric dermatosis: classification by phenotypic and molecular profiles. Am J Clin Pathol. 2007;128:218–29.

107. Cho JH, Lee JD, Kang H, Cho SH. The clinical manifestations and etiologic factors of patients with pigmented purpuric dermatoses. Korean J Dermatol. 2005;43:45–52.

108. Dai HK, Soo HS, Hyo HA, Young CK, Jae EC. Characteristics and clinical manifestations of pigmented purpuric dermatosis. Ann Dermatol. 2015;27(4):404–10.

109. Steven BP, Peter MM. Raynaud phenomenon. JHS. 2013;38(A):375–8.

110. Ratchford EV, Evans NS. Raynaud's phenomenon. Vasc Med. 2015;20(3):269–71.

111. Criado PR, Faillace C, Magalhães LS, Brito K, Carvalho JF. Livedo reticular: classificação, causas e diagnósticos diferenciais. Acta Reumatol Port. 2012;37:218–25.

112. Gibbs MB, English JC 3rd, Zirwas MJ. Livedo reticularis: an update. J Am Acad Dermatol. 2005;52(6):1009–19.

Rash

59

Isadora da Rosa Hoeffel, Marina Resener de Moraes, and Barbara Lovato

Key Points

- Rashes are the main dermatologic presentation responsible for patients visiting a doctor
- The rash is a sudden skin eruption that usually results from multiple etiologic factors, and exanthem is defined as any eruptive skin rash associated with fever or other constitutional symptoms
- During childhood, infections are the most important cause of rash, and adverse reactions to drugs are the most important cause in adults
- For correct diagnostic elucidation, a complete anamnesis and physical examination are required, as well as identification of the related symptoms and characterization of the rash

I. da Rosa Hoeffel (✉) • B. Lovato
Dermatology Service of UFCSPA,
Porto Alegre, Brazil
e-mail: isadorahoeffel@yahoo.com.br

M.R. de Moraes
Irmandade Santa Casa de Misericórdia de Porto
Alegre, Porto Alegre, Brazil

Concept

If a rash is a sudden skin eruption often resulting from an overlying disease, an exanthem is defined as any eruptive skin rash associated with fever or other constitutional symptoms. Usually rashes represent a diagnostic challenge for general practitioners, emergency physicians, and even dermatologists, since different diseases can clinically yield very similar rashes, while the same disease can be differently displayed on the skin [1]. In addition, many of these diseases require prompt and accurate diagnosis for immediate therapeutic management.

The accurate diagnosis of a rash requires detailed anamnesis and physical examination [2, 3]. Data such as patient age, occupation, recent travel, contact with sick people, medication use (ongoing or occasional), immunization status, immunosuppressive condition (drugs, splenectomy, solid-organ transplantation, human immunodeficiency virus [HIV] infection) must be determined. Furthermore, the onset of presentation has to be verified and the presence of associated signs and symptoms, such as fever, cough, rhinorrhea, conjunctivitis, myalgia, arthralgia, headache, gastrointestinal changes, and lymphadenomegaly, has to be questioned. The patient's general condition is another crucial aspect to be determined since some conditions are potentially fatal, for example, meningococcemia, which

© Springer International Publishing Switzerland 2018
R.R. Bonamigo, S.I.T. Dornelles (eds.), *Dermatology in Public Health Environments*,
https://doi.org/10.1007/978-3-319-33919-1_59

evolves rapidly with worsening of the general condition, demanding prompt therapeutic intervention.

Characterization of rash is key to the correct clinical diagnosis. Rashes can be either monomorphic or polymorphic, and many exanthems display exclusive presentation forms. Lesion location can be a major diagnostic clue (e.g., palmar-plantar lesions frequently occur in secondary syphilis). Presence of pruritus is also a key factor in the diagnosis and rules out a great number of diseases. Rash presentation (e.g., papular, vesicular, purpuric rash) is decisive in determining the cause of the rash; therefore, how the basic skin lesions are classified is essential, as are the characterization of the rash according to these definitions and its inclusion into differential diagnosis groups, thus limiting most causes of the exanthem. By describing the patient and the features of the exanthem one can define more or less probable differential diagnoses for each case.

Drug adverse reactions are the main cause of rash and exanthem in the adult population. Infections, usually viral, account for the greater number of these occurrences in the pediatric population [1]. In this chapter the causes of exanthem are divided into adult and pediatric causes to make research and diagnostic clarification easier. However, it is noteworthy that this division is for didactic reasons only, as many diseases, despite their characteristics and frequency in one age range, are not unique for that population, being possible at any stage of life.

Current Condition of the Disease

Rashes are the most common dermatologic sign that lead patients to seek medical attention, regardless of their cause. They are often a major diagnostic challenge because many diseases yield clinically similar exanthems and varied skin manifestations [4]. Despite being less frequent and sometimes rare nowadays, traditional exanthematous diseases, such as measles and rubella, are still prevalent in some countries. Even with the eradication of some of these diseases, new infectious agents are detected and involved in exanthemous presentations each year. Moreover, many diseases with benign behavior, such as infections by some enteroviruses, have been responsible for outbreaks that lead to serious and sometimes fatal forms of exanthematous disease.

Owing to the advance of microorganism detection and isolation technologies, many diseases have had their etiology verified, although many of these diagnostic tests are very expensive and available for research use only. Nevertheless, an etiologic diagnosis should be attempted whenever possible.

Clinical Presentation

Rash is defined as a skin eruption resulting from an underlying disease [1, 2]. Such eruptions can be either localized or diffuse, and display varied clinical forms. Knowledge of the primary skin lesions (Table 59.1) is essential in rash characterization, since one can include each case in a specific group of exanthems, and limit the number of differential diagnoses (e.g., a patient who only displays vesicles is diagnosed with vesicle exanthem and is included in the group of diseases resulting in this kind of eruption).

Table 59.1 Primary skin lesions and their definitions

Macula	Flat nonpalpable lesions, less than 1 cm wide, showing inconspicuous texture and/or color change
Patch	Flat nonpalpable lesions, more than 1 cm wide, showing discrete texture and/or color change
Papule	Circumscribed palpable lesion, above skin surface, less than 1 cm wide
Plaque	Palpable and raised lesion, above skin surface, more than 1 cm wide
Nodule	Palpable raised and indurated lesion usually deeper than the papule
Vesicle	Raised lesion, less than 1 cm wide, with internal light liquid content
Blister	Raised lesion, more than 1 cm wide, with internal liquid content
Pustule	Raised surface lesion with internal yellow content (pus)

Rash: Children

> **Box 59.1 Etiology of Rash in Children**
> In childhood, the most important causes are hand-foot-mouth disease, erythema infectiosum, exanthema subitum, scarlet fever, varicella, measles, rubella, Kawasaki disease, staphylococcal scalded skin syndrome, Gianotti–Crosti syndrome, miliaria, and meningococcemia.

Hand-Foot-Mouth Disease

Hand-foot-mouth disease (HFMD) is a highly contagious disease worldwide that usually affects children. It is caused by enteroviruses, mainly the A6, A10, A16 Coxsackie viruses, and the 71 enterovirus. It is transmitted by interhuman contact, the fecal–oral route, or respiratory droplets [5]. Despite an often benign and self-limited evolution, many fatal cases have been recently reported, mostly in Asia [5–7].

Following a 3- to 10-day incubation period, patients start having fever and odynophagia, rapidly followed by the classic presentation of erosive stomatitis mainly in the palate and oropharynx, and a papular-vesicular exanthem in the palmar-plantar region (Fig. 59.1) [6]. The gluteal region and the perineum are also commonly affected, and atypical HFMD cases with papular-vesicular and purpura presentations reaching the scalp, face, arms, and torso have been recently reported and associated with A6 Coxsackie virus infection [7]. The associated symptoms are generally mild, including low to moderate fever, headache, arthralgia, and myalgia. However, during a major outbreak in Singapore in 2000, many patients displayed evidence of pneumonia, meningitis, and myocarditis, some with a fatal outcome [5, 8].

Erythema Infectiosum

Erythema infectiosum, also known as the Fifth Disease, is a very common exanthemous disease in childhood caused by the parvovirus B19 (PB19) and transmitted by contact with respiratory secretions and blood transfusion [9, 10]. After the PB19 infection an inconspicuous

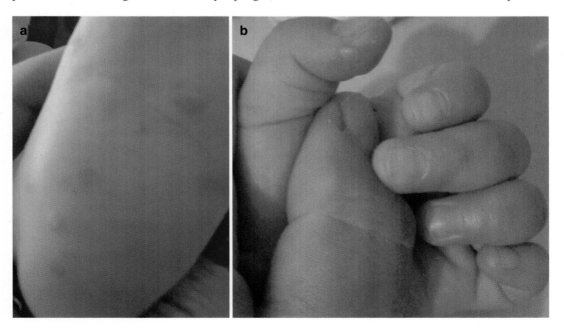

Fig. 59.1 (**a**) Hand-foot-mouth disease. A papular-vesicular rash in the palmar-plantar region. (**b**) Note the vesicle involving the first toe (Courtesy of Ana Elisa Kiszewski Bau, M.D., PhD, Porto Alegre, Brazil)

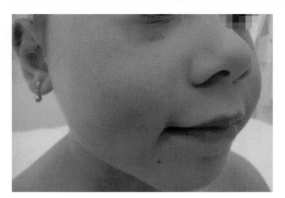

Fig. 59.2 Erythema infectiosum. "Slapped cheek". The characteristic erythematous rash that affects the malar region of children infected with PB19

prodromal period occurs, characterized by fever and unspecific flu symptoms, followed by skin manifestations. During childhood, the most common clinical presentation includes a macular or macular-papular erythematous rash mostly seen on the face, torso, and limbs. On the face, the noticeable malar rash (Fig. 59.2) is traditionally known as "slapped cheek," and an enanthem in the palatal region can be also noticed. The rash usually becomes more evident when the patient is exposed to the sun during physical activities or heavy heat.

In the adult population, the infection is frequently asymptomatic or with often unnoticed mild symptoms. In symptomatic infections articular involvement is the main clinical presentation, occurring in up to 50% of the involved adult patients. It presents as a form of arthralgia or symmetric arthritis in the patient's hands, and occasionally in the ankles, knees, and wrists [11]. It can mimic clinical presentations of rheumatoid arthritis, and it can even present a positive rheumatoid factor. Cutaneous manifestations in this population show significant variation, which make this a more heterogeneous group regarding signs. The most common presentation is a papular-purpuric eruption on the patient's feet and hands, also known as papular-purpuric gloves and socks

syndrome [12]. Palpable purpuric cases can also be seen, and are similar to the systemic dermatomyositis/lupus erythematosus, acral petechiae, and vesicular pustular rash [13].

A significant manifestation of the parvovirus B19 infection is the transient aplastic crisis. This is a condition whereby a direct invasion of the virus into the bone marrow occurs, and since the PB19 displays tropism by the erythroid progenitor cells there may be destruction of these cells with resulting disruption of red cell production for about 5–10 days. There is no clinical repercussion in healthy patients who show a normal life cycle of red blood cells. In patients with chronic hemolytic anemias, however, such as sickle cell disease and thalassemia, a sudden fall of hemoglobin levels and an acute anemia can occur, thus characterizing the transient aplastic crisis. This acute condition can lead to presentations of congestive heart failure, cerebrovascular accident, and death. Platelet and white blood cell levels can also eventually decrease [14, 15].

Another population at risk for PB19 infection is immunosuppressed patients, such as solid-organ transplant recipients and HIV-infected patients. In these groups the infection period is longer and goes beyond the maximum life cycle of the red blood cells, resulting in acute and chronic anemia [14, 15].

Exanthema Subitum

Largely resulting from infection with the human herpesvirus type 6 (HHV-6) and type 7 (HHV-7), exanthema subitum (also called roseola infantum) is very common during childhood and is characterized by high fever and later onset of cutaneous eruption. It predominantly occurs between 6 months and 2 years of age, with up to 90% of the population being infected over the first 2 years of life; it is transmitted via respiratory secretions [16, 17].

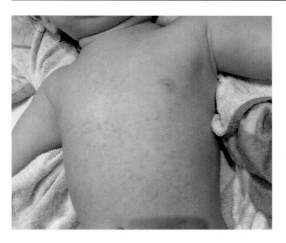

Fig. 59.3 Exanthema subitum. A macular-papular ery-thematous exanthem on the torso, abdomen, neck, and limbs in a 9-month-old infant (Courtesy of Fabiane Kumagai Lorenzini, M.D., Porto Alegre, Brazil)

The clinical presentation is characterized by high fever (39–40 °C) lasting from 3 to 5 days, often in children being nursed and in good health. This is followed by macular-papular erythematous cutaneous eruption on the torso, neck, and proximal parts of the limbs (Fig. 59.3), when the fever typically subsides. Enanthem of the soft palate and uvula, symptoms of upper respiratory tract infection, otitis media, cervical and occipital lymphadenopathy, and fontanelle vault can be noticed. This latter symptom results from central nervous system involvement, which can result in encephalitis and aseptic meningitis. The most frequent complication of the exanthema subitum includes febrile seizures, present in about 10% of cases [18]. The condition often resolves spontaneously in a few days with no sequelae. A virus reactivation can be seen with immunosuppression [19], and usually occurs with unspecific clinical symptoms such as fever, malaise, and cutaneous rash; however, acute situations, such as hepatitis, encephalitis, interstitial pneumonia, and bone marrow failure, can occur.

Scarlet Fever

Scarlet fever, or scarlatina, is an acute infectious disease caused by the Group A β-hemolytic streptococci (*Streptococcus pyogenes*), a pyrogen-producing bacterium transmitted through saliva and nasopharyngeal secretions and, rarely, through contaminated water and food [20]. It usually infects individuals between 5 and 18 years old, being rare in those younger than 3 years old. The disease incubation period lasts from 2 to 5 days, and transmission begins with the early symptoms [21]. Many people can be asymptomatic carriers, and the individual who develops scarlatina is required to lack both *Streptococcus* immunity (specific-type immunity) and pyrogenic exotoxin immunity [22, 23].

The disease usually starts with a sore throat, associated with high fever, asthenia, anorexia and generalized malaise. Some patients also have vomiting, abdominal pain and convulsions. Around 12–48 h after symptoms onset, patients develop a micro papular exanthem on their torso, cervical region and axillae that disappear under digital pressure. The rough and erythematous skin resembles sandpaper, and petechiae develop in the flexural fold areas, known as Pastia's lines. Facial frontal and malar hyperemia occur in contrast with paleness in the perioral region (Filatov's sign) (Fig. 59.4).

Concomitant with the cutaneous eruption, patients develop pharyngoamygdalitis with purulent exudate, cervical lymphadenopathy, and oral mucosa enanthem. The tongue is initially white, with hypertrophied papillae, after which the white layer detaches, making an erythematous and bright tongue evident, known as "raspberry tongue." Between 7 and 10 days of infection onset, diffuse skin scaling occurs, more intense over the palmar and plantar regions, lasting from 2 to 6 weeks.

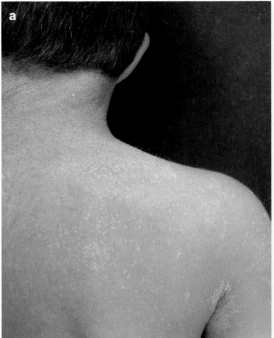
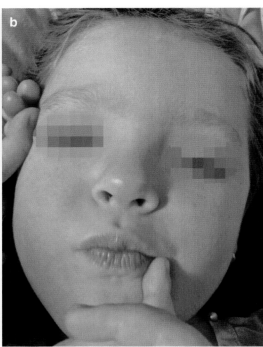

Fig. 59.4 (**a**) Scarlet fever. A micropapular exanthem on the torso, cervical region, and axillae. The rough skin resembles sandpaper. (**b**) Filatov sign, the characteristic paleness of perioral region that occurs in contrast to facial hyperemia (Courtesy of Raquel Bonfa, M.D., Porto Alegre, Brazil)

Varicella

Popularly known as chickenpox, varicella is a primary acute and extremely contagious disease characterized by generalized vesicular exanthem on the skin and mucosa. It usually shows a benign, self-limited course, mainly during childhood; however, during adulthood it can have a worse and unfavorable evolution. It results from the primary infection of the varicella zoster virus (VZV), of the Herpesviridae family, transmitted via contact with airborne particles from the upper respiratory tract or contact with lesions of infected patients [24].

The disease incubation period ranges from 10 to 21 days, and the prodromic symptoms generally can be seen from 1 to 2 days before cutaneous eruption. During childhood these symptoms may often go unnoticed; when they occur, their characteristics include low fever, nausea, anorexia, and headache [25]. The rash usually begins on the head, reaching the patient's scalp and face, rapidly spreading through the torso and limbs in a centripetal distribution. Besides pruritus, a very noticeable characteristic is lesion polymorphism; i.e., surface maculae, papules, vesicles, and damaged lesions and crusts are seen practically at the same time (Fig. 59.5) [26]. Airways and mucosa can also be affected. Increases in transaminase levels and thrombocytopenia can also often occur [24]. In general, up to 20 days from symptom onset residual crusts fall off, and the occurrence of secondary infection or early crust removal can yield typical depressing scars.

Although a benign and self-limited evolution occurs during childhood, the disease can have a more acute and symptomatic course during adult life, even in the immunocompetent patient, with high fever, marked exanthem, and possible death, likely resulting from pneumonia. This is the most acute and frequent

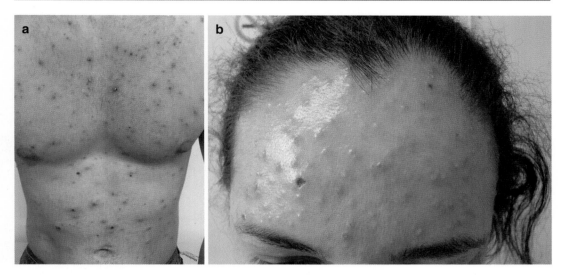

Fig. 59.5 (**a**) Varicella. Lesion polymorphism: maculae, papules, vesicles, and crusts are seen at the same time. (**b**) Vesicles usually begin on the face and scalp

complication, especially in pregnant women, elderly individuals, and immunocompromised patients [24]. Secondary bacterial infection can occur in cutaneous lesions, from simple cases of impetigo to more serious complications, such as cellulitis and erysipelas. Hematologic complications are rare and include leukopenia, fulminant thrombocytopenic purpura, and hemophagocytic syndrome. Involvement of the central nervous system is uncommon, although cerebellar ataxia, meningitis, meningoencephalitis, and cerebral vasculopathy can be seen [24].

Measles

Measles is a highly contagious disease resulting from infection with the measles virus, an RNA virus transmitted through respiratory droplets [27]. Despite the fact that 85% of the children receive at least one dose of the vaccine against measles around the globe annually, the World Health Organization (WHO) estimates that in 2013 there were more than 145,000 deaths from this disease, mostly on the African continent [28]. In many developed countries the disease is still present, and recent outbreaks both in Europe and the United States, where hundreds of cases were reported in 2015, still show the significance of this disease and its potential morbidity and mortality [29, 30].

Following an early incubation period which lasts from 10 to 14 days, the patient shows prodromic symptoms such as fever, nasal discharge, conjunctivitis, and cough. About 2–4 days from this stage the exanthematous presentation begins, consisting of erythematous maculae and papules, beginning on the forehead (especially along the hair line and behind their ears), progressing in the cephalocaudal direction. The exanthematous presentation recedes in about 3–5 days, disappearing first from the head [31]. Besides the rash, pathognomonic Koplik spots can be noticed: small white lesions in the oral mucosa that can be seen even before the rash.

In noncomplicated cases, the general health condition improves with the emerging rashes. However, up to 40% of patients can develop clinical complications, and presentations tend to be more acute in the very elderly and immunocompromised patients, such as pregnant women and malnourished individuals. The respiratory tract is the most frequently affected location. Pneumonia, otitis media, and tracheobronchitis are the most frequent complications. Besides pneumonia, encephalitis is also potentially fatal, occurring in about 0.2% of the patients, mainly older children and adults, with a 10% mortality rate. This condition is usually seen 2 weeks after rash onset, presenting with fever, seizures, and variable neurologic changes. Abdominal pain, diarrhea, and elevated liver function tests often occur, despite frank hepatitis being unusual [32]. Contrary to rubella, there are no reports of congenital malformation cases associated with measles, although the typical immunosuppression of pregnancy can more often lead to maternal complications [31].

Rubella

Rubella, also called the Third Disease or German measles, is an exanthematous disease with a viral etiology, transmitted through respiratory droplets, with an often mild self-limited evolution both in children and adults. In 2015 the disease was considered eradicated on the American continent thanks to an extensive immunization program, and since 2009 only imported cases have been reported. However, it still remains a significant cause of congenital malformation, with approximately 100,000 congenital rubella cases around the world each year [33, 34].

Following around 14–21 incubation days, a mild prodromic phase begins, consisting of conjunctivitis, headache, fever, and upper respiratory symptoms. Over 1–5 days a maculopapular exanthem appears firstly on the face, progressing in a cephalocaudal direction. Concomitant with the rash, painful lymphadenopathy on the occipital, retroauricular and cervical regions is seen, often persisting for many days. After 3 days, in general, the skin eruption tends to disappear following the initial presentation order [33].

Complications in adults and children include arthralgia, arthritis, hepatitis, myocarditis, pericarditis, hemolytic anemia, and thrombocytopenic purpura [31]. The major danger presented by rubella is infection in a nonimmune pregnant woman over the first trimester, when there is a risk for the virus to be transmitted to the fetus and the consequent development of congenital rubella syndrome.

Kawasaki Disease

Kawasaki disease (KD) is an acute systemic vasculitis mainly affecting children younger than 5 years. Despite many studies, the etiology remains unknown [35], although the infectious etiology theory is the most accepted nowadays. No agent has yet been isolated, but the disease shows seasonal variation, is seldom seen in children being nursed under 6 months, and has infrequent recurrences. The main concern regarding the disease is that it represents the main cause for acquired heart disease in developed countries, and it is estimated that aneurysms or ectasia of the coronary arteries develop in up to 25% of nontreated patients [36].

The clinical manifestations of KD are also used as the diagnostic criteria [37, 38]. They include at least five of the six conditions described in Table 59.2.

The exanthem is usually polymorphic and seen up to the fifth day of the disease. It has no pruritus, and shows variation from maculopapular erythematous-like and diffuse lesions, the most usual form, to the hives-like form, scarlatina-like form, erythrodermic-like form, purpuric-like form, erythema multiform-like form, and, rarely micropustules on the limb extensor surfaces [36]. It is often seen on the trunk and limbs, with

Table 59.2 Diagnostic criteria for the Kawasaki disease. At least 5 out of the 6 mentioned findings are necessary to make the diagnosis

1. Fever lasting more than 5 days
2. Bilateral conjunctive and nonpurulent inflammation
3. Limb changes, such as erythema and/or edema on the hands and/or the feet during the acute phase, as well as scaling of the digital pulp during the recovery phase
4. Cervical lymphadenopathy
5. Lips and oral cavity changes such as edema, erythema and lip cracks, raspberry tongue, and oropharyngeal hyperemia
6. Polymorphous exanthem

noticeable preference for the groin and perineal regions.

Organs other than the skin can also be attacked by vasculitis. During the acute phase, besides the diagnostic criteria, arthritis and arthralgia (30%), uveitis (17%), diarrhea (15%), hepatic dysfunction (10–25%), aseptic meningitis (10–25%), and later on neurosensory deafness can occur. However, heart impairment is the major concern regarding cases of KD. Its most usual form involves the coronary arteries, affecting 15–25% of the nontreated patients, and includes aneurysms, ectasia, and stenoses of the coronary arteries, which can lead to acute myocardial infarction. Moreover, myocarditis, pericarditis, endocarditis, and heart valve and coronary damage, with hemodynamic repercussion and a 2% mortality rate can occur [36].

Staphylococcal Scalded Skin Syndrome

The staphylococcal scalded skin syndrome (SSSS) is an infectious and exfoliative disease that affects mainly newborns and children younger than 6 years, and eventually adults (especially immunodepressive or chronic renal failure patients) [39]. The disease is part of an infection range mediated by toxins produced by the *Staphylococcus aureus* bacterium. Most cases of SSSS are caused by exfoliative toxin types A and B, which affect the epidermis granular layer, specifically in the desmoglein glycoproteins 1, and cause their disruption, with the resulting sterile skin blistering and exfoliation. Despite a good prognosis in childhood, with a mortality rate of about 3–4%, this rate increases in adulthood to more than 60% [40].

The disease often presents a prodromal phase characterized by fever, irritability, odynophagia, hypersensitivity, and skin discomfort [41]. A light macular rash begins and quickly progresses to an orange-erythematous color to become confluent, swollen, and scaly. Periorificial, flexural, and friction skin areas wrinkle with blistering and scaling. The Nikolsky sign, a slight friction on the perilesional skin and consequent detachment of the most superficial skin layer, is positive. Another distinctive characteristic is the presence of radial fissures, periorificial crusts, and varying facial edema (Fig. 59.6). One or 2 days after their appearance, the blisters and the perilesional skin detach, and areas of thin

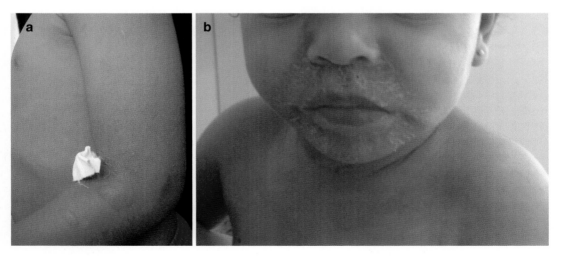

Fig. 59.6 (**a**) SSSS. Flexural skin areas with blistering and scaling. (**b**) Characteristic radial fissures, periorificial crusts, and facial edema

and moist skin of varying sizes remain. Often the primary focus of the *S. aureus* infection is not identified, although some patients can present rhinorrhea, conjunctivitis, or other skin pyogenic foci.

Gianotti-Crosti Syndrome

The Gianotti-Crosti syndrome (GCS), also known as infantile papular acrodermatitis, is a rare disorder, characterized by a papular exanthem affecting mainly the face and limbs of children from 6 months to 14 years old. It is seen as a cutaneous reaction self-limited to many infections, mainly the viral ones, and to some vaccines [42]. The main virus already related to GCS are the Epstein–Barr virus the HHV-6, parvovírus B19, cytomegalovirus, A and B hepatitis viruses, syncytial respiratory virus, and rubella virus.

Commonly the GCS is preceded by mild constitutive symptoms, such as fever, lymphadenopathy, and upper respiratory symptoms, followed by a sudden eruption of erythematous or brownish, sometimes lichenoid, asymptomatic, monomorphic papules, symmetrically distributed throughout the face, the gluteal region, and the limbs (Fig. 59.7), with some patients showing lesions reaching the torso, or limited to the face [43, 44]. A high erythrocyte sedimentation rate, as well as lymphocytosis with atypical lymphocytes in the hemogram, is apparent in some patients. Lesions spontaneously disappear in 2–8 weeks, and cases persisting for up to 6 months are uncommon.

Miliaria

Miliaria is a disorder that affects the eccrine sweat glands, generally occurring as a result of high moisture and heat. On such occasions the

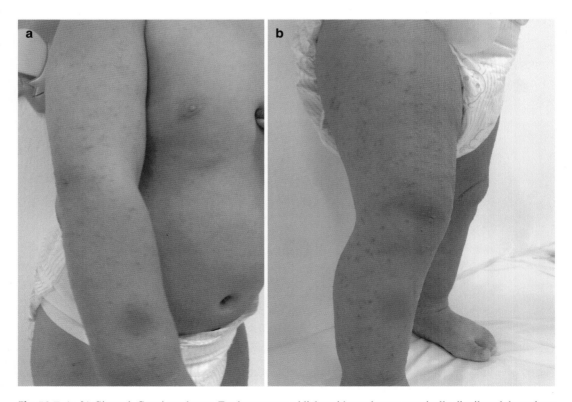

Fig. 59.7 (**a**, **b**) Gianotti–Crosti syndrome. Erythematous and lichenoid papules symmetrically distributed throughout the limbs

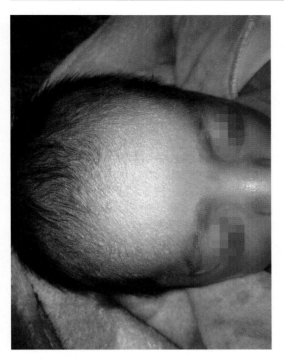

Fig. 59.8 Crystalline miliaria in a newborn. Numerous micropapules and microvesicles

eccrine ducts become obstructed at different skin depths. It can be often found in young children, mainly newborns, whose ducts are not totally formed, but can be also found in adults who live or work under hot and moist conditions. Often the condition develops after episodes of fever, and some drugs have also been associated with miliaria development [45].

There are three basic types of miliaria. In crystalline miliaria, the ducts are obstructed at the corneal stratum level, and tiny vesicles of transparent content can be seen mainly on children's and adults' face and upper torso (Fig. 59.8); they are easily disrupted. Miliaria rubra is characterized by duct obstruction at the level of the mid epidermis layer, and is the most common subtype. It manifests as small papules and erythematous plaques, covered by punctiform vesicles mainly found on the cervical region and the torso. It can cause pruritus and itching, sometimes with sterile pustules [46]. When the miliaria rubra is relapsing or chronic it can result in the third type of miliaria, known as miliaria profunda. In this case a duct obstruction occurs at the

dermoepidermal junction, and although asymptomatic the patient is at significant risk for thermoregulation problems [47].

Meningococcemia

Caused by the *Neisseria meningitides* bacterium, meningococcemia is an acute and potentially fatal disorder that mainly affects small children (6 months to 1 year old), and young adults worldwide. The infection is most frequently seen in the winter and the beginning of spring, occurring more in males than females. It is already known that patients with congenital or acquired immunodeficiencies, as well as asplenic patients, carry a greater risk for the development of meningococcemia [49, 50].

About 1–14 days after contamination and development of the bacterium in the nasopharynx, the prodromal symptoms of fever, anorexia, nausea, vomiting, torpor, headache, arthralgias, myalgias, and limb changes (cold and violet-like) begin. Nuchal rigidity is typically absent, contrary to cases of meningococcal meningitis. A usual occurrence and one which may immediately raise meningococcemia suspicion is the quick evolution of sepsis, characterized by high fever, tachycardia, tachypnea, and eventual hemodynamic instability.

However, the key manifestation is cutaneous: up to half of the patients display a petechial and purpuric eruption; fewer patients can also develop an inconspicuous and transient morbilliform rash on the torso [51]. The major concern regarding meningococcemia is its progression to disseminated intravascular coagulation, known as purpura fulminans. The petechiae, in these cases, progress to hemorrhagic blisters, ecchymoses, ischemic necrosis of the limbs, and adrenal gland hemorrhage and hypotension. The prognosis of such patients' is reserved, and death can occur within 24 h even when patients undergo amputation of the affected limb.

Table 59.3 lists the main differential diagnoses of rashes in childhood and their key characteristics.

Table 59.3 Main differential diagnoses of rashes in childhood and their key characteristics

Disease	Incubation	Exanthem/related symptoms	Key characteristics/diagnosis
Hand-foot-mouth disease	3–10 days	Low fever and odynophagia followed by erosive stomatitis and papular-vesicular exanthem on palms and soles	Good general condition Gluteal and perineal regions also frequently attacked Clinical diagnosis
Erythema infectiosum (fifth disease)	5–4 days	Discrete prodromal period followed by macular or macular-papular, erythematous exanthem that is seen mainly face, torso and limbs, worst in exposed-to-light areas	Exuberant bilateral malar rash, known as "slapped fascia" In the adult population, the most often seen presentation is a papular-purpuric eruption on their feet and their hands, known as "papular-purpuric gloves and socks syndrome," related to arthralgias IgM + parvovirus B19
Exanthema subitum (roseola infantum or sixth disease)	10–15 days	High fever lasting from 3 to 5 days in <3 years, with no other symptoms Abrupt fever recession when macular-papular erythematous exanthems appear on the torso, neck, and upper and lower limbs' proximal parts	High fever (>39 °C) in babies being nursed, in good general health condition Fever recession concomitant of the rash emergence IgM + HHV-6, or HHV-7
Scarlet fever (scarlatina)	2–5 days	High fever + odynophagia + general malaise Micropapular erythematous diffuse exanthem, with rough and scaly skin, resembling "sandpaper"	Pastia sign: linear petechiae in flexural areas Filatov sign: perioral paleness "raspberry tongue" Oropharynx culture or serum antibody detection (e.g., ASLO)
Varicella	10–21 days	Rash usually starts on the face and scalp, rapidly progressing onto the torso and limbs Presence of vesicle on erythematous papule	A remarkable rash feature is the lesion polymorphism: excoriated macular, papular, vesicular surface lesions; excoriated pustules, crusts, and lesions seen virtually at the same time PCR / IgM + varicella zoster
Measles	10–14 days	Prodromes of fever, coryza, conjunctivitis, and cough Erythematous maculae and papules start on the face, mainly at the hair line and retroauricular region, progressing to a cephalocaudal direction. They remain for 5 days at least. Light scaling can occur	Koplik spots: small white lesions on the mucosa (can be seen even before the rash) IgM + measles/increase at least 4× of the IgG titter
Rubella	14–21 days	Mild prodromes of conjunctivitis, headache, fever, and respiratory symptoms Macular-papular erythematous exanthem starting on the face, in cephalocaudal progression	Painful lymphadenopathy in the occipital, retroauricular, and cervical regions PCR oropharyngeal secretions, urine, blood, or liquor Specific IgM + /increase of at least 4× of the IgG titter
Kawasaki disease	Not known	Fever for at least 5 days 1. Polymorphous exanthem 2. Bilateral conjunctival nonpurulent inflammation 3. Limb alterations 4. Cervical lymphadenopathy 5. Lips and oral cavity changes	Very frequent heart impairment ECG + echocardiogram Clinical diagnosis: fever + 4 of the 5 previously described findings

Table 59.3 (continued)

Disease	Incubation	Exanthem/related symptoms	Key characteristics/diagnosis
SSSS	48 hours average	Fever, bad mood, odynophagia, discomfort, and skin hypersensitivity Erythematous-edematous scaly rash	Skin hypersensitivity Radial fissures and periorificial crusts Noticeable impairment of the flexural areas Nikolski sign +
Meningococcemia	1–14 days	Fever, lack of appetite, vomiting, torpor, headache, cold extremities There can be morbiliform discrete transient rash on the torso, followed then by the typical petechial and purpuric eruption	Sudden onset and quick progression into sepsis PCR/bacteriologic/blood, cutaneous lesions, and liquor bacterioscopy to identify the *N. meningitides*
Gianotti-Crosti syndrome	Variable	Sudden eruption of erythematous or mousy, monomorphic, and asymptomatic papules	Noticeable symmetrical extremities impairment: face, gluteal region, and limbs There is no specific test
Miliaria	Not known	Miliaria rubra is the most frequent and clinically important Small papules and erythematous plaques, covered by a punctiform vesicle involving predominantly the cervical region and the torso	Related pruritus and/or itching History of excessive sudoresis or heat and moisture exposure

Rash: Adults

Box 59.2 Etiology of Rash in Adults
The main causes of rash during adulthood discussed in this chapter are drug eruptions, contact dermatitis, syphilis, and the emerging dermatologic viral diseases.

Drug Eruptions

Adverse drug reactions usually occur on the skin and are the main cause of diffuse rash in the adult population [1]. These reactions are often unexpected and occur in 2–3% of the general population, increasing to 10–20% in nosocomial environments [52, 53]. Most of them have a benign course, although they can also lead to significant morbidity and even death in the most acute cases, with rates varying from 0.2% to 29.3% depending on the study [54].

The most usual mechanism of action is tardive hypersensitivity. The administered drug is processed and promoted to the Langerhans cells, acting as haptens and inducing the cellular and humoral response. The drug-triggered process can be either unexpected or a genetic or acquired predisposition

Table 59.4 More commonly involved drugs in pharmacodermias

Class	Commonly involved drugs
Antibiotics	Penicillins Sulfamethoxazole Cephalosporins Quinolones Isoniazid
Antipyretics/ anti-inflammatories	Acetylsalicylic acid Sodic dipyrone Acetaminophen Sodic dicoflenac and diclofenac potassium Piroxicam
Anticonvulsants/ antidepressives	Barbiturates Valproates Carbamazepine Phenytoin Lamotrigine
Antihypertensives	Furosemide Thiazíds
Others	Allopurinol Oral contraceptives Propiltiouracil

by the individual, and the most commonly involved drugs are antibiotics, anti-inflammatories, and anticonvulsants [55, 56] (Table 59.4).

Some risk factors were found in research studies, most of them involving an unexpected response in patients older than 60 years, women, and obese individuals. It is more often seen in patients with autoimmune diseases or with an active viral infection who have been given high doses of drug, although the reactions are not necessarily dose-dependent [57, 58].

When facing a rash in an adult patient a possible pharmacodermia must always be considered. Exanthems are the most usual clinical form of polymorphic manifestation as erythematous macules that can be associated with small papules. At first, the lesions are seen on the torso and upper limbs and can then become confluent, with an unaffected mucosa in most cases. Pruritus and low fever are usual [59].

The rash usually occurs between the first and the second week after drug administration, or even some days after drug interruption; therefore, it is important to list all the drugs used and, if possible, in chronological order. Patients using many drugs make the identification of the causative drug difficult, and often the patients cannot recall the drugs they use or do not mention drugs they sometimes take (not on a daily basis) such as analgesic and anti-inflammatory drugs.

Some clinical aspects signal more acute reactions, such as facial edema, peripheral hypereosinophilia, mucosal lesions, and painful or grayish lesions [60]. These presentations can lead to considerable morbidity and mortality requiring hospital admission. Drug reaction with eosinophilia and systemic symptoms (DRESS) syndrome, acute generalized exanthematous pustulosis (AGEP), Stevens–Johnson syndrome (SJS), and toxic epidermal necrolysis (TEN) are among the most acute presentations (Figs. 59.9 and 59.10).

DRESS syndrome is often triggered after the first use of the drug. Erythematous macules with superficial pustules upon them are apparent, as well as facial edema in certain cases. Many organs are also affected, simultaneously or after the skin manifestations, frequently represented by significant peripheral eosinophilia and higher hepatic enzyme levels. Patients usually show fever and lymphadenopathy during physical examination. When the drug is discontinued the symptoms can still be seen for some weeks. Only seven classes of drugs can trigger this syndrome: anticonvulsants, sulfonamides, allopurinol, nevirapine, abacavir, dapsone, and minocycline [61, 62].

The SJS and TEN are extremely acute forms of drug reaction with a high mortality rate. From 1% to 10% of the skin in SJS and more than 30% in TEN are affected by detachment of the skin. The rash can begin as macules that develop into papules, vesicles, urticarial plaques, confluent erythema, and often bullae. After detachment of the skin, it becomes susceptible to secondary infection. Mucosal lesions are usually displayed, as well as fever and variable systemic changes. The most common causative drugs include allopurinol, anticonvulsants, antiretrovirals, anti-inflammatories, and antibiotics [61, 62].

Acute generalized exanthematous pustulosis (AGEP) usually begins 48 h after drug use. Clinically it shows hundreds of sterile nonfollicular pustules mainly on the torso and intertriginous areas associated with pruritus. When the mucosa is involved it occurs only in one area (the most usual sites include the mouth and the lips). It presents systemic symptoms associated with fever, leukocytosis, and renal, pulmonary, and hepatic dysfunction. Mortality rate is less than 5% [62].

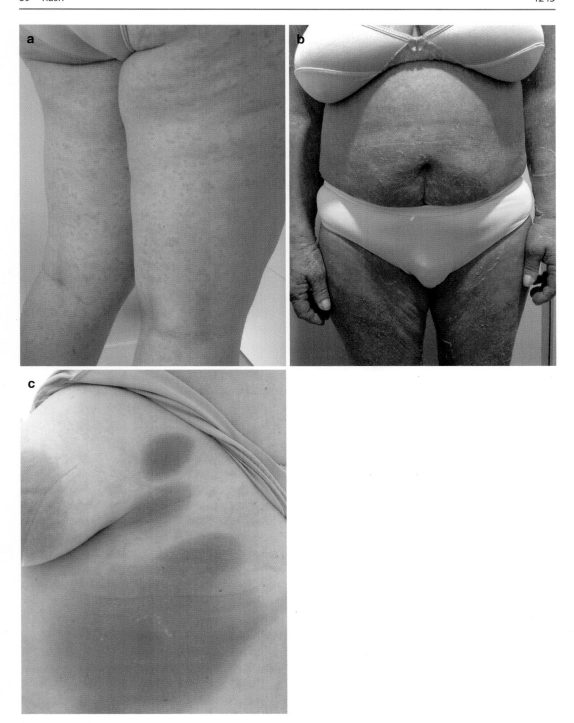

Fig. 59.9 (**a**) Urticarial rash from oral codeine. (**b**) Diffuse erythema and desquamation of skin resulting from ingestion of diclofenac. (**c**) Fixed drug eruption. It is a special type of pharmacodermia, and characteristically recurs in the same site or sites each time a particular drug (in this case ibuprofen) is taken

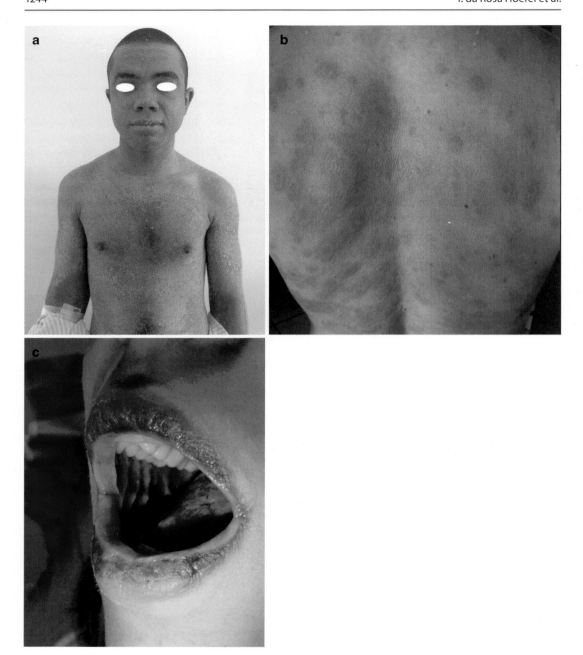

Fig. 59.10 (**a**) DRESS due to phenobarbital. Diffuse involvement of the face, trunk, and upper limbs. (**b**) NET. Target lesions progressing to bullae. (**c**) SJS. Mucosal erosions

Contact Dermatitis

Contact dermatitis is an inflammatory response in skin resulting from contact with external agents. It occurs in about 15–20% of the population, being rare in children. Regarding etiopathogenesis, contact dermatitis is classified as: (1) irritant contact dermatitis; (2) allergic contact dermatitis; (3) phototoxic contact dermatitis, and (4) photoallergic contact dermatitis. In daily clinical practice the most relevant forms include allergic contact dermatitis (ACD) and irritant contact dermatitis (ICD) [64, 65].

ACD is a delayed-type hypersensitivity reaction (Gell–Coombs type IV), resulting from repeated exposure to the allergen after individual sensitization at the first contact. For example, contact dermatitis to chromium and cobalt (found in cement) has been identified in building construction workers. With regard to photoallergic contact dermatitis, the concomitant presence of allergen and radiation is necessary to trigger the immunologic process.

ICD accounts for up to 80% of contact dermatitis cases; it can result from a single or a repeated exposure to aggressive agents, triggered by direct damage caused by the chemical agent, for which the action does not have the participation of immunologic events. A classic example is the individual inadvertently coming into contact with solvents, detergents, and acids used in industry. Similar to ACD, in phototoxic contact dermatitis there is no immunologic response but, in order for

it to occur, the susceptible individual must be exposed to a sufficient amount of agents and light. This latest example can be seen, for example, when a patient has contact with lemon juice or leaf before being exposed to solar radiation. Apart from the type of contact dermatitis, this condition is affected by the triggering chemical substance and the length and the nature of the contact, besides individual predisposition [65, 66].

The clinical manifestation depends on contact type and place, duration of exposure to the allergen, and evolution (Fig. 59.11). The initial phase corresponds to acute eczema, characterized by erythema, edema, papules, vesicles, and even blisters. There is a prevalence of only erythema and edema on specific sites, such as the eyelids and the genital area. In ICD, depending on the contact route, lesions can display necrosis; they

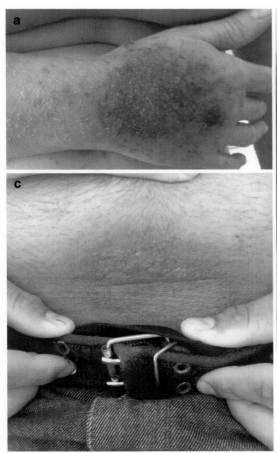

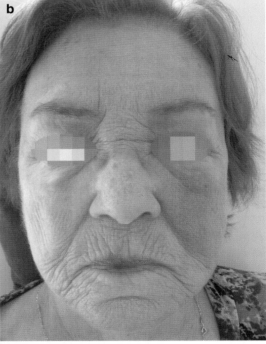

Fig. 59.11 (**a**) Irritant contact dermatitis due to contact with the *Euphorbia milli* plant. (**b**) Acute eczema characterized by edema and erythema due to ketoconazole shampoo. (**c**) Lichenified erythematous plaque characteristic of chronic contact dermatitis to nickel (note the lesion restricted to the belt contact area)

usually occur where the substance exposure occurred, although it can follow a diffuse route in ACD. The irritant form is more common in children and is usually on the legs, hands, and face.

In subacute eruptions, the presence of exudation and crusts is noticed; the chronic form occurs when the contact continues, or the dermatitis remains even without contact. It is characterized by lichenified erythematous plaques, peeling and, eventually, fissures, with pruritus as the main symptom. There is no trend to disseminate, being restricted to the substance contact areas. In ICD it usually occurs in locations experiencing light friction trauma [66, 67].

Pityriasis Rosea

Pityriasis rosea (PR) is an acute inflammatory skin disease of benign and self-limited evolution, characterized by distinctive lesions on oval and desquamative plaques. It usually affects patients

from 10 to 35 years old, with an estimated prevalence of 0.3–1.4% of the general population. Its etiology is still unknown despite many studies suggesting an infections or reactive cause [68].

In its classical presentation, the disease is characterized by the appearance of an initial lesion known as the "herald plaque" or "mother patch," consisting of an oval or round, erythematous–squamous single plaque of centrifugal growth, with a diameter of 2–10 cm. The center of the "mother patch" tends to be lighter, with the outer edge showing a more conspicuous erythema and a thin, scaling peripheral collarette. About 7–14 days after the onset of the "mother patch" the period known as secondary rash or eruptive period begins, when multiple lesions similar to the "mother plaque" appear, smaller but in great quantity, spread over the torso, neck, and limb root (Fig. 59.12). On the torso, the lesions often spread along the skin cleavage lines, giving the typical aspect of a "Christmas tree" pattern. Pruritus is a common symptom of PR, although of low intensity [69]. A few patients

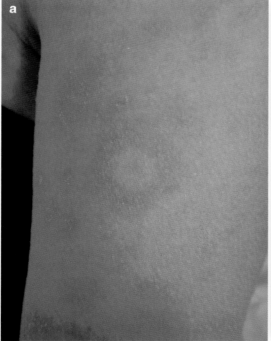
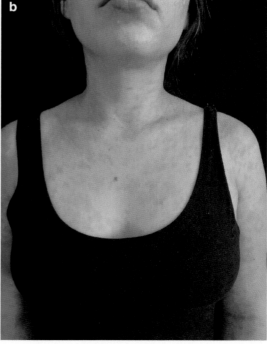

Fig. 59.12 (**a**) Pityriasis rosea. "Herald plaque" or "mother patch." An oval erythematous-squamous single plaque of centrifugal growth, with the lighter center and the outer edge showing a more conspicuous erythema and a thin scaling peripheral collarette. (**b**) Secondary rash of pityriasis rosea (note the herald plaque in the left arm)

develop atypical presentations, such as uncommon distribution, long evolution, rash recurrence, and absence of the mother patch, ranging from mild cases to severe symptoms. Generally the secondary rash spontaneously recedes in 2–4 weeks, with a mean total disease duration of 5–8 weeks [70], with remission with no sequelae.

Secondary Syphilis

Syphilis is a contagious disease caused by the *Treponema pallidum* spirochete; its incidence is worldwide and has shown a steady increase over the second half of the twentieth century, mainly in men with other men as sexual partners [71, 72]. It is transmitted through sex or intrauterine (vertical transmission), and estimates point to about 10.6 million cases a year, most of them in developing countries [73]. Traditionally syphilis is divided into the primary stage (chancre), secondary stage (syphilitic roseola and syphilides), latent period (asymptomatic), and tertiary stage (gumma, neurosyphilis, and cardiovascular, hepatic, renal, or bone lesions). Another classification, which considers treatment, degree of infectivity, and risk for neurologic involvement, organizes the clinical presentations into two major groups, early syphilis and late syphilis [73, 74], a division that also determines the treatment according to the WHO (Table 59.5). Here we focus only on secondary syphilis, since it is a significant differential diagnosis of rashes in the population.

Around 6–8 weeks after the appearance of the primary chancre the secondary manifestations of the disease arise, which result from the spread of the hematogenic pathogen. This secondary phase is characterized by a roseoliform exanthem which shows nonconfluent erythematous macules with little pruritus, usually on the torso, periumbilical region, and internal surfaces of the limbs, rapidly spreading throughout the rest of the body. The lesions are pink to chestnut red in color and eventually can be lightly raised or itchy. Concomitantly generalized adenopathy is noticed. The exanthem is self-limited, and disappears some days or weeks later, possibly leaving some residual hyperpigmentation. A new eruption can arise 3–6 months after appearance of the chancre: they are small, raised, pink- or coppery-colored infiltrating papules that are hard to the touch [74–76]. Papules can be smooth or show an adhered scale which may display a peripheral scaling collarette if more noticeable (Biett collarette). Those lesions are mainly seen on the face, torso, cubital fossa, and popliteal region, although they may affect other parts of the body. Characteristically palmoplantar, red-yellowish, painful macules and papules are noticed (Fig. 59.13). Less often seen are pustulous lesions, and flat or raised plaques known as condyloma lata. Around 5% of secondary syphilis is accompanied by an irregular alopecia, and nearly one-third of patients display a related mucous involvement. Typical syphilis mucous lesions consist of round and flat erosions covered with a grayish membrane, possibly found in the oral cavity or the genital region. Not uncommonly the patient may have pharyngitis, tonsillitis, laryngitis, or areas on the tongue devoid of gustatory papillae. Secondary syphilis lesions may fall into remission after treatment or spontaneously when the recurrence rate can reach 25% [74–76]. After lesion disappearance the disease begins a clinical latency stage, although serologic tests remain positive.

Table 59.5 Syphilis division into early and tardive forms and respective treatments

Classification	Clinical forms	Characteristics	Treatment
Early syphilis	Primary stage Secondary stage Early latent stage	High infectivity Low risk for neurological sequelae	Benzathine benzylpenicillin 2.400.000 UI, by intramuscular injection, at a single session (because of the volume involved, this dose is usually given as two injections at separate sites)
Late syphilis	Late latent stage Tertiary stage	Low infectivity High risk for neurological sequelae	Benzathine benzylpenicillin 2.400.000 UI, intramuscular, once weekly for 3 consecutive weeks Aqueous benzylpenicillin 12–24 million UI by intravenous injection, administered daily in doses of 2–4 million IU every 4 h for 14 days

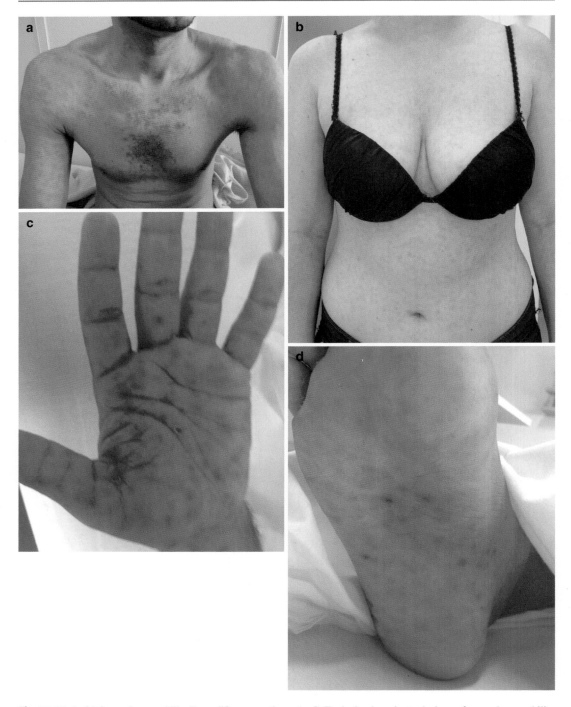

Fig. 59.13 (**a**, **b**) Secondary syphilis. Roseoliform exanthem. (**c**, **d**) Typical palmoplantar lesions of secondary syphilis

Emerging Dermatologic Viral Diseases

Recently diseases thus far displaying an essentially benign character have become a more acute problem in public health, resulting in global actions by the scientific community and the WHO. This section focuses on the three main recently emerging dermatologic viral diseases: dengue fever, Zika, and chikungunya. These are all diseases basically transmitted by the bite of a mosquito belonging to the *Aedes* species (mainly *A. aegypti* and *A. albopictus*), although vertically transmitted (mother–baby), blood and sexually transmitted cases have been reported. The mosquito has diurnal and domestic habits, lives inside people's homes, and feeds on human blood, mainly during early morning and early night. Reproduction takes place in clean and still water through the female's oviposition, and only females bite the humans.

Dengue fever results from the DEN-1, DEN-2, DEN-3, and DEN-4 serotypes of the dengue virus, an RNA virus of the Flaviviridae family. The disease infection may vary from asymptomatic to acute forms, and even death, all depending on the host and the virus conditions. Estimates nowadays refer to 50–100 million dengue fever cases a year in the world [77]. In addition, the viral infection does not guarantee permanent protection, and the same patient may be repeatedly infected [78]. Traditionally the disease is divided into dengue fever and dengue hemorrhagic fever. In classical dengue fever, after the 5- to 7-day average incubation stage there is abrupt fever onset, general malaise, arthralgia, myalgia, and retro-orbital pain. Cephalea, nausea, vomiting, and cutaneous manifestations are usual findings. Cutaneous involvement is seen in 50–80% of the patients, usually as a patchy exanthematous eruption on the face, neck, and torso, coincident with the fever or not. Maculopapular eruption is also frequent, mainly on the torso. Small petechiae and ecchymoses can also occur, mainly in the conjunctiva and the palatum, although they are more often found in dengue hemorrhagic fever, the most severe form [79]. Dengue hemorrhagic fever has an onset similar to that of classical dengue, but evolves with high fever and hemorrhagic phenomena, secondary to an increase in vascular permeability, plasma extravasation, thrombocytopenia, platelet function changes, and disseminated vascular coagulation. Multiple petechiae and ecchymoses are often seen, as well as cavitary effusions, gastrointestinal bleeding, hepatosplenomegaly, and circulatory failure.

Besides dengue fever, another virus transmitted by the *Aedes* mosquito species is the Zika virus, which also belongs to the RNA type of the Flaviviridae family. It was named after the place where it was found for the first time, the Zika Forest, in Uganda, in 1947. Only 20% of the virus-infected patients develop a clinically evident disease, and the absolute majority of infected patients show a mild form of the disease, with symptom disappearance over 3–7 days. Cephalea, low fever, arthralgias, cutaneous rash, pruritus, and conjunctival erythema are the main symptoms. Other less frequent symptoms include limb edema, odynophagia, coughing, and vomiting. The rash displayed in most of the patients is generally maculopapular and erythematous, predominantly involving the torso and the upper limbs. Despite the usually benign course of the disease, it has recently been given great relevance because of a suspected association of the infection with pregnant women and the possible occurrence of microcephaly in newborn babies. At the end of 2015 Brazil registered a very significant increase of microcephaly cases, mainly in the northeast region where, at the beginning of the year, many Zika cases were registered. Initially the presence of viral RNA in the amniotic liquid was shown in two fetuses with microcephaly, an event consistent with intrauterine viral transmission [80]. More recently, the presence of the virus in the brain of a fetus with acute microcephaly was shown, whose mother had been in Brazil by the end of the first gestational trimester and had developed a clinical presentation compatible with the Zika infection. In that report the virus had not been found in any other fetal organ but the central nervous system, and its genome was totally recognized and decoded. A difference in the sequence of two amino acids in relation to the previously known sequence was observed in the viral genome, something that may be merely an accidental event or a virus adaptation to the new environment [81].

Certainly new studies are necessary to confirm such an association. Another significant fact is that, just like dengue, cases of neuropathies and Guillain–Barré syndrome were also associated with Zika infection, a still unproven fact.

The third emerging dermatologic viral disease results from an RNA alphavirus of the Togaviridae family and causes a disease named after it: chikungunya. Just like dengue and Zika, it is transmitted by the *Aedes* species of mosquitoes, and following the incubation stage from 2 to 4 days the clinical manifestations of the disease begin. They are characterized by sudden onset of high fever, cephalea, myalgia, back pain, and arthralgia which is sometimes disabling. A cutaneous involvement occurs in 40–50% of the cases [82], and erythematous and pruriginous maculopapular rash can occur involving mainly the torso, besides facial edema. A vesicular-bullous edema can occur in children, with noticeable skin scaling related to petechiae and gingival bleeding. Hemorrhagic fever is uncommon but can occur. Contrary to dengue, the individual acquires permanent immunity after being infected by the virus.

Table 59.6 lists the main differential diagnoses of rashes in the adult population.

Table 59.6 Main differential diagnoses of rashes in adult population

Disease	Exanthem/related symptoms	Key characteristics/diagnosis
Pharmacodermias	Polymorphous exanthem often with presence of erythematous, confluent macules and papules that make up plaques Vesicles and blisters may occur The rash often begin on the torso and upper limbs Pruritus is a very common symptom. Low fever is also frequent	The rash usually occurs between the first and second weeks after drug use Always consider all medications being used by the patient, either the drugs of continuous and intermittent use Alertness signs for acute reactions: facial edema, peripheral hypereosinophilia, painful or grayish lesions, mucosal involvement
Contact dermatitis	Acute eczema: erythem, edema, papules, vesicles and even blisters Subacute eczema: exudation, crusts Chronic eczema: erythematous and lichenified plaques, scaling, and sometimes fissures	Focus on location – initially lesions occur in areas of allergen contact Pruritus and burning are usual symptoms Ask the patients about their occupation, hobbies, usual cosmetics, contact with plants and fruits, solar radiation
Pityriasis rosea	Multiple small lesions with 1–2 cm average, erythematous and scaling, oval lesions scattered on the torso, neck, and limb root Pruritus is a common symptom although of low intensity	Presence of a "mother patch" or "herald plaque": single oval or round erythematous scaling 2–10 cm plaque, displaying a typical peripheral scaling collarette on the outer margin On the torso, the lesions usually disseminate along the skin cleavage lines and display the typical appearance of "Christmas tree" pattern
Secondary syphilis	Roseoliform exanthem characterized by erythematous nonconfluent macules, with little or absence of pruritus, at first on the torso, periumbilical area and inner surface of limbs, rapidly disseminating to the rest of the body Generalized adenopathy is common. Fever, arthralgias, myalgias, alopecia, hoarseness, mucosal involvement may occur	The distinctive characteristic is the palmoplantar involvement with erythematous yellowish hardened and sometimes painful macules and papules Treponemal tests, such as the FTA-abs and the MHA-TP, and nontreponemal tests, such as the VDRL and the RPR, are positive for secondarism
Emerging dermatological viral diseases – dengue, Zika, chikungunya	Main transmission through the *Aedes* species insect bite Erythematous maculopapular exanthem prevailing on the torso and upper limbs. Face and neck may be sometimes involved Fever, malaise, myalgias, arthralgias, retro-orbital pain More common hemorrhagic phenomena in dengue	Rash is almost always found in Zika, very common in the chikungunya, and less common in dengue fever Origin or recent trips to endemic areas should raise suspicion PCR and serologies positive for the 3 viruses

Diagnosis

Because of the lack of specificity of most exanthems, their correct and precise diagnosis is often very difficult to make. When a diagnosis is not so obvious the physician must first characterize the rash according to the cutaneous primary lesions to limit the majority of the differential diagnoses. Flowchart 59.1 proposes a process of thought to make rash assessment easier.

After classification one must pay attention to lesion location, color (drug reactions tend to show a darker and more conspicuous color), presence of pruritus (it is generally present in most of pharmacodermias and absent in viral exanthems), pain (frequent in some pharmacodermias and KD), fever (related to infectious exanthems), lymphadenopathy (important in rubella and KD), diarrhea (common in exanthems caused by rotavirus and picornavirus), and the patient's general health condition (requiring prompt intervention when impaired). Also, the patient's history of contact with sick persons or recent travel (imported cases of diseases, such as measles and even rubella, are not uncommon) must be investigated.

Benign exanthems during childhood are often only clinically diagnosed, as is the case for hand-foot-mouth disease, infectious erythema, sudden exanthem, scarlatina, and varicella. Nevertheless, when in doubt about the diagnosis, specific tests are available most of the time, and when suspicious about any of those diseases additional tests must be carried out by the physician.

The diagnosis of measles, especially during outbreak periods, is usually easy. The Koplik spots are especially useful for diagnosis because, besides being pathognomonic, they are often present even before the exanthem. Since many countries have shown rare and sporadic cases of the disease, it is important for measles to be included in the differential diagnosis for all patients displaying fever and exanthem. According to the WHO, all patients displaying fever and macular-papular exanthem (not vesicular exanthem), related with cough, coryza, or conjunctivitis, must raise the suspicion of measles. Laboratory diagnosis can be made in different ways; the most used method being antibody detection of the immunoglobulin M (IgM) class against the measles virus in serum or oral mucosa secretions, usually positive for the early days of cutaneous eruption. Another diagnostic method is a four-fold or more increase in the virus-specific IgG titers. A single sample of positive IgG is not diagnostic, since it can simply represent a previous infection. Virus isolation through culture of nasopharyngeal, urinary, or

Flowchart 59.1 Diagnosis of rash in childhood

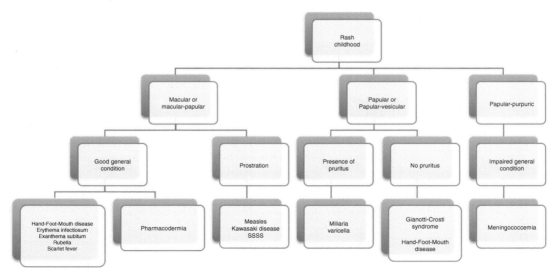

blood secretions, as well as magnification of the viral RNA through the polymerase chain reaction (PCR), can also be used, although they are more expensive and slower technologies [83].

The exanthem found in rubella is unspecific and common to other diseases, so laboratory tests are usually required. The gold-standard diagnostic method is viral RNA research in oropharyngeal and nasal secretions, urine, blood, or liquor using PCR, which can be positive up to a week before rash onset. However, serologic tests are more often used because of their widespread availability and low cost. Therefore, IgM and IgG antibody research are still very useful. IgM antibody positivity is commonly found from 4 to 30 days after disease onset, although it can be negative before the fifth day of rash development, with its repetition suggested after that period. A four-time increase in the IgG titers can be also considered diagnostic [33].

When meningococcemia is suspected diagnostic tests must be required, although they cannot postpone treatment implementation. Blood cultures must be collected before beginning antibiotic use, and hemodynamically stable patients may undergo lumbar puncture. With regard to cutaneous lesions, *Neisseria meningitidis* can be seen on Gram stain in up to 70% of cases. Latex agglutination tests using urine and liquor samples show low sensitivity despite their specificity. The PCR technique has been increasingly used because of its high sensitivity and specificity, despite not being widely used to date.

The SSSS diagnosis is based on clinical suspicion, although the *S. aureus* can be found and cultivated from skin, conjunctiva, nasopharynx, and pyogenic foci of feces. Skin biopsy sometimes can be useful to distinguish other disorders, and KD, TEN, primary sunburn, and extensive bullous impetigo are among the main differential diagnoses of the disorder. Table 59.7 lists the main diagnostic examinations for infectious diseases resulting in exanthem presentations.

GCS and miliaria are basically clinically diagnosed, and there are no specific diagnostic tests. However, in GCS attention must be paid to a history of systemic symptoms or recent infections as well as vaccination. Since the infectious agent spectrum related to GCS is affected by typically regional epidemiologic factors there is no universal

Table 59.7 Diagnostic laboratory tests when infectious diseases resulting in child rash are suspected

Disease	Diagnostic tests
Hand-foot-mouth disease	Oropharynx discharge, palmar-plantar lesions, and feces PCR
Exanthema subitum	IgM + / 4× increase of IgG levels against serum HHV-6 or HHV-7 Immunofluorescence, PCR blood mononuclear cells culture
Erythema infectiosum	Serum IgM + Parvovírus B19
Scarlet fever	Leukocytosis with prevalence of young and eosinophilic forms Antistreptolysin, antihyaluronidase, and antifibrolysin antibodies Oropharynx culture with growth of hemolytic Streptococcus β of group A
Rubella	Oropharynx and nasal secretions, urine, blood, and liquor PCR IgM + / a 4× increase in the IgG levels against the serum rubella virus
Measles	Discharge culture/PCR of the nasopharynx, urine, and blood IgM + / a 4× increase in the IgG levels against serum measles virus and the oral mucosa
Varicella	IgM + /a 4× increase in the IgG levels against the varicella zoster virus
Meningococcemia	Bacterioscopy and culture of cutaneous lesions, blood, and liquor Latex agglutination test
SSSS	Clinical diagnosis Pyogenic foci culture of skin, conjunctiva, nasopharynx, and feces

Table 59.8 Association between lesion location and probable cause of contact dermatitis

Location	Cause
Scalp	Hair coloring substances, shampoo, hair straightening products
Eyelids	Nail polish, make up products
Face	Cosmetics used on the face, hands, and hair
Ears	Earrings, perfume, shampoo
Lips	Lipstick, toothpaste, dyeing substances
Neck	Perfume, bijou
Armpits	Deodorants, fabrics
Genitals	Cosmetics, fabrics, condoms (latex)
Hands	Soaps, detergents, gloves, cosmetics, occupational exposure substances, plants
Feet	Shoes, socks, occupational exposure substances

recommendation regarding the pathogens to be investigated. In general, however, it is known that the Epstein–Barr virus, HHV-6, parvovírus B19, cytomegalovirus, A and B hepatitis viruses, syncytial respiratory virus, and rubella virus have already often been related to the disorder, as well as vaccines.

In drug eruption cases, the diagnosis is made through the clinical history, the patient's characteristics, and the physical examination. Laboratory tests help to assess the patient's systemic involvement, and the anatomopathologic test of the cutaneous injury, although unspecific, can help the diagnosis.

To diagnose ACD a deep anamnesis and clinical presentation are indispensable and often are sufficient to elucidate the dermatitis type and cause (Table 59.8). Patient evaluation must show possible exposures to substances in the patient's occupation, sports, and personal care; for children, the caregiver's history must be assessed. In ACD cases, the most effective method is the contact test or the epicutaneous test to confirm the etiologic diagnosis [63], indicated when this kind of contact dermatitis is suspected, and in all other cases of occupation-related contact dermatitis and chronic dermatitis not controlled by the most often used topical drugs [84]. The provocation test of use and the open test are other available modalities, although they need to be used with caution.

Pityriasis rosea is a disease with an eminently clinical diagnosis because there is no specific laboratory test for this condition. However, the differential diagnosis is required with secondary syphilis at the secondary rash stage; therefore, a nontreponemal triage test, such as the Venereal Disease Research Laboratory test (VDRL), is indicated.

When facing a clinical suspicion of syphilis at any stage, laboratory investigation is mandatory. Serologic tests are divided into nontreponemal (VDRL and rapid test reagin (RPR)) and treponemal (fluorescent treponemal antibody absorption (FTA-abs) and microhemagglutination treponema pallidum test (MHA-TP)). The FTA-abs becomes positive 7–10 days after cancer onset, the MHA-TP after 10 days, and the VDRL after 15 days [73–75]. Hence, for secondary syphilis the nontreponemal tests are markedly positive, and should be confirmed through a treponemal test because of the various clinical situations that may yield a false-positive nontreponemal test (lupus, hanseniasis, hepatitis, pregnancy). Another noteworthy fact is that syphilis may increase the risk for HIV transmission; thus, HIV triage is strongly recommended for patients diagnosed with syphilis.

The emerging dermatologic viral disease diagnosis is made based on clinical and laboratory findings. Dengue fever, Zika, or chikungunya can be diagnosed through PCR research and the specific IgM and IgG serologic tests for each virus. In dengue cases when the occurrence of hemorrhagic disease is more common, the tourniquet test must be made: a 2.5-cm square (or an area around the thumb distal phalanx) is drawn, a blood pressure cuff is applied and inflated to the midpoint between the systolic and diastolic blood pressures for 5 min, then the number of petechiae that arise within the drawn square is count. The proof is considered positive when 20 or more petechiae are counted, and even in the negative cases a complete blood count is indicated.

Moreover, attention must be paid to changes in coagulation tests, platelet count, hematocrit, leukopenia, and hepatic enzymes. When Zika infection is suspected in a pregnant woman, the patient must be referred for possible fetal evaluation [80].

Therapeutic Approach

When facing an exanthem presentation, and after making a diagnostic hypothesis and possible differential diagnoses, the initial treatment of the patient is decided by the physician. Most exanthems are benign and self-limited, although some patients require careful monitoring and treatment, and even isolation and precautionary measures must be promptly initiated.

Viral exanthems, in general, do not require specific treatment; they only need support and symptomatic measures. Therefore, hand-foot-mouth disease, sudden exanthem, rubella, GCS, and miliaria generally require only symptomatic treatment.

Infectious erythema needs special treatment only for aplastic transient crisis, which involves supportive measures and blood transfusion, and for immunosuppressed patients. In these cases the use of standard human Ig is the treatment of choice besides immunosuppression correction.

For scarlatina cases the treatment of choice is penicillin, which can be started up to 8 days after presentation onset. Penicillin-allergic patients can receive erythromycin as well as macrolides [23].

For measles there is no effective antiviral therapy against the virus, but there is an indication for supplementary use of vitamin A. Thus, all measles-diagnosed children must receive 200,000 IU of vitamin A every 24 h for 2 days [28]. This was shown to be an effective measure to decrease the incidence of blindness and death, according to the WHO. In secondary bacterial infection cases mainly resulting in acute otitis media and pneumonia, antibiotic therapy must be initiated.

For varicella, immunocompromised children undergo symptomatic treatment, mainly antihistamines. However, antiretroviral therapy is indicated for specific cases when there is greater risk of disease aggravation. Acyclovir has been the preferred drug to treat varicella, but alternative drugs such as valacyclovir and famciclovir can be used. Acyclovir must be initiated preferably over the first 24 h for the following patients [26]:

- All patients older than 12 years old
- Patients with cutaneous or chronic pulmonary disorder
- Patients undergoing corticosteroid or long-term salicylate treatment

The usual acyclovir dose for children is 20 mg/kg, oral route, four times a day, not more than 800 mg/day, over 5 days. The adult dose is 800 mg/day, oral route, five times a day, over 5 days. Acute cases require intravenous acyclovir. Postexposure prophylaxis for the virus-exposed and immune-depressed patients under the same condition can be implemented through vaccination or use of immunoglobulin. Studies have shown that early vaccine use (up to 96 h post-exposure) is effective to prevent disease development and occurrence of its acute configurations. Intravenous human Ig (IVIG) must be used for the virus-nonimmune patients who cannot receive the vaccine and who are also at risk for developing acute varicella [26]. Therefore, intravenous human Ig is indicated for immunosuppressed patients, pregnant women, newborns whose mothers developed varicella 5 days before or 2 days after childbirth, and premature babies exposed to the varicella virus (specifically patients born with gestational age of 28 weeks or more whose mothers displayed no evidence of immunity against the virus, or patients of gestational age less than 28 weeks, and/or weighing less than 1,000 g).

Patients diagnosed with KD should receive IVIG at 2 g/kg, single infusion, for 10–12 h.

Related to the IVIG, acetylsalicylic acid must be started early at a dosage of 80–100 mg/kg/day, divided into four ingestions, and kept for at least 72 h following fever cessation (although some centers of excellence have kept a low dose for a long time) [38]. Studies recommend the use of corticosteroids (methylprednisolone pulse therapy) only for patients who had received two IVIG doses with no reaction whatsoever).

SSSS treatment depends on the extension and gravity of each case. Patients with confirmed disease and displaying good general condition can receive oral treatment against the *S. aureus*. β-lactamase-resistant antibiotics, such as cephalexin and flucloxacillin, given for at least 7 days [40, 41]. Also, the detached skin areas can be initially lubricated with mild moisturizer, and *S. aureus*-colonized patients must undergo topical antibiotic therapy. Acute patients must be taken to hospital, often in need of some time in the intensive therapy unit. The antibiotic of choice is intravenous oxacillin or vancomycin (mainly in areas showing a high rate of methicillin-resistant *S. aureus* or MRSA) [40, 41].

When meningococcemia is suspected, antibiotic therapy must be immediately initiated. Crystalline penicillin G is the antibiotic of choice, at 500,000 U/kg/day, divided into six doses. Cefotaxime 200 mg/kg/day, divided into three doses, or ceftriaxone 100 mg/kg/day, one or two doses, can be given [48]. Attention must be paid to individuals in contact with meningococcemia patients, since they must undergo appropriate chemoprophylaxis. Rifampicin, every 12 h, for 2 days, is indicated for children and adults. Single doses of ciprofloxacin and ceftriaxone can be also used for adults [48, 49].

The basic treatment of patients with a cutaneous drug eruption consists in symptom control and interruption of the drug responsible for the clinical presentation. After assessment of the used drugs, all of them must be discontinued. When the drug under suspicion is necessary for the patient, the potential risk/benefit has to be considered. In general, topical corticosteroids alleviate the pruritus and are often used in more circumscribed lesions. On the other hand, patients with acute forms of pharmacodermia usually need a systemic corticosteroid and even IVIG [54]. Hospital admission to improve monitoring is an indication for the acute and severe cases.

To treat contact dermatitis one must first try to identify the cause and, therefore, avoid repeat exposures. The adoption of protective measures, such as use of appropriate clothes, gloves, and barrier cream, is very helpful, and in some cases diet changes may be necessary, mainly in cases of nickel allergy; improvement can be seen when its ingestion is decreased [62]. In cases of acute eczema, wet packs soaked into 1/10 or 1/20 Burrow liquid or Alibour water can be used, and topical corticosteroids in gel, lotion, or cream may also be used. Extensive and acute cases can be treated with oral corticosteroids for a short time (usually 1 mg/kg/day over 3–14 days) [63]. For the chronic forms, topical corticosteroids as ointment are the usual choice; in some cases occlusive corticosteroids are used [84]. Calcineurin inhibitors, such as tacrolimus and pimecrolimus, are another option [85]. Oral antihistamines are useful for pruritus control only; when the lesions improve, treatments to recover the skin barrier are important.

In pityriasis rosea, the treatment in most cases involves patient education about the course of the disease and its self-limited character. Topical corticosteroids and, rarely, oral corticosteroids may be used in patients displaying extensive and pruritus-associated injuries. Phototherapy is another useful therapeutic procedure for disease control [86]. In recent years, studies have used systemic erythromycin, azithromycin, and acyclovir [87, 88], given that there may be evidence for acyclovir to have some benefit in disease control.

All syphilis cases, regardless of form, have penicillin as the drug of choice. In the early forms, benzathine benzylpenicillin, 2.4 million

IU by intramuscular injection, at a single session is recommended. There are protocols that associate a second dose 1 week later in secondary syphilis and early latent syphilis. For patients with tardive forms, three doses of penicillin benzathine are indicated: benzathine benzylpenicillin, 2.4 million IU also by intramuscular injection, once weekly for three consecutive weeks (Table 59.5). The alternative for allergic patients involves the use of tetracycline or doxycycline, although it is important to underscore that HIV-positive patients or pregnant women have an indication of desensitization to use the first-choice drug [75, 76, 89, 90]. Serologic post-treatment follow-up is conducted with nontreponemal tests, since treponemal tests remain positive regardless of treatment, and it is expected for the early forms to show a decrease of at least two titrations from the starting value up to 6 months after treatment has ended.

There is no specific treatment for dengue, Zika, and chikungunya. All patients must go through powerful rehydration therapy and be given symptomatic drugs with no acetylsalicylic acid. Signs of acute hemorrhagic disease and shock demand hospital admission and eventually intensive care [78].

Future Perspectives

The advance of technology and the body of knowledge in recent years concerning many diseases has yielded a significant increase of diagnostic accuracy in the cases of rash. Many laboratory tests nowadays, either serologic or viral load detection tests, are available in many healthcare clinics around the world. There is an increased ability to determine the cause of a rash and approach it the best possible way.

Many diseases already controlled and even eradicated in some parts of the world have now once again become part of the differential diagnoses of exanthem following recent outbreaks in both underdeveloped and developed countries, such as the case of measles. This reasserts the need for constant alertness and massive immunization for the appropriate control of many infectious diseases. In addition, the emerging dermatologic viral diseases have become a major world concern because of their high morbidity rate, with dengue fever, Zika, and chikungunya among their number.

Besides the infectious causes, pharmacodermias are still, and will continue to be an important cause of rash in the adult and pediatric population. Every year new drugs are developed, mainly chemotherapeutic, antihipertensive, and antimicrobial, and the physician must be fully aware of the possible adverse effects of such new drugs. Moreover, since health care systems are being perfected, more patients have had access to medical assistance and consequently to these drugs, which makes the possible occurrence of pharmacodermias even more important.

Thus, the knowledge and the correct management of the main causes of rash are increasingly more significant and necessary, given that cases of rash will probably continue to happen for many different reasons.

Glossary

Biett's collarette A syphilitic symptom characterized by a thin white ring of scales on the surface of a macule or papule.

Filatov sign A typical sign of scarlet fever characterized by paleness around the mouth and congestion of the cheeks.

Koplik spots Spots characterized by clustered, small, white lesions on the buccal mucosa (opposite the upper first and second molars), pathognomonic for measles. The spots resemble tiny grains of white sand, each surrounded by a red ring.

Papular-purpuric gloves and socks syndrome An acute dermatosis characterized by a papular-purpuric edematous rash in a distinct "gloves and socks" distribution often accompanied by fever, asthenia, and lymphadenopathies. It is mainly caused by parvovirus B19 (B19V) although other viruses and drugs may be involved.

Pastia's lines A clinical sign whereby pink or red lines formed of confluent petechiae occur in areas of skin creases, such as the axilla, the neck, the antecubital fossa, and the popliteal fossa. This is a typical sign of scarlet fever.

Primary skin lesions Blister: Raised lesion, more than 1 cm wide, with internal liquid content.Macula: Flat nonpalpable lesions, less than 1 cm wide, showing inconspicuous texture and/or color change.Nodule: Palpable raised and indurated lesion usually deeper than the papule.Patch: Flat nonpalpable lesion, more than 1 cm wide, showing discrete texture and/ or color change.Papule: Circumscribed palpable lesion, above skin surface, less than 1 cm wide.Plaque: Palpable and raised lesion, above skin surface, more than 1 cm wide.Pustule: Raised surface lesion with internal yellow content (pus).Vesicle: Raised lesion, less than 1 cm wide, with internal light liquid content.

References

1. Drago F, Rampini P, Rampini E, Rebora A. Atypical exanthems: morphology and laboratory investigations may lead to an aetiological diagnosis. About 70% of cases. Br J Dermatol. 2002;147:255–60.
2. Ely JW, Stone MS. The generalized rash: differential diagnosis. Am Fam Physician. 2010;81(6 Pt 1):735–9.
3. Ely JW, Stone MS. The generalized rash: diagnostic approach. Am Fam Physician. 2010;81(6 Pt 2):726–34.
4. Fleischer AB, Feldman SR, Bullard CN. Patients can accurately identify when they have a dermatologic condition. J Am Acad Dermatol. 1999;41:784–6.
5. Chan KP, Goh KT, Chong CY, Teo ES, Lau G, Ling AE. Epidemic hand, foot and mouth disease caused by human enterovirus 71, Singapore. Emerg Infect Dis. 2003;9(1):78–85. doi:10.3201/eid1301.020112.
6. Stock I. Hand, foot and mouth disease -more than a harmless "childhood disease". Med Monatsschr Pharm. 2014;37(1):4–10. quiz 11-2
7. Chatproedprai S, Tempark T, Wanlapakorn N, Puenpa J, Wananukul S, Poovorawan Y. Unusual skin manifestation of hand, foot and mouth disease associated with coxsackievirus A6: cases report. Springer Plus. 2015;4:362. doi:10.1186/s40064-015-1143-z.
8. Chang L-Y, et al. Clinical features and risk factors of pulmonary edema after enterovirus-71-related hand, foot, and mouth disease. Lancet. 1999;354:1682–6.
9. Neal S, Young MD, Kevin E, Brown MD. Parvovirus B19. N Engl J Med. 2004;350:586–97.
10. Azzi A, Morfini M, Mannucci PM. The transfusion-associated transmission of par- vovirus B19. Transfus Med Rev. 1999;13:194–204.
11. Naides SJ. Rheumatic manifestations of parvovirus b19 infection. Rheum Dis Clin N Am. 1998;24(2):375–401.
12. Magro CM, Dawood MR, Crowson N. The cutaneous manifestations of humanparvovirus B19 infection. Hum Pathol. 2000;31(4):488–97.
13. Naides SJ, Piette W, Veach LA, Argenyi Z. Human parvovirus B19-induced vesiculopustular skin eruption. Am J Med. 1988;84(5):968–72.
14. Brown KE, Young NS. Parvovirus B19 infection and hematopoiesis. Blood Rev. 1995;9(3):176–82.
15. Setúbal S, Adelmo GHD, Nascimento JP, Oliveira SA. Aplastic crisis caused by parvovirus B19 in an adult patient with sickle-cell disease. Rev Soc Bras Med Trop. 2000;33(5):477–81. [online] [acesso 23 Sep 2015].
16. Stoeckle MY. The spectrum of human herpesvirus 6 infection: from roseola infantum to adult disease. Annu Rev Med. 2000;51:423–30.
17. Zerr DM, et al. A population-based study of primary human herpesvirus 6 infection. N Engl J Med. 2005;352:768–76.
18. Sadao S, Kyoko S, Masaru I, Tetsushi Y, Yuji K, Takao O, et al. Clinical characteristics of febrile convulsions during primary HHV-6 infection. Arch Dis Child. 2000;82:62–6.
19. Larry J, Strausbaugh MT, Caserta DJM, Stephen D. Human herpesvirus 6. Clin Infect Dis. 2001;33(6):829–33.
20. Chiou CS, et al. Epidemiology and molecular characterization of *Streptococcus pyogenes* recovered from scarlet fever patients in central Taiwan from 1996 to 1999. J Clin Microbiol. 2004;42(9):3998–4006.
21. Escarlatina: orientações para surtos. Boletim Epidemiológico Paulista. [online] [acesso em em Mar 09] SES; 49(46). Disponível em http://periodicos. ses.sp.bvs.br/pdf/bepa/v4n46/v4n46a03.pdf. ISSN 1806.423-X, n.d.
22. Stevens DL. Severe group A streptococcal infections associated with a toxic shock-like syndrome and scarlet fever toxin A. N Engl J Med. 1989;321:1–7.
23. Dong H, et al. β-Haemolytic group A streptococci *emm*75 carrying altered pyrogenic exotoxin A linked to scarlet fever in adults. J Infect. 2008;56(4):261–7.
24. Lobo IM, Santos ACL, Júnior JAS, Passos RO, Pereira CU. Vírus varicela zoster. RBM rev. bras. med. 2015;72(6):231–38.
25. Oliveira MJC, et al. Frequency of measles, rubella, dengue and erythema infectiosum among suspected cases of measles and rubella in the State of Pernambuco between 2001 and 2004. Rev Soc Bras Med Trop. 2008;41(4):338–44.
26. American Academy of Pediatrics. Varicella-zoster infections. In: Pickering LK, editor. Red book: 2012 report of the committee on infectious diseases, vol. 2012. 29th ed. Elk Grove Village: American Academy of Pediatrics. p. 774–89.
27. Moss WJ, Griffin DE. Measles. Lancet. 2012;379(9811):153–64.
28. World Health Organization. Measles. 2015. [online]. Disponível em URL: http://www.who.int/ mediacentre/factsheets/fs286/en./.
29. Centers for Disease Control and Prevention. Measles United States. 2015 Jan 4/Apr 2.[acesso Mar 9];

Centers for Disease Control and Prevention, Atlanta. Disponível em URL:http://www.cdc.gov/mmwr/preview/mmwrhtml/mm6414a1.htm.

30. Muscat ML, Bang H, Wohlfahrt J, Glismann S, Molbak K. Measles in Europe: an epidemiological assessment. Lancet. 2009;373(9661):383–9.

31. Rosa C. Rubella and rubeola. Semin Perinatol. 1998;22(4):318–22.

32. Orenstein WA, Perry RT, Halsey NA. The clinical significance of measles: a review. J Infect Dis. 2004;189(Suppl 1):S4–16.

33. Lambert N, Strebel P, Orenstein W, Icenogle J, Poland GA. Rubella. Lancet. 2015;385(9984):2297–307.

34. Centers for Disease Control and Prevention. Manual for the surveillance of vaccine-preventable diseases, Atlanta. 2012. Disponível em URL: http://www.cdc.gov/vaccines/pubs/surv-manual/chpt14-rubella.html.

35. Kawasaki T. Kawasaki disease. Int J Rheum Dis. 2014;17:597–600.

36. Castro PA, Urbano LMF, Costa IMC. Doença de Kawasaki. An Bras Dermatol. 2009;84(4):317–31.

37. Ayusawa M, Sonobe T, Uemura S, Ogawa S, Nakamura Y, Kiyosawa N, et al.; Kawasaki Disease Research Committee. Revision of diagnostic guidelines for Kawasaki disease (5th revised edition). Pediatr Int. 2005;47:232–34.

38. Newburger JW, Takahashi M, Gerber MA, Gewitz MH, Tani LY, Burns JC, et al. Diagnosis, treatment, and long-term management of Kawasaki disease: a statement for health professionals from the Committee on Rheumatic Fever, Endocarditis and Kawasaki Disease, Council on Cardiovascular Disease in the Young. Am Heart Assoc. 2004;110(17):2747–71.

39. Brewer JD, et al. Staphylococcal scalded skin syndrome and toxic shock syndrome after tooth extraction. J Am Acad Dermatol. 2008;59(2):342–6.

40. Patel GKL, Finlay AY. Staphylococcal scalded skin syndrome: diagnosis and management. Am J Clin Dermatol. 2003;4(3):165–75.

41. Patel NN, Patel DN. Staphylococcal scalded skin syndrome. Am J Med. 2010;123(6):505–7.

42. Caputo R, Gelmetti C, Ermacora E, et al. Gianotti-Crosti syndrome: a retrospective analysis of 308 cases. J Am Acad Dermatol. 1992;26:207–10.

43. Chuh AA. Diagnostic criteria for Gianotti-Crosti syndrome: a prospective case-control study for validity assessment. Cutis. 2001;68:207–13.

44. Lima DA, Rocha DM, Miranda MFR. Gianotti-Crosti syndrome: clinical, laboratorial features, and serologic profiles of 10 cases from Belém, State of Para, Brazil. An Bras Dermatol. 2004;79(6):699–707. Rio de Janeiro.

45. Nguyen TA, Ortega-Loayza AG, Stevens MP. Miliaria-rash after neutropenic fever and induction chemotherapy for acute myelogenous leukemia. An Bras Dermatol. 2011;86(4 Suppl 1):104–6.

46. Al-Hilo MM, Al-Saedy SJ, Alwan AI. Atypical presentation of miliaria in Iraqi patients attending Al -Kindy Teaching Hospital in Baghdad: a clinical descriptive study. Am J Dermatol Venereol. 2012;1(3):41–6.

47. Kirk JF, Wilson BB, Chun W, Cooper PH. Miliaria profunda. J Am Acad Dermatol. 1996;35(5 Pt 2):854–6.

48. Rosenstein NE. Meningococcal disease. N Engl J Med. 2001;344:1378–88.

49. Dwilow R, Fanella S. Invasive meningococcal disease in the 21st century – an update for the clinician. Curr Neurol Neurosci Rep. 2015;15(3):2.

50. Sabatini C, et al. Clinical presentation of meningococcal disease in childhood. J Prev Med Hyg. 2012;53:116–9.

51. Hill WR, Kinney TD. The cutaneous lesions in acute meningococcemia: a clinical and pathologic study. JAMA. 1947;134(6):513–8.

52. Mockenhaupt M. Epidemiology of cutaneous adverse drug reactions. Chem Immunol Allergy. 2012;97:1–17.

53. Borch JE, Andersen KE, Bindslev-Jensen C. The prevalence of acute cutaneous drug reactions in a Scandinavian university hospital. Acta Derm Venereol. 2006;86:518–22.

54. Roujeau JC, Stern RS. Severe adverse cutaneous reactions to drugs. N Engl J Med. 1994;331:1272–84.

55. Hernandez-Salazar A, Ponce-de-Leon Rosales S, Rangel-Frausto S, et al. Epidemiology of adverse cutaneous drug reactions: a prospective study in hospitalized patients. Arch Med Res. 2006;37:899–902.

56. Sharma VK, Sethuraman G, Kumar B. Cutaneous adverse drug reactions: clinical pattern and causative agents – a 6 year series from Chandigarh, India. J Postgrad Med. 2001;47:95–9.

57. Zaraa I, Jones M, Trojjet S, Cheikh Rouhou R, El Euch D, Mokni M, et al. Severe adverse cutaneous drug eruptions: epidemiological and clinical features. Int J Dermatol. 2011;50:877–80.

58. Bolognia JL, Jorizzo JL, Rapini R. Dermatologia. Reações a medicamentos. 2nd . Rio de Janeiro: Elsevier Saunder; 2012. p. 301–320. Cap. 22.

59. Grando LR, Schmitt TAB, Bakos RM. Severe cutaneous reactions to drugs in the setting of a general hospital. An Bras Dermatol. 2014;89(5):758–62.

60. Djien V, Bocquet H, Dupuy A, et al. Symptomatology and markers of the severity of erythematous drug eruptions. Ann Dermatol Venereol. 1999;126:247–50.

61. Marzano AV, Borghi A, Cugno M. Adverse drug reactions and organ damage: the skin. Eur J Intern Med. 2015;7(15):00414–8. pii: S09536205.

62. Szatkowski J, Schwartz RA. Acute generalized exanthematous pustulosis (AGEP): a review and update. J Am Acad Dermatol. 2015;73(5):843–8.

63. Duarte IAG, Lazzarini R, Bedikrow RB, Pires MC. Contact dermatitis. An Bras Dermatol. 2000;75(5):529–48.

64. Peiser M, Tralau T, Heidler J, et al. Allergic contact dermatitis: epidemiology, molecular mechanisms, in vitro methods and regulatory aspects. Current knowledge assembled at an international workshop at BfR, Germany. Cell Mol Life Sci. 2012;69(5):763–81. doi:10.1007/s00018-011-0846-8. Epub 2011 Oct 14.

65. Martin SF. New concepts in cutaneous allergy. Contact Dermatitis. 2014;72:2–10.

66. Bolognia JL, Jorizzo JL, Rapini R. Dermatologia. Local New York: Publisher Elsevier 2nd ed; 2012. p. 209–30. Cap.15 e 16.

67. Brasch J, Becker D, Aberer W, et al. Guideline contact dermatitis. Allergo J Int. 2014;23:126–38.

68. Chuh AA, Chan HH. Prospective case-control study of chlamydia, legionella and mycoplasma infections in patients with pityriasis rosea. Eur J Dermatol. 2002;12:170–3.

69. Bitencourt MSM, Delmaestro D, Miranda PB, Filgueira AL, Pontes LFL. Pityriasis rosea. An Bras Dermatol. 2008;83(5):461–9.

70. Stulberg DL, Wolfrey J. Pityriasis rosea. Am Fam Physician. 2004;69(1):87–91.

71. Fuente MJ. Syphilis a resurgent disease. Actas Dermosifiliogr. 2010;101(10):817–9.

72. Gállego-Lezáun C, Arrizabalaga Asenjo M, González-Moreno J, et al. Syphilis in men who have sex with men: a warning sign for HIV infection. Actas Dermosifiliogr. 2015;106(9):740–5.

73. Tuddenham S, Ghanem KG. Emerging trends and persistent challenges in the management of adult syphilis. BMC Infect Dis. 2015;15:351.

74. James WD, Berger T, Elston D. Andrew's doenças da pele – dermatologia clínica. 10th ed. Rio de Janeiro: Elsevier Editora Ltda; 2007.

75. Dupin N, Farhi D. Syphilis. Presse Med. 2013;42(4 Pt 1):446–53.

76. Dylewski J, Duong M. The rash of secondary syphilis. CMAJ. 2007;176(1):33–5.

77. World Health Organization. Dengue control. 2016. Disponível em URL: http://www.who.int/denguecontrol/en/.

78. Centers for Disease Control and Prevention. Dengue. Clinical guidance. Atlanta. 2014. Disponível em URL: http://www.cdc.gov/dengue/clinicalLab/clinical.htmlhttp://www.cdc.gov/dengue/clinicalLab/clinical.html.

79. Lupi O, Carneiro CG, Coelho ICB. Manifestações mucocutâneas da dengue. An Bras Dermatol. 2007;82(4):291–305.

80. Oliveira Melo AS, Malinger G, Ximenes R, Szejnfeld PO, Alves Sampaio S, Bispo de Filippis AM. Zika virus intrauterine infection causes fetal brain abnormality and microcephaly: tip of the iceberg? Ultrasound Obstet Gynecol. 2016;47:6–7.

81. Mlakar J, et al. Zika virus associated with microcephaly. N Engl J Med. 2016;374(10):951–8.

82. Pialoux G, Gaüzère B, Jauréguiberry S, Strobel M. Chikungunya, an epidemic arbovirosis. Lancet Infect Dis. 2007;7:319–27.

83. Bellini WJ, Helfand RF. The challenges and strategies for laboratory diagnosis of measles in an international setting. J Infect Dis. 2003;187(Suppl 1):S283–90.

84. Levin C, Maibach HI. An overview of the efficacy of topical corticosteroids in experimental human nickel contact dermatitis. Contact Dermatitis. 2000;43:317–21.

85. Saripalli YV, Gadzia JE, Belsito DV. Tacrolimus ointment 0.15 in the treatment of nickel-induced allergic contact dermatitis. J Am Acad Dermatol. 2003;49:477–82.

86. Eritro Leenutaphong V, Jiamton S. UVB phototerapy for pityriasis rosea: a bilateral comparison study. J Am Acad Dermatol. 1995;33:996–9.

87. Bukhari IA. Oral erythromycin is ineffective in the treatment of pityriasis rosea. J Drugs Dermatol. 2008;7(7):625.

88. Drago F, Vecchio F, Rebora A. Use of high-dose acyclovir in pityriasis rosea. J Am Acad Dermatol. 2006;54(1):82–5.

89. Morales-Múnera CE, Fuentes-Finkelstein PA, Vall MM. Update on the diagnosis and treatment of syphilis. Actas Dermosifiliogr. 2015;106(1):68–9.

90. World Health Organization. Guidelines for the management of sexually transmitted infections. Geneva: World health organization; 2003.

Suggested Literature

Allmon A, Deane K, Martin KL. Common skin rashes in children. Am Fam Physician. 2015;92(3):211–6.

Bahrani E, Nunneley CE, Hsu S, Kass JS. Cutaneous adverse effects of neurologic medications. CNS Drugs. 2016. doi:10.1007/s40263-016-0318-7.

Blair JE. Evaluation of fever in the international traveler. Unwanted 'souvenir' can have many causes. Postgrad Med. 2004;116(1):13–20, 29.

Browning JC. An update on pityriasis rosea and other similar childhood exanthems. Curr Opin Pediatr. 2009;21(4):481–5. doi:10.1097/MOP.0b013e32832db96e.

Carneiro SC, Cestari T, Allen SH, Ramos e-Silva M. Viral exanthems in the tropics. Clin Dermatol. 2007;25(2):212–20.

Chang C, Ortiz K, Ansari A, Gershwin ME. The Zika outbreak of the 21st century. J Autoimmun. 2016. pii:S0896-8411(16)30008-7. doi:10.1016/j.jaut.2016.02.006.

Ely JW, Stone MS. The generalized rash: part I. Differential diagnosis. Am Fam Physician. 2010;81(6):735–9.

Ely JW, Stone MS. The generalized rash: part II. Diagnostic approach. Am Fam Physician. 2010;81(6):726–34.

McKinnon HD Jr, Howard T. Evaluating the febrile patient with a rash. Am Fam Physician. 2000;62(4):804–16.

Pigmented Lesions

60

José Carlos Santos Mariante
and Gabriela Fortes Escobar

Introduction

Pigmented moles and nevi are the most common neoplasms found in humans [1]. The incidence of melanocytic nevi in newborns is slightly more than 1% [2]. The incidence increases in infancy and adulthood, with a peak at puberty and adolescence. The size and pigmentation of these lesions also increase during adolescence, pregnancy, or after estrogen and corticosteroid therapy. Between the second and third decades of life, most Caucasians acquire their maximum number of lesions, and later in life most lesions tend to fade and eventually disappear.

Skin tumors can be differentiated into several groups: epidermal surface; epidermal appendages; fibrous, neural, vascular, fatty, muscular, and osseous tissues; melanocytic; and malignant. The term *nevus* refers to a circumscribed congenital abnormality of any type present at birth. When this term is used, it is important to include a qualifying adjective (epidermal, melanocytic, pigmented, vascular) to specify the particular cell of origin. Being in common use this term is also used in a loose manner to refer to a benign tumor of pigmented cells [1].

In contrast, moles are pigmented cutaneous lesions not present at birth that are apparently hereditarily predetermined. In general, moles appear during childhood and adolescence and are flat or slightly elevated. In adulthood they tend to be polypoid or dome-shaped, sessile, or papillomatous [1].

Pigmented lesions may comprise melanocytes or nevus cells. Both are of neural origin. A melanocyte is a dendritic cell that produces melanin and transfers it to the keratinocytes and hair cells, supplying the pigment to skin and hair. It originates in the neural crest and early in fetal life it migrates with the nerves to the skin. Many types of skin lesions may appear because of the melanocytic cells remaining in the dermis after birth, such as Mongolian spots, blue nevi, and the nevi of Ota and Ito [1].

Theories suggest that nevus cells arise from a bipotential precursor cell that develops into a melanoblastic or schwannian nevoblast. In this theory, the nevoblasts develop into epidermal nevus cells that give rise to the junctional and compound nevi. In addition, the schwannian nevoblasts develop into neural nevi cells and intradermal nevi [3]. In the most popular theory, nevus cells have a dual derivation and develop from the melanocytes in the epidermis and Schwann cells of the neural sheath [4]. A line of Schwann cells in the peripheral nerves appear to form a pathway between the central nervous

J.C.S. Mariante
Dermatology of Mãe de Deus Center,
Porto Alegre, Brazil
e-mail: jcmariante@gmail.com

G.F. Escobar
Dermatology Service of Hospital
de Clínicas de Porto Alegre,
Porto Alegre, Brazil

© Springer International Publishing Switzerland 2018
R.R. Bonamigo, S.I.T. Dornelles (eds.), *Dermatology in Public Health Environments*,
https://doi.org/10.1007/978-3-319-33919-1_60

system and the skin. These cells migrate to the dermis and give rise to a number of dermal tumors. Nevus cells, therefore, may locate at the dermal–epidermal junction (junction nevi), within the dermis (intradermal nevi), or be a combination of both (compound nevi) [1].

In the clinical evaluation the most important step is to differentiate the pigmented lesions from others. Using this approach it is often difficult to establish the melanocytic origin. Lesions such as basocellular carcinoma or seborrheic keratosis sometimes require better knowledge about other methods of evaluation, such as dermoscopy and pathology. Although dermoscopy and confocal microscopy are discussed in detail in a specific chapter elsewhere in this book, the description of lesions in this chapter some mentions details about these instruments. Some structures described in dermoscopy, such as aggregated globules, typical pigmented network, pseudonetwork, branched streaks, and parallel pattern, are the most important features for the diagnosis of benign melanocytic lesions [5]. Pathology is the gold-standard method of diagnosis to differentiate melanocytic from non-melanocytic lesions, and anatomopathologic characteristics for each lesion will be described. The use of immunohistochemistry as a complementary method of diagnosis can improve this evaluation.

Nevocellular or Common Pigmented Nevi

Concepts Nevocellular or pigmented nevi are lesions comprising nevus cells. Based on the location of the nevus cells, they are subdivided and described as junctional, intradermal, or compound lesions. Intradermal moles and nevi only have nests cells in the dermis. In junctional nevi, nevus cell nests are confined to the dermal–epidermal junction, and compound nevi have nevus cells nests in both locations.

Clinical Presentation and Diagnosis Pigmented nevi have a wide range of clinical appearances and locations. The prevalence varies with age, race, and perhaps genetic and environmental factors. Few nevi are present at birth or childhood;

they progressively increase in number, reaching a peak at the third and fourth decades of life, and then disappear with age. The most important factors related to number, development, and growth of nevi are skin color, race, genetic and familial occurrence, sun exposure, systemic immunosuppression, pregnancy, and hormonal diseases [6].

Pigmented nevi are usually well circumscribed, round or ovoid, regular and symmetric with a size ranging between 2 and 6 mm. They may occur anywhere on the skin surface (Fig. 60.1) and vary from flat to slightly elevated or dome shaped, nodular, verrucous, polypoid, or papillomatous. Junctional nevi are commonly hairless macules with color ranging from light to dark brown or brownish black. Most of them are circular, elliptical, or oval with few variations in colors and shapes. They are more common in children and located on palms, soles, and genitalia [1]. Compound nevi are more common in older children and adults, tend to be elevated with shades of brown, and may have coarse hairs within the lesion. In adolescence they frequently tend to increase in thickness and pigmentation. Intradermal nevi are seen most frequently in adults after the third decade of life and tend to fade with maturation, when nevus cells are often destroyed and replaced by fibrous or fatty tissue. They are

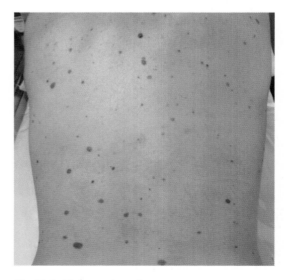

Fig. 60.1 Melanocytic nevi

usually dome shaped, sessile, or pedunculated and range in size from a few millimeters to 1 cm or more. The color varies from nonpigmented to brown or black [1].

Depending of the characteristics of the nevi, sometimes it may be very difficult to distinguish them from other lesions such as seborrheic keratosis, dermatofibromas, and neurofibromas. The most important differential diagnoses are dysplastic nevi and melanoma. Common nevi usually appear to be smaller and show clinical characteristics such as symmetry, regularity in shape, and well-defined borders. Furthermore, colors such as red, blue, gray, and black are more common in dysplastic nevi and melanomas.

Congenital Melanocytic Nevi

Concepts Congenital melanocytic nevi are moles present at birth. They consist of intraepidermal, dermal, or both benign melanocytic proliferations with a wide range of sizes, locations, and clinical appearances. Although it has been suggested that the increased incidence of malignant melanoma in large nevi may be related to the increased number of cells, studies suggest that small congenital nevi also have an increased risk of malignant degeneration [7]. Small congenital nevi (less than 1.5 cm in diameter), occur in 1% of all newborns and have an estimated lifetime risk of developing melanoma of 2.6–4.9% [8]. The risk of developing melanoma in medium-sized congenital nevi (measuring 1.5–20 cm in diameter) is uncertain; and large or giant congenital pigmented nevi, measuring greater than 20 cm in diameter, are believed to have 6.3% lifetime risk for developing malignant melanoma [7, 9].

Clinical Presentation and Diagnosis Small and medium-sized congenital nevi usually are oval or round, flat, pale tan to light brown macules or papules. Others are well-circumscribed lesions with mottled freckling. With time they become elevated, and coarse dark brown hairs may or not become prominent. Giant nevi frequently lie in the distribution of a dermatome

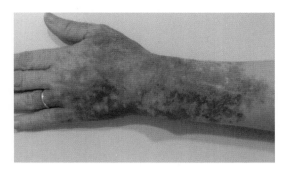

Fig. 60.2 Giant melanocytic nevi in arm and hand

and vary in size. Furthermore, they may cover limbs or extensive areas of trunk (Fig. 60.2). Their color ranges from dark brown to black and over 95% have a hairy component consisting of large coarse terminal hairs [1]. It is common to also observe a verrucous or papillomatous surface and an irregular margin. Almost invariably satellite nevi appear at the periphery of the lesion, and numerous other pigmented nevi coexist elsewhere on the body. Giant hairy nevi, particularly those on the scalp and neck, may be associated with leptomeningeal melanocytosis and neurologic disorders such as epilepsy or other focal neurologic abnormalities. Those that overlie the vertebral column may be associated with spina bifida or meningomyelocele [1].

Characteristically dermoscopy demonstrates a target network, focal thickening of network lines, target globules, skin furrow hypopigmentation, focal hypopigmentation, hair follicles, perifollicular hypopigmentation, vessels, and target vessels.

Halo Nevus

Concepts and Clinical Presentation Halo nevus (Sutton's nevus or leukoderma acquisitum centrifugum) consists of a single or multiple pigmented skin lesion centrally placed surrounded by a 1- to 5-mm halo of depigmentation (Fig. 60.3). This common disorder occurs between 3 and 45 years of age, usually with onset in late adolescence [1]. Compound and intradermal nevi are the most frequently

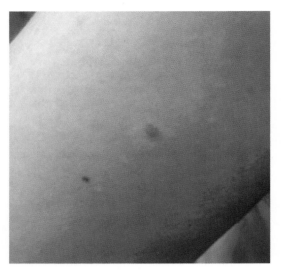

Fig. 60.3 Halo nevi

associated melanocytic lesions. However, it may also occur with blue nevi, neuromas, neurofibromas, melanomas, metastatic lesions, seborrheic keratoses, angiomas, molluscum contagiosum, warts, basal cell carcinoma, and congenital nevi. The cause appears to be related to an immunologic destruction of melanocytes and nevus cells. About 30% of patients with halo nevi have a tendency to vitiligo. It may occur on almost any cutaneous surface and is usually asymptomatic. The natural course tends to a spontaneous resolution and disappearance of the central lesion. Later, complete resolution leads to repigmentation of the site [1].

Diagnosis Dermoscopy reveals in the center of these lesions usually a regular pigmented network, dots and globules, an amorphous area, or a pseudonetwork pattern when lesions are located on the face. During involution, these structures disappear. The histologic examination reveals reduction or absence of melanin and dense inflammatory infiltrate around the central lesion.

Therapeutic Approach The prognosis for benign lesions is excellent, but attention must be directed to the rare cases in which a malignant melanoma or metastatic lesions of this tumor

may be the affected lesion [1]. The correct management consists in the clinical and the dermatoscopic observation of central lesion. With benign characteristics (color, regularity, shape, development) and its permanence over the consultations, the lesion may be observed until it has resolved. Lesions with unusual appearance and evolution require surgical excision of the central tumor and its surrounding halo [1].

Nevus Spilus

Concepts and Clinical Presentation Nevus spilus (speckled lentiginous nevus, zosteriform lentiginous nevus) is a solitary, flat, brown patch dotted by smaller dark brown to blackish brown freckle-like areas of pigmentation ranging from 1 to 6 mm of diameter (Fig. 60.4). These dots vary from junctional and compound nevi to Spitz and blue nevi. Nevus spilus may vary from 1 to 20 cm in diameter and appear on any area of the face, trunk, or extremities without relation to sun exposure. Larger lesions may be unilateral or segmental, or follow Blaschko lines affecting substantial parts of the skin (a limb, trunk). It is a common disorder, usually presenting at birth, although it may appear at any age and persists indefinitely. Males and females are equally affected. Nevus spilus should be considered with the same potential for neoplastic change as any other pigmented nevus.

Diagnosis The dermoscopy presents a thin and bright reticular background and outbreaks with pigmented network and aggregated globules.

Therapeutic Approach There are reports about dysplastic transformation or melanomas appearing from these lesions. For this reason, periodic clinical and photographic observation is recommended. In addition, biopsy and surgical excision is necessary for lesions with typical dysplasia or a clearly documented onset [10].

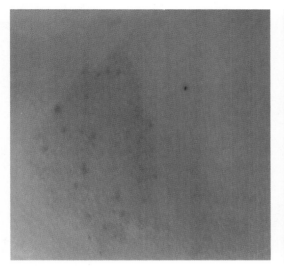

Fig. 60.4 Nevus spilus

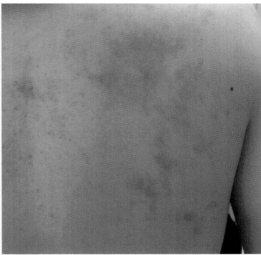

Fig. 60.5 Becker's nevus on the back

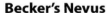

Becker's Nevus

Concepts Becker's nevus (pigmented hairy nevus or nevus spilus tardus) may begin in childhood or shortly after puberty. It is six times more common in males than in females and may occur in all races [11]. The pathogenesis is unclear, but the clinical features seen in individuals with this disorder suggest a localized increase in androgen sensitivity. Furthermore, a familial occurrence seen in some patients demonstrates a genetic influence [12]. The association with other abnormalities (such as unilateral breast, areolar hypoplasia, pectus carinatum, spina bifida) suggests an organoid nevus, as a part of the spectrum of epidermal nevi and the epidermal nevus syndrome [13]. There are no nevus cells and no increases in the number of melanocytes; therefore, malignant transformation does not occur.

Clinical Presentation and Diagnosis Becker's nevus is a relatively frequent and asymptomatic disorder. Usually it begins as a grayish brown pigmentation, unilateral on the chest, back, or upper arm, that spreads in an irregular format until it reaches an area 10–15 cm in diameter (Fig. 60.5), often surrounded by islands of blotchy pigmentation. It has been reported on other areas of the trunk, face, neck wrist, buttocks, and shins. After 1–2 years coarse hairs appear in the region. The hairy area does not necessarily coincide with the pigmented area. The hyperpigmentation and hypertrichosis tend to persist for life. Acneiform lesions have been described in association with Becker's nevus.

Histopathologic features reveal epidermal thickening, elongation of the rete ridges, and hyperpigmentation of the basal layer. Network, focal hypopigmentation, skin furrow hypopigmentation, hair follicles, perifollicular hypopigmentation, and vessels are the main dermoscopic features. Differential diagnosis includes congenital melanocytic nevus, plexiform neurofibroma, and smooth muscle hamartoma.

Therapeutic Approach The treatment of this disorder is purely cosmetic (electrolysis, depilation, camouflage), and therapy with lasers have also been described (Q-switched, Nd:YAG) [14].

Freckles

Concepts, Clinical Presentation, and Diagnosis Freckles (ephelides) are red or light brown circumscribed macules, round, oval, or irregular, usually less than 5 mm in diameter. These lesions appear in early childhood, generally between 2 and 4 years of age, especially on sun-exposed areas of the skin (face, shoulders, upper back), and tend to fade during the winter and in adult life (Fig. 60.6) [1]. It appears to be inherited as an autosomal dominant trait linked with a tendency to fair skin and red or reddish-brown hair. There is seasonal variation in their appearance. They become darker and more confluent during the summer and are smaller and lighter during the winter [1]. The sun increases the melanogenesis and the transport of melanosomes to keratinocytes. Freckles do not have tendency to malignant transformation.

Histopathologic features include increased melanin pigmentation of the basal layer without an increase in the number of melanocytes, which are more arborized and reactive to dopa than adjacent skin and also contain more melanosomes [1].

Therapeutic Approach The treatment is based on avoidance of sun exposure and covering makeup. Sunscreens permit a more uniform tan whereby freckling is less pronounced. Peeling, cryotherapy, and hydroquinone use may be partially effective. Laser therapy also is effective.

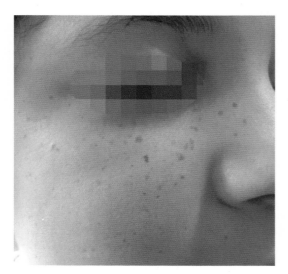

Fig. 60.6 Freckles

Lentigines

Lentigines are seen in all races and equally in both sexes. They are small, tan, dark brown or black, flat, oval, or circular lesions. They usually begin in childhood and may increase in number during adult life. They vary from 1 to 5 mm in diameter and may occur on any cutaneous surface or, occasionally, on the mucous membrane or conjunctiva of the eyes. The pigmentation is uniform and darker than that seen in ephelides, and the color is unaffected by sun exposure [1]. They may occur as a single lesion or be multiple. Generalized or multiple lentigines can be an isolated phenomenon with no disease involved, present at birth or later in childhood or adult life. However, lentigines may be seen genetic diseases with other multiple clinical manifestations, such as leopard syndrome, Peutz–Jeghers syndrome.

In mucous membranes lentigines often have nonhomogeneous irregular borders, with areas lacking pigmentation and varying in size and number. These lesions may grow slowly during months or years and also present with or without variations in pigmentation.

Solar Lentigines (Senile Lentigines, Liver Spots)

Concepts and Clinical Presentation Solar lentigines are multiple light or dark brown macules related to solar explosion. They usually appear in the Caucasian population older than 60 years and are located on the forearms, face, chest, neck, and dorsal area of the hands (Fig. 60.7). However, they may also be observed in younger adults with heavy solar exposure. The shape of these lesions is well circumscribed or confluent, oval to round, varying from 3 mm to 2 cm in diameter. They may slowly disappear with sun protection. Solar lentigines are an independent risk factor for the development of melanoma.

Diagnosis For the evaluation of these lesions it may be necessary to use Wood's lamp, dermoscopy, and histopathologic examination. Differential diagnosis includes junctional and compound melanocytic nevi, ephelides, actinic

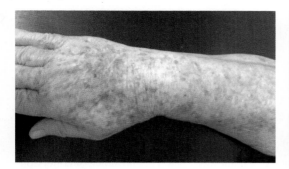

Fig. 60.7 Solar lentigines

keratosis, pigmented actinic keratosis, seborrheic keratosis, hemangioma, cutaneous hemorrhage, and cutaneous melanoma.

Dermoscopy demonstrates a faint pigmented network, fingerprint structures, or uniform pigmentation.

Histopathologic features include an increase in the number of melanocytes just above the basal layer, and an increase of melanization of the keratinocytes of the basal layer. The etiology is unknown but seems to be related to genetic modifications of the neural crest.

Therapeutic Approach Treatment other than for cosmetic purposes is ordinarily not indicated. For senile lentigines, it is important to monitor for melanoma or nonmelanoma cutaneous cancer. Clarifying agents are not effective, although cryotherapy and laser surgery may help. Prevention with sun protection is necessary [1, 6].

Café-au-Lait Spots

Concepts, Clinical Presentation, and Diagnosis Café-au-lait spots are large flat lesions, round or oval, of light brown to dark brown pigmentation, found in 10–20% of normal individuals. They may occur anywhere on the skin and are frequently present at birth. In addition, they may be unique or multiple, often increasing in number and size with age. They vary from 1.5 cm or less to 15–20 cm in diameter (Fig. 60.8). The average size varies from 2 to 5 cm in adults. These macules may be a sign of neurofibromatosis and may be associated with other neurocutaneous disease, for example McCune–Albright

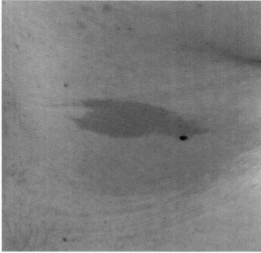

Fig. 60.8 Café-au-lait spot on the back

syndrome. There is no risk of malignancy. Multiple lesions are rare in the normal population and should alert the physician to the possibility of an associated disease [1].

Café-au-lait spots occur in 90% of patients with neurofibromatosis. Characteristically, six or more lesions greater than 1.5 cm in diameter may be observed in this disease. Smaller spots in the axilla, called axillary freckling, may also serve as a valuable diagnostic sign of neurofibromatosis (Crowe's sign). In addition there is an increased incidence of café-au-lait spots in patients with tuberous sclerosis, epidermal nevus syndrome, Bloom's syndrome, Sylver's syndrome, basal cell nevus syndrome, Gaucher's disease, ataxia-telangiectasia, and Turner's syndrome [6].

Histopathologic examination reveals an increase in pigment in the basal layer of the epidermis. Ultrastructural examination may reveal giant pigmented granules in the keratinocytes and melanocytes, particularly in those of individuals with neurofibromatosis [1]. The number of melanocytes per unit area in patients with neurofibromatosis may be increased, decreased, or equal to that in normal-appearing surrounding skin [15]. Differential diagnosis includes nevus spilus, Becker's melanosis, mastocytoma, postinflammatory hyperpigmentation, acquired melanocytic nevus, congenital nevus, and lentigines.

Therapeutic Approach Treatment is unnecessary [1]. The results with hydroquinone and laser therapy are poor with a high risk of hyperpigmentation. Camouflage can help for cosmetic appearance.

Dermal Melanocytic Lesions

Mongolian Spots

Concepts, Clinical Presentation, and Diagnosis Mongolian spots are flat dark brown to gray or blue-black large macular lesions, poorly circumscribed and reaching more than 20 cm. They may present as a single or multiple lesions, usually located over the lumbosacral area, buttocks, lower limbs, and shoulders of normal infants (Fig. 60.9). It may be seen in all races, especially in blacks, Asians, Indians, Hispanics, and less frequently in Caucasians (9.8%) [1]. The spots develop in utero, present at birth, in both sexes, and often fade during the first 1 or 2 years of life [1]. Occasionally they persists into adulthood, although these lesions usually disappear by 7–13 years of age [16].

The color seen is a result of the presence of melanocytes located deep in the dermis, probably as a result of an arrest during their embryonic migration from neural crest to the epidermis where they suffer cellular death. The blue color depends on the Tyndall effect (a phenomenon whereby light passing through skin is scattered as it strikes particles of melanin). Colors of shorter wavelengths (blue, indigo, and violet) are scattered to the side and backward to the skin surface, thus creating the blue-black or slate-gray discoloration [1].

Clinical morphology aids the differential diagnosis with nevus of Ota and nevus de Ito, maculous blue nevus, trauma, and hemangiomas. When in doubt, the diagnosis may be confirmed by histopathologic examination of lesions. Histopathology shows the presence of collections of elongated, slender, spindle-shaped, dopa-positive melanocytes that run in parallel to the skin surface, deep within the dermis or around the cutaneous appendages.

Therapeutic Approach Treatment is unnecessary. Cosmetic camouflage and laser therapy may help [1, 6].

Nevus of Ota

Concepts, Clinical Presentation, and Diagnosis Nevus of Ota (nevus fuscoceruleus ophthalmomaxillaris) represents a bluish gray discoloration of the skin of the face, usually unilateral. Size and shape may vary (round, oval, serrated) and the lesion is located on the skin supplied by the first and second divisions of the trigeminal nerve, especially the periorbital region, the forehead, nose, malar area, and temple (Fig. 60.10). In 5–15% of patients nevus of Ota may be bilateral,

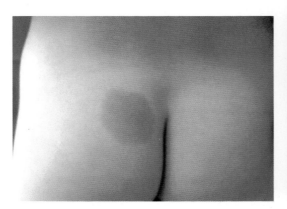

Fig. 60.9 Mongolian spot

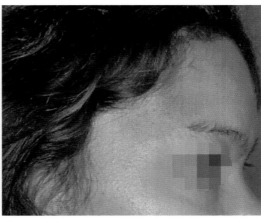

Fig. 60.10 Nevus of Ota

and in many cases the lips, palate, pharynx, eardrum, and nasal mucosa are involved. About two-thirds of patients have a patchy bluish discoloration of the sclera of the ipsilateral eye, occasionally also affecting the conjunctiva, cornea, retina, iris, and optic nerve. It may grow with time and generally persists throughout life (although some have been observed to fade over the course of years). Malignant transformation and sensorineural deafness are rare [1].

Approximately 50% of lesions are congenital; the remainder appear during the second decade (puberty) or are associated with pregnancy. Most commonly seen in Asians and blacks, it has been described also in Caucasians. It is more commonly seen in females (80% occur in females) [1].

The characteristic color is due to the production of melanin from dendritic and elongated melanocytes located in dermis, especially in the upper-third portion, scattered among the collagen bundles.

Considering the colors, shapes, and histopathologic features, the nevus of Ito (nevus fuscoceruleus acromiodeltoideus), differs from nevus of Ota by its location. It tends to involve the shoulder, supraclavicular areas, sides of the neck, and the upper arm, scapular, and deltoid regions. It may occur alone or be seen in conjunction with the nevus of Ota.

Mongolian spots, blue nevus, facial melasma, nevus spilus, and vascular malformations are part of differential diagnosis.

Therapeutic Approach Monitoring of glaucoma and ocular melanoma by the ophthalmologist is important. Cosmetic camouflage is necessary in many cases. Successful treatment has been obtained with laser ablation by Q-switched ruby, alexandrite, and Nd:YAG lasers [17, 20].

Blue Nevi

Concepts, Clinical Presentation, and Diagnosis Blue nevi (blue nevi of Jadassohn–Tièche) usually are acquired in childhood and adolescence, although 25% appear in adult life. They are benign tumors constituted by dermal melanocytes. These lesions represent hamartomas

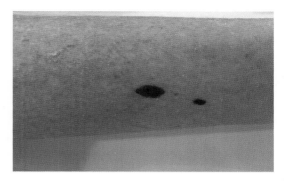

Fig. 60.11 Blue nevi in arm

that result from the arrested embryonal migration of melanocytes limited to the dermal–epidermal junction. Their color is the result of the Tyndall phenomenon. Blue nevi may be divided in two groups: common and cellular.

Common blue nevi are small, round or oval, dark blue or bluish black, smooth-surfaced and sharply circumscribed lesions (Fig. 60.11). In addition, they may be a slightly elevated dome-shaped nodule or plaque ranging from 2 to 10 mm in diameter. Usually isolated, they may occur on any part of the body. Areas of predilection include the buttocks, dorsal aspect of the hands and feet, scalp, and extensor surfaces of the forearms. Blue nevi usually remain unchanged and persist throughout life. Malignant degeneration of this type is rare. Dermoscopy of common blue nevi is characterized for its grayish blue or blackened blue homogeneous pigmentation [1].

Histopathologic examination reveals compactly arranged and elongated spindle-shaped, flattened, or fusiform melanocytes grouped in irregular bundles, mainly in the middle and lower third of the dermis. These cells have long dendritic processes, with their long axes parallel to the epidermis. Occasionally the melanocytes may extend to subcutaneous layer or epidermis. The amount of collagen is usually increased, giving a fibrous appearance [6].

Cellular blue nevi are less common and larger than common blue nevi, generally measuring more than 1 cm in diameter. They present as blue or grayish blue, smooth-surfaced nodules or plaques occasionally with an irregular surface. Cellular blue nevi appear in a relatively high incidence over the buttocks, sacrococcygeal areas, and dorsal aspect of hands and feet, although common blue nevi are five times more common. There is a low risk of malignant transformation, which should be suspected if the following features are observed: sudden increase in size with multinodular appearance, asymmetry, infiltrative changes, and ulceration. They are locally aggressive, more common on the scalp, and in about 5% may present with the risk of producing regional lymph node metastases. Except for the local involvement, patients may be asymptomatic for many years after the primary tumor excision [1].

Histopathology reveals nodular islands composed of densely packed, large, rounded, or spindle-shaped cells with variously shaped nuclei and abundant pale cytoplasm. Round islands of these melanocytes are often seen in the subcutaneous layer and may appear atypical with nuclear pleomorphism.

Traumatic tattoos, vascular lesions, primary melanoma and its metastasis, atypical nevi, dermatofibroma, pigmented basal cell carcinoma, apocrine hidrocystoma, nevi of Ota, hamartomas, and spindle cell nevus are part of the differential diagnosis of blue nevi.

Therapeutic Approach The treatment for lesions of less than 1 cm diameter is conservative. Larger lesions with atypical characteristics, a multinodular or patch aspect, asymmetry, or undergoing any transformation should be considered for histopathologic examination. Many authors consider the treatment of choice for both types of blue nevus to be conservative surgical excision with careful histologic examination. Patients who have cellular blue nevi should be examined for the presence of regional lymphadenopathy [1].

Pigmented Lesions Important in the Differential Diagnosis of Melanoma (See Also Chap. 14)

Spitz Nevus

Concepts, Clinical Presentation, and Diagnosis Spitz nevus (spindle cell nevus, spindle

and epithelioid nevus) is a benign lesion of melanocytic origin that can occur anywhere on the cutaneous surface, more often on the face, usually the cheek of children and adolescents. It is believed that about 1% of lesions surgically removed from children exhibited histologic characteristics of Spitz nevus, in any age group and in both sexes. These lesions have certain histologic features that may resemble malignant melanoma and may be a cause of concern to physicians and pathologists [18]. No etiologic factors have been identified, but eruptive cases have been identified in immunosuppressed patients and pregnancy.

Clinically the lesions present as a smooth-surfaced, hairless, dome-shaped papule or nodule with a distinctive reddish brown color, usually single or less often multiple. Spitz nevi may vary in size from a few millimeters to several centimeters, usually ranging from 0.6 to 1 cm in diameter (Fig. 60.12). In some lesions, particularly those on the extremities, the reddish color is replaced by a mottled brown to tan or black appearance, often with a verrucous surface and an irregular margin [1]. Multiple or disseminated cases may be seen with hundreds of lesions of sudden onset, on any part of the body, with the exception of palms, soles, and mucous membranes. These cases tend to be polymorphic, more often in adults, with a possibility of spontaneous regression and no reported cases of malign transformation [1].

Atypical cases have one or more characteristics that differ from conventional lesions, such as larger size, asymmetry, ulceration, pagetoid

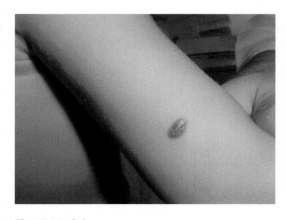

Fig. 60.12 Spitz nevus

dissemination, or high density of melanocytes in dermis.

The histologic pattern of this disorder appears to be a variant of the compound nevus. The nevus cells are pleomorphic and generally consist of spindle-shaped and, less frequently, polygon-shaped epithelioid cells. Multinucleated giant cells and mitotic figures complete the histopathologic features. This benign tumor can be differentiated from malignant melanoma by the presence of spindle and giant cells, and absence or sparseness of melanin, edema, and telangiectasia of the stroma and increased maturation of the tumor cells in the deeper aspect of the dermis. Important characteristics that aid the diagnosis are recognition that the cells are larger than those of common melanocytic nevi and the coalescent eosinophilic globules resembling colloid bodies (Kamino bodies), which are present in the basal layer above the tips of dermal papillae [1, 19, 20].

The differential diagnosis includes intradermal nevi, pyogenic granulomas, juvenile xanthogranulomas, hemangiomas, adnexal tumors, dermatofibromas, mastocytomas, and malignant melanomas.

Therapeutic Approach There is controversy regarding the management of these lesions. Some authors take a conservative approach, because the histopathologic appearance of incompletely removed lesions or biopsied lesions that leave a slight residual cellular or vascular component may be misinterpreted as malignant melanoma. Total conservative surgical excision is frequently recommended. In addition, other authors recommend removal with at least 1 cm of margin for atypical lesions and a periodic evaluation every 6 or 12 months.

Reed Tumor

Concepts, Clinical Presentation, and Diagnosis Reed tumor represents a pigmented form of Spitz nevus. They are less common than Spitz nevi and are seen especially in women of a mean age of 25 years. These lesions present with a mottled brown to tan or black appearance and

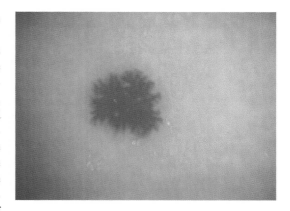

Fig. 60.13 Reed tumor

are uniform in color, often with a verrucous surface and irregular margin (this lesion may easily be confused with a malignant melanoma). In addition, Reed tumors may be flat or slightly elevated in shape, usually measuring an average of 4 mm (variation at 1.5–10 mm), particularly on the extremities. Dermoscopy often demonstrates a dark central area without structures, with globules or pseudopodia on the periphery, symmetrically arranged (Fig. 60.13). Variations in this pattern are seen in atypical cases [1, 6].

The differential diagnosis includes melanoma, atypical nevus, blue nevus, angiokeratoma, and pigmented basal cell carcinoma.

The principal histologic characteristics are ribbons of thin and uniform fusiform cells closely organized with granular melanin and streaky tissue slits. The nuclear appearance is homogeneous with subdued chromatin. The histopathologic examination is essential for the correct diagnosis [1, 6].

Therapeutic Approach The natural evolution is unknown. The knowledge about the association of atypical variants with melanoma is evidence of this rare transformation. The recommended treatment is total surgical excision with free margins to avoid recurrence. The pathologic characteristics of Reed tumor are extremely difficult to distinguish from melanoma. When atypical characteristics are seen, surgical excision is recommended with margins between 5 and 10 mm and medical monitoring for 6 or 12 months [1, 6].

Recurrent Nevus

Concepts and Clinical Presentation A recurrent or a persistent nevus is the development of a melanocytic lesion where a previous benign nevus was removed [21]. Many times it may clinically, dermoscopically, and histologically resemble melanoma, for which reason it has been called "pseudomelanoma." However, many authors find this term confusing and misleading, since recurrent nevi are benign and should not be mistaken for recurrent melanomas.

Recurrent nevi occur after incomplete removal of a melanocytic nevus. It may be observed after shave biopsies, electrocoagulation, or laser therapy [21]. The occurrence of this phenomenon can be explained by the reminiscent melanocytes in the adnexal structures, which migrate into the regenerating epithelium [22, 23]. During the healing process and scar formation, these melanocytes may be stimulated to proliferate [21].

Clinically, recurrent nevi are characterized by dark brown to black pigment in the scar, often exhibiting bizarre forms [21, 24]. Lesions may also display asymmetry (Fig. 60.14) [21, 24]. Various reports have stated that when recurrence of pigmentation is confined to the scar, this is a sign of benignity, such as recurrent nevi. Usually pigmentation of recurrent nevi develops for a limited period and stabilizes, sometimes even fading over time [25].

Recurrent nevi occur more frequently in females under the age of 40 years and in lesions excised on the back, followed by the abdomen and extremities [22, 26]. Usually the pigmentation

recurs within 6 months after the initial procedure [22, 27]. The majority of recurrent nevi may be observed after removal of ordinary nevi, followed by dysplastic nevus [22, 26]. Additional studies have shown that in 23% of cases of recurrent nevi the primary lesion appeared to be completely removed in the histopathologic report [22] and that only 75% of recurrent nevi had previous positive margins [26].

The most important differential diagnosis with recurrent nevi is recurrent melanoma (Tables 60.1 and 60.2) [25]. With the objective of studying the diagnostic differences between these lesions, a multicenter study was conducted in 2014 [28]. The authors found that patients with recurrent melanoma had a longer time interval between the procedures (median 25 months), while recurrent nevi occurred more quickly (median 8 months) [28]. Also, to help differentiation between both entities, the study defined dermoscopic characteristics for recurrent nevi and recurrent melanomas. Recurrent nevi were characterized by radial lines, symmetry, and a centrifugal growth pattern. Meanwhile, recurrent melanomas showed eccentric pigmentation at the periphery, a chaotic and noncontinuous growth pattern, and pigmentation beyond the scar's edge. In addition, it was found that recur-

Table 60.1 Clinical differences between recurrent nevi and melanoma [23–25, 28]

Recurrent nevi	Recurrent melanoma
Usually occurs with 6 months of the procedure	Usually occurs within a longer interval (median 24 months)
Usually fades over time	Progressive growth

Table 60.2 Dermoscopic differences between recurrent nevi and melanoma [23–25, 28]

Recurrent nevi	Recurrent melanoma
Pigmentation within scar area	Pigmentation extends beyond scar's edge
Centrifugal growth pattern	Chaotic growth pattern
Segmental Radial lines	Circles (especially visualized in facial lesions)
Symmetry	Asymmetry
–	Eccentric pigmentation at the periphery

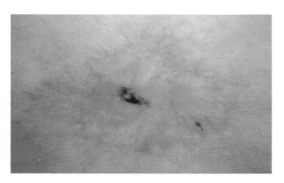

Fig. 60.14 Recurrent nevus

rent melanomas may display a circular pattern; however, most lesions included in this subgroup were on the face, a possible confounder [28]. Also, authors found that the presence of globules and heterogeneous pigmentation were the strongest dermoscopic findings related to recurrent nevi, followed by irregular network and absence of streaks [28].

Another differential diagnosis to recurrent nevi is reactive pigmentation. This entity tends to extend perpendicular to the main axis of the scar, and shows a regular pigmented network and thin continuous streaks [29].

Three zones may be seen in histology: intraepidermal alterations that can be mistaken for melanoma, as a junctional melanocytic component with varying degrees of pigmentation; fibrotic scar tissue; and below this, the residual intradermal component of the melanocytic lesion may be seen [21]. It is possible to observe a histologic overlap with primary melanoma in some cases, especially when a retiform epidermis and atypical features are found, such as a confluent growth pattern, pagetoid spread, and cytologic spread [22].

Immunohistochemical analysis may be useful to help differentiate atypical recurrent nevi and melanoma. In recurrent nevi, labeling for gp100 (with HMB-45) is strong only in the junctional portion, while in melanomas it is found to be strong in both the junctional and deep dermal components [31]. Furthermore, tyrosinase and Ki-67 demonstrate a maturation pattern in recurrent nevi, whereby the strongest labeling is seen in the junctional component, with a progressive reduction throughout the dermis. The Ki-67 junctional proliferation rate is also found to be less than 5%. By contrast, melanoma expresses tyrosinase throughout the whole lesion and the proliferation rate is much higher [30].

Diagnosis To confirm the exact diagnosis of a recurrent nevus and exclude the possibility of recurrent melanoma, it is recommended to review the original histopathologic slides [21]. The importance of analyzing the first original sections lies in the fact that in only 67% of cases is it possible to correctly predict the original melanocytic lesion [26].

Therapeutic Approach In cases where there is no previous histopathologic diagnosis, excision and histopathologic examination are mandatory to rule out melanoma. With the confirmation of a benign nevus, no further treatment is necessary.

Whenever melanoma is suspected or the diagnosis is unclear, the lesion should be completely excised [21]. Partial biopsies may be problematic when trying to differentiate recurrent nevi from atypical melanocytic proliferations and melanoma. Cases in which biopsies were thought to represent recurrent nevi but the re-excised lesion showed unequivocal melanoma have been described [22].

Atypical Nevus

Concepts Atypical nevi, also known as Clark nevi, are benign melanocytic lesions that may share clinical and dermoscopic features with melanoma [31]. To date, the correct terminology between atypical and dysplastic nevus has been controversial. Often the term "atypical nevus" is clinically used to describe potentially suspicious lesions, which could present with histologic dysplasia. However, there is not always a clinical and histologic correlation [32, 33]. Therefore, many authors encourage the use of the term "atypical nevi" in the clinical setting, while "dysplastic nevi" is used as a histologic description [21, 34].

In 1992, an expert panel organized by the NIH Consensus Development Conference proposed abandoning the term "dysplastic nevus" and reinforced the terms "atypical nevus" [35]. This approach was justified based on two common errors: viewing different grading steps of dysplasia as a progression toward melanoma or stating that dysplastic nevus would be a "premalignant lesion" [32]. Many have even advocated the term "Clark nevus" to honor its first descriptor, as referred below, and to reaffirm the idea that it is simply a nevus variant [32]. In addition, many also use the term "nevus with architectural disorder" [32].

The first description regarding atypical nevi and melanoma was introduced by Clark and coworkers in 1978, termed the B-K mole syndrome [36]. The letters B and K stood for the initials of the two affected families [36]. Later, Lynch et al. characterized the familiar atypical multiple mole melanoma syndrome (FAMMM), referring to patients with a similar phenotypic nevus in a melanoma-prone family [37]. In addition, Elder et al. [38] described the "dysplastic nevus syndrome" with familiar and sporadic variants. Later on, Rigel et al. [39] created a melanoma risk classification for patients with dysplastic nevus syndrome, according to their personal and family history of melanoma. Thus, both groups showed that there is a broad melanoma risk spectrum regarding this syndrome, ranging from isolated cases of individuals with only atypical moles to the description of FAMMM syndrome [40].

The exact prevalence of dysplastic nevus is unknown, because the majority of studies do not include histologic confirmation. Regarding the clinical classification, the estimated frequency of atypical nevi is 2–10% of the population [21, 41].

Diagnosis Atypical nevi usually appear during puberty, although they may develop throughout life [32]. Often atypical nevi are located in intermittently sun-exposed areas, such as the trunk and extremities. However, they may also appear in sun protected areas [31].

Many clinical criteria for atypical nevi overlap with those of early melanomas [21]. Tucker et al. clinically defined atypical nevus characteristics: variable pigmentation, irregular or asymmetric outline, indistinct borders, diameter over 5 mm, and a macular component [42].

Analyzing dermoscopic aspects, Hoffman-Wellenhof et al. identified six patterns, including reticular, globular, homogeneous, reticuloglobular, reticular-homogeneous, and globular-homogeneous (Fig. 60.15). Additionally the distribution of pigmentation was classified into six groups: central hyperpigmentation or hypopigmentation, eccentric peripheral hyperpigmentation or hypopigmentation, and multifocal hyperpigmentation or hypopigmentation. Similarly to common nevi, the authors found that most individuals had one predominant type of

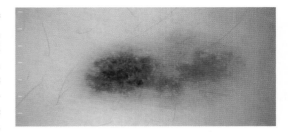

Fig. 60.15 Dermoscopy of atypical nevus

atypical nevi, also known as the signature nevi. Moreover, it was observed that eccentric peripheral hyperpigmentation is a rare (7.5%) finding in atypical nevi and should be evaluated to rule out melanoma [43].

Atypical nevi may be observed as isolated lesions or also can occur in the "atypical or dysplastic mole syndrome," which presents a broad clinical spectrum. Patients may have atypical/dysplastic nevus with no personal or family history of melanoma, while others may present with FAMMM syndrome [31]. According to the NIH Consensus statement published in 1992, the diagnosis of FAMMM or dysplastic nevus syndrome requires: occurrence of melanoma in one or more first or second degree relatives; presence of a large quantity of nevi (>50), some of which are clinically atypical; and nevi with distinct histologic features [35]. Compared with the general population, FAMMM carriers have a 150-fold greater risk of developing melanoma.

Histologic criteria for classification of dysplastic nevus may be divided into architectural and cellular [21]. Regarding architectural aspects, atypical nevus may display irregular nests at the junctional zone, bridging (horizontal anastomosis) between these nests, and the "shoulder phenomenon," which occurs when junctional nests extend beyond the dermal component [21]. Furthermore, lamellar or concentric fibroplasia (a dense extracellular matrix around the epidermal ridges) may be observed, as well as initial migration of single cell elements or nests through the epidermis [21]. At the cellular level, atypical melanocytes, nuclear polymorphism, and shift of the nucleus/plasma ratio may be seen [21].

In an attempt to standardize the histologic classification of dysplastic nevus, the World Health Organization enumerated major and minor criteria [44]. For establishment of the diagnosis it is necessary to have both major criteria and at least two minor criteria [44]. The major criterion is basilar proliferation of atypical melanocytes, which must extend at least three rete ridges beyond the dermal component and organization of this proliferation in a lentiginous or epithelioid-cell pattern. The minor criteria include the presence of lamellar fibrosis or concentric eosinophilic fibrosis, neovascularization, an inflammatory response, and the fusion of rete ridges [44].

There is controversy over whether dysplastic nevi may be melanoma precursors, as it is known that most do not progress to melanoma [21, 34]. Tsao et al. estimated the individual risk of a nevus (including a dysplastic nevus) transforming to melanoma is 1 in 10,000 during a lifetime [45]. In addition, only 20–30% of melanomas arise from nevi [46]. Of these nevus-derived melanomas, it appears that the incidence between common and dysplastic nevus is similar [47].

However, it is well established that atypical nevus is a phenotypic risk marker for melanoma [32]. The presence of atypical nevus, regardless of the total number of moles, increases the melanoma risk ten-fold compared with their absence [41].

Therapeutic Approach Prophylactic excision of atypical nevi is not indicated, since there is lack of evidence that the procedure reduces melanoma risk [48, 49, 50]. Also, unnecessary excisions increase costs and morbidity. Atypical lesions should only be removed when there is doubt regarding its differential diagnosis with melanoma [34, 49]. As in common nevi, atypical nevi may be removed by several techniques such as elliptical resection, shaving, or cauterization. Whenever possible, full excision should be attempted, so that the whole lesion can be assessed histologically. Therefore, a narrow excisional biopsy with 1- to 3-mm margins beyond the clinically visible pigmentation is recommended, as well as a depth sufficient to avoid transection [34]. It is known that dysplastic nevus may demonstrate heterogeneous histopathology and that melanoma may be missed through a sampling error [34, 51]. When these techniques are not possible, it is acceptable to carry out incisional punch biopsy or shaving of a more suspicious dermoscopic area [34].

The necessity of re-excision of dysplastic nevus is very controversial and there are no strong and formal recommendations. Some physicians decide to re-excise to prevent recurrence and the pseudomelanoma phenomenon. However, greater consensus exists regarding re-excision of severely dysplastic nevus, independently of margins, because of the difficulty of distinguishing it from melanoma [49]. In 2014, a panel of specialists summarized the results of several studies and established management recommendations for atypical nevus/dysplastic nevus [52, 53]. This report, authors stated that: (1) mildly and moderately dysplastic nevus with clear margins do not need to be re-excised; (2) mildly dysplastic nevus with positive margins and without clinical recurrence may be observed; (3) moderately dysplastic nevus with positive margins and without clinical recurrence possibly may be observed, although there is a lack of more formal data to verify this recommendation; (4) in cases with severe dysplasia and positive margins, re-excision is recommended with a 2–5-mm clinical margin [52, 53].

The follow-up of patients with atypical nevus includes clinical and dermoscopic evaluation every 3–6 months, which can be spaced to semi-annually or annually if lesions remain stable [54]. Patients who are at higher risk, such as those with multiple atypical lesions and personal or family history of melanoma, benefit from total body photography and digital dermoscopy [31, 54]. In addition, patients should be advised to perform self-examinations periodically and to use regular sun protection. In patients with dysplastic nevus syndrome or FAMMM, some consensus indicates annual eye examination, as there could be a greater risk of developing ocular melanoma.

Glossary

Cryotherapy A technique that uses an extremely cold liquid or instrument to freeze and destroy abnormal skin cells that require removal.

Electrolysis Electrochemical process whereby current is passed between two electrodes through an ionized solution (electrolyte) to deposit positive ions (anions) on the negative electrode (cathode) and negative ions (cations) on the positive electrode (anode). It is used for removing unwanted hair by destroying the hair root.

Hydroquinone An aromatic organic compound that is a type of phenol, having the chemical formula $C_6H_4(OH)_2$. It is prescribed to reduce pigmentation of the skin in certain conditions whereby an excess of melanin causes hyperpigmentation.

HMB-45 A monoclonal antibody that reacts against an antigen present in melanocytic tumors such as melanomas. The use of immunohistochemistry with melanocytic markers such as HMB-45 and Melan A, increases the detection rate of micrometastases.

Ki-67 The Ki-67 protein (also known as MKI67) is a cellular marker for proliferation. It is strictly associated with cell proliferation.

Leptomeningeal melanocytosis The excessive deposit of melanin by increasing the number of melanocytes, usually seen as a signal in the convexities of subarachnoid spaces, or brain parenchyma such as cerebellum, temporal lobes, pons, and medulla on noncontrast images.

Melanocytic A type of lesion that contains nevus cells (a type of melanocyte).

Peeling Peeling skin, called desquamation in medical terms, can be caused by different conditions. Very often, skin peels following chemical, thermal, or sunburn, with the latter being the most common cause.

Pseudopodia Cytoplasmic structures found in some eukaryotes. Pseudopods are one of the three locomotion modes of unicellular organisms (together with flagella and cilia). Pseudopods can also capture prey by phagocytosis.

Tyrosinase An oxidase that is the rate-limiting enzyme for controlling the production of melanin.

References

1. Hurwitz S. Cutaneous tumors in childhood. In: Hurwitz S (Org.). Clinical pediatric dermatology: a textbook of skin disorders of childhood and adolescence. Philadelphia: W.B. Saunders Company; 1993. p. 198–241.
2. Walton RG, Jacobs AH, Cox AJ. Pigmented lesions in newborn infants. Br J Dermatol. 1976;95:389–96.
3. Mishima Y. Macromolecular changes in pigmentary disorders. Arch Dermatol. 1965;91:519–57.
4. Masson P. My conception of cellular nevi. Cancer. 1951;4:9–38.
5. Braun RP, Rabinovitz HS, Oliviero M, Kopf AW, Saurat JH. Dermoscopy of pigmented skin lesions. J Am Acad Dermatol. 2005;52:109–21.
6. Barnhill RL, Rabinovitz H. Neoplasias Melanocíticas Benignas. In: Bolognia JL, Jorizzo JL, Rapini RP (Org.). Dermatologia. São Paulo: Elsevier; 2011. p. 1713–40.
7. Rhodes AR, Sober AJ, Day CL. The malignant potential of small congenital nevocellular nevi: Na estimate based on histologic study of 234 primary cutaneous melanomas. J Am Acad Dermatol. 1982;6:230–41.
8. Illig L, Weidner F, Hundeiker M, et al. Congenital nevi <10 cm as precursors to melanoma. Arch Dermatol. 1985;121:1274–81.
9. Hurwitz S. Pigmented nevi: semin. Dermatology. 1988;7:17–25.
10. Rhodes AR, Mihm MC Jr. Origin of cutaneous melanoma in a congenital dysplastic nevus spilus. Arch Dermatol. 1990;126:500–5.
11. Cohen PR. Becker's nevus. Am Fam Physician. 1988;37:221–6.
12. Fretzin DF, Whitney D. Familial Becker's nevus. J Am Acad Dermatol. 1985;12:589–90.
13. Glinick SE, Alper JC, Bogaars H, et al. Becker's melanosis: associated abnormalities. J Am Acad Dermatol. 1980;9:509–14.
14. Tse Y, Levine VJ, McClain SA, Ashinoff R. The removal of cutaneous pigmented lesions with the Q-switched ruby laser and the Q-switched Nd:YAG laser: a comparative study. J Dermatol Surg Oncol. 1994;20:795–800.
15. Jimbow K, Szabo G, Fitzpatrick TB. Ultrastructure of giant pigment granules (macromelanosomes) in cutaneous pigmented macules of neurofibromatosis. J Invest Dermatol. 1973;61:300–9.
16. Cole HN Jr, Hubler WR, Lund HZ. Persistent, aberrant Mongolian spots. Arch Dermatol Syph. 1950;61:244–60.
17. Chan HH, Ying SY, Ho HS, et al. An in vivo trial comparing the clinical efficacy and complications of Q-switched 755 nm alexandrite and Q-switched 1064 nm Nd:YAG lasers in treatment of nevus of Ota. Dermatol Surg. 2000;26:919–22.
18. Spitz S. Melanomas of childhood. Am J Pathol. 1948;24:591–602.

19. Arbuckle S, Weedon D. Eosinophilic globules in the Spitz nevus. J Am Acad Dermatol. 1982;7:324–7.

20. Paniago-Pereira C, Maize JC, Ackerman AB. Nevus of large spindle and/or epithelioid cells (Spitz's nevus). Arch Dermatol. 1978;114:1811–23.

21. Hauschild A, Egberts F, Garbe C, Bauer J, Grabbe S, Hamm H, et al. Melanocytic nevi. J Dtsch Dermatol Ges. 2011;9(9):723–34.

22. King R, Hayzen BA, Page RN, Googe PB, Zeagler D, Mihm MC Jr. Recurrent nevus phenomenon: a clinicopathologic study of 357 cases and histologic comparison with melanoma with regression. Mod Pathol. 2009;22:611–7.

23. Fox JC, Reed JA, Shea CR. The recurrent nevus phenomenon: a history of challenge, controversy, and discovery. Arch Pathol Lab Med. 2011;135:842–6.

24. Tschandl P. Recurrent nevi: report of three cases with dermatoscopic-dermatopathologic correlation. Dermatol Pract Concepts. 2013;3:29–32.

25. Kelly JW, Shen S, Pan Y, Dowling J, McLean CA. Postexcisional melanocytic regrowth extending beyond the initial scar: a novel clinical sign of melanoma. Br J Dermatol. 2014;170:961–4.

26. Sommer LL, Barcia SM, Clarke LE, Helm KF. Persistent melanocytic nevi: a review and analysis of 205 cases. J Cutan Pathol. 2011;38:503–7.

27. Dummer R, Kempf W, Burg G. Pseudomelanoma after laser therapy. Dermatology. 1998;197:71–3.

28. Blum A, Hofmann-Wellenhof R, Marghoob AA, Argenziano G, Cabo H, Carrera C, et al. Recurrent melanocytic nevi and melanomas in dermoscopy: results of a multicenter study of the International Dermoscopy Society. JAMA Dermatol. 2014; 150:138–45.

29. Botella-Estrada R, Nagore E, Sopena J, Cremades A, Alfaro A, Sanmartín O, et al. Clinical, dermoscopy and histologic correlation study of melanotic pigmentations in excision scars of melanocytic tumours. Br J Dermatol. 2006;154:478–84.

30. Hoang MP, Prieto VG, Burchette JL, Shea CR. Recurrent melanocytic nevus: a histologic and immunohistochemical evaluation. J Cutan Pathol. 2001;28:400–6.

31. Bolognia JL, Schaffer JV, Duncan KO, Ko CJ. Neoplasms of the skin. In: Bolognia JL, Schaffer JV, Duncan KO, Ko CJ, editors. Dermatology essentials. EUA: Elsevier; 2014. p. 892–928.

32. Duffy K, Grossman D. The dysplastic nevus: from historical perspective to management in the modern era: part I. J Am Acad Dermatol. 2012;67:1.e1–16.

33. Antonio JR, Soubhia RM, D'Avila SC, Caldas AC, Trídico LA, Alves FT. Correlation between dermoscopic and histopathologic diagnoses of atypical nevi in a dermatology outpatient clinic of the Medical School of São José do Rio Preto, SP, Brazil. An Bras Dermatol. 2013;88:199–203.

34. Kim CC, Swetter SM, Curiel-Lewandrowski C, Grichnik JM, Grossman D, Halpern AC, et al. Addressing the knowledge gap in clinical recommendations for management and complete excision of clinically atypical nevi/dysplastic nevi: pigmented lesion subcommittee consensus statement. JAMA Dermatol. 2015;151:212–8.

35. NIH Consensus Development Conference. Diagnosis and treatment of early melanoma. Consens Statement. 1992;10:1–25.

36. Clark WHJ, Reimer RR, Greene M, Ainsworth AM, Mastrangelo MJ. Origin of familial malignant melanomas from heritable melanocytic lesions: "The B-K mole syndrome". Arch Dermatol. 1978;114:732–8.

37. Lynch HT, Fusaro RM, Pester J, Lynch JF. Familial atypical multiple mole melanoma (FAMMM) syndrome: genetic heterogeneity and malignant melanoma. Br J Cancer. 1980;42:58–70.

38. Elder DE, Goldman LI, Goldman SC, Greene MH, Clark WH Jr. Dysplastic nevus syndrome: a phenotypic association of sporadic cutaneous melanoma. Cancer. 1980;46:1787–94.

39. Rigel DS, Rivers JK, Friedman RJ, Kopf AW. Risk gradient for malignant melanoma in individuals with dysplastic naevi. Lancet. 1988;1:352–3.

40. Reimer RR, Clark WH Jr, Greene MH, Ainsworth AM, Fraumeni JF Jr. Precursor lesions in familial melanoma. A new genetic preneoplastic syndrome. JAMA. 1978;239:744–6.

41. Gandini S, Sera F, Cattaruzza MS, Pasquini P, Abeni D, Boyle P, et al. Meta-analysis of risk factors for cutaneous melanoma: I. Eur J Cancer. 2005;41:28–44.

42. Tucker MA, Halpern A, Holly EA, Hartge P, Elder DE, Sagebiel RW, et al. Clinically recognized dysplastic nevi. A central risk factor for cutaneous melanoma. JAMA. 1997;277:1439–44.

43. Hofmann-Wellenhof R, Blum A, Wolf IH, Piccolo D, Kerl H, Garbe C, et al. Dermoscopic classification of atypical melanocytic nevi (Clark nevi). Arch Dermatol. 2001;137:1575–80.

44. Clemente C, Cochran AJ, Elder DE, Levene A, MacKie RM, Mihm MC, et al. Histopathologic diagnosis of dysplastic nevi: concordance among pathologists convened by the World Health Organization Melanoma Programme. Hum Pathol. 1991;22:313–9.

45. Tsao H, Bevona C, Goggins W, Quinn T. The transformation rate of moles (melanocytic nevi) into cutaneous melanoma: a population-based estimate. Arch Dermatol. 2003;139:282–8.

46. Lin WM, Luo S, Muzikansky A, Lobo AZ, Tanabe KK, Sober AJ, et al. Outcome of patients with de novo versus nevus-associated melanoma. J Am Acad Dermatol. 2015;72:54–8.

47. Fuller SR, Bowen GM, Tanner B, Florell SR, Grossman D. Digital dermoscopic monitoring of atypical nevi in patients at risk for melanoma. Dermatol Surg. 2007;33:1198–206.

48. Arumi-Uria M, McNutt NS, Finnerty B. Grading of atypia in nevi: correlation with melanoma risk. Mod Pathol. 2003;16:764–71.

49. Duffy K, Grossman D. The dysplastic nevus: from historical perspective to management in the modern era: part II. J Am Acad Dermatol. 2012;67:19. e1–12.

50. Halpern AC, Guerry D 4th, Elder DE, Trock B, Synnestvedt M, Humphreys T. Natural history of dysplastic nevi. J Am Acad Dermatol. 1993;29:51–7.
51. Barr RJ, Linden KG, Rubinstein G, Cantos KA. Analysis of heterogeneity of atypia within melanocytic nevi. Arch Dermatol. 2003;139:289–92.
52. Strazzula L, Vedak P, Hoang MP, Sober A, Tsao H, Kroshinsky D. The utility of re-excising mildly and moderately dysplastic nevi: a retrospective analysis. J Am Acad Dermatol. 2014;71:1071–6.
53. Hocker TL, Alikhan A, Comfere NI, Peters MS. Favorable long-term outcomes in patients with histologically dysplastic nevi that approach a specimen border. J Am Acad Dermatol. 2013;68:545–51.
54. Silva JH, Sá BC, Avila AL, Landman G, Duprat Neto JP. Atypical mole syndrome and dysplastic nevi: identification of populations at risk for developing melanoma – review article. Clinics (Sao Paulo). 2011;66:493–9.

Suggested Literature

Farber MJ, Heilman ER, Friedman RJ. Dysplastic nevi. Dermatol Clin. 2012;30:389–404.
Kittler H, Tschandl P. Dysplastic nevus: why this term should be abandoned in dermatoscopy. Dermatol Clin. 2013;31:579–88.
Marghoob AA. Recurrent (persistent) nevi. In: Marghoob AA, Malvehy J, Braun RP, editors. Atlas of dermoscopy. London: Informa Healthcare; 2012. p. 198–202.
Nestle FO, Halpern AC. Melanoma. In: Bolognia JL, Jorizzo JL, Rapini RP (Org.). Dermatology. EUA: Elsevier; 2008. p. 1745–70.
Rosendahl CO, Grant-Kels JM, Que SK. Dysplastic nevus: fact and fiction. J Am Acad Dermatol. 2015;73:507–12.

Pruritus

61

Magda Blessmann Weber
and Fernanda Oliveira Camozzato

"Itch is an unpleasant sensation which evokes the desire to scratch"

Samuel Hafenreffer, 1660

Key Points

- Pruritus is the most common dermatologic symptom and is the main symptom of several dermatoses; it also frequently occurs in systemic diseases
- It may manifest many years before systemic diseases, including malignant ones. In some cases, it is the first symptom of malignant systemic diseases
- Several etiopathologic mechanisms may cause pruritus with peripheral or central origin
- Patient assessment includes complete clinical history, detailed history of pruritus, and additional tests
- Patient management requires treatment of symptoms and underlying diseases
- Providing follow-up and orientation is essential in the management of patients with chronic pruritus. Psychological assessment is required for these patients.

M.B. Weber, MD, PhD (✉)
Dermatology Service of Federal University of Health Sciences of Porto Alegre, Porto Alegre, Brazil
e-mail: mbw@terra.com.br

F.O. Camozzato
Brazilian Center for Studies in Dermatology, Porto Alegre, Brazil

Concepts

Pruritus was defined by Samuel Hafenreffer in 1660 as an unpleasant sensation that causes the desire or reflex to scratch [1]. This condition is the most frequent symptom of dermatologic diseases and also the one that better defines these diseases; additionally, it may be present in several systemic diseases. Pruritus may be disseminated or localized, affecting the skin surface; the squamous epithelium of the conjunctiva, mouth, nose, pharynx, and anogenital region; and the ciliated epithelium of the trachea [2, 3]. This symptom may be intense, even when patients have no visible skin changes. Pruritic areas around the primarily stimulated site that itch even after very weak stimuli are defined as areas of alloknesis [4].

Pruritus may be acute or chronic, the latter occurring, by definition, when the symptom lasts for 6 months or more [5]. Acute pruritus, because it occurs with pain, is a defense mechanism against external harmful agents. Chronic pruritus is difficult to ignore, leading to difficulties concentrating, sleep disorders, absence from school or work, and sometimes suicide attempts in patients with more severe symptoms [3, 6]. Additionally it is associated with a considerable reduction in quality of life and may be as debilitating as chronic pain [7].

In addition to biological pruritus, triggered by several chemical mediators, itch may be also a psychosocial manifestation resulting from mechanisms of frustration, similar to what happens in nonhuman social animals (grooming) [8].

Epidemiology

Statistical data on the epidemiology of pruritus are scarce, possibly leading to an underestimation of its prevalence. This is because many studies, especially those outside the field of dermatology, do not collect data on pruritus, even when the symptom is considered as relevant by patients.

Pruritus is more common in women than in men and is more frequently diagnosed in Asians than in Caucasians [9–11]. The prevalence of pruritus increases with age, because the elderly population not only usually presents with xeroderma but also has a higher prevalence of systemic problems that cause pruritus [12, 13]. Pruritus is more prevalent among individuals of low socioeconomic status and low income [9].

A cross-sectional study including almost 19,000 adults found a prevalence of 8–9% of acute pruritus in the study population [9] and an association between pruritus and chronic pain [14]. Recent research shows that the prevalence of chronic pruritus is around 13.5% in the general adult population [10] and around 16.8% in a sample of company employees attending a routine medical appointment [12]. In a study of 18,137 individuals with skin diseases, 42% reported having pruritus [15].

Few studies evaluated the frequency of pruritus in the primary health care setting. According to data from the Bettering the Evaluation and Care of Health (BEACH) Program for the Australian population, pruritus is the main complaint at 0.6% of medical visits, excluding perianal, periorbital, or auricular pruritus [16]. The Fourth National Study of Morbidity Statistics from General Practice [17], conducted in Great Britain with 502,493

patients, found that pruritus and related conditions are reported in 1.04% of appointments (0.73% for men and 1.33% for women).

The origin of pruritus, whether dermatologic or systemic, could not be established in 8–15% of patients [13]. However, in systemic diseases that cause pruritus its prevalence may be very high, as is the case with hemodialysis patients, who may present with pruritus in up to 90% of cases [18]. This symptom may be present in up to 50% of patients with cholestasis, in 80–100% of those with primary biliary cirrhosis, in up to 80% of those with cutaneous T-cell lymphoma, in up to 50% of those with polycythemia vera, and in up to 30% of those with Hodgkin's lymphoma [6]. In dermatologic diseases, the frequency of pruritus is relevant and depends on the underlying disease; it is present, for example, in all patients with urticaria and atopic dermatitis [19].

Classification

Pruritus may be of peripheral or central origin, and the perception of this symptom depends on the neurophysiologic and psychological changes it causes. Patients may report different sensations to define pruritus, such as itch, bite, tingle, perforation, pinch, and burn [6].

A neurophysiologic classification of the type of pruritus was proposed and is important both for patient management and for understanding of disease mechanisms. More than one form of pruritus may coexist in the same patient, for example, atopic individuals who present with neurogenic and pruritoceptive pruritus. In 2003 Twycros et al. [3] proposed a neurophysiologic classification:

(a) Pruritoceptive or dermal pruritus: induced by stimulation of C-nerve fibers by different pruritogens. It originates in the skin and may be caused by inflammatory mechanisms, xeroderma, or direct skin damage. It is present in scabies, urticaria, and insect bites

(b) Neuropathic pruritus: resulting from lesions at any point of the afferent nervous pathway, such as occurs in postherpetic neuralgia, multiple sclerosis, and brain tumors

(c) Neurogenic pruritus: of central origin, but there are no lesions to nervous fibers. It results from an increase in the concentration of endogenous opioids, as in cholestasis and after the administration of exogenous opioids

(d) Psychogenic pruritus: triggered by psychiatric diseases such parasitophobia or by psychological factors such as anxiety disorders

Another classification of pruritus was defined by the International Forum for the Study of Itch (IFSI) in 2007 [5]. This classification is divided into two parts and gives priority to the clinical manifestations of pruritus, distinguishing between disorders with or without skin lesions and whether these lesions are primary or secondary.

In the first part of classification, three groups of conditions are defined according to history and symptoms in the skin of patients with pruritus.

- *First group*: includes pruritus in primary skin diseases represented by pruritic dermatoses (inflammatory, infectious and autoimmune diseases, genodermatosis, reaction to drugs, dermatoses of pregnancy, and skin lymphomas), all of which lead to specific skin changes
- *Second group*: includes pruritus in normal skin resulting from systemic diseases (endocrine, hematologic and metabolic disorders, infections, lymphoproliferative diseases, solid neoplasms, neurologic diseases, psychiatric diseases, and drug-induced pruritus)
- *Third group*: includes chronic lesions secondary to scratching, such as prurigo nodularis or simple chronic lichen

In the second part of the classification, patients were categorized according to their underlying disease, which was divided into several categories:

I. Dermatologic disease: pruritus caused by "skin diseases" such as psoriasis, atopic dermatitis, dry skin, scabies, or urticaria

II. Systemic disease: pruritus caused by "systemic diseases" other than those affecting the skin, such as hepatic diseases (primary biliary cirrhosis), renal diseases (chronic kidney disease), hematologic diseases (Hodgkin's disease), and multifactorial causes such as metabolic or drug-induced

III. Neurologic disease: pruritus caused by "diseases of the central or peripheral nervous system" such as nerve compression, nerve damage, or nerve irritation

IV. Psychogenic or psychosomatic disease: pruritus caused by "psychiatric or psychosomatic disease"

V. Mixed: pruritus caused by the overlap and coexistence of several diseases

VI. Pruritus of undetermined origin

This classification aims to avoid unnecessary laboratory and imaging studies, as is the case in patients with typical clinical history suggestive of dermatosis-induced pruritus, when usually there is no need for further investigation.

Neurophysiology

The neuronal basis of the mechanisms underlying pruritus is complex and has been elucidated by new discoveries in the field. Skin, conjunctiva, and mucosa are the peripheral tissues that may produce a sensation of pruritus. In the skin, sensory nerves innervate epidermis, dermis, and subcutaneous adipose tissue. Free nerve endings for pruritus are located mainly at the dermoepidermal junction [20]. Electrophysiology studies of peripheral nerves in humans and animal models show that the chemical mediators of pruritus elicit action potentials in a subset of nociceptors, the pruriceptive nociceptive neurons (or pruriceptors), which are mainly amyelinic C fibers [21].

Pruritoceptors carry impulses toward the dorsal horn of the spinal cord, where they make a synapse with the secondary neuron. The axons of this neuron cross to the contralateral spinothalamic tract (STT) through the anterolateral funiculus and continue into the thalamus to terminate in the somatosensory cortex, reaching areas involved in the processes of evolution, sensation, emotion, reward, and memory, which are superposed to the areas activated by painful stimuli [22]. The transection of this ascending pathway impairs itch as well as pain and temperature sensations [23].

Electrophysiologic studies of the neurons of the STT in animal models show that nearly two-thirds of the nociceptive neurons of this tract are not pruritogenic and the other third is. Nonpruritogenic neurons of the STT are activated by mechanical stimuli, heat, or capsaicin, and pruritogenic neurons are activated both by painful stimuli such as heat or capsaicin and by pruritic stimuli such as histamine. It is still unclear whether there are specific pruritogenic neurons, i.e., that transmit only the sensation of pruritus [24, 25]. However, a recent study found that, in a genetically engineered mouse with restricted expression of the capsaicin receptor, selective activation of a class of pruriceptors by capsaicin elicits itch-like and not pain-like behavior, showing that there may be a neurologic distinction between nerve cells that cause pain and cells that cause itching [26].

As a hypothesis, itch may result from activity in the pruriceptive neurons in the absence of sufficient activity in nonpruriceptive neurons. The neural circuitry hypothesized to evaluate the relative activity in pruriceptive and nonpruriceptive neuronal populations and to decode itch from pain is unknown, but is likely to reside in suprasegmental regions of the brain [21].

Mediators of Pruritus

Pruritus is triggered by pharmacologic mediators that act on nerve endings, the so-called pruritogenic agents. These pruritogens may be located both peripherally and centrally, and many of them act synergistically, by means of a myriad of mechanisms summarized in Table 61.1.

Histamine is the main peripheral mediator of pruritus, having been acknowledged for more than 60 years, and is secreted by degranulated mast cells and circulating basophils. This substance causes pruritus by directly stimulating nerve endings and also by interacting with H1 receptors present in C fibers [27], leading to vasodilation and edema [27]. There are other histamine receptors, such as H2 and H3, but these are not linked to the mediation of pruritus, although there has been

Table 61.1 Itch mediators and corresponding antipruritic agents

Mediators of pruritus	Antipruritic agent
Histamine	Antihistamines
Serotonin	Paroxetine, fluoxetine, mirtazapine, sertraline, citalopram, ondansetron
Substance P	Aprepitant
Prostaglandins	Nonsteroidal anti-inflammatory drugs, aspirin
Opioids	Naloxone, naltrexone, nalfurafine, butorphanol
TRPV1 receptor	Capsaicin
TRPM8 receptor	Menthol
Interferon-α	Thalidomide
GABA (γ-aminobutyric acid)	Gabapentin, pregabalin
Acetylcholine	Doxepin, oxybutynin
Leukotrienes	Zafirlukast, zileuton

Adapted from Hassan and Haji [118]

an improvement of pruritus in patients with urticaria with the use of some H2 blockers. Histamine type 4 receptor (H4), present in dendritic cells, mast cells, and eosinophils, is involved in allergic inflammation [28] and also may be involved in the mediation of pruritus, making this receptor a possible new target in the management of pruritus, especially in atopic dermatitis [28]. The role of histamine in pruritic diseases such as urticaria, reactions to insect bites, skin mastocytosis, and some drug eruptions has already been established [2, 3]. However, this substance is not the main pruritogenic agent in systemic diseases, which is evidenced by the low response of patients with these diseases to antihistamine therapy [29].

Serotonin is a less potent pruritogenic agent than histamine. Its peripheral action is due to the release of histamine from mast cells [30], and its central action probably involves the neurotransmitter system of opioids and the activation of $5HT_3$ receptors, which are not found in the skin. Serotonin is also found in great amounts in platelets, a fact that may explain the presence of pruritus in hematologic diseases with platelet involvement [3].

Substance P is synthesized in the body of C-type neurons and transported through peripheral nerve endings. Intradermal injection of substance P causes pruritus, edema, and erythema, resulting in the release of tumor necrosis factor α (TNF-α), leukotriene B4, histamine, and prostaglandin D2 [31]. In atopic dermatitis, serum levels of substance P are elevated and correlated to disease severity [32]. This neuropeptide acts through the neurokinin 1 (NK1) receptor pathway. A study conducted by Costa et al. showed that aprepitant, the NK1 receptor antagonist, was tested as a potential antipruritic agent in Sézary syndrome [33]. Depletion of this substance by capsaicin is one of the mechanisms of controlling pruritus and pain [24].

Prostaglandins, considered in isolation, are not pruritogenic agents, but may potentiate the effect of histamine and of other mediators of pruritus [35]. The use of cyclooxygenase inhibitors does not improve pruritus in the general patient population, but appears to be useful in patients with human immunodeficiency virus (HIV). The use of aspirin improves pruritus in patients with polycythemia vera, probably due to the action of this drug on platelet adhesiveness rather than on the formation of prostaglandins [36].

Cytokines: The involvement of *interleukin 2* (IL-2) in the development of pruritus is based on the observation of generalized pruritus in patients using high doses of recombinant IL-2 for the treatment of cancer [37]. Patients with atopic dermatitis using cyclosporine, an IL-2 inhibitor, experience a considerable relief of pruritus. It is not clear whether this process is directly mediated by receptors or indirectly mediated by mast cells and endothelial cells. High levels of *interleukin-31* (IL-31) are present in the skin of patients with atopic dermatitis and prurigo nodularis, indicating that this substance may be a possible cause of pruritus in patients with these conditions [38, 39].

Opioid peptides may trigger pruritus by leading both to degranulation of mast cells and activation of opioid receptors, either central or peripheral. Intradermal morphine causes pruritus, which may be inhibited by topic pretreatment with doxepin (H1 antihistamine agent) [40] but may be only partially inhibited by the μ-receptor antagonist (naloxone). Intraspinal μ-opioid agonists induce segmental pruritus, a condition that may be inhibited by μ-receptor antagonists [41], but is not affected by antihistamines [41]. Additionally it has been demonstrated that the stimulation of κ-opioid receptors blocks the effect of μ-receptor agonists [42], showing that opioid-induced pruritus may be the balance of the interaction between the system of receptors μ and κ. Opioid peptide antagonists have been used in the treatment of pruritus-associated diseases in chronic kidney disease and cholestasis.

Proteolytic enzymes: Human mast cells produce two proteases: tryptase and chymase. These enzymes act on G proteins coupled to PAR-2 receptors expressed in afferent C-fiber neurons [43]. When activated, these fibers secrete substance P, which activates mast cells, thus closing the cycle that stimulates pruritus [4]. Upregulation of PAR-2 receptors has been observed in patients with atopic dermatitis [43].

Transient receptor potential channels (TRP): These molecules are calcium-permeable channels that sense temperature, osmotic, and mechanical changes. TRPV1 is present on nociceptive C neurons and is activated by capsaicin and endogenous substances (endovanilloids). Other TRPVs (TRPV2, TRPV3, TRPV4, TRPM8) are activated at specific temperatures [44]. Evidence suggests that TRPV1 is a fundamental integrating element in pruritic and pain pathways. It has been discovered that sensory neuronal activation by histamine and PAR2 receptor also involves the activation/sensitization of TRPV1, that TRPV1 expression is amplified in keratinocytes of prurigo nodularis, and that stimulation of TRPV1 channels releases multiple pruritoceptive mediators such as interleukins and neuropeptides [45]. It has been postulated that TRPV3 might be a regulator and/or cotransducer of TRPV1-mediated pruritus and pain. A study by Stokes et al. [46] showed mast cell degranulation upon thermal and physical activation of TRPV2. In addition, mast cells also express TRPV1 and TRPV4. TRP melastatin 8 (TRPM8) is expressed selectively by C-type neurons. Menthol and its analogs as well as icilin stimulate TRPM8 [47];

Neurotrophin and nerve growth factor (NGF) is overexpressed in prurigo nodularis and its therapeutic administration is pruritogenic [48]. In atopic dermatitis, NGF is released by keratinocytes, mast cells, and fibroblasts, and plasma levels of NGF are also elevated and correlate with disease activity [49]. In addition, expression of neurotrophin-4 is elevated in the cutaneous lesions of patients with atopic dermatitis and prurigo nodularis [48, 49].

Endocannabinoids and cannabinoid receptors: Cannabinoid receptors are expressed on skin nerve fibers and may have a role in pruritus. For instance, cannabinoid receptor (CB1) agonist HU210 diminishes histamine-induced excitation of nerve fibers and thereby reduces itching. [50] This suggests that CB1 signaling may be involved in initiation of itch.

Corticotropin-releasing hormone (CRH) and its analog, urocortin, lead to histamine release upon intradermal injection [51]. CRH is also involved in mast cell degranulation occurring during periods of acute stress. The exact function played by leukotrienes in itch is unclear. Studies have reported the use of leukotriene receptor antagonists zileuton and zafirlukast for antipruritic action in atopic dermatitis [52]

Calcitonin gene-related peptide: Many neurons of the dorsal root ganglion coexpress substance P, calcitonin gene-related peptide (CGRP), and PAR2. CGRP plays a modulatory role in inflammation and pruritus. It would seem that CGRP has an inhibitory effect on substance P-induced itching as it prolongs itch latency following injection [53], but increased levels of CGRP are seen in atopic dermatitis, nummular eczema. and prurigo nodularis [53]. Like substance P, CGRP-mediated itch may result from mast cell activation.

Acetylcholine (ACh) is a neurotransmitter which binds to both muscarinic and nicotinic receptors. In mice, activation of the muscarinic M3 receptors causes pruritus [54]. Intracutaneously injected ACh caused itch in atopic eczema [55]. Histamine-sensitive as well as histamine-insensitive C-nerve fibers are stimulated by ACh. Atopic dermatitis patients are more sensitive to ACh and less sensitive to histamine than normal subjects [54].

Clinical Presentation

Pruritus in Systemic Diseases

In systemic diseases, the skin may appear normal or have skin lesions induced by scratching, and a diagnosis may be difficult to establish. In these cases pruritus is usually symmetric and extensive and has an insidious onset; in addition, its intensity is not directly related to the severity of under-

lying disease. Moreover, localized forms may be transformed into generalized forms during disease progression. Only 50% of patients complaining of pruritus and without apparent dermatologic lesions at the time of the medical visit have its etiology identified [56], showing that pruritus may precede the diagnosis of the underlying disease by years.

There are many etiologic hypotheses for the several manifestations of pruritus in systemic diseases, some of which have not yet been confirmed. This is one of the main reasons why the treatment of this symptom is still difficult and often does not give a definitive solution for the patient. Patient follow-up and a good doctor–patient relationship are essential to manage this symptom, which in most cases is extremely debilitating and has no curative treatment. Symptoms are summarized in Table 61.2.

Table 61.2 Systemic diseases that can induce pruritus (examples)

Metabolic and endocrine diseases	Chronic renal disease
	Liver diseases with or without cholestasis
	Hyperparathyroidism
	Hyper- and hypothyroidism
	Carcinoid syndrome
	Iron deficiency
Infective diseases	HIV and AIDS
	Parasitoses
Hematologic disorders	Polycythemia vera
	Leukemia
	Lymphoma (Hodgkin's lymphoma, cutaneous lymphoma)
Neurologic diseases	Multiple sclerosis
	Brain tumors
	Notalgia paresthetica
	Brachioradial pruritus
	Postzosteric neuralgia
Psychiatric or psychosomatic diseases	Depression
	Affective disorders
	Hallucinosis
	Obsessive and compulsive disorders
	Schizophrenia
	Eating disorders

Adapted from Weisshaar et al. [85]

Pruritus in Chronic Kidney Diseases

The pathophysiology of pruritus associated with chronic kidney diseases is unknown. However, some mechanisms have been suggested, including skin conditions such as moderate to severe xeroderma, dialysis, medications taken by the patient, metabolic factors, dysfunction of peripheral or central nerves, involvement of opioid receptors (μ and κ), and microinflammation in uremia [57, 58]. Pruritus is not related to the etiology of renal failure nor to age, gender, skin color, or time on dialysis.

The number of mast cells is greater in uremic patients than in normal patients [59], and the skin of uremic patients produces several pruritogenic cytokines that stimulate the nerve endings of fibers carrying the sensation of pruritus. Additionally an increase in the concentration of calcium, magnesium, phosphates, and mast cells was observed in hemodialysis patients with symptoms of pruritus [57]. Although plasma concentrations of histamine are higher in uremic patients than in nonuremic patients, these values are not related to the severity of pruritus, and antihistamines did not resolve the symptoms. Serum serotonin is high in hemodialysis patients; however, randomized, placebo-controlled, double-blind trials did not observe an improvement in pruritus among patients treated with ondansetron, an antagonist of $5HT_3$ receptors [60]. Studies obtained controversial results on the improvement of chronic kidney disease-associated pruritus with the use of opioid antagonists. Ultraviolet B (UVB) phototherapy has been used with good results. Systemic changes resulting from dialysis, such as decreased erythropoietin, and hyperparathyroidism were also related to pruritus and should be corrected in patients with these conditions.

A total of 22–90% of patients with severe renal failure complains of pruritus, especially those who are undergoing dialysis. This complaint has declined in recent years, probably due to the use of highly permeable membranes during dialysis. Patients with more intense pruritus have worse prognosis for renal disease and have higher mortality rates.

Pruritus in Liver Disease

Pruritus is a frequent symptom in patients with liver diseases caused by cholestasis, mechanical obstruction, metabolic disorders, or inflammatory diseases [62], and is less frequent in patients with infectious liver disease (hepatitis B or C) or alcoholic liver disease.

Pruritus is an initial symptom of cholestasis and affects 20–50% of patients with jaundice; additionally its intensity is not related to the severity of cholestasis. The onset of this type of pruritus occurs in the palmoplantar region, but most patients present with the generalized form, with symptoms worsening at night [63]. In addition to pruritus, these patients show postinflammatory hyperpigmentation on their back, which spares the central region, and the characteristic "butterfly" sign. Other clinical findings related to cholestasis may also be present, such as xanthelasma secondary to hypercholesterolemia, jaundice, ascites, and hepatomegaly. Sometimes pruritus is so intense that it leads the patient to think about suicide and becomes one of the indications for liver transplantation [62].

Diseases causing intrahepatic cholestasis that may lead to pruritus are primary biliary cirrhosis, pruritus gravidarum, sclerosing cholangitis, viral hepatitis, and drug-induced cholestasis. In primary biliary cirrhosis, pruritus occurs in almost 100% of patients and is the initial symptom of disease in nearly 50% of the cases. The symptom may be severe and may precede the diagnosis of primary biliary cirrhosis by years [64]. In pruritus gravidarum, pruritus occurs in the third trimester of pregnancy, being more common in multiple pregnancies. The symptom disappears immediately after delivery and may recur in subsequent pregnancies and with the use of oral contraceptives. Drug-induced cholestasis may be very symptomatic and may be caused mainly by phenothiazine, estrogens, and tolbutamide. Extrahepatic bile duct obstruction may also cause pruritus [2, 62].

Several hypotheses have been suggested to explain the cause of cholestatic pruritus, such as the stimulation of skin fibers by toxic bile salts, pruritogens derived from destroyed hepatic cells, changes in the metabolism of bile salts in the intestine, steroid hormones, accumulation of endogenous opioids, and plasma accumulation of substances produced in the liver [65]. Recent studies showed that increased serum levels of autotaxin (ATX), the enzyme responsible for metabolizing lysophosphatidylcholine into lysophosphatidic acid (LPA) and increasing the levels of this acid, is a specific finding for cholestatic pruritus but not for other types of systemic pruritus [66]. Rifampicin significantly reduces the intensity of pruritus by decreasing ATX activity in patients with cholestatic pruritus. The therapeutic action of rifampicin may be partially explained by the binding of this drug to the pregnane X receptor, which inhibits ATX expression [66].

The treatment of cholestasis recommended in guidelines includes anion-exchange resins (cholestyramine), pregnane X receptor agonists, opioid antagonists (naltrexone, naloxone), and serotonin reuptake inhibitors (sertraline). In patients with severe pruritus and unresponsive to standard therapy, experimental approaches should be considered, such as UVB phototherapy, extracorporeal albumin dialysis, nasobiliary drainage, and liver transplantation [65].

Pruritus in Hematologic Diseases

Several hematologic diseases evolve into symptoms of pruritus, which are often severe. Most of these diseases are malignant, including tumors, bone marrow diseases, and lymphoproliferative diseases. The mechanisms leading to pruritus in these diseases may consist of toxic products released by the tumor, allergic reactions to the released components, and direct damage to brain nerves, in the case of tumors located in this area [67, 68].

Iron deficiency anemia: The most common symptom is generalized pruritus, with no direct relationship to the severity of anemia. Some patients may present with localized pruritus, especially in the vulvar and perianal regions. Laboratory abnormalities may be observed only for ferritin levels, with normal levels of serum iron. The causes of this deficiency should be investigated and corrected [69].

Polycythemia vera: Approximately 50% of patients with polycythemia vera complain of pruritus [70] characterized by the sensation of "biting" and usually triggered by contact with water (aquagenic pruritus). Pruritus may precede the clinical disease by years. Studies suggest that the mechanism of pruritus in polycythemia vera is related to platelet aggregation leading to the secretion of serotonin and other pruritogenic agents [70]. Other studies show that the release of high levels of histamine resulting from the increased number of basophil granulocytes may trigger pruritus [68]. Pruritus appears to be more pronounced in patients with the JAK2V617 mutation [71].

Hodgkin's disease: Pruritus is present in up to 30% of patients with Hodgkin's disease and may precede the disease by up to 5 years [68, 69]. It is described as producing a burning sensation that usually becomes more severe at night, affects the lower half of the body, and tends to evolve into generalized pruritus. Dermatologic lesions may be present and resemble ichthyosiform changes. Patients with more severe pruritus and exhibiting poor therapeutic response are those with the worst prognosis of disease progression [69]. Several factors, such as the secretion of leukopeptidases and bradykinin, histamine, and high immunoglobulin E levels deposited in the skin, may contribute to pruritus in lymphomas [68, 69].

Leukemia: Pruritus is not a frequent complaint in patients with leukemia, but when present it is usually disseminated. Skin infiltrates may produce localized itch at the site of the lesion [69].

Systemic mastocytosis: Causative agents of degranulation of mast cells cause generalized pruritus in these patients [68].

Cutaneous T-cell lymphoma (*CTCL*) encompasses a diverse group of diseases characterized by malignant T lymphocytes that initially home to the skin. Mycosis fungoides is the most common variant and Sézary syndrome the rarest [72]. A characteristic hallmark of CTCL, especially Sézary syndrome, is pruritus, the sensation of itch which is repeatedly observed in various CTCL types [73, 74]. In an outpatient setting, approximately one-third of the patients with the diagnosis of CTCL complain of itch that accompanies the disease, and in some cases pruritus was the only symptom in a patient leading to the diagnosis of a CTCL [73, 74]. Pruritus as a symptom is almost invariably present in CTCL progressing into generalized erythrodermic mycosis fungoides and Sézary syndrome. It may be speculated that T cells homing to the skin provoke the release of inflammatory cytokines, but the precise molecular mechanism is still unknown. Pruritus in CTCL seems to be both a blessing and a curse: a blessing in those patients in whom it may lead to early diagnosis, and a curse for those who are resistant to therapy. Further research is mandatory to unravel the molecular mechanisms and provide more specific treatment of pruritus in CTCL [75].

Pruritus in Endocrinologic Diseases

Pruritus is present in several endocrinologic diseases such as hyperthyroidism, hypothyroidism, diabetes mellitus, multiple endocrine neoplasia, carcinoid syndrome, and hyperparathyroidism [69].

Hyperthyroidism: Four percent to 11% of patients with thyrotoxicosis present with pruritus [76, 77]. Triggering mechanisms may include: (1) activation of kinins in the skin; (2) decrease of itch threshold due to vasodilation; and (3) changes of bile acids in the blood. The correction of disease improves pruritus, which may be the main complaint in some patients with hyperthyroidism.

Hypothyroidism: Pruritus is related to xeroderma, a characteristic symptom of patients with hypothyroidism. The use of emollients, as well as the correction of the underlying disease, improves the symptoms [76].

Diabetes mellitus: Nearly 3% of these patients present with pruritus. In this case, the mechanisms involved in the development of pruritus are peripheral neuropathy, uremia secondary to chronic renal failure, and anatomic dysfunction [78].

Carcinoid syndrome: Patients with carcinoid syndrome may present with pruritus combined with flushing, diarrhea, and cardiac symptoms [76].

Primary hyperparathyroidism: A substantial number of patients with primary hyperparathyroidism complain of pruritus [77]. The pathophysiology of pruritus in this disease is not well known, although these patients usually present with deficiency of vitamin D and minerals such as zinc, which may contribute to pruritus.

Pruritus in Psychiatric Diseases

Psychiatric diseases such as depression, anxiety, and some psychoses may include severe pruritus as one of their symptoms [6]. The accurate diagnosis of these patients is important, because treatment requires a psychiatric approach. In this case there are no primary skin lesions but rather lesions secondary to itching, ranging from superficial excoriations to major lichenifications. Currently it is estimated that one-third of patients seeing a dermatologist have emotional and psychosocial factors involved in their disease; however, there is still great reluctance to include psychiatric treatment as part of the management of dermatoses [3, 7]. It is extremely important to raise awareness of these diseases and to provide appropriate guidance to patients, despite their reluctance.

Pruritus in Neurologic Diseases

Neurologic diseases such as multiple sclerosis, focal lesions, tumors, abscesses, and stroke may include pruritus as part of their clinical picture. Localized neurologic lesions, such as tumors and brain abscesses, may result in unilateral pruritus.

Brachioradial pruritus: Located in the dorsal and lateral regions of upper limbs, this type of pruritus especially affects patients in the sixth decade of life and is more common in summer months, being classified by several authors as a photodermatosis. An investigation for associated neuropathies should always be made, because current studies show that up to 57% of these patients present with radiculopathies in the cervical region. Treatment with antihistamines, topical capsaicin, and topical corticosteroids may lead to an improvement in these patients. Therapy regimens for neuropathies may also relieve symptoms [79].

Pruritus in HIV Infection

Pruritus is a very common complaint in patients with HIV and is sometimes the first manifestation of disease. The intensity of pruritus may range from mild to very severe presentations. It is associated with most common dermatoses in patients with HIV, but may be present even when there is no dermatologic change. Pruritic dermatoses associated with HIV disease include pruritic papular eruption and eosinophilic folliculitis.

These dermatoses may be easily diagnosed through skin inspection and physical examination, and have a high positive predictive value for the diagnosis of HIV infection [80, 81].

In these patients, chronic pruritus may lead to skin changes such as excoriations, lichenification, prurigo nodularis, pigmentation changes, and secondary infection. Intense xeroderma is found in patients with AIDS and leads to a physicochemical action on the endings of C fibers in the skin. In addition, systemic complications such as liver diseases and renal failure may also worsen pruritus in these patients. Finally, the drugs used in the specific treatment of this disease often trigger pruritus [80].

Treatment of these patients includes the treatment of xeroderma, with the daily use of emollients and basic care to avoid the worsening of skin dryness.

Pruritus in Dermatologic Diseases

Dermatologic diseases often evolve into pruritus, which may be located in the area of skin lesion or sometimes be generalized. Many dermatoses cause this symptom, such as atopic dermatitis, urticaria, irritative and allergic contact dermatitis, seborrheic dermatitis, stasis eczema, prurigus, and lichen planus, but analyzing the specific approaches for these diseases beyond the remit of this chapter.

Pruritus Ani

Anal and perianal pruritus affects 1–5% of the general population in the proportion of four males to one female [82]. Its symptoms have an insidious onset and may last for years before the patient seeks treatment. This type of pruritus may be primary, with no apparent dermatologic lesion, or secondary to hemorrhoids, anal fistulas and fissures, psoriasis, contact eczema, lichen sclerosus, sexually transmitted diseases, parasitosis, and neoplasms. Primary causes include dietary factors such as increased intake of coffee, poor personal hygiene, and psychogenic dis-

eases. Anxiety and depression increase pruritus ani. Patients with mild pruritus ani respond to general care such as hip baths and cold compresses, avoidance of abrasives and soaps in the area, and corticosteroid therapy with low-potency corticosteroids [82]. Patients with severe pruritus require high-potency corticosteroids and sometimes topical immunomodulators such as tacrolimus [69].

Genital Pruritus

The characteristics of vulvar and scrotal pruritus are very similar to those of perianal pruritus. However, less than 10% of patients with genital pruritus symptoms present with psychogenic pruritus; thus, a detailed investigation should be conducted to find the triggering agent. The management of these patients is similar to that of patients with pruritus ani [69].

Scar Pruritus

During the time when scars are healing, which ranges from 6 months to 2 years, patients commonly present with pruritus triggered by nerve regeneration and chemical and physical stimuli. However, the formation of keloids and hypertrophic scars may prolong the duration of pruritus. The treatment is performed with emollients, topical and injectable corticosteroids, interferon, topical retinoids, gels, and silicone strips [69].

Drug-Induced Pruritus

Almost all drugs have the potential of inducing pruritus by several mechanisms; therefore, the use of medications should always be addressed in medical history taking [83]. Drugs may induce pruritus by causing skin lesions such as urticarial and morbilliform rash, by producing systemic changes such as hepatotoxicity or cholestasis, or by causing xeroma or phototoxicity [84]. Drugs that may induce or maintain chronic pruritus are listed in Table 61.3.

Table 61.3 Drugs that may induce or maintain chronic pruritus (without a rash)

Class of drug	Substance (examples)
ACE inhibitors	Captopril, enalapril
Antiarrhythmic agents	Amiodarone, disopyramide, flecainide
Antibiotics	Amoxicillin, ampicillin, cefotaxime, ceftriaxone, chloramphenicol, ciprofloxacin, clarithromycin, clindamycin, cotrimoxazole, erythromycin, gentamycin, metronidazole, minocycline, ofloxacin, penicillin, tetracycline
Antidepressants	Amitriptyline, citalopram, clomipramine, doxepin, fluoxetine, fluvoxamine, imipramine, lithium, mirtazapine, nortriptyline, paroxetine, sertraline
Antidiabetic drugs	Glimepiride, metformin
Antihypertensive drugs	Clonidine, doxazosin, hydralazine, methyldopa, prazosin, reserpine
Anticonvulsants	Carbamazepine, clonazepam, gabapentin, lamotrigine, phenobarbital, phenytoin, topiramate, valproic acid
Anti-inflammatory drugs	Acetylsalicylic acid, celecoxib, diclofenac, ibuprofen, indomethacin, ketoprofen, naproxen, piroxicam
AT II antagonists	Irbesartan, telmisartan, valsartan
β-Blockers	atenolol, bisoprolol, metoprolol, nadolol, pindolol, propranolol
Bronchodilators, mucolytic agents, respiratory stimulants	Aminophylline, doxapram, ipratropium bromide, salmeterol, terbutaline
Calcium antagonists	Amlodipine, diltiazem, felodipine, nifedipine, nimodipine, verapamil
Diuretics	Amiloride, furosemide, hydrochlorothiazide, spironolactone, triamterene

Table 61.3 (continued)

Class of drug	Substance (examples)
Hormones	Clomifene, danazol, oral contraceptives, estrogens, progesterone, steroids, testosterone and derivatives, tamoxifen
Immunosuppressive drugs	Cyclophosphamide, cyclosporine, methotrexate, mycophenolate mofetil, tacrolimus, thalidomide
Antilipids	Clofibrate, fenofibrate, fluvastatin, lovastatin, pravastatin, simvastatin
Neuroleptics	Chlorpromazine, haloperidol, risperidone
Tranquilizers	Alprazolam, chlordiazepoxide, lorazepam, oxazepam, prazepam
Uricostatics	Allopurinol, colchicine, probenecid

Adapted from Weisshaar et al. [85]

Diagnosis

The first step in the therapeutic approach of pruritus is attempting to evaluate whether itch is attributed to a dermatologic cause or to an underlying disease. In a practical approach, patients with pruritus may be divided into the following groups: (1) patients with primary pruritic dermatologic disease; (2) patients with dermatologic lesions secondary to pruritus; (3) patients with pruritus and without dermatologic lesions [85]. In most cases, no systemic diseases are found in patients with generalized pruritus, who are classified as patients with pruritus sine materia [85, 86] (Tables 61.4 and 61.5).

In patients with pruritic dermatologic disease, the diagnosis and management of pruritus aims to treat the dermatosis [85–90]. However, in individuals who have no dermatologic lesions or in those whose lesions are secondary to scratching, a detailed assessment should be made, including patient's history, clinical characteristics of pruritus, thorough physical examination, laboratory screening, and imaging studies to investigate systemic diseases that cause pruritus [85–90].

Table 61.4 Clinical evaluation of patients with pruritus

1. Patient's clinical history: including hygiene habits that may dry the skin, contact with animals, occupation, leisure activities, infectious and parasitic diseases
2. Patient's history: allergies; renal, hepatic, hematologic, and psychiatric diseases
3. Family history of allergic and systemic diseases
4. Use of topical and systemic drugs

Table 61.5 Medical history taking for the assessment of pruritus

1. Occurrence of progression of previous episodes
2. Onset of current symptoms (acute, progressive)
3. Period of the day when the disease worsens (day/night)
4. Triggering agents (baths, clothes, room temperature)
5. Sensation caused by pruritus (bite, burn)
6. Frequency (continuous, intermittent)
7. Location (localized, generalized)
8. Association with daily activities (interference, triggering)
9. Patient's perception about pruritus (the extent to which it affects quality of life)

Patient's clinical history: A detailed past and current medical history should be taken with the purpose of identifying symptoms of systemic diseases, and family history should be taken to identify factors that predispose to systemic diseases [85–90]. It is also important to investigate the use of drugs that may trigger pruritus, possible allergenic agents, infectious diseases such as scabies, parasitological diseases, patient's occupation and lifestyle, and personal and family history of atopy and other allergic diseases. Personal and family psychiatric history of the patient should also be investigated.

Some factors also should be considered in pruritus evaluation [85]. When several family members are affected, scabies or other parasites should be considered. The relationship between pruritus and special physical activities are suggestive of cholinergic pruritus. Pruritus provoked by skin cooling after bathing should prompt consideration of aquagenic pruritus and may be associated with polycythemia vera or myelodysplastic syndrome. Nocturnal generalized pruritus associated with chills, fatigue, tiredness, and "B" symptoms (weight loss, fever, and nocturnal sweating) raises the possibility of Hodgkin's disease.

Somatoform pruritus rarely disturbs sleep but most other pruritic diseases cause nocturnal wakening. Seasonal pruritus frequently presents as "winter itch," which may also be the manifestation of pruritus in the elderly due to xerosis cutis and asteatotic eczema (Table 61.4).

History of pruritus: A detailed evaluation of pruritus may lead to the differential diagnosis of this condition. It is important to investigate how disease onset occurred, the period of the day when the disease worsens, whether pruritus is intermittent or continuous, and the sensation that pruritus causes, as well as duration of symptoms, severity, location, relationship with daily activities, triggering factors, and patient's perception about the symptoms [85, 86] (Table 61.5).

Measurement of pruritus: Pruritus is a subjective symptom that can be fully assessed only by the individual suffering from this symptom. However, several methods of assessment and measurement of pruritus have been developed in order to enable a better investigation of both the etiology of pruritus and the results of therapeutic studies. Visual analog scales and measures of scratching activity have been used for this assessment. A questionnaire developed by Yosipovitch et al. [19] evaluates the intensity, affective, and sensory dimensions of pruritus and may be extremely useful for the measurement of pruritus in systemic diseases.

Patient physical examination involves the search for dermatologic lesions that characterize pruritic dermatosis, xeroderma, jaundice, weight loss, hematomas, and excoriations caused by scratching [85–87]. General physical examination also should include palpation of the liver, kidneys, spleen, and lymph nodes.

Laboratory tests: Complete blood count, platelet, ferritin, serum iron, fasting glucose, stool test, erythrocyte sedimentation rate, evaluation of renal, hepatic, thyroid, and parathyroid function, hepatitis B and C markers, anti-HIV, and qualitative urine test. Other tests, such as immunoelectrophoresis, may also be performed in cases of clinical suspicion of the disease [85, 86].

Imaging tests: Chest X-ray and full abdominal ultrasound. Other tests may be requested according to clinical suspicion or medical judgment [85].

Histopathologic tests may sometimes elucidate the diagnosis, but are not routinely performed [85].

Patients with generalized pruritus and normal test results should be periodically monitored because they may present with malignant disease or other systemic diseases later in life, with pruritus as the initial symptom. In some cases, such as in patients with skin lymphoma, pruritus may persist for many years before the onset of clinical and laboratory manifestations of the disease and the possibility of diagnosis.

Therapeutic Approach

Considering that pruritus has various causes, there is no standardized recommendation for treatment. Topical and systemic therapies should be individualized, taking into account age, previous diseases, current medications, allergies, pruritus severity, and impact on quality of life [88, 89]. According to recent studies, the therapy should also address both cutaneous and central mechanisms of pruritus (Fig. 61.1).

The first step in pruritus treatment is focused on the diagnosis of an underlying disease and on how to control it. Depending on the underlying cause, the appropriate therapy may vary considerably, including treatment for a specific dermatosis, nonexposure to contact allergens, discontinuation of a medication, treatment of systemic, neurologic, or psychiatric diseases, and even surgical treatments for removal of an underlying tumor [88, 89]. Pruritus caused, for example, by hyperthyroidism or cutaneous T-cell lymphoma resolves with an effective treatment for these diseases.

When the cause cannot be determined, knowing the characteristics of the pruritus, such as intense itching hours and triggering agents, is extremely important for the therapeutic approach [88]. We should keep in mind that, in some cases, there is no totally effective therapy for itch relief. Therefore, patient counseling on measures for relieving pruritus is essential. Xeroderma occurs in a great number of these patients and should

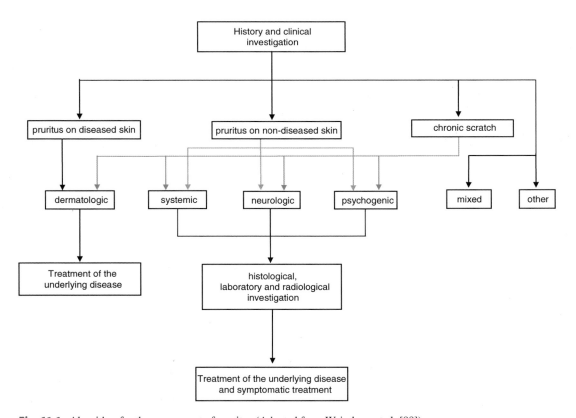

Fig. 61.1 Algorithm for the assessment of pruritus (Adapted from Weisshaar et al. [88])

always be addressed with the use of emollients. Being careful with active substances that may cause skin irritation and increase pruritus is also important. Itching causes traumatic skin lesions, which may be avoided by keeping fingernails trimmed. Elevated body temperature may increase pruritus. Measures such as wearing light clothes, staying in cooled areas, taking warm showers, and avoiding intake of alcohol and spicy foods help alleviate the symptom [88, 89]. It should be considered that chronic pruritus is often caused by several factors and may be intensified by many cofactors, suggesting a multifactorial origin [90].

Care of patients, particularly those with chronic pruritus, may often extend for a long time, with periods of diagnostic uncertainty, therapeutic failures, and psychological stress. Physicians should discuss treatment duration and diagnostic investigation with patients to increase adherence to treatment and establish a good doctor–patient relationship. In all cases, however, early treatment and patient counseling may prevent nerve sensitization and, thus, pruritus chronification.

Topical Treatment

Emollients: Topical emollients are the first-line therapy for mild or localized pruritus and for xeroderma. In hemodialysis patients with intense xeroderma, the use of emollients associated with other therapies is indicated [85]. These agents are likely to reduce pruritus by softening the sharp edges of the outermost layer of dry skin (stratum corneum) and by improving skin barrier function. In inflammatory diseases the skin barrier function is insufficient, and repetitive itching intensifies this problem, facilitating the entry of irritating substances. "Wet wrap" therapy may be useful and soothing in cases of extensive inflammation, such as in severe atopic dermatitis [91]. In this instance, the patient should first apply an emollient and a low-potency topical glucocorticoid on the affected area and then wear water-soaked cotton pajamas at night. This treatment should be limited to short periods (<1 week at a time) because of the associated risks of infection and

absorption of topical glucocorticoids in excess. High pH solutions, such as alkaline soaps, may increase the secretion of serine proteases, which intensify itching and should be avoided in those patients. Conversely, moisturizers and skin care products with low pH (4.5–6.0) can be used [92].

Corticosteroids are not antipruritic agents, acting only in situations where the pruritus is caused by inflammatory skin reaction. In randomized clinical trials, moderate- to high-potency glucocorticoids have been proved to be an effective treatment for inflammatory skin diseases, such as atopic eczema, psoriasis, lichen planus, and genital lichen sclerosus et atrophicus [85]. High-potency glucocorticoids have also been used in medical practice in cutaneous manifestations secondary to chronic pruritus, such as prurigo nodularis and lichen simplex chronicus.

Capsaicin acts locally by desensitizing peripheral nerve fibers through depletion of substance P [93]. Usually its concentration varies from 0.025 % to 0.075 %. However, irritation on the injection site is a side effect, greatly limiting its utilization. Topical capsaicin is proven as an effective treatment for notalgia paresthetica and for hemodialysis patients with localized pruritus, as well as for patients with brachioradial pruritus [34, 79].

Menthol: Topical menthol relieves itching by activating cold-sensitive Aδ fibers, which are responsible for transmitting a cool sensation through the activation of a transient receptor potential cation channel subfamily M member 8 (TRPM8) [47]. Clinical experience has suggested that this substance may be effective in skin-care creams with concentrations varying from 1 % to 5 %, applied several times a day. Higher concentrations tend to cause skin irritation [94].

Calamine: Oil-based lotions and aqueous creams are effective in relieving pruritus. Patients often refuse to use it because of its pinkish color, and some formulations may cause skin dryness with water evaporation [3].

Topical anesthetics: Preparations such as pramoxine 1 % or 2.5 % cream and lidocaine 2.5 % and prilocaine 2.5 % cream were effective in alleviating neuropathic, facial, and anogenital pruritus in a number of cases. In a randomized clinical trial with chronic kidney disease-associated pruritus, pramoxine 1% cream significantly reduced pruritus when compared with the isolated vehicle [95]. The long-term safety of these agents is still unknown.

Calcineurin inhibitors relieve itching in inflammatory diseases, such as psoriasis, eczema, seborrheic dermatitis, and anogenital pruritus [96]. However, a common adverse effect of these agents is a burning sensation that begins a few days after repeated application of the product.

Doxepin 5% cream, a tricyclic antidepressant with H1-receptor inhibitory properties, was effective in reducing the sensation of itching in patients with atopic eczema and contact dermatitis [97]. Potential adverse events include sleepiness and allergic contact dermatitis.

Systemic Treatment

Antihistamines: Sedating antihistamines, which are H1-receptor antagonists, are the most often used drugs in medical practice as a first-line therapy for pruritus, despite the shortage of clinical trials proving their efficacy for pruritic diseases, with the exception of urticaria. The benefit observed in medical practice may result from the sedative action of these medications, which can help patients with sleeping problems and relieve the symptoms. Nonsedating histamine H1- and H2-receptor antagonists have limited efficacy in the treatment of chronic pruritus [85, 98]. Antihistamines have little effect on hemodialysis patients and patients with cholestatic disease [57, 61].

Neuroactive drugs: Structural analogs to the neurotransmitter γ-aminobutyric acid, such as gabapentin and pregabalin, are an effective treatment for some types of pruritus. In randomized clinical trials in patients with chronic kidney disease, low-dose gabapentin (100–300 mg administered three times a week) was effective in controlling pruritus when compared with placebo [99]. Case reports show that these drugs may also be used in the treatment of postherpetic neuralgia, brachioradial pruritus, and prurigo nodularis [86]. The most common adverse events are constipation, weight gain, sleepiness, ataxia, and blurred vision.

Opioid agonist-antagonists: In patients with chronic urticaria, atopic eczema, and cholestasis,

μ-opioid antagonists (naltrexone, nalmefene, and naloxone) have shown antipruritic effects [100]. Naltrexone and naloxone were effective for resistant itching associated with uremia and cholestasis. In randomized controlled trials conducted in Japan, nalfurafine hydrochloride (a κ-opioid agonist) significantly reduced itching in hemodialysis patients with chronic kidney disease [101, 102]. However, some studies involving patients with chronic kidney disease have shown inconsistent results [103, 104]. According to reports, butorphanol, a μ-opioid antagonist and κ-opioid agonist administered via intravenous route and approved by Food and Drug Administration for migraine treatment, reduced intractable pruritus associated with non-Hodgkin lymphoma, cholestasis, and the use of opioids [105]. Initial adverse effects of these agents, such as nausea, loss of appetite, abdominal colic, diarrhea, and insomnia, limit their utilization.

Tricyclic antidepressants: Serotonin reuptake inhibitors (paroxetine, sertraline, fluvoxamine, and fluoxetine) have been used to reduce psychogenic pruritus and various types of generalized pruritus [106]. A double-blind study demonstrated the efficacy of sertraline (daily dose of 100 mg) for the treatment of cholestatic pruritus [107]. Studies have suggested that the antidepressant mirtazapine (daily dose of 15 mg) may relieve nocturnal itching related to some types of cancer [108]. In several cases of intractable pruritus related to cutaneous T-cell lymphoma, patients treated with a combination of low-dose mirtazapine and gabapentin or pregabalin showed improvement of symptoms [109]. Tricyclic antidepressants, such as amitriptyline, have also been used in the treatment of chronic pruritus (neuropathic and psychogenic forms, for example) [85]. Paroxetine, a selective serotonin reuptake inhibitor, seems to have positive effects in low doses (5–10 mg a day). However, these effects tend to decrease after 4–6 weeks of use [3]. Ondansetron, a serotonin receptor antagonist, has been used for controlling pruritus in patients with cholestasis and hemodialysis patients. Case reports have shown important benefits, while randomized controlled trials have not demonstrated the same relevance.

Sodium cromoglycate: A mast cell stabilizer that has effects on the improvement of pruritus in patients with Hodgkin's lymphoma [110].

Rifampicin is indicated for the treatment of severe pruritus in patients with primary biliary cirrhosis and patients with cholestasis. Recent reports of drug-induced hepatitis caused by this medication reduce its therapeutic indication [111].

Cholestyramine reduces the levels of bile salts through chelation in the intestinal lumen. It is indicated in the treatment of cholestatic pruritus, but does not work when there is bile duct obstruction. It may also be used in hemodialysis patients [112].

Activated charcoal has shown positive results in relieving pruritus in hemodialysis patients with pruritus, at a daily dose of 6 g [112].

Thalidomide it is used for pruritus treatment in several pruritic diseases, such as eczema, psoriasis, senile pruritus, and liver diseases, and has an effect on hemodialysis patients, who have shown an improvement of more than 50% [113, 114].

Phototherapy: Observational studies have suggested that narrow-band UVB (NB-UVB) phototherapy, either isolated or in combination with ultraviolet A (UVA) radiation, reduces pruritus caused by chronic kidney disease and alleviates itching in diseases such as psoriasis, atopic eczema, and cutaneous T-cell lymphoma [115, 116]. In a randomized clinical trial involving patients with refractory itch secondary to chronic kidney disease [117], there was no significant difference in terms of efficacy between NB-UVB radiation and UVA radiation.

Liver transplantation and kidney transplantation: Both are indicated in patients with extremely serious pruritus who do not respond to any therapeutic modality [112].

Psychotherapeutic treatments may be used in cases of psychogenic pruritus. Some patients with pruritus that is difficult to control have depressive symptoms and may also benefit from psychotherapeutic treatment.

Glossary

Amyelinic C fibers One of three classes of nerve fiber in the central nervous system and peripheral nervous system. There are a myriad of mediators capable of stimulating these afferent nerves leading to itch, including biogenic amines, proteases, cytokines, and peptides. Some of these mediators can also evoke sensations of pain, and the sensory processing underlying both sensations overlaps in complex ways.

Capsaicin An active component of chili peppers, which are plants belonging to the genus *Capsicum*. Capsaicin is used to help relieve a certain type of pain known as neuralgia.

JAK2V617 mutation The *JAK2*V617 mutated allele is present in virtually all patients with polycythemia vera (PV) and in about 60% of those with essential thrombocythemia (ET) and primary myelofibrosis (PMF), which are the other two main clinical entities included within the group of myeloproliferative neoplasms. The presence of the mutation, and/or the burden of *JAK2*V617 allele, has been found to correlate with defined laboratory abnormalities and clinical features in the different myeloproliferative neoplasms.

References

1. Hafenreffer S. De pruritu, in Nosodochium, in quo cutis, eique adharetium partuim, affectus omnes, singulari methodo, et cognoscendi et curandi fidelissime traduntur. Ulm, B Kühn, 1660, p. 98–102. Apud Wahlgren C-F. Measuremento of Itch. Seminars in Dermatol. 1995;14(4):277–84.
2. Etter L, Myers SA. Pruritus in systemic disease: mechanisms and management. Dermatol Clin. 2002;20(3):459–72.
3. Twycross R, Greaves MW, Handwerker H, Jones EA, Libretto SE, Szepietowski, et al. Itch: scratching more than the surface. QJM. 2003;96(1):7–26.
4. LaMotte RH. Subpopulations of "nocifensor neurons" contributing to pain and allodynia, itch and alloknesis. Am Pain Soc J. 1992;1:115–26.
5. Ständer S, Weisshaar E, Mettang T, Szepietowski JC, Carstens E, Ikoma A, et al. Clinical classification of itch: a position paper of the international forum for the study of itch. Acta Derm Venereol. 2007;87:291–4.
6. Yosipovitch G, Greaves M, Schmelz M. Itch. Lancet. 2003;361:690–4.
7. Yamamoto Y, Yamazaki S, Hayashino Y, et al. Association between frequency of pruritic symptoms and perceived psychological stress: a Japanese population based study. Arch Dermatol. 2009;145:1384–8.
8. Adler HM. Might a psychosocial approach improve our understanding of itching and scratching? Int J Dermatol. 2003;42:160–3.

9. Dalgard F, Svensson A, Holm JO, Sundby J. Self-reported skin morbidity in Oslo. Associations with sociodemographic factors among adults in a cross-sectional study. Br J Dermatol. 2004;151:452–7.

10. Matterne U, Apfelbacher CJ, Loerbroks A, et al. Prevalence, correlates and characteristics of chronic pruritus: a population based cross-sectional study. Acta Derm Venereol. 2011;91:674–9.

11. Stander S, Stumpf A, Osada N, Wilp S, Chatzigeorgakidis E, Pfeiderer B. Gender differences in chronic pruritus: women present different morbidity, more scratch lesions and higher burden. Br J Dermatol. 2013;168(6):1273–80. (Epub ahead of print).

12. Stander S, Schäfer I, Phan NQ, et al. Prevalence of chronic pruritus in Germany: results of a cross-sectional study in a sample working population of 11,730. Dermatology. 2010;221:229–35.

13. Weisshaar E, Dalgard F. Epidemiology of itch: adding to the burden of skin morbidity. Acta Derm Venereol. 2009;89:339–50.

14. Dalgard F, Dawn AG, Yosipovitch G. Are itch and chronic pain associated in adults? Results of a large population survey in Norway. Dermatology. 2007;214:305–9.

15. Wolkenstein P, Grob JJ, Bastuji-Garin S, Ruszczynski S, Roujeau JC, Revuz J. French people and skin diseases: results of a survey using a representative sample. Arch Dermatol. 2003;139:1614–9.

16. Britt H, Pan Y, Miller GC, Valenti L, Charles J, Knox S, et al. Presentations of 'itch' in Australian general practice. Aust Fam Physician. 2004;33:488.

17. McCormick A, Fleming D, Charlton J. Morbidity statistics from general practice. Fourth national study 1991–1992. London: Her Majestic's Stationery Office; 1995.

18. Szepietowski JC, Salomon J. Uremic pruritus: still an important clinical problem. J Am Acad Dermatol. 2004;51:842–3.

19. Yosipovitch G, Goon AT, Wee J, Chan YH, Zucker I, Goh CL. Itch characteristics in Chinese patients with atopic dermatitis using a new questionnaire for the assessment of pruritus. Int J Dermatol. 2002;41:212–6.

20. Ikoma A, Steinhoff M, Ständer S, Yosipovitch G, Schmelz M. The neurobiology of itch. Nat Rev Neurosci. 2006;7:535–47.

21. LaMotte RH, Dong X, Ringkamp M. Sensory neurons and circuits mediating itch. Nat Neurosci. 2014;15:19–31.

22. Davidson S, Giesler GJ. The multiple pathways for itch and their interactions with pain. Trends Neurosci. 2010;33:550–8.

23. Hyndman OR, Wolkin J. Anterior cordotomy: further observations on the physiologic results and optimum manner of performance. Arch Neurol Psychiatr. 1943;50:129–48.

24. Davidson S, et al. The itch-producing agents histamine and cowhage activate separate populations of primate spinothalamic tract neurons. J Neurosci. 2007;27:10007–14.

25. Davidson S, et al. Pruriceptive spinothalamic tract neurons: physiologic properties and projection targets in the primate. J Neurophysiol. 2012;108:1711–23.

26. Han L, Ma C, Liu Q, Weng H-J, Cui Y, et al. A subpopulation of nociceptors specifically linked to itch. Nat Neurosci. 2013;16:174–82.

27. Han SK, Mancino V, Simon MI. Phospholipase Cβ 3 mediates the scratching response activated by the histamine H1 receptor on C-fiber nociceptive neurons. Neuron. 2006;52:691–703.

28. Huang JF, Thurmond R. The new biology of histamine receptors. Curr Allergy Asthma Rep. 2008;8:21–7.

29. Greaves MW, Wall PD. Pathophysiology of itching. Lancet. 1996;348:938–40.

30. Weisshaar E, Ziethen B, Rohl FW, Gollnick H. The antipruritic effect of a 5HT3 receptor antagonist (tropisetron) is dependent on mast cell depletion: an experimental study. Exp Dermatol. 1999;8:254–60.

31. Cocchiara R, Lampiasi N, Albeggiani G, Bongiovanni A, Azzolina A, Geraci D. Mast cell production of TNF-alpha induced by substance P: evidence for a modulatory role of substance P-antagonists. J Neuroimmunol. 1999;101:128–36.

32. Toyoda M, Nakamura M, Makino T, Hino T, Kaqoura M, Morohashi M. Nerve growth factor and substance P are useful plasma markers of disease activity in atopic dermatitis. Br J Dermatol. 2002;147:71–9.

33. Costa SK, Starr A, Hyslop S, Gilmore D, Bran SD. How important are NK1 receptors for influencing microvascular inflammation and itch in the skin? Studies using Phoneutria nigriventor venom. Vasc Pharmacol. 2006;45:209–14.

34. Nolano M, Simone DA, Wendelschafer-Crabb G, Johnson T, Hazen E, Kennedy WR. Topical capsaicin in humans: parallel loss of epidermal nerve fibres and pain sensation. Pain. 1999;81:135–45.

35. Hagermark O, Strandberg K. Pruritogenic activity of prostaglandin E2. Acta Derm Venereol. 1977;57:37–43.

36. Greaves MW, McDonald-Gibson W. Itch: role of prostaglandins. Br Med J. 1973;3:608–9.

37. Gaspari AA, Lotze MT, Rosenberg SA, Stern JB, Katz SI. Dermatologic changes associated with interleukin 2 administration. JAMA. 1987;258:1624–9.

38. Wahlgren CF, Tenvall Linder M, Hagermark O, Scheynius A. Itch and inflammation induced by intradermally injected interleukin-2 in atopic dermatitis patients and healthy subjects. Arch Dermatol Res. 1995;287:572–80.

39. Neis MM, Peters B, Dreuw A, Wenzel J, Bieber T, Mauch C, et al. Enhanced expression levels of IL-31 correlate with IL-4 and IL-13 in atopic and allergic contact dermatitis. J Allergy Clin Immunol. 2006;118:930–7.

40. Heyer G, Dotzer M, Diepgen TL, Handwerker HO. Opiate and H1 antagonist effects on histamine induced pruritus and alloknesis. Pain. 1997;73:239–43.

41. Saiah M, Borgeat A, Wilder-Smith OH, Rifat K, Suter PM. Epidural morphine induced pruritus: propofol vs naloxone. Anesth Analg. 1994;78:1110–3.

42. Umeuchi H, Togashi Y, Honda T, Nakao K, Okano K, Tanaka T, et al. Involvement of central mu-opioid system in the scratching behavior in mice and the suppression of it by the activation of kappa-opioid system. Eur J Pharmacol. 2003;477:29–35.

43. Steinhoff M, Neisius U, Ikoma A, Fartasch M, Heyer G, Skov PS, et al. Proteinase-activated receptor-2 mediates itch: a novel pathway for pruritus in human skin. J Neurosci. 2003;23:6176–80.

44. Peier AM, Reeve AJ, Andersson DA, Moqrich A, Earley TJ, Hergarden AC, et al. A heat-sensitive TRP channel expressed in keratinocytes. Science. 2002;296:2046–9.

45. Ständer S, Moormann C, Schumacher M, Buddenkotte J, Artuc M, Shpacovitch V, et al. Expression of vanilloid receptor subtype 1 in cutaneous sensory nerve fibers, mast cells, and epithelial cells of appendage structures. Exp Dermatol. 2004;13:129–39.

46. Stokes AJ, Shimoda LM, Koblan-Huberson M, Adra CN, Turner H. A TRPV2-PKA signaling module for transduction of physical stimuli in mast cells. J Exp Med. 2004;200:137–47.

47. Peier AM, Moqrich A, Hergarden AC, Reeve AJ, Andersson DA, Story GM, et al. ATRP channel that senses cold stimuli and menthol. Cell. 2002;108:705–15.

48. Aloe L. *Rita* Levi-Montalcini: the discovery of nerve growth factor and modern neurobiology. Trends Cell Biol. 2004;14:395–9.

49. Groneberg DA, Serowka F, Peckenschneider N, Artuc M, Grutzkau A, Fischer A, et al. Gene expression and regulation of nerve growth factor in atopic dermatitis mast cells and the human mast cell line-1. J Neuroimmunol. 2005;161:87–92.

50. Dvorak M, Watkinson A, McGlone F, Rukwied R. Histamine induced responses are attenuated by cannabinoid receptor agonist in human skin. Inflamm Res. 2003;52:238–45.

51. Theoharides TC, Singh LK, Boucher W, Pang X, Letourneau R, Webster E, et al. Corticotropin-releasing hormone induces skin mast cell degranulation and increased vascular permeability, a possible explanation for its proinflammatory effects. Endocrinology. 1998;139:403–13.

52. Zabawski EJ Jr, Kahn MA, Gregg LJ. Treatment of atopic dermatitis with zafirlukast. Dermatol Online J. 1999;5:10.

53. Weidner C, Klede M, Rukwied R, Lischetzki G, Neisius U, Skov PS, et al. Acute effects of substance P and calcitonin gene-related peptide in human skin – a microdialysis study. J Invest Dermatol. 2000;115:1015–20.

54. MiyamotoT NH, Kuraishi Y. Intradermalcholinergic agonists induce itch-associated response via M3 muscarinic acetylcholine receptors in mice. Jpn J Pharmacol. 2002;88:351–4.

55. Rukwied R, Lischetzki G, McGlone F, Heyer G, Schmelz M. Mast cell mediators other than histamine induce pruritus in atopic dermatitis: a dermal microdialysis study. Br J Dermatol. 2000;142:1–8.

56. Zirvas MJ, Seraly MP. Pruritus of unknown origin: a retrospective study. J Am Acad Dermatol. 2001;45:892–6.

57. Urbonas A, Schwartz RA, Szepietowski JC. Uremic pruritus – an update. Am J Nephrol. 2001;21(5):343–50.

58. Mettang T, Pauli-Magnus C, Alscher DM. Uraemic pruritus new perspectives and insights from recent trials. Nephrol Dial Transplant. 2002;17:1558–63.

59. Szepitowski JC, Morita A, Tsuji T. Ultraviolet B induces mast cell apoptosis: a hypotjetical mechanism of ultraviolet B treatment for uremic pruritus. Med Hypotheses. 2002;58(2):167–70.

60. Murphy M, Reaich D, Pai P, Finn P, Carmichael AJ. A randomized, placebo-controlled, double-blind trial of andonsetron in renal itch. Br J Dermatol. 2003;148:314–7.

61. Szepitowski JC, Schwartz RA. Uremic pruritus. Int J Dermatol. 1998;37:247–53.

62. Bergasa NV. The pruritus of cholestasis. J Hepatol. 2005;43:1078–88.

63. Cacoub P, Poynard T, Ghillani P, Charlotte F, Olivi M, Piette JC, et al. Extrahepatic manifestations of chronic hepatitis C. MULTIVIRC group. Multidepartment virus C. Arthritis Rheum. 1999;42:2204–12.

64. Bergasa NV, Mehlman JK, Jones EA. Pruritus and fatigue in primary biliary cirrhosis. Baillieres Best Pract Res Clin Gastroenterol. 2000;14:643–55.

65. Bolier R, Oude Elferink RPJ, Beuers U. Advances in pathogenesis and treatment of pruritus. Clin Liver Dis. 2013;17:319–29.

66. Kremer AE, Dijk RV, Leckie P, Schaap FG, Kuiper EM, Mettang T, et al. Serum autotaxin is increased in pruritus of cholestasis, but not of other origin and responds to therapeutic interventions. Hepatology. 2012;56:1391. (Epub ahead of print).

67. Zylicz Z, Twycross R, Jones EA. Pruritus in advanced disease. Oxford: Oxford University Press; 2004.

68. Krajnik M, Zylicz Z. Pruritus in advanced internal diseases. Pathog Treat Neth J Med. 2001;58:27–40.

69. Weisshaar E, Kucenic MJ, Fleischer Jr AB, Bhard JD. Pruritus and dysesthesia. In: Bolognia JL, Jorizzo J, Rapini RP, editors. Spain: Dermatology. Mosby; 2015. p. 95–110.

70. Diehn F, Tefferi A. Pruritus in polycythaemia vera: prevalence, laboratory correlates and management. Br J Haematol. 2001;115:619–21.

71. Pieri L, Bogani C, Guglielmelli P, Zingariello M, Rana RA, Bartalucci N, et al. The JAK2V617 mutation induces constitutive activation and agonist hypersensitivity in basophils from patients with polycythemia vera. Haematologica. 2009;94:1537–45.

72. Willemze R, Jaffe ES, Burg G, et al. WHO-EORTC classification for cutaneous lymphomas. Blood. 2005;105:3768–85.

73. Bowen GM, Stevens SR, Dubin HV, Siddiqui J, Cooper KD. Diagnosis of Sezary syndrome in a patient with generalized pruritus based on early molecular study and flow cytometry. J Am Acad Dermatol. 1995;33:678–80.

74. Pujol RM, Gallardo F, Llistosella E, et al. Invisible mycosis fungoides: a diagnostic challenge. J Am Acad Dermatol. 2002;47:S168–71.

75. Tobias Görge, Meinhard Schiller. Chapter 18 Cutaneous T-cell lymphoma. Misery L, Ständer S, editors. Pruritus. London: Springer-Verlag London Limited; 2010. p. 121–4.

76. Jabbour SA. Cutaneous manifestations of endocrine disorders: a guide for dermatologists. Am J Clin Dermatol. 2003;4:315–31.

77. Caravati CM Jr, Richardson DR, Wood BT, Cawley EP. Cutaneous manifestations of hyperthyroidism. South Med J. 1969;62:1127–30.

78. Neilly JB, Martin A, Simpson N, MacCuish AC. Pruritus in diabetes mellitus: investigation of prevalence and correlation with diabetes control. Diabetes Care. 1986;9:273–5.

79. Goodkin R, Wingard E, Bernhard JD. Brachioradial pruritus: cervical spine disease and neurogenic/neurogenic pruritus. J Am Acad Dermatol. 2003;48(4):521–4.

80. Gelfand JM, Rudikoff D. Evaluation and treatment of itching in HIV-infected patients. Mt Sinai J Med. 2001;68(4–5):298–308.

81. Eisman S. Pruritic papular eruption in HIV. Dermatol Clin. 2006;24:449–57.

82. Daniel GL, Longo WE, Vernava AM III. Pruritus ani. Causes and concerns. Dis Colon Rectum. 1994;37:670–4.

83. Reich A, Ständer S. Drug-induced pruritus: a review. Acta Derm Venereol. 2009;89:236–44.

84. Kaplan AP. Drug-induced skin disease. J Allergy Clin Immunol. 1984;74:573–9.

85. Weisshaar E, Szepietowski JC, Darsow U, et al. European guideline on chronic pruritus. Acta Derm Venereol. 2012;92:563–81.

86. Yosipovitch G, Bernhard JD. Chronic pruritus. N Engl J Med. 2013;368:1625–34. 17 nejm.org april 25.

87. Yosipovitch G, David M. The diagnosis and therapeutic approach to idiopatic generalized pruritus. Int J Dermatol. 1999;38:881–7.

88. Weisshaar E, Kucenic MJ, Fleischer AB. Pruritus: a review. Acta Derm Venereol. 2003;213(Suppl):5–32.

89. Ständer S, Streit M, Darsow U, et al. Diagnostic and therapeutic measures in chronic pruritus. J Dtsch Dermatol Ges. 2006;4:350–70.

90. Sommer F, Hensen P, Böckenholt B, et al. Underlying diseases and cofactors in patients with severe chronic pruritus: a 3-year retrospective study. Acta Derm Venereol. 2007;87:510–6.

91. Bingham LG, Noble JW, Davis MD. Wet dressings used with topical corticosteroids for pruritic dermatoses: a retrospective study. J Am Acad Dermatol. 2009;60:792–800.

92. Ali SM, Yosipovitch G. Skin pH: from basic science to basic skin care. Acta Derm Venereol. 2013;93:261. (Epub ahead of print).

93. Papoiu AD, Yosipovitch G. Topical capsaicin: the fire of a "hot" medicine is reignited. Expert Opin Pharmacother. 2010;11:1359–71.

94. Patel T, Ishiuji Y, Yosipovitch G. Menthol: a refreshing look at this ancient compound. J Am Acad Dermatol. 2007;57:873–8.

95. Young TA, Patel TS, Camacho F, et al. A pramoxine-based anti-itch lotion is more effective than a control lotion for the treatment of uremic pruritus in adult hemodialysis patients. J Dermatolog Treat. 2009;20:76–81.

96. Suys E. Randomized study of topical tacrolimus ointment as possible treatment for resistant idiopathic pruritus ani. J Am Acad Dermatol. 2012;66:327–8.

97. Drake LA, Fallon JD, Sober A. Relief of pruritus in patients with atopic dermatitis after treatment with topical doxepin cream. J Am Acad Dermatol. 1994;31:613–6.

98. O'Donoghue M, Tharp MD. Antihistamines and their role as antipruritics. Dermatol Ther. 2005;18:333–40.

99. Gunal AI, Ozalp G, Yoldas TK, Gunal SY, Kirciman E, Celiker H. Gabapentin therapy for pruritus in haemodialysis patients: a randomized, placebo-controlled, double-blind trial. Nephrol Dial Transplant. 2004;19:3137–9.

100. Phan NQ, Bernhard JD, Luger TA, Ständer S. Antipruritic treatment with systemic μ-opioid receptor antagonists: a review. J Am Acad Dermatol. 2010;63:680–8.

101. Kumagai H, Ebata T, Takamori K, Muramatsu T, Nakamoto H, Suzuki H. Effect of a novel kappa-receptor agonist, nalfurafine hydrochloride, on severe itch in 337 haemodialysis patients: a phase III, randomized, double-blind, placebo-controlled study. Nephrol Dial Transplant. 2010;25:1251–7.

102. Wikström B, Gellert R, Ladefoged SD, et al. Kappa-opioid system in uremic pruritus: multicenter, randomized, double blind, placebo-controlled clinical studies. J Am Soc Nephrol. 2005;16:3742–7.

103. Peer G, Kivity S, Agami O, et al. Randomised crossover trial of naltrexone in uraemic pruritus. Lancet. 1996;348:1552–4.

104. Pauli-Magnus C, Mikus G, Alscher DM, et al. Naltrexone does not relieve uremic pruritus: results of a randomized, double-blind, placebo-controlled crossover study. J Am Soc Nephrol. 2000;11:514–9.

105. Dawn AG, Yosipovitch G. Butorphanol for treatment of intractable pruritus. J Am Acad Dermatol. 2006;54:527–31.

106. Ständer S, Böckenholt B, Schürmeyer-Horst F, et al. Treatment of chronic pruritus with the selective serotonin re-uptake inhibitors paroxetine and fluvoxamine: results of an open-labelled, two-arm proof of concept study. Acta Derm Venereol. 2009;89:45–51.

107. Mayo MJ, Handem I, Saldana S, Jacobe H, Getachew Y, Rush AJ. Sertraline as a first-line treatment for cholestatic pruritus. Hepatology. 2007;45:666–74.

108. Hundley JL, Yosipovitch G. Mirtazapine for reducing nocturnal itch in patients with chronic pruritus: a pilot study. J Am Acad Dermatol. 2004;50:889–91.

109. Demierre MF, Taverna J. Mirtazapine and gabapentin for reducing pruritus in cutaneous T-cell lymphoma. J Am Acad Dermatol. 2006;55:543–4.

110. Suchin KR. Pruritus of unknown etiology including senile pruritus. In: Lebwohl M, Heymann WR, Berth-Jones J, Coulson I, editors. Treatment of skin disease – comprehensive therapeutic strategies. Mosby: EUA; 2002. p. 519–22.

111. Prince MI, Burt AD, Jones DEJ. Hepatitis and liver dysfunction with rifampicin therapy for pruritus in primary biliary cirrhosis. Gut. 2002;50:436–9.

112. Suchin KR, Suchin EJ. Pruritus of renal and liver disease. In: Lebwohl M, Heymann WR, Berth-Jones J, Coulson I editors. Treatment of skin disease – comprehensive therapeutic strategies. Mosby: EUA; 2002. p. 515–8.

113. Daly BM, Shuster S. Antipruritic action of thalidomide. Acta Derm Venereol. 2000;80:24–5.

114. Moraes M, Russo G. Thalidomide and its dermatologic uses. Am J Med Sci. 2001;321(5):321–6.

115. Rivard J, Lim HW. Ultraviolet phototherapy for pruritus. Dermatol Ther. 2005;18:344–54.

116. Gilchrest BA, Rowe JW, Brown RS, Steinman TI, Arndt KA. Ultraviolet phototherapy of uremic pruritus: long-term results and possible mechanism of action. Ann Intern Med. 1979;91:17–21.

117. Ko MJ, Yang JY, Wu HY, et al. Narrowband ultraviolet B phototherapy for patients with refractory uraemic pruritus: a randomized controlled trial. Br J Dermatol. 2011;165:633–9.

118. Hassan I, Haji MI. Understanding itch: an update on mediators and mechanisms of pruritus. Indian J Dermatol Venereol Leprol. 2014;80:106–14.

Prurigo

62

Daniel Lorenzini, Fabiane Kumagai Lorenzini, Karen Reetz Muller, and Sabrina Dequi Sanvido

Key Points
- Establishment of prurigo nomenclature and its differential diagnoses
- Presentation of the probable etiologies of chronic prurigo by showing the importance of the patient's clinical assessment
- Update of the therapeutic options for prurigo management

Concepts

The word *prurigo* has been used to designate a heterogeneous group of dermatoses that have papular eruption and pruritus as common aspects. Prurigo can be seen as a reactive clinical pattern, and 20% of the cases are still regarded as idiopathic. This term has been used whether the cause is known or unknown.

The clinical aspect of the lesions may vary and includes papules and nodules with excoriation, erosion, lichenification, crust-covered papules, and seropapules. Scars and residual hyperchromia can be found.

Clinical Presentation

The different types of prurigo had been described and designated by eponyms, with a confusing terminology. Greither [1] and Jorizzo et al. [2] classified the previously reported groups into acute, subacute, and chronic, as shown in Box 62.1. In addition to this division, we may include other varieties of prurigo in the classification, such as the prurigo of pregnancy, prurigo pigmentosa, and actinic prurigo [3, 4].

Box 62.1 Classification of Prurigo and Synonyms

Acute prurigo	Strophulus, prurigo mitis, papular urticaria, prurigo Hebra (prurigo "ferox"), prurigo simplex acuta Brocq, prurigo temporanea Tommasoli
Subacute prurigo	Prurigo subacuta Kogoj, prurigo vulgaris Darier, prurigo multiforme Lutz, lichen urticatus Vidal, prurigo simplex subacuta, urticaria papulosa chronica perstans, neurotic excoriation
Chronic prurigo	Prurigo nodularis Hyde, keratosis verrucosa, lichen obtusus corneus, urticaria perstans verrucosa, eczema verrucocallosum

D. Lorenzini (✉)
Federal University of Health Sciences from Porto Alegre, School of Medicine, Porto Alegre, Brazil
e-mail: daniellorenzini@gmail.com

F.K. Lorenzini • K.R. Muller
Santa Marta Health Center,
Porto Alegre, Brazil

S.D. Sanvido
Irmandade Santa Casa de Misericórdia de Porto Alegre, Porto Alegre, Brazil

© Springer International Publishing Switzerland 2018
R.R. Bonamigo, S.I.T. Dornelles (eds.), *Dermatology in Public Health Environments*,
https://doi.org/10.1007/978-3-319-33919-1_62

Other	Besnier's prurigo
	Prurigo of pregnancy
	Dermographic prurigo
	Prurigo pigmentosa
	Actinic prurigo
	Hutchinson prurigo

Adapted from Wallengren [3] and González et al. [4]

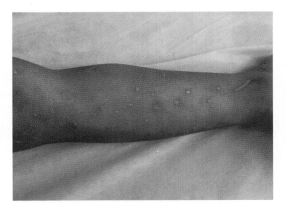

Fig. 62.1 Residual hypochromia surrounded by hyperpigmentation on a lower limb of a patient with strophulus

Acute Prurigo

Most often found in childhood, 86% of cases occur during the first 3 years of life. It is common among the economically lower classes, especially during summer [4].

Acute Prurigo: Simplex

Also known as strophulus, prurigo mitis, lichen urticatus, and papular urticaria, acute prurigo (simplex) is characterized by papules, vesicles, and/or urticaria during the early years of life, lasting for about a week. Hypersensitivity to arthropod bites, such as mosquitoes, ants, and fleas, is the main cause. Association with food allergies and psychological and infectious factors have also been described [5, 6]. Patients with acute prurigo show greater sensitivity to insect antigens during skin tests. Patient improvement in adulthood may correspond to desensitization resulting from repetitive bites [4]. On superficial blood vessels, granular deposits of C1q, C3, and immunoglobulin M were found, suggesting that dissemination is mediated by the immune complex [7].

It has sudden onset, with a small pruriginous vesicle/papule, which breaks up if scratched, being covered by a crust. It is believed that the early lesions primarily result from insect bites and that the subsequent symmetric and disseminated lesions are probably due to hematogenic dissemination of the bite-inoculated antigen [4].

Erosions, lichenification, and secondary infection may also be noticed. Lesions may show themselves as erythematous-edematous plaques, vesicles, and blisters, with blisters more often seen on the limbs. The papules persist over a week, with the development of new, nonconflu-

ent lesions; lesions of varying stages may coexist, sometimes leaving scars, hyperchromia, or residual hypochromia as seen in Fig. 62.1. The trunk and the limbs are the main locations; lesions are seldom seen on the face. The genital, perineal, and axillary regions are usually spared [4]. It is more frequently seen in children of 2–7 years of age, also being associated with the presence of atopy [3, 8].

The histopathologic examination is unspecific and shows the presence of perivascular inflammatory infiltrate, with lymphocytes and eosinophils, acanthosis, spongiosis with intraepidermal vesicle, and parakeratosis.

The diagnosis is clinical, based on lesion and pruritus history, location, and aspect. Epicutaneous tests can be helpful.

The differential diagnoses may include scabies, body pediculosis, herpetiform dermatitis, varicella, and urticaria.

Acute Prurigo: Simplex: Adulthood

Prurigo simplex temporanea Tommasoli has a presentation similar to that of strophulus, except that it occurs in young adults. The clinical presentation is characterized by papules on the extensor surfaces of the upper limbs and the anterolateral surfaces of the lower limbs. It has an insect-bite hypersensitivity, but may be related to hormonal factors, and infectious and parasite foci. In persistent lesions, systemic causes, such as diabetes, hepatopathies, nephropathies, and neoplasms, must be assessed. The diagnosis is clinical, and the differential diagnosis includes herpetiform dermatitis and scabies [1, 2].

Prurigo Hebra

Known as prurigo "ferox", it displays pruriginous, eczematous, impetiginous, and lichenified papules, with lymphadenopathy mainly in atopic children. It occurs mainly in geographic areas lacking sanitation and good nutritional conditions [3]. The histopathology is the same as described for prurigo simplex.

Subacute Prurigo

Prurigo subacuta Kogoj, prurigo vulgaris Darier, prurigo multiforme Lutz, lichen urticatus Vidal, urticaria papulosa chronica perstans, and neurotic excoriations are multiple entities that share the same clinical and histologic presentation. It mainly affects middle-aged women, being related to emotional and psychogenic factors. Atopy, dermographism, and seborrheic dermatitis are also associated [9].

Subacute prurigo shows papules, excoriations, and symmetric urticariform plaques on the trunk, extensor surfaces of the limbs, face, and scalp, but not on the palms and the foot plantar region, as seen in Fig. 62.2. The pruritus develops in successive flares, and may be precipitated by exercise, heat, or emotional status [4].

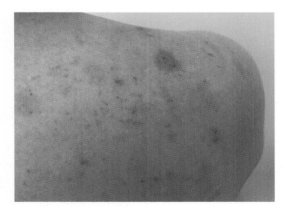

Fig. 62.2 Subacute prurigo: papules, excoriation on the back of a male patient

The differential diagnosis includes herpetiform dermatitis, transient and persistent acantholytic dermatitis, and scabies.

The histologic examination shows acanthosis, hyperkeratosis, proliferation of nervous fibers, focal spongiosis, and perivascular and perifollicular inflammatory infiltrate.

Chronic Prurigo

Chronic prurigo includes prurigo nodularis, keratosis verrucosa, lichen obtusus corneus, and urticaria perstans verrucosa.

Prurigo Nodularis

Prurigo nodularis is the most characteristic representative of chronic prurigo in the terminology, described in 1909 by Hyde as nodules on the extensor surface of a woman's arms and legs, relatively rare and difficult to treat. Similar cases were reported by Hardaway in 1880 [10] and Brocq in 1900 [11]. In 1934, Pautrier showed the presence of dermal neural hyperplasia, known as Pautrier's neuroma [12].

Lichen simplex chronicus and lichen amyloidosis may correspond to the same disease spectrum given their similar clinical presentation and histopathologic findings, according to Weyers in 1995 [13]. Many authors regard prurigo nodularis as an atypical form of circumscribed dermatitis [14]; nevertheless, the indirect immunofluorescence of nerve bundles in prurigo nodularis showed increased immunoreactivity for substance P and the calcitonin gene-related peptide (CGRP) [15].

Prurigo nodularis shows symmetric, hardened, hyperkeratous, very pruriginous nodules and papules mainly on the extensor surfaces of the limbs, more often found in middle-aged women (Fig. 62.3). The lesions may show variation in quantity, and may affect the sacral region in 50% of patients and the abdominal region in 44%; palms, soles, and face are rarely affected [16]. Lesion onset is insidious, with chronic evolution. The pruritus is intense and intermittent, relieved by scratching to the point of skin mutilation and bleeding. In chronic lesions

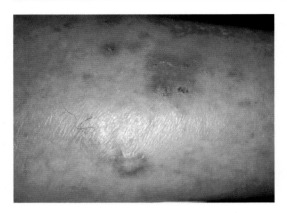

Fig. 62.3 Prurigo nodularis: pruriginous nodules and excoriations on the extensor face of the lower limb of a female patient

verrucous papules, lichenoid plaques, and excoriation may be noticed, as well as postinflammatory hyperchromia and scars. The papular distribution mainly follows the cleavage lines but not Blaschko lines [17].

The cause is unknown, although emotional factors may be present, and 65–80% of the patients are atopic [16]. Metabolic changes (such as anemia, hepatopathies, uremia, and myxedema), trauma, and neuronal etiology were suggested as related to prurigo nodularis [2, 16]. Focal causes of pruritus, such as insect bites, venous stasis, folliculitis, and nummular eczema are also related to this condition. Gluten-driven enteropathy with prurigo nodularis was already described by some authors, with improvement of both presentations when food is restricted [18–22].

Histopathology shows acanthosis, hyperkeratosis with proliferation of small vessels, and unspecific inflammatory infiltrate on the dermis (histiocytes, lymphocytes, mastocytes, and eosinophils). Fibroblast proliferation occurs, possible findings including a subepidermal fibrin deposit [2, 23, 24], papillomatosis, and irregular epidermal proliferation. The histologic findings may be similar to those of chronic eczema or persistent reaction to insect bite [16, 23]. Some authors believe the detected neural and vascular hyperplasia may result from mechanical trauma [25].

The diagnosis is clinical, according to the lesion history, location, and clinical aspect. Histologic examination may complement the diagnosis.

The differential diagnosis includes lichen simplex chronicus, hypertrophic lichen planus, pemphigoid nodularis, pruriginous epidermolysis bullosa, multiple keratoacanthoma, epidermal cysts, disseminated cutaneous cytomegalovirus in HIV-positive patients, and botryomycosis [26].

Endogenous and Exogenous Factors Related to Prurigo

Box 62.2 shows the main factors related to prurigo onset [3].

Box 62.2 Endogenous and Exogenous Factors Related to Prurigo

Endogenous	Exogenous
Atopy	Infections and parasitoses
Internal diseases	Contact allergy and drug reactions
Malabsorption	Light eruption
Malignancy	
Emotional factors	
Pregnancy	
Ethnic predisposition	
Adapted from Wallengren [3]	

Atopy

The term Besnier's prurigo is used to designate the chronic papular and lichenified form of atopic dermatitis as seen in Fig. 62.4. Many cases of Hebra prurigo have possibly involved patients living under poor social conditions. This pruriginous form of atopic dermatitis is less frequent and found in 9% of young adults who have had the disease during childhood [27].

Internal Diseases

Many internal diseases associated with pruritus may yield skin lesions that simulate prurigo nodularis resulting from scratching. Pruritus is a very common symptom in patients suffering from chronic renal failure who undergo hemodialysis. Perforating folliculitis with overlaying nodular prurigo has been described [28].

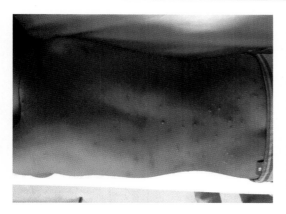

Fig. 62.4 Lichenified papules on the back of an atopic dermatitis patient

Diabetes mellitus, disseminated lupus erythematosus, systemic scleroderma, and deficiency of α1-antitrypsin may be associated with prurigo nodularis or prurigo-like lesions [29, 30].

Malabsorption

The association of prurigo nodularis with malabsorption was described in 1962 in a patient with celiac disease. Some other cases have been described since then in association with therapy-resistant enteropathies and prurigo nodularis. After some months of gluten-free diet, complemented with vitamins and iron, the intestinal symptoms improved and the skin lesions reduced or disappeared [31]. Anorexia nervosa and prurigo were associated because pruritus is one of the characteristics resulting from low weight. Once the weight is normalized, the prurigo lesions improve [32].

Malignancy

Pruritus and excoriations may be a nonspecific marker of internal malignant disease. Prurigo has been associated with T cell lymphoma and esophageal visceral, ventricular, rectal, hepatic, and biliary duct neoplasia. In a patient with lymphoma, the prurigo may appear before the symptoms of malignancy [33]. Prurigo may also be a warning sign for malignant change in patients with early tumors diagnosed as benign. In malignant cases prurigo nodules possibly result from scratching [34].

Emotional Factors

In clinical studies of patients with nodular prurigo, 50% of the subjects showed depression, anxiety, or some other psychological disease, and 72% of the patients reported that psychological problems were relevant to the skin disease [16].

Prurigo of Pregnancy

Prurigo of pregnancy, prurigo gestationis Besnier, is a pregnancy-specific, benign, self-limited dermatosis that affects 1 out of 300 pregnant women [35–43]. Earlier classified as pregnancy dermatosis of exclusion, it has now been reclassified as a subtype of atopic gestational eruption [43]. There are no risks for either the baby or the mother. Box 62.3 reports a related case.

> **Box 62.3 Case Report: Prurigo of Pregnancy**
> In 2010, Fan Wen-Ge and Qu Yun reported a case of a pregnant woman with a clinical presentation compatible with prurigo of pregnancy which, in 1995, resulted in fetal death. At that time the woman and baby underwent investigation whereby both showed no laboratory or chromosomal alterations, anomalies, or illnesses. In 2005 the same woman presented with gestational prurigo, underwent follow-up, and was treated with topical and intravenous corticosteroids to aid the baby's lung maturation; the gestational process was interrupted in the 34th week, with both being healthy [37].

It is considered the second most common gestational-specific dermatosis, although its etiology is unknown [41]. The trigger could involve some immunity-related change resulting from the pregnant condition: a decrease in cellular immunity and T-helper 1 (Th1) cytokine production compared with an increase in Th2 cytokine production through humoral immunity [36]. There seems to be a correlation with atopy, and some authors believe that it is the severe gestational pruritus in atopic patients [40–42]. Small 0.5- to 1-cm papules, extremely pruriginous, erythematous, and even hyperchromic, which evolve into nodules on the extensor surface of the limbs may be noticed. Eventually they may spread; they usually appear as excoriated lesions more often occurring between the 25th and the 30th gestational weeks, although they are not limited to the period between those 2 weeks. The condition subsides some weeks postpartum, or may last for up to 3 months [42]. No vesicles or bullae are noticed [41].

Considered an exclusion diagnosis, it is based on clinical and normal laboratory tests, except for a possible increased IgE [36, 39–41]. The anatomopathologic examination is unspecific; it may present a perivascular lymphocytic infiltrate on the upper dermis, possibly affecting the epidermis. Direct and indirect immunofluorescence is negative.

Differential diagnoses are other gestational dermatoses, such as cholestasis and pruritic urticarial papules and plaques of pregnancy (PUPP), besides atopic dermatitis, arthropod bites, scabies, and drug reactions.

Ethnic Predisposition

Prurigo pigmentosa, or Nagashima's disease, is a rare condition in the Western world, more common in young Japanese women aged 23–27 years [44], although male cases and other ethnic background cases have been reported [45]. The etiopathogenesis remains uncertain. There are hypotheses of an association with ketosis, type 1 diabetes mellitus, anorexia nervosa, *Helicobacter pylori* infection, and atopy. It is not clear whether the highest incidence on Japanese women results from environmental factors or genetic predisposition [45]. It is severely manifested as intense pruriginous erythematous papules and papules/vesicles [45]. The lesions usually concentrate on the back, chest, and cervical region [46]. With evolution, the lesions heal and scars are seen as hyperchromic macules with a reticular pattern [45]. The clinical course oscillates, with both exacerbations and remissions [47].

The diagnosis is based on clinical and histopathologic manifestations. There is variation in the anatomopathology according to the stage of lesion evolution. The most recent lesions show a superficial perivascular neutrophilic infiltrate while the well-established lesions show spongiosis and many necrotic keratinocytes. Eventually, the late lesions display a predominantly lymphocytic infiltrate, with melanophages in the papillary dermis [45].

The differential diagnoses in the severe phase are herpetiform dermatitis, acute erythematous lupus, and linear IgA dermatosis; in regard to the remission phase, Ashy dermatosis, macular amyloidosis, and confluent and reticulated papillomatosis (Gougerot–Carteaud syndrome) must be excluded [45].

Infections and Parasitic infections

The organ most affected by HIV is the skin [48]. An average 90% of HIV-positive patients will present some form of dermatosis during their lives [48–50]. The HIV pruritic-papular eruptions result in high morbidity and are difficult to treat [51]. It is a noninfectious chronic dermatosis, more often seen in highly immunologically affected patients [48, 52–54].

It is a chronic, recurrent condition with papular lesions, papulopustules, and/or nodules mainly affecting the distal region. There is intense pruritus and high recurrence. Eventually it disseminates [48]. Multiple lesions (more than 100) represent the usual pattern, although one or two lesions have been reported [50]. A linear disposition is common, usually evolving with dyschromias [50]. Both men and women are affected [50]. The etiopathogenesis is not well known and in HIV patients the treatment is challenging [53, 54]. Some authors believe there may be some hypersensitivity to arthropod bites [54, 55]. By virtue of the HIV there would be greater stimulus of B lymphocytes, inversion of the CD4/CD8 relationship, decrease in number and function of Langerhans cells, alteration of macrophage function, d IgE increase, possibly leading to a hypersensitivity reaction, more common in higher phototypes and CD4 cell count <50 [48, 50, 56]. Some research studies show lower levels of interleukin-2 and interferon-γ [54]. It is less often seen in Europe and North America [54, 55]. Firstly we must exclude causes leading to pruritus and, therefore, prurigo lesions. Also, infectious and neoplastic diseases such as lymphoma and hepatic, renal, and neurologic diseases must be excluded. Eosinophilia and increased serum IgE may be found in laboratory tests [54, 57]. The anatomopathologic examination is usually unspecific; there is perivascular inflammatory infiltrate mainly comprising lymphocytes, with or without eosinophils. There must be hyperkeratosis, acanthosis, and papillomatosis with dermal fibrosis [50].

Differential diagnosis includes syphilis, drug eruption, scabies, folliculitis, demodicidosis, and tuberculids [54].

Strophulus prurigo may be caused by flea, mosquito, and tick bites. Lyme disease, mycobacteriosis, skin toxoplasmosis, and *H. pylori* infection have also showed an association with prurigo [3].

Contact Allergy and Drug Reactions

Contact allergy is usually related to intense itch, and can occur together with prurigo secondary to scratching. Patients with already established prurigo may develop a contact allergy to the drugs used to manage the condition. In a study at the Mayo Clinic, 29 out of 199 patients with prurigo who underwent contact tests were positive to neomycin, fragrance, and nickel. Many patients reported improvement after removal of the allergen [58].

Some drugs, such as etanercept, may induce acute prurigo; carbamazepine may induce subacute prurigo, and etretinate may induce nodular prurigo-like reactions [3].

Light Eruption

Actinic prurigo, also known as Hutchinson summer prurigo, is a photoinduced dermatosis, with the collaboration of hereditary and geographic components. It is more common among Native Americans and is seldom seen in Europe, Asia, and Oceania [59]. A possible relationship with the presence of HLA-DR4 has been investigated, and it is more frequent in higher-altitude inhabitants (1,000 m above sea level) [61]. Women are more affected than men [61], and actinic prurigo usually starts during childhood [62]. It may be induced by solar exposition, with higher incidence in the summer and spring, with possible remission in fall and winter [60]. Some authors have suggested that actinic prurigo may be a specter of polymorphous light eruption [63, 64].

The etiopathogenesis is unknown. Exposure to solar radiation has been suggested as the main trigger, which would yield the production of self-antigens and a consequent immune reaction in genetically predisposed individuals [59]. It manifests as flat papules, which may coalesce to create plaques and nodules in photoexposed areas, mainly the face, cervical region, upper torso, extensor aspect of the forearms, and dorsum of the hands. On the face the lesions tend to concentrate on areas of more direct incidence of light, such as the forehead, nasal dorsum, and malar regions. The lesions are heavily pruriginous, leading to the development of excoriations and possible scars. They are usually associated with cheilitis (mainly on the lower lip), conjunctivitis, and eyebrow alopecia [59, 60, 65].

The diagnosis is based on the clinical and histopathologic manifestations. Regarding the anatomopathology, the recent lesions usually show spongiosis while the older lesions are similar to prurigo nodularis [66]. The finding of HLA-DR4 favors the diagnosis. A photoprovocation test may be carried out [60]. Differential diagnoses include polymorphous light eruption, prurigo nodularis, cutaneous lupus erythematosus, and porphyria [60, 62].

Diagnosis

The diagnosis of prurigo is usually clinical. Additional investigation is important to define the related factors [67]. Box 62.4 synthesizes the basic assessment for prurigo when its cause cannot be established by early clinical assessment.

Box 62.4 Additional Examinations in Prurigo Investigation
- Complete blood count
- Urea, creatinine, and electrolytes
- Liver function
- Blood sugar
- Hepatitis serology

- HIV serology
- Total serum IgE
- Protein electrophoresis
- Thyroid/parathyroid function
- Chest X-ray or computed tomography/ magnetic resonance imaging
- Skin biopsy
- Patch test

Therapeutic Approach

When assessing a patient with a prurigo nodularis, it is important to search for the underlying cause. Acute prurigo also has inflammation and heavy pruritus that can be treated with topical corticosteroids and antihistamines. Subacute prurigo is a relapsing disease which demands treatment during its exacerbation periods. The courses of nodular and secondary prurigo are long. The chronic and persistent forms are treatment resistant, which force patients to go through many kinds of therapeutic experiences. Encouraging the patient to avoid scratching the lesions is important, since lesion manipulation worsens the symptoms [68].

Topical Treatments

The use of moisturizer must be encouraged because xerosis may exacerbate the pruritus [67].

Topical corticosteroids, preferably with occlusive membrane on the lesions, are very useful in acute and subacute injuries. In the case of more chronic lesions, the application of an intralesional corticosteroid is more effective. Coal tar with antipruritic and antibacterial properties is used during the severe phases in patients showing many excoriations. Calcipotriol is also effective for prurigo nodularis [69].

Cryotherapy has been recommended, since it induces thermal damage to peripheral sensory nerves. The application time varies from 10 to 30 s for two to four cycles. If postprocedural improvement of the lesion occurs, a topical corticosteroid must be applied. Intralesional lidocaine

and capsaicin cream are also effective. Menthol cream at 1% and camphor at 2% are good antipruritic applications [70–72].

Calcineurin inhibitors, such as pimecrolimus and tacrolimus, have been successful in decreasing pruritus in the investigated patients [73].

Systemic Treatments

Hydroxyzine (or similar sedative antihistamine of first generation) is very important for pruritus control, at 10–50 mg/day (or 0.5–1 mg/kg/day), every 6 or 12 h [3].

Systemic psoralen combined with ultraviolet A in research studies was effective, although it may lose efficacy after some time [74]. Narrowband ultraviolet B has also been proposed as an effective option [3].

Azathioprine 50 mg, twice a day, over 6–12 months, decreased pruritus and nodules in patients with prurigo nodularis. Relapses can occur between 2 months and 3 years after treatment interruption. Its efficacy in decreasing actinic prurigo symptoms has also been shown [75, 76].

Cyclosporine must to be used at high doses (3–4.5 mg/kg/day) over 6–9 months, resulting in pruritus decrease after 2 weeks. Pruritus and nodules may decrease and disappear during the period of treatment, although the condition relapses only 1 month after interruption [77].

Dapsone is the drug of choice to treat prurigo pigmentosa. Relapse occurs after treatment interruption. In Japan, minocycline 100–200 mg/day seemed to have anti-inflammatory action and provided a quick disappearance of pruritus, papules, and erythema; hyperchromia usually persists, being difficult to treat [44–46].

Naltrexone was successfully used to treat pruritus at a daily dose of 50 mg, with the possibility of doubling the dose in a few weeks. Naltrexone has a considerable antipruritic effect, thus playing a role in improving prurigo nodularis lesions [78].

Gabapentin and pregabalin inhibited neurotransmitters that provoke pruritus in prurigo nodularis patients [79, 80]. In a study with pregabalin, 23 out of 30 patients (77%) showed complete remission of pruritus and prurigo lesions at a dose of 25 mg, three times a day, over 3 months. The maintenance dose is 50 mg/day for up to 2 years [80].

In 1973 the successful treatment of prurigo nodularis with thalidomide was described, since when it has been implemented [81]. Pruritus decreased in a few weeks while lesion involution took a few months. When there was drug interruption the pruritus took 2 months to reoccur and became severe in 4 months. The authors suggested a long-term treatment at a dose of 200 mg/day, possibly higher [82]. In patients with HIV prurigo, thalidomide has been signaled to have a promising role considering that it is not an immunosuppressive drug. However, one-third of the investigated patients developed peripheral neuropathy [51].

Thalidomide should not be used in women within fertility range if they do not use a satisfactory contraceptive method, because of the drug's teratogenicity.

Glossary

Erosion Erosion is caused by loss of the surface of a skin lesion; it is a shallow moist or crusted lesion.
Excoriation A scratch mark. It may be linear or a picked scratch (prurigo). Excoriations may occur in the absence of a primary dermatosis.
Lichenification Lichenification is caused by chronic rubbing, which results in palpably thickened skin with increased skin markings and lichenoid scale. It occurs in chronic atopic eczema and lichen simplex.
Nodule An enlargement of a papule in three dimensions (height, width, length). It is a solid lesion.
Papules Small palpable lesions. The usual definition is that they are less than 0.5 cm diameter, although some authors allow up to 1.5 cm. They are raised above the skin surface, and may be solitary or multiple.
Plaques A palpable flat lesion greater than 0.5 cm in diameter. Most plaques are elevated, but a plaque can also be a thickened area without being visibly raised above the skin surface. They may have well-defined or ill-defined borders.
Vesicles Small fluid-filled blisters less than 0.5 cm in diameter. They may be single or multiple.

References

1. Greither A. On the different forms of prurigo. Pruritus-Prurigo. Curr Probl Dermatol. 1970;3:1–30.
2. Jorizzo JL, Gatti S, Smith EB. Prurigo: a clinical review. J Am Acad Dermatol. 1981;4:723–8.
3. Wallengren J. Prurigo: diagnosis and management. Am J Clin Dermatol. 2004;5(2):85–95.
4. González FU, Moya ES, Saba CM, Salas RS. Prurigos. La Medicina Hoy. Available from: http://apps.elsevier.es/watermark/ctl_servlet?_f=10&pident_articulo=15305&pident_usuario=0&pcontactid=&pident_revista=1&ty=86&accion=L&origen=zonadelectura&web=www.elsevier.es&lan=es&fichero=1v60n75me2.pdf.
5. Derbes VJ. Papular urticaria. Cutis. 1972;9:779–81.
6. Rook A. Papular urticaria. Pediatr Clin N Am. 1961;8:817–83.
7. Heng MCY, Kloss SG, Haberfelde GC. Pathogenesis of popular urticaria. J Am Acad Dermatol. 1984;10:1030–4.
8. Maruani A, Samimi M, Lorette G. Les Prurigos. Presse Med. 2009;38:1099–105.
9. Mali JWH. Prurigo simplex subacuta. A group of cases with atopic background. Acta Dermatol Venereol (Stockh). 1967;47:304–8.
10. Hardaway WA. A case of multiple tumors of the skin accompanied by intense itching. Arch Dermatol. 1880;6:129–32.
11. Brocq LAJ. Lichen obtusus corneus. Prat Dermatol. 1900;3:201.
12. Pautrier LM. Le néurome de la lichénification circonscrite nodulaire chronique (lichen ruber obtusus corné prurigo nodularis). Ann Dermatol Syph. 1934;7:897–919.
13. Weyers W. Lichen amyloidosus. Krankheitsentität oder Kratzeffekt. Hautarzt. 1995;46:165–72.
14. Pillsbury DM. Eczema. In: Moschella SL, Pillsbury DM, Hurley HJ, editors. Dermatology. Philadelphia: WB Saunders; 1975.
15. Vaalasti A, Suomalainen H, Rechardt L. Calcitonin gene-related peptide immunoreactivity in prurigo nodularis: a comparative study with neurodermatitis circumscripta. Br J Dermatol. 1989;120:619–23.
16. Payne CM, Wilkinson JD, McKee PH, Jurecka W, Black MM. Nodular prurigo – a clinicopathologic study of 46 patients. Br J Dermatol. 1985;113(4):431–9.
17. Wollina U, Simon D, Knopf B. Prurigo nodularis Hyde – Bevorzugung der Hautspaltlinien. Dermatol Mon Schr. 1990;176:469–73.
18. Wells GC. Skin disorders in relation to malabsorption. Br Med J. 1962;4:937–43.

19. Howell R. Exudative nummular prurigo with idiopathic malabsorption syndrome. Br J Dermatol. 1967;79:357.

20. McKenzie AW, Stubbing DG, Elvy BL. Prurigo nodularis and gluten enteropathy. Br J Dermatol. 1976;95:89–92.

21. Goodwin PG. Nodular prurigo associated with gluten enteropathy. Proc R Soc Med. 1977;70:140–1.

22. Suárez C, Pereda JM, Moreno LM, García-González F, Gómez-Orbaneja J. Prurigo nodularis associated with malabsorption. Dermatologica. 1984;169:211–4.

23. Lever WF, Schaumburg-Lever G. Histopathology of the skin. 7th ed. Philadelphia: JB Lippincott; 1990. p. 155–6.

24. Wong E, MacDonald DM. Localized subepidermal fibrin deposition – a histopathologic feature of friction induced cutaneous lesions. Clin Exp Dermatol. 1982;7:499–503.

25. Doyle JA, Connolly SM, Hunziker N, Winkelmann RK. Prurigo nodularis: a reappraisal of the clinical and histologic features. J Cutan Pathol. 1979;6:392–403.

26. Accioly-Filho JW, Nogueira A, Ramos-e-Silva M. Prurigo nodularis of Hyde: an update. JEADV. 2000;14:75–82.

27. Kissling S, Wuthrich B. Sites, types of manifestation and micro manifestations of atopic dermatitis in Young adults: a personal follow-up 20 years after diagnosis in childhood. Hautarzt. 1994;45(6):368–71.

28. White CR Jr, Heskel NS, Pokorny DJ. Perforating folliculitis of hemodialysis. Am J Dermatopathol. 1982;4(2):109–16.

29. Sass U, Forton F, Dequenne P, et al. Acquire reactive perforating collagenosis. J Eur Acad Dermatol Venereol. 1995;5:110–4.

30. Heng MC, Allen SG, Kim A, et al. Alpha 1-antitrypsin deficiency in a patient with widespred prurigo nodularis. Aust J Dermatol. 1991;32(3):151–7.

31. Well GC. Skin disorders in relation to malabsortion. BMJ. 1962;4:937–43.

32. Morgan JF, Lacey JH. Scratching and fasting: a study of pruritus and anorexia nervosa. Br J Dermatol. 1999;140(3):453–6.

33. Pagliuca A, Williams H, Salisbury J, et al. Prodromal cutaneous lesions in adult T-cell leucemia/lymphoma [letter]. Lancet. 1990;335(8691):733–4.

34. Dereure O, Guilhou JJ. Multifocal hepatocellular carcinoma presenting as prurigo: two cases. Br J Dermatol. 2000;143(6):1331–2.

35. Alves GF, Black MM. Dermatoses Específicas da Gravidez. An Bras Dermatol. 1998;73(4):353–9.

36. Bergman H, Melamed N, Koren G. Pruritus in pregnancy. Can Fam Physician. 2013;59:1290–4.

37. Wen-Ge F, Qu Y. Images for diagnosis prurido gestationis. Chin Med J. 2010;123(5):638–40.

38. Massod S, Rizvi DA, Tebassum S, Akhtar S, Alvi RU. Frequency and clinical variants of specific dermatoses in third trimester of pregnancy: a study from a tertiary care centre. JPMA. 2012;62:244.

39. Soutou B, Aractingi S. Dermatoses de la grossesse. La Rev Méd Internet. 2015;36:198–202.

40. Roth MM. Pregnancy dermatoses diagnosis, management, and controversies. Am J Clin Dermatol. 2011;12(1):25–41.

41. Bolognia JL, Jorizzo J, Rapini R. Dermatologia, Segunda edição. Rio de Janeiro: Eselvier; 2011.

42. Alves GF, Nogueira LSC, Varella TCN. Dermatologia e gestação. Bras Dermatol. 2005;80(2):179–86.

43. Lehrhoff S, Pomeranz MK. Specific dermatoses of pregnancy and their treatment. Dermatol Ther. 2013;26:274–84.

44. Shannon JF, Weedon D, Sharkey MP. Prurigo pigmentosa. Aust J Dermatol. 2006;47:289–90.

45. Hijazi M, Kehdy J, Kibbi AG, Ghosn S. Prurigo pigmentosa: a clinicopathologic study of 4 cases from the Middle East. Am J Dermapathol. 2014;36(10):800–6.

46. Schedel F, Schürmann C, Metze D, Ständer S. Prurigo: klinische definition und klassifikation. Hautarzt. 2014;65:684–90.

47. Lapeere H, Boone B, De Shepper S, Verhaeghe E, Ongenae K, Van Geel N, Lambert J, Brochez L, Naeyaert LM. Hypomelanoses and hypermelanoses. In: Wolff K, Goldsmith LA, Katz SI, Gilchrest BA, Paller AS, Leffell DJ, editors. Fitzpatrick's dermatology in general medicine. Seventh ed. New York: McGraw-Hill; 2008. p. 622–40.

48. Porro AM, Yashioka MCN. Dermatologic manifestation of HIV infection. An Bras Dermatol. 2000;75(6):665–91.

49. Zancanaro PCQ, McGirt LY, Mamelak AJ, Nguyen R, Martins C. Cutaneous manifestations of HIV in the era of highly active antiretroviral therapy: an institutional urban clinic experience. J Am Acad Dermatol. 2006;54(4):581–8.

50. Shanonn N, Cockerell CJ. Prurigo nodular in HIV infected individuals. Int J Dermatol. 1998;37:401–9.

51. Maurer T, Poncelet A, Berger T. Thalidomide treatment for prurigo nodularis in human immunodeficiency virus-infected subjects: efficacy and risk of neuropathy. Arch Dermatol. 2004;140:845–9.

52. Huang X, Li H, Chen D, Wang X, Li Z, Wu Y, Zhang T, et al. Clinical analysis of skin lesions in 796 Chinese HIV-positive patients. Acta Derm Venereol. 2011;91:552–6.

53. Unemori P, Kieron S, Maurer T. Persistent prurigo nodularis responsive to initiation of combination therapy with raltegravir. Arch Dermatol. 2010;146(6):682–3.

54. Resneck JS, Van Beek M, Furmanski L, Oyugi J, LeBoit PE, Katabira E, et al. Etiology of pruritic papular eruption with HIV infection in Uganda. JAMA. 2004;292(21):2614–21.

55. Rieger A, Chen TM, Cockerell CJ. Manifestações cutâneas do HIV. In: Bolognia JL, Jorizzo J, Rapini R, editors. Dermatologia, Segunda edição. Rio de Janeiro: Elsevier; 2011. p. 1173–4.

56. Maurer T. Dermatologic manifestations of HIV infection. Top HIV Med. 2005;13(5):149–54.

57. Cardoso F, Ramos H, Lobo M. Dermatoses in HIV infected patients with different degrees of immunosuppression. An Bras Dermal. 2002;77(6):669–80.

58. Zelickson BD, McEvoy MT, Fransway AF. Patch testing in prurigo nodularis. Contact Dermatitis. 1989;20:321–5.

59. Valbuena MC, Muvdi S, Lim HW. Actinic prurigo. Dermatol Clin. 2014;32:335–44.
60. Hawk JLM, Ferguson J. Abnormal responses to ultraviolet radiation: idiopathic, probably immunologic, and photo-exacerbated. In: Wolff K, Goldsmith LA, Katz SI, Gilchrest BA, Paller AS, Leffell J, editors. Fitzpatrick's dermatology in general medicine. 7th ed. New York: McGraw-Hill; 2008. p. 816–27.
61. Rébora I. El prurigo actínico:características clínicas, histopatológicas y consideraciones sobre su inmunología, fotobiología y genética, Parte I. Arch Argent Dermatol. 2009;59:89–95.
62. Londoño F. Prurigo Actínico. An Bras Dermatol. 1984;59(3):137–41.
63. Grabczynska SA, McGregor JM, Kondeatis E, et al. Actinic prurigo and polymorphic lighteruption: common pathogenesis and the importance of HLA-DR4/DRB1*0407. Br J Dermatol. 1999;140(2):232–6.
64. Grabczynska SA, Hawk JL. What is actinic prurigo in Britain? Photodermatol Photoimmunol Photomed. 1997;13(3):85–6.
65. Lim HW, Hawk JLM. Photodermatoses. In: Bolognia JL, Jorizzo J, Rapini R, editors. Dermatologia. 2nd ed. Rio de Janeiro: Elsevier; 2011. p. 1333–51.
66. Rapini RP. Outras doenças não-neoplásicas. In: Rapini RP, editor. Dermatologia Prática. Rio de Janeiro: Di Livros; 2005. p. 221–31.
67. Lee MR, Shumack S. Prurigo nodularis: a review. Aust J Dermatol. 2005;46:211–20.
68. Vaidya DC, Schartz RA. Prurigo nodularis: a benign dermatoses derived from a persistente pruritus. Acta Dermatovenerol Croat. 2008;16(1):38–44.
69. Wong SS, Goh CL. Double-blind, right/left comparison of calcipotriol ointment and bethamethasone ointment in the treatment of prurigo nodularis [letter]. Arch Dermatol. 2000;136(6):807–8.
70. Waldinger TP, Wong RC, Taylor WB, et al. Cryotherapy improves prurigo nodularis. Arch Dermatol. 1984;120(12):1598–600.
71. Stoll DM, Fields JP, King LE Jr. Treatment of prurigo nodularis: use of cryosurgery and intralesional steroids plus lidocaine. J Dermatol Surg Oncol. 1983;9(11):922–4.
72. Stander S, Luger T, Metze D. Treatment of prurigo nodularis with topical capsaicin. J Am Acad Dermatol. 2001;44(3):471–8.
73. Ständer S, Luger TA. Antipruritic effects of pimecrolimus and tacrolimus. Hautarzt. 2003;54:413–7.
74. Clark AR, Jorizzo JL, Fleischer AB. Papular dermatitis (subacute prurigo,"itchy red bump" disease): pilot study of phototherapy. J Am Acad Dermatol. 1998;38(6 pt1):929–33.
75. Lear JT, English JS, Smith AG. Nodular prurigo responsive to azathioprine [letter]. Br J Dermatol. 1996;134(6):1151.
76. Lestarini D, Khoo LS, Goh CL. The clinical features and management of actinic prurigo: a retrospective study. Photodermatol Photoimmunol Photomed. 1999;15(5):183–7.
77. Berth-Jones J, Smith SG, Graham-Brown RA. Nodular prurigo responds to cyclosporine. Br J Dermatol. 1995;132(5):795–9.
78. Metze D, Reimann S, Beissert S, et al. Efficacy and safety of naltrexone, an oral opiate receptor antagonist, in the treatment of pruritus in internal and dermatologic diseases. J Am Acad Dermatol. 1999;41:533–9.
79. Genconglan G, Inanir I, Gunduz K. Therapeutic hotline: treatment of prurigo nodularis and lichen simplex chronicus with gabapentin. Dermatol Ther. 2010;23:194–8.
80. Mazza M, Guerriero G, Marano G, et al. Treatmentof prurigo nodularis with pregabalin. J Clin Pharm Ther. 2013;38:16–8.
81. Mattos O. Prurigo nodular de Hyde tratado com talidomida. Bol Div Nac Lepra. 1973;32:71–7.
82. Winkelmann RK, Connoly SM, Doyle JA, Gonçalves AP. Thalidomide treatment of prurigo nodularis. Acta Derm Venereol (Stockh). 1984;64:412–7.

Urticaria

63

Roberta Fachini Jardim Criado and Paulo Ricardo Criado

Key Points

- Urticaria is a vascular pattern of response to immune and nonimmune stimulation of mast cells and basophils
- Based on the disease course, urticaria is classified as acute urticaria (less than 6 weeks since onset) or chronic urticaria (longer than 6 weeks of evolution)
- Urticaria can be induced by recognized stimuli, and in this clinical setting is called induced urticaria (e.g., water, cold, pressure, dermographism); in most cases there is no apparent cause and the urticaria is named spontaneous urticaria
- Nowadays, activation of the coagulation system has been demonstrated in at least 50% of patients with acute and chronic urticaria. D-dimer and F1+2 prothrombin fragment blood levels are directly related with the severity of the urticaria and/or angioedema in these patients
- The first step in the treatment of urticaria is the use of antihistamines per os. According to international consensus the new second-generation antihistamines must be used as a standard dose and in refractory cases to four-fold dose is recommended
- The second step in the treatment is add on to antihistamine treatment other drugs as omalizumab, cyclosporine or montelukast

Introduction

Acute urticaria (AU) and angioedema can be part of the clinical spectrum of anaphylaxis, and thus present a lethal risk if left untreated [1]. Chronic urticaria (CU) on the other hand is a disease with major negative impact on patients' daily activities and can therefore worsen their quality of life.

Over the past decade, European consensus has regulated the classification, diagnosis, and treatment of this group of diseases, based on critical analysis of evidence-based medicine [2].

This chapter approaches relevant aspects of the "Position Paper of the Fourth International Consensus Meeting on Urticaria, Urticaria

R.F.J. Criado (✉)
Department of Dermatology,
Scholl of Medicine – ABC, Santo André, Brazil
e-mail: roberta2201@gmail.com

P.R. Criado
Department of Dermatology, School of Medicine,
Sao Paulo University, São Paulo, Brazil
e-mail: prcriado@uol.com.br

© Springer International Publishing Switzerland 2018
R.R. Bonamigo, S.I.T. Dornelles (eds.), *Dermatology in Public Health Environments*,
https://doi.org/10.1007/978-3-319-33919-1_63

2012," etiologic factors, and pathophysiologic mechanisms associated with CU in the literature that were deemed relevant in the new millennium [2]. Another important position paper about urticaria management was published by the Joint Task Force on Practice Parameters, representing the American Academy of Allergy, Asthma & Immunology during 2014, and added relevant observation in urticaria study and practice [3].

Acute Urticaria

AU and angioedema are differentiated from CU practically on the basis of the duration of illness. The protagonist cell in both types of urticaria is the mast cells (Fig. 63.1) and basophils and their mediators (presynthesized, in their intracytoplasmic granules, or neosynthesized, such as leukotrienes, prostaglandins, and several types of cytokines) (Fig. 63.2a, b).

Urticaria and angioedema with duration of less than 6 weeks is termed AU [3]. If urticaria of less than 6 weeks' duration has features suggesting it might progress to CU, such patients should be periodically re-evaluated until a diagnosis is clarified [3].

AU and angioedema should be differentiated from anaphylaxis [3]. Urticaria/angioedema associated with signs and symptoms in organs other than the skin, such as the pulmonary tract (wheezing and cough), gastrointestinal system (vomiting and diarrhea), nervous system (dizziness and loss of consciousness), or cardiac system (changes in blood pressure or heart rate), can occur in patients with anaphylaxis [3]. Therefore, all patients who attend medical consultation showing wheals (Fig. 63.3a) and/or angioedema (Fig. 63.3b) must submit to a complete physical examination to detect extracutaneous signs, which can signal an anaphylaxis.

In many cases of AU, no specific cause is found [4]. Pite et al. [4] suggested that overall, success in identifying a cause in pediatric AU varies widely in the literature, from approximately 20% to 90%. This is mainly justified by different patient recruitment (e.g., from emergency departments, hospitalized or specialized units/departments), diagnostic testing performed, and criteria used for establishing a cause [4]. The possibility that a specific combination of several triggers is required to elicit AU could be one explanation for why symptoms may never reappear [4], and why most cases of AU do not remain as CU. Infections and drug and food hypersensitivity have been

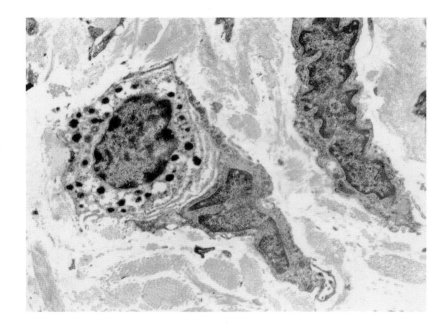

Fig. 63.1 Mast cell (*left*) and dermal dendrocyte (*right*) in acute drug-induced urticaria (electron microscopy, 25.000×).

reported as common potential triggers of AU in children [4]. In adults, AU often is trigged by infections or drug exposition [5].

Many etiologic factors or causes can be involved in AU [5]:

(i) Idiopathic
(ii) Viral agents (adenovirus, cytomegalovirus, enterovirus, Epstein–Barr virus, hepatitis A, B, or C, HIV, herpes simplex, influenza A, parvovirus B19, respiratory syncytial virus, rotavirus, varicella/zoster virus)
(iii) Bacterial pathogens (group A β-hemolytic streptococci, *Haemophilus influenzae*, *Staphylococcus aureus*)
(iv) Drugs: angiotensin-converting enzyme inhibitors (isolated angioedema), antibiotics (especially penicillin and cephalosporin), nonsteroidal anti-inflammatory drugs and acetylsalicylic acid, opiates, tramadol, paracetamol, dipyrone, proton pump inhibitors, isotretinoin, hyaluronidase, vaccination, etc.
(v) Food (especially, protein antigens): cow's milk, egg, fish and seafood, fruit (peach, kiwi), tomato and other vegetables, wheat, yeast
(vi) Other conditions, substances, or parasites: *Anisakis simplex*, insect bites or stings, scabies in children, mycoplasma, Malaria, *Strongyloides*, *Ascaris*, latex, iodine radiocontrast, gadolinium-containing radiocontrast media, thyroid papillary carcinoma or other thyroid disease, sinus tract infection, urinary infection, systemic lupus erythematosus

During an attack of AU, wheals are variable in number and size [5]. More than 50% of the body

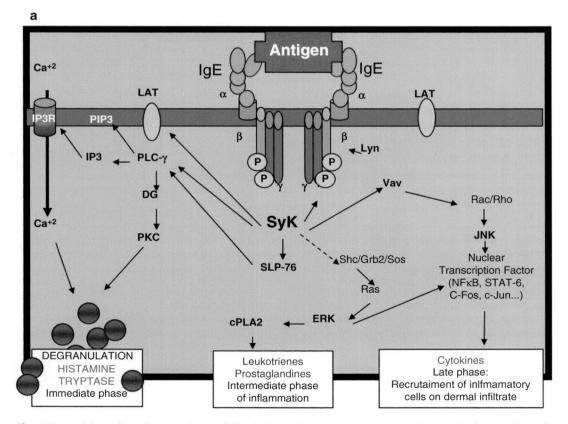

Fig. 63.2 (**a**) Mast cell mediators under anaphylactic degranulation (acute response) and neosynthesized mediators in late response to trigger stimulation. (**b**) Mast cell stimulation and preformed and neosynthesized mediators

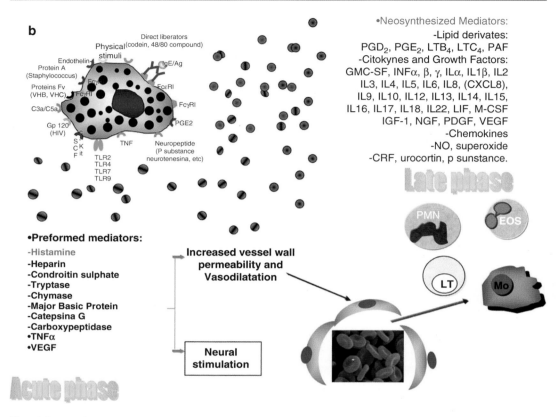

Fig. 63.2 (continued)

surface area may be involved, and in one study the rash was described as generalized in 48% patients [5]. Urticarial wheals may occur alone or with angioedema [4, 5]. Coexistent angioedema has been reported in 16–31% of patients [5] but may be more common in children younger than 3 years (60%), who may also develop hemorrhagic wheals [5], suggesting a clinical setting of multiform urticaria or urticaria vasculitis. Systemic symptoms occur in up to a quarter of patients [5]. Wheezing, breathlessness, cough, rhinorrhea, dizziness, flushing, gastrointestinal upset (nausea, vomiting, diarrhea, or abdominal pain), headache, fever, tachycardia, joint pain, or conjunctivitis can occur with an attack of AU [5]. Rapid onset of such symptoms may indicate anaphylaxis [5].

Epinephrine should be prescribed if the diagnosis of anaphylaxis has not been excluded [3]. If the urticaria is part of an anaphylactic reaction, national guidelines and local protocols for anaphylaxis should be followed [54]. Intramuscular epinephrine, intravenous antihistamines, intravenous corticosteroids, oxygen therapy, salbutamol, fluid replacement, and other supportive treatment may be needed [5].

AU and angioedema are often but not always related to mast cell and basophil activation from multiple triggers, which include immunoglobulin (Ig) E–mediated and non-IgE-mediated mechanisms [3].

These cells play a broad critical role in the innate and acquired immune response because they express multiple receptors responding to specific antigens, as well as complement fragments, circulating immune complexes binding IgG and IgM, cytokines, changes in blood pressure, and immunologic activation [3].

Thus it is likely that mast cell activation in patients with AU and angioedema occurs through multiple pathways in addition to IgE [3]. The presence of a specific mast cell or basophil receptor for

Fig. 63.3 (a) Acute urticaria due to a nonsteroidal anti-inflammatory drug. (**b**) Angioedema (Courtesy of Dr. Renan Bonamigo)

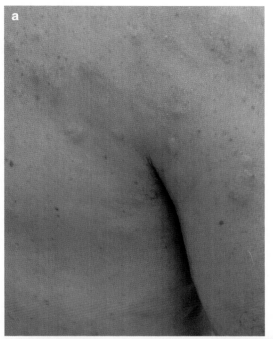

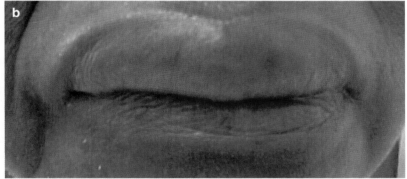

proteases might account for IgE-independent activation of these cells through proteases in aeroallergens, foods, and enzymes, as well as by proteases generated by the complement response to infectious agents [3].

AU and angioedema are more frequently associated with identifiable conditions [3], as described above [4]. When this disorder becomes chronic, it is less likely to be associated with an identifiable cause [1, 3].

Because AU and angioedema usually resolve spontaneously, laboratory evaluation for chronic illness is not required unless supported by the clinical history or physical examination [1, 3].

Furthermore, empiric elimination diets (not guided by history and testing) are not recommended [3]. The presence of alimentary allergy can be signaled if there is a direct correlation among certain food protein ingestion and development of signs including wheals and/or angioedema, wheezing, or gastrointestinal symptoms after minutes or a few hours.

Although many cases of AU are caused by viral or other infectious illnesses, extensive evaluation for specific viral pathogens or antiviral therapy is not indicated unless suggested by the clinical history [3]. For AU, skin testing or immunoassays to identify specific triggers for AU and angioedema can be helpful if an allergic cause is suggested by history [3].

Skin testing in this scenario would usually be done after the resolution of AU and after suspension of antihistamines or through serologic testing in the presence of significant dermatographism [3]. Cutaneous biopsies might occasionally be useful for differentiating this condition from other inflammatory disorders [3] such as urticarial vasculitis.

Common causes of AU and angioedema, including medications and foods, should be identified by a detailed history and eliminated, if possible [3].

For the treatment of AU and angioedema, antihistamines are efficacious in most cases and recommended as first-line therapy [3]. Although first-generation antihistamines are rapidly acting and effective, in both pediatric and adult patients, they can be associated with sedation and impaired cognitive skills due to their ability to cross the blood–brain barrier, whereas these impairments are less evident or not evident with second-generation antihistamines as a class [3].

When agents that can cause drowsiness or impair performance are prescribed, adult patients and parents of child patients should be made aware of this potential side effect [3]. In patients with a poor response to antihistamines, a brief course of oral corticosteroids might also be required while attempting to eliminate suspected triggers and develop an effective treatment plan [3]. In our practice, we treat patients with AU under a scheme of prednisone or prednisolone 0.5–1 mg/kg/day for 7 days combined with at least 20–30 days of antihistamine use, after remission of signs and symptoms.

Chronic Urticaria

The duration of CU varies considerably [3]; however, physical urticaria tend to persist the longest, often for many years [3]. The prevalence of CU in the general population has been estimated to range from 0.5% to 5% [3]; however, the true point prevalence, cumulative prevalence, and lifetime prevalence of CU have not been established

[3]. The incidence of CU has been estimated at 1.4% per year [3]. Some patients with CU might have both urticaria and angioedema, occurring simultaneously or separately [3].

Pathogenically, the skin mast cells are the most important cell in patients with CU, and histamine is the predominant mediator, although other cells and mediators also play a key role [3, 6]. A predominantly lymphocytic infiltrate can be found in the lesions of both patients with acute and those with chronic types of urticaria [3]. However, many patients demonstrate urticarial lesions that have a mixed cellular infiltrate: a mixture of lymphocytes, polymorphous nuclear cells (PMNs, such as eosinophils, neutrophils, basophils) [3], and other inflammatory cells, such as dermal dendrocytes [7].

Physiopathologic Mechanisms/ Etiologic Factors

Urticaria is a cutaneous reaction characterized by a sudden pruriginous rash accompanied by erythema and edema, and defined borders, location, size, and shapes that lasts for a few hours and is linked to the release of chemical mediators, mainly histamine, from mast cells in the dermis [1]. It is thus a heterogeneous group of diseases caused by or related to various factors, marked by the pattern of response with skin wheals and/or angioedema. According to its evolution over time, it can be classified as acute (<6 weeks) or chronic (>6 weeks) [2].

Several etiologic factors have been associated with CU throughout history: thyroid diseases, pseudoallergens, actual allergens, *Helicobacter pylori* infection, other infections/infestations, and autoimmunity/autoreactivity.

Helicobacter pylori **infection and its relation to CU** Hizal et al. demonstrated the positivity of autologous serum skin test (ASST) and high levels of IgG against *H. pylori* among patients with CU and concluded that the link between autoimmunity and infection by *H. pylori* warranted further studies [8].

Federman et al. [9], in an attempt to try and resolve this controversy, performed a literature review and selected ten relevant studies published in English that fulfilled the following criteria: (i) patients with CU only, (ii) exclusion of other known causes of urticaria through specific tests, (iii) initial diagnosis of *H. pylori* infection established by serology, urea test, or endoscopy, and (iv) complete treatment of *H. pylori* with antibiotics [9]. The authors observed that the resolution of CU was more likely after the *H. pylori* treatment had been completed, than if the pathogen was not eradicated. About 50% of the population has serologic evidence of past or present *H. pylori* infections and at least 30% of CU patients are infected with this agent, but in general the treatment of this bacterium does not influence the course of CU [9].

Greaves [10] suggested that *H. pylori* infection might have an indirect role in CU pathogenesis. Because of the immunogenicity of the pathogen's cell envelope, it could be linked to the production of autoantibodies against Lewis X and Y blood group polysaccharide antigens, similar to that which occurs through molecular mimicry in *Campylobacter jejuni* infections and during Guillain–Barré syndrome. Therefore, *H. pylori* can have an indirect involvement in the etiology of CU by reducing the immune tolerance and inducing the formation of autoantibodies, including the production of autoantibodies to anti-FcεRIα [11].

Based on these data, there is still no overall consensus that the investigation of *H. pylori* should be performed as a routine or that when it is present the treatment might influence the course of CU.

Chronic Urticaria: Food as a Cause of Pseudoallergic Reactions

Tharp et al. [12] suggested that gastrin, a 17-amino-acid peptide released by G cells in the gastric antrum and proximal duodenum immediately after feeding, may be involved in anaphylactic reactions and urticaria reported after the ingestion of certain foods. This is corroborated by the observation that it is not always possible to establish a direct correlation between clinical symptoms and the detection of antigen-specific IgE antibodies in cases of suspected food allergy [12].

In recurring CU, it is assumed that there might be histamine intolerance caused by an excessive dose of histamine in the diet and/or by abnormal histamine metabolism (diamine oxidase deficiency) [13]. Diamine oxidase is the main enzyme involved in the degradation of histamine, acting predominantly in the intestinal mucosa. Alcohol and some medications may decrease the activity of this enzyme and determine a higher sensitivity to histamine-rich or histamine-producing foods. Several experiments have demonstrated deficiency of diamine oxidase in enterocytes of patients with recurrent CU [13].

Certain fishes (tuna, sardines, anchovies), cheeses (Emmenthal, Gouda), salami, sausage, certain fruits and vegetables (tomatoes), wine, and beer are histamine-rich foods [14]. Drugs that may inhibit the intestinal activity of diamine oxidase and determine a higher concentration of histamine in general are imipenem, dobutamine, pancuronium, pentamidine, salazosulfapyridine, verapamil, isoniazid, clavulanic acid, dihydralazine, chloroquine, cycloserine, acetylcysteine, metoclopramide, and cefuroxime [14, 15].

Food additives such as preservatives, dyes, and natural salicylates may trigger or aggravate urticaria through pseudoallergic non-IgE-dependent mechanisms [6]. These additives are sodium metabisulfite, sodium benzoate, monosodium glutamate (MSG), sodium nitrate, tartrazine, erythrosine, sorbic acid, and butylated hydroxyanisole [15]. Regarding MSG, there is still no definitive conclusion about its causal relation to CU, despite the existence of controlled studies [16].

Di Lorenzo et al. [17] studied pseudo-food allergy in 838 patients with chronic/recurrent idiopathic urticaria and found it present in about 1.0–3.0% of their population. The provocation tests with a double-blind placebo-controlled technique were performed using the following substances: tartrazine (E102), erythrosine (E127), monosodium benzoate (E211), *p*-hydroxybenzoate (E218), metabisulfite (E223), and MSG (E620). The authors recommend considering the possibility of exclusion diets and provocation tests with food additives in cases of CU/refractory angioedema that fail to fully respond to H1-antihistamine treatment. The general consensus is that, regarding CU, although food additives can aggravate the disease they are rarely its sole cause.

Dental Infections and Urticaria

The connection between dental infections and CU remains unclear [18]. There have been reports of transient urticaria with high fever outbreaks after dental treatment, suggesting that bacteremia and/or toxemia arising from treatment would induce urticaria through immune and nonimmune mechanisms. Histamine release by mast cells, secondary to lipopolysaccharides from oral flora Gram-negative bacteria such as *Veilonella* sp., could be relevant as a pathogenic factor in urticaria outbreaks in patients with odontogenic infection; furthermore, these anaphylotoxins can have an acute direct vasodilatory effect that determines urticaria outbreaks [18]. We believe that patients with urticaria should have their dental condition assessed.

Hepatitis B and C Infection

The fact that hepatitis B may be the cause of wheals or hives, particularly AU or CU, is already well established [19]. It has been widely debated that hepatitis C can cause hives. We concur with the opinion of Siddique et al. that patients with urticaria living in areas of high prevalence of hepatitis C infection should be screened for hives [20].

Helminthic Parasites and Infestations

The association of AU and angioedema or CU with infestations by parasites, protozoa, ectoparasites, and helminths has been postulated for many decades. In fact the literature is replete with case reports or case series, but there are few case–control studies or meta-analyses on this subject. The association of urticaria with the following parasites has been reported: *Giardia lamblia*, *Fasciola hepatica*, *Toxocaracanis*, *Echinococcus*

granulosus, *Strongyloides stercoralis*, *Hymenolepis nana*, *Blastocystis hominis*, *Ascaris lumbricoides*, *Anisakis simplex*, *Cimex lectularius* (bedbug), and *Argas reflexus* (bird tick) [21–30].

The association between parasitism and urticaria has been better established with *A. simplex* and recently with *B. hominis*. *A. simplex*, also known as *Pseudoterranova decipiens*, *Terranova decipiens*, or *Phocanema decipiens*, belongs to the Anisakidae family [31]. These nematodes have been described in infestations affecting humans after the ingestion of raw or not fully cooked seafood [31]. Anisakiasis is the term used to describe the acute form of the disease in humans. Seafood is the main source of larval infection. Aside from urticaria and anaphylaxis, other manifestations such as rheumatic symptoms, contact dermatitis, Crohn's disease, eosinophilic gastroenteritis, conjunctivitis, and asthma have been reported [31]. Sensitization to *A. simplex* can be investigated through specific RAST test in peripheral blood.

The prevalence of *B. hominis* ranges from 10% in developed countries to 50% in those in process of development [32]. Several authors have correlated different *B. hominis* genetic subtypes, especially subtype 3, with cases of CU and AU, a fact that not confirmed by other researchers [32]. Apparently the subtype identified may vary according to the different regions of the world, climate or seasonal changes, and source of infection [32]. Therefore, cases of CU in highly endemic geographic areas should be investigated for *B. hominis* in the stool and if the diagnosis is confirmed, treatment should be prescribed with metronidazole.

Chronic Urticaria and Thyroid

Hashimoto's thyroiditis and Graves' disease are associated with idiopathic CU [33, 34]. Antithyroid antibodies are found in 27% of patients with idiopathic CU and 19% of patients have abnormal thyroid function [35]. In such CU cases, high titers of antithyroid antibodies (antithyroglobulin and antiperoxidase) can be detected, whereas it occurs in only about 3–4% of the general population without thyroid diseases [36].

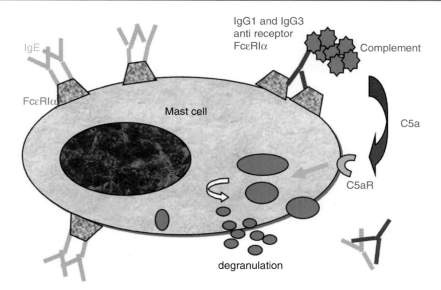

Fig. 63.4 Autoimmunity/autoreactivity in chronic spontaneous urticaria (CSU). Antibodies IgG1 and IgG3 are directed to high-affinity receptor for IgE in mast cells and basophils. After binding to receptor in membrane cell, this interaction stimulates an interaction among two IgE and antigen (allergen) and active intracellular pathways for degranulation and neoformation of lipid derivatives (leukotriene and prostaglandin) and cytokines. Besides this mechanism, some authors demonstrated the presence of IgE autodirected to circulating thyroid peroxidase antigens and double-stranded DNAs

The simultaneous occurrence of antithyroid antibodies and anti-FcεRIα in some patients with so-called idiopathic urticaria seems to indicate the existence of a disease or a "state" secondary to an underlying autoimmune process and/or a disruption of immune regulation. Rottem (2003) reinforces this concept, suggesting that there are no data to support a connection between the presence of antithyroid antibodies and CU pathogenesis, and that these are most likely parallel events, as occurs with autoimmune diseases [37]. In conclusion, tests for antithyroid antibodies and thyroid function should be performed in all CU cases in order to detect early those thyroid dysfunctions that require follow-up and treatment [37].

Autoimmune/Autoreactive Chronic Urticaria

About 50% of the cases of CU are considered autoimmune diseases, owing to the presence of circulating histamine-releasing autoantibodies, especially directed against IgE high-affinity receptors (FcεRIα) present in the cytoplasmic membrane of mast cells and basophils or anti-IgE autoantibodies (Fig. 63.4) [38].

There is clear evidence for a genetic predisposition to develop CU, i.e., there is a strong association between human leukocyte antigen (HLA)/familial inheritance and autoimmune etiology in some cases, especially those with a positive autologous serum skin test (ASST) [38]. There are reports suggesting a connection between CU with a positive ASST and autoimmune diseases, such as autoimmune thyroiditis, celiac disease, rheumatoid arthritis, Graves' disease, and type 1 diabetes mellitus, in addition to a higher frequency of autoimmunity serum markers such as rheumatoid factor, antinuclear antibody, and antithyroid antibody [33]. Patients with CU and positive ASST have a high frequency of HLA-DRB1*04 and its associated allele DQB1*0302 when compared with the healthy population and patients with CU and negative ASST [38–40].

Unfortunately, we still lack a routine laboratory test to detect anti-FcεRIα and/or circulating and functionally active anti-IgE. ASST autoantibodies have been considered an in vivo test to confirm both the presence of these autoantibodies and histamine release in basophils [38, 40].

In a retrospective study performed in Israel, Confino-Cohen et al. [40] analyzed data from 12,778 patients with CU during a period of 17 years and compared clinical and laboratory data with 10,714 control patients without CU. There was a definite increase in the odds ratio of hypo- or hyperthyroidism and the presence of antithyroid antibodies among patients with CU. Female patients with CU had a higher incidence of rheumatoid arthritis, Sjögren's syndrome, celiac disease, type 1 diabetes mellitus, and systemic lupus erythematosus during their lifetime, and those illnesses were diagnosed mainly in the 10 years following the diagnosis of CU. Increases in mean platelet volume, and positivity for rheumatoid factor and antinuclear antibodies were more prevalent and significant among patients with CU [6, 40]. Probably the presence of a chronic inflammatory process, implied by the increased mean platelet volume, shares a common pathogenic pathway with autoantibody formation in patients with CU. However, 50–60% of CU cases remain idiopathic, the so-called spontaneous CU [2, 40].

Recently, some authors demonstrated the activation of the coagulation system in patients with CU via thrombin generation, initiated by the increased expression of coagulation tissue factor on eosinophils [41–43]. This determines a potential contribution to the increase in capillary permeability. These patients often have elevated coagulation and fibrinolysis serum markers, such as fragment 1+2 prothrombin and D-dimer, whose levels seem to correlate with the severity of CU [41–43]. In animal models, thrombin shows increased capillary permeability by direct action on the endothelium and indirectly by inducing the release of proinflammatory mediators by mast cells, increasing C5a in the absence of C3, and bypassing the first part of the complement cascade [41–43]. It is possible that a synergy between the action of autoantibodies and the coagulation cascade exists in some patients with CU [41].

An article defining and proposing criteria for the diagnosis of autoimmune urticaria, by the European Academy of Allergy and Clinical Immunology, was published in 2013 [44]. The following criteria were proposed as the gold standard for autoimmune CU [44]: (a) presence of a positive in vitro biological test to demonstrate the autoantibodies' functionality (basophil histamine release test or the expression of a basophil activation marker such as CD63 or, better still, CD203c during flow cytometry) AND (b) positive autoreactivity (positive ASST) in order to demonstrate the in vivo relevance of mast cell degranulation and the increase in capillary permeability, AND (c) a positive immunologic assay for autoantibodies against FcεRIα receptors (western blot or ELISA) to demonstrate the autoantibodies' specificity.

In daily practice, however, most physicians have only the autologous serum skin test available, and its positivity in a patient with CU can only suggest "autoreactivity" [6]. Unfortunately, in Brazil we do not yet have the other tests indicated for the diagnosis of autoimmune CU [6].

Chronic Urticaria and Allergic Etiology

The link between CU, IgE sensitization, aeroallergens, and allergy has been much discussed but seldom studied [45].

Between 2006 and 2008 in France, Augey et al. [45] studied 128 adult patients with CU under the aspects of IgE sensitization and allergy. These authors considered CU an allergic disease if: (i) there was a high correlation of positive prick tests (skin puncture tests) to an allergen that was clinically relevant in the patient's medical history, and (ii) a complete remission of urticaria occurred within the first 2 months after the allergen was removed. Among 105 patients with interpretable puncture tests, 46.7% were sensitized by IgE. Two patients had clinically relevant puncture tests; however, their CU had many other triggering factors and there was no remission after withdrawal from allergen exposure. The authors concluded that the rate of IgE sensitization is higher among patients with CU compared with the general adult population [45]. However, these CU cases cannot be considered as an expression of IgE-mediated allergies, but as a chronic inflammatory disease that is more common in IgE-sensitized subjects and induced by many factors, among which IgE-mediated allergy is the least frequent [45].

The relevance of allergic sensitization to dust mites in the etiology and treatment of CU is still unknown. In Turkey, Caliskaner et al. [46] studied 259 patients with CU and angioedema, without respiratory allergic diseases (rhinitis and/or asthma) and compared their results with 300 healthy controls and 300 atopic patients. Immediate cutaneous reactivity to one or more allergens was detected in 71 cases of CU and angioedema (27.4%). The most commonly detected allergen was residential house dust (24.7%) [46]. Positive prick tests (skin puncture tests) were correlated with other aeroallergens, including pollen, mold, and cockroaches in 7.7%, 0.4%, and 0.8% of patients, respectively. In the healthy control group, 7% of cases were considered atopic regarding the prick test results [46]. Pollen (6%) and house dust (4.7%) were the most commonly found allergens in the healthy control group. In the atopic control group, pollen and dust mites were the allergens most commonly detected in the prick test (62% and 50.3%, respectively) [46]. The difference between patients with CU and the control group was statistically significant regarding the presence of atopy and sensitivity to mites ($p < 0.001$) [46]. The proportion of skin tests that were positive to house dust was higher in the CU group than among healthy cases, but not as high as in atopic patients [46]. Furthermore, the rate of cutaneous reactivity to other aeroallergens did not differ from the healthy group. The authors concluded that urticaria, as an isolated clinical manifestation in patients who are sensitive to dust, was not common in this study [6].

Therefore, it is well established that CU is not included in the indications for immunotherapy with allergy desensitization [46]. In our opinion, therefore, the systematic practice of skin prick test reading should not be routinely performed during the investigation of CU, unless there is a definite correlation between episodes of CU worsening and data from the patient's medical history.

Definition, Classification, and Course of the Disease

Urticaria is characterized by the sudden appearance of wheals, which may be accompanied by angioedema [47, 48]. Superficial dermal edema is called wheals or hives, while edema in the deep dermis, hypodermis, and gastrointestinal tract is known as angioedema [47, 49]. Diagnosis is mainly clinical [1].

Wheals have three typical features: (i) central edema of variable size, almost always surrounded by a reflex erythema, (ii) association with pruritus and sometimes a burning sensation, and (iii) ephemeral nature, with the skin returning to its regular appearance in usually 1–24 h. Angioedema is characterized by: (i) a sudden, pronounced edema of the deep dermis and subcutaneous tissue, (ii) pain more often than pruritus, (iii) frequent involvement of mucous membranes, and (iv) resolution of symptoms in about 72 h, more protracted than in the case of wheals [1].

It is well known that the spectrum of clinical manifestations of the different subtypes of urticaria is very broad. Moreover, two or more subtypes of urticaria can coexist in the same patient. During the Fourth International Consensus Meeting on Urticaria 2012, the adoption of a clinical classification (shown in Chart 63.1) was proposed [2].

Undoubtedly, this classification is not perfect since there are still some inconsistencies, e.g., physical urticaria also has a chronic nature [46]. However, physical urticarias are grouped as a result of the special nature of their causal factors, while in AU and CU, lesions appear spontaneously without external physical stimuli [3].

In 2001, Kozel et al. [47] published a study, conducted in the Netherlands, of 220 adults diagnosed with urticaria. Of these, 72 cases (33.2%) had physical urticaria, 24 (10.9%) had a combination of physical urticaria and idiopathic CU,

Chart 63.1 Classification and subtypes of urticaria

Type of urticaria	Duration
Spontaneous urticaria:	
1. Acute urticaria	1. Less than 6 weeks
2. Chronic urticaria	2. More than 6 weeks
Unknown etiology	
Induced urticaria:	
(i) Dermographism	(i) Application of mechanical forces to the skin (wheals appear in 1–5 min)
(ii) Delayed pressure urticaria	(ii) Vertical pressure (wheals appear after 3–8 h of latency)
(iii) Urticaria secondary to cold	(iii) Cold air/water/wind
(iv) Urticaria secondary to heat	(iv) Localized heat
(v) Solar urticaria	(v) Ultraviolet (UV) and or visible light
(vi) Urticaria/vibratory angioedema	(vi) Vibratory forces, usually pneumatic devices
(vii) Aquagenic urticaria	(vii) Contact with water, regardless of its temperature
(viii) Cholinergic urticaria	(viii) Stress, perception of body temperature elevation by the hypothalamus
(ix) Contact urticaria	(ix) Allergic or pseudoallergic

Adapted from Zuberbier et al. [2]

Chart 63.2 Urticaria Activity Score (UAS): daily evaluation during the most prominent number of lesions and intensity of itching

Score[a]	Wheals	Pruritus
0	Absence of wheals	Absence of symptoms
1	Light (<20 wheals/24 h)	Light
2	Moderate (21–50 wheals/24 h)	Moderate
3	Severe (>50 wheals/24 h or large confluent areas with wheals)	Intense

[a]Maximum score is 6 (3 points for number of wheals and 3 points for pruritus intensity)

inspections (visualization of the skin) should be made periodically (Urticaria Activity Score (UAS) 0–6 points) to increase the accuracy of the score; the sum of points scored over 7 days (UAS 7, 0–42 points) is currently being used in clinical studies [48]. In general, larger wheals indicate outbreaks that are more intense and more difficult to treat [48].

Diagnosis

Spontaneous UC is a disease that causes a serious impact on patients along with high direct and indirect costs to the health system, as well as extensive socioeconomic implications, since it delays by about 20–30% the return of productive individuals to the work force [2]. Due to the wide heterogeneity of this group of diseases called urticaria, routine investigation should include a thorough history, extensive physical examination, quests for information on possible causal factors, and important data on the nature of urticaria [2]. The next step is laboratory testing to exclude significant systemic diseases, provided they are warranted by clinical history and physical examination [2].

Skin biopsy of wheals must be performed if there is suspicion of vasculitis or urticaria vasculitis, which usually persists for more than 24 h in the same location and can leave hyperchromic or purplish residual lesions, although this does not always occur [2, 6, 49]. Furthermore, burning symptoms isolated or coupled with pruritus may be reported by these

and 78 (36%) had idiopathic CU; 20 cases (9.0%) were induced by drugs, 15 (6.8%) by food, four (1.8%) by infections, and 3 (1.4%) by internal diseases; and 2 (0.9%) were urticaria due to contact. Causality was established in 53.1% of the cases. Thirty-five percent of the cases were free of symptoms after 1 year and in 28.9% there was an improvement of symptoms. Spontaneous remission occurred in 47.4% of patients in whom no causal agent was identified and only in 16.4% of cases with physical urticaria. In this study, patients with physical urticaria had the worst prognosis regarding disease duration, as 84% of them still had symptoms after 1 year [47]. Another important factor in urticaria is to classify the intensity and activity of the disease. Młynek et al. [48] proposed a classification, later validated in 2008, which was easy to adhere to by both physicians and patients in their daily activities (Chart 63.2) [9].

Due to the variable intensity pattern of urticaria throughout the day, sequential dermatologic patients. Skin biopsy of wheals is also indicated in cases that are refractory to treatment with antihistamines [2, 49].

Considerations on Autologous Serum Skin Test

In 1946, Malmros published the first report on the likelihood of autologous serum (from patients with urticaria) triggering positive skin tests, although this hypothesis was disregarded for decades [50].

The ASST is an in vivo test that measures the autoreactivity of an individual [44, 51]. This autoreaction is characterized by the formation of wheals and pruritus in response to an intradermal injection of autologous serum (obtained from the patient during the clinical activity of urticaria, or crisis), which acts indirectly through the release of mediators from mast cells/other cells or directly by acting on the skin's microvasculature [44, 51]. It should be stressed that autoreactivity does not define, nor does it imply the presence of, autoimmune urticaria, but may be an indication of mast cell activation by the autoantibodies present in the autologous serum of patients with CU and positive ASST [44, 51].

The frequency of positive ASST in adults with CU ranges from 4.1% to 76.5% depending on different criteria for positivity, including confirmation by histamine release test (HRT) [44]. The discrepancy in results can be attributed to patient selection bias, severity of illness, methodology, and interpretation of the results or even the actual prevalence of autoimmune urticaria in the population tested [44]. The frequency of positive ASST is 45.5% (95% confidence interval (CI), 24.7–74.4%) when establishing a 1.5-mm difference in diameter between the response obtained with cases tested with saline (negative control) and 43.5% (95% CI, 34.8–62.1%) when the difference is 2 mm [46]. A positive ASST result on a CU case could mean an autoreactive CU [44].

Current recommendations to establish the methodologic standardization for ASST are summarized in Fig. 63.5 [44]. In order to perform an ASST it is necessary to take the patient off any medication with antihistamine activity for a variable period of time before testing, as depicted in Chart 63.3 [44].

Considerations on the Autologous Plasma Skin Test

The ASST is based on intradermal injection of autologous serum, and merely represents a diagnostic procedure used in autoimmune CU [52, 53]. The plasma used in the autologous plasma skin test (APST) also contains coagulation factors and sodium citrate. Therefore, the positivity occurring in the APST may be due both to autoantibodies that induce thrombin activity and/or to the sodium citrate [52].

In a study with 96 patients with CU, Asero et al. [53] found that 51 of 96 patients (53%) were ASST positive, and 61 of 71 (86%) were APST positive. Asero's group in Italy advocates that the APST increases the sensitivity of diagnosis in cases of autoreactive CU, since it indicates the activation of the coagulation cascade in the presence of autoantibodies. These autoantibodies, when degranulating mast cells and basophils, activate eosinophils, which in turn release tissue factor, thus stimulating the coagulation cascade and compensatory fibrinolysis. The latter will generate thrombin, which will induce the activation of more mast cells and the vascular endothelium; D-dimers are also detected at higher levels as a final result of fibrinolysis.

In another multicenter study [52], the positivity rate was 37.5% for ASST and 43% for APST among 200 patients with CU (146 women and 54 men).

Yildiz et al. [52] studied 42 patients (19 males, 23 females; mean age 35.7, range 28–76 years) and 35 healthy volunteers (19 males, 16 females; mean age 30.28, range 20–80 years). The authors performed APST, ASST, negative control with saline and sodium citrate, and positive control with histamine. In terms of positivity, no statistically significant difference between APST and ASST was found [52]. Therefore, the authors concluded that APST to assess autoreactivity in clinical practice was not superior to ASST, and

Fig. 63.5 Steps for performing autologous serum skin test (ASST)

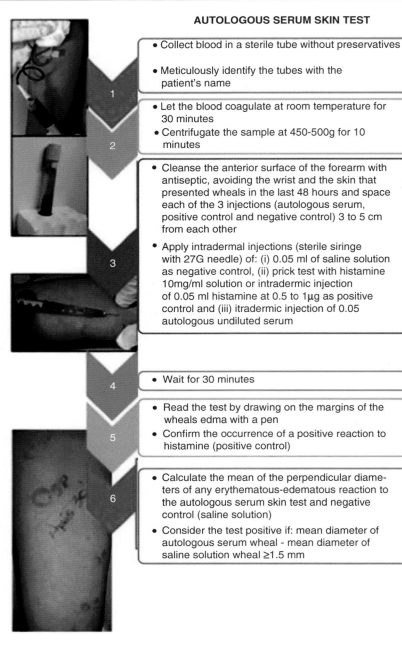

AUTOLOGOUS SERUM SKIN TEST

1
- Collect blood in a sterile tube without preservatives
- Meticulously identify the tubes with the patient's name

2
- Let the blood coagulate at room temperature for 30 minutes
- Centrifuge the sample at 450-500g for 10 minutes

3
- Cleanse the anterior surface of the forearm with antiseptic, avoiding the wrist and the skin that presented wheals in the last 48 hours and space each of the 3 injections (autologous serum, positive control and negative control) 3 to 5 cm from each other
- Apply intradermal injections (sterile siringe with 27G needle) of: (i) 0.05 ml of saline solution as negative control, (ii) prick test with histamine 10mg/ml solution or intradermic injection of 0.05 ml histamine at 0.5 to 1µg as positive control and (iii) itradermic injection of 0.05 autologous undiluted serum

4
- Wait for 30 minutes

5
- Read the test by drawing on the margins of the wheals edma with a pen
- Confirm the occurrence of a positive reaction to histamine (positive control)

6
- Calculate the mean of the perpendicular diameters of any erythematous-edematous reaction to the autologous serum skin test and negative control (saline solution)
- Consider the test positive if: mean diameter of autologous serum wheal - mean diameter of saline solution wheal ≥1.5 mm

further studies should be conducted to corroborate these findings [6].

Treatment

The treatment of urticaria includes pharmacologic and nonpharmacologic interventions [55, 56]. Nonpharmacologic interventions for phys-

ical urticaria are limited to reduction of stress levels and sun exposure, and diminished alcohol intake. There is little evidence that reducing drug intake and exposure to pseudoallergens would improve urticaria in these patients, except in cases of spontaneous CU, which is aggravated by nonsteroidal anti-inflammatory drugs (especially aspirin) in 25–30% of patients with urticaria [55]. Cooling lotions, such as 1%

Chart 63.3 Different antihistamines and time of dropout to perform the autologous serum skin test

Drug/daily dose	Elimination $T_{1/2}$ (h)	Length of suppression of urticarial response secondary to histamine prick test	
		Single dose (h)	Continuous use (days)
Acrivastine 8 mg	1.4–3.1	8	UD
Azelastine	22	12	7
Cetirizine 10 mg	7–11	≥24	3
Cyproheptadine 8 mg	UD	UD	11
Dexchlorpheniramine 4 mg	UD	UD	4
Diphenhydramine	9.2 ± 2.5	UD	UD
Ebastine 10 mg	10.3 ± 19.3	≥24	3
Fexofenadine 60 mg	14.4	24	2[a]
Hydroxyzine 0.7 mg/kg	20 ± 4.1	26	UD
Loratadine 10 mg	7.8 ± 4.2	24	7
Mizolastine 10 mg	12.9	24	UD
Levocetirizine 5 mg	7 ± 1.5	UD	4
Desloratadine 5 mg	27	UD	UD
Doxepin 25 mg	17	4–6 (days)	UD

UD unavailable data
[a]Similar length of suppression with 120 or 180 mg

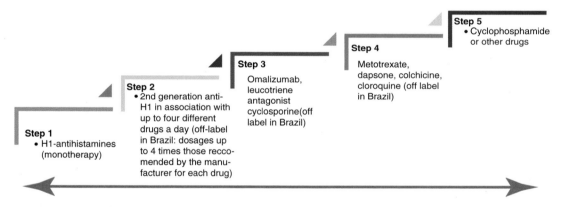

Fig. 63.6 Treatment schedule proposed for chronic spontaneous urticaria patients in Brazil

menthol, can be useful to many patients with very active urticaria [55].

In our opinion, it is important in the treatment of CU to make the patient understand the need for continuous, and not intermittent treatment, in order to achieve the proper control of the disease; and also to explain that this is a chronic condition that requires uninterrupted medication similarly to hypothyroidism or diabetes mellitus, although unlike these two diseases urticaria tends to go into remission over time [6].

Treatment of wheals outbreaks is sequential or made in steps, but its main cornerstone is the use of antihistamines (Fig. 63.6) [55]. Therefore, H1

antihistamines (anti-H1) are crucial in the treatment of urticaria [55, 56]. Nevertheless, some CU cases may present a marked inflammatory cell infiltration, which can be somewhat refractory to anti-H1 and respond satisfactorily to oral corticosteroids or second-line agents (montelukast, dapsone, or colchicine) [55–57].

Criado et al. [58] studied 22 CU patients unresponsive to conventional antihistamine treatment. The patients had uncontrolled urticaria even with multiple combinations of antihistamines at maximum doses and corticosteroids for short cycles (prednisone 20–40 mg, orally, once a day, 3–7 days per month). Cutaneous biopsies of the wheals were performed. The findings were classified as: (i) dermal perivascular mixed inflammatory infiltrate composed of lymphocytes, monocytes, and neutrophils and/or eosinophils; (ii) inflammatory infiltrate formed mainly by neutrophils; and (iii) inflammatory infiltrate composed mainly of eosinophils. According to histopathologic results, patients were subjected to one of the following regimens: class A, antihistamine associated with dapsone; class B, colchicine or dapsone; class C, montelukast. Four patients in class A, eight in class B, and seven in class C showed complete remission of urticaria after 12 weeks of treatment; one patient in class B and two in class C did not respond to therapy. Two years after treatment discontinuation, 16 patients remained urticaria free. The authors concluded that dapsone or colchicine might be effective adjuvant drugs in the presence of intense neutrophilic infiltrate, as could montelukast in cases with eosinophilic infiltrate [58].

H1-antihistamines have been used in the treatment of urticaria since 1950 [59]. Although first-generation drugs have a relatively lower cost than second-generation ones, the former have pronounced anticholinergic effects, with sedative action on the central nervous system (CNS) that lasts 12 h, while their antipruritic effects last between 4 and 6 h [59]. As a consequence, there have been many reports on interactions between first-generation anti-H1 drugs, alcohol, and medications (analgesics, hypnotics, sedatives, and antidepressant drugs) that cause unwanted effects in the CNS [59, 60]. In addition, monoamine oxidase inhibitors may prolong and intensify the anticholinergic effects of first-generation H1-antihistamines [59].

The most used first-generation, anti-H1 drugs to treat CU belong to the groups of ethanolamines (diphenhydramine, clemastine), piperazines (hydroxyzine, dexchlorpheniramine), and piperidines (cyproheptadine and ketotifen) [59]. Some randomized studies compared the effects of cetirizine versus hydroxyzine and loratadine in the treatment of CU and demonstrated similar clinical efficacy but a superior safety profile for cetirizine in comparison with hydroxyzine. The main differences

Chart 63.4 Differences between first and second generation of antihistamines [6]

First-generation H1 antihistamines	Second-generation H1 antihistamines
Usually given 3–4 times a day	Usually given once or twice a day
Cross the blood–brain barrier (they are lipophilic substances, have low molecular weight and are not substrates of the P-glycoprotein efflux pump system)	Do not cross the blood–brain barrier (they are lipophobic substances, have high molecular weight, and are substrates of the P-glycoprotein efflux pump system)
Cause several adverse events (sedation, hyperactivity, insomnia, and seizures)	Do not cause significant adverse events in the absence of drug interactions
Case reports on toxicity are regularly published	Reports on serious toxicity events are virtually nonexistent
Absence of placebo-controlled, randomized, double-blind clinical trials	Some placebo controlled, randomized, double-blind clinical trials, even in children
Lethal dose already identified in infants and children	No report of fatality due to overdose

Adapted from De Benedictis et al. [110]

between first- and second-generation anti-H1 antihistamines are listed in Chart 63.4 [60, 61].

Second-generation H1-antihistamines are the only drugs for the treatment of CU supported by high levels of scientific evidence, from the perspective of evidence-based medicine, as there are prospective, randomized, and double-blind controlled studies published [2, 60]. Therefore, these medications are indicated as first-line treatment for symptomatic CU [2]. Second-generation antihistamines provide moderate to good control for 44–91% of all types of urticaria and 55% of patients with CU [62]. In general, all H1-antihistamines are effective in reducing pruritus in urticaria, although less often affecting the number and size of wheals [63]. Therefore, there is a sizable group of patients with CU for whom H1-antihistamines in doses usually recommended on-label are not able to control disease symptoms.

Some authors propose that in young adults without associated disease, the doses of second-generation anti-H1 should be increased up to four times those recommended by manufacturers on the label, before substituting the drug or adding another medication in the treatment of CU (not approved by the National Health Surveillance Agency (ANVISA) in Brazil) [2, 56, 57, 64].

A study using cetirizine in 22 patients with CU confronted these recommendations, given that no improvement was observed after 2 weeks of treatment with 30 mg of cetirizine, although this may have been due to the limited observation period during the study [62].

Weller et al. [65] conducted a retrospective questionnaire survey on 319 patients diagnosed with spontaneous CU. The aim of this study was to establish the patients' perception on the effectiveness and adverse events of treatment with H1-antihistamines, both at standard and higher doses. Of the total population, 121 patients received questionnaires from their doctors or hospitals and 198 were informed about the research over the Internet, at the *Allergie-Centrum-Charité* homepage or at the *Urticaria Network* (www.urtikaria.net) web page. The latter group completed the questionnaire online [65]. Both questionnaires were identical. All surveys were completed anonymously and no Internet Protocol was retrieved. The only prerequisite for participation was that subjects had spontaneous CU (spontaneous wheals recurring for more than 6 weeks) and that they were adults, over 18 years of age. Participants agreed that the usual doses of second-generation antihistamines (recommended by the manufacturer) were significantly more effective than those of the first-generation drugs ($p < 0.005$) [65]. Furthermore, they found that second-generation drugs caused significantly fewer side effects ($p < 0.001$) and less sedation than first-generation antihistamine medications ($p < 0.001$) [65]. Three-quarters of the patients reported that they had increased the doses of second-generation antihistamines, and 40%, 42%, and 54% of the subjects reported significantly higher benefits by taking two, three, or four tablets per day, respectively [65]. The number of reports on adverse events and sedation with higher doses was not significantly different from those reported with usual doses [65].

In a literature review study, Sánchez-Borges et al. [66] concluded that the use of higher doses of second-generation anti-H1 increased the proportion of patients who achieved the control of urticaria symptoms, without producing higher rates of adverse events, including somnolence [66].

Despite the small number of studies, the best results seem to be those obtained with cetirizine, levocetirizine, and desloratadine; regarding dosage increase, there were mixed results with rupatadine and one study with fexofenadine failed to show greater improvement with higher doses [66].

Overall, studies comparing various second-generation anti-H1 drugs in the treatment of CU observed no significant difference regarding symptom control, quality of life, and safety profile, and all of them are designated as first-line agents in the treatment of CU [2, 61]. Chart 63.5 summarizes the recommendations for the treatment of urticaria, according to the Fourth Consensus Meeting, Urticaria 2012 held in Berlin.

An ample variety of H1-antihistamines available on the market, their dosage, and recommended doses can be seen in Chart 63.6. A recent review performed by Fedorowicz et al. [67] for the Cochrane Skin Group Specialized Register concluded that the presence of few studies and small case series in the literature regarding the use of anti-H2 (cimetidine and ranitidine) in the

Chart 63.5 Summary of the European Consensus of Chronic Urticaria (4th Consensus Meeting, Urticaria 2012) [6]

Terminology and classification	Chronic urticaria may occur as "chronic spontaneous urticaria" or "inducible chronic urticaria." The inducible group includes physical, cholinergic, contact, and aquagenic urticarias; the term "idiopathic" chronic urticaria should be avoided
Differential diagnoses	Differential diagnoses should include bradykinin-related angioedema (hereditary angioedema and angioedema secondary to angiotensin conversion inhibitors) and urticarial syndromes associated with interleukin-1 (autoinflammatory syndromes or diseases, urticaria vasculitis)

(continued)

Chart 63.5 (continued)

Determination of disease activity	(a) New methods and tools area available
	(b) Disease activity: UAS (urticaria activity score), AAS (angioedema activity score), triggering threshold of inducible urticaria
	(c) Quality of life: CU-Q2oL (chronic urticaria quality of life survey chronic urticaria), AE-QoL (angioedema quality of life survey – quality of life questionnaire for patients with angioedema)
Diagnosis	(a) In spontaneous chronic urticaria there are two steps to the diagnosis:
	Routine diagnosis (exclusion of serious underlying diseases in all patients): erythrocyte sedimentation rate or C-reactive protein, complete blood count, suspend the use of nonsteroidal anti-inflammatory drugs or substitute them
	Complementary diagnosis (to identify and treat possible causes in patients with persistent disease and/or severe spontaneous urticaria): based overall on the patient's medical history, detection of autoreactivity, intolerance, and infection
	(b) In inducible chronic urticaria, the diagnosis is limited (usually) to determining the triggering factor and the tolerance threshold to stimuli
Treatment	Treatment is indicated in three steps:
	Step 1: nonsedating, second-generation antihistamines
	Step 2: doses up to four times those recommended on the label of nonsedating, second-generation antihistamines
	Step 3: Omalizumab, cyclosporine A, montelukast

treatment of urticaria preclude any conclusion on their effectiveness in treating the disease.

Other Pharmacologic Interventions in Chronic Urticaria (Third-Line Agents)

While antihistamine treatments with high-dose second-generation anti-H1 (up to four times the recommended doses) can control the symptoms in most patients, alternative treatments may be required for the remaining unresponsive population [2]. Since the intensity of CU fluctuates, and spontaneous remission may occur in 50% of patients within 6 months of diagnosis, it is advisable to re-evaluate the need for continued treatment or alternative therapies every 3–6 months, although in our opinion patients should be assessed at interval periods no longer than 2 months [2]. There are numerous studies on alternative drugs for the treatment of CU, either in combination with H1-antihistamines or as monotherapy, albeit with low levels of scientific evidence [2]. Examples for this strategy include ketotifen, montelukast, warfarin, nifedipine, tranexamic acid, colchicine, dapsone, sulfasalazine, methotrexate, plasmapheresis, intravenous immunoglobulin, hydroxychloroquine, biological agents, danazol/stanozolol, and cyclophosphamide, among others [9]. Even with low levels of scientific evidence, many of these drugs are used in antihistamine-resistant patients with CU, and we will therefore discuss them further.

Immunosuppressors

Cyclosporine

Most studies on cyclosporine used 5 mg/kg/day doses for periods ranging from 8 to 16 weeks with good results, varying from approximately 64–95%. Some studies used smaller doses (2–5 mg/kg/day) [68–71]. At these doses, side effects occur less frequently than at higher ones. In these cases in particular there have been reports on infections, hypertension, nephrotoxicity, and increased malignancy [72, 73]. Other less severe side effects include hirsutism, headache, nausea, paresthesia, abdominal pain, and hypertension. For this reason it is necessary to monitor blood pressure, renal function, and cyclosporine levels, and even glycemia and lipidemia [72, 75].

Methotrexate

This drug has anti-inflammatory and immunosuppressive activities, although much of its mechanisms of action are unknown. It is known

Chart 63.6 Antihistamine drugs in the Brazilian market, doses for children and adults, time of action, metabolizing, drug interactions, and dose adjustment if necessary [6]

Generation	Drugs	Dose for children (day)	Dose for adults (day)	T_{max}*	Time to action (h)**	Hepatic metabolism	Drug interactions	Dose adjustment
1st	Chlorpheniramine (Dex◆)	0.15 mg/kg/day	2–8 mg/day÷3 doses	2.8 ± 0.8	3	Yes	Likely	ND
	Clemastine◆	0.5 ml/kg/day	2 mg	ND	2	Yes	Likely	ND
	Cyproheptadine◆	0.125 mg/kg/day	2–8 mg	ND	ND	Yes	Likely	LF
	Diphendhydramine	5 mg/kg ÷ 3–4 times/day	50–400 mg	1.7 ± 1.0	2	Yes	Likely	LF
	Doxepin◆	Not used	10–100 mg	2	ND	Yes	Likely	LF
	Hydroxyzine◆	1–2 mg/kg/day	10–200 mg	2.1 ± 0.4	2	Yes	Likely	LF
2nd	Acrivastine	Unavailable	Unavailable	1.4 ± 0.4	1	<50%	Unlikely	ND
	Bilastine◆	Unavailable (only >12 years old)	20 mg	1.0–1.5	1	No	Unlikely	
	Ketotifen◆	0.05 mg/kg/day	1–2 mg	3.6 ± 1.6	ND	Yes (?)	ND	LF and KF
	Cetirizine◆	2–6 years, 2.5 mg; 6–12 years, 5 mg; 2×/day	10 mg	1.0 ± 0.5	1	<40%	Unlikely	IH and IR
	Loratadine◆/ Descarboethoxyloratadine	2–6 years, 2.5 mg, 6–12 years, 5 mg; 1×/day	10 mg	1.2 ± 0.3 / 1.5 ± 0.7	2	Yes	Very unlikely	LF and KF
	Ebastine◆/Carebastine	2–6 years, 2.5 mg, 6–12 years, 5 mg;1×/day	60/180 mg	2.6 ± 5.7	2	Yes	Likely	LF and KF
	Fexofenadine◆	>12 years, 60 mg 2×/day	(6 months to 2 years: 2.5 ml q. 12 h) (2–11 years: 5 mg q 12 h)	26	2	<8% Yes	Yes (P-glycoprotein)	KF
	Mizolastine	Unavailable	Unavailable	1.5	1	Yes	Likely	ND
	Levocetirizine◆	<2–6 years: 5 drops q 12 h or (0.25 mg/kg/day); >6 years: 5 mg	5 mg	0.8 ± 0.5	1	<15%	Unlikely	LF and KF
	Desloratadine◆	6 months–1 year: 1 mg; 1–6 years: 1.25 mg; 6–12 years: 2.5 mg; 1×/day	5 mg	1–3	2	Yes	Unlikely	LF and KF
	Rupatadine◆	Unavailable	10 mg	0.75	2	Yes	Unlikely	

LF liver failure, *KF* kidney failure, *ND* not defined

that methotrexate increases adenosine levels, inducing the apoptosis of CD4 lymphocytes and inhibiting neutrophil chemotaxis [74, 75]. It has been used in doses of 10–15 mg per week in cases that were resistant to antihistamines and systemic corticosteroids, with results achieved after 3–6 weeks of treatment [74, 75]. It is considered a corticosteroid-sparing alternative. Gastrointestinal side effects, stomatitis, headache, fatigue, and hematologic alterations may occur at low doses [74, 75]. Since there is a risk of hepatotoxicity and myelosuppression, laboratory surveillance is mandatory, especially of hepatic function [74, 75].

Cyclophosphamide

Prescribed usually in cases of extreme treatment resistance, cyclophosphamide it has been used orally at 100-mg doses (equivalent to 1.5 mg/kg for 5 days, every week) associated with 600 mg/day acetylcysteine to reduce bladder toxicity, with good results [76]. It should be used sparingly because of its many potential adverse events [76].

Biologic Agents

Omalizumab

This is an anti-IgE monoclonal antibody approved for the treatment of moderate to severe asthma. Omalizumab decreases free IgE and inhibits the expression of high-affinity IgE receptors on mast cells and basophils [6]. Applied subcutaneously, it was one of the first biopharmaceuticals on the market indicated to treat severe allergic asthma. When treating CU, one must take into consideration the presence of IgE autoantibodies [80, 81]. Good results have been reported in idiopathic and cholinergic CU, urticaria secondary to sun or cold exposure, dermographism, and angioedema [80, 81].

A randomized multicenter, double-blinded study evaluated 90 patients aged 12–75 years with chronic spontaneous urticaria unresponsive to antihistamines, for whom good control of the disease was achieved with one dose of omalizumab [82]. The improvement obtained with the medication versus placebo was statistically significant at 300- and 600-mg doses, but not at 75 mg; complete

resolution of urticaria was achieved in the first 2 weeks in 36% of patients in the 300-mg group, 28.6% in the 600-mg group, 4.4% in the 75-mg group, and 0% in the placebo group [82]. Recently, a randomized multicenter study with 323 patients treated every 4 weeks observed, at week 16, a 44% improvement in the 300-mg group, 22% in the 150-mg group, 16% in the 75-mg group, and 5% in the placebo group [83].

Therefore, the use of omalizumab at 300- or 600-mg doses seems to be a rapid and effective treatment for patients with CU who are persistently symptomatic despite the use of anti-H1 medications [83, 84].

Recently, omalizumab treatment for urticaria has been approved in Brazil at a dose of 300 mg per month.

Intravenous Immunoglobulin

Intravenous immunoglobulin has immunomodulatory activities, including complement and cell adhesion modulation, and acts at the level of cytokines and autoantibodies. This drug has been used with good results in CU, at a dose of 0.4 mg/kg/day for 5 consecutive days, or in other schemes, also used subcutaneously [77–80]. Anaphylactoid reactions, aseptic meningitis, and renal failure are reported as rare adverse events and, despite being relatively safe, this is a very high-cost treatment.

Anti-CD20 Drugs (Rituximab and Others)

A chimeric monoclonal antibody against CD20 protein, anti-CD20 is expressed mainly on B cells (lymphocytes) [84]. Rituximab destroys B lymphocytes and decreases the production of autoantibodies. In three case reports, the drug was effective in two patients with H1-antihistamine-resistant CU and in another case it was ineffective [85–87].

Anti-Tumor Necrosis Factor α (TNF-α) Agents

Wilson et al. [88] treated six patients with CU who had unsuccessfully received a combination of H1-antihistamines and immunosuppressants, with different anti-TNF agents (four with etanercept, one infliximab, and one adalimumab) based on previous studies that had shown elevated serum and cutaneous TNF-α in patients with CU compared with controls [89, 90]. The authors reported improvement on the urticaria, with length of remission varying from months to years, and three patients continuing in long-lasting remission even after all medications were withdrawn [88].

Corticosteroids

Corticosteroids are known to be effective in the treatment of CU in patients who are unresponsive to anti-H1 medications [84]. Nonetheless, controlled studies on the subject are still lacking. Clinical effects may be evident at 25-mg doses in the early days of treatment; however, given the potential adverse events associated with the chronic use of corticosteroids (diabetes mellitus, hypertension, osteoporosis, and gastrointestinal bleeding), oral corticosteroids should be used for short periods of time (3–7 days per month) and at the smallest effective dose [2, 84].

Drugs with Anti-inflammatory Effects

These medications are generally safe and affordable to the majority of the population and have still limited evidence of effectiveness in the literature, but can be used in the treatment of CU before more expensive or toxic drugs are considered [84].

Hydroxychloroquine

Reeves et al. [91] studied 18 patients with CU who were treated with hydroxychloroquine for 12 weeks. The treatment significantly improved the quality of life of patients, although the levels of urticaria activity were scarcely influenced. This drug is relatively safe, although it can cause retinopathy, usually after 5 years of continuous use [84].

Colchicine

There are two studies published in the indexed literature, a prospective one by Criado et al. [58] and a retrospective analysis by Pho et al. [92], evaluating the use of colchicine in the treatment

of CU. The drug acts by precluding the formation of the apparatus that extrudes granules from mast cells and basophils [6]. Both studies found partial or complete response in at least half of the patients [6]. Adverse events are bearable, including diarrhea, leukopenia, and hematuria; furthermore, it is a low-cost medication [6]. Colchicine should not be used in pregnant women [6].

Dapsone

Dapsone has been reported to be effective in the treatment of CU/angioedema at doses of 25–50 mg per day [57, 58, 84, 93]. In a study in association with desloratadine and as monotherapy, it showed higher rates of remission, although urticaria activity scores were not reduced [89]. According to Noda et al. [93], dapsone's anti-inflammatory activity occurs by inhibiting the chemotactic migration of neutrophils, protecting cells from neutrophil- and eosinophil-mediated damage, reducing the release of prostaglandins and leukotrienes, and reducing the integrin-mediated neutrophil adherence, which inhibits the migration of these cells into the extravascular compartment [93].

Although generally well tolerated, dapsone can induce dose-dependent anemia and, less frequently, peripheral neuropathy, exanthema, DRESS syndrome (drug rash with eosinophilia and systemic symptoms), gastrointestinal symptoms, hepatotoxicity, and methemoglobinemia. Monitoring serum levels of glucose-6-phosphate dehydrogenase is necessary, owing to the risk of severe hemolysis in patients lacking this enzyme [84].

Sulfasalazine

The recommended dose is 2 g orally, daily, with results usually seen within a month [84]. Adverse events such as nausea, dyspepsia, headache, proteinuria, hepatotoxicity, and hematologic abnormalities have been reported [84], [94].

Leukotriene Receptor Antagonist (Montelukast)

Montelukast is used at 10 mg per day in adults, as an adjuvant drug to the antihistamine treatment, with excellent safety profile [58, 84]. Leukotrienes C4, D4, and E4 play an important role in the process of allergic inflammation, warranting this drug as an adjunct in the treatment of CU. Khan and Lynch [95] achieved CU control in 48% of 25 patients treated with montelukast associated with anti-H1 and anti-H2, whereby 11 had no improvement and in two patients the urticaria worsened after the drug was introduced. Adverse events included upper respiratory tract symptoms, diarrhea, nausea, vomiting, exanthema, elevated transaminases, and, exceptionally, psychiatric disorders [95].

Anticoagulants

Frequently patients with CU show an increase in plasma markers of thrombin generation and fibrinolysis during periods of disease exacerbation, perhaps as a consequence of tissue factor expression on the plasma membrane of activated eosinophils [84, 96]. The activation of coagulation and fibrinolysis decreases as the disease enters remission [84]. The exact role of this phenomenon (activation of coagulation and fibrinolysis) acting as the centerpiece of the disease's pathophysiology or epiphenomenon, acting as an amplifier of inflammation, is not yet elucidated.

According to Asero et al. [84] it seems reasonable to use anticoagulant or antifibrinolytic agents in patients with CU, since the disease's activity runs parallel to this phenomenon. Reports on the use of oral anticoagulation, warfarin (keeping international normalized ratio >2), and heparin have been published for the last decade [97–100]. However, the use of these drugs is still not routinely recommended in the treatment of CU [84].

Levothyroxine

The association between thyroid autoimmunity and CU is well established. Karaayvaz et al. [101] conducted a study with 60 patients with UC, divided into two groups matched for sex and age, using ketotifen or levocetirizine. The group using ketotifen achieved symptom relief while taking the medication, but relapsed after drug withdrawal. Eighteen patients in the group using levothyroxine achieved complete remission and three had partial improvements; furthermore, symptoms did not recur in those with complete response [101].

Treatment with levothyroxine takes at least 10 days to demonstrate an effect; 0.1 mg/kg/day for 4 weeks is usually appropriate and does not cause alterations in thyroid function [101]. It is advisable to approach these cases in conjunction with an endocrinologist, especially in situations where no control of CU associated with thyroid autoimmunity was obtained with other pharmacologic interventions and provided there are no contraindications to thyroid hormone replacement therapy [101].

It is hypothesized that patients with autoimmune thyroiditis have autoantibodies against thyroid proteins (antithyroglobulin and antiperoxidase), which induce inflammation and cytokine release that will subsequently bind to C4, activate the complement system, and stimulate the release of histamine by basophils and mast cells [102]. Thus, antithyroid and anti-FcεRIα antibodies activate the complement in a synergic manner, increasing the release of vasoactive amines and leading to urticaria [6].

Therapeutic Strategies in Clinical Practice

In our understanding, the treatment of CU should be customized according to patients' lifestyles (profession, social interactions, and recreational activities), their socioeconomic level, and understanding of disease and treatment. A basic principle is to avoid known aggravating or triggering agents, such as alcohol and indiscriminate use of cyclooxygenase inhibitors and nonsteroidal anti-inflammatory drugs. Each therapeutic intervention cannot be assessed as to its effectiveness before 2–4 weeks, at the earliest. If disease control is not achieved with a certain drug, as long as there is no contraindication for an association, it should be maintained at least until the illness is controlled.

Patients with CU tend to develop psychological/psychiatric problems, some even preceding the initial event of urticaria, such as post-traumatic stress disorder, alexithymia (marked difficulty in verbalizing emotions, describing feelings or bodily sensations), anxiety (particularly phobias) and depression, which may affect up to 48% of patients with spontaneous CU [103–105]. Thus, psychological and/or psychiatric support, beside positive attitudes from the health care team, can always be helpful to the treatment.

The quality of life of patients with CU is greatly affected, as patients suffer with pruritus and wheals, and present fatigue caused by sleep disorders and adverse events of medications [106]. The disease affects many realms of the patient's life, also having an economic impact for the patient and the health system [106]. In tertiary referral centers, the impact on quality of life for these patients is comparable with that experienced by older subjects with severe ischemic heart disease and overall, in various dimensions, with the impact suffered by patients with psoriasis and atopic dermatitis [106].

Therefore, facing up to the reality of medical practice in Brazil, we adopted a strategy of sequential treatment (in steps), ranging from the use of anti-H1 as standard initial drugs, to second-line agents (leukotrienes and corticosteroids in short courses), third-line medications (omalizumab, cyclosporine, methotrexate; anti-inflammatory drugs, such as dapsone, hydroxychloroquine, and colchicine), and fourth-line drugs (immunosuppressants that are more toxic), considering that in most cases progression to the next level of therapy also implies an increase in direct or indirect costs, as well as greater risks of adverse events (Fig. 63.6) [84].

Chronic Urticaria: Severity Markers and Disease Prognosis

Rabelo-Filardi et al. [107], in a systematic review of 34 studies published on spontaneous CU, concluded that the clinical severity of CU can forecast disease duration, and laboratory parameters such as elevation of serum levels of fragments 1+2 prothrombin, D-dimer, and C-reactive protein may reflect the gravity of the disease, and perhaps its resistance to conventional treatment. Patients with more severe symptoms may have more persistent disease courses [108]. Spontaneous remissions occur in 30–50% of patients within a year of disease evolution, and another 20% within 5 years [108]. About 20% of patients with CU remain ill after 5 years of evolution [108]. Nearly half of patients with CU lasting 6 months will probably still have the disease 10 years later [108].

A Korean study of 131 patients with CU evaluated the presence of signs of metabolic syndrome (MetS), disease activity score, and serum markers for inflammatory activity [109]. Thirty-nine patients (28.9%) had MetS compared with 17.8% of subjects in the matched control group ($p = 0.001$). Patients with CU and metabolic syndrome were older, had higher mean scores of disease activity, and higher levels of serum eosinophil cationic protein (ECP), TNF-α, and complement system factors, besides higher frequency of negative tetrachlorosalicylanilide when compared with patients with CU without MetS. Logistic regression showed that an urticaria activity score $\geq$13 ($p = 0.025$) and the presence of MetS ($p = 0.036$) were independent predictors of a likely difficult-to-treat CU [109]. Therefore, both CU and MetS may share low-grade chronic inflammation, involving TNF-α, ECP, and C3, which may be mutually triggering or exacerbating the disease [109]. Future studies will better elucidate subsequent disorders in patients with CU, since the disease may course with coexisting MetS, activation of coagulation/fibrinolysis, and chronic inflammation, which may represent potential cardiovascular diseases and diabetes mellitus during the life of these patients.

Summary
- CU is currently classified as spontaneous or induced by physical stimuli. Convention determined that the term "idiopathic" should be avoided

- Studies with larger samples should be conducted in the future to assess the value of screening and treatment of infectious and parasitic agents in the course of CU, especially in endemic areas
- The presence of autoreactivity in patients with spontaneous CU can be demonstrated in 50% of cases, in a simple manner, by the autologous serum skin test;
- The vast majority of CUs are not IgE-mediated allergic diseases
- The diagnosis of autoimmune CU should be based on strict criteria established by the European consensus
- The link between inflammation and coagulation, boosting the mediator release cascade, was demonstrated in a group of patients with CU and high levels of eosinophilic activation
- First-line treatment of CU in the first decade of this century is based on second-generation antihistamines; however, in some patients it is necessary to combine these with anti-inflammatory or immunosuppressive drugs, besides the promising use of immunobiological agents such as omalizumab

Similar to some cases of psoriasis, spontaneous CU can have a major impact on patients' quality of life, and also in the various realms of the psyche. Further studies will confirm or deny the progressive course of metabolic syndrome and cardiovascular complications among patients with long lasting spontaneous CU.

References

1. Cousin F, Philips K, Favier B, Bienvenu J, Nicolas JF. Drug-induced urticaria. Eur J Dermatol. 2001;11:181–7.
2. Zuberbier T, Aberer W, Asero R, Bindslev-Jensen C, Brzoza Z, Canonica GW, et al. The EAACI/GA(2) LEN/EDF/WAO Guideline for the definition, classification, diagnosis, and management of urticaria: the 2013 revision and update. Allergy. 2014;69:868–87.
3. Bernstein JA, Lang DM, Khan DA, Craig T, Dreyfus D, Hsieh F, Sheikh J, Weldon D, Zuraw B, Bernstein DI, Blessing-Moore J, Cox L, Nicklas RA, Oppenheimer J, Portnoy JM, Randolph CR, Schuller DE, Spector SL, Tilles SA, Wallace D. The diagnosis and management of acute and chronic urticaria: 2014 update. J Allergy Clin Immunol. 2014;133:1270–7.
4. Pite H, Wedi B, Borrego LM, Kapp A, Raap U. Management of childhood urticaria: current knowledge and practical recommendations. Acta Derm Venereol. 2013;93(5):500–8.
5. Sabroe RA. Acute urticaria. Immunol Allergy Clin North Am. 2014;34(1):11–21.
6. Criado PR, Criado RF, Maruta CW, Reis VM. Chronic urticaria in adults: state-of-the-art in the new millenium. An Bras Dermatol. 2015;90(1):74–89.
7. Criado PR, Jardim Criado RF, Sotto MN, Pagliari C, Takakura CH, Vasconcellos C. Dermal dendrocytes FXIIIA+ phagocytizing extruded mast cell granules in drug-induced acute urticaria. J Eur Acad Dermatol Venereol. 2013;27(1):e105–12.
8. Hizal M, Tuzun B, Wolf R, Tuzun Y. The relationship between *Helicobacter pylori* IgG antibody and autologous serum test in chronic urticaria. Int J Dermatol. 2000;39:443–5.
9. Federman DG, Kirsner RS, Moriarty JP, Concato J. The effect of antibiotic therapy for patients infected with *Helicobacter pylori* who have chronic urticaria. J Am Acad Dermatol. 2003;49:861–4.
10. Burova KP, Mallet AI, Greaves MW. Is *Helicobacter pylori* a cause of urticaria? Br J Dermatol. 1999;51:42.
11. Greaves MW. Chronic idiopathic urticaria and *H pylori*: not directly causative but could there be a link? ACI Int. 2001;13:23–6.
12. Tharp MD, Thirlby R, Sullivan TJ. Gastrin induces histamine release from human cutaneous mast cells. J Allergy Clin Immunol. 1984;74:159–65.
13. Lessof MH, Gant V, Hinuma K, Murphy GM, Dowling RH. Recurrent urticaria and reduced diamine oxidase activity. Clin Exp Allergy. 1990;20:373–6.
14. Maintz L, Novak N. Histamine and histamine intolerance. Am J Clin Nutr. 2007;85:1185–96.
15. Asero R. Multiple intolerance to food additives. J Allergy Clin Immunol. 2002;110:531–2.
16. Simon RA. Additive-induced urticaria: experience with monosodium glutamate(MSG). J Nutr. 2000;130:1063S–6S.
17. Di Lorenzo G, Pacor ML, Mansueto P, Martinelli N, Esposito-Pellitteri M, Lo Bianco C, et al. Food-additive-induced urticaria: a survey of 838 patients with recurrent chronic idiopathic urticaria. Int Arch Allergy Immunol. 2005;138:235–42.
18. Goga D, Vaillant L, Pandraud L, Mateu J, Ballon G, Beutter P. The elimination of dental and sinusal infectious foci in dermatologic pathology. A double-blind study in 27 cases confined to chronic urticaria. Rev Stomatol Chir Maxillofac. 1988;89:273–5.
19. Vaida GA, Goldman MA, Bloch KJ. Testing for hepatitis B virus in patients with chronic urticaria and angioedema. J Allergy Clin Immunol. 1983;72:193–8.

20. Siddique N, Pereira BN, Hasan AS. Hepatitis C and urticaria: cause and effect? Allergy. 2004;59:668.

21. Nenoff P, Domula E, Willing U, Herrmann J. *Giardia lamblia* – cause of urticaria and pruritus or accidental association? Hautarzt. 2006;57:518–20. 521–2

22. Demirci M, Yildirim M, Aridogan BC, Baysal V, Korkmaz M. Tissue parasites inpatients with chronic urticaria. J Dermatol. 2003;30:777–81.

23. Ismail MA, Khalafallah O. *Toxocara canis* and chronic urticaria in Egyptian patients. J Egypt Soc Parasitol. 2005;35:833–40.

24. Gulalp B, Koseoglu Z, Toprak N, Satar S, Sebe A, Gokel Y, et al. Ruptured hydatid cyst following minimal trauma and few signs on presentation. Neth J Med. 2007;65:117–8.

25. Pattison DA, Speare R. Strongyloidiasis in personnel of the Regional Assistance Mission to Solomon Islands (RAMSI). Med J Aust. 2008;189:203–6.

26. Marseglia GL, Marseglia A, Licari A, Castellazzi AM, Ciprandi G. Chronic urticaria caused by *Hymenoleptis nana* in an adopted girl. Allergy. 2007;62:821–2.

27. Zuel-Fakkar NM, Abdel Hameed DM, Hassanin OM. Study of *Blastocystis hominis* isolates in urticaria: a case-control study. Clin Exp Dermatol. 2011;36:908–10.

28. Kaji K, Yoshiji H, Yoshikawa M, Yamazaki M, Ikenaka Y, Noguchi R, et al. Eosinophilic cholecystitis along with pericarditis caused by Ascaris lumbricoides: a case report. World J Gastroenterol. 2007;13:3760–2.

29. Criado PR, Belda Junior W, Criado RF, Vasconcelos e Silva R, Vasconcellos C. Bedbugs (Cimicidae infestation): the worldwide renaissance of an old partner of human kind. Braz J Infect Dis. 2011;15:74–80.

30. Spiewak R, Lundberg M, Johansson G, Buczek A. Allergy to pigeon tick (*Argas reflexus*) in Upper Silesia, Poland. Ann Agric Environ Med. 2006;13:107–12.

31. Armentia A, Martin-Gil FJ, Pascual C, Martin-Esteban M, Callejo A, Martinez C. *Anisakis simplex* allergy after eating chicken meat. J Investig Allergol Clin Immunol. 2006;16:258–63.

32. Daschner A, De Frutos C, Valls A, Vega F. *Anisakis simplex* sensitization-associated urticaria: short-lived immediate type or prolonged acute urticaria. Arch Dermatol Res. 2010;302:625–9.

33. Leznoff A, Josse RG, Denburg J, Dolovich J. Association of chronic urticaria and angioedema with thyroid autoimmunity. Arch Dermatol. 1983;119:636–40.

34. Leznoff A, Sussman GL. Syndrome of idiopathic urticaria and angioedema with thyroid autoimmunity: a study of 90 patients. J Allergy Clin Immunol. 1989;84:66–71.

35. Zauli D, Grassi A, Ballardini G, Contestabile S, Zucchini S, Bianchi FB. Thyroid autoimmunity in chronic idiopathic urticaria. Am J Clin Dermatol. 2002;3:525–8.

36. Turktas I, Gokcora N, Demirsoy S, Cakir N, Onal E. The association of chronic urticaria and angioedema with autoimmune thyroiditis. Int J Dermatol. 1997;36:187–90.

37. Rottem M. Chronic urticaria and autoimmune thyroid disease: is there a link? Autoimmun Rev. 2003;2:69–72.

38. Konstantinou GN, Asero R, Maurer M, Sabroe RA, Schmid-Grendelmeier P, Grattan CE. EAACI/GA(2) LEN task force consensus report: the autologous serum skin test in urticaria. Allergy. 2009;64:1256–68.

39. Tedeschi A, Cottini M, Asero R. Simultaneous occurrence of chronic autoimmune urticaria and nonallergic asthma: a common mechanism? Eur Ann Allergy Clin Immunol. 2009;41:56–9.

40. Confino-Cohen R, Chodick G, Shalev V, Leshno M, Kimhi O, Goldberg A. Chronic urticaria and autoimmunity: associations found in a large population study. J Allergy Clin Immunol. 2012;129:1307–13.

41. Cugno M, Marzano AV, Asero R, Tedeschi A. Activation of blood coagulation in chronic urticaria: pathophysiologic and clinical implications. Intern Emerg Med. 2010;5:97–101.

42. Asero R, Tedeschi A, Riboldi P, Griffini S, Bonanni E, Cugno M. Severe chronic urticaria is associated with elevated plasma levels of D-dimer. Allergy. 2008;63:176–80.

43. Takahagi S, Mihara S, Iwamoto K, Morioke S, Okabe T, Kameyoshi Y, et al. Coagulation/fibrinolysis and inflammation markers are associated with disease activity in patients with chronic urticaria. Allergy. 2010;65:649–56.

44. Konstantinou GN, Asero R, Ferrer M, Knol EF, Maurer M, Raap U, et al. EAACI taskforce position paper: evidence for autoimmune urticaria and proposal for defining diagnostic criteria. Allergy. 2013;68:27–36.

45. Augey F, Gunera-Saad N, Bensaid B, Nosbaum A, Berard F, Nicolas JF. Chronic spontaneous urticaria is not an allergic disease. Eur J Dermatol. 2011;21:349–53.

46. Caliskaner Z, Ozturk S, Turan M, Karaayvaz M. Skin test positivity to aeroallergens in the patients with chronic urticaria without respiratory disease. J Investig Allergol Clin Immunol. 2004;14:50–4.

47. Kozel MM, Mekkes JR, Bossuyt PM, Bos JD. Natural course of physical and chronic urticaria and angioedema in 220 patients. J Am Acad Dermatol. 2001;45:387–91.

48. Młynek A, Zalewska-Janowska A, Martus P, Staubach P, Zuberbier T, Maurer M. How to assess disease activity in patients with chronic urticaria? Allergy. 2008;63:777–80.

49. Grattan CEH. The urticaria spectrum: recognition of clinical patterns can help management. Clin Exp Dermatol. 2004;29:217–21.

50. Malmros H. Auto serum test. Nord Med. 1946;29:150–1.

51. Sabroe RA, Greaves MW. Chronic idiopathic urticaria with functional autoantibodies: 12 years on. Br J Dermatol. 2006;154:813–9.

52. Yıldız H, Karabudak O, Doğan B, Harmanyeri Y. Evaluation of autologous plasma skin test

in patients with chronic idiopathic urticaria. Br J Dermatol. 2011;165:1205–9.

53. Asero R, Tedeschi A, Riboldi P, Cugno M. Plasma of patients with chronic urticaria shows signs of thrombin generation, and its intradermal injection causes wheal and-flare reaction much more frequently than frequently than autologous serum. J Allergy Clin Immunol. 2006;117:1113–7.

54. Metz M, Gimenez-Arnau A, Borzova E, Grattan CE, Magerl M, Maurer M. Frequency and clinical implications of skin autoreactivity to serum versus plasma in patients with chronic urticaria. J Allergy Clin Immunol. 2009;123:705–6.

55. Criado PR, Criado RFJ, Maruta CW, Martins JEC, Rivitti EA. Urticaria. An Bras Dermatol. 2005;80:613–30.

56. Criado PR, Criado RFJ, Maruta CW, Machado CDA. Histamine, histamine receptors and antihistamines: new concepts. An Bras Dermatol. 2010;85:195–210.

57. Pires JS, de Ue APF, Furlani EJ, de Souza PK, Rotta O. Dapsone as an alternative to the treatment of chronic urticaria nonresponsive to antihistamines. An Bras Dermatol. 2008;83:413–8.

58. Criado RF, Criado PR, Martins JE, Valente NY, Michalany NS, Vasconcellos C. Urticaria unresponsive to antihistaminic treatment: an open study of therapeutic options based on histopathologic features. J Dermatolog Treat. 2008;19:92–6.

59. Jauregui I, Ferrer M, Montoro J, Davila I, Bartra J, del Cuvillo A, et al. Antihistamines in the treatment of chronic urticaria. J Investig Allergol Clin Immunol. 2007;17:41–52.

60. Kalivas J, Breneman D, Tharp M, Bruce S, Bigby M. Urticaria: clinical efficacy of cetirizine in comparison with hydroxyzine and placebo. J Allergy Clin Immunol. 1990;86:1014–8.

61. Zuberbier T, Bindslev-Jensen C, Canonica W, Grattan CE, Greaves MW, Henz BM, et al. EAACI/GA2LEN/EDF. EAACI/GA2LEN/EDF guideline: management of urticaria. Allergy. 2006;61:321–31.

62. Asero R. Chronic unremitting urticaria: is the use of antihistamines above the licensed dose effective? A preliminary study of cetirizine at licensed and above-licensed doses. Clin Exp Dermatol. 2007;32:34–8.

63. Black AK, Greaves MW. Antihistamines in urticaria and angioedema. Clin Allergy Immunol. 2002;17:249–86.

64. Kozel MM, Sabroe RA. Chronic urticaria: aetiology, management and current and future treatment options. Drugs. 2004;64:2515–36.

65. Weller K, Ziege C, Staubach P, Brockow K, Siebenhaar F, Krause K, et al. H1-antihistamine updosing in chronic spontaneous urticaria: patients' perspective of effectiveness and side effects – a retrospective survey study. PLoS One. 2011;6:e23931.

66. Sanchez-Borges M, Caballero-Fonseca F, Capriles-Hulett A. Treatment of recalcitrant chronic urticaria with nonsedating antihistamines: is there evidence for updosing? J Investig Allergol Clin Immunol. 2013;23:141–4.

67. Fedorowicz Z, van Zuuren EJ, Hu N. Histamine H2-receptor antagonists for urticaria. Cochrane Database Syst Rev. 2012;3:CD008596.

68. Grattan CE, O'Donnell BF, Francis DM, Niimi N, Barlow RJ, Seed PT, et al. Randomized double-blind study of cyclosporine in chronic 'idiopathic' urticaria. Br J Dermatol. 2000;143:365–72.

69. Hollander SM, Joo SS, Wedner HJ. Factors that predict the success of cyclosporine treatment for chronic urticaria. Ann Allergy Asthma Immunol. 2011;107:523–8.

70. Di Leo E, Nettis E, Aloia AM, Moschetta M, Carbonara M, Dammacco F, et al. Cyclosporine-A efficacy in chronic idiopathic urticaria. Int J Immunopathol Pharmacol. 2011;24:195–200.

71. Vena GA, Cassano N, Colombo D, Peruzzi E, Pigatto P, Neo-I-30 Study Group. Cyclosporine in chronic idiopathic urticaria: a double-blind, randomized, placebo-controlled trial. J Am Acad Dermatol. 2006;55:705–9.

72. Neverman L, Weinberger M. Treatment of chronic urticaria in children with antihistamines and cyclosporine. J Allergy Clin Immunol Pract. 2014;2:434–8.

73. Kessel A, Toubi E. Cyclosporine-A in severe chronic urticaria: the option for long term therapy. Allergy. 2010;65:1478–82.

74. Sagi L, Solomon M, Baum S, Lyakhovitsky A, Trau H, Barzilai A. Evidence for methotrexate as a useful treatment for steroid-dependent chronic urticaria. Acta Derm Venereol. 2011;91:303–6.

75. Perez A, Woods A, Grattan CE. Methotrexate: a useful steroid-sparing agent in recalcitrant chronic urticaria. Br J Dermatol. 2010;162:191–4.

76. Asero R. Oral cyclophosphamide in a case of cyclosporine and steroid-resistant chronic urticaria showing autoreactivity on autologous serum skin testing. Clin Exp Dermatol. 2005;30:582–3.

77. O'Donnell BF, Barr RM, Black AK, Francis DM, Kermani F, Niimi N, et al. Intravenous immunoglobulin in autoimmune chronic urticaria. Br J Dermatol. 1998;138:101–6.

78. Pereira C, Tavares B, Carrapatoso I, Loureiro G, Faria E, Machado D, et al. Lowdose intravenous gammaglobulin in the treatment of severe autoimmune urticaria. Eur Ann Allergy Clin Immunol. 2007;39:237–42.

79. Mitzel-Kaoukhov H, Staubach P, Muller-Brenne T. Effect of high-dose intravenous immunoglobulin treatment in therapy-resistant chronic spontaneous urticaria. Ann Allergy Asthma Immunol. 2010;104:253–8.

80. Maurer M, Altrichter S, Bieber T, Biedermann T, Brautigam M, Seyfried S, et al. Efficacy and safety of omalizumab in patients with chronic urticaria who exhibit IgE against thyroperoxidase. J Allergy Clin Immunol. 2011;128:202–209.e5.

81. Khan DA. Alternative agents in refractory chronic urticaria: evidence and considerations on their selection and use. J Allergy Clin Immunol Pract. 2013;1:433–440.e1.

82. Saini S, Rosen KE, Hsieh HJ, Wong DA, Conner E, Kaplan A, et al. A randomized, placebo-controlled, dose-ranging study of single-dose omalizumab in patients with H1-antihistamine-refractory chronic idiopathic urticaria. J Allergy Clin Immunol. 2011;128:567–73.e1.

83. Maurer M, Rosen K, Hsieh HJ, Saini S, Grattan C, Gimenez-Arnau A, et al. Omalizumab for the treatment of chronic idiopathic or spontaneous urticaria. N Engl J Med. 2013;368:924–35.

84. Asero R, Tedeschi A, Cugno M. Treatment of chronic urticaria. Immunol Allergy Clin N Am. 2014;34:105–16.

85. Chakravarty SD, Yee AF, Paget SA. Rituximab successfully treats refractory chronic autoimmune urticaria caused by IgE receptor autoantibodies. J Allergy Clin Immunol. 2011;128:1354–5.

86. Arkwright PD. Anti-CD20 or anti-IgE therapy for severe chronic autoimmune urticaria. J Allergy Clin Immunol. 2009;123:510–1.

87. Mallipeddi R, Grattan CE. Lack of response of severe steroid-dependent chronic urticaria torituximab. Clin Exp Dermatol. 2007;32:333–4.

88. Wilson LH, Eliason MJ, Leiferman KM, Hull CM, Powell DL. Treatment of refractory chronic urticaria with tumor necrosis factor-alfa inhibitors. J Am Acad Dermatol. 2011;64:1221–2.

89. Piconi S, Trabattoni D, Iemoli E, Fusi ML, Villa ML, Milazzo F, et al. Immune profiles of patients with chronic idiopathic urticaria. Int Arch Allergy Immunol. 2002;128:59–66.

90. Hermes B, Prochazka AK, Haas N, Jurgovsky K, Sticherling M, Henz BM. Upregulation of TNF-alpha and IL-3 expression in lesional and uninvolved skin indifferent types of urticaria. J Allergy ClinImmunol. 1999;103:307–14.

91. Reeves GE, Boyle MJ, Bonfield J, Dobson P, Loewenthal M. Impact of hydroxychloroquine therapy on chronic urticaria: chronic autoimmune urticaria study and evaluation. Intern Med J. 2004;34:182–6.

92. Pho LN, Eliason MJ, Regruto M, Hull CM, Powell DL. Treatment of chronic urticaria with colchicine. J Drugs Dermatol. 2011;10:1423–8.

93. Noda S, Asano Y, Sato S. Long-term complete resolution of severe chronic idiopathic urticaria after dapsone treatment. J Dermatol. 2012;39:496–7.

94. Engin B, Ozdemir M. Prospective randomized non-blinded clinical trial on the use of dapsone plus antihistamine vs. antihistamine in patients with chronic idiopathic urticaria. J Eur Acad Dermatol Venereol. 2008;22:481–6.

95. Khan S, Lynch N. Efficacy of montelukast as added therapy in patients with chronic idiopathic urticaria. Inflamm Allergy Drug Targets. 2012;11:235–43.

96. Criado PR, Antinori LC, Maruta CW, Reis VM. Evaluation of D-dimer serum levels among patients with chronic urticaria, psoriasis and urticarial vasculitis. An Bras Dermatol. 2013;88:355–60.

97. Asero R, Tedeschi A, Cugno M. Heparin and tranexamic acid therapy may be effective in treatment-resistant chronic urticaria with elevated d-dimer: a pilot study. Int Arch Allergy Immunol. 2010;152:384–9.

98. Samarasinghe V, Marsland AM. Class action of oral coumarins in the treatment ofa patient with chronic spontaneous urticaria and delayed-pressure urticaria. Clin Exp Dermatol. 2012;37:741–3.

99. Chua SL, Gibbs S. Chronic urticaria responding to subcutaneous heparin sodium. Br J Dermatol. 2005;153:216–7.

100. Parslew R, Pryce D, Ashworth J, Friedmann PS. Warfarin treatment of chronic idiopathic urticaria and angio-oedema. Clin Exp Allergy. 2000;30:1161–5.

101. Karaayvaz M, Calişkaner Z, Turan M, Akar A, Ozturk S, Ozanguc N. Levothyroxine versus ketotifen in the treatment of patients with chronic urticaria and thyroid autoimmunity. J Dermatol Treat. 2002;13:165–72.

102. Temboury Molina C, Alins Sahun Y, Cerecedo CI. Recurrent urticaria and autoimmune thyroiditis: the influence of thyroxin treatment on the outcome of the urticaria. An Pediatr (Barc). 2012;77:66–7.

103. Gupta MA, Gupta AK. Chronic idiopathic urticaria and post-traumatic stress disorder (PTSD): an under-recognized comorbidity. Clin Dermatol. 2012;30:351–4.

104. Hunkin V, Chung MC. Chronic idiopathic urticaria, psychological comorbidity and posttraumatic stress: the impact of alexithymia and repression. Psychiatr Q. 2012;83:431–47.

105. Staubach P, Dechene M, Metz M, Magerl M, Siebenhaar F, Weller K, et al. High prevalence of mental disorders and emotional distress in patients with chronic spontaneous urticaria. Acta Derm Venereol. 2011;91:557–61.

106. O'Donnell BF. Urticaria: impact on quality of life and economic cost. Immunol Allergy Clin N Am. 2014;34:89–104.

107. Rabelo-Filardi R, Daltro-Oliveira R, Campos RA. Parameters associated with chronic spontaneous urticaria duration and severity: a systematic review. Int Arch Allergy Immunol. 2013;161:197–204.

108. Sanchez-Borges M, Asero R, Ansotegui IJ, Baiardini I, Bernstein JA, Canonica GW, et al. Diagnosis and treatment of urticaria and angioedema: a worldwide perspective. World Allergy Organ J. 2012;5:125–47.

109. Ye YM, Jin HJ, Hwang EK, Nam YH, Kim JH, Shin YS. Coexistence of chronic urticaria and metabolic syndrome: clinical implications. Acta Derm Venereol. 2013;93:156–60.

110. De Benedictis FM, De Benedictis D, Canonica GW. New oral H1 antihistamines in children: facts and unmeet needs. Allergy. 2008;63:1395–404. doi:10.1111/j.1398–9995.2008.01771.x.

Erythema Nodosum

64

Débora Sarzi Sartori, Lara Mombelli,
and Natalia Sarzi Sartori

Key Points

- Erythema nodosum (EN) is the most frequent form of panniculitis
- EN is mainly idiopathic, but can be a reaction pattern from a wide variety of etiologic agents
- The lesions are subcutaneous nodules clinically manifested as erythematous and painful patches located symmetrically on the anterior surface of the lower extremities
- Histologically EN is characterized by a predominantly septal panniculitis without vasculitis
- EN prevails in women between 15 and 30 years of age
- Early diagnosis in primary care is necessary to guide investigation and treat the underlying cause

D.S. Sartori (✉)
Service of Dermatology, UFCSPA,
Porto Alegre, Brazil
e-mail: desarzisartori@yahoo.com

L. Mombelli
Service of Dermatology, UFCSPA,
Rio Grande do Sul, Porto Alegre, Brazil

N.S. Sartori
Service of Rheumatology,
Federal Univesity of Rio Grande do Sul,
Porto Alegre, Brazil

Introduction

Panniculitis is inflammation of the subcutaneous adipose tissue and is an uncommon pathology characterized by sudden inflammatory patches or nodules under the skin. Erythema nodosum (EN) is the most common clinical presentation of panniculitis, affecting 1–5 per 100,000 persons per year. The highest incidence is in young women from 15 to 30 years of age, and the male-to-female ratio is 1:6 [12]. In children the ratio between the genders is 1:1 [10, 11].

EN is nowadays considered a reaction pattern resulting from a wide variety of etiologic agents [1, 2]. About 55% of EN are classified as idiopathic [1, 18]. Infections are the most common etiology of EN in children, mainly streptococcal pharyngitis, and the main causes in the adult population are medicaments, systemic inflammatory diseases (sarcoidosis, inflammatory bowel disease), pregnancy, and malignancy.

The classic clinical presentation of EN is painful and symmetric nodules of imprecise limits on the tibial anterior surface. Characteristically the nodules are more palpable than visible. Frequently it consists of a

© Springer International Publishing Switzerland 2018
R.R. Bonamigo, S.I.T. Dornelles (eds.), *Dermatology in Public Health Environments*,
https://doi.org/10.1007/978-3-319-33919-1_64

potentially grave systemic disease manifestation, and for this reason it must be promptly recognized so that the etiologic investigation and correct treatment can be instigated as early as possible.

Concepts

Currently there is a tendency to classify EN not as a disease itself but as a nonspecific pattern of reaction from different types of antigens. Many different immunologic patterns are involved in its immunopathology, the most important of them being delayed type 4 hypersensitivity.

Despite exhaustive investigation more than 50% of cases remain without related etiology, being classified as idiopathic. The main causes of EN are listed in Table 64.1.

The main recognizable cause of EN is streptococcal pharyngitis (caused by group A β-hemolytic streptococci), which is more likely to occur in the young. The skin lesions appear from 2 to 4 weeks after the pharyngeal infection and are accompanied by high levels of antistreptolysin O (ASLO) and/or anti-DNase B. Other possible streptococcal infections should be searched for, such as impetigo, cellulitis, intertrigo (axilla, perineum), vulvovaginitis, balanitis, and infection of the perianal area. Group A β-hemolytic *Streptococcus* can also be found by rapid diagnostic testing or collection of a secretion culture from the suspected areas.

EN can often be the first sign of a systemic disease such as tuberculosis, profound fungal infection, sarcoidosis, inflammatory bowel disease, and malignancy [13].

Many single case reports document other possible associations, including reports of EN in the setting of vaccinations [1, 8, 23, 24].

Table 64.1 Causes of EN

Common	Rare (<1%)
Idiopathic (up to 55%)	Vaccine
	Tuberculosis, cholera, hepatitis B, human papillomavirus, malaria, rabies, smallpox, typhoid, tetanus–diphtheria–acellular pertussis (Tdap)
Infections	Infections
Bacterial:	Bacterial:
Streptococcal pharyngitis (28–48%), tuberculosis, yersiniosis, *Mycoplasma*, *Chlamydia*	*Salmonella*, *Campylobacter*, *Shigella*, brucellosis, psittacosis, *Rickettsia*, syphilis
Fungal:	Fungal:
Histoplasmosis, coccidioidomycosis	Blastomycosis, sporotrichosis, dermatophytosis
	Viral:
	Infectious mononucleosis, hepatitis B, hepatitis C, herpes simplex virus, human immunodeficiency virus
	Parasitosis:
	Amoebiasis, giardiasis, ascariasis
Systemic disease:	Systemic disease:
Sarcoidosis (11–25%)	Behcet's disease
With bilateral hilar adenopathy	
Enteropathies (1–4%):	
Ulcerative colitis and Crohn's disease	
Drugs (3–10%):	Drugs:
Antibiotics (e.g., sulfonamides, penicillin), oral contraceptives, bromides, iodide	Minocycline, gold salts, salicylates
Pregnancy (2–5%)	Malignancies:
	Hodgkin's lymphoma, non-Hodgkin lymphoma, leukemia, renal cell carcinoma
	Miscellany:
	Vitamin B12 deficiency

Clinical Presentation

EN is characterized by painful, erythematous, and symmetric subcutaneous nodules of imprecise limits. The size of the lesions varies from 0.5 to 10 cm in diameter [2]. The most frequent location is the tibial anterior surface, but the extensor surface of forearms, thighs, chest, and even the face can also be involved (Fig. 64.1).

The nodules are of sudden appearance. Individually they tend to decline in 2 weeks, although new outcroppings persist for up to 6 weeks. Complete healing often takes 1–2 months when the nodules assume a bruise-like appearance, also known as "erythema contusiformis." They can leave local hyperchromia but no atrophy or scars because there is no ulcer formation.

EN usually occurs at the end of the winter and the beginning of spring. Prodromal symptoms such as low-grade fever (60%), malaise (67%), arthralgias (64%), arthritis (31%) [1], cough, and weight loss may often precede the onset of the lesions by 1–3 weeks. Arthralgias can also persist for up to 2 years after the resolution of the cutaneous lesions, causing nonspecific destructive joint changes [2].

Rare clinical variants of the disease are recognized [2]. EN migrans consists of persistent but minimally symptomatic unilateral nodules that tend to migrate centrifugally. Subacute nodular migratory panniculitis can reach 20 cm in diameter by confluence of the nodules on the legs. Another rare form of EN is seen in children after physical activity and affects unilaterally the palmoplantar surface.

The earlier the diagnosis is made, the earlier the underlying disease can be investigated and found.

Some clinical symptoms and physical findings should draw attention to causes associated with EN. The main symptoms are listed in Box 64.1.

Box 64.1 Findings Suggestive of Erythema Nodosum with Systemic Cause

Arthritis/synovitis

Diarrhea

History of previous upper respiratory infection

Rising ASLO titers, positive throat swab culture, or rapid test for group A *Streptococcus*

Abnormal chest X-ray

Positive skin tuberculin test

Diagnosis

The syndromic diagnosis is clinical, taking into account the sudden onset of the pretibial painful nodular lesions, generally associated with constitutional symptoms (Box 64.2).

Box 64.2 Clinical Criteria for Diagnosis of Erythema Nodosum

1. Painful erythematous or purple nodules or patches, with irregular and poorly defined borders, from 1 to 5 cm

2. Symmetric tibial anterior surface lesions, reaching or not reaching other skin areas

3. Lesions of sudden appearance, each one lasting less than 8 weeks

4. Resolution without ulceration or scars

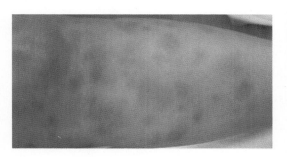

Fig. 64.1 Erythema nodosum: erythematous nodules (Courtesy of Dermatology Service of UFCSPA)

Histopathologic examination can help in doubtful cases and rule out other diseases such as other kinds of panniculitis, but it is not pathognomonic. The microscopic aspects vary considerably according to the evolutionary stage of the lesions, although the local and type of inflammation can vary between different samples of the same panniculitis regardless of the time of evolution of the disease. Therefore, currently there is a tendency to classify panniculitis as predominantly septal panniculitis and predominantly lobular panniculitis. Other anatomopathologic data that help to guide the diagnosis are the presence or absence of fat necrosis, type of necrosis, presence or absence of vascular alteration (vasculitis, thrombosis) and presence or absence of other findings such as sclerosis and infectious agents [12].

The specimen for histopathology must be obtained through profound incisional or excisional biopsy, since punch biopsy produces inadequate samples for subcutaneous tissue visualization [10]. The histopathologic findings of EN include inflammation of the subcutaneous septum (septal panniculitis, Fig. 64.2), and perivascular inflammatory infiltrate with neutrophil predominance, edema, and hemorrhage-determined septum thickening in early lesions. In later stages granulomatous lesions can be seen in the septum (typically radial or Miescher granulomas) [10].

The etiologic investigation must be guided by the clinical symptoms and must include biochemical analysis, serologic testing, streptococcal infection research, culture examination, X-ray, pregnancy test, and Mantoux skin test.

In the pediatric demographic the most prevailing is the infectious diagnosis for EN (up to 68%), in the main being associated with streptococcal pharyngitis. However, as some studies show significant involvement of gastrointestinal infections, a stool test is imperative for children [1, 20].

Increase of nonspecific inflammatory tests such as erythrocyte sedimentation rate and C-reactive protein are regularly seen, associated or not with leukocytosis.

Differential Diagnoses

The main differential diagnoses of EN are listed in Table 64.2. One major differential that must be highlighted is the type II leprosy reactional episode, also called leprosy EN. This reactional episode can be the first manifestation of the disease and usually happens during and after leprosy treatment, with sudden appearances of painful nodular lesions not only in the anterior tibial region but primarily in the arms, abdomen, and lower limbs. Another different feature is that

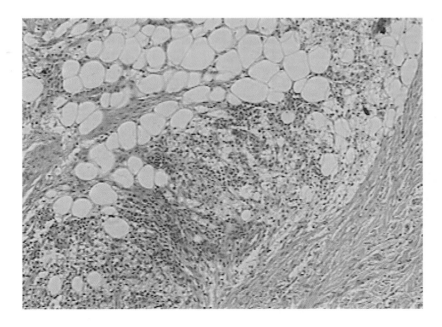

Fig. 64.2
Histopathology of erythema nodosum: septal panniculitis (Courtesy of Dermatology Service of UFCSPA)

Table 64.2 Differential diagnosis of erythema nodosum

Other panniculitis		Other diseases (occasional differential diagnostic)
Panniculitis predominantly lobular:	Other panniculitis predominantly septal	Pretibial myxedema
More common	Polyarteritis nodosa	Necrobiosis lipoidica
α1-Antitrypsin deficiency	Eosinophilic fasciitis	Necrobiotic xanthogranuloma
Cytophagic histiocytic panniculitis (a lymphoma)	Eosinophilia-myalgia syndrome	Gum (tertiary syphilis)
Lupus erythematosus profundus (lupus panniculitis)	Scleroderma	
Nodular fat necrosis	Thrombophlebitis	
Rare		
Cold panniculitis		
Infectious panniculitis		
Leukemic fat infiltrates		
Poststeroid panniculitis		
Povidone panniculitis		
Scleroderma neonatorum		
Sclerosing panniculitis		
Pancreatic panniculitis		
Lipodystrophies		
Subcutaneous fat necrosis of the newborn		
Idiopathic lobular panniculitis (Pfeiffer-Weber-Christian disease)		
Nodular vasculitis (erythema induratum)		

leprosy nodules can evolve with ulceration. It is considered an immune reaction to a multibacillary disease and usually is associated with systemic symptoms such as fever, malaise, and fatigue. It can also affect other organs such as joints, eyes, and testicles [33]. Treatment consists of prednisone and thalidomide (for men and women after childbearing age).

Therapeutic Approach

Since EN is a self-limited condition, whenever possible the treatment should be directed to its etiologic cause.

Symptomatic treatment is based on rest and elevation of the affected extremities. Nonsteroidal anti-inflammatory drugs (NSAIDs) are helpful in relieving the pain, with satisfactory outcome in most of the cases; however, they must be avoided in those cases of EN that are due to Crohn's disease because of the risk of flare and bleeding [6].

More aggressive treatments are restricted to recurrent or difficult cases.

Corticosteroids have a prompt response, but should be initiated only if infection and malignancy are discarded as possible causes of EN (due to the possibility of sepsis and spread). Commonly prednisone is used at a daily oral dose of 60 mg or 1 mg per kg body weight [1, 2].

It is important to bear in mind that prednisone can lead to a false-negative Mantoux skin test and delay the diagnosis of tuberculosis. It should therefore be avoided during early onset of the symptoms, especially in endemic areas.

Potassium iodide can be a therapeutic alternative at a dose of 400–900 mg per day, being more effective the earlier it is started. Attention should be paid to the risk of secondary hyperthyroidism development with prolonged use of this medication [4].

Other treatments can be proposed according to the underlying pathology, such as colchicine for EN associated with Behcet's disease [5, 15] and hydroxychloroquine, thalidomide, cyclosporine, and infliximab in monotherapy or combined with corticosteroids in those cases linked to Crohn's disease [7].

Even in patients with idiopathic EN, the use of tumor necrosis factor α (TNF) inhibitors can be considered in refractory cases. Some case reports indicate a satisfactory and sustained outcome with the use of subcutaneous etanercept at the dose of 25 mg twice a week in patients who had treatment failure with prednisone, potassium iodide, dapsone, NSAIDs, and methotrexate [15, 17, 25].

Other therapeutic options are mycophenolate mofetil and dapsone, depending on the clinical context. Table 64.3 shows the level of evidence regarding management.

Table 64.3 Treatment recommendations for erythema nodosum

Key for clinical practice	Level of evidence	References
Once diagnosed, etiologic search must be made according to clinical symptoms and age group of the patient	C	[1, 12]
In children, up to 68% of the cases are secondary to infectious processes, mainly streptococcal pharyngitis and bacterial gastroenteritis	C	[9, 20]
Histopathologic exam reveals septal panniculitis without vasculitis, but it is not pathognomonic	C	[10, 12, 13]
Painful symptoms are solved in the most cases by rest, elevation of the affected limbs, and use of NSAIDs	C	[1, 2]
Prednisone can be started only after infection and malignancy are discarded as possible causes	C	[1, 2]
Patients who react strongly to a Mantoux skin test must receive treatment for tuberculosis even without evidence of active infectious focus, especially in endemic areas	C	[15, 15]
Anti-TNF drugs are a promising treatment to refractory idiopathic erythema nodosum	C	[17]

A = consistent, good-quality patient-oriented evidence; B = inconsistent or limited-quality patient-oriented evidence; C = consensus, disease-oriented evidence, usual practice, expert opinion, or case series. Levels according to Strength of Recommendation Taxonomy (SORT)

Etiologic Treatment: The Impact of Etiologies Associated with EN

Streptococcal Pharyngitis

Streptococcal pharyngitis is the most identifiable disease related to EN. EN begins about 2–3 weeks after the onset of acute pharyngitis.

Epidemiologically about 15–30% cases of acute pharyngitis in children and teenagers and about 5–10% in adults are caused by group A β-hemolytic streptococci [31, 32]. The etiologic investigation can be made by culture of the throat swab, streptococcal ASLO titers, and rapid antigen detection testing (RADT). In children and teenagers, if RADT is negative, because of its lower sensitivity it is recommended that the diagnosis be confirmed with culture of the oropharynx swab (golden pattern). On the other hand, because of the low incidence of streptococcal pharyngitis in adults, the negative result of RADT in this population is an isolated acceptable alternative [32]. In the case of a positive RADT result, treatment must be initiated because of the high specificity (>95%) of the test.

The treatment of choice for this condition is antibiotics of the penicillin group, because of the high effectiveness, low cost, and safety of these drugs. For patients allergic to penicillin, erythromycin is a suitable choice. First-generation cephalosporins can be used as well, since the patient does not manifest immediate-type hypersensitivity to β-lactam antibiotics. Sulfonamides and tetracycline should be avoided because of evidence of increased rates of bacterial resistance.

Tuberculosis and Atypical Mycobacteriosis

The association between EN and tuberculosis is well established. EN can appear together with primary tuberculosis, in reactivation episodes, associated with latent tuberculosis, BCG vaccination, and after PPD (Mantoux) test [14, 15, 22].

In every case of EN a risk stratification must be made for tuberculosis with X-ray, tuberculin skin test, and direct search for acid-/alcohol-resistant bacilli. The culture examination can also help to diagnose tuberculosis and suspected cases of atypical mycobacteriosis [10, 14].

Some atypical mycobacteria have been associated with EN, such as *Mycobacterium marinum* (common in swimming pools). In this subgroup it is important that the species is identified to provide specific treatment for the causal agent [10, 19].

In a retrospective analysis by Kumar et al. of a total of 52 patients diagnosed with idiopathic EN with a strongly positive Mantoux test (average of 19 mm), after treatment with antitubercular drugs new lesions stopped appearing in 45 patients within 6–8 weeks and subsided in 2 (data could be analyzed in 47 patients). The therapy was well tolerated except for jaundice in one patient and transient urticarial lesions in another.

Because of the strong association between EN and tuberculosis, a positive Mantoux test is an indication to receive antitubercular therapy, even without evidence of identifiable infectious focus, mainly in endemic areas [14].

Sarcoidosis

Sarcoidosis is a systemic inflammatory disease of unknown cause, characterized by noncaseating granulomas that can attack a number of organs.

The systemic clinical manifestations are various, most frequently reaching the respiratory tract, but also often affecting ocular, skin, and musculoskeletal systems.

Skin manifestations of sarcoidosis are divided into specific and nonspecific according to the presence of the noncaseating granulomas. Among the nonspecific manifestations the most common is EN, affecting 10% of patients [27].

EN in sarcoidosis prevails in young women and generally has a benign course.

When EN presents in association with pulmonary manifestations (bilateral hilar lymphadenopathy) and polyarthritis, it is known as Löfgren's syndrome. The Löfgren syndrome tends to be acute and self-limited, and usually resolves within 6–8 weeks.

Acute lesions usually require only symptomatic treatment. When cutaneous lesion is the predominant impairment of sarcoidosis the drug of choice is prednisone, and the dosage regimen should be adjusted according to the progression and severity of the disease [27].

Pregnancy and Oral Contraceptives

The immune mechanism of pregnancy and oral contraceptive use in the induction of EN is not fully elucidated. Immune complexes may play a role in the pathogenesis of EN during pregnancy, or EN may be a hypersensitivity reaction to either estrogens or progesterone [6].

As it is often a self-limited condition and various medications available to treat EN are contraindicated in pregnancy, initial treatment can involve rest, elevation of the limbs, and compression stockings, which often lead to resolution. In more resistant cases the choice of treatment should be made preferably together with obstetrics, with risk/benefit of the treatment being taken into account [3, 6].

When EN is associated with the use of oral contraceptives, the suspension of medication and symptomatic treatment of the skin lesions is recommended.

Inflammatory Bowel Disease (IBD)

IBD is often associated with nonintestinal manifestations. EN is the most observed cutaneous manifestation, predominating in females and varying from 4% to 10% of patients with IBD [28, 30]. In patients with Crohn's disease it is seen more in patients with ileocolonic disease than in those with small intestine disease [28, 30].

EN may precede the onset or follow the course of the disease. The appearance of EN lesions associated with diarrhea and abdominal pain can lead to disease flare. Improvement in the frequency of skin crises may indicate stability of the intestinal disease [29]. There is no association between EN and severity of IBD [28].

Behcet's Disease

Behcet's disease is a systemic vasculitis of unknown cause that affects veins and arteries from small to large caliber. The mucocutaneous manifestations are characteristic of the syndrome and include oral and genital ulcers, pustulosis, and EN [26].

The EN lesions related to Behcet's disease usually present in lower limb extremities, and can evolve with healing to residual skin pigmentation. Histologic examination of these lesions is characterized by elements of vasculitis, which is a sufficient finding to differentiate them from EN related to other etiologies [26].

Colchicine is the drug of choice when EN is the dominant manifestation in Behcet's disease [5, 15]. Manifestations resistant to colchicine may be treated with azathioprine and thalidomide; in more severe cases immunobiological therapy with TNF antagonists are considered [16, 17].

Medications

About 1–3% of EN is credited to medications. The main associated drugs are sulfonamides, penicillin, oral contraceptives, bromides, and iodide.

In cases of EN in patients receiving medications known to be associated with it, the drug should be discontinued whenever possible.

Malignancies

Rarely, neoplastic diseases are implicated as being responsible for triggering EN. In the absence of associated clinical symptoms, more complete diagnostic investigation for malignancies is only justified in cases of refractory EN.

The most frequently associated cancers are leukemia and lymphoma. Neoplasms of solid organs such as carcinoid tumor, colorectal, renal, and pancreatic cancer are eventually seen in association with EN.

Future Perspectives

Multiple causes of EN are currently known. However, as observational studies are conducted, idiopathic EN rates continue to remain high. In line with technological improvements in diagnostic methods, new etiologic agents are emerging as possible causes of EN.

In a case report of chronic EN, lesions without response to NSAIDs in a patient with restricted diet and vitamin B12 deficiency achieved resolution with vitamin replacement. Thus, vitamin B12 deficiency is presented as a new possible cause of EN and should be borne in mind especially in populations at higher risk of vitamin deficiency [21].

For refractory cases, immunobiological therapy with the use of TNF antagonists is emerging as a potential treatment. Case reports indicate an excellent response in more severe and refractory cases to already established drugs [17, 25].

Glossary

Gumma Solid formation characterized by nodules that liquefies in its central portion, and may ulcerate. Typical lesion of tertiary syphilis. Common in skin, but may occur in other organs such as liver, bone, and testis.

Panniculitis Inflammation of the adipose tissue. Also called hypodermitis.

Punch biopsy Skin biopsy performed with cylindrical instruments that can range from 2 to 8 mm.

References

1. Blake T, Manahan M, Rodin K. Erythema nodosum – a review of an uncommon panniculitis. Dermatol Online J. 2014;20(4):3.
2. Schwartz RA, Nervi SJ. Erythema nodosum: a sign of systemic disease. Am Fam Physician. 2007;75(5):695–700.
3. Bombardieri S, Munno O, Punzio C, Pasero G. Erythema nodosum associated with pregnancy and oral contraceptives. Br Med J. 1977;1:1509–10.
4. Marshall JK, Irvine EJ. Successful therapy of refractory erythema nodosum associated nodosum associ-

ated with Crohn's disease using potassium iodide. Can J Gastroenterol. 1997;11:501–2.

5. Yurdakul S, Mat C, Tuzun Y, Ozyazgan Y, Hamuryudan V, Uysal O, et al. A double-blind trial of colchicine in Behcet's syndrome. Arthritis Rheum. 2001;44:2686–92.

6. Acosta KA, Haver MC, Kelly B. Etiology and therapeutic management of erythema nodosum during pregnancy: an update. Am J Clin Dermatol. 2013;14(3):215–22.

7. Tremaine WJ. Treatment of erythema nodosum, aphthous stomatitis, and pyoderma gangrenosum in patients with IBD. Inflamm Bowel Dis. 1998;4(1): 68–9.

8. Cohen PR. Combined reduced-antigen content tetanus, diphtheria, and acellular pertussis (tdap) vaccine-related erythema nodosum: case report and review of vaccine-erythema nodosum. Dermatol Ther (Heidelb). 2013;3(2):191–7.

9. Kakourou T, Drosatou P, Psychou F, Aroni K, Nicolaidou P. Erythema nodosum in children: a prospective study. J Am Acad Dermatol. 2001;44: 17–21.

10. Requena L, Yus ES. Panniculitis. Part I. Mostly septal panniculitis. J Am Acad Dermatol. 2001;45:163–83.

11. Cengiz AB, Kara A, Kanra G, et al. Erythema nodosum in childhood: evaluation of ten patients. Turk J Pediatr. 2006;48:38–42.

12. Diaz Cascajo C, Borghi S, Weyers W. Panniculitis: definition of terms and diagnostic strategy. Am J Dermatopathol. 2000;22:530–49.

13. Requena L, Sanchez YE. Panniculitis. Part II. Mostly lobular panniculitis. J Am Acad Dermatol. 2001;45:325–61.

14. Kumar B, Sandhu K. Erythema nodosum and antitubercular therapy. J Dermatol Treat. 2004;15:218–21.

15. Brodie D, Schluger NW. The diagnosis of tuberculosis. Clin Chest Med. 2005;26:247–71.

16. Hatemi G, et al. EULAR recommendations for the management of Behcet disease. Ann Rheum Dis. 2008;67:1656–62.

17. Boyd AS. Etanercept treatment of erythema nodosum. Skinmed. 2007;6(4):197–9.

18. Cribier B, Caille A, Heid E, Grosshans E. Erythema nodosum and associated diseases. A study of 129 cases. Int J Dermatol. 1998;37:667–72.

19. Garty B. Swimming pool granuloma associated with erythema nodosum. Cutis. 1991;47:314–6.

20. Sota Busselo I, Onate Vergara E, Perez-Yarza EG, Lopez Palma F, Ruiz Benito A, Albisu Andrade Y. Erythemanodosum: etiological changes in the last two decades. Ann Pediatr (Barc). 2004;61: 403–7.

21. Volkov I, Rudoy I, Press Y. Successful treatment of chronic erythema nodosum with vitamin B12. Ann Fam Med. 2005;18(6):567–9.

22. Gupta SN, Flaherty JP, Shaw JC. Erythema nodosum associated with reactivation tuberculous lymphadenitis (scrofula). Int J Dermatol. 2002;41(3): 173–5.

23. Galzerano G, Sorrentini R. Case of erythema nodosum appearing after BCG vaccination. Arch Tisiol Mal Appar Respir. 1958;13:631–41.

24. Longueville C, Doffoel-Hantz V, Hantz S, Souyri N, Nouaille Y, Bedane C, Sparsa A. Gardasil-induced erythema nodosum. Rev Med Interne. 2012;33:17–8.

25. Ramien ML, Wong A, Keystone JS. Severe refractory erythema nodosum leprosum successfully treated with the tumor necrosis factor inhibitor etanercept. Clin Infect Dis. 2011;52(5):133–5.

26. Yurdakul S, Hamuryudan V, Fresko I, Yazici H. Behçet's syndrome. In: Hochberg MC, editor. Rheumatology. 6th ed. Philadelphia: Elsevier; 2015. p. 1328–33.

27. West SG. Sarcoidosis. In: Hochberg MC, editor. Rheumatology. 6th ed. Philadelphia: Elsevier; 2015. p. 1392–400.

28. Farhi D, Cosnes J, Zizi N, et al. Significance of erythema nodosum and pyoderma gangrenosum in inflammatory bowel diseases: a cohort study of 2402 patients. Medicine. 2008;87:281–93.

29. Bernstein CN, Blanchard JF, Rawsthorne P, Yu N. The prevalence of extraintestinal diseases in inflammatory bowel disease: a population based study. Am J Gastroenterol. 2001;96:1116–22.

30. Areias E, Silva LGE. Erythema nodosum and Crohn's disease. Med Cutan Ibero Lat Am. 1984;12(6): 489–95.

31. Bisno AL. Acute pharyngitis. N Engl J Med. 2001;344:205–11.

32. Poses RM, Cebul RD, Collins M, Fager SS. The accuracy of experienced physicians probability estimates for patients with sore throats: implications for decision making. JAMA. 1985;254:925–9.

33. Guerra JG, Penna GO, Castro LCM, Martelli CMT, Stefani MMA, Costa MB. Erythema nodosum leprosum case series report: clinical profile, immunologic basis and treatment implemented in health services. Rev Soc Bras Med Trop. 2004;37(5):384–90.

Suggested Literature

Acosta MB, Dominguez-Munõz JE, Nuñez-Pardo de Vera MC, Lozano-León A, Lorenzo A, Penã S. Relationship between clinical features of Crohn's disease and the risk of developing extraintestinal manifestations. Eur J Gastroenterol Hepatol. 2007;19(1):73–8.

Bisno AL, Gerber MA, Gwaltney JM Jr, Kaplan EL, Schwartz RH. Practice guidelines for the diagnosis and management of group A streptococcal pharyngitis. Clin Infect Dis. 2002;35(2):113–25.

Demirkesen C, et al. Clinicopathologic evaluation of nodular cutaneous lesions of Behçet syndrome. Am J Clin Pathol. 2001;116:341–6.

FrancoParedes C, Diaz-Borjon A, Senger MA, Barragan L, Leonard M. The ever-expanding association between rheumatologic diseases and tuberculosis. Am J Med. 2006;119:470–7.

Fox MD, Schwartz RA. Erythema nodosum. Am Fam Physician. 1992;46:818–22.

McDougal KE, Fallin MD, Moller DR, et al. Variation in the Lymphotoxin-α/Tumor Necrosis Factor Locus Modifies Risk of Erythema Nodosum in Sarcoidosis. The Journal of investigative dermatology. 2009;129(8):1921–26. doi:10.1038/jid.2008.456.

Moraes AJ, Soares PM, Zapata AL, et al. Panniculitis in childhood and adolescence. Pediatr Int. 2006;48:48–53.

Leg Ulcers and Lymphedema

65

Luciana Patrícia Fernandes Abbade
and Hélio Amante Miot

Chronic Leg Ulcers

Introduction

Chronic leg ulcer is defined as an ulcer in the skin below the level of the knee persisting for more than 6 weeks and showing no tendency to heal after 3 or more months. It is a relatively common condition among adults, with multiple causes (Charts 65.1 and 65.2), the main ones being venous disease, arterial disease, and neuropathy [1].

These ulcers affect large portion of the adult population and cause a significant social and economic impact in terms of medical and nursing care, absence from work, and adverse impact on patients' quality of life.

Venous Ulcer

Epidemiology

Venous ulcer (VU), the most advanced stage of chronic venous disease, is a common problem in Western countries and represents the most com-

mon entity, accounting for 51–70% of all chronic leg ulcers [2]. The prevalence of VU varies between 0.06% and 2%, occurring in approximately 4% of adults over 65 years [3].

Complications arising from VU are diverse, primarily related to its chronicity and high rates of relapse after healing. In addition, the physical, social, economic, and emotional burdens are sizable [4, 5]. The overall costs of treatment of patients with VUs in most Western countries constitutes approximately 1% of the entire health care budgets [6].

Etiopathogenesis

VU is caused by a dysfunction in the muscular pump of the calf, which is the primary mechanism for the return of blood from the lower limbs to the heart. It comprises calf muscles, the deep venous system, the superficial venous system, and the perforating/communicating vein system. Pump dysfunction can result from deep venous insufficiency (primary or post-thrombotic), deep venous obstruction, perforating insufficiency, superficial venous insufficiency, arteriovenous fistulas, neuromuscular dysfunction, or a combination of these factors. However, the two main causes of dysfunction in the calf muscle pump are primary varicose diseases and late effects of deep venous thrombosis (post-thrombotic or postphlebitic syndrome) [7].

L.P.F. Abbade (✉) • H.A. Miot
Department of Dermatology,
UNESP, Botucatu, Brazil
e-mail: lfabbade@fmb.unesp.br;
heliomiot@fmb.unesp.br

© Springer International Publishing Switzerland 2018
R.R. Bonamigo, S.I.T. Dornelles (eds.), *Dermatology in Public Health Environments*,
https://doi.org/10.1007/978-3-319-33919-1_65

Chart 65.1 Main aspects of the three main causes of chronic leg ulcers

Chronic leg ulcers	Features
Venous ulcer	The most common entity accounting for 51–70% of all chronic leg ulcers It occurs in the distal portion of the legs The surrounding skin is erythematous or hyperpigmented with variable degrees of induration Varicose veins and ankle edema are common The pulses of the lower limbs are usually normal, and ABI greater than 0.9 Compression therapy: the main methods for healing
Arterial ulcer	10–25% of cases of chronic leg ulcers Ulcers occur mainly on bony prominences of the feet, ankles, and heels The main symptom associated is intermittent claudication and pain during resting The affected limb is often colder, with pallor during lifting and flushing when pending; absence of peripheral pulses ABI (ankle-brachial index) below 0.9 Assessment of the vascular surgeon; limbs with critical ischemia may benefit from bypass surgery or angioplasty Drug treatments: aspirin, clopidogrel, and cilostazol
Neuropathic ulcers	Main causes are *diabetes mellitus* and leprosy It occurs particularly in trauma sites; the perforating plantar ulcer is the typical representative and it is painless ulcer, deep with calloused edges The test of Semmes-Weinstein: If the patient is unable to detect the test when using monofilaments in the plantar region, this is considered with loss of protective sensation Management: preventive, local treatment of ulcer, and measures to reduce plantar pressure

Chart 65.2 Main aspects of the less common causes of chronic leg ulcers

Chronic leg ulcers less common	Features
Hypertensive ischemic ulcer (Martorell ulcer)	Patients with uncontrolled arterial hypertension The ulcers often are extremely painful, located in the anterolateral and posterior portions of the legs, and may have purplish color or erythema in the periphery of the ulcer Peripheral pulses are palpable and ABI (ankle-brachial index) is greater than 0.9 The reduction and control of blood pressure is the best therapeutic measure It is important to replace beta-blockers for other classes of antihypertensive drugs
Pyoderma gangrenosum	It is considered an inflammatory ulcer The pathogenesis remains unknown, but it is probably related to a hyperergic reaction The disease begins as a papule, vesicle, or pustules that quickly ulcerate, generating a very painful injury. The ulcers are necrotic and have purpura and undermined borders It is frequently associated with Crohn's disease, ulcerative colitis, rheumatoid arthritis, and myeloproliferative diseases The treatment is mainly with immunosuppressors as systemic corticosteroids
Rheumatoid arthritis ulcers	Ulcers can be due to chronic venous insufficiency, vasculitis disease activity, or pyoderma gangrenosum
Vasculitis	The lesion begins with purpuric and necrotic areas that later progress to ulceration. Examples: leukocytoclastic vasculitis, cryoglobulinemia, Henoch-Schönlein purpura, polyarteritis nodosa, Churg-Strauss syndrome, and Wegener's granulomatosis The treatment follows the cause

(continued)

Chart 65.2   (continued)

Chronic leg ulcers less common	Features
Thrombophilia	The ulcers are characterized by pain, gangrene, and lower limb ischemia, preceded by livedo reticularis and white atrophy. The antiphospholipid syndrome is the main condition of acquired thrombophilia
Livedoid vasculopathy	Small and recurrent ulcers characterized by painful purple macules and papules that subsequently ulcerate. The ulcers heal over weeks to months resulting in smooth, porcelain-white, atrophic plaque-like areas with surrounding telangiectasia and hyperpigmentation. Treatment: anticoagulants, antiplatelet agents (aspirin, dipyridamole), pentoxifylline, danazol, and other fibrinolytic agents. Additional measures such as rest and compression therapy are also important
Hematological diseases	Sickle cell anemia, thalassemia, thrombotic thrombocytosis, and polycythemia vera are responsible for chronic leg ulcers
Infections	Leishmaniasis: the ulcers are usually circular, with infiltrated borders and granular clean wound bed. Paracoccidioidomycosis: the ulcers may have a wound bed with hemorrhagic dotted appearance
Neoplasia	Squamous cell carcinoma, basal cell carcinoma, and lymphomas as primary neoplastic ulcers. Neoplastic transformation of chronic ulcers such as in long-term venous ulcers, which may undergo malignant transformation into squamous or basal cell carcinoma, and these are called Marjolin's ulcers
Lymphedema	Injuries and subsequent infections can lead to formation of ulcers. The treatment is based on the local care of the ulcer and compression therapy

(continued)

Chart 65.2   (continued)

Chronic leg ulcers less common	Features
Other causes	Ulcers secondary to occlusion vascular due to drugs: warfarin and hydroxyurea. Necrobiosis lipoidica. Ulcers as manifestations of microvascular occlusion syndromes: cryoglobulins, cryofibrinogen, vascular occlusion by cholesterol emboli and oxalate, calciphylaxis, vascular coagulopathy (Sneddon syndrome), vascular invasion by microorganisms (ecthyma gangrenosum, opportunistic fungi, Lucio's phenomenon in leprosy)

Valvular incompetence of the venous system has been implicated as a major factor in the development of VUs, which may compromise the superficial venous system, deep and perforating, alone or in combination. When venous valves are damaged, blood reflux from the deep to the superficial veins occurs and, consequently, venous hypertension develops. This continuous hypertension in veins, venules, and capillaries is responsible for typical alterations associated with VU. However, the mechanism by which this hypertension causes alterations remains unclear despite some theories that attempt to explain its pathogenesis. The most recently advanced theories associate the origin of the ulcer with microcirculatory abnormalities and the generation of an inflammatory response [8].

Other factors described include the inflammatory status, chronic nonhealing VUs, such as excess metalloproteinase (MMP), and cytokine imbalance. MMPs, a family of zinc-dependent endoproteinases, are known for their tissue-remodeling properties. In general this family of enzymes is not expressed in healthy tissue, although in the remodeling processes it does increase. Moreover, tissue inhibitors of metalloproteinases (TIMPs) have been extensively studied because of their ability to avoid excessive breakdown of extracellular matrix [9].

An orchestrated balance between MMPs and TIMPs is necessary for proper healing. Imbalance can lead to accumulation of MMPs, resulting in uncontrolled proteolysis, as seen in chronic inflammatory conditions.

Clinical Presentation

In general, the VU is an irregularly shaped wound, initially superficial, with well-defined borders. The surrounding skin is erythematous or hyperpigmented with variable degrees of induration (acute or chronic lipodermosclerosis). Yellowish exudate is usually observed. The size and site of ulcers vary, but they usually occur in the distal portion of the lower limbs. Varicose veins and ankle edema are common [10] (Fig. 65.1).

The pain is frequent and of variable intensity, generally worsening toward the day's end and in a standing position, and improves with limb ele-

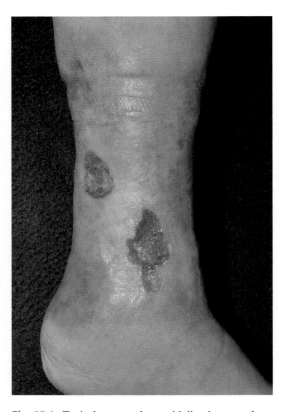

Fig. 65.1 Typical venous ulcers with lipodermatosclerosis and hyperpigmentation (ochre dermatitis) in peripheral wound area

vation. When the pain is very strong, especially with limb elevation, arterial disease as a cause must be ruled out [11].

Between 58% and 86% of patients have eczema around the ulcer, as evidenced by erythema, scaling, and pruritus, and augmented by topical medications, particularly antibiotics and lanolin [12].

The main complications that occur in patients with chronic venous ulcers are infections of soft tissue, critical colonization, contact dermatitis, osteomyelitis and, less frequently, neoplastic transformation.

Complementary Test

The diagnosis of VU is based primarily on clinical criteria. Complementary laboratory tests such as duplex scanning favor the surgical approach of the underlying venous change because it allows differentiation between patients with primary varicose veins, whose changes mainly occur in the superficial venous system, and patients with secondary varicose veins, in whom the deep venous system is the site of pathophysiologic changes.

The pulses of the lower limbs should be palpated, and are usually normal. A decrease in pulse or its absence should make one aware of arterial disease as a cause of ulceration or an association with venous disease, featuring in the latter case ulcers of mixed etiology (venous and arterial) [11].

Doppler ultrasonography should be used to determine systolic index between the ankle and the arm (ankle–brachial index; ABI). The index is calculated with the highest systolic blood pressure of the ankle divided by the systolic blood pressure of the brachial artery. ABI below 0.9 indicates that there is insufficient blood component influencing the development of ulcer [13].

Duplex scanning is a noninvasive method of choice to assess the superficial, deep, and perforating venous system, since the venous change may be located in the superficial, deep, or perforating veins, in isolation or combined. In addition, it provides a functional assessment to identify whether the disease is due to venous reflux, obstruction, or both [14].

Qualitative bacteriologic tests using swabs and bacterial cultures should not be performed in a systematic way because they cannot differentiate whether there is colonization or infection [15].

Treatment

The main methods of VU treatment are compression therapy, local treatment of ulcers, systemic medications, and surgical treatment of venous abnormalities.

Compression Therapy

This approach aims to decrease chronic venous hypertension and its impact on macrocirculation and microcirculation. It is contraindicated in the presence of severe arterial disease. The most commonly used methods are compression bandages and elastic stockings.

The bandages can be inelastic and elastic [16]. Among the more traditional inelastic is Unna's boot, consisting of bandage impregnated with zinc oxide, creating a semi-solid mold for carrying out efficient external compression. The modified Unna's boot (Fig. 65.2) is less rigid and uses a small stretch bandage, for example, Viscopaste® (Smith & Nephew) and Flexdress® (ConvaTec). Both the traditional and modified Unna's boot should remain in place for 7 days, although at the beginning of treatment, when there is large amount of exudate and edema, it can be reapplied more often [17].

Elastic bandages have higher stretch and are widely used in clinical practice. An example is the Surepress® (ConvaTec). It has rectangles on the surface which turn into squares when the stretch reaches proper tension (Fig. 65.3a, b). In general it should be immediately applied when the patient wakes up and be removed at the end of the day. It can be washed but should be discarded as soon as stretch is lost.

The most effective elastic compression is performed by multilayers. With this type of compression, sustained pressure of 40–45 mmHg is achieved at the ankle. An example of this compression is Dynaflex® (Johnson & Johnson), whose first layer of wool and foam is applied in a

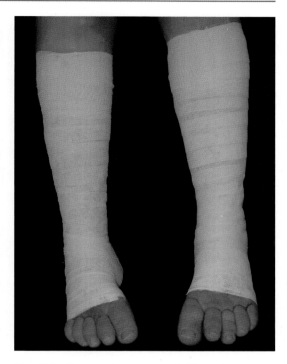

Fig. 65.2 Compression therapy with Unna's boot

spiral, which absorbs the exudate and redistributes the pressure around the ankle; the second layer consists of elastic compression bandage, and the third a layer of adhesive bandage which maintains all of the layers properly (Fig. 65.4a–c). This compression system may remain in place for 7 days [18].

These inelastic and elastic compression bandages may be harmful or useless if not properly used, and their effectiveness can be influenced by the application technique used by doctors, nurses, or patients themselves.

The stockings are generally difficult to use in the active phase because of the difficulty in proper placement for ulcer patients; they are most suitable for the post-healing period to avoid recurrences [19].

Ulcer Treatment

Local treatment should begin with bedside evaluation of the ulcer, which requires systematic and structured assessment in order to detect the possible factors that negatively interfere with the

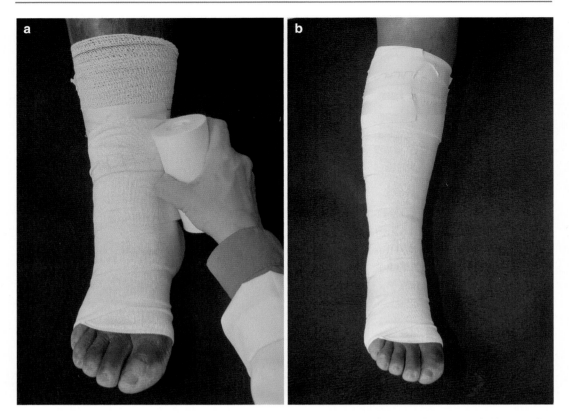

Fig. 65.3 (**a**) Placement of elastic compression with the technique half and half. (**b**) Elastic band applied instep to just below the knee

healing process. To facilitate this evaluation a mnemonic rule using the acronym TIME has been created. The letter T refers to tissue, i.e., assessment for the presence of devitalized or non-viable tissue; I refers to the presence of infection or colonization; M refers to moisture imbalance; and E refers to edge of wound [20].

After this evaluation, cleansing of the ulcer is carried out. This should be performed with physiologic saline solution or tap water, since many antiseptic substances (chlorhexidine, povidone-iodine, acetic acid, sodium hypochlorite, etc.) are cytotoxic and can delay healing.

In the presence of nonviable tissue (TIME letter T) debridement is necessary, as these tissues favor infections, and do not allow the formation of good granulation tissue and proper re-epithelialization [6]. There are basically five types of debridement: autolytic, chemical, mechanical, surgical, and biological. Autolytic debridement can be achieved

with occlusive dressings, through exudate enzyme action that remains in contact with the ulcer. Examples are hydrogel dressings such as Nu-Gel®, Saf-Gel®, Duoderm Gel®, IntraSite Gel®, and Purilon® (Fig. 65.5a–c) and hydrocolloid dressings such as Nu-derm®, Tegasorb®, Comfeel®, and Duoderm® (Fig. 65.6a, b). Chemical debridement is accomplished by application of various enzymes including papain and collagenase. Mechanical debridement can be performed using surgical instruments or by the application of dressings ranging from moist to dry, but the main disadvantage is the inability to be selective when removing viable tissue along with devitalized tissue [21]. Negative pressure therapy (e.g., VAC®) is an alternative whose use has been expanding in recent years [22].

For the approach to infection or colonization of the ulcer bed (Letter I of TIME), it is essential to know the difference between colonization and

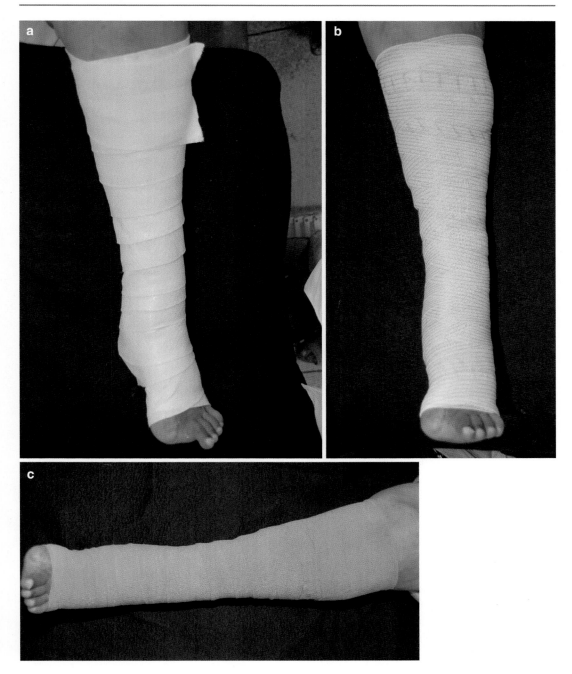

Fig. 65.4 Multilayer compression. (**a**) First layer of wool and foam applied in a spiral. (**b**) Second layer consists of elastic compression bandage. (**c**) Final layer of adhesive bandage

infection of chronic ulcers. The increased number of bacteria in the wound bed does not necessarily mean infection. Ulcer with critical colonization represents increased bacterial load, and these bacteria can form complex structures called biofilms. Biofilms are communities of microorganisms surrounded by a matrix of extracellular polysaccharides. Bacteria in biofilms are

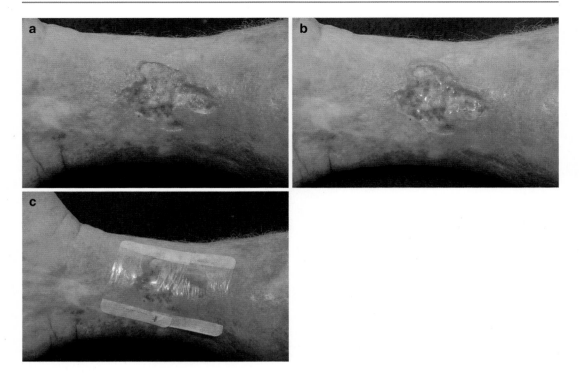

Fig. 65.5 (a) Venous ulcer with wound bed devitalized and little exudate. (b) Hydrogel in wound bed. (c) Secondary dressing with plastic film. This dressing can be left in this ulcer for 2–3 days

better protected and more resistant to the body's defenses, antiseptics, and antibiotics, both topical and systemic. A critically colonized ulcer does not have well granulated tissue, but friable greenish or purplish tissue (Fig. 65.7), with excessive exudation and foul odor; it does not respond to conventional treatment. However, sometimes the only sign of critical colonization is the failure to heal [23].

Local treatment of ulcers with critical colonization can be performed surgically or with chemical debridement. Occlusive dressings with hydrofiber, alginate, and silver are options that control the excess exudate and promote reduction in bacterial load (e.g., activated carbon with silver – Actisorb Plus®, with hydrofiber with silver – Aquacell prata®, alginate – Kaltostat®). These dressings can be changed, according to saturation, after 3–7 days (Fig. 65.8a, b). It must be emphasized that systemic antibiotics are not indicated for failure to act on biofilm.

Soft tissue infections occur when there is penetration of bacteria in periwound tissues, whereby erythema, edema, local heat in tissues surrounding the ulcer, and pain are evident. Treatment should be carried out with systemic antibiotics and debridement of the infected tissue when necessary.

Another important aspect is to maintain the moist environment (letter M of TIME). Excess exudate must be combated because, besides favoring infections, this brings discomfort to the patient. On the other hand, dehydration of the ulcer bed must be avoided and countered because it favors the formation of devitalized tissue. Therefore, to provide an optimal way of healing some occlusive dressings can be specified according to the characteristics of ulcers. Ulcers with excess exudate are best treated with hydrofiber dressing, alginates, carbon and silver, and carbon and alginate (Fig. 65.8). For ulcers with mild to moderate exudate, curative hydrocolloids and hydrogels are indicated (Figs. 65.5 and 65.6). Compression therapy can and should be used where possible with such dressings [6].

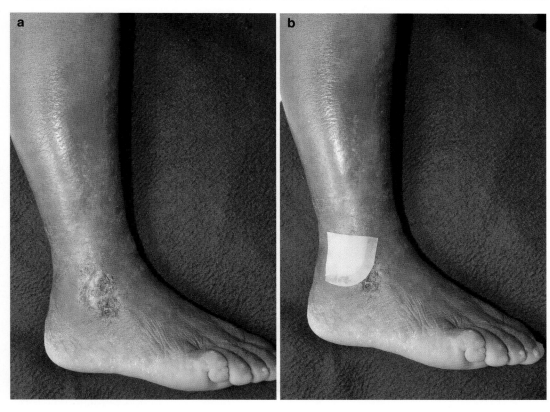

Fig. 65.6 (**a**) Venous ulcer with wound bed with little devitalized tissue and little exudate. (**b**) Hydrocolloid dressing. This dressing can be left in this ulcer for 5–7 days, according to its saturation

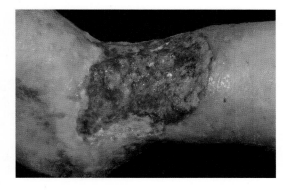

Fig. 65.7 Venous ulcer with critical colonization: part of the wound bed presents itself *greenish* and *grayish*, with clinical features of bacterial burden

Systemic Drug Therapy

For long-standing or large venous leg ulcer, treatment with either pentoxifylline or micronized purified flavonoid fraction used in combination with compression therapy is recommend [6].

Surgical Treatment of Venous Ulcer

Surgical correction of insufficient veins favors ulcer healing and also improves the prognosis by reducing the relapse rate. Patients who benefit most from surgical treatment are those with insufficiency of the superficial venous system, alone or combined with insufficient perforation [6].

Ancillary Measures

The remaining measures must be oriented to decrease venous hypertension. The lower limbs should be elevated above the heart level for 30 min about three to four times each day. The optimum position is achieved by raising the foot above the bed to a height ranging from 15 to 20 cm. Short walks, three to four times a day, should be encouraged. Patients should be instructed to maintain their weight within the normal range and avoid smoking. Manual lymphatic drainage and physiotherapy to improve ankle joint mobility are necessary in some patients.

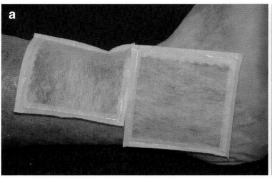
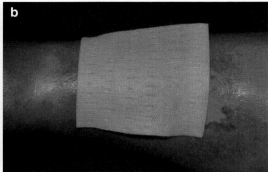

Fig. 65.8 (**a**) Dressing with activated carbon with silver. (**b**) Hydrofiber with silver. These dressings are indicated for ulcers with critical colonization and high exudation

Methods to Prevent Relapses

The rate of relapse after venous ulcer healing is very high. The most necessary measures to reduce the relapse rate are educating the patient about the use of high-compression stockings of high compression and adequate surgical intervention for venous abnormality [24].

Arterial Ulcer

Epidemiology

Arterial ulcer is the second most common cause of leg ulcers, corresponding to 10–25 % of cases [25]. Risk factors for development are age over 45 years, smoking, diabetes mellitus, hyperlipidemia, hypertension, hypercholesterolemia, family history of atherosclerotic disease, and sedentary lifestyle [26].

Etiopathogenesis

The gradual narrowing of the artery lumen as a result of atherosclerotic disease causes gradual obstruction of blood flow and consequent formation of collateral circulation. The reduction in the blood supply results in ischemia, necrosis, and ulceration [27].

Clinical Presentation

The main symptom associated with arterial ulcer is intermittent claudication, i.e., pain in the calf or thigh during walking with improvement after a few minutes of rest. Pain at rest often occurs with progression of the disease, to the point of the patient having to sleep while sitting. Ulcers occur mainly on bony prominences of the feet, ankles, and heels. However they may occur in other sites, especially when initiated by trauma. They are usually deep, with well-defined and undermined edges and devitalized bed, and often necrotic (Fig. 65.9). Exposed tendons and deep tissue may occur more frequently than in venous ulcer. The periulcer area may be erythematous.

Complementary Test

The affected limb is often colder, with pallor during lifting and flushing when bending. The absence of peripheral pulses allied to the clinical manifestations described suggests arterial etiology for the ulcer. Capillary refill time is slow (more than 3–4 s), obtained by hallux compression until becoming white and then released.

Doppler ultrasonography should be used to determine the systolic index between the ankle and the arm (ABI). ABI below 0.9 indicates that there is insufficient blood component influencing the development of the ulcer. ABI below 0.7 is highly significant and, when there is no abnormal vein, can indicate that arterial insufficiency is the only cause of the ulcer. It is important to remember that the absence of distal pulses is also considered indicative of arterial disease, regardless of the value of the index [28].

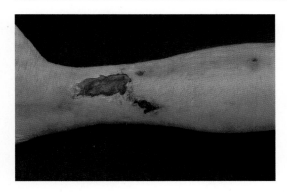

Fig. 65.9 Arterial ulcers with necrosis of the wound bed and erythematous peripheral wound skin. There are no tibial or dorsal pedis pulses palpable, and ABI is <0.6

Arterial duplex scanning is important for treatment planning because it allows assessment of the distribution and extent of arterial disease [28].

Treatment

Assessment by the vascular surgeon is very important. Limbs with critical ischemia with resting pain and low blood pressure in the ankle (below 50 mmHg) may benefit from bypass surgery or angioplasty, or often a combination of both procedures. If the patient has no clinical indication for the procedure or the prospects of improvement with revascularization are poor, amputation should be considered. Drug treatment includes aspirin (due to antiplatelet action), clopidogrel (inhibitor of ADP-inducing platelet aggregation), and cilostazol (phosphodiesterase III inhibitor) [29].

Local treatment of the ulcer is aimed at maintaining wound moisture. Additional therapies include adequate pain control and maintenance of the affected limb.

Neuropathic Ulcers

Neuropathic ulcers occur as a result of sensory loss and trophic changes due to denervation [30]. Among the many causes of peripheral sensory neuropathy in Western countries, the main ones are diabetes mellitus, leprosy, spina bifida, spinal cord injuries, alcohol, drugs, and hereditary sensory and motor neuropathies. Whatever the cause, sensory loss in the feet puts them at risk when traumatized. Ulcers on the feet are the most common cause of hospitalization of diabetic patients from Western countries.

Etiopathogenesis

The two main causes of peripheral neuropathy and neuropathic ulcers are diabetes mellitus and leprosy. Diabetic neuropathy is a chronic, insidious, sensory neuropathy, which also encompasses motor and autonomic neuropathy. The feet lose their sensitivity and therefore may be under pressure. The motor change causes atrophy with change in the intrinsic muscles of the feet, which leads to deformities with increased load, mainly at the base of the metatarsals. Autonomic dysfunction results in dry skin, which is more prone to infections and eczema. This dysfunction also causes changes in the microcirculatory blood flow through interference in arteriovenous shunts. All of these changes lead to the appearance of ulcers especially in the plantar region of diabetic patients, known as perforating plantar ulcers [31].

In leprosy, *Mycobacterium leprae* has particular tropism for peripheral nerves. The lesions in nerve fibers are essentially sensory, motor, and autonomic. In the lower limbs the main nerves affected are the peroneal and posterior tibial. The fibula, when injured, causes "foot drop" and loss of sensation on the dorsum of the feet and outward side of the leg. Lesions of the posterior tibial nerve lead to paralysis of the intrinsic muscles of the foot, hypoesthesia, or anesthesia. Sensory and motor changes are responsible for the pathogenesis of perforating plantar ulcer [32].

Clinical Presentation

Perforating plantar ulcer is the typical sign of diabetic and leprosy neuropathy. It is characterized by a painless ulcer with deep and calloused edges (Fig. 65.10).

Neuropathic ulcers may occur in other locations, particularly in those subject to trauma. Irregularities in the inner linings of shoes or foreign materials such as small stones may go unnoticed and cause ulcers. Osteomyelitis and bacterial soft tissue infections are frequent complications.

Fig. 65.10 Perforating plantar ulcer in patients with diabetes mellitus with important deformities of feet

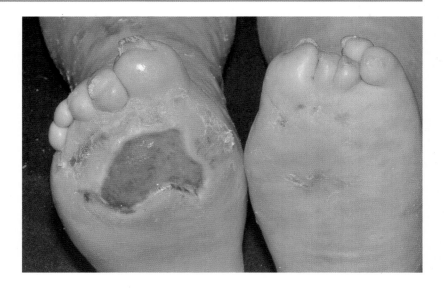

Complementary Test

The test of Semmes–Weinstein is used to test the perception of pressure. If the patient is unable to detect the test when using monofilaments 5.07 (10 g) in the plantar region, this is considered as loss of protective sensation, and therefore an increased risk for ulceration in regions with such presentation [33].

It is necessary to conduct serial radiographs to assess the bone, especially in the case of deep ulcers that affect the bones. Other tests may be needed to confirm osteomyelitis, such as magnetic resonance imaging and bone scintigraphy.

Treatment

The management of patients with peripheral neuropathy should be in three dimensions: preventive, local treatment of ulcer, and measures to reduce plantar pressure.

The basic preventive measures are: orientation in relation to shoes, particularly new shoes, with special attention to the seams and maladjustments; guidance for use of insoles that distribute the weight in the plantar region to reduce high pressure; patients and caregivers should make systematic inspection of the feet looking for initial areas of trauma such as erythema and blisters; in cases of dry skin it is essential to use lotions to prevent fissures; it is important to advise patients not to walk barefoot; guidance regarding weight loss should be provided for overweight and obese patients.

The approach to the treatment of ulcer is as follows. When the ulcer is infectious it requires appropriate systemic antibiotics; in the case of critical colonization, topical antibiotics can be used for reduction of bacterial flora in the granulation tissue, but for short periods, to avoid cytotoxic effects and resistance; dressings such as hydrofiber, activated carbon, and silver are indicated. If there is no critical colonization and infection, dressings such as hydrocolloids and hydrogels may be indicated to maintain the moist environment and debridement autolysis. Chemical or surgical debridement of devitalized tissue and callous tissue of the ulcer edges should be made whenever necessary. The selected dressing should also maintain moisture balance and avoid excess exudate, which promotes skin maceration around the ulcer, favoring an increase in the ulcerated lesion and slowing the healing process [34].

Pressure relief, or off-loading, is another key aspect in these patients. Measures to achieve this goal are: orthoses that promote the reduction of pressure on the ulcerated sites and calluses; in cases of major orthopedic deformities, specially made shoes customized to allow greater width and depth; crutches and walkers; and even total deprivation of contact. The choice of off-loading modality should be determined by the patient's physical characteristics and the ability to comply with treatment, as well as by the location and severity of the ulcer [34].

In the case of osteomyelitis, treatment consists in removal of infected bone, accompanied by 2–4 weeks of systemic antibiotics. However, when this is not possible, antibiotics should be prescribed for long periods [35].

Less Common Causes of Chronic Leg Ulcers

Hypertensive Ischemic Ulcer (Martorell Ulcer)

Hypertensive ischemic ulcer is a rapidly progressive and extremely painful ulcer that is frequently underdiagnosed, and which should not be confused with arterial ulcers. In arterial ulcer there is involvement of micro- and macrocirculation, whereas a hypertensive ulcer involves only the microcirculation. Failure of vasodilation in response to arteriolar narrowing caused by hypertension determines the reduction of skin perfusion that results in formation of a hypertensive ischemic ulcer. The physiopathology of an arterial ulcer is different because here the reduction in skin perfusion pressure is due to reduction of the arterial flow in the macrocirculation [36].

It occurs in patients with arterial hypertension that is difficult to control, and was first described by Martorell, Hines, and Farber in the 1940s. These ulcers occur most commonly in women, especially after the sixth decade.

Clinical Presentation

These ulcers often are located in the anterolateral and posterior portions of the legs and may have purplish color or be erythematous in the periulcer region (Fig. 65.11). In general they are very painful disproportionately to the size of the ulcer and are often refractory to standard therapy for chronic ulcers [37]. Peripheral pulses are palpable, and ABI is greater than 0.9 [36].

Treatment

Hypertensive ulcers do not respond to local treatment. The reduction and control of blood pressure is the best therapeutic measure. The most commonly used antihypertensive drugs are calcium channel blockers and angiotensin-converting enzyme inhibitors. Many patients with hypertensive ulcer use

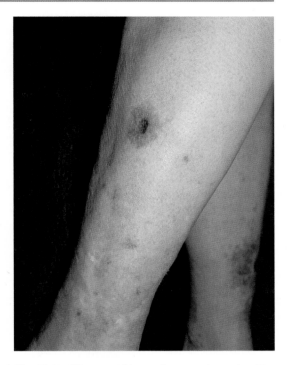

Fig. 65.11 Woman with severe hypertension and sudden onset of painful hypertensive leg ulcers. Palpable peripheral pulses and ABI = 1.0

β-blockers for blood pressure control, but these should be replaced with other antihypertensive classes since they may aggravate vasoconstriction and therefore impair healing [38].

Pyoderma Gangrenosum

Pyoderma gangrenosum is a rare, ulcerative, cutaneous condition. First described in 1930, the pathogenesis of pyoderma gangrenosum remains unknown, but is probably related to a hyperergic reaction and is considered an inflammatory ulcer. Usually the disease begins as a papule, vesicle, or pustules that quickly ulcerate, generating a very painful injury. It occurs most often in lower limbs but can occur elsewhere. It usually is necrotic with purpura and undermined borders (Fig. 65.12). It is frequently associated with systemic diseases such as Crohn's disease, ulcerative colitis, rheumatoid arthritis, and myeloproliferative diseases [39].

The treatment is mainly systemic corticosteroids (1 mg/kg). Local care of the ulcer is important. In the initial phase, which can involve critical colonization

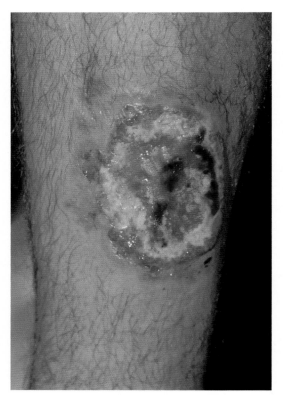

Fig. 65.12 Pyoderma gangrenous on the side of the leg. Ulcer with infiltrated and purplish edge

and exudation, the use of dressings with activated carbon/silver or hydrofiber with silver and alginates, with changes every 3 days, is recommended. In the following stages, hydrogels and hydrocolloid dressings promote autolytic debridement and accelerate healing. Surgical debridement should be avoided because of the pathergy phenomenon, i.e., onset or worsening of injury by trauma [40].

Leg Ulcers in Rheumatoid Arthritis

Ulcers associated with rheumatoid arthritis may occur in the lower limbs and are multifactorial. Many are due to chronic venous insufficiency, because patients have deformities in the regions of the ankle, worsening function of the calf muscle pump via difficulty in dorsiflexion, and therefore have similar venous ulcers (Fig. 65.13). Less often the ulcer is associated with vasculitis disease activity with high titers of rheumatoid factor. Pyoderma gangrenosum is another possible consequence of chronic ulcers of the lower limbs in patients with rheumatoid arthritis [40].

Treatment is a challenge and depends on the main cause of the ulcer. Elastic compression with an Unna's boot is useful since it is often associated with venous insufficiency. Local care of the ulcer is also very important and follows the principles of treatment of venous ulcers previously described.

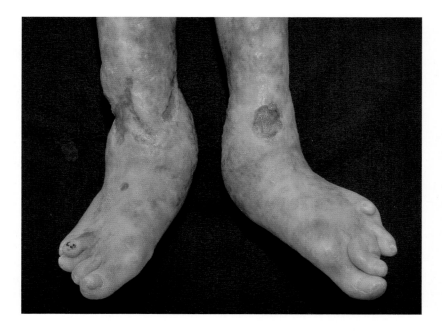

Fig. 65.13 Chronic ulcers in patients with rheumatoid arthritis with deformities in the feet and joints

Leg Ulcers due to Vasculitis

Vasculitis of small and medium vessels can result in leg skin ulcerations. They begin with purpuric and necrotic areas that later progress to ulceration. Examples include leukocytoclastic vasculitis (Fig. 65.14), cryoglobulinemia, Henoch–Schönlein purpura, polyarteritis nodosa, Churg–Strauss syndrome, and Wegener's granulomatosis [40].

Leg Ulcers due to Thrombophilia

Thrombophilia is defined as abnormalities in the blood coagulation and/or the fibrinolytic cascade leading to hypercoagulability states. It can be inherited or acquired and predisposes to venous and/or arterial thrombosis at relatively young ages.

Thrombophilia can cause ulcers in the lower limbs indirectly as a result of deep vein thrombosis, or directly through the formation of thrombi in arteries, arterioles, capillaries, and venules. Microthrombotic ulcers are characterized by pain, gangrene, and lower limb ischemia, preceded by livedo reticular and white atrophy. Usually the feet are warm and distal pulses are palpable [40].

The antiphospholipid syndrome is the main condition of acquired blood hypercoagulability. Patients may have a history of cerebrovascular accident, myocardial infarction, deep vein thrombosis, recurrent fetal loss, and pulmonary thromboembolism. Treatment is aimed at control of thromboembolic events with anticoagulants and antiplatelet agents. [41]

Livedoid Vasculopathy

Livedoid vasculopathy occurs mainly in middle-aged women. It is involved in the pathogenesis local or systemic coagulation changes leading to the formation of fibrin thrombi in the dermal vessels. In general, there is formation of small and recurrent ulcers in the leg, characterized by painful purple macules and papules that subsequently ulcerate. The ulcers heal over weeks to months resulting in smooth, porcelain-white, atrophic plaque-like areas with surrounding telangiectasia and hyperpigmentation (Fig. 65.14) [42].

Treatment is a real challenge and many therapies are cited in the literature. The treatment is based on the use of anticoagulants such as warfarin (especially when associated with antiphospholipid syndrome, factor V Leiden), antiplatelet agents (aspirin, dipyridamole), pentoxifylline, danazol, and other fibrinolytic agents. Other therapies described include the use of niacin, psoralen combined with ultraviolet A, and intravenous immunoglobulins. Additional measures such as rest and compression therapy are also important [43].

Leg Ulcers Associated with Hematologic Diseases

Some hematologic diseases such as sickle cell anemia, thalassemia, thrombotic thrombocytosis, and polycythemia vera are responsible for chronic leg ulcers. In most cases, ulcers develop secondary to deep venous thrombosis and capillary thrombosis [1].

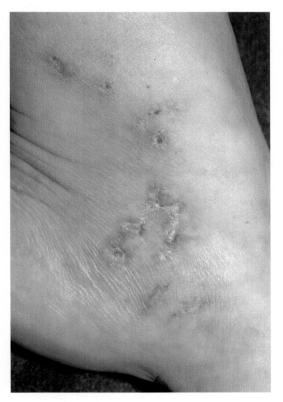

Fig. 65.14 Livedoid vasculopathy characterized by small and superficial ulcers. There are also purple macules and porcelain-white, atrophic plaques

Leg Ulcer due to Infections

Infectious diseases such as cutaneous leishmaniasis and paracoccidioidomycosis can cause chronic ulcers of the lower limbs. The ulcers of leishmaniasis usually are circular, with infiltrated borders and granular clean wound beds (Fig. 65.15). The ulcer in paracoccidioidomycosis may have a wound bed with hemorrhagic dotted appearance (Fig. 65.16). The diagnosis should be based on clinical, epidemiologic, and laboratory abnormalities.

Leg Ulcer of Neoplastic Origin

Squamous cell carcinoma, basal cell carcinoma, and lymphomas may present as chronic leg ulcers and are therefore primary neoplastic ulcers [44]. Another situation is neoplastic transformation of chronic ulcers such as in long-term venous ulcers, which may undergo malignant transformation into squamous or basal cell carcinoma; these are called Marjolin's ulcers (Fig. 65.15). In the latter situation, in general the tumor begins at the edge of the ulcer or scar and grows slowly and only a portion of the ulcer suffers malignant transformation, increasing the chance of false-negative histopathology. To confirm the diagnosis of suspicious lesions multiple biopsies should be performed, preferably

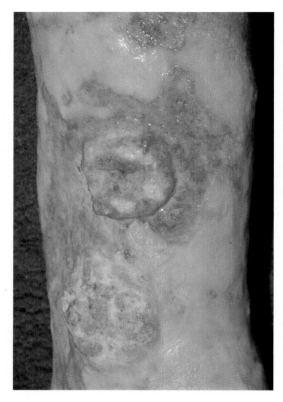

Fig. 65.15 Neoplastic transformation of chronic venous ulcers to squamous cell carcinoma (Marjolin's ulcer). Hypertrophy of granulation tissue is noticeable

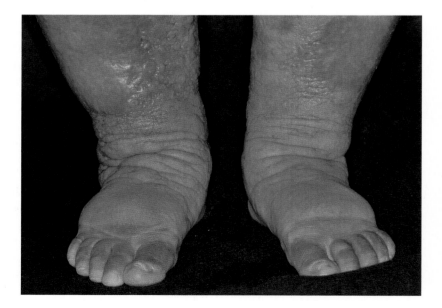

Fig. 65.16 Chronic bilateral lymphedema of lower limbs

in the edges of the lesion. Treatment should be complete excision of the tumor with adequate surgical margins and subsequent reconstruction with grafts and skin flaps. Limb amputation is indicated in cases of extensive invasion of local tissues and involvement of the joint or bone [45].

Leg Ulcer due to Lymphedema

This is rare when not associated with venous insufficiency. Injuries and subsequent infections can lead to formation of ulcers. Treatment is based on local care of the ulcer and compression therapy.

Other Causes of Chronic Leg Ulcers

Other rare causes of chronic leg ulcers are the drugs warfarin and hydroxyurea, as they may cause vascular occlusion with subsequent formation of ulcers in the legs; necrobiosis lipoidica, ulcers as manifestations of microvascular occlusion syndromes, cryoglobulins, cryofibrinogen, vascular occlusion by cholesterol emboli and oxalate, calciphylaxis, vascular coagulopathy (Sneddon syndrome), and vascular invasion by microorganisms (ecthyma gangrenosum, opportunistic fungi, Lucio phenomenon (in leprosy)).

Lymphedema

Lymphedema is defined as a functional or anatomic disorder of the lymphatic system that causes accumulation of protein-rich fluid and subsequent inflammation, adipose tissue hypertrophy, and fibrosis. As lymphatic drainage accounts for 1–10% of interstitial drainage, most lymphedemas have a chronic and progressive course, and adequate treatment rarely improves it but lengthens this progression [46, 47].

There are congenital (primary) and acquired (secondary) causes of lymphedema (Chart 65.3). Nevertheless, the progressive swelling and skin induration inflict limitations on mobility and function that favor recurrent infection and skin ulcers, and significantly decrease overall quality of life [46, 48].

The real prevalence of lymphedema per se is not known and varies according to the causes and

Chart 65.3 Main causes of lymphedema

Primary lymphedema	Milroy's disease
	Meige's disease
	Amniotic band
	Proteus syndrome
	Yellow nail syndrome
	Neurofibromatosis
	Vascular malformation
Secondary lymphedema	Wuchereriosis
	Soft tissue infection (erysipelas)
	Trauma
	Obesity
	Neoplastic obstruction (lymphangitis, external compression, or lymphatic metastasis)
	Iatrogenic (lymphadenectomy or lymphatic resection/transection)
	Radiotherapy
	Podoconiosis

population of study. The rates of arm lymphedema after mastectomy range from 4% to 50% according to the surgical technique. Acquired lymphedema and the association with venous insufficiency is the most prominent picture. In a British community, the overall prevalence was about 0.01% of the population, with a predominance of older women. Primary lymphedema is extremely rare [46, 49].

The clinical presentation of lymphedema can vary according to the cause, severity, and topography. Adequate anamnesis should be taken to characterize the evolution time, familiar occurrence, and precipitating factors such as infection, trauma, surgical procedure, radiotherapy, weight gain, and malignancy.

Initial (Stage 0), swelling is not clinically evident, merely the lymphatic transportation being impaired. At Stage I there is mild, pitting edema that resolves with limb elevation. In a later Stage II, pitting is not present and swelling does not revert with limb elevation. At Stage III there is a patent skin induration with lymphostatic elephantiasis, and pitting is absent. Trophic skin changes, such as acanthosis, fat deposits, and warty overgrowths (mossy foot), are noticeable (Figs. 65.16, 65.17, and 65.18). On the lower limbs the Kaposi–Stemmer sign – digital pinch at the base of the second toe – is usually present, and complications such as ulcers and chronic lipodermosclerosis can arise [46, 50].

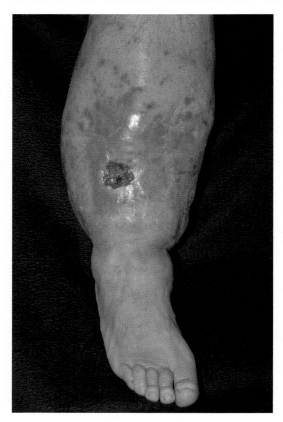

Fig. 65.17 Chronic ulcer in a lymphedematous limb

In general, the diagnosis of lymphedema occurs frequently at later stages (Stage II or III) because mild swelling is generally asymptomatic. There is usually no great difficulty in establishing the diagnosis after clinical examination, but computed tomography and lymphoscintigraphy can help in the confirmation of lymph node stasis.

Despite its rarity, clinicians should be aware that chronic lymphedema is associated with the development of lymphangiosarcoma (e.g., Stewart–Treves syndrome), Kaposi sarcoma, or lymphoma [51].

Postoperative or post-trauma lymphedema should be treated with precocious lymphatic drainage, elevated limb at rest, and compression stockings.

A multidisciplinary team that includes a vascular surgeon, physiotherapist, nurse, and dermatologist should manage chronic lymphedema.

Conservative treatment with compression is the first option for mild to moderate cases. Multilayer inelastic band or controlled compression therapy reduces the edema volume in up to 46% of cases. Additional physical therapy (e.g., lymphatic drainage and exercises) are recommended.

Diuretics and benzopyrones are prescribed in selected cases. Surgical therapy is effective in decompression (debulking of the compressive

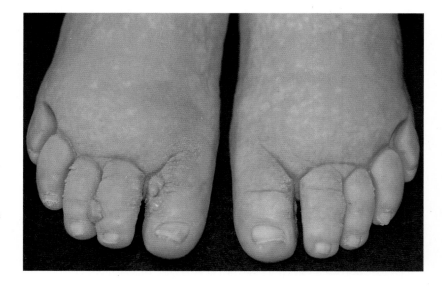

Fig. 65.18 Hypertrophic acral papillomatosis due to chronic lymphedema, leading to a mossy foot appearance

tissue and liposuction). Microsurgery (lympho-venous anastomosis) is not widely performed, and the results are as favorable as those for compressive regimens. The recommendation for amputation in severe cases and multiple complications due to lymphedema should be discussed with patients.

Areas with lymphedema should be protected from trauma, burn, and venipuncture; moreover, patients should be made aware of adequate moisturizing and cautionary nail care without pushing back cuticles. All patients with chronic lymph-edema benefit from 1,200,000 IU penicillin, intramuscularly, every 3 weeks for prevention of soft tissue infection [52].

Glossary

Lipodermosclerosis Considered a type of panniculitis (inflammation of subcutaneous fat). Literally means "scarring of the skin and fat" and is a slow process that occurs over a number of years. It is a condition that affects the skin just above the ankle in patients with long-standing venous disease resulting in chronic venous insufficiency. The end result of untreated lipodermosclerosis is ulcer formation with high incidence of delayed healing and infection.

Lymphedema An abnormal collection of high-protein fluid just beneath the skin. It usually develops when lymph vessels are damaged or lymph nodes are removed (secondary lymphedema) but can also be present when lymphatic vessels are missing or impaired due to a hereditary condition (primary lymphedema).

Vasculitis Inflammation of the blood vessels. It causes changes in the walls of blood vessels, including thickening, weakening, narrowing, and scarring. These changes restrict blood flow, resulting in organ and tissue damage.

References

1. Agale SV. Chronic leg ulcers: epidemiology, aetiopathogenesis and management. Ulcers. 2013;2013:e1–9.
2. Jockenhöfer F, Gollnick H, Herberger K, et al. Aetiology, comorbidities and cofactors of chronic leg ulcers: retrospective evaluation of 1 000 patients from 10 specialised dermatological wound care centers in Germany. Int Wound J. 2016;13(5):821–8.
3. Rabe E. Epidemiology of varicose veins. In: Phlebolymphology. 2010;17(1):19.
4. Park SH, Ferreira K, Santos VL. Understanding pain and quality of life for patients with chronic venous ulcers. Wounds Compend Clin Res Pract. 2008;20:309–20.
5. Lal BK. Venous ulcers of the lower extremity: definition, epidemiology, and economic and social burdens. Semin Vasc Surg. 2015;28:3–5.
6. Donnell TFO Jr, Passman MA, Marston WA, et al. Management of venous leg ulcers: clinical practice guidelines of the society for vascular surgery Ò and the American Venous Forum. J Vasc Surg. 2014;60:3–59.
7. Meissner MH. Venous ulcer care: which dressings are cost effective? Phlebol J Venous Dis. 2014;29:174–80.
8. Wilkinson LS, Bunker C, Edwards JCW, Scurr JH, Smith PDC. Leukocytes: their role in the etiopathogenesis of skin damage in venous disease. J Vasc Surg. 1993;17:669–75.
9. Liu YC, Margolis DJ, Isseroff RR. Does inflammation have a role in the pathogenesis of venous ulcers? A critical review of the evidence. J Invest Dermatol. 2011;131:818–27.
10. Abbade LPF, Lastoria S, Rollo HDA. Venous ulcer: clinical characteristics and risk factors. Int J Dermatol. 2011;50:405–11.
11. Zimmet SE. Venous leg ulcers: modern evaluation and management. Dermatol Surg. 1999;25:236–41.
12. Beldon P. Avoiding allergic contact dermatitis in patients with venous leg ulcers. Br J Commun Nurs. 2006;11:S6. s8, s10–2
13. Vowden P. Understanding the ankle brachial pressure index to treat venous ulceration. Wounds UK. 2012;8:10–5.
14. Malgor RD, Labropoulos N. Diagnosis of venous disease with duplex ultrasound. Phlebology. 2013;28:158–61.
15. Souza JM, Vieira ÉC, Cortez TM, Mondelli AL, Miot HA, Abbade LPF. Clinical and microbiologic evaluation of chronic leg ulcers: a cross-sectional study. Adv Skin Wound Care. 2014;27:222–7.
16. Stücker M, Link K, Reich-Schupke S, Altmeyer P, Doerler M. Compression and venous ulcers. Phlebology. 2013;28(Suppl 1):68–72.
17. de Lima EL, Salome GM, Rocha M, Ferreira LM. The impact of compression therapy with Unna's boot on the functional status of VLU patients. J Wound Care. 2013;22:558–61.
18. Mauck KF, Asi N, Elraiyah TA, et al. Comparative systematic review and meta-analysis of compression modalities for the promotion of venous ulcer healing and reducing ulcer recurrence. J Vasc Surg. 2014;60:71s–90s.
19. Raju S, Hollis K, Neglen P. Use of compression stockings in chronic venous disease: patient compliance and efficacy. Ann Vasc Surg. 2007;21:790–5.

20. Schultz GS, Barillo DJ, Mozingo DW, et al. Wound bed preparation and a brief history of TIME. Int Wound J. 2004;1:19–32.

21. Schultz GS, Sibbald RG, Falanga V, et al. Wound bed preparation: a systematic approach to wound management. Wound Repair Regen. 2003;11:S1–S28.

22. Runkel N, Krug E, Berg L, et al. Evidence-based recommendations for the use of negative pressure wound therapy in traumatic wounds and reconstructive surgery: steps towards an international consensus. Injury. 2011;42:s1–s12.

23. Sibbald RG, Orsted H, Schultz GS, Coutts P, Keast D. Preparing the wound bed 2003: focus on infection and inflammation. Ostomy Wound Manag. 2003;49:23–51.

24. Nelson EA, Bell-Syer SEM. Compression for preventing recurrence of venous ulcers. Cochrane Database Syst Rev. 2014;(9):CD002303.

25. Pannier F, Rabe E. Differential diagnosis of leg ulcers. Phlebology. 2013;28(Suppl 1):55–60.

26. Grey JE, Harding KG, Enoch S. Venous and arterial leg ulcers. BMJ Br Med J. 2006;332:347–50.

27. Weir GR, Smart H, van Marle J, Cronje FJ. Arterial disease ulcers, part 1: clinical diagnosis and investigation. Adv Skin Wound Care. 2014;27:421–8.

28. Dean S. Leg ulcers: causes and management. Aust Fam Physician. 2006;35:480–4.

29. Hankey GJ, Norman PE, Eikelboom JW. Medical treatment of peripheral arterial disease. JAMA. 2006;295:547–53.

30. Bakker K, Schaper NC, Apelqvist J. Practical guidelines on the management and prevention of the diabetic foot 2011. Diabetes Metab Res Rev. 2012;28(Suppl 1):225–31.

31. Vinik AI, Nevoret M-L, Casellini C, Parson H. Diabetic neuropathy. Endocrinol Metab Clin N Am. 2013;42:747–87.

32. Nascimento OJM. Leprosy neuropathy: clinical presentations. Arq Neuropsiquiatr. 2013;71:661–6.

33. Feng Y, Schlösser FJ, Sumpio BE. The Semmes Weinstein monofilament examination is a significant predictor of the risk of foot ulceration and amputation in patients with diabetes mellitus. J Vasc Surg. 2011;53:220–6.

34. Frykberg RG, Zgonis T, Armstrong DG, et al. Diabetic foot disorders: a clinical practice guideline (2006 revision). J Foot Ankle Surg. 2006;45:S1–66.

35. Alavi A, Sibbald RG, Mayer D, et al. Diabetic foot ulcers: Part II. Management. J Am Acad Dermatol. 2014;70:e1–21.

36. Alavi A, Mayer D, Hafner J, Sibbald RG. Martorell hypertensive ischemic leg ulcer: an underdiagnosed entity. Adv Skin Wound Care. 2012;25:563–72.

37. Blanco González E, Gago Vidal B, Murillo Solís D, Domingo Del Valle J. Martorell's ulcer: an unusual complication of long-term hypertension. Hipertens Riesgo Vasc. 2011;28:211–3.

38. Vuerstaek JDD, Reeder SWI, Henquet CJM, Neumann HAM. Arteriolosclerotic ulcer of Martorell. J Eur Acad Dermatol Venereol. 2010;24:867–74.

39. Ruocco E, Sangiuliano S, Gravina AG, Miranda A, Nicoletti G. Pyoderma gangrenosum: an updated review. J Eur Acad Dermatol Venereol. 2009;23:1008–17.

40. Panuncialman J, Falanga V. Basic approach to inflammatory ulcers. Dermatol Ther. 2006;19:365–76.

41. Ruiz-Irastorza G, Crowther M, Branch W, Khamashta MA. Antiphospholipid syndrome. Lancet. 2010;376:1498–509.

42. Gonzalez-Santiago TM, Davis MDP. Update of management of connective tissue diseases: livedoid vasculopathy. Dermatol Ther. 2012;25:183–94.

43. Kerk N, Goerge T. Livedoid vasculopathy – current aspects of diagnosis and treatment of cutaneous infarction. J Dtsch Dermatol Ges. 2013;11:407–10.

44. Yesilada AK, Sevim KZ, Sucu DO, et al. Marjolin ulcer: clinical experience with 34 patients over 15 years. J Cutan Med Surg. 2013;17:404–9.

45. Pavlovic S, Wiley E, Guzman G, Morris D, Braniecki M. Marjolin ulcer: an overlooked entity. Int Wound J. 2011;8:419–24.

46. Warren AG, Brorson H, Borud LJ, Slavin SA. Lymphedema: a comprehensive review. Ann Plast Surg. 2007;59(4):464–72.

47. Clodius L. Lymphatics, lymphodynamics, lymphedema: an update. Plast Surg Outlook. 1990;4:1.

48. Smeltzer DM, Stickler GB, Schirger A. Primary lymphedema in children and adolescents: a follow-up study and review. Pediatrics. 1985;76:206–18.

49. Moffatt CJ, Franks PJ, Doherty DC, et al. Lymphoedema: an underestimated health problem. QJM. 2003;96:731–8.

50. Pannier F, Hoffmann B, Stang A, Jöckel KH, Rabe E. Prevalence of Stemmer's sign in the general population. Phlebologie. 2007;36:287–342.

51. Ruocco V, Schwartz RA, Ruocco E. Lymphedema: an immunologically vulnerable site for development of neoplasms. J Am Acad Dermatol. 2002;47:124–7.

52. Thomas KS, Crook AM, Nunn AJ, et al. Penicillin to prevent recurrent leg cellulitis. N Engl J Med. 2013;368:1695–703.

Xerosis

Clarice Gabardo Ritter

Key Points
- Xerosis is a very common disorder in the general population
- Dry skin can be caused or aggravated by factors such as age, associated dermatosis, genetic background, and environmental factors
- Moisturizers are effective in reducing dry skin symptoms

Abbreviations

AD   Atopic dermatitis
NMF   Natural moisturizing factor
SC   Stratum corneum
TEWL   Transepidermal water loss

Introduction

Xerosis, or dry skin, is a cutaneous reaction indicative of abnormal desquamation resulting in a rough texture and appearance of the skin. Skin

---

C.G. Ritter
Dermatology of Hospital Nossa Senhora da Conceição, Porto Alegre, Brazil
e-mail: clariceritter@gmail.com

becomes dehydrated when the stratum corneum (SC) is unable to retain water and loses moisture faster than it is replenished. It is a very common condition among the general population, especially the elderly, in whom the prevalence can reach from 30% to 60% [1–3]. Dry skin can occur in association with many other dermatoses and unfavorable environmental factors.

Dry skin can affect the patient's quality of life and work productivity because it can cause discomfort, pain, and itching, and repetitive scratching can result in secondary lesions. Severe xerosis can lead to the onset of a type of eczema characterized by intensely itchy, fissured, and cracked skin called xerotic eczema or eczema craquelé.

Emollients are central to the management of xerosis, and the aim of treatment with emollients is primarily to restore epidermal differentiation, leading to the restoration of normal skin. However, dry skin is often the result of a combination of etiologic factors, so the treatment involves multiple actions, such as bath and soap care and control of other environmental factors.

State of the Art

Besides xerosis being a common symptom of a great number of skin conditions, only fairly recently has more progress been made toward elucidating the structure and function of the SC and the mechanisms that result in xerosis.

© Springer International Publishing Switzerland 2018
R.R. Bonamigo, S.I.T. Dornelles (eds.), *Dermatology in Public Health Environments*,
https://doi.org/10.1007/978-3-319-33919-1_66

Nowadays we have a better understanding of the complex pathophysiology of epidermis and SC, and it is believed that disturbed epidermal differentiation is a root cause of dry skin [4]. The disturbance of epidermal differentiation can include a wide range of etiologic factors that often work together, such as genetic background, metabolic causes, and environmental triggers.

The treatment of xerosis with emollients has scientific evidence of efficacy. This approach can prevent flares of atopic dermatitis and psoriasis, and manifest anti-inflammatory properties, and it can improve patients' quality of life and reduce prescription costs [5].

The traditional use of simple emollients using nonphysiologic lipids such as petrolatum and mineral oil create a fine occlusive layer, thereby reducing water loss from the SC. Current knowledge supports the use of additional ingredients, such as humectants and physiologic lipids, which rapidly penetrate the epidermis and have more physiologic actions to restore epidermal differentiation [4, 5].

A recent systematic review about skin care in the aged demonstrated that application of moisturizers containing humectants such as lactic acid, urea, glycerin, and α-hydroxy acids is clearly effective in reducing dry skin conditions and enhancing the skin barrier function. However, there is no evidence that one humectant-containing moisturizer is superior to another [6].

Pathogenesis of Dry Skin

The epidermis is a stratified keratinized epithelium and is the main affected skin layer in the xerosis process. The most important function of the epidermis lies in the SC, a cornified layer of epidermis that provides physical protection against water loss and prevents the passage of soluble substances into the body from outside.

The principal acellular components of the SC are the structural proteins, the intercellular lipids, the natural moisturizing factor (NMF), and the enzyme systems. The success in maintaining epidermal homeostasis depends on coordinate actions between these elements. Epidermal

enzyme activity promotes synthesis of lipids and the subsequent degradation of intercellular bonds to produce physiologic desquamation. This enzymatic activity is modulated by several factors including pH, temperature, and hydration. If, for some reason, a decrease in lipid content occurs, there will be an increase in insensible transepidermal water loss (TEWL), which in turn will destabilize the optimum environment for epidermal enzyme activity. These events will culminate in a disruption of the process of corneocyte maturation and inhibition of cell desquamation in a self-perpetuating cycle of dry skin. In summary, xerosis is the result of an impairment of epidermal desquamation [4, 7].

The barrier function and skin hydration depend on two essential elements: the lipids present in the SC and the levels of NMF. The lipids are formed on stratum granulosum and then migrate upward into the SC during the process of epidermal differentiation. Their intercellular component is arranged in bilayers between the corneocytes. Through an enzymatic process, these lipids are transformed on nonpolar lipids such as ceramides, free fatty acids, and cholesterol. A lipid deficiency destabilizes SC hydration, affecting the elasticity and flexibility of healthy skin [8].

The NMF is a water-retaining substance, composed of a mixture of amino acids and salts generated by filaggrin hydrolysis. This substance is highly water soluble and has great water-retention capacity. It is responsible for retaining the turgidity of corneocytes and preventing skin cracking and desquamation. The water content of a healthy SC under normal conditions is 15–20% [9]. When the water content of the cornified layer falls below 10%, visible scales form and the skin acquires a rough, dry appearance.

Aquaporin-3, an epidermal water/glycerol transporter, is also the subject of recent studies about the pathogenesis of xerosis. These channels are responsible for carrying glycerol into the SC, where it acts as an endogenous humectant. The expression of the aquaporin-3 in human skin is strongly affected by aging and chronic sun exposure. The high prevalence of xerosis in these clinical situations may be justified by the lower levels of these channels [4].

The SC contains other moisturizing components, such as hyaluronic acid and lactate. These components also play a role in maintaining the physical properties of the epithelial barrier [10].

Epidemiology and Clinical Aspects of Xerosis

Most people have experienced xerosis, a very common skin condition, at some point in their lives. The available epidemiologic data are generally related to elderly patients. One study of community-dwelling individuals found prevalence as high as 38.9% [11], and a recent cross-sectional study in a primary care setting showed that in patients >65 years 56% experienced at least some degree of xerosis [3]. Other long-term care studies found prevalence to range from 29.5% to 58.3% [12–14].

A physical examination will reveal rough, dry skin to the touch. There may be scaling, dry white patches, flakes, and even fissures. If the xerosis worsens, there may be redness and cracking (eczema craquelé) (Fig. 66.1), and severe cases may appear ichthyotic or fish-scale like (Fig. 66.2). The patient may complain of a

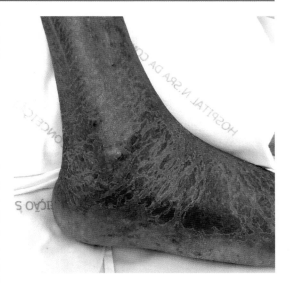

Fig. 66.2 Severe xerosis in a critically ill patient

feeling of uncomfortably tight skin and of symptoms such as itch, pain, stinging, or tingles.

Pruritus is an important clinical condition related to xerosis. The prevalence of pruritus in the elderly can be as high as 40% [11], and xerosis is the most common cause of pruritus in older adults [15]. Scratching the skin can lead to complications such as secondary infection or ulceration and chronic wounds. Managing dry skin and maintaining moisture is of utmost importance to prevent these complications.

Skin Diseases and Conditions Related to Xerosis

Dry skin is often the result of a combination of etiologic factors (Table 66.1), in particular genetic abnormalities, but also metabolic and environmental triggers. The following are the most important situations in which dry skin may be a result or a symptom.

Environmental Humidity and Temperature

It is broadly accepted that skin barrier functions may be negatively affected by climatic conditions [16]. A recent systematic review studied the neg-

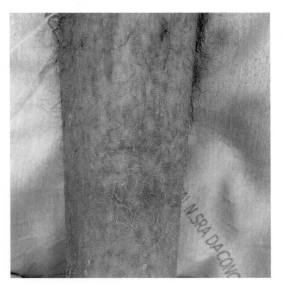

Fig. 66.1 Eczema craquelé: severe xerosis with fissures and erythema

Table 66.1 Factors that contribute to xerosis

Genetic predisposition

Age

Concomitant skin diseases: atopic dermatitis, ichthyosis, psoriasis, chronic hand eczema

Comorbid diseases: hypothyroidism, diabetes, nutritional deficiency, renal disease

Medications: statins, diuretics, retinoids, targeted anticancer therapies

Environmental conditions: temperature, humidity, exposure to sunlight

Exposure to chemical agents: soaps and detergents, lotions, and perfumes

Physical insult: friction, abrasion, and radiation

ative effects of low humidity, low temperatures, and different seasons on the skin barrier and on the risk of dermatitis [17].

Meta-analysis of 99 selected studies concluded that low humidity and low temperatures lead to a general decrease in skin barrier function and increased susceptibility toward mechanical stress. As proinflammatory cytokines and cortisol are released by keratinocytes and the number of dermal mast cells increases, the skin also becomes more reactive toward skin irritants and allergens [17].

Human skin that is exposed to low relative humidity (32%) appears to be more susceptible to mechanical stress and fracture than skin in high relative humidity (96%). The exposure of healthy volunteers to very low humidity (10%) causes a decrease in skin hydration and clinically drier skin [18]. Furthermore, on experimental studies of the effect of air humidification, participants reported significantly fewer skin symptoms under higher absolute and relative humidity [19, 20]. Optimal relative humidity for lipids and protein organization is 60% [21].

The effects of cold temperature and the resulting winter xerosis have been investigated by several studies, which have identified a decrease in SC lipids and NMFs components, and an increase in SC pH and stiffness during winter [9, 22–24]. Drier skin and increased reaction to skin irritants suggest that the skin becomes more fragile and permeable in winter. The warm dry air produced by central heating systems aggravates winter xerosis [4].

Surfactant-Related Xerosis

In daily life, substances that include chemicals such as surfactants and solvents potentially perturb the SC barrier. Certain anionic surfactants such as sodium lauryl sulfate affect not only the barrier itself but also the underlying viable cell layers. For instance, sodium dodecyl sulfate upregulates intercellular adhesion molecules or vascular endothelial growth factor, suggesting that this class of surfactant has an intrinsic ability to induce epidermal hyperplasia and irritation [25, 26].

Aging

Some epidemiologic studies estimate that generalized and diffused xerosis affects between 30% and 60% of individuals over 65 years of age and is the most common cause of itching in this age group [27–29]. A history of atopy, especially atopic dermatitis, is associated with an increased risk of xerosis in the elderly [3].

There are many possible causes of dry skin in older people: a lower rate of epidermal proliferation than in a younger healthier skin, a decline in gonadal and adrenal androgens associated with decreased synthesis of sebum and ceramides, and lower levels of filaggrin, the protein from which the components of NMF are derived [7, 30]. These progressive intrinsic changes of aged skin combine synergistically with cumulative environment insults to produce structural and functional disturbances causing xerosis.

Atopic Dermatitis

Atopic dermatitis (AD) is a chronic inflammatory skin disorder characterized by recurrent eczema and severe pruritus. It is a multifactorial condition associated with genetic abnormalities and environmental conditions that give rise to immunologic imbalance and skin disturbances. Xerosis is almost a rule in AD, and the skin of patients with atopic eczema is characterized by low ceramide levels [31], increased transepidermal water loss [32] and decreased water-binding capacity [33].

Xerosis is such an important feature of AD that it is one of the diagnostic criteria for this dermatosis [34]. Researchers have discussed whether xerosis is secondary to skin inflammation or if skin barrier abnormalities occur first, causing increased allergen sensitization through an impaired skin barrier and creating the conditions leading to the development of AD. Generalized xerosis, whether acquired or inherited, is also associated with other common skin disorders such as hand eczema, contact sensitization, and even asthma [35, 36].

In young children with AD, treating xerosis improves quality of life [37], decreases the risk of developing percutaneous sensitization [38] and improves AD as demonstrated by a decrease in objective AD scores [39]. In addition, a number of clinical trials have shown that treating xerosis decreases symptoms and signs of AD, including pruritus, erythema, fissuring, and lichenification [40–42]. The correct use of moisturizers can reduce inflammation and AD severity.

Ichthyosis

Ichthyosis belongs to a large group of genetic skin disorders characterized by xerosis caused by defects in the formation and function of the epithelial barrier.

Ichthyosis vulgaris is the most prevalent form of the disease (prevalence 1 in 100), and is characterized by abnormalities in the formation of keratohyalin granules and, consequently, in filaggrin. This abnormality leads to the formation of an SC deficient in many of the components of NMF. Impaired corneodesmolysis caused by defective water binding in the SC and alterations in skin pH give rise to visibly abnormal desquamation [7, 43].

Systemic Diseases and Drugs

The presence of some concomitant disease states, therapies, and medications makes individuals more susceptible to xerosis. Some of these pre-existing situations include radiation, end-stage renal disease, nutritional deficiency (especially zinc and essential fatty acids), thyroid disease, neurologic disorders with decreased sweating, HIV (human immunodeficiency virus), and malignancies. Xerosis is one of the earliest and most common signs of diabetes and is found in up to 22% of patients with type 1 diabetes mellitus [44].

Certain medications can exacerbate xerosis or eczema by interfering with skin barrier function. For example, HMG-CoA reductase inhibitors (statins) have been demonstrated to promote xerosis cutis mimicking asteatotic irritant dermatitis. Barrier dysfunction in this case is believed to be a consequence of inhibition of cholesterol biosynthesis and the resultant decrease in the production and distribution of lipids in the skin that are essential for maintaining the barrier [45, 46].

Many targeted therapies used in the treatment of some cancers can lead to the development of xerosis, and this is an important side effect of this type of therapy [47].

Other medications associated with xerosis include diuretics, antiandrogenic therapies, and retinoids [14].

Treatment

Prevention

A recent insight in the treatment of dry skin is the importance of prophylaxis between episodes of xerosis. It is suggested that preventive strategies be practiced in situations that potentially lead to dry skin, such as patients with atopic dermatitis, those with occupational contact dermatitis, and the elderly. Prevention or treatment of xerosis follows the same principles: avoidance of aggravating factors, epidermal hydration, and repair of the barrier function. Studies suggest that the skin barrier and integrity can be improved by using low-irritation cleansing products and humectant-containing moisturizers, stressing that these are the main preventive measures [6].

General Measures

Many general measures can be used to improve xerosis (Table 66.2), and consist in altering ambient humidity, changing bathing habits, and applying emollients.

As described earlier, ambient humidity can play an important role in xerosis severity. Humidity levels of less than 10% cause the SC to lose moisture, and the use of humidifier with a setting of 45–60% humid air output can prevent this occurrence.

Table 66.2 General recommendations for skin care in xerosis

Reduce the frequency and duration of bathing and use warm (not hot) water
Minimize the use of soap and use a nonirritating soap
Avoid harsh skin cleansers and powders that act as drying agents
Apply moisturizers directly to skin that is still damp
Consider using a humidifier during the winter to ensure a relative humidity setting of 45–60%
Avoid friction from washcloths, rough clothing, and abrasives

Table 66.3 Ingredients used on emollients

Ingredient	Action
Lipids (e.g., mineral, vegetable oil)	Replace the lost natural skin lipids
Physiologic lipids (e.g., ceramides, cholesterol)	Epidermal differentiation and repair of structural elements in the SC
Humectants (e.g., glycerol, urea, lactic acid)	Balance the water content of SC and restore barrier function
Antipruritic agents (e.g., glycine)	Break the itch-scratch cycle
Others (e.g., dexpanthenol)	Fibroblast proliferation and migration, epidermal differentiation

When treating patients with xerosis, it is very important to spend a long time discussing bathing habits. Water, soap, and detergent skin-washing liquids are generally the most common irritants applied to the skin. When xerosis is accompanied by itching, the application of water gives temporary relief and reduces the feeling of dryness. Therefore, it is important to convince patients to reduce excess contact with water that, in the long term, is damaging to the skin.

Topical Treatment

Emollients are essential to the management of xerosis and should be used by all patients suffering from dry skin. The aim of treatment with emollients is primarily to restore epidermal differentiation, leading to the production of normal skin. Secondly, emollient therapy should also aim to soothe the affected skin, help break the itch-and-scratch cycle, and thus prevent further physical damage to skin.

An ideal emollient should contain a combination of ingredients (Table 66.3) to protect the skin from further damage by reducing TEWL, irritation, and itching, and stimulate the production of normal skin by restoring epidermal differentiation [5]. Among these possible ingredients are occlusive lipids, physiologic lipids, humectants, and antipruritic agents.

Application of lipids to the skin surface produces skin hydration by several mechanisms, the most conventional of which is occlusion, which implies a simple reduction of the loss of water from the outside of the skin. Examples of lipids with these properties are petrolatum, lanolin, and mineral oil.

On the other hand, physiologic lipids such as ceramides, cholesterol, and free fatty acids, naturally found in the SC, seem to replenish and restore the intercellular lipid matrix [48, 49]. The application of physiologic lipids has been suggested to be more efficient compared with nonphysiologic molecules because they penetrate the SC more easily, function as structural elements in the epidermal barrier, and restore proper epidermal differentiation. However, trials between specific moisturizing products are few in number, and until now there has been no evidence of the superiority of physiologic lipids over traditional emollients [50].

Humectants, such as urea, lactic acid, and glycerol, attract and hold water in the SC, and therefore compensate for the reduced levels of NMF and other natural humectants in skin [51–53]. Applications of urea with concentrations up to 10% and lactic acid 5% reduced skin dryness, increased SC hydration, and decreased transepidermal water loss (TEWL) compared with lotions containing no humectant or no treatment [4, 5]. Based on substantial evidence, the use of emollients combined with humectants seems to be the best strategy for treating xerosis.

Many other substances with possible benefits in the treatment of xerosis are under study. Glycerol, in particular, seems to play an important role in stimulating the expression of epidermal aquaporin-3. The better function of these aquaporins results in improvement of skin barrier function and skin hydration [53, 54]. Antipruritic agents, such as glycine, which can block histamine release from mastocytes, seem to be useful in breaking the itch–scratch cycle. Finally, some topical formulations include an active ingredient that stimulates cell proliferation and lipid synthesis: dexpanthenol is an example of this class of ingredient [54, 55].

Various emollient formulations, including lotions, creams, and ointments, are available, and attention to patient need is important to secure compliance. The choice of the emollient should be ideally discussed with the patient, and may be driven by cosmetic acceptability, cost, oil content, and adjuvant properties such as humectant and/or anti-itching properties. Patients may require different types of emollient product, depending of the area of the body to be treated, the patient's lifestyle, and seasonal factors.

The benefits of emollient use on health economics are many: they help to control flares of AD, reduce referrals, and improve the quality of life of patients. To obtain these objectives emollient products should remain on prescription, and prescribers should be aware of the costs and properties of the various emollients. Humectant-containing products can produce greater barrier repair per gram than an emollient without humectants [5].

Emollients should be applied correctly and generously; sufficient quantities must therefore be prescribed, and patient education is crucial for maximum effect of therapy. They should be routinely applied by being gently rubbed into the skin after a bath or shower because there is some evidence that this will help trap moisture in the skin. Ideally, emollients should be applied several times a day to keep the skin hydrated.

If inflammation becomes severe, topical corticosteroids may be needed for short-term use. Emollients should be continued while the patient is on corticosteroid therapy.

Adverse Effects of Topical Treatment for Xerosis

Serious reactions are rare, and the most common adverse effects of topical treatment are irritant and allergic contact dermatitis. Irritant contact dermatitis is more common and is caused by frequent and prolonged use of preparations containing potential irritants such as sodium lauryl sulfate. Contact allergic dermatitis is a delayed hypersensitivity reaction to an allergen whereby the initial sensitization exposure must occur first in order to activate immune system response. It is important, therefore, to avoid skin sensitizers such as wound-care agents in patients with xerosis, in whom the cutaneous barrier is impaired. Table 66.4 lists common skin sensitizers found in emollients that should be avoided, if possible.

Humectants such as urea and lactic acid are associated with a subjective sensation of mild burning in some individuals, but are generally tolerable [56, 57].

Table 66.4 Common skin sensitizers that may be found in emollients

| Balsam of Peru |
| Lanolin |
| Propylene glycol |
| Parabens |
| Formaldehyde |
| Fragrance |
| Vitamin E |
| Aloe vera |
| Methylchloroisothiazolinone/methylisothiazolinone (Kathon CG) |

Future Perspectives

The growing knowledge of the mechanisms involved in the xerosis process makes it increasingly possible to choose the most appropriate emollient for an individual patient based on specific epidermal disarrangement.

Considering the great number of emollients available today, it is of absolute importance to develop studies that compare different active substances. Only through such studies will the choice of treatment be based on better efficacy.

Finally, because the recent advances in our understanding of the pathogenesis of xerosis, the development of new classes of compounds will be an imminent reality in the next few years.

Glossary

Ceramide The basic unit of the sphingolipids, consisting of sphingosine (unsaturated amino alcohol) or a related base attached via its amino group to a long-chain fatty acid anion. A lipid molecule that plays a fundamental role in skin water.

Emollients Complex mixtures of chemical agents specially designed to make the external layers of the skin (epidermis) softer and more pliable. They increase the skin's hydration (water content) by reducing evaporation. Emollients work by forming an oily layer on the top of the skin that traps water in the skin.

Humectants Substances that absorb water from the atmosphere and also from the lower layers of the skin, making more moisturized the upper skin that is palpable.

References

1. Norman R. Xerosis and pruritus in the elderly: recognition and management. Dermatol Ther. 2003;16:254–9.
2. Farage MA, Miller KW, Berardesca E, Maibach HI. Clinical implications of aging skin: cutaneous disorders in the elderly. Am J Clin Dermatol. 2009;10:73–86. doi:10.2165/00128071-200910020-00001.
3. Paul C, Maumus-Robert S, Mazereeuw-Hautier J, Guyen CN, Saudez X, Schmitt AM. Prevalence and risk factors for xerosis in the elderly: a cross-sectional epidemiological study in primary care. Dermatology. 2011;223:260–5. doi:10.1159/000334631.
4. Proksch E, Lachapelle JM. The management of dry skin with topical emollients–recent perspectives. J Dtsch Dermatol Ges. 2005;3:768–74.
5. Moncrieff G, Cork M, Lawton S, Kokiet S, Daly C, Clark C. Use of emollients in dry-skin conditions: consensus statement. Clin Exp Dermatol. 2013;38:231–8. doi:10.1111/ced.12104.
6. Kottner J, Lichterfeld A, Blume-Peytavi U. Maintaining skin integrity in the aged: a systematic review. Br J Dermatol. 2013;169:528–42. doi:10.1111/bjd.12469.
7. Barco D, Gimenez-Arnau A. Xerosis: a dysfunction of the epidermal barrier. Actas Dermosifiliogr. 2008;99:671–82.
8. Elias PM. Stratum corneum defensive functions: an integrated view. J Invest Dermatol. 2005;125:183–200.
9. Nakagawa N, Sakai S, Matsumoto M, Yamada K, Nagano M, Yuki T, et al. Relationship between NMF (lactate and potassium) content and the physical properties of the stratum corneum in healthy subjects. J Invest Dermatol. 2004;122:755–63.
10. Rawlings AV, Matts PJ. Stratum corneum moisturization at the molecular level: an update in relation to the dry skin cycle. J Invest Dermatol. 2005;124:1099–110.
11. Kiliç A, Gül U, Aslan E, Soylu S. Dermatological findings in the senior population of nursing homes in Turkey. Arch Gerontol Geriatr. 2008;47:93–8.
12. Smith DR, Sheu HM, Hsieh FS, Lee Y, Chang SJ, Guo YL. Prevalence of skin disease among nursing home patients in southern Taiwan. Int J Dermatol. 2002;41:754–9.
13. Smith DR, Atkinson R, Tang S, Yamagata Z. A survey of skin disease among patients in an Australian nursing home. J Epidemiol. 2002;12:336–40.
14. White-Chu EF, Reddy M. Dry skin in the elderly: complexities of a common problem. Clin Dermatol. 2011;29:37–42.
15. Haroun MT. Dry skin in the elderly. Geriatr Aging. 2003;6:41–4.
16. Denda M, Sato J, Tsuchiya T, et al. Low humidity stimulates epidermal DNA synthesis and amplifies the hyperproliferative response to barrier disruption: implication for seasonal exacerbations of inflammatory dermatoses. J Invest Dermatol. 1998;111:873–8.
17. Engebretsen KA, Johansen JD, Kezic S, Linneberg A, Thyssen JP. The effect of environmental humidity and temperature on skin barrier function and dermatitis. J Eur Acad Dermatol Venereol. 2016;30:223–49. doi:10.1111/jdv.13301.
18. Egawa M, Oguri M, Kuwahara T, et al. Effect of exposure of human skin to a dry environment. Skin Res Technol. 2002;8:212–8.
19. Reinikainen LM, Jaakkola JJK. The effect of air humidification on symptoms and perception of indoor air quality in office workers: a six-period cross-over trial. Arch Environ Health. 1992;47:8–15.
20. Reinikainen LM, Jaakkola JJ. Significance of humidity and temperature on skin and upper airway symptoms. Indoor Air. 2003;13:344–52.
21. Vyumvuhore R, Tfayli A, Duplan H, et al. Effects of atmospheric relative humidity on stratum corneum structure at the molecular level: ex vivo Raman spectroscopy analysis. Analyst. 2013;138:4103–11.
22. Andersen F, Andersen K, Kligman A. Xerotic skin of the elderly: a summer versus winter comparison based on biophysical measurements. Exog Dermatol. 2004;2:190–4.
23. Rogers J, Harding C, Mayo A, et al. Stratum corneum lipids: the effect of ageing and the seasons. Arch Dermatol Res. 1996;288:765–70.
24. Ishikawa J, Shimotoyodome Y, Ito S, et al. Variations in the ceramide profile in different seasons and regions of the body contribute to stratum corneum functions. Arch Dermatol Res. 2013;305:151–62.
25. Grunewald AM, Gloor M, Gehring W, Kleesz P. Damage to the skin by repetitive washing. Contact Dermatitis. 1995;32:225–32.
26. Harding CR. The stratum corneum: structure and function in health and disease. Dermatol Ther. 2004;17:6–15.
27. Yalçin B, Tamer E, Toy GG, Oztaş P, Hayran M, Alli N. The prevalence of skin diseases in the elderly:

analysis of 4099 geriatric pa- tients. Int J Dermatol. 2006;45:672–6.

28. Polat M, Yalçin B, Calişkan D, Alli N. Complete dermatologic examination in the elderly: an exploratory study from an outpatient clinic in Turkey. Gerontology. 2009;55:58–63.

29. Seyfarth F, Schliemann S, Antonov D, Elsner P. Dry skin, barrier function, and irritant contact dermatitis in the elderly. Clin Dermatol. 2011;29:31–6.

30. Engelke M, Jensen JM, Ekanayake-Mudiyanselage S, Proksch E. Effects of xerosis and ageing on epidermal proliferation and differentiation. Br J Dermatol. 1997;137:219–25.

31. Imokawa G, Abe A, Jin K, Higaki Y, Kawashima M, Hidano A. Decreased levels of ceramides in stratum corneum of atopic dermatitis: an etiological factor in atopic dermatitis. J Invest Dermatol. 1991;96:523–6.

32. Werner Y, Lindberg M. Transepidermal water loss in dry and clinically normal skin in patients with atopic dermatitis. Acta Derm Venereol. 1985;65:102–5.

33. Thune P. Evaluation of the hydration and water binding capacity in atopic skin and so-called dry skin. Acta Derm Venereol. 1989;144(Suppl):133–5.

34. Williams HC, Burney PG, Pembroke AC, Hay RJ. The U.K. working party's diagnostic criteria for atopic dermatitis. III. Independent hospital validation. Br J Dermatol. 1994;131:406–16.

35. Thyssen JP, Johansen JD, Zachariae C, Menné T, Linneberg A. Xerosis is associated with atopic dermatitis, hand eczema and contact sensitization independent of filaggrin gene mutations. Acta Derm Venereol. 2013;93:406–10. doi:10.2340/00015555-1539.

36. Engebretsen KA, Linneberg A, Thuesen BH, Szecsi PB, Stender S, Menné T, Johansen JD, Thyssen JP. Xerosis is associated with asthma in men independent of atopic dermatitis and filaggrin gene mutations. J Eur Acad Dermatol Venereol. 2015;29:1807–15. doi:10.1111/jdv.13051.

37. Giordano-Labadie F, Cambazard F, Guillet G, et al. Evaluation of a new moisturizer (Exomega milk) in children with atopic dermatitis. J Dermatol Treat. 2006;17:78–81.

38. Boralevi F, Hubiche T, Leaute-Labreze C, et al. Epicutaneous aeroallergen sensitization in atopic dermatitis infants – determining the role of epidermal barrier impairment. Allergy. 2008;63:205–10.

39. Boralevi F, Saint Aroman M, Delarue A, Raudsepp H, Kaszuba A, Bylaite M, Tiplica GS. Long-term emollient therapy improves xerosis in children with atopic dermatitis. J Eur Acad Dermatol Venereol. 2014;28:1456–62. doi:10.1111/jdv.12314.

40. Breternitz M, Kowatzki D, Langenauer M, Elsner P, Fluhr JW. Placebo-controlled, double-blind, randomized, prospective study of a glycerol-based emollient on eczematous skin in atopic dermatitis: biophysical and clinical evaluation. Skin Pharmacol Physiol. 2008;21:39–45.

41. Korting HC, Schollmann C, Cholcha W, Wolff L. Efficacy and tolerability of pale sulfonated shale oil cream 4% in the treatment of mild to moderate atopic eczema in children: a multicentre, randomized vehicle-controlled trial. J Eur Acad Dermatol Venereol. 2010;24:1176–82.

42. Grimalt R, Mengeaud V, Cambazard F. The steroid-sparing effect of an emollient therapy in infants with atopic dermatitis: a randomized controlled study. Dermatology. 2007;214:61–7.

43. Traupe H, Fischer J, Oji V. Nonsyndromic types of ichthyoses – an update. J Dtsch Dermatol Ges. 2014;12:109–21. doi:10.1111/ddg.12229.

44. Torres BE, Torres-Pradilla M. Cutaneous manifestations in children with diabetes mellitus and obesity. Actas Dermosifiliogr. 2014;105:546–57.

45. Garibyan L, Chiou AS, Elmariah SB. Advanced aging skin and itch: addressing an unmet need. Dermatol Ther. 2013;26:92–103.

46. Krasovec M, Elsner P, Burg G. Generalized eczematous skin rash possibly due to HMG-CoA reductase inhibitors. Dermatology. 1993;186:248–52.

47. Valentine J, Belum VR, Duran J, Ciccolini K, Schindler K, Wu S, Lacouture ME. Incidence and risk of xerosis with targeted anticancer therapies. J Am Acad Dermatol. 2015;72:656–67. doi:10.1016/j. jaad.2014.12.010.

48. Chamlin SL, Kao J, Frieden IJ, et al. Ceramide-dominant barrier repair lipids alleviate childhood atopic dermatitis: changes in barrier function provide a sensitive indicator of disease activity. J Am Acad Dermatol. 2002;47:198–208.

49. Msika P, De Belilovsky C, Piccardi N, et al. New emollient with topical corticosteroid-sparing effect in treatment of childhood atopic dermatitis: SCORAD and quality of life improvement. Pediatr Dermatol. 2008;25:606–12.

50. Eichenfield LF, Tom WL, Berger TG, Krol A, Paller AS, Schwarzenberger K, et al. Guidelines of care for the management of atopic dermatitis. Part 2: management and treatment of atopic dermatitis with topical therapies. J Am Acad Dermatol. 2014;71:116–32. doi:10.1016/j.jaad.2014.03.023.

51. Bissonnette R, Maari C, Provost N, et al. A double-blind study of tolerance and efficacy of a new urea-containing moisturizer in patients with atopic dermatitis. J Cosmet Dermatol. 2010;9:16–21.

52. Wiren K, Nohlgard C, Nyberg F, et al. Treatment with a barrier-strengthening moisturizing cream delays relapse of atopic dermatitis: a prospective and randomized controlled clinical trial. J Eur Acad Dermatol Venereol. 2009;23:1267–72.

53. Draelos ZD. Modern moisturizer myths, misconceptions, and truths. Cutis. 2013;91:308–14.

54. Schrader A, Siefken W, Kueper T. Effects of glyceryl glucoside on AQP3 expression, barrier function and hydration of human skin. Skin Pharmacol Physiol. 2012;25:192–9.

55. Gehring G, Gloor M. Effect of topically applied dexpanthenol on epidermal barrier function and stratum corneum hydration. Drug Res. 2000;50(2):659–63.

56. Proksch E, Nissen HP. Dexpanthenol enhances skin barrier repair and reduces inflammation after sodium

lauryl sulphate-induced irritation. J Dermatol Treat. 2002;13:173–8.

57. Pan M, Heinecke G, Bernardo S, Tsui C, Levitt J. Urea: a comprehensive review of the clinical literature. Dermatol Online J. 2013;19(11):20392.

Suggested Literature

Kirkup MEM. Xerosis and stasis dermatitis. In: Norman RA, editor. Preventive dermatology. London: Springer; 2010. p. 71–9.

Kottner J, Lichterfeld A, Blume-Peytavi U. Maintaining skin integrity in the aged: a systematic review. Br J Dermatol. 2013;169:528–42. doi:10.1111/bjd.12469.

Moncrieff G, Cork M, Lawton S, Kokiet S, Daly C, Clark C. Use of emollients in dry-skin conditions: consensus statement. Clin Exp Dermatol. 2013;38:231–8. doi:10.1111/ced.12104.

Hyperhidrosis

Doris Hexsel and Fernanda Oliveira Camozzato

Key Points
- Sweating is a normal and important mechanism of thermoregulation which is essential for survival. When excessive, it is called hyperhidrosis.
- It is necessary to understand the biology of eccrine, apocrine, and apoeccrine sweat glands to understand hyperhidrosis.
- Hyperhidrosis can be primary (idiopathic/essential) or secondary to another condition. Hyperhidrosis can be further classified as focal or generalized.
- Primary hyperhidrosis is most often focal, affecting the palms, soles, and axillae. Thighs and gluteal and inguinal regions may also be involved. One or more regions can be affected in the same patient.
- Secondary hyperhidrosis must be ruled out before a diagnosis of primary hyperhidrosis is made. A variety of conditions can induce hyperhidrosis.
- There are many treatments for hyperhidrosis, including aluminum compounds, iontophoresis, botulinum toxin, drugs, microfocused ultrasound, and endoscopic thoracic sympathectomy.

Introduction

Hyperhidrosis is a chronic autonomic disorder whereby the production of sweat exceeds the amount required for thermoregulation. This condition is not merely characterized by excessive sweating but also by any amount of sweating that causes physical, emotional, and social discomfort for the patient [1]. Hyperhidrosis may impair the ability to perform daily functions and, in some cases, may increase the risk of cutaneous infections because of the continuous dampness of the skin [2]. Patients with hyperhidrosis have a decreased quality of life, which is comparable with that observed in patients with acne vulgaris or psoriasis [3, 4].

Hyperhidrosis can be classified as a primary or secondary disorder, and may have focal or generalized manifestations [5]. Primary hyperhidrosis

D. Hexsel (✉)
Brazilian Center for Studies in Dermatology,
Porto Alegre, Brazil

Hexsel Dermatology Clinic,
Porto Alegre, Rio de Janeiro, Brazil
e-mail: doris@hexsel.com.br

F.O. Camozzato
Brazilian Center for Studies in Dermatology,
Porto Alegre, Brazil

© Springer International Publishing Switzerland 2018
R.R. Bonamigo, S.I.T. Dornelles (eds.), *Dermatology in Public Health Environments*,
https://doi.org/10.1007/978-3-319-33919-1_67

is most often focal and usually causes idiopathic, symmetrically bilateral excessive sweating [6]. Secondary hyperhidrosis manifests most often as generalized excessive sweating related to an underlying medical condition or to the use of a medication [5]. The cause of hyperhidrosis should always be investigated and treated whenever possible.

Epidemiology

Currently hyperhidrosis affects about 1–3% of the population [7, 8]. One epidemiologic survey estimated that 0.5% of the US population may be suffering from the effects of hyperhidrosis, with major interference in daily activities [6]. However, this number may be underestimated, because hyperhidrosis is underreported by patients and underdiagnosed by healthcare professionals [6]. A study conducted in the United States to determine the prevalence of hyperhidrosis sent a survey inquiring about excessive sweating to 150,000 US households and concluded that 2.8% of the US population is affected by hyperhidrosis [6].

Data suggest no difference in the incidence between men and women [6]. However, studies in Japan [7] and Germany [8] found that the incidence of hyperhidrosis is higher in men than in women: 16.66% versus 10.66% and 18.1% versus 13.3%, respectively. Men reported higher intensity of hyperhidrosis symptoms than women in a study of Polish students [9], but in a study of Canadian patients, women reported being more severely affected than men [10]. Another study found that the most patients with hyperhidrosis (93%) had primary hyperhidrosis [5].

The onset of primary hyperhidrosis usually takes place between the ages of 14 and 25 years. When the onset happens at a prepubertal age, normally the palmar or plantar areas are affected, with presentations in the axillary, facial, or abdominal and dorsal regions less likely. A postpubertal onset is more often associated with an axillary distribution [10].

A positive family history is present in 35–56% of patients with hyperhidrosis. The inheritance pattern has a variable penetrance and is most likely autosomal dominant [2, 6, 10]. However, one study found a higher association with a positive family history in patients with primary palmar hyperhidrosis, with 65% of patients having a positive family history [11]. Earlier age at onset (<20 years of age) also correlated with a positive family history [10].

Hyperhidrosis is potentially underdiagnosed and undertreated. To properly diagnose this condition the physician should question the patients, during a routine review of systems, about sweating and how it affects the patient's quality of life.

Etiopathogenesis

The skin appendages are composed of the eccrine and apocrine sweat glands, the hair follicles, the sebaceous glands, and the nails. All of these are embryonically derived from buds of epidermis that grow down into the dermis to form these specialized structures.

Eccrine sweat glands are distributed all over the body surface, except in the external auditory conduit, vermilion border, nail bed, clitoris, and labia minora [12]. These glands are most numerous on the palms, soles, face, axilla, and, to a lesser extent, the back and chest [13]. The number varies greatly with site, occurring more densely on the soles compared with the thighs, and also vary in size from person to person [12]. Histologically, the eccrine gland is divided into three subunits with a snarled secretory portion located at the dermal–hypodermal junction or lower dermis; in an intradermal sweat conduit, which also constitutes half of the basal layer; and in an intraepidermal sweat conduit [14]. The secretory portion consists of an external layer of contractile myoepithelial cells that mobilize sweating secretion. These cells secrete a hypotonic saline solution and are innervated by cholinergic postganglionic sympathetic nerve fibers [15, 16] responding to the cholinergic stimuli. There is no relationship between the density of eccrine glands in normal individuals and the density of eccrine glands in those who suffer from focal hyperhidrosis [17].

Apocrine sweat glands (ASG) are part of the pilosebaceous unit [15] that is composed of hair follicles and sebaceous glands. Apocrine glands are specialized sweat glands that secrete a solution with high oil content and are under adrenergic control [18]. Apocrine glands are usually restricted to a few regions such as axillae, anogenital region, periumbilical region, perimammary area, prepuce, scrotum, in a modified form of glands in the external auditory conduit (ceruminous glands), eyelids (Moll glands), and mamma (mammary glands) [18, 19]. In the normal axillary region, apocrine glands outnumber eccrine glands by approximately 10 to 1 [13]. Histologically, ASG may be divided in three segments: a secretory portion, an intradermal channel, and an intraepidermal channel [17]. The secretory portion is composed of a single layer of columnar cells whose size reflects their secreting activity [18]. These glands release a portion of their cytoplasm into the glandular lumen, which is called decapitation secretion [18]. Proteins, ammonia, sugars, fatty acids, and sometimes chromogens constitute the apocrine secretion. The secretion is odorous, and it is assumed that the odor is due to products excreted by local bacterial skin flora [19]. The function of apocrine glands in humans is not fully elucidated, although it is thought that they may be important for body odor and pheromones [17]. They are activated after reaching sexual maturity.

A third type of gland, described by Sato et al., was termed *"apoeccrine"* because they contain morphologic features common to the other two types [20]. Histologically this gland is subdivided into three portions, with a secretory portion, which features an irregular dilated segment and another nondilated segment; an intradermal channel; and an intraepidermal channel. Secreting cells resemble the eccrine gland light cells in the nondilated segment; however, they resemble apocrine glands in the dilated region [20]. Ductal opening occurs at the epidermal level, as is the case for eccrine glands [21]. Apoeccrine glands receive sympathetic innervation and respond to cholinergic stimuli and epinephrine. They apparently develop after adolescence in both sexes [20]. These glands produce copious, watery fluid and can represent 10–45% of all axillary glands [19].

The degree to which each gland type is involved in hyperhidrosis is unknown, but is believed to be of eccrine origin because of its profuse nature and watery consistency [17, 21]. This fact, however, does not exclude the possibility that other glands may be involved [17, 21].

The cause of hyperhidrosis is unknown, but it has been postulated that this condition occurs as a primary process of autonomic neuronal dysfunction, as the sweat glands and their innervation do not show any histologic abnormalities. This dysfunction tends to occur in areas where there is a higher concentration of eccrine glands such as the palms, soles, and axillae, which are sweat-producing glands. Less common sites are the scalp or face [15].

A central sudomotor efferent pathway is suggested for hyperhidrosis with the following connections: (1) cerebral cortex to hypothalamus; (2) hypothalamus to medulla; (3) fibers crossing in the medulla oblongata and travelling to the lateral horn of the spinal cord; (4) the lateral horn to sympathetic ganglia; and (5) sympathetic ganglia to sweat glands as postganglionic C fibers [15]. Sweat gland innervation is sympathetic and postganglionic, with acetylcholine as primary neurotransmitter [18]. These fibers consist of unmyelinated class C fibers [15]. Norepinephrine and vasoactive intestinal peptide (VIP) may play a role, but neither of these amplifies cholinergic sweat secretion [22].

Emotional stimuli alone can activate sweat glands. Frontal and premotor projections to the hypothalamus probably promote sweating during enhanced emotions [18]. The hypothalamic sweat center, which is in charge of the palms, soles, and in some individuals the axilla, seems to be distinct from the other hypothalamic sweat centers and is actually under exclusive control of the cortex, with no input from the thermosensitive elements. Because emotional sweating does not occur during sleep or sedation, one of the criteria for primary hyperhidrosis is that the individual does not experience sweating during sleep. Sympathetic cholinergic nerves activate both thermoregulatory and emotional sweating and are controlled by different central nervous system neurons. It is possible that primary hyperhidrosis is due to abnormal central control of emotional sweating, given that it affects the same body areas as those affected in emotional sweating (hands, feet, and axillae) [23].

Classification

Primary Hyperhidrosis

Primary hyperhidrosis is excessive sweating in specific regions of the body, the sweating itself being the medical problem [5]. *Primary hyperhidrosis* is usually symmetric, starts in childhood or in the second decade of life, and is often hereditary. This form of hyperhidrosis is not secondary to medical conditions or medications, and the diagnostic criteria are shown in Table 67.1.

Table 67.1 Criteria for diagnosis of Hyperhidrosis [5, 54, 67]

Primary hyperhidrosis	Excessive sweating focal and visible of at least 6 months' duration without any apparent cause and at least two of the following:
	Bilateral and relatively symmetric
	Impairs daily activities
	At least one episode per week
	Age of onset <25 years
	Family history of hyperhidrosis
	Cessation of focal sweating during sleep
	Exclusion of secondary causes of excessive sweating
Secondary generalized hyperhidrosis	Generalized excessive sweating attributable to a definitive underlying medical cause: most commonly drugs, cardiovascular disorders, respiratory failure, infections, malignancies, endocrine disease, metabolic disorders, neurologic disease, among others
Secondary focal hyperhidrosis	Excessive sweating in typical anatomic sites as palms, soles, axillae, craniofacial, or in a well-defined anatomic distribution such as trunk, inguinal folds, buttocks, legs, submammary folds, neck, or wrist *and* identification of a definitive underlying cause; most commonly Frey syndrome, eccrine nevus, social anxiety disorder, neurologic disorder, or tumor

Adapted from Walling [5]

When excessive sweating affects only a specific part of the body it is called localized hyperhidrosis [1]. Common focal sites for primary hyperhidrosis include palms, soles, axillae, craniofacial area, inguinal area, and gluteal region. Palmar, plantar, and axillary hyperhidrosis are the most common [5, 6]. Patients with primary hyperhidrosis may have one or multiple sites of involvement, as palmar hyperhidrosis alone, palmar and axillary hyperhidrosis, or various other combinations of focal involvement [6, 24].

Axillary Hyperhidrosis

Axillary hyperhidrosis (AH) is excessive sweating specifically in the area of the axillae and usually presents with a bilateral pattern. While it can be continuous, it is more commonly phasic. It may be precipitated by heat, mental stress, or exercises [25] and is associated with dermatologic complications including pompholyx, contact dermatitis, bromhidrosis, chromhidrosis, and intertrigo [26]. Its onset is usually after puberty.

Plantar and Palmar Hyperhidrosis

In palmoplantar hyperhidrosis the feet and hands are often cold because of perspiration evaporation, which also stimulates the sympathetic nervous system and contributes to aggravating hyperhidrosis [27]. This form of hyperhidrosis constitutes a substrate for the establishment of fungal infection and contact dermatitis. It fosters the appearance of bacterial infections and keratolysis plantare sulcatum, whereas palmar hyperhidrosis may be associated with dyshidrosis.

Inguinal Hyperhidrosis or Hexsel's Hyperhidrosis

Hexsel's hyperhidrosis is often associated with other forms of hyperhidrosis [28]. It symmetrically affects the groin region, including the suprapubic area, the shallow depression that lies immediately below the fold of the groin, the medial surfaces of the upper inner thighs, and the genital area. It may also include the lower part of the gluteus maximus, gluteal fold, and natal cleft [29]. Patients with this condition have difficulty in concealing the often-embarrassing sweat-drenched clothing in this area that typically results from having the disorder.

Prevalence is largely unknown because of under-reporting, but the condition appears less frequently than other forms of focal hyperhidrosis. Fifty percent of patients with Hexsel's hyperhidrosis have a positive family history of some form of hyperhidrosis, suggesting an inherited mechanism [29].

Localized Unilateral Hyperhidrosis

Localized unilateral hyperhidrosis is usually seen as a sharply demarcated region of sweating on the forearm or forehead restricted to less than 10 × 10 cm. Most cases are idiopathic with no triggering factors. The pathogenesis is unclear [30], and one case report suggests that there is a hypohidrotic element to the disorder [31]. Fewer than 40 cases have been reported in the literature [31].

Secondary Hyperhidrosis

Secondary hyperhidrosis is usually generalized and is due to an underlying cause. This condition can be further classified as focal or generalized.

Secondary Generalized Hyperhidrosis

Secondary generalized hyperhidrosis is caused by a medication or a medical condition. Conditions that may cause secondary hyperhidrosis can be physiologic, such as pregnancy, menopause, fever, excessive heat; or pathologic, including malignancy, lymphoma, carcinoid syndrome, diabetes mellitus, thyrotoxicosis, diabetes insipidus, hyperthyroidism, pheochromocytoma, tuberculosis, HIV (human immunodeficiency virus), endocarditis, and autonomic dysreflexia, among others [5, 32, 33]. There are many drugs that are known to cause secondary hyperhidrosis, including antidepressants, hypoglycemic agents, tryptans, antipyretics, cholinergics, sympathomimetic agents, and many others. Psychiatric disorders can also present with hyperhidrosis. Secondary hyperhidrosis is a clinical feature in 32% of persons with social anxiety disorder [34, 35]. Some debate exists, however, over whether the relationship between these two entities is causal [36].

Secondary causes of hyperhidrosis must be ruled out before diagnosing primary hyperhidrosis [5, 32]. This is best accomplished by a complete review of systems and additional follow-up as appropriate based on the patient response. Some clinical features help distinguish between primary and secondary types of hyperhidrosis and include onset of the disease, characteristics of the sweating, and associated symptoms [5]. The onset of symptoms in patients with secondary hyperhidrosis is more likely later than in patients with primary hyperhidrosis. Patients with secondary hyperhidrosis are more likely to exhibit unilateral or asymmetric sweating, or be generalized, and to have symptoms during sleep ("night sweats"). Secondary hyperhidrosis is less often associated with positive family history [5].

Secondary Focal Hyperhidrosis

Although rare, multiple types of focal secondary hyperhidrosis exist.

Gustatory Sweating

Gustatory sweating is characterized by profuse sweating of the face, scalp, and neck [37]. A physiologic type of gustatory sweating occurs as bilateral facial sweating secondary to heat or to the ingestion of hot or spicy foods. Nonphysiologic types of gustatory sweating are caused by sympathetic nerve damage from neoplasm or sympathectomy, auriculotemporal nerve syndrome, diabetic neuropathy, or infection [37–39].

Gustatory sweating is a common postsurgical complaint occurring in patients after parotidectomy, usually for adenoma. It can be a component of Frey's syndrome, which also includes parotid flushing. Frey's syndrome may occur in up to 60% of patients after parotidectomy with facial nerve dissection [39]. Auriculotemporal nerve syndrome can occur sporadically as a familial trait or be due to a preceding trauma to the nerve. Diabetic gustatory sweating may occur as a by-product of sympathetic denervation, which is compensated by innervation of aberrant parasympathetic fibers [38]. These fibers stem from the minor petrous nerve and innervate the parotid gland, causing sweating when salivation is induced. This finding is seen in 69% of patients with diabetic nephropathy and 36% of patients with diabetic neuropathy [37]. Gustatory sweating may also occur after infection, most commonly secondary to herpes zoster infection [33].

Cutaneous Disorders

Secondary focal hyperhidrosis may be seen in conjunction with a variety of cutaneous disorders, although a causal relationship has not been established. Disorders include eccrine nevus, pachyonychia congenita, palmoplantar keratodermas, glomus tumor, blue rubber bleb nevus syndrome, nevus sudoriferous, POEMS (polyneuropathy, organomegaly, endocrinopathy, M protein, skin changes) syndrome, speckled lentiginous nevus syndrome, Riley–Day syndrome, pachydermoperiostosis, Gopalan syndrome, pretibial myxedema, Buerger disease, eccrine pilar angiomatous hamartoma, local injury, and increased size of eccrine glands [40, 41].

Eccrine nevus or nevus sudoriferous can cause localized hyperhidrosis in an area of skin with increased numbers of eccrine glands [42]. Associated hypertrichosis and comedones can be seen in the area. A similar lesion, eccrine angiomatous hamartoma [43], shows an abundance of eccrine glands and a proliferation of vascular channels. Because of clinical and histologic similarities, these lesions may share a similar genetic pathway.

Pachyonychia congenita is a rare autosomal dominant genodermatosis that is often associated with focal palmar and plantar hyperhidrosis. One study found hyperhidrosis in 51.5% of all patients with pachyonychia congenita and in 22.7% of children with the disorder [44].

Other Forms of Secondary Hyperhidrosis

Some types of secondary hyperhidrosis are characterized by anhidrosis in one area with compensatory hyperhidrosis in another area. Most commonly the condition is iatrogenic, in the form of compensatory sweating following surgical treatment of primary focal hyperhidrosis. It may also manifest as part of Ross syndrome or in one of several neurologic conditions [45, 46].

Compensatory hyperhidrosis is a known potential complication of endoscopic thoracic sympathectomy (ETS), which occurs in areas that do not present abnormal preoperative sweating. Its intensity varies [47] and can worsen with climate changes and heat, as well as with psychological and emotional alterations. It can affect the inferior portion of the chest (generally below the nipple), dorsal and lumbar region, abdomen, pelvic waist, popliteal fossa, and lower limbs. An expert consensus of the Society of Thoracic Surgeons reported that 3–98% of patients having had ETS develop iatrogenic compensatory hyperhidrosis [48]. One large-scale study found that only 55% of patients developed compensatory sweating [49].

Ross syndrome is a rare nervous system disorder, with about 50 case reports in the literature [50] characterized by a tonic pupil ("Adie pupil"), deep tendon hyporeflexia, and unilateral or bilateral anhidrosis [46]. It can present with associated segmental hyperhidrosis. Recent studies suggest that Ross syndrome may have autoimmune etiology [45].

Secondary regional hyperhidrosis may be related to stroke, spinal cord lesion, neoplasm, or peripheral neuropathies [51, 52]. One pathophysiologic explanation for this phenomenon is that the primary lesion causes impairment of preganglionic neurons and subsequent anhidrosis, but bladder distension and other visceral stimuli enter the spinal cord distal to the lesion, causing a spinal dysreflexia that manifests as abnormal sweating. The phenomenon has also been called "perilesionary hyperhidrosis" or "border-zone sweating" [51]. Hyperhidrosis can also be associated with syringomyelia and other central nervous system diseases [53].

Associated Factors and Conditions

Heat, stress levels, and physical activities can aggravate hyperhidrosis. Other possible aggravating factors are sexual activity, excessive intake of liquids, weight increase, premenstrual tension, prolonged sitting, and wearing synthetic clothing. Cold acts as an attenuating factor. Some patients also refer to the absence of stress as an attenuating factor.

Hyperhidrosis can also be a triggering and a sustaining factor of other diseases in the affected sites. Besides the excessive sweating, these associated diseases can be aggravated by contact with clothing or products used in the area to decrease perspiration [11], or by the increase in local moisture, with consequent skin maceration and proliferation of microorganisms. The most frequent associated diseases are bacterial and fungal infections, but pompholyx, contact dermatitis [26], folliculitis, erythrasma, and dermatitis can occur. Patients suffering from hyperhidrosis frequently mention bromhidrosis, chromhidrosis, and skin color changes in the inguinal region.

Diagnosis

The criteria for diagnosis of hyperhidrosis are summarized in Table 67.1 [5, 54]. Patient history usually provides all the information required to differentiate common primary hyperhidrosis from potentially worrisome causes (Fig. 67.1) [55].

Asymmetric hyperhidrosis should prompt an investigation for a neurologic lesion. Generalized primary hyperhidrosis is rare, and the diagnosis is made after causes of secondary sweating are excluded.

Some tools are useful for the diagnosis and assessment of hyperhidrosis severity. The Minor test is an important instrument to localize the hyperactive sweat glands in different forms of hyperhidrosis and to assess the response to treatment. This test does not quantify the severity of hyperhidrosis [56], but identifies different sweating intensities. Hexsel and coworkers proposed the Sweating Intensity Visual Scale to classify the sweating intensity. This is a visual 6-grade scale based on the final color resulting from the Minor test: Grade 0 = minimal or no sweating; Grade I = initial, discrete sweating; Grade II = mild sweating; Grade III = moderate sweating; Grade IV = intense sweating; and Grade V= excess sweating [57]. There are also other tools for the assessment of

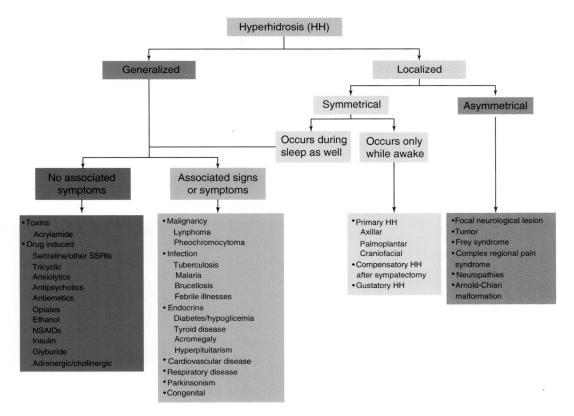

Fig. 67.1 Diagnostic algorithm for evaluation of the patient with pruritus (Adapted from Vary [55])

hyperhidrosis severity, such as the 4-point single-question Hyperhidrosis Disease Severity Scale [56], gravimetry, [58] and the Hyperhidrosis Area and Severity Index [59].

Therapeutic Approach

Depending on the type, location, and severity of the hyperhidrosis, different treatments can be used, including topical, oral, and iontophoretic treatments, botulinum neurotoxin (BoNT) injections, and surgery. To date, an established level of evidence (level A, two or more class I papers) [60] exists only for BoNT-A treatment of axillary hyperhidrosis. Some nonpharmacologic treatments can control the disease.

The Canadian Hyperhidrosis Advisory Committee designed an algorithm to guide the treatment of hyperhidrosis [56]. Mild axillary, palmar, and plantar hyperhidrosis should firstly be treated with topical aluminum chloride. In case of failure, BoNT-A or iontophoresis should be considered. In severe cases, BoNT-A and topical aluminum chloride are first-line therapy. For palmar and plantar hyperhidrosis, iontophoresis is also first-line therapy. First-line therapies for craniofacial hyperhidrosis, regardless of disease severity, include oral medications, BoNT-A, or topical aluminum chloride. Local surgery and endoscopic thoracic sympathectomy should be considered in severe cases of hyperhidrosis, mainly when the patient fails to respond to all other treatment options [56].

Nonpharmacologic Treatment

Weight control In general, an increase in body mass index is associated with an increased need to sweat. Therefore, keeping body mass index within the normal range helps patients with hyperhidrosis [47].

Nonthermogenic diet Some foods activate the sympathetic nervous system, leading to metabolic and endocrine responses after their intake. Such foods include certain legumes, pepper, garlic, coriander, cinnamon, ketchup, salt, ginger, chocolate, coffee, pork, viscera, red meat, milk, milk derivatives, strawberries, cola-based soft drinks, and mate (*Ilex paraguariensis*) infusion, as well as black, green, and chamomile tea [47]. Regarding the diet composition, proteins are the highest contributors to activating the sympathetic nervous system (i.e., they activate thermogenesis), followed by carbohydrates. The intake of food supplements with high quantities of proteins and carbohydrates can also trigger increased sweating.

Physical exercise A daily 30-min walk can help avoid weight increase in sedentary individuals, and additional exertion is sufficient to lose weight and reduce the body mass index.

Clothing Clothes, either social or professional, have to be tolerable to the patient. A thin dry-fit T-shirt or cotton shirt can help distribute the sweat more evenly when used under the clothes [47]. Changing clothes one or more times a day is often necessary, especially on hot, humid days.

Weather conditions Ambient temperature plays an important role in cooling the human body. The thermal sensation of heat increases when the environment is hotter, more humid, and less ventilated, with a consequent increase in sweating intensity. The patients present improvement of the symptoms in cold environments with low humidity and good ventilation [47].

Topical Treatments

Aluminum salts are the main topical agents for hyperhidrosis. Their mechanism of action is attributed either to an interaction between aluminum chloride and keratin in the sweat ducts or to a direct action on the excretory eccrine gland epithelium [61]. Solutions of aluminum chloride concentrations vary between 12% and 20% formulations. Higher concentrations of aluminum chloride and higher salt content in preparations commonly cause irritation or burning, which can limit use. The sweat glands of primary hyperhidrosis are less active during sleep, allowing the metal salts to remain in place when applied at night [62]. Topical agents can be used in all forms of hyperhidrosis (axillary, palmoplantar, and gustatory), although these are more commonly used for axillary and palmar hyperhidrosis. These solutions are effective in milder [62] and severe cases [56] of hyperhidrosis as the duration of effect is often limited to 48 h.

Newer topical preparations have shown an improvement in tolerability, such as a combination of 15% aluminum chloride with 2% salicylic acid gel [63]. The addition of salicylic acid may improve tolerability by hydrating and mitigating the drying effect of alcohol, and may also act synergistically with aluminum chloride given its astringent and antiperspirant properties. Tolerability may also be improved with use of a 20% aluminum chloride spray in a silicone base [63].

Topical anticholinergic preparations such as topical glycopyrrolate improved sweating in certain patients, but efficacy is not consistent [64, 65]. Furthermore, some evidence suggest that the effect may involve systemic absorption of the anticholinergic medication [66–68].

Oral Treatments

Oral treatments can offer significant benefit, but the doses required for clinically meaningful effect cause significant and undesired side effects. Anticholinergic agents (glycopyrrolate, menthatheline bromide, oxybutynin, atropine, and scopolamine) and α-adrenergic agonists (clonidine) are the most used in clinical practice. Anticholinergic agents work by inhibiting the production of acetylcholine at muscarinic receptors [69].

Oxybutynin chloride is a promising medication. This drug can be of great help in the control of primary hyperhidrosis or in compensatory hyperhidrosis when patients tolerate its side effects. The use of oxybutynin has been reported as a therapeutic option in children with hyperhidrosis [70, 71]. It is effective for 6–10 h, or even up to 24 h if continuous-use formulations are taken. The lowest dose of oxybutynin is 5 mg at bedtime, at which dosage patients are not likely to present side effects. Generally the effective dosage requires the intake of 15 mg a day: three intakes of 5 mg fractionated over the course of the day.

A retrospective study [72] included 110 patients with hyperhidrosis treated with oxybutynin. After 3 months of treatment, 79% responded. After 12 months, 62% continued to respond, and the response was considered excellent in 50%. Most of the patients who responded at 3 and 12 months reported mild adverse events. No serious adverse events were observed. Uptitrating the dosing regimen resulted in higher treatment adherence rates than a fixed-dose regimen.

In some cases, the side effects of anticholinergic drugs result in noncompliance with treatment, leading many patients to use these drugs only on social occasions and at the lowest necessary dose. Side effects can be very disabling and include dry mouth, blurring of vision, urinary hesitancy, dizziness, tachycardia, and confusion [69]. Contraindications include myasthenia gravis, pyloric stenosis, narrow-angle glaucoma, and paralytic ileus. Gastroesophageal reflux disease, glaucoma, bladder outflow obstruction, and cardiac insufficiency are relative contraindications.

Oral agents can be used in all subtypes of hyperhidrosis such as axillary, palmoplantar, craniofacial/gustatory, and generalized. However, double-blind studies are available only for axillary and palmoplantar hyperhidrosis. Current evidence indicates that both oxybutinin (one class I study and one class II study) and menthatheline bromide (two class II studies) are probably effective, with level B evidence. Retrospective studies suggested oral glycopyrrolate and clonidine are also effective. Collectively, oral agents have level B evidence (probably effective) with one class I study and three class II studies present in the literature [73].

Iontophoresis

Iontophoresis is the introduction of an ionized substance through application of a direct current on intact skin [74]. Although the exact mechanism of action is unknown, this technique facilitates transdermal movement of solute ions by generation of an electrical potential gradient. This process decreases the perspiration production in the treated areas, partially improving the symptoms [75, 76]. Repeated treatments are required [76]. Although there are devices with special configurations to treat the axilla, palm, and sole regions, there is no special configuration for the inguinal region. Devices for home use are very cost-effective after the initial investment. Tap water over the metal plates improves contact with the skin and provides a source of ions. Iontophoresis is performed initially every 2–7 days, until a therapeutic effect is achieved, after which the treatment can be performed once every 2–3 weeks [74]. Implantable electronic devices such as pacemakers or defibrillators, artificial joints, and application in pregnant women are contraindications.

Botulinum Neurotoxin Type A (BoNT-A) Treatment

BoNT-A is one of the most effective therapies for localized hyperhidrosis. BoNT-A is an inhibitor of acetylcholine release from the presynaptic membranes of neuromuscular junctions, thus preventing cholinergic transmission to postganglionic neuroreceptors. The treatment is applied in focal sites of localized hyperhidrosis such as axilla, palms, soles, face, and scalp. Compensatory hyperhidrosis can be also treated with BoNT-A [47]. Side effects include pain and possible transitory muscle weakness.

As a painful procedure, anesthetic creams and local or truncal anesthesia are useful to increase patient comfort. Trichotomy of the region may be necessary. Minor's test performed in the hyperhidrosis zone delimits the area. Bearing in mind that the sweat glands are located about 2.5 mm below the skin [77], the application should be intradermic, preferably using fine-gauge needles, such as 30-gauge. A simple technique to avoid overly deep injections is to use a cut needle lid over the needle as a shield [78]. Minor's test can be repeated about 1 month after the procedure to identify any residual perspiring areas.

The field of anhidrotic effects of BoNT-A does not vary significantly when the same doses in different dilutions and depths are injected on the back of patients suffering from compensatory hyperhidrosis [79]. However, areas of more intense sweating such as midline demand higher doses to achieve a similar field of anhidrotic effects [79]. These results support that dose is more important than brand, usual dilutions, and depths in determining the size or area of the field of anhidrotic effects [79]. Ideal doses have been the focus of discussion, aiming to obtain more efficacious and lasting results Table 67.2 lists some articles and the proposed doses for the treatment of axillary, inguinal, and palmar hyperhidrosis and the average duration of effects.

Lasers and Microwave-Based Treatment

The efficacy of laser treatments for hyperhidrosis remains unclear. A pilot study evaluated a long-pulsed neodynium yttrium aluminum garnet (1,064 nm Nd:YAG) laser and showed improvement of sweating in patients with axillary hyperhidrosis for up to 9 months compared with the control group [89]. However, another study of Nd-YAG laser hair removal therapy showed a side effect of hyperhidrosis in the treated areas [90].

Microwave energy is a new technology and a nonsurgical option for hyperhidrosis treatment [91–93]. It targets the skin and subcutaneous tissue interface, which causes irreversible thermolysis of eccrine glands. Nestor and Park [94] reported the results of two randomized double-blind, sham-controlled pilot studies with the Ulthera® system (Ulthera, Mesa, AZ, USA) to treat patients with axillary hyperhidrosis. The results showed significant and long-lasting reductions in baseline sweat production, high levels of patient satisfaction, and only minor transient discomfort during treatment [94].

Surgical Therapy

Surgical approaches for focal hyperhidrosis include excision of sweating areas, curettage, liposuction, and thoracic sympathectomy [48]. These procedures are typically reserved for patients who have failed conservative therapy or are not candidates for previously described therapies [56].

Table 67.2 Proposed dose regimens for the treatment of axillary, inguinal, and palmar hyperhidrosis

Authors	HH area	Study design	Patients	Treatment	Results	Duration
Heckmann [80]	Axillary	R, DB, PC, multicenter	158	200 U (ABO) unilaterally vs placebo. Placebo-treated side received 100 U (ABO) after 2 weeks	Equal reductions in sweating with the two doses	26 weeks for both groups
Naumann and Lowe [81]	Axillary	R, DB, PC, parallel group	320	50 U (ONA) vs placebo	Response at week 4: 94% (active group) vs 36% (placebo). At week 16: 82% (active) vs 21% (placebo),	16 weeks
Saadia et al. [23]	Palmar	R, SB comparison of 2 doses, intraindividual	24	50 U (ONA) vs 100 U (ONA) in each palm	At 1 month: significant decrease in sweating. At 6 months: anhidrotic effect evident in both dose groups	6 months
Odderson [82]	Axillary	R, DB, PC	18	100 U (ONA) vs placebo	At 2 weeks: sweat production decreased 91.6% in BoNT ($p < 0.05$). At 5 months: 88.2% reduction in BoNT	5 months
Simonetta Moreau et al. [83]	Palmar	R, DB, active comparator, intra-individual comparison	8	69 U (ONA) or 284 U (ABO) (mean dose)	At 1 month: decrease in mean palmar sweating area: 76.8%, ABO vs 56.6% ONA	17 weeks ABO 18 weeks ONA
					At 3 months: decrease in sweating area was 69.4%, ABO and 48.8%, ONA	
Hexsel [29]	Inguinal	Case series	26	100 U (ONA) 60 and 80 U (ONA) can be used to treat less severe cases	Improvement showed for inguinal HH for first time	6–8 months
Lowe [84]	Axillary	R, DB, PC, multicenter, parallel-group	322	50 or 75 U (ONA) or placebo	At 4 weeks: 75% of subjects in active groups vs 25% from placebo	197 days in the 75-U group and 205 days in 50-U group
Vadoud-Seyedi and Simonart [85]	Axillary	R, DB, side by side	29	100 U (ONA) total dose in both axillae, reconstituted in saline or lidocaine	Similar time of onset and duration of effect, and decrease in sweating. Significantly lower pain in axillae treated with lidocaine-BoNT (29.3 vs 47.5)	8 months

(continued)

Table 67.2 (continued)

Authors	HH area	Study design	Patients	Treatment	Results	Duration
Talarico [86]	Axillary	DB, R, prospective	10	50 U (ONA) in one axilla and 150 U (ABO) in the other	Sweat rate decreased 97.7% in ONA axilla and 99.4% in ABO axilla	260 days for ONA and 290 days for ABO
Gregoriou [87]	Palmar and plantar	Open label	36	100 U (ONA) per palm	Significant improvement in palmar HH	6.2 months
Dressler and Adib Saberi [88]	Axillary	DB, intra-individual comparison	51	First: 100 U (ONA) bilaterally; then: direct comparison 100 U (ONA) unilaterally vs 50 U (ONA) contralaterally	Both doses had similar effects	3–4 months

ABO abotulinumtoxin A, *BoNT* botulinum neurotoxin, *DB* double-blind, *HH* hyperhidrosis, *ONA* onabotulinumtoxin A, *PC* placebo-controlled, *R* retrospective, *SB* single-blind

Curettage or liposuction cannula and surgical excision of glands are mainly indicated for axillary hyperhidrosis. Insertion of a liposuction cannula or curette via a small incision allows near-complete removal of the glands. Local hematoma, seroma, or necrosis can occur, as well as recurrence [95]. In other focal forms, these procedures may result in unacceptable scars.

ETS is mostly indicated for palmar, craniofacial, or axillary hyperhidrosis. This technique interrupts signaling to the sweat glands by disrupting or destroying a portion of the sympathetic trunk at the thoracic level [96, 97]. The main complications are compensatory hyperhidrosis, Horner's syndrome, hemothorax, neuralgia, pneumothorax, and lesion in the phrenic nerve [47].

Glossary

Apocrine sweat glands Larger sweat glands that occur in hair follicles. They appear after puberty.

Apoeccrine sweat glands Contain morphological features common to the eccrine and apocrine sweat glands.

Eccrine sweat glands Small sweat glands that produce a fluid secretion without removing cytoplasm from the secreting cells and that are restricted to the human skin.

Hyperhidrosis Sweating greater than necessary for the maintenance of normal body thermoregulation.

Primary hyperhidrosis Excessive sweating in specific regions of the body and not caused by other medical conditions or by medications.

Secondary hyperhidrosis Excessive sweating caused by medications or medical conditions.

Sympathectomy Procedures that break the sympathetic innervation, thereby blocking stimulation of eccrine glands.

References

1. Leung AK, Chan PYH, Choi MCK. Hyperhidrosis. Int J Dermatol. 1999;38:5617.
2. Walling HW. Primary hyperhidrosis increases the risk of cutaneous infection: a case control study of 387 patients. J Am Acad Dermatol. 2009;61(2):242–6.
3. Lasek RJ, Chren MM. Acne vulgaris and the quality of life of adult dermatology patients. Arch Dermatol. 1998;134:454–8.
4. Higaki Y, Kawamoto K, Kamo T, Horikawa N, Kawashima M, Chren MM. The Japanese version of Skindex-16: a brief quality-of-life measure for patients with skin diseases. J Dermatol. 2002;29:693–8.
5. Walling HW. Clinical differentiation of primary from secondary hyperhidrosis. J Am Acad Dermatol. 2011;64(4):690–5.
6. Strutton DR, Kowalski JW, Glaser DA, Stang PE. US prevalence of hyperhidrosis and impact on individuals with axillary hyperhidrosis: results from a national survey. J Am Acad Dermatol. 2004;51:241–8.

7. Fujimoto T, Kawahara K, Yokozeki H. Epidemiological study and considerations of primary focal hyperhidrosis in Japan: from questionnaire analysis. J Dermatol. 2013;40:886–90.

8. Augustin M, Radtke MA, Herberger K, Kornek T, Heigel H, Schaefer I. Prevalence and disease burden of hyperhidrosis in the adult population. Dermatology. 2013;227:10–3.

9. Stefaniak T, Tomaszewski KA, Proczko-Markuszewska M, Idestal A, Royton A, Abi-Khalil C. Is subjective hyperhidrosis assessment sufficient enough? Prevalence of hyperhidrosis among young Polish adults. J Dermatol. 2013;40:819–23.

10. Lear W, Kessler E, Solish N, Glaser DA. An epidemiological study of hyperhidrosis. Dermatol Surg. 2007;33:S69–75.

11. Ro KM, Cantor RM, Lange KL, Ahn SS. Palmar hyperhidrosis: evidence of genetic transmission. J Vasc Surg. 2002;35(2):382–6.

12. Quinton PM, Elder HY, Jenkinson DME, et al. Structure and function of human sweat glands. In: Laden K, editor. Antiperspirants and deodorants. New York: Marcel Dekker; 1999. p. 17–57.

13. Bovell DL, Clunes MT, Elder HY, Milsom J, Jenkinson DM. Ultrastructure of the hyperhidrotic eccrine gland. Br J Dermatol. 2001;145:298–301.

14. Dobson RL. The human eccrine gland. Arch Environ Health. 1965;2:423–9.

15. Sato K, Kang WH, Saga K, Sato KT. Biology of sweat glands and their disorders. I. Normal sweat glands function. J Am Acad Dermatol. 1989;20:537–63.

16. Hurley HJ, Witkowski JA. The dynamics of the eccrine sweating in man. I. Sweat delivery through myoepithelial contraction. J Invest Dermatol. 1962;39:329–38.

17. Lonsdale-Eccles A, Leonard N, Lawrence C. Axillary hyperhidrosis: eccrine or apocrine? Clin Exp Dermatol. 2003;28:2–7.

18. Lakraj AD, Moghimi N, Jabbari B. Hyperhidrosis: anatomy, pathophysiology and treatment with emphasis on the role of botulinum toxins. Toxins (Basel). 2013;5:821–40.

19. Elder DE, Elenitsas R, Rosenbach M, Murphy GF, Rubin AI, Xu X. Lever's histopathology of the skin. 11th ed. Philadelphia: Press: Lippincott Williams & Wilkins; 2014.

20. Sato K, Ohtsuyama M, Samman G. Eccrine sweat gland disorders. J Am Acad Dermatol. 1991;24(6):1010–4.

21. Naumann M. Hypersecretory disorders. In: Moore P, Naumann M, editors. Handbook of botulinum toxin treatment. 2nd ed. Oxford: Blackwell-Science; 2003. p. 343–59.

22. Sato K, Sato F. Effect of VIP on sweat secretion and cAMP accumulation in isolated simian eccrine glands. Am J Phys. 1987;253:R935–41.

23. Saadia D, Voustianiouk A, Wang AK, Kaufmann H. Botulinum toxin type a in primary palmar hyperhidrosis: randomized, single-blind, two-dose study. Neurology. 2001;57:2095–9.

24. Smith FC. Hyperhidrosis. Vasc Surg. 2013;31(5):251–5.

25. Schnider P, Binder M, Kittler H, Birner P, Starkel D, Wolff K, et al. A randomized, double-blind, placebo-controlled trial of botulinum a toxin for severe axillary hyperhidrosis. Br J Dermatol. 1999;140:677–80.

26. Champion RH. Disorders of sweat glands. In: Champion RH, Burton JL, Ebling FJG, eds. Textbook of Dermatology. 5th edn. Oxford: Blackwell, 1992;3: 1758–9.

27. Almeida AT, Boraso RZ. Palmar hyperhidrosis. In: Almeida AT, Hexsel D, editors. Hyperhidrosis and botulinum toxin. São Paulo: Author's Edition; 2003. p. 167–74.

28. Hexsel D, Ave BR, Hexsel C, Dal Forno T. Inguinal hyperidrosis. In: Almeida AT, Hexsel D, editors. Hyperhidrosis and botulinum toxin. São Paulo: Author's Edition; 2003. p. 181–5.

29. Hexsel DM, Dal'Forno T, Hexsel CL. Inguinal, or Hexsel's hyperhidrosis. Clin Dermatol. 2004;22:53–9.

30. Kreyden OP, Schmid-Grendelmeier P, Burg G. Idiopathic localized unilateral hyperhidrosis. Case report of successful treatment with Botulinum Toxin Type A and review of the literature. Arch Dermatol. 2001;137:1622–5.

31. Kocyigit P, Akay BN, Saral S, Akbostanci C, Bostanci S. Unilateral hyperhidrosis with accompanying contralateral anhidrosis. Clin Exp Dermatol. 2009;34:e544–6.

32. Glaser DA, Herbert AA, Pariser DM, Solish N. Primary focal hyperhidrosis: scope of the problem. Cutis. 2007;79(5):5–17.

33. Chopra KF, Evans T, Severson J, Tyring SK. Acute varicella zoster with postherpetic hyperhidrosis as the initial presentation of HIV infection. J Am Acad Dermatol. 1999;41:119–21.

34. Connor KM, Cook JL, Davidson JR. Botulinum toxin treatment of social anxiety disorder with hyperhidrosis: a placebo-controlled double-blind trial. J Clin Psychiatry. 2006;67:30–6.

35. Davidson JR, Foa EB, Connor KM, Churchill LE. Hyperhidrosis in social anxiety disorder. Prog Neuro-Psychopharmacol Biol Psychiatry. 2002;26:1327–31.

36. Ruchinskas R. Hyperhidrosis and anxiety: chicken or egg? Dermatology. 2007;214:195–6.

37. Shaw JE, Parker R, Hollis S, Gokal R, Boulton AJ. Gustatory sweating in diabetes mellitus. Diabet Med. 1996;13:1033–7.

38. Blair D, Sagel J, Taylor I. Diabetic gustatory sweating. South Med J. 2002;95(3):360–2.

39. de Bree R, Van der Waal I, Leemans R. Management of Frey syndrome. Head Neck. 2007;29(7):773–8.

40. Baskan EM, Karli N, Baykara M, et al. Localized unilateral hyperhidrosis and neurofibromatosis type I: case report of a New Association. Dermatology. 2005;211:286–9.

41. Almeida AT, Boraso RZ. Palmar hyperhidrosis. In: Almeida AT, Hexsel D, editors. Hyperhidrosis and

botulinum toxin. São Paulo: Author's Edition; 2003. p. 41–56.

42. Dua J, Grabczynska S. Eccrine nevus affecting the forearm of an 11-year-old girl successfully controlled with topical glycopyrrolate. Pediatr Dermatol. 2014;31(5):611–2.

43. Sen S, Chatterjee G, Mitra PK, Gangopadhyay A. Eccrine angiomatous naevus revisited. Indian J Dermatol. 2012;57(4):313–5.

44. Shah S, Boen M, Kenner-Bell B, Schwartz M, Rademaker A, Paller AS. Pachyonychia congenital in pediatric patients: natural history, features and impact. JAMA Dermatol. 2014;150(2):146–53. epublished:E1–7.

45. Biju V, Sawhney MP, Vishal S. Ross syndrome with ANA positivity: a clue to possible autoimmune origin and treatment with intravenous immunoglobulin. Indian J Dermatol. 2010;55(3):274–6.

46. Ballestero-Diez M, Garcia-Rio I, Dauden E, Corrales-Arroyo M, García-Díez A. Ross Syndrome, an entity included within the spectrum of partial disautonomic syndromes. J Eur Acad Dermatol Venereol. 2005;19:729–31.

47. Lyra Rde M, Campos JR, Kang DW, Loureiro MP, Furian MB, Costa MG, et al. Guidelines for the prevention, diagnosis and treatment of compensatory hyperhidrosis. J Bras Pneumol. 2008;34(11):967–77.

48. Cerfolio RJ, Milanez de Campos JR, Bryant AS, Connery CP, Miller DL, de Camp MM, et al. The Society of Thoracic Surgeons expert consensus for the surgical treatment of hyperhidrosis. Ann Thorac Surg. 2011;91:1642–8.

49. Drott C, Gothberg G, Claes G. Endoscopic transthoracic sympathectomy: an efficient and safe method for the treatment of hyperhidrosis. J Am Acad Dermatol. 1995;33:78–81.

50. Yazar S, Aslan C, Serdar ZA, Demirci GT, Tutkavul K, Babalik D. Ross syndrome: Unilateral hyperhidrosis, Adie's tonic pupils and diffuse areflexia. J Dtsch Dermatol Ges. 2010;8:1004–6.

51. Saito H, Sakuma H, Seno K. A case of traumatic high thoracic myelopathy presenting dissociated impairment of rostral sympathetic innervations and isolated segmental sweating on otherwise anhidrotic trunk. J Exp Med. 1999;188:95–102.

52. Nishimura J, Tamada Y, Iwase S, Kubo A, Watanabe D, Matsumoto Y. A case of lung cancer with unilateral anhidrosis and contralateral hyperhidrosis as the first clinical manifestation. J Am Acad Dermatol. 2011;65(2):438–40.

53. Smith CD. A hypothalamic stroke producing recurrent hemihyperhidrosis. Neurology. 2001;56:1394–6.

54. Hornberger J, Grimes K, Naumann M, Glaser DA, Lowe NJ, Naver H, et al. Recognition diagnosis, and treatment of primary focal hyperhidrosis. J Am Acad Dermatol. 2004;51(2):274–86.

55. Vary JC Jr. Selected disorders of skin appendages – acne, alopecia, hyperhidrosis. Med Clin N Am. 2015;99(6):1195–211.

56. Solish N, Bertucci V, Dansereau A, Hong HC, Lynde C, Lupin M, et al. A comprehensive approach to the recognition, diagnosis, and severity-based treatment of focal hyperhidrosis: recommendations of the Canadian Hyperhidrosis Advisory Committee. Dermatol Surg. 2007;33:908–23.

57. Hexsel D, Rodrigues TC, Soirefmann M, Zechmeister-Prado D. Recommendations for performing and evaluating the results of the minor test according to a sweating intensity visual scale. Dermatol Surg. 2010;36:120–2.

58. Steiner D. Quantitative sweats tests: iodine-starch and gravimetry. In: Almeida ART, Hexsel DM, editors. Hyperhidrosis and botulinum toxin. São Paulo: Edition of authors; 2004. p. 59–61.

59. Bahmer F, Sachse M. Hyperhidrosis area and severity index. Dermatol Surg. 2008;34:1744–5.

60. French J, Gronseth G. Lost in a jungle of evidence: we need a compass. Neurology. 2008;71:1634–8.

61. Shelley WB, Hurley HJ Jr. Studies on topical antiperspirant control of axillary hyperhidrosis. Acta Derm Venereol. 1975;55:241–60.

62. Walling HW, Swick BL. Treatment options for hyperhidrosis. Am J Clin Dermatol. 2011;12:285–95.

63. Flanagan KH, Glaser DA. An open-label trial of the efficacy of 15% aluminium chloride in 2% salicylic acid gel base in the treatment of moderate-to-severe primary axillary hyperhidrosis. J Drugs Dermatol. 2009;8:477–80.

64. MacKenzie A, Burns C, Kavanagh G. Topical glycopyrrolate for axillary hyperhidrosis. Br J Dermatol. 2013;69:483–4.

65. Baker D. Topical glycopyrrolate spray 2% reduces axillary hyperhidrosis to a similar extent as Botox injections. Br J Dermatol. 2013;169(Suppl. 1):4.

66. Panting KJ, Alkali AS, Newman WD, Sharpe GR. Dilated pupils caused by topical glycopyrrolate for hyperhidrosis. Br J Dermatol. 2008;158:187–8.

67. Johnson C, Smereck J. Unilateral mydriasis due to a topical 'antisweat' preparation. J Emerg Med. 2013;44:673–5.

68. Madan V, Beck MH. Urinary retention caused by topical glycopyrrolate for hyperhidrosis. Br J Dermatol. 2006;155:634–5.

69. Glaser DA. Oral medications. Dermatol Clin. 2014;32:527–32.

70. Wolosker N, De Campos JRM, Kauffman P, et al. A randomized placebo controlled trial of oxybutynin for the initial treatment of palmar and axillary hyperhidrosis. J Vasc Surg. 2012;55:1696–700.

71. Wolosker N, Schvartsman C, Krutman M. Efficacy and quality of life outcomes of oxybutynin for treating palmar hyperhidrosis in children younger than 14 years old. Pediatr Dermatol. 2014;31:48–53.

72. Millán-Cayetano JF, Boz J, Rivas-Ruiz F, Blázquez-Sánchez N, Ibáñez CH, Troya-Martín M. Oral oxybutynin for the treatment of hyperhidrosis: outcomes after one-year follow-up. Australas J Dermatol 2017;58(2): e31–5.

73. Stolman LP. Hyperhidrosis: medical and surgical treatment. Eplasty. 2008;8:e22.
74. Stolman LP. Treatment of excess sweating of the palms by iontophoresis. Arch Dermatol. 1987;123:893–6.
75. Togel B, Greve B, Raulin C. Current therapeutic strategies for hyperhidrosis: a review. Eur J Dermatol. 2002;12:219–23.
76. Karakoc Y, Aydemir EH, Kalkan MT, Unal G. Safe control of palmoplantar hyperhidrosis with direct electrical current. Int J Dermatol. 2002;41:602–5.
77. Almeida AT, Cernea SS. Tratamento da hiperidrose. In: Hexsel D, Almeida AT, editors. Uso cosmético da toxina botulínica. Porto Alegre: AGE; 2002. p. 226–7.
78. Hexsel DM, Soirefmann M, Rodrigues TC, do Prado DZ. Increasing the field effects of similar doses of *Clostridium botulinum* type A toxin-hemagglutinin complex in the treatment of compensatory hyperhidrosis. Arch Dermatol. 2009;145(7):837–40.
79. Hexsel D, Soirefmann M, Porto MD, Schilling-Souza J, Siega C. Fields of anhidrotic effects of abobotulinumtoxin A in patients with compensatory hyperhidrosis. Dermatol Surg. 2015;41:S93–S100.
80. Heckmann M, Ceballos-Baumann AO, Plewig G. Botulinum toxin a for axillary hyperhidrosis (excessive sweating). N Engl J Med. 2001;344:488–93.
81. Naumann M, Lowe NJ. Botulinum toxin type a in treatment of bilateral primary axillary hyperhidrosis: randomised, parallel group, double blind, placebo controlled trial. BMJ. 2001;323:596–9.
82. Odderson IR. Long-term quantitative benefits of botulinum toxin type A in the treatment of axillary hyperhidrosis. Dermatol Surg. 2002;28:480–3.
83. Simonetta Moreau M, Cauhepe C, Magues JP, Senard JM. A double-blind, randomized, comparative study of Dysport vs Botox in primary palmar hyperhidrosis. Br J Dermatol. 2003;149:1041–5.
84. Lowe NJ, Glaser DA, Eadie N, Daggett S, Kowalski JW, Lai PY. Botulinum toxin type a in the treatment of primary axillary hyperhidrosis: a 52-week multicenter double-blind, randomized, placebo-controlled study of efficacy and safety. J Am Acad Dermatol. 2007;56:604–11.
85. Vadoud-Seyedi J, Simonart T. Treatment of axillary hyperhidrosis with botulinum toxin type A reconstituted in lidocaine or in normal saline: a randomized, side-by-side, double-blind study. Br J Dermatol. 2007;156:986–9.
86. TalaricoFilho S, Mendonça do Nascimento M, Sperandeo de Macedo F, De Sanctis Pecora C. A double-blind, randomized, comparative study of two type a botulinum toxins in the treatment of primary axillary hyperhidrosis. Dermatol Surg. 2007;33:S44–50.
87. Gregoriou S, Rigopoulos D, Makris M, Liakou A, Agiosofitou E, Stefanaki C, Kontochristopoulos G. Effects of botulinum toxin-a therapy for palmar hyperhidrosis in plantar sweat production. Dermatol Surg. 2010 Apr;36(4):496–8.
88. Dressler D, Adib SF. Towards a dose optimisation of botulinum toxin therapy for axillary hyperhidrosis: comparison of different Botox(®) doses. J Neural Transm. 2013;120(11):1565–7.
89. Letada PR, Landers JT, Uebelhoer NS, et al. Treatment of focal axillary hyperhidrosis using a long pulsed Nd: YAG 1064 nm laser at hair reduction settings. J Drugs Dermatol. 2012;11:59–63.
90. Aydin F, Pancar GS, Senturk N, et al. Axillary hair removal with 1064-nm Nd:YAG laser increases sweat production. Clin Exp Dermatol. 2010;35:588–92.
91. Hong HC, Lupin M, O'Shaughnessy KF. Clinical evaluation of a microwave device for treating axillary hyperhidrosis. Dermatol Surg. 2012;38:728–35.
92. Lee S, Chang K, Suh D, et al. The efficacy of a microwave device for treating axillary hyperhidrosis and osmidrosis in Asians: a preliminary study. J Cosmet Laser Ther. 2013;15:255–9.
93. Glaser DA, Coleman WP, Fan LK, et al. A randomized, blinded clinical evaluation of a novel microwave device for treating axillary hyperhidrosis: the dermatologic reduction in underarm perspiration study. Dermatol Surg. 2012;38:185–91.
94. Nestor MS, Park H. Safety and efficacy of microfocused ultrasound plus visualization for the treatment of axillary hyperhidrosis. J Clin Aesthet Dermatol. 2014;7(4):14–21.
95. Feldmeyer L, Bogdan I, Moser A, Specker R, Kamarashev J, French LE, et al. Short- and long-term efficacy and mechanism of action of tumescent suction curettage for axillary hyperhidrosis. J Eur Acad Dermatol Venereol. 2015;29(10):1933–7.
96. Ojimba TA, Cameron AE. Drawbacks of endoscopic thoracic sympathectomy. Br J Surg. 2004;91:264–9.
97. Bell D, Jedynak J, Bell R. Predictors of outcome following endoscopic thoracic sympathectomy. ANZ J Surg. 2014;84:68–72.

Alopecia

68

Giselle Martins, Isabella Doche, Laura Freitag, Maria Miteva, and Patricia Damasco

Key Points Summary
- Knowledge about of different types of scarring and nonscarring alopecia is very important
- Dermoscopy and scalp biopsy are tools to aid the etiologic diagnosis of alopecia
- The treatment of alopecia must be individualized

G. Martins (✉)
Irmandade Santa Casa de
Misericódia de Porto Alegre, Porto Alegre, Brasil
e-mail: gisellempinto@yahoo.com.br

I. Doche
University of Sao Paulo, Sao Paulo, Brazil

University of Minnesota, Minneapolis, MN, USA
e-mail: isabelladoche@gmail.com

L. Freitag
Private Clinic, Santa Maria,
Brazil
e-mail: md.laurafreitag@gmail.com

M. Miteva
Department of Dermatology and Cutaneous Surgery,
University of Miami, Miami, USA
e-mail: mmiteva@med.miami.edu

P. Damasco
Dermatology, Hospital Regional Asa Norte/Private
Office, Brasilia, Brazil
e-mail: patdamasco@gmail.com

Concepts The word *alopecia* has been used to designate all kinds of hair loss; however, the most important differentiation is between scarring and nonscarring alopecia. This concept is important in helping to find the correct diagnosis and establish the prognosis.

Hair Shaft Disorders

Hair shaft abnormalities encompass a group of congenital or acquired alterations that can lead to variations in hair appearance, texture, density, and growth capacity with or without increased hair fragility [1]. These changes may be occasional findings or important clues for the diagnosis of systemic or localized disorders and genetic syndromes [2, 3].

Dermoscopy, optic microscopy, and polarized light microscopy of hair shafts, in addition to a complete anamnesis and physical examination, are essential to a correct diagnosis. To treat the cause and minimize hair shaft damage are the mean aims for these conditions.

Structural hair abnormalities associated with increased hair fragility comprise monilethrix, trichorrhexis invaginata, trichorrhexis nodosa, pili torti, and trichothiodystrophy. However, some hair shaft disorders are not associated with increased hair fragility, for example, pili annuati and woolly hair.

© Springer International Publishing Switzerland 2018
R.R. Bonamigo, S.I.T. Dornelles (eds.), *Dermatology in Public Health Environments*,
https://doi.org/10.1007/978-3-319-33919-1_68

Monilethrix

Introduction and Etiopathogenesis Monilethrix is a rare hereditary autosomal dominant human hair disorder in which affected fragile hairs have a unique beaded morphology. It is caused by mutations in type II hair cortex keratins KRT86 (most of all), KRT81, and KRT83, and chromosome 12q13 [3]. In addition, autosomal recessive mutations have been found in the gene that encodes desmoglein 4.

Clinical Presentation and Diagnosis The monilethrix phenotype is variable even among members of the same family; in the mildest forms dystrophic hair may be confined to the occiput, but more severely affected individuals have near total alopecia [2]. Hair is usually normal at birth and is replaced with abnormal hair within the first few months of life. Hair is beaded and fragile, which tends to break at points of narrowing, thus leading to short, stubby hair, especially at the sites of friction such as the nape and occipital areas. In more extensive cases the eyebrows, eyelashes, pubic area, axillary area, arms, legs, and nails may be involved (especially koilonychia). Perifollicular erythema, follicular keratosis of the affected scalp, and keratosis pilaris are also typical [4, 5].

Dermoscopy shows hair abnormalities of terminal and vellus hair, with uniform and elliptical nodes and intermittent constrictions, leading to hair thickness variations [6]. The nodes are the normal diameter of the shaft and the internodes represent atrophic parts [2]. The hairs are bent at regular intervals and usually break in constricted areas [6], as seen in Fig. 68.1.

In the differential diagnosis pseudomonilethrix, pili torti, and "monilethrix-like" shafts must be excluded. Pseudomonilethrix is a developmental hair shaft defect characterized by irregular nodes along the hair shaft, with fragility and hair breakage resulting in partial baldness. No follicular papule can be seen. On electron microscopy, the pseudomonilethrix nodes appear to be an optical illusion, and the constriction sites show real indentations protruding beyond the normal shaft [2]. Monilethrix-like shafts show similar ovoid hair shaft constrictions without characteristic typical regularity. They can be found in alopecia areata and lichen planopilaris, and after chemotherapy [6].

Therapeutic Approach Counseling the patient and avoiding hair trauma represent the most effective treatment. Oral acitretin and topical minoxidil can help in some cases.

Trichorrhexis Invaginata

Introduction and Etiopathogenesis Trichorrhexis invaginata (bamboo hair) is a follicular abnormality with hair shaft fracture resulting from invagination of the shaft's distal portion into the proximal portion, due to a cornification defect. It is pathognomonic of Netherton syndrome, a rare autosomal recessive disease that combines ichthyosis linearis circumflexa, erythroderma, growth retardation, failure to thrive, and atopic state [2, 7]. The disorder results from mutation with function lost on the *SPINK5* gene, which codes LEKT1, a serine protease inhibitor [5].

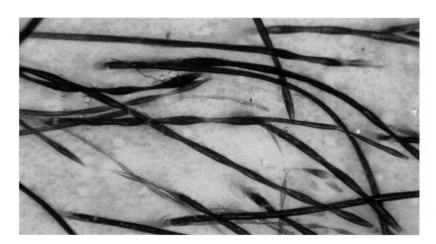

Fig. 68.1 Monilethrix: uniform elliptical nodes and intermittent constrictions (Courtesy of Dr. Giselle Martins Pinto, Porto Alegre, Brazil)

Clinical Features and Diagnosis The hair abnormality usually becomes evident in infancy, showing patchy hair thinning and sometimes complete alopecia. Eyelashes and eyebrows are sparse or absent [2]. Hair shafts tend to be dry, short, sharp, and brittle.

On dermoscopy, trichoscopy shows a hair shaft telescoping into itself (invagination) at several points along the shaft, typical of "bamboo hair" and "golf tee hair." At lower magnifications this may appear as nodular structures located along the hair shaft [8, 9].

The differential diagnosis includes trichorrhexis nodosa, monilethrix, and black piedra [9].

Therapeutic Approach Oral retinoid therapy seems to improve keratinization and hair appearance. In adults the scalp hair tends to improve, but the eyebrow and eyelash alterations tend to persist [2].

Trichorrhexis Nodosa

Introduction and Etiopathogenesis Trichorrhexis nodosa is the most common hair structure abnormality and is not specific for a disease. It consists of hair shaft fracture with splayed individual cortical cells, and their fragments resemble two brushes pushed together [2]. Most cases are acquired and are related to hair trauma or associated with genetic syndromes (i.e., Netherton syndrome, acrodermatitis enteropathica, biotinidase deficiency, argininosuccinic aciduria, citrullinemia, Menkes disease,

and ectodermal defects). Congenital trichorrhexis nodosa is rare.

Clinical Features and Diagnosis Hair shafts seem dry and brittle, with evident hair breaks leaving variable lengths of broken hair and even partial alopecia. There may be intense itching in the affected areas.

Dermoscopy at low magnification shows nodular thickening along hair shafts, which appear as light-colored nodules or gaps, as seen in Fig. 68.2a, b. High-magnification trichoscopy shows hair fibers with typical brush-like ends [8].

The differential diagnosis includes trichorrhexis invaginata, monilethrix, and black piedra.

Therapeutic Approach Reducing trauma and mild cosmetic procedures are the aspects essential to treatment. Early recognition and specific treatment of inherited causes are mandatory.

Pili Torti

Introduction and Etiopathogenesis In pili torti the hairs are flattened and, at irregular intervals, completely rotated through 180° around their long axis [10]. It can be associated with copper deficiency (i.e., Menkes disease) and ectodermal disorders [2]. This hair shaft disorder can be congenital, sporadic, or acquired.

Clinical Features and Diagnosis The classic, inherited, form can be autosomal dominant or

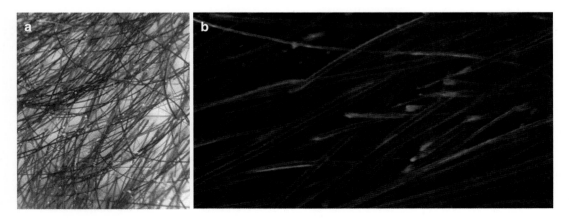

Fig. 68.2 (**a, b**) Trichorrhexis nodosa on dermoscopy: see the white structures along the hair shaft (Courtesy of Dr. Giselle Martins Pinto, Porto Alegre- Brazil)

recessive, beginning in childhood between the third month and third year of life. It is more common in blond-haired girls, and the typical appearance predominates at friction areas, especially temporal and occipital, occasionally affecting eyebrows and eyelashes [2, 11]. The later type, an autosomal dominant disorder, begins after puberty and involves predominately dark hairs. The acquired form of pili torti is related to repetitive trauma, oral retinoids, cicatricial alopecia, and scleroderma. Menkes disease, or trichopoliodystrophy, is a lethal X-linked disease of copper metabolism caused by mutations in ATP7A, a gene that encodes a copper-transporting ATPase. It affects males with classical pili torti, neurodegenerative symptoms, and connective tissue disturbances. Hair is sparse in density, depigmented, lusterless, and feels like steel wool [5]. The most important clue is a marked reduction in blood copper and ceruloplasmin levels. However, these levels may be normal within the first weeks of age, with great reduction after the fourth week [2]. Hair is brittle and breaks easily at different lengths with a spangled appearance in reflected light. There may be only a short coarse stable or circumscribed baldness, irregularly patchy or occipital. The scalp area, less subject to trauma, can be spared [10].

Dermoscopy at high magnification light microscopy reveals a flattened hair shaft twisted through 180° on its own longitudinal axis, irregularly along the hair shaft. Only some shafts and some parts of shafts are affected.

The main differential diagnosis is Bjornstad syndrome, an autosomal recessive disease caused by mutation of the gene BCSIL with associated pili torti and neurosensorial deafness. Isolated twisted hairs can be found in a normal scalp [2].

Therapeutic Approach The conditions usually improve after puberty. Patients should avoid additional traumas. Menkes disease has a poor prognosis and most of the patients die within the first 3 years of life. When diagnosis have been made early, especially before neurologic manifestation, copper-histidine injection may be useful to a certain extent [2].

Pili Annulati

Introduction and Etiopathogenesis Pili annulati is a hair shaft disorder that causes a distinct appearance of the hair with intermittent light and dark bands [2]. The condition may be sporadic or autosomal dominant, and the genetic defect maps to chromosome 12q [11].

Clinical Features and Diagnosis Pili annulati is visualized at birth or in the first year of age. Hair appears bright and without increased fragility, and there may be some additional fragility at lighter areas. The bright bands are subtle, opaque, and shorter than dark bands. Usually 20–80% of hairs are affected. The bright appearance of the bands is due to air-filled cavities within the cortex that scatter the light [2]. Lighter areas extend to 50–100% hair thickness [11, 12].

Trichoscopy shows hair shafts with alternate light and dark bands. In other respects, hair is normal.

For the differential diagnosis, pseudopili annulati is a condition where the alternate-band clinical appearance is an optical effect caused by partial twisting of the hair shaft. Pili torti and fragmented or intermittent medulla must be excluded.

Therapeutic Approach Generally treatment is not necessary, although avoidance of additional hair trauma is desirable.

Trichothiodystrophy

Introduction and Etiopathogenesis The term trichothiodystrophy (TTD) covers a range of phenotypes, with low-sulfur, fragile hair representing the central defining criterion [10]. This is a neuroectodermal complex disturbance, with heterogeneous clinical manifestations and autosomal recessive inheritance. Currently there are three disease types: (1) the photosensitive type, which has mutation at genes encoding transcription-DNA factor IIH (TFIIH) subunits (XPD, XPB, p8/TTDA); (2) the nonphotosensitive type with TTDN1 mutation, and (3) the nonphotosensitive type without TTDN1 mutation and without known genetic basis [11, 13, 14].

Clinical Features and Diagnosis Patients with TTD share the distinctive features of short, sparse, and brittle hair and variable degrees of alopecia. The abnormalities are inversely proportional to the sulfur content. Trauma may lead to transverse break (trichoschisis) or nodes resembling trichorrhexis nodosa [2, 10]. The presence of low sulfur content in hairs and one of trichoschisis, tiger-tail pattern by polarizing light microscopy, or severe cuticular damage are mandatory for diagnosing TTD [2]. Clinical features are variable; persistent alopecia is often found and other body hairs may be affected. Physical and mental impaired and nail and dental dysplasia are frequent. TTD syndromes include BIDS (Brittle hair, Intellectual impairment with low IQ, Decreased fertility, Short stature) and the variants PIBDS (BIDS plus Photosensitivity and ichthyosis) and IBIDS (BIDS with ichthyosis).

Trichoscopy has limited value in TTD, although sometimes it can show trichoschisis. The diagnosis is made by polarizing light microscopy, with the tiger-tail pattern with alternating light and dark bands along the hair shaft. This is not a specific signal but highly suspicious.

For the differential diagnosis, any hair shaft disease associated with increased hair fragility, such as monilethrix, must be considered.

Therapeutic Approach There is no specific treatment. In photosensitive types it is important to avoid solar exposure.

Woolly Hair

Introduction and Etiopathogenesis Woolly hair is a structural hair abnormality not associated with increased hair fragility. It can occur over the entire scalp or part of it as a woolly hair nevus [10]. Its inheritance may be congenital, autosomal dominant, or recessive.

Clinical Features and Diagnosis Tight coiling, fractures, and knots are common. Microscopic examination reveals ovoid or elliptical cross-sections and 180° axial twisting of the hair shaft. Woolly hair is found in association with palmoplantar keratoderma and cardiomyopathy syndromes: Naxos (mutation in the gene for plakoglobin) and Carvajal (mutation in the gene for desmoplakin). In addition, there are autosomal dominant forms associated with ichthyosis and deafness, an acquired type, and a localized woolly hair nevus, a nevoid condition showing different hair texture and color [10].

Trichoscopy demonstrates a hair shaft with waves at very short intervals. The appearance of variable hair shaft thickness results from twists [6].

As differential diagnoses one must consider trichorrhexis nodosa and pili annulati, which sometimes can coexist.

Therapeutic Approach There is no specific treatment.

Inflammatory Scalp Diseases

Psoriasis

Introduction and Etiopathogenesis Psoriasis is a very common inflammatory skin dermatosis affecting 2–3% of the general population. Although the scalp is frequently affected in this condition, few reports of permanent alopecia have been described to date [15, 16]. Itching and scaling are very frequent and can be the sole presentation of the disease, making it difficult to differentiate from seborrheic dermatitis. The precise pathogenesis of psoriasis is unknown [17]. Similarly to other autoimmune diseases, a complex interaction of genetic and environmental factors leading to self-sustained and chronic immune response seems to be critical. Scales are a result of hyperproliferative status of the epidermis with premature maturation of keratinocytes and incomplete cornification, with retention of nuclei in the stratum corneum [18]. More recently, the role of some lipid mediators and neuropeptides, such as substance P, have been studied in the setting of this disease [19, 20].

Clinical Features and Diagnosis Alopecia may be directly related to the psoriasis itself, and can affect both the scalp and other parts of the body. It is characterized by sharply circumscribed erythematosquamous plaques with silvery scales usually extending over the hairline (Fig. 68.3). Immunocompromised patients may present more severe lesions. Psoriatic alopecia most commonly affects lesional skin, but may present as a generalized telogen effluvium. In most cases there is regrowth of hair, but in rare cases it can cause scarring alopecia.

Regarding pathology, classic plaques of scalp psoriasis show psoriasiform acanthosis (regular hyperplasia) with confluent parakeratosis, neutrophils in the stratum corneum (Munro microabscesses), and dilated vessels with perivascular infiltrate in the upper dermis. Necrotic keratinocytes can be found in the epidermis. The sebaceous glands show atrophy and present as epithelial stands of underdeveloped lobules (mantle structures), as seen on Fig. 68.4 [21].

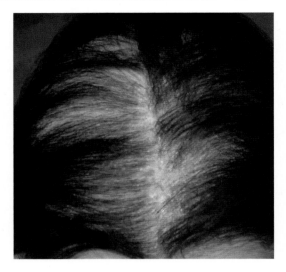

Fig. 68.3 Psoriatic alopecia: erythema, scales, and decreased hair density (Courtesy of the Division of Dermatology, Hospital das Clinicas, University of São Paulo, Brazil)

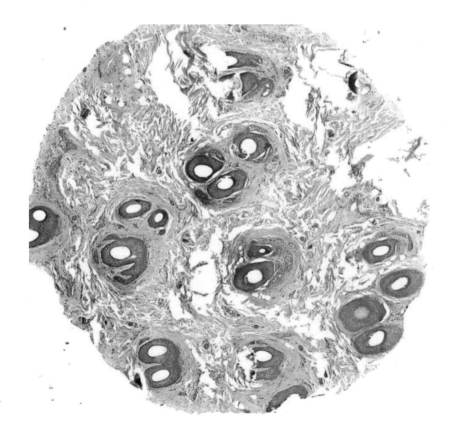

Fig. 68.4 Scalp psoriasis: horizontal sections at the isthmus level. The sebaceous glands are absent and replaced by mantle structures (Courtesy of Dr. Maria Miteva Pinto, Miami, USA)

Since telogen effluvium is a common presentation in scalp psoriasis, there is an increased telogen count in horizontal sections. Prominent eosinophils and plasma cells have been found in scalp biopsies of patients who developed psoriatic alopecia (alopecia areata like) reactions after treatment with tumor necrosis factor α (TNF-α) inhibitors [22].

Dermoscopy of psoriatic alopecia shows interfollicular twisted red loops characteristic of scalp psoriasis, and lack of follicular openings (Fig. 68.5). Silvery scales with keratin casts along the hair shafts can also be noted.

In the differential diagnosis, other causes of flacking include seborrheic dermatitis, contact dermatitis, tinea capitis, and pityriasis amiantacea. Other infrequent conditions include ichthyosis, pityriasis rubra pilaris, zinc deficiency, Langerhans cell histiocytosis, and Wiskott–Aldrich syndrome [23].

Therapeutic Approach Various topical treatment options including steroids, keratolytic agents, and coal tar, and calcineurin inhibitors are available for scalp psoriasis [24]. In some cases, psoriasis treatments may also contribute to hair loss. Application of topical preparations may cause hair loss through friction, and many of the systemic treatments used for psoriasis can also cause hair problems. Treatment with anti-TNF-α agents can precipitate de novo psoriasis and subsequent psoriatic alopecia [25].

Seborrheic Dermatitis

Introduction and Etiopathogenesis Seborrheic dermatitis (SD) is an inflammatory condition of the skin which affects 1–3% of immunocompetent adults [26]. It is more frequent in adolescents and young adults, although a high incidence can be noted in patients older than 50 years. Typical lesions commonly occur on the scalp, face, and chest. SD can worsen during winter time and be more prevalent in patients with immunodeficiencies and neurologic conditions. Dandruff is a mild presentation of the disease, resulting in fine scaling of the scalp. The cause of SD is unknown. Many factors such as sebum production, *Malassezia* sp. colonization, and individual immune response are thought to play an important role in its pathogenesis. The current understanding of dandruff is that while some degree of increased cell turnover may contribute to the amount of flaking, this is not a primary hyperproliferative condition. Rather, any increased cell production is a consequence of inflammation [27].

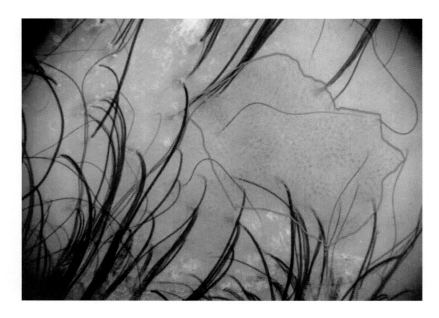

Fig. 68.5 Scalp psoriasis: area of interfollicular twisted red loops (Courtesy of the Division of Dermatology, Hospital das Clinicas, University of São Paulo, Brazil)

Clinical Features and Diagnosis Clinical lesions of SD are characterized by yellowish moist scales over the scalp, and oily areas such as eyebrows, sideburns, and beard, and alar, nasolabial, and postauricular creases. Variable erythema and pruritus may occur. Dandruff is marked by white-grayish tiny flakes that can accumulate and fall from the scalp onto the shoulders. Usually it is not inflamed or pruritic.

In dermoscopy, the most specific trichoscopic features of scalp SD are multiple thin arborizing vessels and yellowish perifollicular and interfollicular scaling (Fig. 68.6) [28, 29].

Regarding pathology, classic SD is rarely biopsied for diagnostic purposes. It may be encountered as a concomitant finding in the scalp biopsies from patients with other primary hair disorders. The main findings are acanthosis (sometimes psoriasiform) with spongiosis and peri-infundibular (shoulder) parakeratosis (Fig. 68.7). There is mild perivascular lymphocytic infiltrate in the upper dermis. Yeast

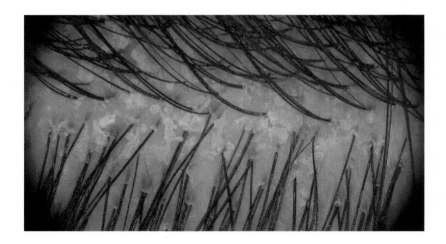

Fig. 68.6 Seborrheic dermatitis: yellowish perifollicular and interfollicular scaling (Courtesy of Dr. Patricia Damasco, Brasilia, Brazil)

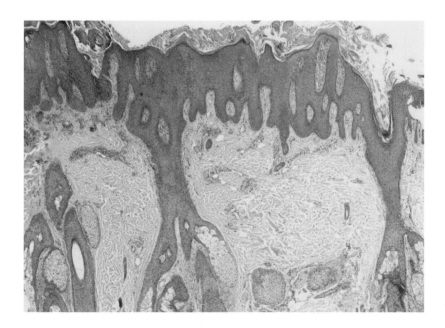

Fig. 68.7 Seborrheic dermatitis: psoriasiform acanthosis with parakeratosis mostly in perinfundibular pattern (Courtesy of Dr. Maria Miteva, Miami, USA)

Fig. 68.8 Seborrheic dermatitis: horizontal section at the level above the isthmus. Note dilated sebaceous canals, spongiosis and parakeratosis in the follicular epithelium, as well as lymphocytic inflammatory infiltrate (Courtesy of Dr. Maria Miteva, Miami, USA)

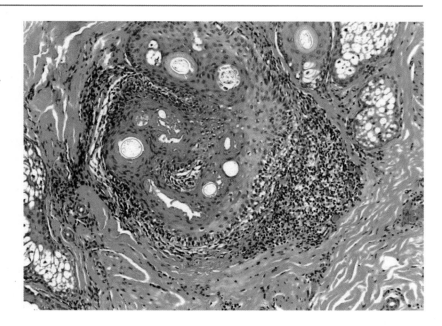

Table 68.1 Treatment of seborrheic dermatitis

Antidandruff and antiseborrheic shampoos (ketoconazole, ciclopirox, selenium sulfide, zinc pyrithione, coal tar)
Topical keratolytics (salicylic acid or urea)
Topical antifungal medications (miconazole or ketoconazole)
Topical low-potency steroids (hydrocortisone, betamethasone, mometasone)
Topical calcineurin inhibitors (tacrolimus, pimecrolimus)
Oral ketoconazole, itraconazole, or terbinafine

forms of *Pityrosporum* can be found in the stratum corneum. The sebaceous ducts are dilated and the sebaceous glands show hypertrophy (Fig. 68.8).

The clinical differential diagnosis includes psoriasis, atopic dermatitis, tinea capitis, discoid lupus erythematosus, and contact dermatitis.

Therapeutic Approach Although there is no cure for SD, patients may be aware that this is a relapsing condition that may require maintenance treatment. SD can be treated with a large number of agents such as antidandruff shampoos, topical low-potency steroids, and oral therapy for resistant cases, as seen in Table 68.1 [30].

Infections Scalp Disease

Syphilitic Alopecia

Introduction and Etiopathogenesis Syphilis is a chronic systemic, sexually transmitted infection caused by the spirochete *Treponema pallidum*. Syphilis can mimic many diseases through its pattern of scalp alopecia. Alopecia is an uncommon clinical manifestation of secondary syphilis, ranging from 2.9% to 7% [31]. The precise pathogenesis of this condition is still unknown. The spirochetes pass through the mucous membranes or minor abrasions of the skin to the lymphatics and bloodstream within a few hours of inoculation. After local proliferation of the causative agent, there is formation of chancre, the primary lesion of the disease. Usually the lesion is rarely noted and cellular immunity results in healing of this primary stage. If not treated, the disseminated organisms result in the late stages of the disease, with essentially underlying vasculitis.

Clinical Features and Diagnosis Syphilitic alopecia can present patterned hair loss such as "moth-eaten," diffuse, or both. The "moth-eaten" pattern is the most common type and is considered to be a pathognomonic manifestation of secondary syphilis [31–33]. The alopecia, which is nonscarring, can occasionally affect hair-bearing areas other than scalp [31, 33]. Alopecia syphilitica often is associated with other mucocutaneous symptoms of secondary syphilis, but the hair loss as a unique clinical presentation is extremely rare [32]. Two basic patterns of secondary syphilitic alopecia have been described in the literature, symptomatic and essential syphilitic alopecia. The first type presents with either a patchy or diffuse pattern associated with skin lesions of secondary syphilis on the scalp or elsewhere over the body (Fig. 68.9). However, the essential alopecia has the same hair loss pattern as symptomatic alopecia but without any other cutaneous feature of syphilis [33].

In dermoscopy, trichoscopic features in syphilitic alopecia are unspecific with few reports in the literature. Decreased hair density, yellow dots, and broken hairs are the most frequent findings [34, 35]. The lack of specific markers such as "exclamation-mark" hairs and comma hairs on trichoscopy can help to rule out alopecia areata and tinea capitis.

Pathologically, in a scalp biopsy from the moth-eaten-like patches of nonscarring alopecia in secondary syphilis there is a markedly reduced number of anagen follicles and an increased number of catagen and telogen follicles [36]. The pathology can be indistinguishable from acute-stage alopecia areata, as the presence of peribulbar lymphocytic infiltrate has been observed in both. Scattered plasma cells when present may indicate the diagnosis. Immunohistochemistry can highlight the *T. pallidum* in in the hair follicles, usually in the perifollicular and peribulbar regions, and helps in the diagnosis.

For the differential diagnosis, syphilitic alopecia can mimic alopecia areata both on clinical and histopathologic examinations [32, 37]. Trichotillomania, tinea capitis, and systemic lupus must be excluded as well. Serologic treponemic tests are fundamental to confirm the disease. It is important to include syphilitic alopecia as a cause of diffuse hair shedding.

Therapeutic Approach Penicillin is the drug of choice for treating all stages of syphilis. A single shot of 2.4 million units of benzathine penicillin

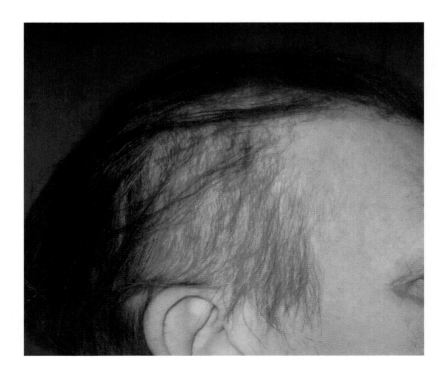

Fig. 68.9 Syphilis: diffuse pattern of alopecia in a patient with secondary syphilis (Courtesy of the Division of Dermatology, Hospital das Clinicas, University of Sao Paulo, Brazil)

G is highly effective for the treatment of primary and secondary infection. In cases of penicillin allergy, tetracycline hydrochloride, 500 mg every 6 h or doxycycline 100 mg, twice daily for 15 days can be used. Treatment for late latent syphilis, tertiary syphilis, or latent disease of unknown duration require a longer duration of therapy.

Tinea Capitis

Introduction and Etiopathogenesis Tinea capitis is a fungal infection that usually affects children between the ages of 4 and 7 years and immunocompromised individuals. Nowadays, the etiology and pattern of the lesions are considered to vary with age, as well with gender and general health condition. The incidence of tinea capitis in the general population seems to be increasing, particularly among African American children who account for more than 80% of the cases [38]. The epidemiology of this disease varies widely, ranging from antropophilic, zoophilic, and geophilic dermatophytes. The main causative organisms of tinea capitis belong to two genera, *Microsporum* and *Trichophyton*, although the organisms responsible for superficial scalp fungal infections also vary considerably with geography [39]. Dermatophytes cause superficial fungal infections by the attachment of the hyphae to the keratinized surfaces including the perifollicular stratum corneum. The organism produces arthroconidia after it easily penetrates the cortex of the hair by way of keratinase enzymes. The hairs that are filled with arthroconidia become fragile and tend to break at the surface of the scalp. Microscopically, ectothrix arthroconidia can be observed in the surface of plucked hairs, while endothrix arthroconidia are localized within the hair shaft.

Clinical Features and Diagnosis The pattern of clinical findings with tinea capitis infection depends on the causative organism and the host inflammatory response. The most common presentation is single or multiple patches of alopecia associated with variable inflammation, scale, and pruritus (Fig. 68.10). Special forms of tinea capitis are kerion celsi and favus. Kerion celsi is a highly inflammatory and suppurative form of tinea capitis, usually caused by zoophilic fungi. It can cause scarring alopecia if not aggressively treated. Favus, also known as tinea favosa, is a rare but severe presentation of tinea capitis, characterized by the chronic fungal infection in endemic regions. In the late phase of the disease it can also cause scarring hair loss. The diagnosis of tinea capitis is based on microscopic examination of infected hairs. Mycologic culture is fundamental for a precise identification of the causative organism. Wood's lamp examination may also be useful in some forms of tinea (Table 68.2).

Dermoscopy is an inexpensive and useful tool that can provide an easy and rapid diagnosis of tinea capitis. The presence of specific trichoscopy features, such as comma and corkscrew hairs, may help to differentiate tinea capitis from other scalp conditions (Fig. 68.11). Comma hairs may be found in both endothrix and ectothrix

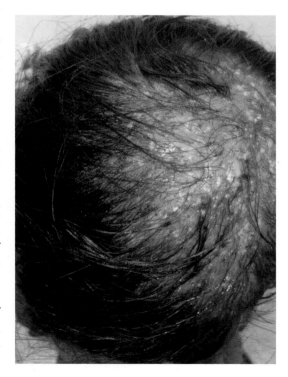

Fig. 68.10 Tinea capitis: inflammation and pustules on the scalp (Courtesy of Dr. Giselle Martins Pinto, Porto Alegre, Brazil)

infections [40]. Corkscrew hairs were first described in black patients with *Trichophyton soudanense*, although a recent publication described this finding in a white adult patient [41, 42]. Broken hairs, although very common, are not specific and may be present also in trichotillomania, chemotherapy, and alopecia areata [43].

Table 68.2 Hair invasion patterns of dermatophytes

Ectothrix infections

Most common organisms: *Microsporum* spp. and *Trichophyton rubrum*

Clinical presentation: annular scaling plaque with less inflammation and scale

Wood's lamp fluorescence: fluorescent (*Microsporum* spp.) or nonfluorescent (*T. rubrum* and *Microsporum gypseum*)

Endothrix infections

Most common organisms: *Trichophyton* spp.

Clinical presentation: multiple plaques with less inflammation and scale

Wood's lamp fluorescence: nonfluorescent

Kerion celsi

Most common organisms: *T. verrucosum*, *T. mentagrophytes*, and *M. gypseum*

Clinical presentation: suppurative, boggy, nodular deep folliculitis with fistulas and pus secretion. Regional lymphadenopathy, fever, and headache may occur

Wood's lamp fluorescence: nonfluorescent

Favus

Most common organisms: *T. schoenleinii*

Clinical presentation: presence of scutulas (small, yellow, scaly crusts) with musky odor. Purulent discharge may occur

Wood's lamp fluorescence: fluorescent

Pathologically, in tinea capitis caused by ectothrix infection (*Mycobacterium canis*) the hyphae and spores cover the outside surface of the hair shaft, which results in destruction of the cuticle. In tinea capitis caused by endothrix infection (*Trichophyton tonsurans*), the inside of the hair shaft is invaded only by rounded and box like arthrospores and not by hyphae (Fig. 68.12).

In inflammatory tinea capitis (kerion) caused by *M. canis*, *T. mentagrophytes*, *T. tonsurans*, *T. rubrum*, and *M. gypseum*, there is dense mixed cell inflammatory infiltrate of neutrophils, plasma cells, eosinophils, lymphocytes, and histiocytes as well as giant cells. The infiltrate involves the follicles and the surrounding dermis and subdermis (suppurative granulomatous folliculitis) (Fig. 68.13). The special stains may be falsely negative [44].

The differential diagnosis of many scalp conditions may mimic tinea capitis, including SD, atopic dermatitis, psoriasis, and trichotillomania. Alopecia areata typically presents as bare scalp patches with no erythema or scale. Pustular and inflamed lesions may rule out bacterial infections and decalvans folliculitis. Dissecting folliculitis may also resemble tinea capitis, but the lack of comma hairs and follicular ostia may lead to the correct diagnosis.

Therapeutic Approach Systemic antifungals should be initiated upon clinical suspicion of tinea capitis, as topical medications alone are ineffective. The most effective drugs are griseofulvin, terbinafine, and the azoles (Table 68.3).

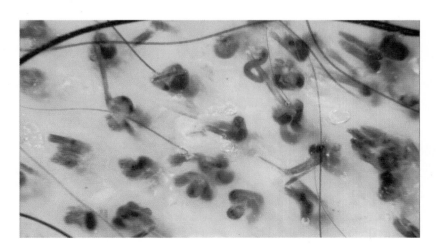

Fig. 68.11 Tinea capitis: dermoscopy shows corkscrew hairs and broken hairs (Courtesy of Dr. Giselle Martins Pinto, Porto Alegre, Brazil)

Fig. 68.12 Inflammatory tinea capitis: horizontal sections at the level of the bulb: there is dense (abscess like) mixed cell infiltrate which extends from the bottom to the surface (Courtesy of Dr. Maria Miteva, Miami, USA)

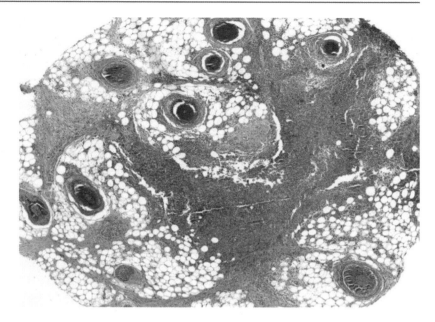

Fig. 68.13 Tinea capitis: the hair shaft is loaded with fungal spores (Courtesy of Dr. Maria Miteva, Miami, USA)

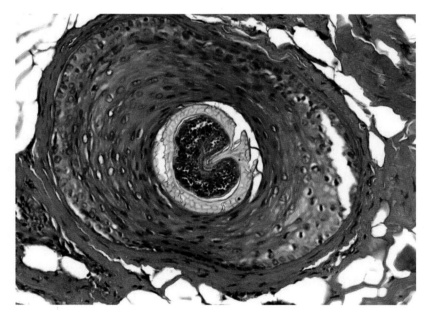

Topical medications such as ketoconazole 2% and zinc pyrithione 1% shampoos should be used to decrease the viability of fungal spores present on the hair, as well as for all household contacts, to prevent infection or eliminate the carrier state [45]. Children can return to school once appropriate treatment has been initiated. Personal hair items should be disinfected or discarded. If a zoophilic organism is isolated, cats and pets should also be treated. Kerion celsi may require oral steroids in the management of inflammation if no response is achieved after 2 weeks of systemic antifungal therapy. Tinea favosa requires that all family members should be treated simultaneously because of its chronic and endemic infection pattern.

Table 68.3 Systemic drugs used for the treatment of tinea capitis

Griseofulvin (first-line therapy for adults and children)
Dosage: 10–15 mg/kg/day (maximum: 500 mg/day) or 20–25 mg/kg/day for microsized formulation
Duration: 6–8 weeks/ continue 2 weeks after resolution of the lesions
Side effects: headache, gastrointestinal discomfort and, rarely, rash and elevated liver enzymes
Notes: better absorption with fatty meals. Eczematous id reaction may occasionally occur in the beginning of the treatment
Terbinafine
Dosage: 3–6 mg/kg/day based on weight
10–20 kg: 62.5 mg/day
20–40 kg: 125 mg/day
>40 kg: 250 mg/day
Duration: 2–4 weeks continuously or 2–4 1-week pulses, 3–4 weeks between pulses
Side effects: headache, gastrointestinal discomfort, rash
Notes: *M. canis* may require longer course
Itraconazole
Dosage: 5 mg/kg/day in capsules
Duration: 2–4 weeks continuously or 2–4 1-week pulses, 2–3 weeks between pulses
Side effects: headache, gastrointestinal discomfort, rash, dysgeusia
Note: Capsules should be taken with food for better absorption. *M. canis* may require longer course. Suspension is not recommended as it has shown increased incidence of pancreatic adenocarcinomas in rats
Fluconazole
Dosage: 6 mg/kg/day
Duration: 2–4 weeks
Side effects: headache and gastrointestinal discomfort
Note: Absorption not affected by the presence of the food

Acquired Nonscarring Alopecia

Acute Telogen Effluvium

Introduction and Etiopathogenesis This condition was first described by Kligman in 1961, as an acute and diffuse hair loss due to a variety of triggers [46]. The normal hair follicle activity is cyclical, consisting of anagen (hair growth phase), catagen (involution phase), telogen (resting phase), and exogen (release phase occurring in late telogen or early anagen) [47]. On the scalp, hairs remain in anagen for 2–6 years, whereas telogen lasts for approximately 100 days [48]. An average normal scalp has 100,000 hairs, with approximately 85% being in anagen, 15% in telogen, and only a few follicles in the transitional or catagen phase [48]. By definition, telogen effluvium (TE) is a nonscarring, diffuse hair loss from the scalp that occurs around 3 months after a triggering event, and is usually self-limiting within 6 months [48]. TE occurs if a significant number of anagen hairs are triggered to stop growing prematurely by any stimulus and subsequently enter catagen phase, followed by telogen phase. After about 2–3 months there is excessive hair shedding [49]. A wide variety of potential triggers have been implicated in the pathogenesis of TE. Postfebrile, postpartum, crash diet, drugs (oral contraceptives, antithyroid drugs, anticonvulsants, β-blockers, oral retinoids), and severe emotional distress are among the most common causes [50].

There are five functional types of TE described by Headington [48].

1. Immediate anagen release, whereby the follicles are stimulated to leave anagen and enter telogen prematurely, resulting in increased TE 2–3 months later. This can accompany physiologic stress, severe illness, and drug-induced hair loss.

2. Delayed anagen release due to prolongation of anagen, resulting in delayed but synchronous onset of heavy telogen shedding. This type typically occurs in postpartum hair loss (telogen gravidarum) or after discontinuation of contraceptive pills.

3. Immediate telogen release occurs with drug-induced shortening of telogen, leading to follicles re-entering anagen prematurely. This type of hair shedding usually occurs 2–8 weeks after initiation of therapy with minoxidil.

4. Short anagen syndrome is characterized by inability to grow long hair because of an idiopathic short anagen phase.

5. Delayed telogen release is characterized by prolonged telogen and delayed transition to anagen. This may be responsible for seasonal hair loss in humans.

Clinical Features and Diagnosis Patients generally present with complaints of visible and diffuse increased hair loss. It can produce thinning of hair all over the scalp and bitemporal recession. Loss is normally not more than 50% of the scalp hair, and the daily rate of shedding can be up to 300 hairs [48].

Dermoscopically, trichoscopy has limited value in diagnosing effluvium. Frequent findings include the presence of empty hair follicles, peripilar sign (perifollicular discoloration), upright regrowing hairs (Fig. 68.14), and increase of follicular units within one hair. The frontal and occipital areas show no significant difference on the trichoscopy findings [51].

Differential diagnosis of TE must include androgenetic alopecia, diffuse alopecia areata, and psychogenic pseudoeffluvium.

Pathologically, the diagnosis of nonscarring alopecia requires horizontal sections of 4-mm punch biopsies. The horizontal sections provide the pathologist with an overview of the follicular architecture and follicular counts performed at several levels from the bulb to the infundibulum [52]. Nonscarring alopecia is characterized by preserved follicular architecture; the follicular units are composed of terminal and vellus follicles and sebaceous glands [53]. Acute TE is rarely biopsied since the condition is self-resolving. There is an increase in telogen count of more than 15%.

Therapeutic Approach Detailed history and clinical examination help to detect the cause of TE. If the cause is not obvious from the patient's history, iron studies, thyroid function tests, syphilis serology, and antinuclear antibody titer should be performed [48]. The most important aspect in the management of TE is counseling the patient about the natural history of the condition. Attempts should be made at identifying and correcting the cause. Hair shedding takes 3–6 months to stop, after which regrowth can be noted 3–6 months after removal of the trigger.

Chronic Telogen Effluvium

Introduction and Etiopathogenesis Chronic telogen effluvium (CTE) presents as a diffuse shedding of telogen hairs that persists more than 6 months. Although some cases of CTE may follow acute telogen effluvium with a known trigger, in most cases a specific trigger cannot be identified [53]. The pathogenesis of CTE is unknown,

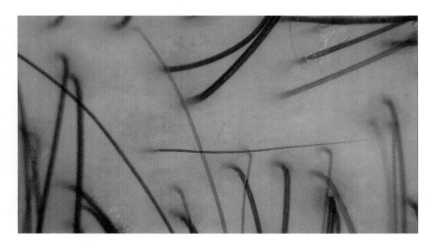

Fig. 68.14 Telogen effluvium: upright regrowing hair and follicle unites with one hair. Note that the terminal hairs are uniform in thickness (Courtesy of Dr. Patricia Damasco, Brasilia, Brazil)

although it has been suggested that it is due to a reduction in the duration of anagen growth phase without hair follicle miniaturization [54, 55].

Clinical Features and Diagnosis Features include an insidious onset and a fluctuating course lasting for several years [55]. It typically affects middle-aged women. On examination there is some bitemporal recession and a positive hair-pull test equally over the vertex and occiput [48]. There is no widening of the central part, and shorter regrowing hairs can be noted in the frontal and bitemporal areas [47]. It is important to reassure patients that this condition represents exaggerated shedding rather than actual hair loss.

Dermoscopy produces results similar to those for acute TE.

Pathologically, a scalp biopsy from CTE is indistinguishable from the normal scalp. There is no or a slight decrease in the number of hairs with normal, and even increased terminal/vellus ratio of 9:1, as well as normal telogen count (up to 15%) [55] (Fig. 68.15).

Differential diagnosis includes androgenetic alopecia, diffuse alopecia areata, psychogenic pseudoeffluvium, and acute TE.

Therapeutic Approach The condition can spontaneously resolve after a decade or so [56].

Alopecia Areata

Introduction and Etiopathogenesis Alopecia areata is an autoimmune disease that presents as a nonscarring hair loss affecting children and adults [57]. Even though it is potentially reversible, it can lead to complete baldness of the scalp and the entire body. In the United States, alopecia areata was estimated to occur in 0.1–0.2% of the general population [57]. Although the exact pathogenesis of the disease remains to be clarified, the genetics of an individual may play roles at multiple levels in the development of alopecia areata. It is regarded as a T-cell-mediated autoimmune disease of the hair follicle

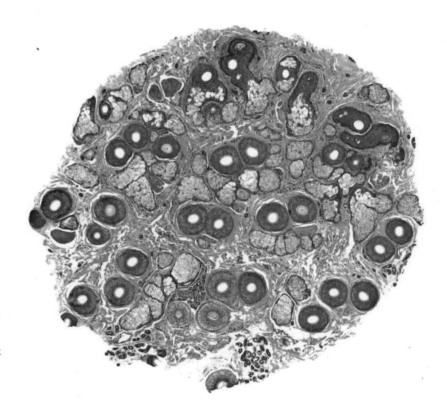

Fig. 68.15 Chronic telogen effluvium: horizontal section at the isthmus level. There is preserved follicular architecture. There are 34 terminal follicles and 3 vellus follicles (terminal/vellus ratio 11:1). The telogen count is 3% (Courtesy of Dr. Maria Miteva, Miami, USA)

that is mediated by CD4[+] and CD8[+] T lymphocytes. Alopecia areata most likely has a polygenic character, whereby susceptibility is dictated by several major genes and the phenotype may be modified by numerous minor genes [58]. An association with other autoimmune diseases has also been reported, such as thyroiditis and atopy [59]. Coexpression of vitiligo and alopecia areata has also been reported at between 4% and 9% [58].

Clinical Features and Diagnosis Alopecia areata can occur virtually in any hair-bearing area, affecting more commonly the scalp. It can present as single or multiple delimited patches of hair loss or diffuse scalp alopecia. In alopecia totalis there is a 100% loss of scalp hair, and if it involves additionally body hair it is called alopecia universalis [57, 59]. The pattern hair loss observed in alopecia areata can vary, including: reticular patches of hair loss; ophiasis type (band-like hair loss in parieto-temporo-occipital area); sisaipho type (reverse of ophiasis pattern, occurring on fronto-parieto-temporal area); and the diffuse variant of alopecia areata, characterized by global decrease in scalp hair density.

Classic alopecia areata lesions are circular patches of hair loss without any accompanying symptoms. The skin is usually normal on examination, but it is not uncommon to see slightly peach or reddened color [60]. The course is unpredictable and typically characterized by phases of acute hair loss followed by spontaneous hair regrowth. However, in severe forms hair loss can persist for many years (Fig. 68.16) [58].

Nail involvement may be observed in alopecia areata, and includes trachyonychia, Beau lines, transverse leukonychia, and red spotted lunulae [61].

Dermoscopically, the features of alopecia areata are regularly distributed yellow dots, micro-exclamation-mark hairs (Fig. 68.17), tapered hairs, black dots, broken hairs, and regrowing upright or regrowing coiled hairs (Fig. 68.3). Depending on disease activity, severity, and duration, the trichoscopic findings may differ [62]. Black dots, tapered hairs, and broken hairs correlates positively with disease activity [63]. Pohl–Pinkus constrictions with variable activity can be seen during the course of a disease (Fig. 68.18).

Pathologically, the findings in alopecia areata depend on the stage of the disease. In acute-stage alopecia areata there is peribulbar lymphocytic infiltrate ("swarm of bees") around terminal follicles in early episodes and around vellus follicles in repeated episodes (Fig. 68.19a) [64]. The infiltrate is composed of both CD4[+] and CD8[+] T-cell lymphocytes, with CD8[+] NKG2D[+] T-cell lymphocytes being the predominant portion. In subacute alopecia areata, there is decreased follicular

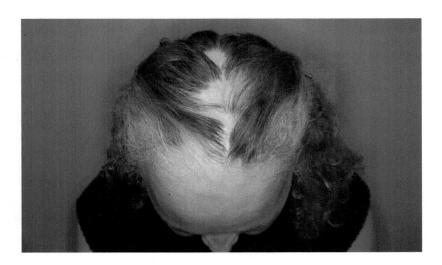

Fig. 68.16 Alopecia areata: multiple patches of hair loss on the scalp (Courtesy of Dr. Patricia Damasco, Brasilia, Brazil)

Fig. 68.17 Alopecia areata: micro-exclamation-mark hairs in alopecia areata (*white arrow*). These hairs are thin at the proximal end and thicker at the distal end (Courtesy of Dr. Patricia Damasco, Brasilia, Brazil)

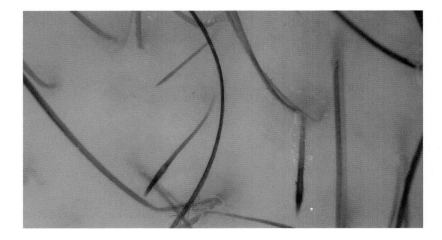

Fig. 68.18 Alopecia areata: black dots, Pohl–Pinkus constrictions, and regrowing upright hairs (Courtesy of Dr. Patricia Damasco, Brasilia, Brazil)

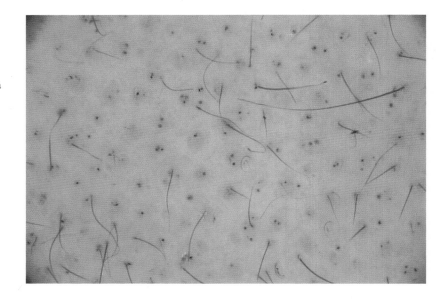

density with a reduced number of anagen and increased number of telogen follicles. The telogen count may be significantly increased, and is composed of catagen and telogen follicles and telogen germinal units (Fig. 68.19b). In the chronic stage there is a decreased number of terminal and an increased number of miniaturized follicles (decreased terminal/vellus ratio), and the biopsies may resemble those of androgenetic alopecia. There is usually no inflammation (Fig. 68.19c).

Trichotillomania and tinea capitis are the most important differential diagnoses. The differentiation of diffuse alopecia areata from TE can be challenging. Lupus and secondary syphilis may also be considered in the differential diagnosis of patchy alopecia areata.

Therapeutic Approach There is still no approved drug in the United States for the treatment of alopecia areata [59] although many are used, for example contact sensitizers, intralesional or topical steroids, systemic steroids, and immunosuppressors. Considering the possibility of spontaneous remission, especially for those in the early stages of the disease, the option of not being treated therapeutically may be an alternative way of dealing with this condition [58].

Fig. 68.19 (**a**) Alopecia areata, acute stage: dense lymphocytic infiltrate affecting the follicular matrix of an anagen follicle. A telogen follicle is noted in the vicinity (Courtesy of Dr. Maria Miteva, Miami, USA). (**b**) Alopecia areata, subacute stage: note the increased number of telogen follicles in this horizontal section (telogen count of 50%) (Courtesy of Dr. Maria Miteva, Miami, USA). (**c**) Alopecia areata, chronic stage: there are only four vellus follicles and no terminal follicles in this biopsy. Note the fibrous streamers in the dermis (Courtesy of Dr. Maria Miteva, Miami, USA)

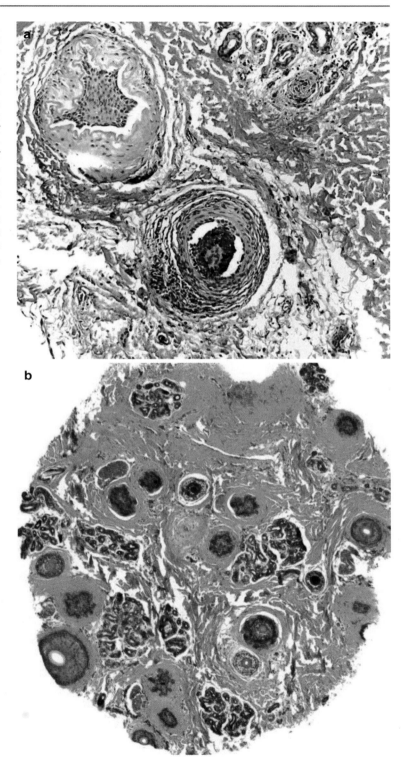

Fig. 68.19 (continued)

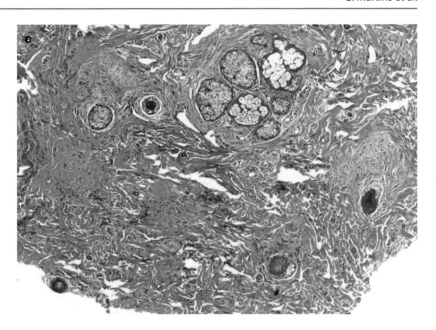

Androgenetic Alopecia or Female and Male Pattern Hair Loss

Introduction and Etiopathogenesis Androgenetic alopecia (AGA) affects both genders and is an androgen-related condition that develops in genetically predisposed individuals [65]. There is a progressive reduction in the average duration of the anagen phase (the growth period) at each hair cycle and, for this reason, the hair follicles become progressively smaller and the hair shorter and thinner. There is also an increase of the physiologic kenogen interval (period between the loss of the hair in telogen and its replacement with new hair), causing empty follicles [66, 67]. The pathogenesis of this disease is polygenic, and in men is particularly related to dihydrotestosterone (DHT). The concentration of DHT levels and 5α-reductase activity are increased on balding areas of the scalp in these patients. In women, the term female pattern hair loss (FPHL) is the preferred appellation, because not all women with this condition present a clear genetic and androgenic trait [68]. Signs of hyperandrogenism (hirsutism, irregular periods) or hyperandrogenemia occur in a subset of women with FPHL, but most women with FPHL have neither [69].

Clinical Features and Diagnosis In the majority of men, balding is patterned, the two major components being frontotemporal recession and loss of hair over the vertex. Hamilton classified male AGA into several stages, and his classification was subsequently revised by Norwood. A small proportion of men show a diffuse pattern of hair loss, similar to FPHL [70]. In FPHL, terminal, thick hair follicles, mainly localized in the frontal parietal scalp and vertex, become thinner, shorter, and less pigmented, and appear very similar to vellus hairs [68].

Dermoscopically male and female AGA share similar trichoscopic features, including hair shaft thickness heterogeneity, thin hairs, yellow dots, peripilar sign (brown perifollicular discoloration), an increased proportion of vellus hairs, and a large number of follicular units with one hair shaft. Honeycomb pigmentation can be observed, which is due to increased sun exposure of an unprotected scalp [71]. In trichoscopy of AGA the abnormalities are more pronounced in the frontal than in the occipital area, as seen on Figs. 68.20 and 68.21.

Pathologically, the main finding is the presence of follicular miniaturization. There is a decreased terminal/vellus ratio of less than 2:1.

Fig. 68.20 Androgenetic alopecia: hair shaft thickness heterogeneity, with multiple vellus hairs, increased proportion of follicular units with one hair, and honeycomb hyperpigmentation (Courtesy of Dr. Patricia Damasco, Brasilia, Brazil)

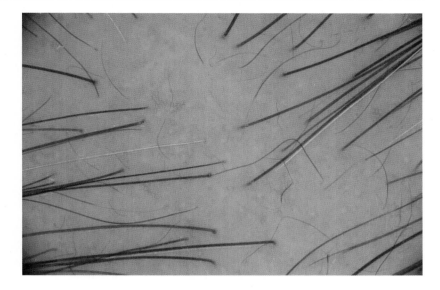

Fig. 68.21 Androgenetic alopecia: yellow dots, thin wavy hair (Courtesy of Dr. Patricia Damasco, Brasilia, Brazil)

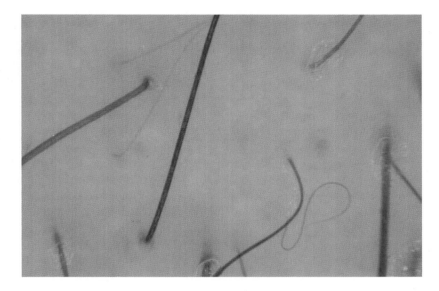

The telogen count may be slightly increased to about 19–20% (Fig. 68.22).

Differential diagnosis includes alopecia areata incognita, frontal fibrosing alopecia with fronto-temporal onset, fibrosing alopecia in a pattern distribution, and psychogenic alopecia; TE can resemble AGA.

Therapeutic Approach Topical minoxidil and finasteride (5α-reductase type II inhibitor) are the only treatments approved by the US Food and Drug Administration (FDA) for male androgenetic alopecia. In women, the only FDA-approved drug is topical minoxidil [68]. Oral antiandrogens and other therapeutic options can be used as adjuvants to prevent the progression of hair loss and stimulate partial regrowth of hair. Combining medications with different mechanisms of action enhances the efficacy. Surgical treatment of follicular unit hair transplantation is an option in cases that have failed medical treatment.

Fig. 68.22 Androgenetic alopecia: horizontal section at the isthmus/infundibulum level. There are 8 terminal follicles and 15 the vellus follicles (terminal/vellus ratio 0.6:1) (Courtesy of Dr. Maria Miteva, Miami, USA)

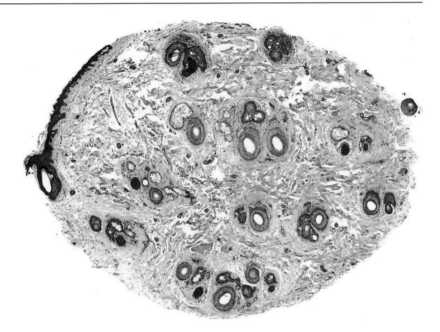

Trichotillomania

Introduction and Etiopathogenesis Trichotillomania (TTM) is a psychiatric disorder characterized by an irresistible urge to pull out one's hair [72]. The condition most affects children from 9 to 13 years, although adult onset may be secondary to underlying psychiatric disturbances and has a long-lasting course [73]. Usually hair pulling is preceded by mounting tension and consequently brings relief or gratification [74]. Patients frequently experience co-occurring anxiety disorders, depressive disorders, and other body-focused repetitive behaviors [75].

Clinical Features and Diagnosis Patients present with single or multiple, usually irregular, hairless areas, predominantly in the parietal and vertex regions of the scalp. However, any area of the body can be affected.

Pathologically the biopsy of trichotillomania shows increased telogen count of up to 70%. The majority are catagen follicles, which may be arranged in groups. The differential diagnosis with alopecia areata, particularly with the subacute stage, can be difficult but the presence of trichomalacia (fragmented or distorted hair shafts in the follicular canal) and pigmented casts can indicate the diagnosis of trichotillomania [76]. The pigmented casts are black clumps of melanin usually with a weird shape, and are encountered at different follicular levels (Fig. 68.23).

Trichoscopy shows decreased hair density, broken hairs at different lengths, short hairs with trichoptilosis, irregular coiled hairs, flame hairs, V-sign, hair powder, upright regrowing hairs, and black dots (Fig. 68.24a–c) [77, 78].

Differential diagnosis includes alopecia areata, androgenetic alopecia, and tinea capitis. Sometimes alopecia areata and trichotillomania can coexist in the same patient, making trichoscopic differential diagnosis even more challenging [77].

Therapeutic Approach Treatment options include specialized age-adapted behavioral therapy, such as habit reversal training, and psychiatric medications [75]. More recently, *N*-acetylcysteine (NAC) has been evaluated in the treatment of TTM. Although offering promise for some individuals, the small number of randomized controlled trials limits inferences about NAC's efficacy for TTM [75, 79].

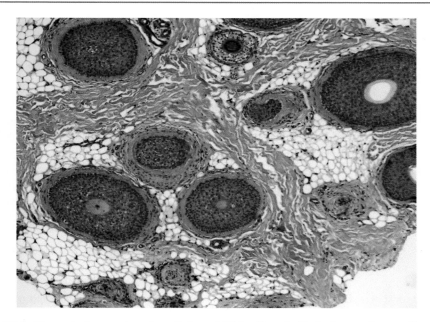

Fig. 68.23 Trichotillomania: increased number of telogen follicles. Note the black pigmented casts with trichomalacia in the follicular canals of two affected follicles (Courtesy of Dr. Maria Miteva, Miami, USA)

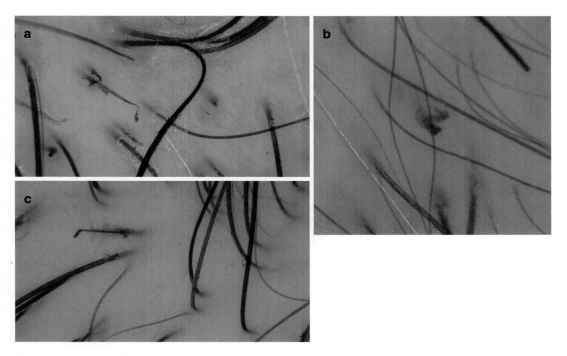

Fig. 68.24 (**a**) Trichotillomania: coiled hairs, flame hair, and broken hairs (Courtesy of Dr. Patricia Damasco, Brasilia, Brazil). (**b**) Trichotillomania: V-sign is created when two or more hairs emerging from one follicular unit are pulled simultaneously and break at the same length (Courtesy of Dr. Patricia Damasco, Brasilia, Brazil). (**c**) Trichotillomania: hair powder in trichotillomania (Courtesy of Dr. Patricia Damasco, Brasilia, Brazil)

Primary Cicatricial Alopecia

Scarring and cicatricial alopecia are synonymous, and mean that hair follicles are replaced by connective tissue. This event occurs because stem cells of bulges are damaged. Some scarring alopecia has a biphasic pattern; the early phase of injury is nonscarring alopecia, and with the time it confers permanent damage, as seen in traction alopecia and discoid lupus erythematosus alopecia. The opposite occurs, for example, in nonscarring alopecia such as androgenetic alopecia, which in time can become cicatricial alopecia.

It is important to understand that in primary alopecia the focus of damage is the hair follicles. However, there are secondary scarring alopecias, such as radiation dermatitis, morphea, and chronic infections, whereby the hair damage is secondarily affected by the damage to surrounding tissue.

Lichen Planopilaris

Introduction and Etiopathogenesis Lichen planopilaris (LPP) is an inflammatory lymphocyte cicatricial alopecia, and is considered the most frequent cause of adult primary scarring alopecia [80]. There are three variants of LPP: classic LPP, frontal fibrosing alopecia (FFA), and Graham-Little-Piccardi-Lasseur syndrome (GLPLS) [80–82]. Some authors consider fibrosing alopecia in a pattern distribution (FAPD) a fourth variant of the disease [80–82]. Women between the ages of 40 and 60 years are more frequently affected [81]. Classic LPP can be associated with nonscalp lichen planus in 50% of cases during the course of disease [83]. The cause of LPP remains unknown. The antigenic trigger remains unidentified, and the inflammatory infiltration occurs around the bulge area, mediated by T lymphocytes activated by Langerhans cells [81].

Clinical Features and Diagnosis Classic LPP is the most common variant of LPP and usually involves the vertex, as seen in Fig. 68.25. However, it can occur on any part of the scalp as a solitary or multiple areas of baldness, with patches stretched centrifugally [84]. The symptoms are hair shedding, scales, scalp tenderness, or pruritus, although patients sometimes do not complain of any symptoms [84].

Dermoscopically, there are different trichoscopic features of classic LPP in active and inactive lesions. Usually active lesions show perifollicular scaling that tends to form tubular structures in hair casts (tubular hyperkeratosis), violaceous areas, and elongated linear blood vessels, as seen

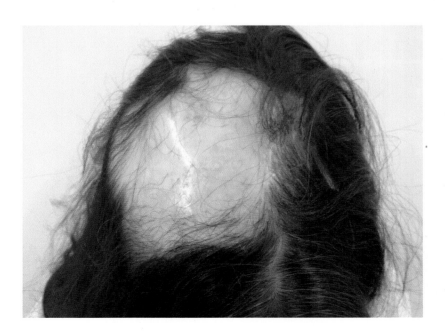

Fig. 68.25 Lichen planopilaris: single patch on the vertex area (Courtesy of Dr. Giselle Martins Pinto, Porto Alegre, Brazil)

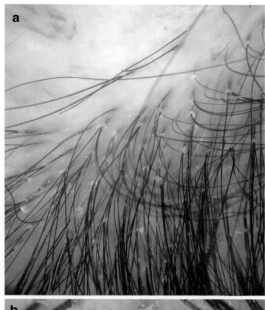

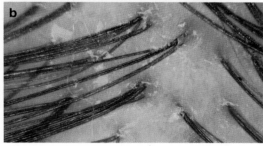

Fig. 68.26 (**a**, **b**) Dermoscopy of lichen planopilaris: cicatricial alopecia and keratosis perifollicularis, tufted hairs (Courtesy of Dr. Giselle Martins Pinto, Porto Alegre, Brazil)

on Fig. 68.26a, b [80]. In inactive lesions one observes white areas, irregular and large white dots (fibrotic white dots), milky red areas (strawberry ice cream color), and tufted hairs [80].

Pathologically, primary cicatricial alopecia is characterized by altered follicular architecture with decreased follicular density and eventual loss of the follicular units (follicular dropout) due to their replacement by scar tissue. Dermoscopy-guided biopsies and horizontal sections are helpful in detecting focal involvement [85]. The sebaceous glands are usually absent or diminished. In the early active stage, there is follicular inflammation which, depending on the type of predominant cells, can be primarily lymphocytic (primary lymphocytic cicatricial alopecia) or of mixed cell type (primary neutrophilic cicatricial alopecia). There is altered follicular architecture with areas of follicular dropout and absence of sebaceous glands (Fig. 68.27). The main pathologic finding is the presence of perifollicular lichenoid lymphocytic infiltrate, which can be encountered at the lower follicular levels but is most pronounced at the level of the isthmus. The infiltrate can invade the outer root sheath in a more interfaced pattern. There is perifollicular concentric fibrosis. In FFA there are usually more apoptotic cells in the outer root sheath (Fig. 68.28) [86].

Fig. 68.27 Lichen planopilaris: In this horizontal section at the isthmus level there are compound follicular structures ("goggles") showing perifollicular inflammation and fibrosis. Note the absence of sebaceous glands (Courtesy of Dr. Maria Miteva, Miami, USA)

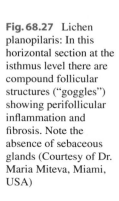

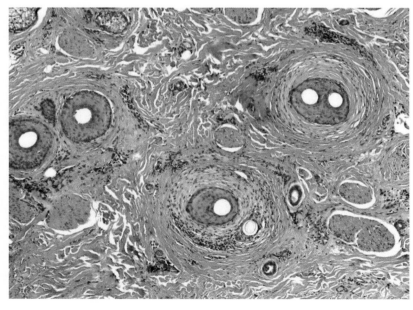

Differential diagnosis includes psoriasis, SD, folliculitis decalvans, FFA, and cicatricial pemphigoid, among others.

Therapeutic Approach Therapy is often not satisfactory [81]. Topical and intralesional corticosteroids are usually helpful. Systemic treatment can include oral corticosteroids, cyclosporine, antimalarials, mycophenolate mofetil, and thalidomide as second-line therapy. Excimer laser treatment may be attempted if any of these medications fail to control the disease [87].

Frontal Fibrosing Alopecia

Introduction and Etiopathogenesis FFA is a primary lymphocytic cicatricial alopecia that more frequently affects postmenopausal women [80]. Only 7.6% of all cases of FFA are premenopausal women and 1.9% are men [88]. FFA is considered a variant of LPP, but some authors believe FFA to be a different disease. The pathogenesis is uncertain, although an androgen effect has been speculated because of the strong association with postmenopausal status [89].

Clinical Features and Diagnosis A progressive frontotemporal symmetric band of alopecia is the most common presentation, as seen on Fig. 68.29

[89]. The skin at the recession area is smooth and shiny, contrasting with the rest of facial skin and indicating where the former hairline used to be [84]. FFA can cause mild pruritus or be asymptomatic. There is a very interesting association with eyebrow loss. In some patients the alopecia is associated with lichen planus pigmentosus of the face, and facial papules that usually show vellus follicle involvement or hyperplasia of sebaceous glands [90, 91].

Dermoscopically there is lack of follicular openings, perifollicular erythema, and scaling on a homogeneous ivory-colored background [80]. The important clue for dermoscopy is the loss of hair vellus on the hairline, as seen on Fig. 68.30.

Pathologically, FFA and LPP are the same; see the description above of LPP.

In the differential diagnosis it is important to bear in mind that some diseases can be clinically similar to FFA, such as ophiasic alopecia areata, lupus erythematosus, traction alopecia and androgenetic alopecia.

Therapeutic Approach Usually FFA is treated as classic LPP, although finasteride has been reported to halt the progression of this disease [92]. Hair transplants can be proposed after no disease improvement for at least 1–2 years [80].

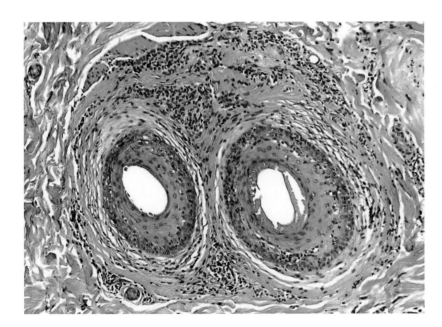

Fig. 68.28 Frontal fibrosing alopecia: follicular lichenoid and interface lymphocytic infiltrate and fibrosis. Note the apoptotic cells in the outer root sheath (Courtesy of Dr. Maria Miteva, Miami, USA)

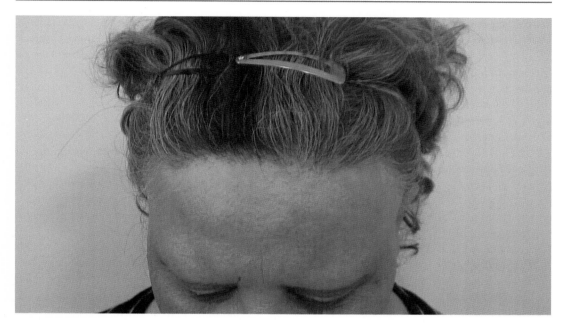

Fig. 68.29 FFA: progressive frontotemporal symmetric band of alopecia (Courtesy of Dr. Giselle Martins Pinto, Porto Alegre, Brazil)

Fig. 68.30 FFA: lack of follicular openings, erythema and scaling, and loss of hair vellus on hair (Courtesy of Dr. Giselle Martins Pinto, Porto Alegre, Brazil)

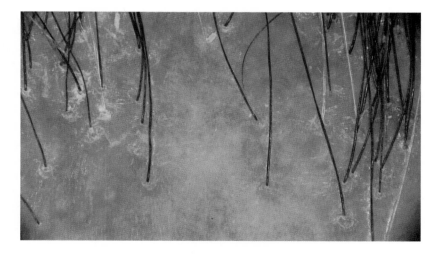

Graham-Little-Piccardi-Lasseur Syndrome

Introduction and Etiopathogenesis GLPLS is a rare disease, affecting women between 30 and 60 years of age. Some authors consider this disease a variant of LPP [80, 93].

Clinical Features and Diagnosis The triad of progressive scarring scalp alopecia, nonscarring loss of pubic and axillary hair, and disseminated follicular papules with spinous scales is characteristic [84]. The scalp disease clinically and histopathologically resembles classic LPP.

Trichoscopy of the scalp is similar to that of classic LPP, although the pubic and axillary areas do not show the dermoscopy signs of LPP, merely thin hairs [80].

Pathologically, GLPLS is the same as LPP.

The main differential diagnosis is classic LPP, although lupus erythematosus must be considered.

Therapeutic Approach Treatment is similar to LPP treatment.

Fibrosing Alopecia in a Pattern Distribution

Introduction and Etiopathogenesis FAPD was for the first time described in 2000. This new form of cicatricial alopecia is not yet well recognized as a variant of LPP, a variant of androgenetic alopecia, or an authentic entity [81].

Clinical Features and Diagnosis Clinically the patients present a pattern similar to that of androgenetic alopecia. The hair loss is limited to the area of androgenetic alopecia.

Dermoscopically, perifollicular erythema and hyperkeratosis is universally seen.

Pathologically, FAPD is consistent with features of LPP with follicular miniaturization.

The differential diagnosis includes AGA, LPP; sometimes AGA and LPP can coexist in the same patient.

Therapeutic Approach Some authors have reported improvement with agents such as finasteride and minoxidil; however, many clinicians prefer drugs used for classic LPP, such as topical or systemic corticosteroids.

Discoid Lupus Erythematosus Alopecia

Introduction and Etiopathogenesis Discoid lupus erythematosus (DLE) alopecia is seen more frequently in young women. Usually it is considered a local disease, as less than 5% of DLE patients have systemic disease [84]. DLE alopecia is classified as primary lymphocytic cicatricial alopecia; however at the beginning of the disease, because the target is not the hair follicles, the alopecia can be reversed with the appropriate treatment. The pathogenesis of DLE involves interaction between genetic, environmental, and host factors [84].

Clinical Features and Diagnosis DLE alopecia begins as a well-demarcated round or oval purplish macule or papule, and enlarges into an alopecic patch with follicular plugging, erythema, and adherent scaling [80]. Commonly it is seen in the vertex, as a single or multiple patches [94]. Symptoms include pruritus, scalp tenderness, hair shedding, burning, and, less commonly, pain [80]. Long-standing DLE alopecia has fibrotic atrophic and white plaques with lack of hair openings.

Dermoscopically, in active lesions one sees thick arborizing vessels, large yellow dots that correspond to follicular keratotic plugs, and fine interfollicular scaling, as seen in Fig. 68.31 [81]. Red dots indicate dilated infundibula surrounded by dilated vessels and extravasated erythrocytes, and represent a good prognosis and chance of hair regrowth [95]. The blue-gray dots seen on dark or sun-exposed skin correlate with pigment incontinence secondary to interface dermatitis [96]. In long-standing inactive lesions one sees loss of follicular openings, pink areas, white areas, arborizing vessels, and yellow dots containing thin spider vessels in prefibrotic lesions [80].
Pathologically, at the level of the bulb in the subcutaneous fat there is perivascular and periadnexal (perieccrine and perifollicular) infiltrate of

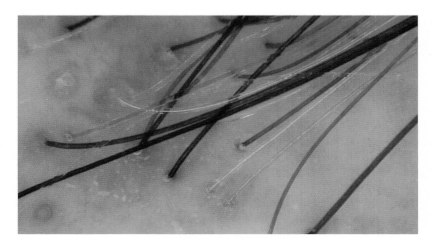

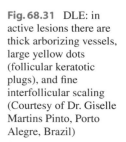

Fig. 68.31 DLE: in active lesions there are thick arborizing vessels, large yellow dots (follicular keratotic plugs), and fine interfollicular scaling (Courtesy of Dr. Giselle Martins Pinto, Porto Alegre, Brazil)

Fig. 68.32 (**a**) DLE: in this vertical section the epidermis is slightly atrophic. The sebaceous glands are only focally present and hypoplastic. There is lymphocytic infiltrate in perivascular and periadnexal distribution. Note the interface changes at the other root sheaths of the follicles which also show infundibular keratin plugs (courtesy of Dr. Maria Miteva, Miami, USA). (**b**) DLE: the dilated infundibula are plugged by keratin material. Note the pigment incontinence in perifollicular distribution (Courtesy of Dr. Maria Miteva, Miami, USA)

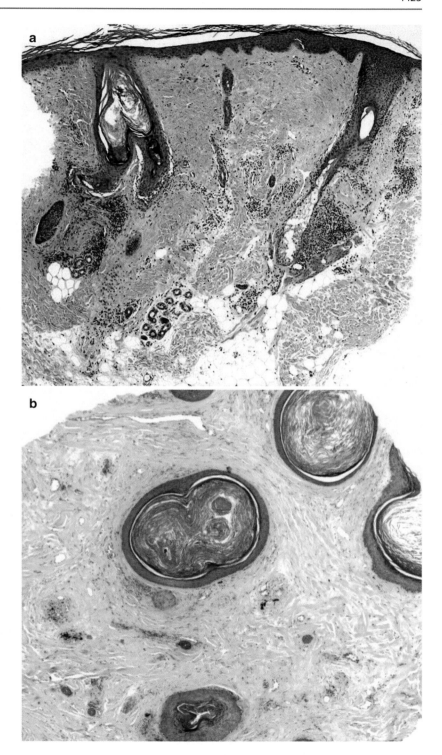

lymphocytes and plasmacytoid cells, which can aggregate in germinal center-like collections (Fig. 68.32a). The infiltrate also affects the upper follicular levels in an interface follicular pattern. The sebaceous glands are absent, but there is no prominent perifollicular fibrosis as seen in lichen planopilaris. There is interface dermatitis along the dermoepidermal junction with pigment incontinence and thickened basement membrane. The follicular infundibula are plugged by keratin (Fig. 68.32b). The dermis and subdermis appear pale and loose because of deposition of mucin.

The most frequent differential diagnosis of DLE alopecia is LPP. However, sometimes one excludes SD, psoriasis, cicatricial pemphigoid, and basal cell carcinoma.

Therapeutic Approach Photoprotection should be advised, as DLE alopecia worsens in upon sun exposure. Topical treatments include potent topical steroids, calcineurin inhibitors, retinoids, and imiquimod, with mixed outcomes. Intralesional steroids are indicated in small areas of alopecia, although there is always a risk of scarring alopecia after the treatment, with depressions on the skin surface. Systemic treatment include antimalarial drugs, systemic steroids, and thalidomide, similar to the treatment of cutaneous lupus erythematosus.

Folliculitis Decalvans

Introduction and Etiopathogenesis Folliculitis decalvans (FD) is a primary neutrophilic scarring alopecia. It is a disease seen in male patients, more commonly in African American men [83]. The pathogenesis of FD is poorly understood; some authors believe that superantigens and an exaggerated immune response might play a role.

Clinical Features and Diagnosis Recurrent follicular pustules involve the vertex and occipital area of the scalp. Patches of alopecia are seen in one or more area. Patients complain of pain, itching, and burning sensation, and the lesions usually are malodorous because of discharge of material from the pustules and hemorrhagic crust lesions. Clinically there are tufts comprising multiple hairs (6–20+ hairs) emerging from one single dilated follicular orifice.

At dermoscopy, active disease shows tufted hairs with more than five hairs in one follicular unit, yellow follicular pustules, yellowish tubular scaling with collar formation, yellow discharge, epidermal hyperplasia and vessels with elongated loops, and concentric perifollicular arrangement, as seen in Fig. 68.33 [80]. Starburst sign consists of yellowish scales and perifollicular epidermal hyperplasia that may be in a starburst pattern [80]. In late-stage or inactive disease, only cicatricial alopecia as white and milky red areas without follicular openings and epidermal hyperplasia are apparent.

Pathologically, in FD there is dense perifollicular but also interfollicular infiltrate of mixed cell origin (lymphocytes, histiocytes, neutrophils, and plasma cells). The main finding is the presence of compound follicular structures (tufts of hairs on clinical examination) arising from the fusion of the outer root sheaths of variable number of follicles but usually of more than 2 (Fig. 68.14). There is perifollicular fibrosis and absence of sebaceous glands. In advanced stages, there is prominent follicular dropout (Fig. 68.34).

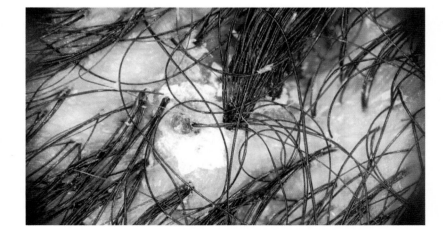

Fig. 68.33 Folliculitis decalvans: dermoscopy shows tufted hairs with more than five hairs in one follicular unit and epidermal hyperplasia (Courtesy of Dr. Giselle Martins Pinto, Porto Alegre, Brazil)

Fig. 68.34 Folliculitis decalvans: compound follicular structures (six packs in this case). Note the dense interfollicular inflammation and the perifollicular fibrosis. The sebaceous glands are absent (Courtesy of Dr. Maria Miteva, Miami, USA)

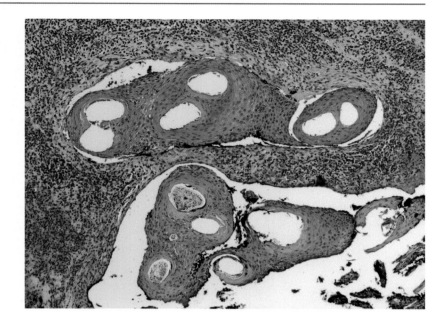

The main differential diagnosis is with disease that causes tufted hairs, such as LPP. Rarely other diseases has tufted hairs, e.g., DLE alopecia, central centrifugal cicatricial alopecia, and dissecting cellulitis.

Therapeutic Approach Various case reports indicate that the use of oral antibiotics in combination may have success as an alternative therapy, such as oral rifampicin and clindamycin, doxycycline, ciprofloxacin, or clarithromycin [97].

Dissecting Cellulite

Introduction and Etiopathogenesis Dissecting cellulite (DC) of the scalp, dissecting folliculites, and perifolliculites capitis abscedens et suffodiens are synonyms, and occur most commonly in young adult men with dark skin phototypes [80]. DC can occur as isolated on the scalp or be part of the follicular occlusion tetrad: DC, pilonidal cyst, hidradenitis suppurativa, and acne conglobata. The pathogenesis of this disease is unknown, although some authors believe there exists a correlation between follicular hyperkeratosis and superinfection.

Clinical Features and Diagnosis DC is a chronic, relapsing, and progressive cicatricial alopecia [80]. Usually the patients complain of perifollicular pustules or firm scalp nodules on the vertex or occiput area. These nodules are firm or fluctuant and can discharge a purulent material. Frequently the material is sterile, but sometimes secondary bacterial infections may occur.

On dermoscopy, active disease shows yellow structureless areas, yellow 3D dots (three-dimensional structures) with or without dystrophic hair shafts, black dots, pinpoint-like vessels with a whitish halo, and cutaneous clefts with emerging hairs and hair tufts [80]. End-stage lesions show white areas with lack of follicular openings.

Pathologically, biopsies from early disease show dense and diffuse mixed cell infiltrate occupying the lower part of the dermis and the subdermis. The infiltrate also contains giant cells. There is edema and red blood cell extravasation. The majority of the follicles are in telogen and the sebaceous glands may still be preserved at that stage (Fig. 68.35). It is distinguished from inflammatory tinea capitis by the fact that infiltrate is mostly in the lower portion of the specimen in DCS.

Fig. 68.35 Dissection cellulitis of the scalp, early disease: the follicular architecture is altered by the presence of dense mixed cell infiltrate with edema and red blood cell extravasation. The telogen count is increased (Courtesy of Dr. Maria Miteva, Miami, USA)

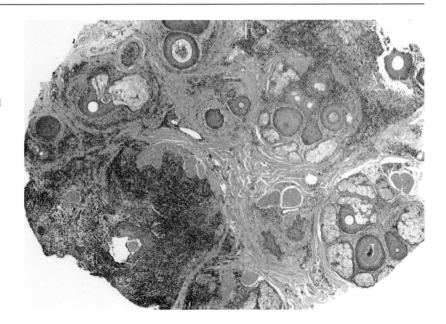

The differential diagnosis of FD includes alopecia mucinosa, tinea capitis, and acne keloidalis nuchae.

Therapeutic Approach The literature has reported the use of isotretinoin as an effective therapy for this disease, although relapses are common. Alternative treatments include intralesional steroids, oral antibiotics, and surgery for specific cases.

Central Centrifugal Cicatricial Alopecia

Introduction and Etiopathogenesis Central centrifugal cicatricial alopecia (CCCA), follicular degeneration syndrome, and hot comb alopecia are synonyms. This disease is the most common scarring alopecia in African American women [98]. Almost all black women of African descent with CCCA have used chemical hair relaxers. However, after discontinuing the use of these chemical treatments the disease can progress. The current hypothesis is that the anatomic abnormality is due to premature desquamation of the inner root sheath [98].

Clinical Features and Diagnosis This disease is a chronic, progressive cicatricial alopecia usually on the vertex or crown. CCCA has a symmetric appearance, with the surrounding zone showing activity similar to that of most common scarring alopecia. Most of the patients have no symptoms, or mild pruritus or tenderness of the involved area. Bacterial superinfections can occur, and in such cases pustules and crusting is described.

The trichoscopic features of CCCA include loss of follicular openings.

Pathologically, there is altered follicular architecture with areas of follicular dropout. The follicular density is decreased and in most cases there is diminished terminal/vellus ratio of about 2:1. The affected follicles show perifollicular concentric fibrosis and, rarely, mild perifollicular lichenoid lymphocytic infiltrate. Often they form compound follicular structures ("goggles") which correspond to pairs of follicles fused by their outer root sheaths and surrounded by concentric fibrosis. The sebaceous glands are focally preserved and often surround vellus follicles [99]. Naked hair shafts are found in the dermis. Premature desquamation of the inner root sheath supports the diagnosis (Fig. 68.36).

Fig. 68.36 CCCA: compound follicular structures ("goggles") showing perifollicular fibrosis but only mild inflammation. The sebaceous glands are focally preserved (Courtesy of Dr. Maria Miteva, Miami, USA)

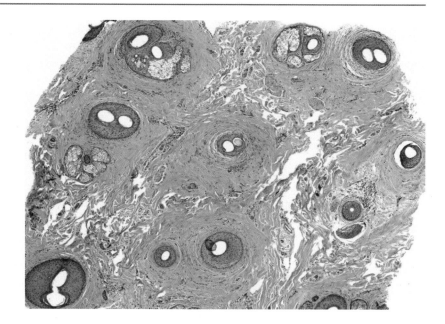

In the differential diagnosis, usually CCCA can be confused with AGA, FD, or LPP.

Therapeutic Approach A combination of oral antibiotics, such as doxycycline or tetracycline, with topical steroids is the most common treatment reported in the literature [98].

Traction Alopecia

Introduction and Etiopathogenesis Traction alopecia (TA) is most commonly caused by hairstyling procedures, and African American women are frequently affected. The most common procedures include ponytails, tight buns, weaves, dreadlocks, cornrows, clips, hair extensions, tight braids, hair relaxers, and stretching of scalp hair.

Clinical Features and Diagnosis TA is a biphasic form of hair loss. In the early phase the alopecia is reversible, and if the traction stops hair regrowth can occur. However, if the traction is maintained for years, the hair loss becomes a permanent area of alopecia. Persistent, bitemporal, or frontal hair loss is the most common pattern, as seen in Fig. 68.37.

Two phases are observed on dermoscopy. First one can observe perifollicular erythema, hair

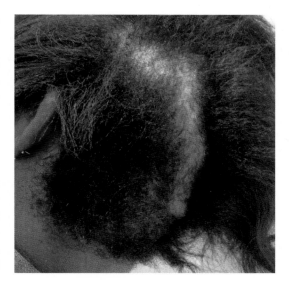

Fig. 68.37 Traction alopecia: linear hair loss and use of hair extensions (Courtesy of Dr. Giselle Martins, Porto Alegre, Brazil)

thinning, focal decrease of hair density, broken hairs, and tulip hairs [80]. Hair casts are characterized by white keratin cylinders around the hair shaft. With progressive traction, perifollicular scarring and cicatricial alopecia ensue.

Pathologically, early cases may show overall preserved follicular architecture with only focal

Fig. 68.38 Traction alopecia: at the level of the isthmus the follicular architecture is preserved overall with only one area of follicular dropout. The sebaceous glands are intact. Only one vellus follicle is present (Courtesy of Dr. Maria Miteva, Miami, USA)

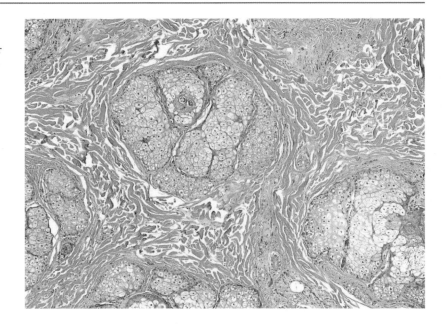

areas of follicular dropout, with no follicular inflammation or fibrosis and intact sebaceous glands. In advanced cases, follicular dropout may dominate. The terminal/vellus ratio is significantly decreased, with vellus follicles outnumbering the terminal follicles (Fig. 68.38).

The differential diagnosis includes TTM, FFA, and LPP.

Therapeutic Approach The most important treatment approach is to stop the traction.

Glossary

Effluvium Shedding of hair.

Endothrix infection Dermatophyte infections of the hair that invade the hair shaft and internalize into the hair cell. The hair shaft is filled with fungal branches (hyphae) and spores (arthroconidia). Endothrix infections do not fluoresce with Woods light.

Pityriasis amiantacea A scalp condition that causes scaling, and can occur in patches anywhere on the scalp. It is an eczematous condition of the scalp resulting in hair loss, whereby thick adherent scale infiltrates and surrounds the base of a group of scalp hairs.

Psoriasiform acanthosis The presence of evenly elongated, thin rete ridges with equally long dermal papillae.

Trichotillomania A disorder that involves recurrent, irresistible urges to pull out hair from the scalp, eyebrows, or other areas of the body, despite trying to stop. Hair pulling from the scalp often leaves patchy bald spots.

Trichoscopy Hair and scalp dermoscopy. May be performed with a handheld dermoscope. This makes it a modern, noninvasive technique.

References

1. Rakowska A, Slowiska M, Kowalska-Oledzka E, Rudnicka L. Trichoscopy in genetic hair shaft abnormalities. J Dermatol Case Rep. 2008;2(2):14–20.
2. Bartels NG, Blume-Peytavi U. Hair loss in children. In: Blume-Peytavi U, Tosti A, Whiting DA, Trueb R, editors. Hair growth and disorders. Berlin: Springer; 2008. p. 273–90.
3. Duverger O, Morasso MI. To grow or not to grow: hair morphogenesis and human genetic hair disorders. Semin Cell Dev Biol. 2014;25-26:22–33.
4. Vora RV, Anjanevan G, Mehta MJ. Monilethrix, a rare inherited hair shaft disorfer in sinblings. Indian Dermatol Online J. 2014;5(3):339–40.
5. Sperling L, Sinclair RD, El Shabravi-Caelen L. Alopecias. In: Bologna JL, Jorizzo JL, Schaffer JV,

editors. Dermatology. third ed. China: Elsevier; 2012. p. 1109–12.

6. Rakowska A, Rudnicka L. Moniletrix, Pseudomoniletrix e Pelos Semelhantes aos da Moniletrix. In: Rudnicka L, Olszewska M, Rakowska A, editors. Atlas de Tricoscopia. Rio de janeiro: Di Livros; 2014. p. 145–52.

7. Rakowska A, Olszewska M, Rudnicka L. Tricorrexe Invaginada e Síndrome de Netherton. In: Rudnicka L, Olszewska M, Rakowska A, editors. Atlas de Tricoscopia. Rio de janeiro: Di Livros; 2014. p. 153–8.

8. Rudnicka L, Olszewska M, Rakowska A, Slowinska M. Trichoscopy update 2011. J Dermatol Case Rep. 2011;5(4):82–8. Published online 2011 Dec 12.

9. Bittencourt MJS, Moure ERD, Pies OTC, Mendes AD, Deprá MM, Mello ALP. Trichoscopy as a diagnostic tool in trichorrhexis invaginata and Netherton syndrome. An Bras Dermatol. 2015;90(1):114–6.

10. Messenger AG, de Berker DAT, Sinclair RD. Disorders of hair. In: Burns T, Breatchnach S, Cox N, Griffiths C, editors. Rook's textbook of dermatology. Chichester: Wiley – Blackwell; 2010. p. 66.1–66.100.

11. Olszewska M, Rakowska A. Pili Torti, Pili Annulati and ricotiodistrofia. In: Rudnicka L, Olszewska M, Rakowska A, editors. Atlas de Tricoscopia. Rio de janeiro: Di Livros; 2014. p. 167–87.

12. Berk DR, Bayliss SJ, Giehl KA. Pili annulati: a report of 2 American families. Cutis. 2013 May;91(5):254–7.

13. Kuschal C, et al. GTF2E2 mutations destabilize the general transcription factor complex TFIIE in individuals with DNA repair-proficient trichothiodystrophy. Am J Hum Genet. 2016;98(4):627–42.

14. Ferrando J, Mir-Bonafé JM, Cepeda-Valdez R, Domínguez A, Ocampo-Candiani J, et al. Further insights in trichothiodistrophy: a clinical, microscopic, and ultrastructural study of 20 cases and literature review. Int JT Int J Trichology. 2012;4(3): 158–63.

15. George SM, Taylor MR, Farrant PB. Psoriatic alopecia. Clin Exp Dermatol. 2015;40(7):717–21.

16. Almeida MC, Romiti R, Doche I, Valente NY, Donati A. Psoriatic scarring alopecia. An Bras Dermatol. 2013;88(6 Suppl 1):29–31.

17. Veale DJ, Ritchlin C, FitzGerald O. Immunopathology of psoriasis and psoriatic arthritis. Ann Rheum Dis. 2005;64(Suppl 2):ii26–9.

18. Nestle FO, Kaplan DH, Barker J. Psoriasis. N Engl J Med. 2009;361(5):496–509.

19. Kutlubay Z, Tüzün Y, Wolf R, Engin B. Inflammatory lipid mediators in common skin diseases. Skinmed. 2016;14(1):23–7.

20. Szepietowski JC, Reich A. Pruritus in psoriasis: an update. Eur J Pain. 2016;20(1):41–6.

21. Werner B, et al. Histopathologic study of scalp psoriasis: peculiar features including sebaceous gland atrophy. Am J Dermatopathol. 2008;30(2):93–100.

22. Doyle LA, et al. Psoriatic alopecia/alopecia areata-like reactions secondary to anti-tumor necrosis factor-alpha therapy: a novel cause of noncicatricial alopecia. Am J Dermatopathol. 2011;33(2):161–6.

23. Dahl M. Management of the scaling scalp. Curr Concepts Skin Dis. 1983;4(4):15–9.

24. van der Kerkhof PC, Kragballe K. Recommendations for the topical treatment of psoriasis. J Eur Acad Dermatol Venereol. 2005;19(4):495–9.

25. Ribeiro LB, Rego JC, Estrada BD, Bastos PR, Piñeiro Maceira JM, Sodré CT. Alopecia secondary to anti-tumor necrosis fator-alpha therapy. An Bras Dermatol. 2015;90(2):232–5.

26. Gupta AK, Bluhm R. Seborrheic dermatitis. J Eur Acad Dermatol Venereol. 2004;18:13–25.

27. Hickman JG. Dandruff and seborrheic dermatitis: use of medicated shampoos. In: McMichael A, Hordisnky MK, editors. Hair and scalp diseases: medical, surgical, and cosmetic treatments. New York: Informa; 2008. p. 73–90.

28. Kim GW, Jung HJ, Ko HC, Kim MB, Lee WJ, Lee SJ, et al. Dermoscopy can be useful in differentiating scalp psoriasis from seborrheic dermatitis. Br J Dermatol. 2011;164(3):652–6.

29. Ross EK, Vincenzi C, Tosti A. Videodermoscopy in the evaluation of hair and scalp disorders. J Am Acad Dermatol. 2006;55(5):799–806.

30. Stefanaki I, Katsambas A. Therapeutic update on seborrheic dermatitis. Skin Ther Lett. 2010;15(5):1–4.

31. Vafaie J, Weinberg JM, Smith B, et al. Alopecia in association with sexually transmitted disease: a review. Cutis. 2005;76:361–6.

32. Bi MY, Cohen PR, Robinson FW, et al. Alopecia syphitica – report of a patient with secondary syphilis presenting as moth-eaten alopecia and a review of its common mimickers. Dermatol Online J. 2009;15:6.

33. Cuozzo DW, Benson PM, Spering LC, et al. Essential syphilitic alopecia revisited. J Am Acad Dermatol. 1995;32:840–3.

34. Ye Y, Zhang X, Zhao Y, Gong Y, Yang J, Li H, Zhang X. The clinical and trichoscopic features of syphilitic alopecia. J Dermatol Case Rep. 2014;8(3):78–80.

35. Piraccini BM, Broccoli A, Starace M, Gaspari V, D'Antuono A, Dika E, Patrizi A. Hair and scalp manifestations in secondary syphilis: epidemiology, clinical features and trichoscopy. Dermatology. 2015;231(2):171–6.

36. Hernandez-Bel P, et al. Syphilitic alopecia: a report of 5 cases and a review of the literature. Actas Dermosifiliogr. 2013;104(6):512–7.

37. Lee JW, Jang WS, Yoo KH, et al. Diffuse pattern essential syphilitic alopecia: an unusual form of secondary syphilis. Int J Dermatol. 2012;51:1006–7.

38. Tack DA, Fleischer A, McMichael A, et al. The epidemic of tinea capitis disproportionately affects school-aged African Americans. Pediatr Dermatol. 1999;16(1):75.

39. Grimalt R. A practical guide to scalp disorders. J Investig Dermatol Symp Proc. 2007;12(2):10–4.

40. Sandoval AB, Ortiz JA, Rodrigues JM, Vargas AG, Quintero DG. Dermoscopic pattern in tinea capitis. Rev Iberoam Micol. 2010;27(3):151–2.

41. Hughes R, Chiaverini C, Bahadoran P, Lacour JP. Corkscrew hair: a new dermoscopic sign for diagnosis of tinea capitis in black children. Arch Dermatol. 2011;147(3):355–6.

42. Neri I, Starace M, Patrizi A, Balestri R. Corkscrew hair: a trichsocopy marker of tinea capitis in an adult White patient. JAMA Dermatol. 2014;149(8):990–1.

43. Slowinska M, Rudnicka L, Schwartz RA, Kowalska-Oledzka E, Rakowska A, Sicinska J, et al. Comma hairs: a dermoscopic marker of tinea capitis: a rapid diagnostic method. J Am Acad Dermatol. 2008;59(5 Suppl):S77–9.

44. Isa-Isa R, et al. Inflammatory tinea capitis: kerion, dermatophytic granuloma, and mycetoma. Clin Dermatol. 2010;28(2):133–6.

45. Roberts BJ, Friedlander SF. Tinea capitis: a treatment update. Pediatr Ann. 2005;34(3):191–200.

46. Kligman AM. Pathologic dynamics of human hair loss, I: telogen effluvium. Arch Dermatol. 1961;83:175–98.

47. Grover C, Khurana A. Telogen effluvium. Indian J Dermatol Venerol Leprol. 2013;79(5):591–603.

48. Trueb RM. Diffuse hair loss. In: Blume-Peytavi U, Tosti A, Whiting DA, Trueb RM, editors. Hair growth and disorders. 1st ed. Berlin: Springer; 2008. p. 259–72.

49. Malkud S. Telogen effluvium: a review. J Clin Diagn Res. 2015;9:9.

50. Sinclair R. Diffuse hair loss. Int J Dermatol. 1999;38(suppl. 1):8–18.

51. Rakowska A, Olszewska M, Rudnicka L. Telogen effluvium. In: Rudnicka L, Olszewska M, Rakowska A, editors. Atlas of trichoscopy – dermoscopy in hair and scalp disease, 1st ed. London: Springer-Verlag; 2012. p. 237e–244.

52. Headington JT. Transverse microscopic anatomy of the human scalp. A basis for a morphometric approach to disorders of the hair follicle. Arch Dermatol. 1984;120(4):449–56.

53. Miteva M. A comprehensive approach to hair pathology of horizontal sections. Am J Dermatopathol. 2013;35(5):529–40.

54. Gilmore S, Sinclair R. Chronic telogen effluvium is due to a reduction in the variance of anagen duration. Australas J Dermatol. 2010;51(3):163–7.

55. Whiting DA. Chronic telogen effluvium: increased scalp hair shedding in middle-aged women. J Am Acad Dermatol. 1996;35(6):899–906.

56. Sinclair R. Chronic telogen efluvium: a study of 5 patients over 7 years. J Am Acad Dermatol. 2005;52:12–6.

57. Alkhalifah A, Alsantali A, Wang E, McElwee KJ, Shapiro J. Alopecia areata update Part I. Clinical picture, histopathology and pathogenesis. J Am Acad Dermatol. 2010;62(2):177–88.

58. Freyschmidt-Paul P, Hoffmann R, McElwee KJ. Alopecia areata. In: Blume-Peytavi U, Tosti A, Whiting DA, Trueb RM, editors. Hair growth and disorders. 1st ed. Berlin: Springer; 2008. p. 311–32.

59. Hordisnky M, Junqueira AL. Alopecia areata update. Semin Cutan Med Surg. 2015;34:72–5.

60. Madani S, Shapiro J. Alopecia areata update. J Am Acad Dermatol. 2000;42:549–66.

61. Gandhi V, Baruah MC, Bhattacharaya SN. Nail changes in alopecia areata: incidence and pattern. Indian J Dermatol Venereol Leprol. 2003;69:114–5.

62. Rudnicka L, Olszewska M, Rakowska A, Czuwara J. Alopecia areata. In: Rudnicka L, Olszewska M, Rakowska A, editors. Atlas of trichoscopy – dermoscopy in hair and scalp disease. 1st ed. London: Springer-Verlag; 2012. p. 205–20.

63. Inui S, Nakajima T, Nakagawa K, Itami S. Clinical significance of dermoscopy in alopecia areata: analysis of 300 cases. Int J Dermatol. 2008;47(7):688–93.

64. Whiting DA. Histopathologic features of alopecia areata: a new look. Arch Dermatol. 2003;139(12):1555–9.

65. Otberg N, Finner AM, Shapiro J. Androgenetic alopecia. Endocrinol Metab Clin N Am. 2007;36(2):379–98.

66. Rinaldi S, Bussa M, Mascaro A. Update on the treatment of androgenetic alopecia. Eur Rev Med Pharmacol Sci. 2016;20:54–8.

67. Guarrera M, Rebora A. Kenogen in female androgenetic alopecia. A longitudinal study. Dermatology. 2005;210(1):18–20.

68. Torres F, Tosti A. Female pattern alopecia and telogen effluvium: figuring out diffuse alopecia. Semin Cutan Med Surg. 2015;34:67–71.

69. Olsen EA. Female pattern hair loss. In: Blume-Peytavi U, Tosti A, Whiting DA, Trueb RM, editors. Hair growth and disorders. 1st ed. Berlin: Springer; 2008. p. 171–96.

70. Messenger A. Male androgenetic alopecia. In: Blume-Peytavi U, Tosti A, Whiting DA, Trueb RM, editors. Hair growth and disorders. 1st ed. Berlin: Springer; 2008. p. 159–70.

71. Rakowska A, Slowinska M, Olszewska M, Rudnicka L. Androgenetic alopecia. In: Rudnicka L, Olszewska M, Rakowska A, editors. Atlas of trichoscopy – dermoscopy in hair and scalp disease. 1st ed. London: Springer-Verlag; 2012. p. 221–35.

72. Johnson J, El-Alfy AT. Review of available studies of the neurobiology and pharmatotherapeutic management of trichotillomania. J Adv Res. 2016;7(20):169–84.

73. Sah DE, Koo J, Price VH. Trichotillomania. Dermatol Ther. 2008;21(1):13–21.

74. Gawlowska-Sawosz M, et al. Trichotillomania and trichophagia – diagnosis, treatment, prevention. The attempt to establish guidelines of treatment in Poland. Psychiatr Pol. 2016;50(1):127–43.

75. McGuire JF, et al. Treating trichotillomania: a meta-analysis of treatment effects and moderators for behavior therapy and serotonin reuptake inhibitors. J Psychiatr Res. 2014;0:76–83.

76. Miteva M, et al. Pigmented casts. Am J Dermatopathol. 2014;36(1):58–63.

77. Rudnicka L, Olszewska M, Rakowska A. Trichotillomania and traction alopecia. In: Rudnicka L, Olszewska M, Rakowska A, editors. Atlas of trichoscopy – dermoscopy in hair and scalp disease. 1st ed. London: Springer-Verlag; 2012. p. 237–44.

78. Rakowska, et al. New trichoscopy findings in trichotillomania: flame hairs, v-sign, hook hairs, hair powder, tulip hairs. Acta Derm Venereol. 2014;94:303–6.

79. Woods DW. Treating trichotillomania across the lifespan. J Am Acad Child Adolesc Psychiatry. 2013;52(3):223–4.

80. Olszewska M, Rakowska A, Slowinska M, Rudnicka L.Classic lichen planopilaris and Graham Little syndrome. In: Rudnicka L, Olszewska M, Rakowska A, editors. Atlas of trichoscopy – dermoscopy in hair and scalp disease. 1st ed. London: Springer-Verlag; 2012. p. 279–94.

81. Assouly P, Reygagne. Lichen planopilaris: update on diagnosis and treatment. Semin Cutan Med Surg. 2009;28(1):3–10.

82. Wiseman MC, Shapiro J. Scarring alopecia. J Cutan Med Surg. 1999;3(Suppl 3):S45–8.

83. Tan E, Martinka M, Ball N, Shapiro J. Primary cicatricial alopecias: clinicopathology of 112 cases. J Am Acad Dermatol. 2004;50(1):25–32.

84. Ramos-e-Silva M, Pirmez R. Red face revisited: disorders of hair growth and the pilosebaceous unit. Clin Dermatol. 2014;32:784–99.

85. Miteva M, Tosti A. Dermoscopy guided scalp biopsy in cicatricial alopecia. J Eur Acad Dermatol Venereol. 2013;27(10):1299–303.

86. Poblet E, et al. Frontal fibrosing alopecia versus lichen planopilaris: a clinicopathologic study. Int J Dermatol. 2006;45(4):375–80.

87. Harries MJ, Sinclair RD, Macdonald-Hull S, Whiting DA, Griffiths CE, Paus R. Management of primary cicatricial alopecias: options for treatment. Br J Dermatol. 2008;159(1):1–22.

88. Chew AL, Bashir SJ, Wain EM, Fenton DA, Stefanato CM. Expanding the spectrum of frontal fibrosing alopecia: a unifying concept. J Am Acad Dermatol. 2010;63(4):653–60.

89. Ross EK, Shapiro J. Primary cicatricial alopecia. In: Blume-Peytavi U, Tosti A, Whiting DA, Trüeb R, editors. Hair growth and disorders. Leipzig: Springer; 2008. p. 187–225.

90. Dlova NC. Frontal fibrosing alopecia and lichen planus pigmentosus: is there a link? Br J Dermatol. 2013;168:439–42.

91. Donati A, Molina L, Doche I, Valente NS, Romiti R. Facial papules in frontal fibrosing alopecia: evidence of vellus follicle involvement. Arch Dermatol. 2011;147(12):1424–7.

92. Tosti A, Piraccini BM, Iorizzo M, Misciali C. Frontal fibrosing alopecia in postmenopausal women. J Am Acad Dermatol. 2005;52(1):55–60.

93. Steglich R, Tonoli RE, Pinto GM, Guarenti IM, Duvellius ES. Graham-Little Piccardi Lassueur syndrome: case report. Ann Braz Dermatol. 2012;87(5):775–7.

94. Hordinsky M. Cicatricial alopecia: discoid lupus erythematosus. Dermatol Ther. 2008;21(4):245–8.

95. Tosti A, Torres F, Misciali C, Vincenzi C, Starace M, Miteva M, Romanelli P. Follicular red dots: a novel dermoscopic pattern observed in scalp discoid lupus erythematosus. Arch Dermatol. 2009;145(12):1406–9.

96. Duque-Estrada B, Tamler C, Sodré CT, Barcaui CB, Pereira FB. Dermoscopy patterns of cicatricial alopecia resulting from discoid lupus erythematosus and lichen planopilaris. An Bras Dermatol. 2010;85(2):179–83.

97. Powell JJ, Dawber RP, Gatter K. Folliculitis decalvans including tufted folliculitis: clinical, histologic and therapeutic findings. Br J Dermatol. 1999;140(2):328–33.

98. Bolognia section 11, chapter 68 – Sperling L. Alopecias. In: Bolognia JL, Jorizzo JL, Rapini RP, editors. Dermatology. 2nd ed. Elsevier; 2008. p. 987–1005.

99. Miteva M, Tosti A. Pathologic diagnosis of central centrifugal cicatricial alopecia on horizontal sections. Am J Dermatopathol. 2014;36(11): 859–864; quiz 865–857.

Nail Diseases

Renan Minotto, Liliam Dalla Corte, Thaís Millán, and Bianca Coelho Furtado

Key Points Summary
- Onychomycosis is one of the most common infections of the nail apparatus via fungi and accounts for more than 50% of nail diseases. In turn, periungual warts are infections caused by the human papilloma virus
- Among the more important inflammatory skin diseases affecting the nails are lichen planus and psoriasis
- Lichen planus is a chronic, inflammatory, autoimmune disease that leads to destruction of basal keratinocytes, causing anonychia and permanent atrophy. Early diagnosis is essential and therapy should start immediately

- Psoriasis is a chronic inflammatory skin disease that can also affect the nails. It is thought that 80–90% of patients with psoriasis will at some point present with nail involvement. Fingernails are more commonly affected than toenails
- Among the nail dyschromias melanonychia, the brown to black color of the nail plate, which requires the important differential diagnoses such as melanoma, is noteworthy
- Ingrown toenails result from an imbalance between nail plate width, nail bed, and lateral nail fold hypertrophy. There are four types of ingrown nails: ingrowing toenail in infancy, lateral and distal nail fold hypertrophy, pincer nails, and juvenile ingrown toenail
- Paronychia is a multifactorial inflammatory disorder affecting proximal and lateral nail folds

This chapter is an approach of clinical interest onychopathies. All photos are of Dr. Renan Minotto's collection.

R. Minotto (✉) B.C. Furtado
Santa Casa Hospital, Porto Alegre, RS, Brazil
e-mail: rminotto@gmail.com;
bcfurtado@hotmail.com

L.D. Corte
Irmandade Santa Casa de Misericórdia de Porto Alegre, Porto Alegre, RS, Brazil
e-mail: ldcorte2009@gmail.com

T. Millán
Service of Dermatology, Federal University of Health Sciences of Porto Alegre, Porto Alegre, Brazil
e-mail: millan_thais@yahoo.com.br

Onychomycosis

Introduction

Onychomycosis is one of the most common fungi-related infections of the nail apparatus and accounts for more than 50% of nail diseases. Several studies have shown its relevance, which can be explained

© Springer International Publishing Switzerland 2018
R.R. Bonamigo, S.I.T. Dornelles (eds.), *Dermatology in Public Health Environments*,
https://doi.org/10.1007/978-3-319-33919-1_69

by factors such as associations with other diseases, increase in life expectancy within the population, and increasing attention to nail conditions by clinicians and patients [1]. Many species of nail fungi exist, and under conditions of moisture and heat these fungi grow quickly. Three groups of fungi cause this disease: dermatophytes, yeasts, and nondermatophyte molds [1, 2].

In certain populations (e.g., soldiers, swimmers, students, runners, sports participants), the prevalence of onychomycosis can be much higher. Several factors have resulted in an increased prevalence of onychomycosis, including wearing of shoes, particularly tight shoes; the use of damp spaces such as locker rooms and gymnasiums; and frequent nail traumas [3].

Concepts

Fungal infection of the nail is considered cosmopolitan and recalcitrant dermatosis. It should not be viewed as a mere aesthetic problem. This condition is known to require prolonged treatment with disappointing results and should be regarded as an important health issue, indicating that it is often associated with physical and psychological distress. It may interfere with the patient's quality of life; therefore, it must be treated seriously and effectively [3, 4].

Fingernails and toenails consist of a protein called keratin, which may provide substrates for the metabolism of fungi and help them to survive, leading to onychomycosis, which is highly prevalent in halluces. Some cases may be difficult to manage, especially in cases of nondermatophytic onychomycosis, even with the recent advances in antifungal drugs. Predisposing factors for onychomycosis include poor peripheral circulation, diabetes, repeated nail trauma, low immune resistance, occupation, inactivity, heat, and humidity [1–4].

Clinical Presentation

Diagnosis of fungal infection of the nails may be difficult since other diseases may clinically mimic onychomycosis. These include psoriasis

and difficulties in identifying the etiologic agent of onychomycosis, and will certainly require different treatments [1, 5].

Four types of onychomycosis are recognized [1, 7]. (1) Distal subungual onychomycosis is the most common form of onychomycosis, characterized by invasion of the nail bed and underside of the nail plate beginning at the hyponychium. It migrates proximally through the underlying nail matrix. (2) White superficial onychomycosis occurs when certain fungi invade directly the superficial layers of the nail plate. It can be favored by previous traumas and occurs primarily in the toenails. (3) Proximal subungual onychomycosis is a relatively uncommon subtype and occurs when organisms invade the nail unit via the proximal nail fold through the cuticle area, penetrate the newly formed nail plate, and migrate distally. Some cases have been reported in human immunodeficiency virus patients. (4) Total dystrophic onychomycosis is used to describe end-stage nail disease caused by dermatophytes, nondermatophytes, or *Candida* sp. The entire nail unit becomes thick and dystrophic.

Nail alterations found in onychomycosis can be seen in other entities, and most of these lesions include onycholysis, subungual hyperkeratosis, color change such as leukonychia and melanonychia, and dystrophies, among others (Figs. 69.1, 69.2, and 69.3). The differential diagnosis should include psoriasis, lichen planus, and traumatic onychopathies [3, 6].

Onycholysis is the separation of the nail from the nail bed. This separation of the nail plate begins at the proximal nail and extends to the free edge, which is seen most often in nail psoriasis. Subungual hyperkeratosis occurs as a result of

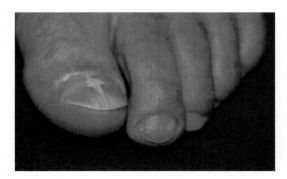

Fig. 69.1 Onychomycosis with irregular spiculated striations

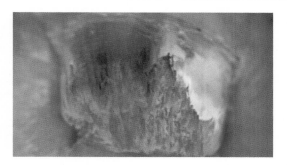

Fig. 69.2 Dermoscopy showing thickly hyperkeratosed nail plate in onychomycosis with ruin aspect

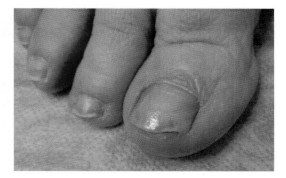

Fig. 69.3 Onycholysis and yellowish appearance of the nail plate

epithelial hyperplasia of the subungual tissues from repeated trauma and exudative skin diseases and may occur with any chronic inflammatory condition (bacterial, viral, and fungal infections) involving this area [1, 2].

Chromonychia refers to an abnormality in color of the substance or the surface of the nail plate or subungual tissues. Nail infection may well appear greenish, black, brown, or various other shades. Pseudoleukonychia caused by fungi is common [5, 6]. The presence of striated melanonychia longitudinal caused by trauma, medications, nevus, melanoma, and fungal and bacterial infection deserves attention. The lesion should be removed for biopsy in the case of suspicion of other diseases, especially melanoma. Partial ungual dystrophies are characterized by fragile, brittle nails with longitudinal or transverse cracks, and even full change of the nail plate. The small changes observed in nails may be age-related, caused by excessive exposure to detergents, nail polish removers, and the use other substances that

can dry out nails [3, 7]. Care should be taken to avoid trauma and the use of detergents, acetone, and chemicals, and to give preference to nail moisturizers that can improve the appearance of the nails. Total ungual dystrophies are commonly associated with other diseases and/or infections.

The most important differential diagnosis should include onychomycosis and psoriasis, which present symptoms such as pitting, nail discoloration, onycholysis, subungual hyperkeratosis, and even total ungual dystrophy in some cases. These two nail abnormalities can be present simultaneously. Lichen planus of nails are associated with nail changes including longitudinal grooming, nail pterygium, nail loss, and subungual hyperkeratosis. Traumatic lesions commonly show onycholysis, leukonychia, bleeding, and pigmentation changes [2, 7].

Diagnosis

Accurate diagnosis requires direct microscopy, fungal culture, and histologic examination when necessary. Direct microscopy of sampled material is necessary to definitively identify whether it is typical of dermatophyte fungi. These structures are then evaluated for morphology and coloration to help determine the clinical laboratory procedure [1, 5]. Filamentous hyaline hyphal elements characteristic of dermatophytes can be observed; the presence of pseudohyphae or tortuous hyphae, irregular, with or without conidia, can reveal nondermatophyte mycelial fungi, which makes it difficult to identify using only direct examination. In turn, the observation of the accumulation oval yeast cell forms with nonpigmented pseudofilaments may suggest *Candida* sp. Culture is the only method by which the causative microorganism can be separated and identified. Caution should be used in analyzing culture results, because nails are nonsterile and fungal and bacterial contaminants may obscure the nail pathogen. Periodic acid-Schiff (PAS) staining of nail clippings, using histopathologic processing, may be used as a complementary method for the diagnosis of onychomycosis. Hyphae are seen between the nail layers and lying parallel to the surface [3, 5].

Fungal nail infections can be caused by three different groups of fungi. Most infections are undoubtedly caused by dermatophytes, usually associated with the involvement of adjacent skin areas; however, nondermatophytic filamentous fungi and yeast also cause onychomycosis. The association between fungi or bacteria in the same nail lesion is very common and can completely change its appearance. To identify the causal agent in each patient and determine cases of multiple etiology are of paramount importance for the treatment, since antifungal drugs have different mechanisms of action [1, 3, 6].

The etiology is variable depending on whether it affects fingernails or toenails. The frequency of yeasts and filamentous fungi (dermatophytes or nondermatophytes) is similar to that found in feet; yeast occurs more frequently in the hands [4, 5].

Tinea unguium (dermatophyte onychomycosis) is caused by dermatophytes. It is an eminently chronic disease characterized by the nail plate detachment from the nail bed, subungual hyperkeratosis, and partial or total destruction of the nail [2, 5, 7]. The species that most often cause onychomycosis are *Trichophyton rubrum* and *Trichophyton mentagrophytes.*

Candida infection of the nail plate most often presents as onycholysis associated with paronychia, although complete destruction of the nail plate and erosion of the distal and lateral nail plate of the fingernails without total nail dystrophy are also seen [1, 2].

Some authors have recommended nail biopsy when it is difficult to diagnose a fungus, mainly when there is a clinical suspicion of saprobic fungus; however, this may not be possible in practice [2].

Therapeutic Approach

The therapeutic advances of recent years with the emergence of drugs for topical, oral, and/or parenteral use, such as amorolfine, ciclopirox, isoconazole, itraconazole, terbinafine, and fluconazole, among others, has promoted treatment success rates, shorter duration of use, and greater safety for patients when compared with the antifungal drugs previously used, such as griseofulvin and ketoconazole. All medications should be prescribed and have its use verified by a dermatologist, since they have the potential to cause adverse effects and more or less severe drug interactions [1, 7].

For the treatment of these diseases it is essential to observe the predisposing and/or aggravating factors that may exist, such as excess moisture, and also to treat any underlying diseases such as diabetes and circulatory problems in the lower limbs [1, 2].

Host factors influencing treatment include age, gender, vascular diseases, diabetes, hypertension, number of toenails infected, infection duration, history of previous treatment, type of onychomycosis, and percentage of nail involvement, nail thickness, presence of dermatophytes, matrix and lateral involvement, and growth rate of the nail [1, 2]. Other factors worth mentioning are inadequate hygiene, frequent traumas on the nails, athlete's foot, prolonged use of moisturizers, excessive sweating, walking barefoot, use of sandals/flip-flops, swimmers' routine, sharing bathrooms and changing rooms, and hot weather. These factors should be taking into account in providing adequate treatment and the need for therapeutic combinations [1, 7].

Onychomycosis that is influenced by host and pathogenic factors requires extensive treatment. The penetration of topical medications into the infected nail bed can be accentuated by the abrasion of the nail or the use of strategies to improve drug permeation using sulfites, hydrogen peroxide, urea, and salicylic acid, among others. Hydrogen peroxide and urea are used in the treatment of nail dermatophytosis and very thick fingernails as well as the abrasion of the affected nail. Slow nail growth caused by tight shoes or circulatory difficulties can be tackled by guidance on the use of proper footwear and hygiene [1, 5].

As onychomycosis treatment may require long-term therapy with oral antifungal and side effects and high costs, it is important to correctly diagnose the infection. Blood tests should be performed and the etiologic agent identified.

Nail Lichen Planus

Introduction

Nail lichen planus (NLP) is a condition that should be diagnosed early. Unless properly treated, it can cause severe scarring. Approximately 10% of patients with lichen planus exhibit ungual alterations, which are commonly found in the nail apparatus. Although it is not pathognomonic, pterygium is very suggestive of lichen planus and indicates fibrosis in the nail matrix, without nail plate formation due to the development of scar tissue [6, 8].

Concepts

Lichen planus lesions can occur in the fingernails or in areas such as the skin and mucous membranes. It is an inflammatory, autoimmune disease that leads to destruction of basal keratinocytes, causing severe irreversible damage to the nail unit. A genetic susceptibility for lichen planus has been reported in familial cases. This condition has a poor therapeutic response and prognosis, affecting the quality of life of the patient. The etiology has yet to be clarified. It can affect the nails only, or may also involve the oral mucosa and the skin in approximately 10–15% of patients. In adults, NPL may often cause scars [4, 6].

Clinical Presentation

NLP may affect both the bed and the nail matrix of one or more digits. Fingernails are more commonly affected than toenails. Its evolution may vary, and the later diagnosis, nail dystrophy, is more severe, leading to irreversible changes. The proximal nail fold can be affected and can lead to erythema and edema, indicating involvement of the matrix [6, 7].

Matrix involvement causes onychodystrophy with a clinical presentation that ranges from mild to severe, depending on the intensity and duration of local inflammatory change. It is characterized by thinning, longitudinal ridging, and distal splitting of the nail plate. The lunula may be irregularly red in a focal or disseminated pattern as a sign of inflammation. Dorsal pterygium, a scarring process whereby there is growth of the proximal nail fold, may occur. Brown or black pigmentation of the nail (melanonychia) may be transient if the symptoms reverse after treatment. The nails become fragile. Longitudinal ridges (onychorrhexis) may occur as the result of surface fragmentation of the nail blade. Evolution may lead to atrophy and consequent loss of the nail plate. Nail bed involvement is rare, and may

present as subungual hyperkeratosis and detachment of the nail plate (onycholysis) [4, 6].

Diagnosis

The prevalence of NLP in the general population ranges from 0.5% to 1%. It occurs in 10% of patients with disseminated disease. Permanent nail change occurs in more than 4% of patients. It is universal, frequent after the third decade of life, and may affect either children or the elderly. Recent studies have shown that women are affected twice as much as men [6, 8].

Although the clinical examination often presents features for the diagnosis, it may be insufficient. A biopsy of the matrix should be used to confirm the diagnosis. The most common nail findings (Figs. 69.4 and 69.5) are changes in nail surface, fragility of free edge with onycholysis, koilonychia, subungual hyperkeratosis, pterygium, and progressive onychatrophia that can evolve into anonychia. Histopathology may show irregular hyperplasia, accentuated acanthosis,

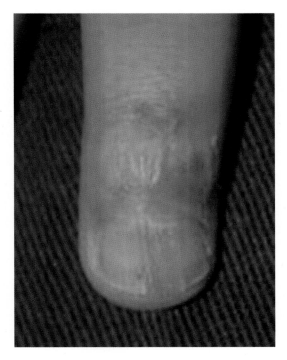

Fig. 69.4 Striae, onychorexis, dorsal pterygium, erythema, and edema of the proximal nail fold in NLP

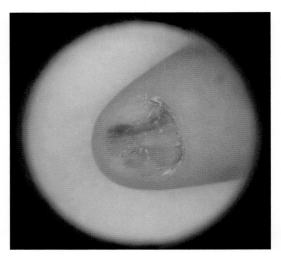

Fig. 69.5 Dermoscopy showing scarring process with pigmentation (melanonychia) in NLP

Clinical Presentation

The clinical features of nail psoriasis depend largely on the type of nail tissue affected by the condition. The effects on the nail matrix include Beau lines, pitting, leukonychia, trachyonychia, and onychorrhexis. Effects on the nail bed include onycholysis, salmon patches, oil spots, dyschromias, splinter hemorrhage, and nail bed hyperkeratosis (Figs. 69.6, 69.7, 69.8, and 69.9).

outbreaks of hypergranulosis, parakeratosis, and vacuolar degeneration of the basal layer. The nail bed can be the site for moderate mononuclear inflammatory infiltrate, with longitudinal ridging and brownish discoloration in the epithelium–nail bed junction [4, 6].

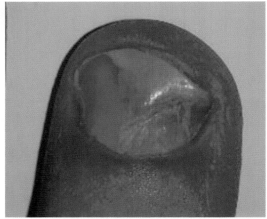

Fig. 69.6 Elkonyxis, onycholysis, and oil spots in a psoriatic nail

Therapeutic Approach

Treatment of NLP involves corticosteroid infiltration or systemic corticosteroids. The prognosis depends on the degree of matrix involvement. Early diagnosis of NPL is of major importance because of its potential aggression. If untreated, the lesions can lead to a permanent and irreversible dystrophy. Therapy may start with clobetasol enamel and pulse therapy with prednisone [4, 6].

Nail Psoriasis

Introduction

Psoriasis is a chronic inflammatory skin disease that can also affect the nails. It is thought that 80–90% of patients with psoriasis will at some point present with nail involvement [6, 9]. Fingernails are more commonly affected than toenails.

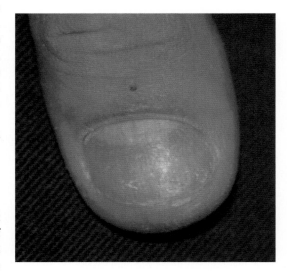

Fig. 69.7 Pitting in a psoriatic nail plate

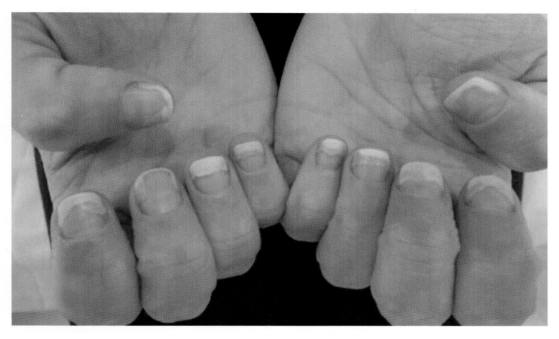

Fig. 69.8 Multiple onycholysis and oil spots in psoriatic nails of fingers

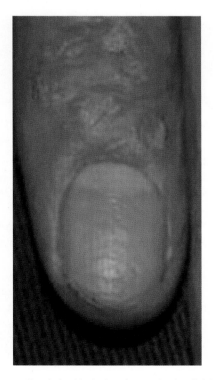

Fig. 69.9 Psoriatic skin lesions in proximal nail fold and pittings in the nail plate

The most common changes that may affect the fingers are pitting, onycholysis, and subungual hyperkeratosis; and the most common in the toes are onycholysis and subungual hyperkeratosis [5].

Diagnosis

The diagnosis is usually clinical. Histopathologic examination may be performed in cases where nail involvement is the only sign. The need for long-term treatment should be considered [11].

All patients should be evaluated for the presence of onychomycosis [6, 10].

Therapeutic

When the disease is limited to the nails, the initial treatment options are high-potency topical corticosteroids, with or without calcipotriol [10].

Clobetasol propionate cream, 0.05% at night [6]

Clobetasol nail lacquer, 0.05–8% three times a week [6]

Triamcinolone acetonide injection (5 mg/mL) into the proximal nail fold, applied monthly [6].

For patients with severe nail disease or for those whose lesions have not responded to treatment, the treatment options are intralesional corticosteroid infiltration or systemic treatment with acitretin, methotrexate, or immunobiological preparations [10].

Periungual Warts

Introduction

This condition is an infectious disease caused by the human papilloma virus (HPV). It is more common in children and adolescents and in persons with onychophagia, in whom the lesions may be multiple [4, 6].

It can evolve into squamous cell carcinoma (SCC). This neoplasm can mimic warts [4].

Clinical Presentation

Periungual warts present as keratotic papules, with black dots representing thrombosed capillaries. When in the nail bed they can cause onycholysis. Wart dissemination occurs by autoinoculation.

Diagnosis

Periungual warts are most often diagnosed by their clinical appearance (Figs. 69.10 and 69.11). The atypical lesions may require histopathologic examination and tests for detection of HPV.

Histopathologic examination should be performed in case of long-lasting warts to exclude SCC [6].

Therapeutic Approach

The choice of treatment modality depends on location, size, number, secondary infection, pain, tenderness, and age.

Topical medications available for the treatment of warts include keratolytic, antivirals, and

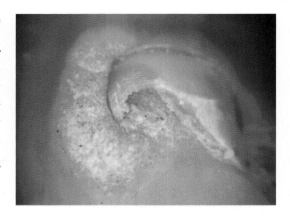

Fig. 69.10 Wart with periungual and subungual hyperkeratosis with black spots microthrombi papillae

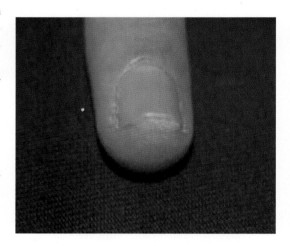

Fig. 69.11 Hyperkeratosis-related subungual wart

immunomodulatory agents. All have been used successfully; however, the keratolytic agent obtained better outcomes [12].

Salicylic acid at concentrations of 10–50% and trichloroacetic acid in solutions of 50–90% used topically promote peeling and removal of mechanistic particles [6].

Imiquimod inhibits viral replication and activates cellular immunity; 5-fluorouracil has an immunostimulatory action, causing destruction of the lesions [6, 13].

Intralesional bleomycin 0.1% has been used with good therapeutic results [6, 13].

Other therapeutic modalities including cryotherapy, chemical cauterization with salicylic acid, and laser have been used safely [12].

Melanocytic Lesions in the Nail Unit

Concepts

Melanonychia is brown or black pigmentation of the nail unit [14–16]. It has varying etiology, from physiologic lesions to malignant neoplasms. Melanonychias may be total or longitudinal. Longitudinal melanonychias are also called striata, and correspond to the melanin deposit in the nail plate. They are more frequent in the African and Asian population. Its incidence is higher in the over-50 age group, and the first and second fingers are most commonly affected [15]. Melanonychia results from melanin produced by melanocytes in the matrix, where melanocytes are usually quiescent, or by increased activation of melanocytes by nevus melanoma (Figs. 69.12, 69.13, and 69.14) [8].

Clinical Presentation

When striated melanonychia occurs in two or more nails, it may be a sign of a widespread disease (AIDS, Addison disease) or, more often, a result of side effects (chemotherapy, azidothymidine, antimalarials, psoralen/ultraviolet A therapy) [8].

Transverse melanonychia is almost always a result of a pharmacologic treatment.

To make the etiological differentiation of the lesions easier, the "ABCDEF" nail rule and dermatoscopy of the nail plate are increasingly used, while nail bed dermatoscopy is a promising test [16, 18].

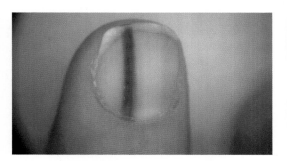

Fig. 69.12 Longitudinal melanocytic nail lesion smaller than 3 mm

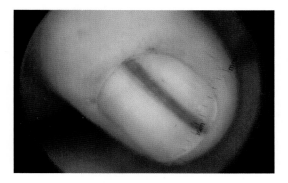

Fig. 69.13 Longitudinal melanocytic nail lesion smaller than 3 mm seen under polarized light dermoscopy (Dermlite)

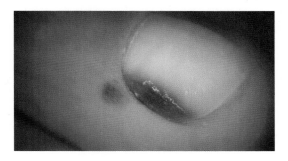

Fig. 69.14 Chromonychia (greenish) affecting the lateral edge of the longitudinal nail plate, suggestive of bacterial contamination. Note a nevus on the lateral nail fold

Diagnosis

The ABCDEF rule is useful for differentiating benign from malign melanonychia (see Box 69.1).

Box 69.1 ABCDEF and Suspect of Malign Melanonychia	
A. Age	50–70 years; African and Asian origin
B. Band	Over 3 mm; brown, black
C. Change	Nail band; nail morphology
D. Digit involved	Thumb, hallux, single
E. Extension	Hutchinson's sign
F. Family and personal history	Dysplastic nevus syndrome or previous melanona

Despite the major assistance of the ABCDEF rule and lesion dermatoscopy, histopathology still is indispensable in cases of uncertainty. The proposed treatment will depend on the etiology of each case.

Tumors in the Nail Unit

Concepts

Tumors are grouped into nonpigmented benign lesions (glomus tumor, myxoid cyst, nail keratoacanthoma) and malignant lesions (SCC and Bowen disease, onychomatricoma, nail melanoma).

Myxoid Cyst

This lesion is found in the distal phalanx of the finger, and may involve the nail matrix. It is sometimes painful and is often associated with degenerative changes in the distal joints and the presence of Heberden nodes, osteoarthritis, and bone spurs. Digital myxoid cysts occur most frequently in persons between the ages of 40 and 70 years (Fig. 69.15). The diagnosis is made by means of anamnesis and clinical examination of characteristic lesions [1]. Differential diagnoses include xanthoma, epidermoid inclusion cyst, and molluscum contagiosum, among others [6].

Some treatment approaches include aspiration with drainage, instillation of corticosteroids, cryosurgery, electrocoagulation, and surgical excision [6]. Surgical complications include infection, recurrence, onychodystrophy, edema, pain, and stiffness [6].

Glomus Tumor

This is a rare benign neoplasm that arises from the neuroarterial structure called a glomus body, an arteriovenous shunt within the dermis that contributes to temperature regulation of the fingers. The branching vessels become surrounded by myoepithelial cells, forming perivascular cuffs called Sucquet-Hoyer channels [6, 19]. They occur in women more than in men [6]. Usually, these tumors present as a small, reddish blue nodule measuring up to 2 cm (Fig. 69.16). Ungual alterations are frequently observed. Clinically the lesions are characterized by intense, pulsating, and debilitating pain. Clinical diagnosis is done by the classical triad of paroxysmal pain, hypersensitivity to temperature changes, and local sensitivity (Box 69.2) [6].

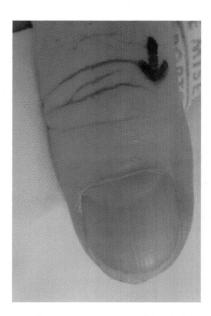

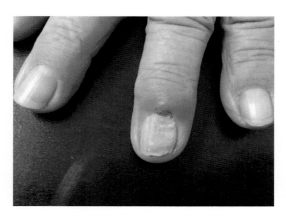

Fig. 69.15 Myxoid cyst. Lesion in dorsal portion of finger

Fig. 69.16 Glomus tumor with reddish painful blue spot in the lunula

Several clinical tests are useful for diagnosing glomus tumors: (1) tourniquet, puncture; (2) radiography; (3) dermatoscopy; (4) ultrasonography; and (5) magnetic resonance imaging (MRI). Histologic assessment of tumors is regarded as the gold standard in this respect. Complete surgical excision (Figs. 69.17 and 69.18) is the recommended treatment for glomus tumors to avoid recurrence [6, 17, 19, 20].

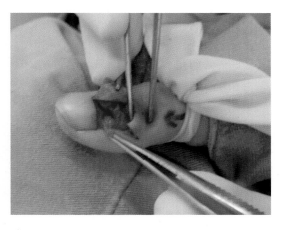

Fig. 69.17 The lobuled tumor is located below the nail bed attached to the bone

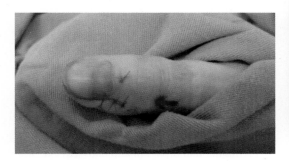

Fig. 69.18 Immediate appearance after suture

Nail Keratoacanthoma

Keratoacanthoma is a low-grade skin tumor that rarely affects the nail apparatus [1]. Middle-aged men are more at risk. It can be solitary, multiple, eruptive, or familial. The clinical feature differs from that of traditional keratoacanthoma, as in the subungual form there is usually pain, early and fast growth, and underlying bone compression [21]. The diagnosis is made by clinical and complementary examinations.

The differential diagnosis of a painful and nodular lesion in the distal phalanx includes dermoid cyst, common wart, subungual exostosis, amelanotic melanoma, SCC, and subungual keratoacanthoma. Radiologically the subungual keratoacanthoma is almost indistinguishable from subungual SCC. Nonetheless, keratoacanthoma causes a lesion in the distal phalanx that has well-defined borders and grows but does not penetrate the bone. Furthermore, keratoacanthoma usually occurs in the fifth decade of life, whereas SCC usually occurs in the seventh decade [21]. Treatment includes curettage and local excision.

Squamous Cell Carcinoma and Bowen's Disease

SCC is a malignant neoplasm originating from the epithelial cells of the skin and mucosa. This neoplasm is characterized by variable clinical features (Fig. 69.19) and an indolent clinical

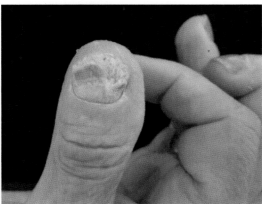

Fig. 69.19 Squamous cell carcinoma of the nail bed causing destruction of the nail plate

course. Bowen disease is a squamous cell carcinoma in situ. It affects all races and is more frequent in males in the fifth and sixth decades of life. The etiopathogenesis has not been confirmed. Several factors are involved: trauma, chronic infections, immune suppression, congenital diseases, exposure to radiation, and infection by the HPV [6].

Biopsy is the gold standard for the diagnosis. The treatment is surgical and may include a limited to digital amputation, depending on the tumor and extension of bone involvement.

Onychomatricoma

Onychomatricomas are rare benign tumors originating from the nail matrix and underlying stroma, affecting middle-aged men and women evenly. It is more prevalent in Caucasians [6].

The condition is usually asymptomatic; however, the key clinical feature for the diagnosis is the presence of a yellowish longitudinal band of variable thickness (Fig. 69.20) [22].

Additional tests may help confirm or rule out the diagnosis, such as dermatoscopy, ultrasonography, and MRI. The biopsy of the lesion is crucial for a definitive diagnosis, which is histologic. Effective treatment is complete surgical excision (Fig. 69.21), and the long-term prognosis is favorable [17, 22].

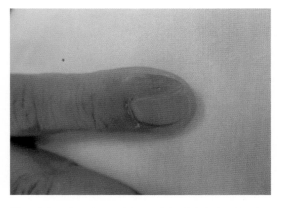

Fig. 69.20 Onychomatricoma of the right index showing yellowish appearance of striations

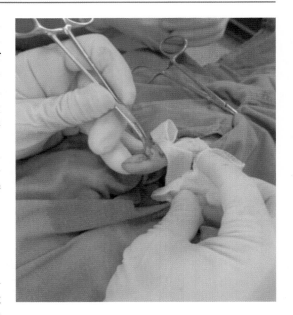

Fig. 69.21 Surgical resection of the tumor

Nail Apparatus Melanoma

Nail apparatus melanoma (NAM) is a rare melanocytic neoplasm, with an average 5-year survival rate of 56% in developing countries [6]. NAM is more commonly seen as longitudinal melanonychia, which can also be a clinical manifestation of other ungual apparatus changes that cause ungual matrix melanocytic activation (Fig. 69.22). The pigmented bands due to continuous growth of the nail plaque can be seen in ungual matrix nevi alongside benign melanocytic hyperplasia and inflammatory, traumatic, and iatrogenic changes.

Hirata et al. have suggested that the use of intraoperative dermatoscopy on the nail bed and matrix with polarized light could result in better visualization of pigmented lesions, since this examines the region of melanin production. Although this is an invasive technique it could give the best level of diagnostic accuracy when compared with clinical examination, ABCDEF rules, and traditional dermatoscopy (Fig. 69.23) [23].

Histopathology is still the gold standard, and biopsy can be incisional or excisional [3]. Although there is no current consensus on managing ungual melanoma in situ, surgical excision

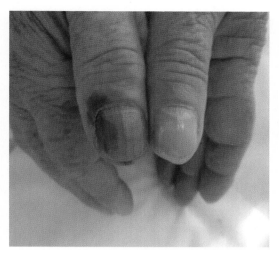

Fig. 69.22 Longitudinal melanonychia on the right distal phalanx of the finger

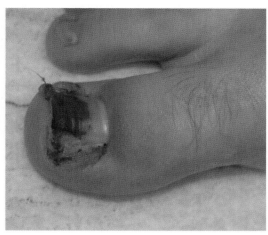

Fig. 69.24 Severe ingrown toenail

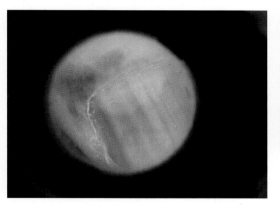

Fig. 69.23 Traditional dermatoscopy shows irregular pigmentation of the nail plate

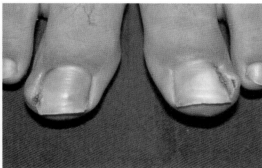

Fig. 69.25 Bilateral ingrown toenail

entails the complete ungual apparatus itself, including the nail plaque, bed, and matrix [17, 23]. The resulting defect can be corrected with a partial or total skin graft.

Ingrown Toenail

Concepts

An ingrown toenail is a multifactorial inflammatory condition that may cause severe discomfort and pain to the patient. Ingrown toenails result from an imbalance between the width of the nail plate, the nail bed, and lateral nail fold hypertrophy [24, 27].

Clinical Presentation

Ingrown toenails (Figs. 69.24 and 69.25) can be classified into four types: ingrowing toenail in infancy, lateral and distal nail fold hypertrophy, pincer nails, and juvenile ingrown toenail.

Ingrown Toenail in Infancy
1. Distal toenail embedding with normally directed nail

This condition consists of congenital hypertrophy of the distal tissue. In most cases, conservative treatment with massage of the distal nail wall in a distal-plantar direction is effective. This condition usually resolves up to 6 years of age [6, 24, 26].

2. Congenital hypertrophic nail fold of the hallux

Most frequently, the medial nail fold is hypertrophic. This condition may resolve spontaneously after several months. In persistent cases, resection of the hypertrophic nail fold is indicated [6, 24, 26].

3. Congenital malalignment of the hallux nail

This condition is characterized by a thickened, triangular, discolored, oyster-shell-like nail.

When the deviation is small, with hardening of the nail, distal locking disappears; when the deviation is severe, surgical rotation of the nail matrix is required [24, 26].

Lateral and Distal Nail Fold Hypertrophy

The nail plate exerts pressure on the nail folds, keeping its anatomic shape. When the nail plate is absent, the pulp of the hallux is dislocated dorsally during foot gait, leading to nail fold hypertrophy. Treatment consists of surgical removal of hypertrophic nail folds, allowing for physiologic growth of the nail plate [24, 26].

Pincer Nails

This condition is characterized by transverse overcurvature of the nail plate. In most cases, the overcurvature is bilaterally symmetric and combined with lateral deviation of the long axis of the nail. Radiography is an essential diagnostic tool, often revealing osteophytes [24, 26].

Juvenile Ingrown Toenail

This condition results from an imbalance between the width of the nail plate and that of the distal portion of the nail bed. Contributing factors include convex nail clipping, overcurvature of the nail plate, toe rotation, and wearing inappropriate shoes [6, 24, 26].

Juvenile ingrown toenail can be classified into three clinical stages [24, 26]

1. Erythema, edema, and pain on pressure
2. Purulent drainage and infection
3. Purulent granulation tissue and lateral nail hypertrophy

Therapeutic Approach

Conservative Treatment

The decision to adopt a conservative treatment approach depends on the clinical aspect of the ingrown toenail. This approach is indicated in the following cases: absence of lateral nail fold hypertrophy, presence of mild distal nail fold hypertrophy, and presence of mild transverse overcurvature of the nail [26].

General measures: wearing wide shoes or walking barefoot and correcting nail trimming [24].

The clip system: a plastic brace is glued crosswise to the nail and maintained for 3–4 weeks. The goal is to correct the transverse overcurvature of the nail. This method promotes fast pain relief [24, 26].

Placing wisps of cotton on lateral nail folds protects the nail spike and allows the nail plate to grow without traumatizing the surrounding tissue [26].

Gutter treatment: consists of inserting a longitudinally sectioned vinyl tube into the lateral nail margin. This procedure is performed under local anesthesia [24].

Tape is used to pull the lateral nail fold laterally. This method should be performed daily [6, 24, 26].

Acrylic artificial nails are placed over ingrown nails to push the lateral nail folds laterally and decrease hypertrophy [24, 26].

Surgical Treatment

Surgery is indicated when conservative treatments fail or in moderate and severe cases.

Definitive Narrowing of the Nail Plate

1. Chemical cauterization

This treatment is indicated for stage 2 and 3 ingrown toenails and for pincer nails at any stage. In the latter, the procedure will relieve the pinching effect on the underlying tissue. In pincer nails with hyperostosis of the distal tuft, this technique is beneficial in the presence of pain on lateral pressure. When pain on downward pressure is present, other techniques are indicated [25, 29].

Phenol cauterization is a simple but highly effective method for treating ingrown nails, with success rates as high as 95% [24, 29]. Phenol is a necrotizing, disinfecting, anesthetic agent. It causes tissue destruction, disinfects the surgical field, and improves postoperative patient comfort (phenol induces demyelination of terminal nerve endings for several weeks) [6].

Distal digital block anesthesia is administered with lidocaine 2% without epinephrine. When granulation tissue is present, it should be removed to improve visualization of the lateral margin of the nail plate. A lateral strip of nail is cut longitudinally and avulsed, allowing access to the lateral horns of the matrix. When necessary, the nail matrix, the nail bed, and the lateral nail folds are gently curetted to remove debris. A tourniquet is applied and a cotton swab with phenol 88% is rubbed vigorously over the area for 1–3 min [24, 25, 27, 30].

Phenol will be inactivated with the blood flow after release of the tourniquet. Some authors use alcohol to do this [6, 28]. Oozing will appear on the third postoperative day and continue for up to 2–4 weeks. Frequent washing of the wound prevents infection and accelerates healing [1, 3]. Antibiotic therapy is indicated when infection is present [24, 25, 27, 28].

2. Wedge resection

This treatment is technically more challenging. A lateral strip of nail is avulsed and an oblique section is performed on the proximal nail fold to allow nail fold elevation and visualization of the lateral horn of the matrix. The horn is then meticulously dissected from the bone. Pain and a high postoperative infection rate (20%) [24, 28] are drawbacks of this technique.

Debulking of Periungual Soft Tissues

This procedure is indicated when an ingrown nail is caused by hypertrophy of the nail folds. There are two main debulking surgical approaches.

1. Howard–Dubois procedure

Distal digital block with lidocaine 2% without epinephrine is administered followed by application of a tourniquet. A crescent of soft tissue is removed with a fish-mount incision performed parallel to the distal groove, around the tip of the toe. The first incision is made 5 mm below the distal and lateral grooves. The second incision is made so as to create a wedge of 3–5 mm at its greatest width in the middle of the distal wall. Both fat and fibrous tissue should be removed. The wound should be closed using simple interrupted stitches (4.0 or 5.0 nylon). The major complication of this procedure is necrosis by overtight suturing. The postoperative period is painful, requiring good pain control. Stitches are removed after 10–14 days [25, 27, 29].

2. Super U procedure

This technique described by Eval Rosa is indicated in cases of severe hypertrophy of nail folds. Eligible patients should be informed of the long healing time (up to 2 months). A U-shaped incision is performed starting at the proximal edge of one of the lateral nail folds, running through to the distal nail fold, and ending on the other side of the lateral nail fold. All hypertrophic tissues are removed. Running locked suture with 3.0 or 4.0 nylon is performed to avoid bleeding [25, 27, 29]. Pain is severe in the first 48 h. Mild opioid-type narcotic pain medications should be prescribed.

Paronychia

Concepts

Paronychia is an inflammatory disorder affecting the proximal and lateral nail folds, usually caused by trauma to the cuticle, which is the physical barrier between the nail plate and nail folds [7, 30]. Trauma can result from ordinary events, such as dishwashing, nail biting, finger sucking, an ingrown nail, or other types of nail manipulation [30, 31]. When the cuticle separates from the nail plate, an inflammatory reaction may occur as a result of the penetration of infectious organisms, allergens, or irritants [30, 31]. The pathogen most commonly associated with paronychia is *Staphylococcus aureus*, but cases infected by *Streptococcus pyogenes*, *Pseudomonas pyocyanea*, and *Proteus vulgaris* have also been reported [30–32].

Paronychia can be classified into acute or chronic. Acute paronychia is characterized by the rapid onset and evolution of symptoms after the trauma. Chronic paronychia is a multifactorial inflammatory reaction lasting longer than 6 weeks [30–32]. Chronic paronychia is common in housewives, bartenders, and kitchen workers, whose work activities require frequent hand contact with water and detergents [6, 30].

Acute Paronychia

Clinical Presentation

The affected digit is painful, showing erythema and swelling of the proximal and lateral nail folds [30, 31]. Patients initially present with accumulation of purulent material under the nail fold. Subungual abscess with pain and inflammation of the nail matrix can occur if the infection remains untreated [6, 30, 31].

Diagnosis

The diagnosis of acute paronychia is based on history of minor trauma and physical examination findings.

The digital pressure test may be useful to detect the condition in early stages. The test is performed by applying light pressure to the distal volar aspect of the affected digit. The increase in pressure within the nail fold (particularly in the abscess cavity) causes blanching of the overlying skin and clear demarcation of the abscess.

In moderate and severe cases, it is important to identify the responsible agent and rule out infections caused by methicillin-resistant *S. aureus* [6, 29, 30].

Therapeutic Approach

Clinical treatment [6, 30, 31]:

1. Soaking the affected digit in warm water and in Burow's solution
2. Mild cases: antibiotic cream (gentamicin, mupirocin, fusidic acid) alone or in combination with topical corticosteroid
3. Persistent lesions: oral antistaphylococcal antibiotic therapy

Surgical treatment is recommended when an abscess is present [6, 7, 21, 30]:

1. Superficial infections: easily drained with a size-11 scalpel or by lifting the nail fold with the tip of a 21- or 23-gauge needle
2. Severe cases: removal of the proximal third of the nail plate

Preventive measures are listed in Box 69.3.

Box 69.3 Recommendations for Preventing Acute and Chronic Paronychia [7, 30]
1. Avoid moist environments, chronic microtrauma, and contact with irritants or allergens (for at least 3 months once the condition is resolved)
2. Wear cotton gloves under rubber gloves during manual work
3. Avoid aggressive nail procedures (e.g., manicuring)
4. Keep nails short
5. Keep affected areas clean and dry

Chronic Paronychia

Clinical Presentation

In chronic paronychia, erythema is less intense than in acute paronychia. Other clinical manifestations include tenderness and swelling, with retraction of the proximal nail fold and absence of the adjacent cuticle (Fig. 69.26). Pus may form bellow the nail fold.

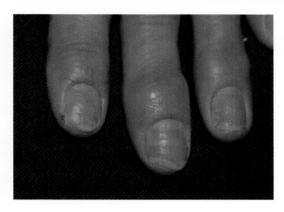

Fig. 69.26 Chronic paronychia, dystrophic nails, and onychomycosis

Usually several fingernails are affected. Colonization by *Candida albicans* or bacteria may occur [6, 30].

Diagnosis

Chronic paronychia is diagnosed based on clinical findings present for at least 6 weeks, history of trauma, frequent contact with detergents or other chemicals, or systemic drug therapy (retinoids, antiretroviral agents, antiepidermal growth factor receptor antibodies) [4, 26, 30].

In cases that do not respond to treatment, differential diagnosis with squamous cell carcinoma, malignant melanoma, and metastases from malignant tumors should be performed.

Therapeutic Approach

Clinical Treatment

Exposure to irritants should be avoided. Topical steroids are the first-line therapy; tacrolimus 0.1% ointment is an alternative option [6, 30].

Topical treatment with a steroid and an antifungal agent combined may be used, but data showing the superiority of this combined treatment in relation to steroid therapy alone are lacking [30, 31].

In refractory cases, monthly intralesional injections of triamcinolone acetonide (2.5 mg/mL) may be used.

Surgical Treatment

Surgery is recommended when the associated fibrosis does not improve with clinical treatment [6, 30, 33].

En bloc excision of the proximal nail fold (4–5 mm) is effective.

Recently, the square flap technique has been proposed to treat chronic fibrosis caused by paronychia. The technique consists of incising the proximal nail fold, exposing the fibrosis, and removing it carefully, so as to prevent damage to the nail matrix [33].

Preventive measures are listed in Box 69.4.

> **Box 69.4 Recommendations for Preventing Acute and Chronic Paronychia** [7, 30]
> 1. Avoid moist environments, chronic microtrauma, and contact with irritants or allergens (for at least 3 months once the condition is resolved)
> 2. Wear cotton gloves under rubber gloves during manual work
> 3. Avoid aggressive nail procedures (e.g., manicuring)
> 4. Keep nails short
> 5. Keep affected areas clean and dry

Glossary

Chromonychia Abnormalities of color depend on the transparency of the nail, its attachments, and the character of the underlying tissue.

Hutchinson's sign Extension of melanocytic pigment to lateral, proximal, and distal folds, adjacent to the nail plate.

Koilonychia A transverse and longitudinal concave nail dystrophy giving a spoon-shaped appearance.

Melanonychia A black or brown discoloration of the nail, usually localized and often longitudinal.

Onychomycosis A fungal infection of the nail apparatus.

Pitting Pits are small erosions in the nail surface.

PUVA therapy PUVA is a combination treatment used for severe skin diseases consisting of psoralens (P) followed by exposure of the skin to UVA (long-wave ultraviolet radiation).

References

1. Gupta AK, Cernea M, Foley KA. Improving cure rates in onychomycosis. J Cutan Med Surg. 2016;20:517–31.
2. Vlahovic TC. Onychomycosis: evaluation, treatment options, managing recurrence, and patient outcomes. Clin Podiatr Med Surg. 2016;33(3):305–18.
3. Gupta AK, Daigle D, Foley KA. Network metaanalysis of onychomycosis treatments. Skin Appendage Disord. 2015;1(2):74–81.
4. Bolognia J, Jorizzo J, Rapini R. Nail disorders. In: Dermatology. 2nd ed. St. Louis: Mosby Elsevier; 2008. p. 1019–142.
5. Natarajan V, Nath AK, Thappa DM, Singh R, Verma SK. Coexistence of onychomycosis in psoriatic nails: a descriptive study. Indian J Dermatol Venereol Leprol. 2010;76(6):723.
6. Baran R, Nakamura R. Doença das Unhas: do diagnóstico ao tratamento. Rio de Janeiro: Elsevier; 2011.
7. Iorizzo M. Tips to treat the 5 most common nail disorders: brittle nails, onycholysis, paronychia, psoriasis, onychomycosis. Dermatol Clin. 2015;33:175–83.
8. Belda W Jr, Di Chiacchio N, Criado PR. Tratado de Dermatologia. Athenaeum. 2014;50:1079–118.
9. Baran R. How to diagnose and treat psoriasis of the nails. Presse Med. 2014;43(11):1251–9.
10. Crowley JJ, Weinberg JM, Wu JJ, Robertson AD, Van Voorhees AS. National Psoriasis Foundation. Treatment of nail psoriasis: best practice recommendations from the Medical Board of the National Psoriasis Foundation. JAMA Dermatol. 2015;151(1):87–94.
11. Grover C, Reddy BS, Uma CK. Diagnosis of nail psoriasis: importance of biopsy and histopathology. Br J Dermatol. 2005;153(6):1153–8.
12. Tosti A, Piraccini BM. Warts of the nail unit: surgical and nonsurgical approaches. Dermatol Surg. 2011;27(3):235–9.
13. Herschthal J, McLeod MP, Zaiac M. Management of ungual warts. Dermatol Ther. 2012;25(6):545–50.
14. Baran R, Kechijian P. Longitudinal melanonychia (melanonychiastriata): diagnosis and management. J Am Acad Dermatol. 1989;21:1165–78.
15. Haneke E, Baran R. Longitudinal melanonychia. Dermatol Surg. 2001;27:580–4.
16. Azulay RD, Azulay DR. Dermatologia. 4th ed. Rio de Janeiro: Guanabara Koogan; 2006. p. 532–48. 653

17. Baran R, Dawber RPR, de Becker D, Haneke E, editors. Baran and Dawber's diseases of the nail and their management. 3rd ed. New York: Blackwell Science; 2001. p. 607–30.
18. Bilemjian APJ, Maceira JP, Barcaui CB, Pereira FB. Melanoníquia: importância da avaliação dermatoscópica e da observação da matriz/leito ungueal. An Bras Dermatol. 2009;84(2):185–9.
19. Di Chiacchio N, Loureiro WR, Di Chiacchio NG, Bet DL. Tumores Glômicos subungueais sincrônicos no mesmo dedo. An Bras Dermatol. 2012;87(3):477–8.
20. Maehara LSN, Ohe EMD, Enokihara MY, Michalany NS, Yamada S, Hirata SH. Diagnóstico do tumor glômico pela dermatoscopia do leito e da matriz ungueal. An Bras Dermatol. 2010;85(2):236–8.
21. Minotto R, Corte LD, Boff AL, Silva MVS, Morais MR. Subungual keratoacanthoma: a case report. Surg Cosmet Dermatol. 2014;6(4):377–9.
22. Baran R, Kint A. Onychomatrixoma: filamentous tufted tumor in the matrix of a funnel-shaped nail: a new entity (report of three cases). Br J Dermatol. 1992;126(5):510–5.
23. Carreno AM, Nakajima SR, Pennini SN, Candido Junior R, Schettini APMS. Nail apparatus melanoma: a diagnostic opportunity. An Bras Dermatol. 2013;88(2):268–71.
24. Haneke E. Nail surgery. Clin Dermatol. 2013;31: 516–25.
25. Di Chiacchio N, Di Chiacchio NG. Best way to treat an ingrown toenail. Dermatol Clin. 2015;33:277–82.
26. Baran R, Rigopoulos D. Cirurgia ungueal. In: Tratamento das doenças da unha. Rio de Janeiro: Di Livros; 2014. p. 147–58. Translated from English.
27. Richert B, Di Chiacchio N, Haneke E. Cirurgia da matriz. In: Cirurgia da unha. Rio de Janeiro: Di Livros; 2012. Translated from English.
28. Richert B. Surgical management of ingrown toenails: an update overdue. Dermatol Ther. 2012;25:498–509.
29. Richert B, Di Chiacchio N, Haneke E. Cirurgia das dobras laterais. In: Cirurgia da unha. Rio de Janeiro: Di Livros; 2012. p. 85–96. Translated from English.
30. Rigopoulos D, Larios G, Gregoriou S, Alevizos A. Acute and chronic paronychia. Am Fam Physician. 2008;77:339–43.
31. Baran R, Rigopoulos D. Paroníquia aguda. In: Tratamento das doenças da unha. Rio de Janeiro: Di Livros; 2014. p. 69–71. Translated from English.
32. Bolognia J, Jorizzo J, Rapini R. Nail disorders. In: Dermatology. 2nd ed. St. Louis: Mosby Elsevier; 2008. p. 1019–36.
33. Ferreira Vieira d'Almeida L, Papaiordanou F, Araújo Machado E, Loda G, Baran R, Nakamura R. Chronic paronychia treatment: square flap technique. J Am Acad Dermatol. 2016. doi: 10.1016/j.jaad.2016.02.1154. [Epub ahead of print].

Metatarsalgia, Calluses, and Callosities of the Feet

Silvio Maffi

Key Points Summary
- Metatarsalgia is localized or diffuse pain in the metatarsal heads
- Metatarsalgia can be classified as primary metatarsalgia resulting from a functional or postural condition, or secondary metatarsalgia resulting from a metabolic, neurologic, traumatic, or iatrogenic condition
- Hyperkeratosis expresses increased activity of keratinocytes in a callus or callosity, where it results from epidermal intermittent mechanical stimulation due to friction or increased pressure
- Callus or heloma is a reactive hyperkeratotic lesion of the skin located in well-defined friction or stress points with well-delimited edges, painful to direct local palpation
- Callosity or tyloma is a larger hyperkeratotic reactive lesion than the callus. It can be seen in larger areas of friction and stress, with more subtle margins, which usually encompass a wider area and show painful and more diffuse symptoms.
- The correct assessment of the etiology and diagnostic differentiation deeply influences the type of therapeutic approach.

Concepts

Metatarsalgia and plantar pain are frequent complaints of modern humanity. Bipedalism, paved ground, footwear and its peculiar variations, and many other evolutionary changes have created an array of factors that favor lesion development, deformities, and pain in the anterior and plantar regions of the human foot.

Calluses and callosity are the most often found hyperkeratotic wounds in the feet. These lesions are strongly related to contact with, friction against, and strain on the feet when individuals walk, jump, and wear shoes. For this reason it is important to distinguish calluses and callosity from other hyperkeratotic lesions that develop on the feet, such as plantar warts, eccrine poroma, arsenical keratosis, plantar keratodermas, and porokeratosis, since the treatment of these lesions requires a totally different approach (Box 70.1).

Metatarsalgia, calluses, and callosities are closely related. They are usually part of the same clinical presentation of the patient's complaint of foot pain and/or hyperkeratosis, as metatarsalgia usually expresses a reactive hyperkeratotic lesion.

S. Maffi
Orthopaedics, Porto Alegre, Brazil
e-mail: silviomaffi@me.com;
clinicaecirurgiadope@gmail.com

© Springer International Publishing Switzerland 2018
R.R. Bonamigo, S.I.T. Dornelles (eds.), *Dermatology in Public Health Environments*,
https://doi.org/10.1007/978-3-319-33919-1_70

Box 70.1 Foot Hyperkeratoses: Main Causes

Bone Causes

Protruding metatarsal condyle

Long metatarsos

Post-traumatic deformities

Congenital foot deformities

Toe deformities

Systemic Diseases

Arthritis rheumatoid

Psoriatic arthritis

Gout

Dermatologic lesions

Plantar warts

Eccrine poroma

Plantar porokeratosis

Keratoderma

Arsenical keratosis

Epithelioma cuniculatum (verrucous carcinoma)

Seborrheic keratosis (stucco keratosis)

Tissular Causes

Plantar fat pad atrophy

Plantar scars

Iatrogenic Causes

Unsuccessful metatarsal surgeries

Unsuccessful toe surgeries

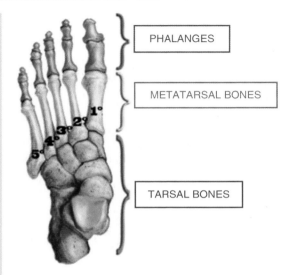

Fig. 70.1 The metatarsal, tarsal, and phalangeal bones

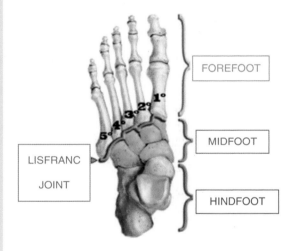

Fig. 70.2 Forefoot, midfoot, and hindfoot

Anatomic and Biomedical Considerations of the Foot

The foot can be anatomically divided into the metatarsal, tarsal, and phalangeal bones. The tarsus encompasses the calcaneus, talus, navicular, and cuboid bones, and the three cuneiform bones. The five metatarsal bones connect the tarsus to the phalanges that make up the foot (Fig. 70.1).

Another anatomic division that takes functionality into account divides the foot into forefoot, midfoot, and hindfoot. The forefoot includes the five toes and the five metatarsal bones; the midfoot includes the navicular, cuboid, and three cuneiform bones; and the hindfoot includes the calcaneus and talus (Fig. 70.2).

It is in the forefoot that most calluses develop, in addition to callosity and plantar warts, since it comprises a large and important foot support area, besides having joint mobility of the toes and many bone prominences that cause direct contact with footwear.

The joint line dividing the midfoot and the forefoot is called the tarsal–metatarsal joint or Lisfranc joint. It is responsible for the movements of plantar flexion, dorsal flexion, and metatarsal pronation and supination (Fig. 70.2).

The metatarsal bones are long bones that show a distal protrusion that joins the toe proximal phalanges, the so-called metatarsal heads. They make up important plantar pressure points, mainly the second and third metatarsal bones, usually longer than the first metatarsal bone.

The metatarsal bone length may show anatomic variation and make up one of the three patterns specified as follows, known as metatarsal formulae:

Index Plus type: $1 > 2 > 3 > 4 > 5$ (Fig. 70.3).

Index Plus-Minus type: $1 = 2 > 3 > 4 > 5$ (Fig. 70.4)

Index Minus type (A): $2 > 1 > 3 > 4 > 5$ (Fig. 70.5) or (B): $2 > 3 > 1 > 4 > 5$ (Fig. 70.6)

The most commonly found pattern in the population is the index minus type (approximately 60%) ($2 > 1 > 3 > 4 > 5$) [1].

Under the metatarsal heads the plantar plaque can be observed, as well as the toe flexor tendons and the plantar fat pad. These structures are important for joint movement and stabilization of the toes, in addition to absorbing the impact and pressure resulting from body weight unloading on the ground. The plantar plaque is a fibrocartilaginous structure included in the metatarsal-phalangeal joint capsule. It hinders toe hyperextension and is extremely resistant to tensile strength involved in the gait mechanism (Fig. 70.7).

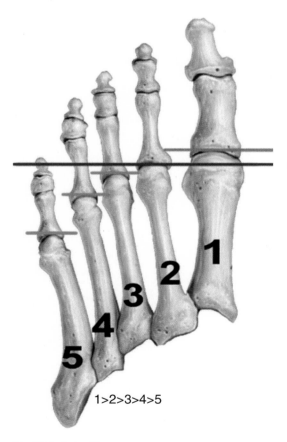

Fig. 70.3 Index Plus type

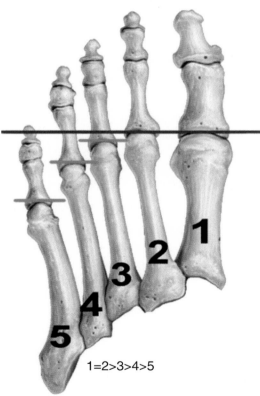

Fig. 70.4 Index Plus-Minus type

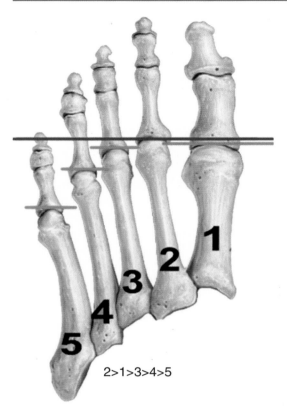

Fig. 70.5 Index Minus type A

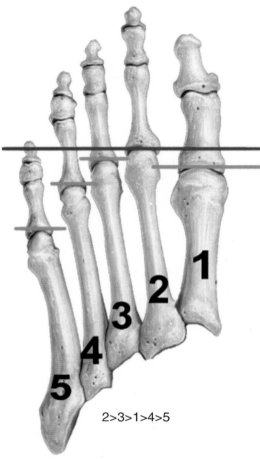

Fig. 70.6 Index Minus type B

The hallux is the great toe which, different from the others, has two sesamoid bones inserted into its plantar plaque, known as the glenosesamoid complex or apparatus. They strengthen the hallux joint stability, act as pulleys for the flexor tendons, and represent two support points under the head of the first metatarsal bone (Fig. 70.8).

The plantar fat pad runs from the calcaneus to the toe bases, displaying a unique septal configuration. Small ligaments cross the fat tissue and connect the skin to the deepest connective tissue, therefore creating resistant compartments that hinder fat displacement when the feet undergo strain (Fig. 70.9).

The biomechanics of the foot are very complex. Bones, muscles, and tendons act in a dynamic mechanism, with oscillations between gait phases. This joint system confers stability, strength, and impulse thus attenuating strain, absorbing impact, and allowing the necessary stability for the feet to adapt to ground irregularities.

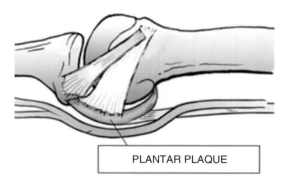

Fig. 70.7 Fibrocartilaginous structure and the gait mechanism

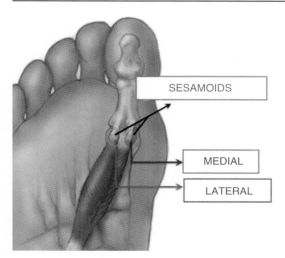

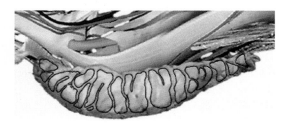

Fig. 70.8 Glenosesamoid complex

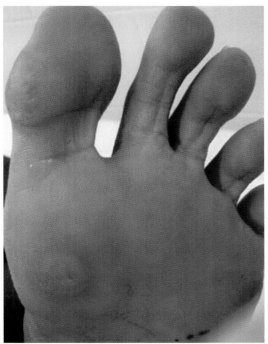

Fig. 70.9 Plantar fat

The hindfoot and midfoot joints have a small movement range that guarantees them mechanical stability and support. The forefoot, however, has the greatest mobility, mainly the fourth and fifth metatarsal bones, an important feature for foot balance and adjustment. On the other hand the first, second, and third metatarsal bones have movements limited at the Lisfranc joint level; they are stronger, more stable, and support a large part of the forefoot. Being longer and firmer, these three metatarsal bones create compression points under their heads that can result in calluses or callosities, depending on the footwear, physical activity, or any other factor that changes the normal distribution of the body weight [2].

During the gait support phase, the center of the plantar pressure moves rapidly from the calcaneus to the metatarsal bones where it remains more than 50% of the time before going toward the toes. Therefore, any change or abnormality of the forefoot, either local or diffused, may result in plantar calluses or callosity development [3].

Clinical Presentation

Metatarsalgia is the localized or generalized pain in the region of the metatarsal heads. It can be classified as primary metatarsalgia, i.e., functional or postural, or secondary metatarsalgia, i.e., metabolic, neurologic, traumatic, or iatrogenic [4, 5]. Hyperkeratosis represents increased activity of keratinocytes, as occurring in a callus or callosity, where hyperkeratosis results from the intermittent mechanical stimulation of the epidermis by friction or increased pressure. Callus, or heloma, is a reactive hyperkeratotic skin lesion located in well-defined friction and pressure points with well-delimited edges, painful to direct local palpation (Fig. 70.10).

Fig. 70.10 Reactive hyperkeratotic skin

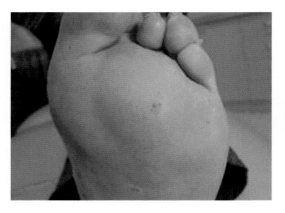

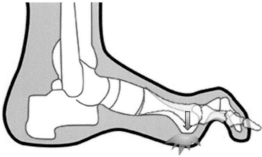

Fig. 70.12 Metatarsal plantar flexion

Fig. 70.11 Callosity (tyloma)

Callosity, or tyloma, is a larger hyperkeratotic reactive lesion than the callus. It is located in larger areas of friction and pressure, with more subtle margins which usually encompass a wider area, and shows painful and more diffuse symptoms (Fig. 70.11).

Metatarsalgia, calluses, and callosities are closely related. They are often seen as a an overall clinical presentation in a patient who complains of pain and/or foot hyperkeratosis, since metatarsalgia expresses a hyperkeratotic reactive lesion.

Primary Metatarsalgia

Primary metatarsalgia includes conditions that alter the metatarsal basic anatomy, the reciprocal relationship of the metatarsal bones, and how they relate to the other toe bones.

The main cause of primary metatarsalgia involves the *Index Minus* type metatarsal pattern, where the second and/or the third metatarsal bones are longer than the hallux and, therefore, more susceptible to the local increased plantar pressure during the gait impulse phase, when there is rolling and detachment of the forefoot.

The second most common cause of primary metatarsalgia is plantar displacement, or

plantar flexion, of one or more metatarsal bones. This changes load distribution and leaves a localized pressure on the flexed head(s), resulting in varied size callosities on the forefoot plantar region. The metatarsal plantar flexion is usually observed as a result of claw deformity in one or more toes which pushes the metatarsal head toward the ground, owing to the anatomic change and imbalanced tendon forces (Fig. 70.12).

Another cause is the congenital postural changes of the feet, such as cavus and equinus deformity of the foot which results in a generalized metatarsal mechanic overload. Cavus deformity results in a decreased support surface that entails an area of plantar hyperpressure (Fig. 70.13). The equinus foot, on the other hand, promotes this increased pressure because of triceps surae muscle contracture that results in forced flexion of the forefoot toward the ground (Fig. 70.14).

Primary metatarsalgia may occur as a result of congenital deformities of the head itself, or the metatarsal condyles. An ill-formed, enlarged head or a more protruding condyle can result in pain and callosity on the plantar aspect.

It is worth noting that together with the causes of primary metatarsalgia, the increased pressure under the metatarsal heads is excessively intensified, with an impact on physical activities and the use of thin-soled or high-heeled shoes.

Fig. 70.13 Normal and
cavus foot

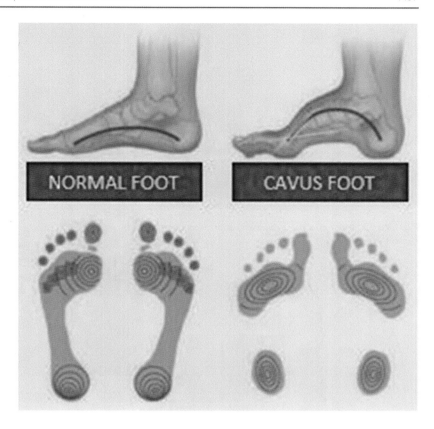

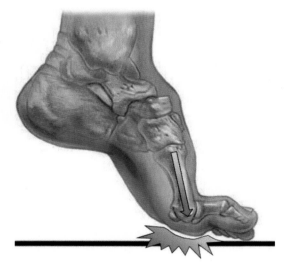

Fig. 70.14 Equinus foot

Secondary Metatarsalgia

Secondary metatarsal pain is caused by different
clinical conditions that indirectly give rise to deformity and generate mechanical overload or inflammatory processes in the forefoot region. However,
secondary metatarsalgia is not always associated
with plantar calluses or callosity development.

Inflammatory diseases, such as rheumatoid
arthritis, psoriatic arthritis, and gout, may cause
chronic synovitis and bursitis that degenerate the
joint capsule and impair the toes. This deformity
brings about the anterior displacement of the
plantar fat pad and leaves the metatarsal heads
unprotected against ground impact. Moreover,
the inflammatory disease itself may cause plantar
fat atrophy, decreasing its thickness (Fig. 70.15).

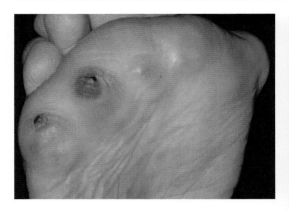

Fig. 70.15 Inflammatory disease and secondary metatarsalgia

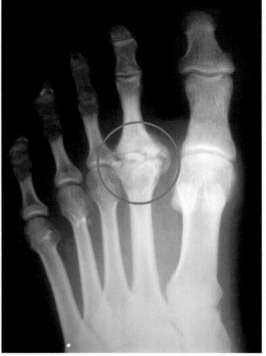

Fig. 70.17 Avascular necrosis (Freiberg's disease)

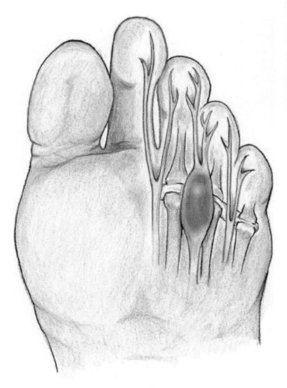

Fig. 70.16 Compressive disorder

Compressive neurologic diseases, such as Morton's neuroma (benign tumoral process of the plantar toe nerve) and tarsal tunnel syndrome (compression of the tibial nerve), may cause pain and paresthesia in the metatarsal plantar region (Fig. 70.16).

Avascular necrosis of the metatarsal head, known as Freiberg's disease, is a local circulatory disease that causes deformity of the metatarsal phalangeal joint and entails pain and movement loss. More frequently it impairs the head of the second metatarsals (Fig. 70.17).

Sequelae of metatarsal fractures, such as fragmented poor alignment, metatarsal shortening, head elevation, or plantar flexion, create hyperpressure points and cause changes in the plantar load distribution.

Iatrogenic metatarsalgia more often occurs after surgical procedures involving osteotomies. Poorly aligned corrections, exaggerated or inappropriate bone resection, and poor consolidation of a bone section may bring about deformities, loss of joint movement, and metatarsal pain. They may also lead to calluses or callosities, frequently noticed after surgeries that change the metatarsal formula and displace support points from one metatarsal bone to the neighboring metatarsal bone, resulting in a condition known as transfer metatarsalgia (Fig. 70.18).

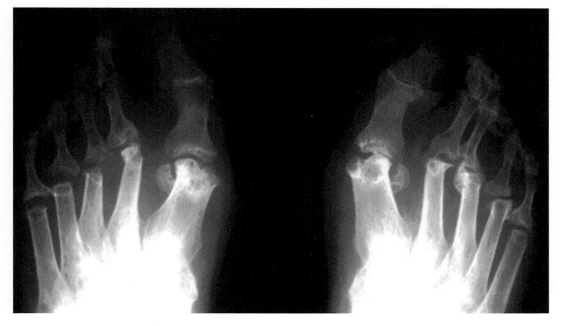

Fig. 70.18 "Transfer" metatarsalgia

Calluses (Helomas)

Calluses may be present in many foot locations. They usually occur where bone protuberances can be noticed, such as the joints and the metatarsal heads, which develop points and mechanical attrition with the ground or footwear. However the attrition of the skin itself between the two faces of the interdigital space, mainly in their most proximal portion, may cause hyperkeratosis, often with secondary tissue maceration and infection, resulting in intertriginous callus.

Many terms to describe calluses have been used: hard callus, heloma durum, clavus durum, and hard corn mainly refer to callosities out of the interdigital space, such as the dorsum toe callosities or lateral callosity of the fifth toe. Soft callus, heloma molle, clavus molle, mirror corn, kissing corn, and soft corn describe interdigital callosities. The intertriginous callus can be mistaken for soft corn, being more precisely termed in English web-space corn. Currently we avoid using the Greek or Latin terms and their difference regarding texture or consistency, since there is no histologic difference among these lesions [6].

Toe Calluses

Clinical Presentation Digital calluses are directly associated with the use of enclosed-toe shoes and joint deformities that occur in the toes. The bunion, or hallux valgus, is the most usual deformity that impairs the big toe. It is a progressive deformity that deviates and rotates the joint during its evolution, thus favoring the growth of a medial protrusion called a bunion. Both rotation and bunion develop contact and attrition points that can create painful calluses, mainly through the use of closed shoes (Fig. 70.19).

Diagnosis Orthopedic changes which will secondarily determine skin alterations are mostly determined by radiologic tests.

Treatment Conservative treatment of bunion is effective for most patients in controlling the related symptoms. Retractors, protective devices, night contention orthosis, footwear change, physical therapy treatment, and anti-inflammatory drugs can be used as alternatives or to postpone surgical procedure. Corrective surgery is indicated when the conservative

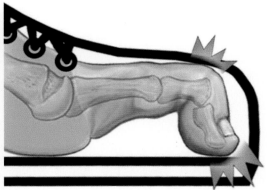

Fig. 70.20 Plantarflexion deformity of the distal interphalangeal joint

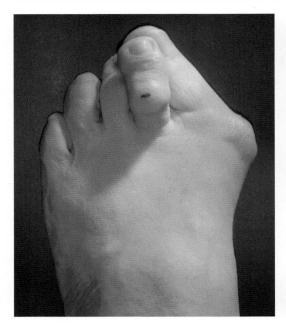

Fig. 70.19 Hallux valgus

treatment fails, the deformity progresses when assessed through serial radiologic tests, and when there is discomfort with or inability to wear appropriate shoes for sports or professional activities. Many techniques are available for surgical treatment.

Orthopedic Deformities in the Toes

Clinical Presentation The three more common deformities that impair the four smaller toes are mallet toe, hammer toe, and claw toe. Mallet toe is plantarflexion deformity of the distal interphalangeal joint. This change brings about the development of a dorsal callus, often painful, resulting from attrition by some part of the shoes and/or a callus on the toe tip that causes nail deformity through contact and direct ground impact. It is more often seen in the Index Minus foot and impairs mainly the second and/or third toe (Fig. 70.20).

Hammer toe is a deformity in the plantarflexion of the proximal interphalangeal joint. It may lead to a painful dorsal callus caused by contact with part of the shoes, although it may also result in a callus on the toe tip and nail deformity. It may

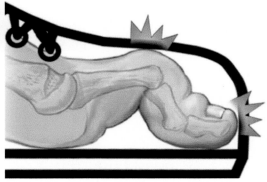

Fig. 70.21 Plantarflexion of the proximal interphalangeal joint

manifest as an isolated deformity or a multiple toe deformity (Fig. 70.21).

Lateral callus of the fifth toe results from attrition and pressure against the lateral edge of the shoe, and can be related to hammer deformity of this toe [6]. The pain can be extremely uncomfortable, mainly when pointed shoes are used (Fig. 70.22).

Claw toe is a more complex deformity and involves hyperextension of the metatarsophalangeal joint and plantarflexion of the proximal and distal interphalangeal joint. This alteration results in painful dorsal calluses and metatarsal pain due to the anterior displacement of the plantar fat pad. It usually impairs multiple toes and is associated with neuromuscular dysfunction (Fig. 70.23).

Fig. 70.22 Dorsal and lateral calluses of the fifth toe

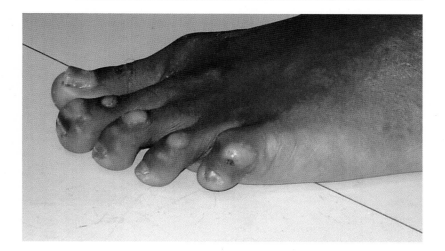

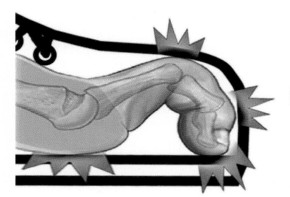

Fig. 70.23   Claw toe

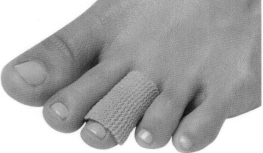

Fig. 70.24   Conservative method for alleviate symptoms

Diagnosis The study of the foot's morphological aspect and its radiologic investigation are the main methods of diagnosis.

Treatment All of these deformities are seen as a rigid or flexible configuration, and this can be assessed by an orthopedist who can better guide the method of treatment to be used. Footwear changes, contention devices, interdigital retractors, and silicone finger coats are conservative methods that may alleviate symptoms, although they do not correct deformities (Fig. 70.24) [7]. Surgical treatment aims at aligning and correcting toe deformities, establishing a more anatomic position, and avoiding footwear attrition and pressure points. There are many surgical techniques that can be used

in isolation or in combination, depending on the deformity intensity, rigidity, and/or associated joint deviations. Osteotomies, condylectomies, arthrodeses, tendon transfers, and lengthenings are among the procedures used by the orthopedic surgeon to correct deformities of the smaller toes.

Interdigital Calluses

Clinical Presentation Interdigital calluses are hyperkeratoses resulting from skin contact and compression between two toes, precisely between two condyles, or between an ungual corner and the condylus, or even between joint osteophytes if there is arthrosis in the interphalangeal joints [8]. They have no relationship with direct attrition with footwear, although footwear compressing the feet laterally, mainly pointed shoes, plays a role in lesion severity and increased pain. Often times they can be mistaken for fungal infections, mainly when lesions are deep and ulcerated [9]. These calluses can be called mirror calluses since both contact faces of the interdigital space display hyperkeratosis, and they are both painful (Figs. 70.25, 70.26, and 70.27).

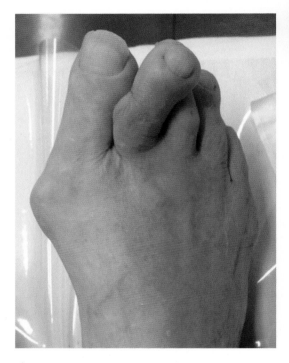

Fig. 70.25 Skin contact and compression

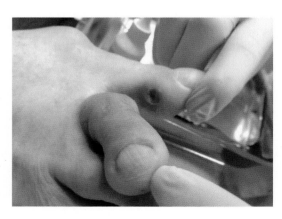

Fig. 70.26 Mirror callus: deep ulcer

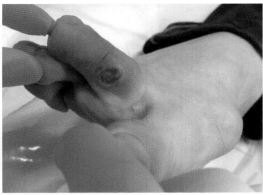

Fig. 70.27 Mirror callus: ulcer (see raised borders)

Treatment Conservative treatment of interdigital calluses aims at symptom alleviation and avoidance of skin ulceration. The use of rounded and larger shoes that provide space for all toes, the use of protective devices or interdigital retractors, and the elimination of local hyperkeratosis growth provide better comfort and prevent worsening of the lesions (Fig. 70.28). There is an indication of surgical treatment if the conservative treatment fails or provides no adaptation, or if the ulcerated lesions display difficult resolution or feet deformities. Joint realignment through resection osteotomies or condylectomies are the main goal of the surgical techniques used to correct interdigital calluses.

Intertriginous Callus

Clinical Presentation Intertriginous callus is observed in the most proximal portion of the interdigital space, mainly between the fourth and fifth toes, and less frequently between the third and fourth toes. Different from the interdigital callus, the hyperkeratosis of the deepest portion of the third or fourth space results from attrition of the skin faces and folds, which entails tissue maceration and fissure. Fungal infection is usually present, favored by the ongoing presence of a humid space and abundant scaling tissue (Fig. 70.29). The association of mechanical hyperkeratosis and tissue mycotic infection promotes lesion deepening at the subcutaneous

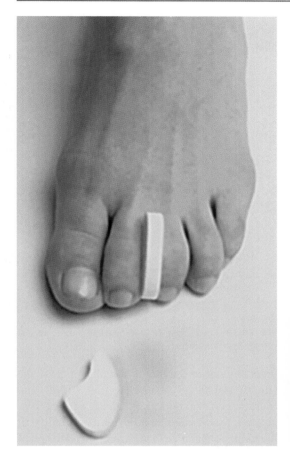

Fig. 70.28 Protective devices

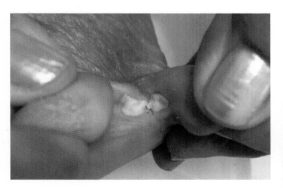

Fig. 70.29 Intertriginous callus and fungal infection

plane, and a fistula track develops that maintains lesion chronicity and leads to bacterial secondary infection (Fig. 70.30).

Diagnosis The clinical presentation helps the diagnosis. Microbiological tests confirm secondary infections.

Treatment Conservative treatment is based on the use of interdigital protective devices, such as foam, gauze, or cotton pads. Drying, antibacterial, and antifungal agents can be useful. The surgical treatment of the intertriginous callus must focus on debridement and local tissue correction. Syndactylization provides interdigital space closure and tissue regularization. Besides correcting and closing the space via a skin plastic procedure, an osteotomy of the condyles of the base of the involved proximal phalanx may be necessary (Figs. 70.31, 70.32, and 70.33) [10].

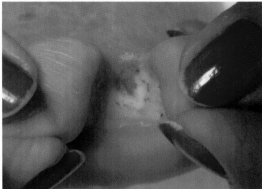

Fig. 70.30 Intertriginous callus and bacterial infection

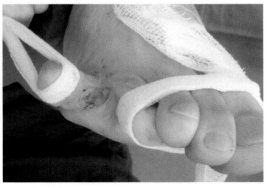

Fig. 70.31 Resection of the intertriginous callus

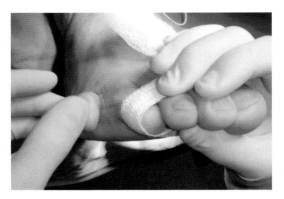

Fig. 70.32 Suture of the fourth space syndactylization

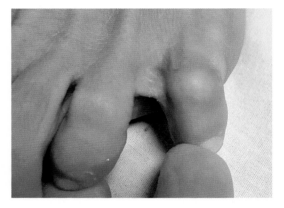

Fig. 70.33 One year after syndactylization

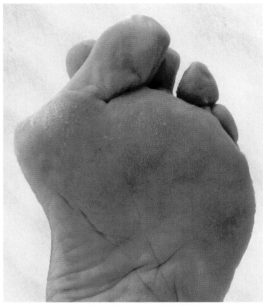

Fig. 70.34 Callosities: deformities and large area of plantar hyperkeratosis

Callosities (Tylomas)

Callosities or tylomas are hyperkeratitic reactive lesions, larger than calluses. They can be seen in areas of more friction and pressure, encompassing a broader area, with more attenuated edges and showing more diffuse painful symptoms.

They are usually related to postural changes of the gait or more complex anatomic alterations of the feet.

Deformities involving more than one metatarsal bone, with no protrusions or specific contact or attrition points, may develop larger areas of plantar hyperkeratosis [11].

The mechanical or anatomic failure of the first ray is an alteration leading to development of diffuse plantar callosities. Deformity evolution in the hallux valgus (bunion) may lead to head support failure of the first ray, thus transferring a

great amount of the foot's frontal support to the lateral metatarsal heads (second, third, and fourth metatarsal bones). Likewise, surgical procedures to shorten or cause joint instability of the hallux unbalance the distribution of the plantar support load and transfer it to the other rays (Fig. 70.34) [11].

Postural changes affecting the foot and the gait may result from many conditions. The most usually associated conditions include genetic deformities, such as idiopathic cavus foot, congenital crooked foot, and tendon shortening; neurologic disorders, such as cerebral palsy, spina bifida, myelomeningocele, poliomyelitis, and Charcot-Marie-Tooth syndrome; and trauma sequelae, such as rachimedullary trauma, peripheral nerve lesion, and severe foot fractures or burns [12].

In postural changes of gait, callosities usually develop through a mechanism of plantar overload in the anterior portion of the foot. The shortened posterior muscle of the leg (gastrocnemius) or the calcaneus tendon (Achilles) continually pushes the frontal portion of the foot against the ground at each step, thus stressing pressure under the metatarsal heads.

Fig. 70.35 Cavus foot

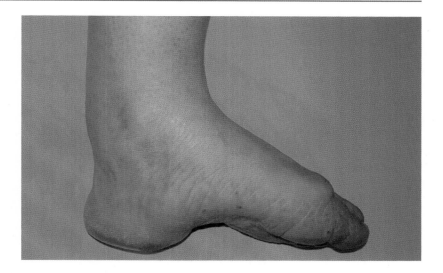

Fig. 70.36 Equinus foot

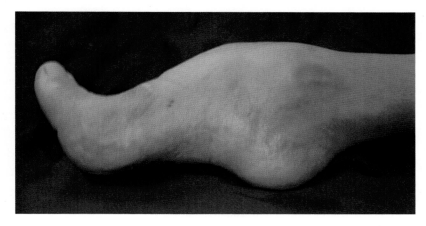

Cavus foot (Fig. 70.35) and equine foot (Fig. 70.36) deformities limit the unloading areas and concentrate the body weight on smaller support surfaces, significantly increasing pressure on the plantar regions in contact with the ground.

Diagnosis The clinical and radiologic presentations are important for diagnostic definition.

Treatment Conservative treatment for plantar callosities aims at providing symptom improvement and comfort when standing or deambulating, with relief of critical support and pressure points. Patients with mild deformities and mild or less symptomatic callosities are encouraged to change footwear and try more anatomic and comfortable footwear

models, with more appropriately comfortable insoles, which may be enough for symptom improvement. Motor physical therapy aiming at stretching, reinforcement, and proprioception enhancement play an important role for patients with muscular imbalances and/or tendon shortening [13]. Hyperkeratosis surface debridement with a scalpel must be conducted by skilled professionals and carefully carried out, without invading the deepest skin layers. Unloading and adaptive insoles may be prescribed for pressure point relief and avoidance of early development of a new hyperkeratotic zone. Keratolytic creams and lotions based on salicylic acid can be used as ancillary agents to treat plantar callosities [14]. The use of orthoses and special footwear acts by adapting more significant deformities, protecting contact and attrition points and balancing possible length discrepancies of the lower limbs. Surgical treatment aims at correcting the current deformities, thus restoring a more anatomically and physiologically possible plantigrade posture. Balance and plantar pressure distribution restoration, provision of appropriate footwear, and even modification of the ability for physical and labor activities are possibly achievable goals [15]. The most significant factor in surgical treatment is the correct choice of the various techniques which can be used for the different types and grades of deformities. Identification and understanding of the primary pathology, as well as the specific aspects of each deformity, are central to foreseeing the reaction and outcome of the indicated surgical treatment [16].

Plantar Wart

Concepts Among the most often seen skin lesions, warts are mainly diagnosed in children, and also affect about 7–10% of the population [17]. A wart is a benign proliferative epithelial lesion that results from infection by the human papillomavirus (HPV). There are many HPV subtypes that account for different clinical presentations of wart, and they also impair different body parts. Both plantar wart and palmar wart result from infection by type 1 and 2 HPV.

Clinical Presentation Plantar warts can manifest according to various impairment patterns, from single small lesions (1–2 mm) to multiple large lesions making up a mosaic of small hyperkeratotic papules (Figs. 70.37 and 70.38). Because this kind of wart impairs the foot sole in areas of constant pressure or contact, it prevents the spontaneous protrusion of the proliferative hyperkeratotic tissue. It thus results in increased intradermal tissue with a significant local compressive effect and an extremely painful lesion.

Diagnosis The most often used method for the diagnosis of plantar warts is the identification of capillary papillae or crests, small intralesional red, brown, or black points. It is sometimes necessary

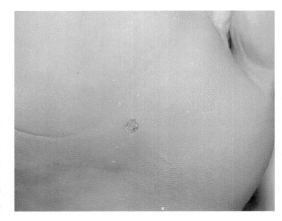

Fig. 70.37 Plantar wart

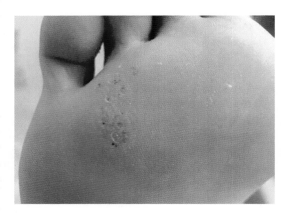

Fig. 70.38 Mosaic pattern of plantar warts

to thin out the wart surface layer with a scalpel for a better visualization of these bleeding points [18]. Dermatoscopy can be successfully used in most cases. Before starting a plantar wart treatment it is worth informing the patient that many warts spontaneously disappear, mainly in children. About 50% of all warts in children disappear within 2 years with no therapy.

Treatment Many methods have been described, mostly through tissue ablation of lesions. The HPV virus is an aggressive intracellular virus, and tissue destruction is the most effective method to eliminate the virus. Treatments to destroy and eliminate the infected tissue include cold cauterization (cryotherapy), heat cauterization (electrocauterization), and cauterization with chemical substances (chemical ablation) [18]. One of the most frequently used treatments for plantar warts is cryotherapy with liquid nitrogen [19]. The lesion has to be deeply thinned out with a number 15 scalpel, followed by two applications of 10 s each, with a 10-s break between each application. Phlyctenae can develop after the applications, and drainage is allowed only when the warts are painful. Wound dressing has to be closed with gauze and antibiotic ointment. The application may be repeated monthly for 2–3 months. In case of numerous or recurring lesions, many topical therapies have been reported as effective [20]. Chemical ablations with phenol, 10% formaldehyde, and 10% formaldehyde with monochloroacetic acid and bleomycin sulfate are described [21, 22]. Topical treatments with cantharidin, salicylic acid, and podophyllotoxin may be applied either in isolation or combined [23, 24]. The use of topical five-fluorouracil, combined or not with salicylic acid, is also described [25]. The pulsed dye laser is also regarded as effective for treating plantar warts [26]. Electrical cauterization or carbon dioxide laser (CO_2) are not recommended, since they can bring about clouds of smoke wherein virus particles may be present [27].

Glossary

Bunion A bony bump that forms on the joint at the base of the big toe. A bunion forms when the big toe pushes against the next toe, forcing the joint of the big toe to get bigger and stick out.

Bursitis Inflammation and swelling of a bursa. A bursa is a fluid-filled sac which forms under the skin, usually over the joints, and acts as a cushion between the tendons and bones.

Condylectomy Excision of a condyle. Plantar condylectomy has been presented as a procedure indicated in the correction of dislocated metatarsophalangeal joints.

Eccrine poroma A benign adnexal neoplasm composed of epithelial cells that show tubular (usually distal ductal) differentiation, derived from sweat glands.

Keratodermia Any skin disorder consisting of a growth that appears horny.

Osteophytes Bony projections that form along joint margins, commonly referred to as bone spurs.

Osteotomy A surgical operation whereby a bone is cut to shorten or lengthen it or to change its alignment.

Paresthesia A sensation of tingling, tickling, pricking, or burning of a person's skin with no apparent physical cause.

Synovitis Inflammation of a synovial (joint-lining) membrane, usually painful, particularly on motion, and characterized by swelling, due to effusion (fluid collection) in a synovial sac.

References

1. Harris RI, Beath T. The short first metatarsal: its a incidence and clinical significance. J Bone Joint Surg. 1949:553.
2. Mann RA, Kaz J. Keratotic disorders of the plantar skin. In: Coughlin MJ, Saltzman CL, Anderson RB, editors. Mann's surgery of foot and ankle. 9th ed. Elsevier Saunders; 2014. p. 425–54.
3. Dockery GL. Evaluation and treatment of metatarsalgia and keratotic disorders. In: Myerson MS, editor. Foot and ankle disorders. 1st ed. Philadelphia: W.B. Saunders Company; 2000. p. 359–77.
4. Scranton, P E Jr, Journal of Bone & Joint Surgery - American Volume. 1980: 723–32.
5. Scranton PE. Metatarsalgia: a clinical review of diagnosis and management. Foot Ankle Int. 1981;1:229.
6. Bonavilla EJ. Histopathology of the Heloma Durum: some significant features and their implications. J Am Podiatr Med Assoc. 1968;58:423–7.
7. Coughlin MJ. Mallet toes, hammer toes, claw toes, and corns. Causes and treatment of lesser-toe deformities. Postgrad Med. 1984;75:191–8.
8. Margo MK. Surgical treatment of conditions of the fore part of the foot. J Bone Joint Surg Am. 1967;49:1665–74.
9. Gillet HC. Interdigital clavus: predisposition is the key factor of soft corns. Clin Orthop. 1979;142:103–9.
10. Marek L, Giacopelli J, Granoff D. Syndactylization for the treatment of fifth toe deformities. J Am Podiatr Med Assoc. 1991;81:247–52.
11. Espinosa N, Brodsky JW, Maceira E. Metatarsalgia. J Am Acad Orthop Surg. 2010;18:474–85.
12. Ibrahim K. Pes cavus. In: Evarts CM, editor. Surgery of the musculoskeletal system. New York: Churchill Livingstone; 1990. p. 4015–34.
13. Tynan MC, Klenerman L, Helliwell TR, et al. Investigation of muscle imbalance in the leg in symptomatic forefoot pes cavus: a multidisciplinary study. J Foot Ankle Cir. 1992;13:189–501.

14. Mann RA, DuVries MD. Intractable plantar keratosis. Orthop Clin North Am. 1973;4:67–73.

15. Guyton G, Mann R. The pathogenesis and surgical management of foot deformity in Charcot-Marie-Tooth disease. Foot Ankle Clin. 2000;5:317–26.

16. Kroon M, Faber FW, van der Linden M. Joint preservation surgery for correction of flexible pes cavovarus in adults. Foot Ankle Int. 2010;31:24–9.

17. Laurent R, Kienzler JL. Epidemiology of HPV infections. Clin Dermatol. 1985;3:64–70.

18. Glover MG. Plantar warts. Foot Ankle Int. 1990;11:172.

19. McCarthy DJ. Therapeutic considerations in the treatment of pedal verrucae. Clin Podiatr Med Surg. 1986;3:433.

20. Gibbs S, Harvey L, Sterling J, Stark R. Local treatments for cutaneous warts. BMJ. 2002;325(7362):461.

21. Jennings MB, Ricketti J, Guadara J, et al. Treatment for simple plantar verrucae. J Am Podiatr Med Assoc. 2006;96:53–8.

22. Salk R, Douglas TS. Intralesional bleomycin sulfate injection for the treatment of verruca plantari. J Am Podiatr Med Assoc. 2006;96:220–5.

23. Kacar N, Tasli L, Korkmaz S, et al. Cantharidin-podophylotoxin-salicylic acid versus cryotherapy in the treatment of plantar warts: a randomized prospective study. J Eur Acad Dermatol Venereol. 2012;26(7):889–93.

24. Bengoa D, Vallejo RB, Iglesias MEL, Gomez-Martin B, et al. Application of canthardin and podophyllotoxin for the treatment of plantar warts. J Am Podiatr Med Assoc. 2008;98:445–50.

25. Young S, Cohen GE. Treatment of verruca plantaris with a combination of topical fluorouracil and salicylic acid. J Am Podiatr Med Assoc. 2005;95:366–9.

26. Borovoy M, Elson LM, Sage M. Flashlamp pulse dye laser (585 nm). Treatment of resistant verrucae. J Am Podiatr Med Assoc. 1996;86:547–50.

27. Gloster HM, Roenigk RK. Risk of acquiring human papillomavirus from the plume produced by the carbon dioxide laser in the treatment of warts. J Am Acad Dermatol. 1995;32:436–41.

Part X

Multidisciplinary Team and Dermatological Care

Dermatologic Assistance in Primary Health Care: A Nursing Approach

Erica Rosalba Mallmann Duarte,
Dagmar Elaine Kaiser, Doris Baratz Menegon,
Silvete Maria Brandão Schneider,
and Alcindo Antônio Ferla

Key Points Summary
- A skin lesion is a public health problem and should be addressed by health professionals within primary health care.
- Considering the increase of the elderly population and the population's life expectancy, the burden of chronic diseases in Brazil is increasing, requiring a new healthcare model, particularly for noncommunicable diseases, classified as cardiovascular diseases, cancer, diabetes, and chronic respiratory diseases.
- The organization of nursing professionals in caring for people with lesions is a challenge because it is characterized by an approach of various dimensions with the establishment of various relationships, and is dependent on user coparticipation.

Introduction

In the past 30 years an increasing number of countries have sought to qualify the concept of primary health care (PHC) or, as it is called in Brazil, basic health care (BHC),[1] to incorporate the principles of sanitary reform. The Brazilian National Health System, Sistema Único de Saúde (SUS), adopted a new care model that seeks to incorporate the concepts of universality and integrality. BHC is developed within this system to be the first contact of the users with health care and to be the site responsible for the organization

E.R.M. Duarte (✉) D.E. Kaiser • A.A. Ferla
School of Nursing from the Federal University of Rio
Grande do Sul (EENF/UFRGS), Porto Alegre, Brazil
e-mail: ermduarte@gmail.com;
dagmar.kaiser@ufrgs.br; ferlaalcindo@gmail.com

D.B. Menegon
Ambulatory Nursing Service and Coordinator of the
Commission for Prevention and Treatment of Wounds
at the HCPA, Brazilian Society of Dermatology
Nursing (SOBENDE), Porto Alegre, Brazil
e-mail: dbmenegon@gmail.com

S.M.B. Schneider
Hospital de Clínicas de Porto Alegre (HCPA),
Porto Alegre, Brazil
e-mail: sschneider@hcpa.edu.br

---

[1] Although they have distinct meanings and epistemological origins, both expressions ("primary" and "basic") will be used in this text, as synonyms, given that, to the subject in question, do not apply the discussion about technological density, cost and nature of the procedure. In this case, it is an act of care that is listed on the scope of practices of the primary health care policy of the Brazilian National Health System and is not developed in all teams, involving matters related to the training of professionals and insufficient technical and material resources, as discussed below.

© Springer International Publishing Switzerland 2018
R.R. Bonamigo, S.I.T. Dornelles (eds.), *Dermatology in Public Health Environments*,
https://doi.org/10.1007/978-3-319-33919-1_71

of the health care of individuals, their families, and the population over their lifetime [1] and for their transfer between the different services that are required to solve their health demands.

The age structure in Brazil is changing very quickly, with the proportion of children and young people decreasing and the proportion of older people and their life expectancy increasing. These changes are quickly creating an age pyramid similar to that of European countries [2]. Analyses of the demographic transition in Brazil indicate that the speed of this transformation has been much faster than in those countries, reaching a growth of the elderly population with an acceleration five times bigger [3]. These changes bring challenges for all areas, imposing the need to rethink the extent of the supply of health services needed for the next decades. It is important to realize that this acute change not only affects public policy, but also the culture, family dynamics, and professional qualifications.

Considering the increase in the elderly population and the population's life expectancy, the burden of chronic diseases in the country is increasing, requiring a new healthcare model, particularly for noncommunicable diseases (NCDs), classified as cardiovascular diseases, cancer, diabetes, and chronic respiratory diseases.

Essential components [4] of the surveillance of NCDs are the monitoring of risk factors; the monitoring of morbidity and specific mortality of the diseases; the response of health systems including management, policies, plans, infrastructure, human resources; and access to essential health services and pharmaceutical care.

By 2022 Brazil [2] will have a population of approximately 209.4 million people and follow a growth course whereby it will reach a ratio of 76.5 elderly for every 100 young people. In this perspective, NCDs will remain at 45.9% of the global burden of disease; in other words, scores will remain similar to the current ones, but with a substantial increase in the number of elderly and onsets, so that today for every three adults in the world one has hypertension, and for every ten, one has diabetes.

Dermatologic nursing care is the theme to be addressed in this chapter, and therefore it is essential to establish the situation to show that this is a public health problem that must be faced by health professionals in the field of primary care (PC). In this context, the nurse, as a member of the multidisciplinary team both in the traditional basic units and in the Health of the Family Teams, effectively acts with education for health, prevention, evaluation, and skin care. According to the National Primary Care Policy (NPCP) of the Brazilian National Health System, PC is developed with a high degree of decentralization and capillarity, and close to the places where people live and work. For care in the SUS, this mode of attention should be the chosen contact of users, the main entrance, the place where most of the problems that affect the population of the area are solved, and the communication center of the entire health care network [5]. Thus, there is a double insertion of the question of skin issues in the nursing routine and the same for other members of the primary care team: the care itself and the management of the user transfer between all necessary services.

Based on the discussions presented, the objective is to discuss and stimulate reflections about the importance of the nurse professional in the care of a patient with skin lesions, emphasizing PHC as a resolute point of attention and the basis for the management flow in the field of skin care.

Figure 71.1 presents the characterization of Brazilian PHC.

Nursing Practice in Skin Care

Cutaneous conditions are responsible for a significant portion of care provided in the diverse health services, regardless of the type of service, basic health units, ambulatory services, or hospital stay. Nursing constantly is faced with people suffering from wounds that are difficult to heal and who have a history of constantly searching for services for skin care. In the scenario of most health facilities in urban centers, as well as people who visit health services there also exists the problem of bedridden people originating from anticipated hospital discharges or even incapacitating chronic diseases. A thorough evaluation is

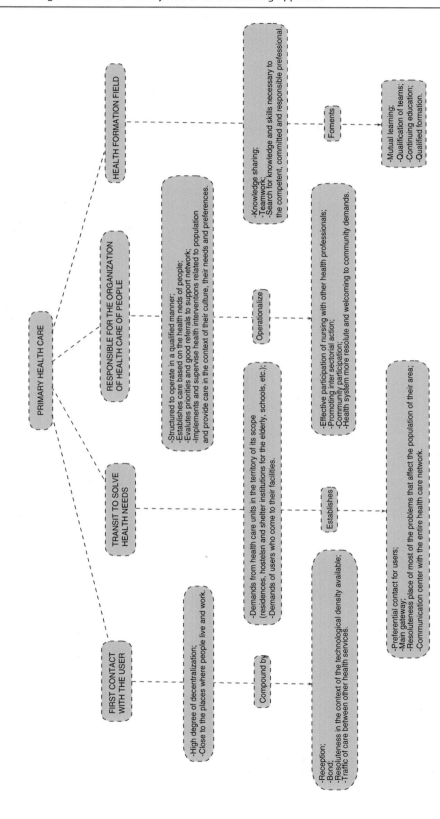

Fig. 71.1 Characterization of Brazilian primary health care

necessary to find important facts that will collate the targeting and the effectiveness of actions to be developed, creating the need for updating of knowledge properly linked to the care of wounds, either in specialized services or by professionals for referral to more specific consultancies.

In Brazil, wound care has always been an everyday activity in nursing practice, and therefore has been designed as a theoretical and scientific framework capable of mediating the complex associations of the needs required by the person with skin lesions. Such practices have enabled the enlargement of a significant knowledge base, consolidated in many manuals and institutional protocols in this field. However, the existence of care capacity for these problems tends to be concentrated in referral services and hospitals.

In this world of complexity, the Health Care Network (HCN) [1], which integrates the SUS, has sought to ensure universal, full, and free access for the entire population. It should be clarified that these are organizational arrangements of health programs and services, which have different technological densities and are integrated through technical, logistical, and managerial support systems in order to guarantee the integrality of care.

These networks can be hybrid productive arrangements that combine the concentration of certain services with the dispersion of others. In general, lower density technology services such as the BHC must be dispersed; on the contrary, the highest technological content services such as hospitals, processing units for clinical pathology tests, imaging equipment, and so forth, tend to be concentrated [1]. Here a critical question concerns the need for access to materials and specialized support in primary care to ensure resolute service.

Care is considered as the object and the essence of nursing, an affective knowledge that relates to distinctive acts. Dermatologic interventions performed by nurses are characterized as care when certain behaviors of care are added, such as respect, kindness, attention, solidarity, and interest [6].

Considering the need for integral and multidisciplinary approach to care for the person with skin lesions, the need to reflect on the organization of the networks, but also aspects of micropolitics of work that are developed in these environments to ensure proper and resolute care of these demands should be emphasized.

Operationally, the HCN consists of five components [1]: the communication center, the primary health care; the sites of attention to secondary and tertiary health care; the diagnostic and therapeutic support systems, the pharmaceutical care, the telemedicine, and the health information systems; the logistics systems such as electronic records on health, access systems regulated to care and health transport systems; and the governance system of the HCN.

The network supports sites of attention designed to ensure the commitment to the health of the population in a horizontal association, in other words, nonhierarchical between different sites, offering continuous service within the different levels of health care. Thus, in the care of people with dermatologic issues, a health unit, with intermediate technological density, but with the ability to operate with lightweight technologies [7], is also important when ensuring the guarantee of health to the person with skin lesions as a center of specialties with different multiprofessional teams, because both of them comply with distinct and important roles to specific and resolute needs. Primary health care usually takes demands from sites of attention in the territory of its scope (residences, hostels and shelter institutions for the elderly, schools, etc.) and users that arrive at their facilities. The importance of lightweight-type technologies (relational) is in the production of user embracement, the bond between patient and health professional, and resoluteness in the context of the technological density available. Equally important is the work mobilized for this type of technology to organize the transit of care through other services.

Considering that primary health care needs to be structured to operate in a qualified manner, resoluteness in skin care requires to be effective in the health unit, reducing the demands for specialized services or avoiding hospital admissions, that usually are responsible for inappropriate overcrowding of the system. For example, a repressed demand in specialty areas such as angiology means that the assessment and the systemic and multidisciplinary approach occur at a time when the lesions are already extant [8]. By contrast, a fragmented organization of the network in dermatology leads to a disorganized work approach in the sites of attention: if the care takes place via an isolated and incommunicable approach between services, everyone will be incapable of paying continuous and effective attention to this population [1], with social, sanitary, and political consequences. The reason for the health care network is the population placed under its health responsibility, precisely the needs of its users. This reinforces the concept of a network with flexible, articulated, and integrated design, which communicate with different levels of technological density from the services, thereby facilitating access for people with skin lesions and the care realized by nurses in different sites of attention.

The interventions of dermatologic nursing should consider multiple aspects, including sociodemographic factors, such as gender, age, level of education, marital status, income and occupation, as these will define the language of approach, the need of social support, and the capacity of sharing involvement in the prevention of complications [8].

From this point of view, dermatologic nursing is an extremely broad specialty, having no limits of age or types of lesion. The person with a skin lesion lives in singular sanitary territories, coexists socially with family and neighbors, and is registered and classified into subpopulations according to social and health risks. Children, adolescents, adults, or the elderly are in need of care that can be clinical, surgical, aesthetic, or psychological. The profound knowledge of the user population by nursing professionals is the basic element which makes it possible to obviate care only based on demand and to establish care centered on health needs, setting priorities and good referrals to the support network. This is a core of knowledge that includes care (preventive and curative aspects, involving the disease, any comorbidities, and risks) and management

(access to greater technological density services, supplies, and support resources).

Figure 71.2, presented below, details the nurse's performance in different sites of attention.

The involvement of the authors with a situation in academic practice, about a woman who had a skin lesion in the lower limb, raised an in-depth study and the creation of a clinical case with an interdisciplinary perspective to be discussed institutionally. It attributed a fictitious name to the woman, Mary, and the other actors involved. The story is presented in its full version in order to transport the reader to the center of this reflection and questioning, from the life experience of the authors in practice that occurred in 2015, setting a path for the teaching and learning of skin care:

Mary, Caucasian, 66 years old, married and mother of three daughters, is a housewife, and follows Evangelical Christianity. Since long ago, 1971, has a skin lesion on the dorsum of the right foot and therefore receives material from the Basic Health Unit (BHU) to execute the skin dressing at home. Nurse Claudia, from Forest BHU, routinely performs Home Visit (HV) at the residence of Mary to assess the need to receive the dressing material provided monthly by the Unit. Her family owns the land where Mary lives; there are three houses there. She lives in the house at the back with John (77 years old), her husband, and Celia (44 years old), who is her eldest daughter. In the house next to Mary's place lives her middle child, named Rita (43 years old), who is married to Jaime (54 years old) and has a 21 year old son, Daniel. The youngest daughter, Joana (41 years old), lives in front of the house. The husband of Mary is retired, but does some freelance jobs. He has a good relationship with Mary and appears to be who most accept the nurse's assistance in the search for help for his wife. However, he is very passive in the situation. Celia, the eldest daughter, is single and has as an occupation the distribution of publicity flyers. She is quite aggressive with health professionals who perform the HV and complains all the time that she has taken care of the mother's skin lesion for 40 years already, and claims that she never had the chance to get married because of this. Insistently refers when the team from the BHU visits that advances are not necessary, because she will not let anyone execute the skin dressing on her mother's foot anymore. For Celia, the skin lesion of Mary only gets worse after treatment performed in the HV. Also prohibits the mother to seek help or

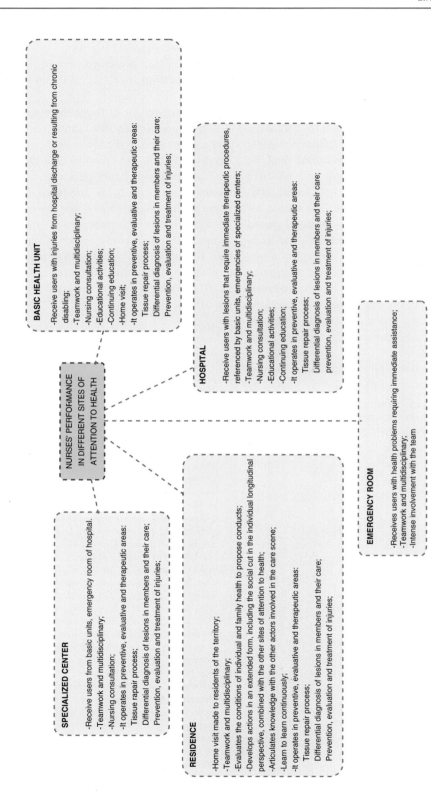

Fig. 71.2 Nurses' performance in different sites of attention to health

make the dressing with this team or any other healthcare service. Rita, the middle child, is married to Jaime, which is retired and has a chronic renal disease, currently waiting for a kidney transplant. Her son, Daniel, does not study and does not work. The couple is in a court fight with Rita's parents, Mary and John, claiming ownership of the house in which they live. They fight continuously with Rita's parents and sisters, complaining that they bullied Jaime, identifying him as wanderer and not as a chronic patient. To block the view by other family members a large yellow canvas covers their house and car. Daniel records with his cellphone the fights they have inside the family, and especially with Rita's younger sister, who spends the day listening to very loud radio. In one of the nurse's visits he showed the recordings that contain shouting and verbal abuse made between family members. Rita makes verbal complaints to the nurse in the presence of her father and mother, claiming that his father ordered from a friend Jaime's death. The youngest daughter, Joana, has lived in the front house for 20 years and remains isolated there without seeing members from her family or anyone else. Her parents provide food to her by the door window. All day long it is possible to hear very loud radio songs coming from Joana's house. Joana also records on her cellphone the fights with her sister Rita, Jaime, and Daniel. In mid-2013 there was a complaint to the prosecutor about Joana's state of health and since then she has been served by the Mental Health Team, with a diagnosis of possible schizophrenia. In one of the HVs, nurse Claudia found through the prescriptions provided by Joana's father that a psychiatrist of the Mental Health Team had accompanied her. In an attempt from the health professionals to approach the family was informed by one of the nursing staff from the Mental Health unit that Joana goes to medical appointments with her father wrapped in a cloth that hides her face. On the ground of the three houses, just in front of Mary's house, there is a lot of garbage accumulated. In one of the HVs, nurse Claudia found Mary in the courtyard, when approaching, Mary did not hesitate to kick, with the injured leg, a dead rat that was on the way to the door of her house. About her skin lesion, Mary knows little and shows no interest in seeking a Specialized Service to carry out treatment, although she is currently in the process to obtain retirement from the INSS because of her injury. At this visit she expressed that it would be a good time to get help and allowed the nurse to photograph the wound and carry out the skin dressing. On the last visit, despite the daughter Celia saying by phone that would not receive the BHU team, the nurse insisted and managed to see the wound, but not execute the skin dressing. Celia as well reminded the nurse that she should not come again

and that she had already said so over the phone. The nurse responded that she had brought the dressing material to deliver to Mary and she was there either to evaluate the wound and the need to continue delivering materials. The daughter asked to just leave the material, but the nurse insisted that without seeing and evaluating the wound she was not going to leave the material and could likewise cancel the request of material. This information triggered discomfort in Mary who then allowed the dressing change; the wound was had the same appearance as ever. It was agreed with Mary and Celia that care for the wound with guidance made by the nurse would take place at a new HV set for the next week to reassess the injury and execute a new dressing change, leaving for the moment the materials with the family. About 30 minutes after the return of the nurse to the BHU, Celia came with different clothes, saying that the BHU team were no longer allowed the visit her mother. Again she was told that the dressing material would be suspended, but if they needed help they could seek the BHU to talk. Facing this, the nurse...

This learning situation becomes a unique opportunity to resume and increase the interdisciplinary care concepts and their applicability in the daily practice of nurses. To attend a woman with a skin lesion, the consequences of which strongly affect her body, whose signs reveal her pain and deserve special consideration, ensures we are facing a unique story while at the same time resembling so many other experiences in the everyday care of people with skin lesions.

Thus, nursing care practices in the healthcare network gain significance, as it is in this field that many contexts express themselves clearly, reflected through the social and cultural approach to the population. Consequently, the health needs are identified on the spot, which can provide the development of more coherent and effective care practices [6].

Figure 71.3, below, shows the social and health inclusion of Mary and considers paths taken at different sites in the network's attention.

From the perspective of an articulated organization and inside a network, whose action can facilitate user access to different levels of complexity, the effective participation of nursing with other health professionals is essential, promoting intersectional actions that encourage community participation, seeking to make the health system

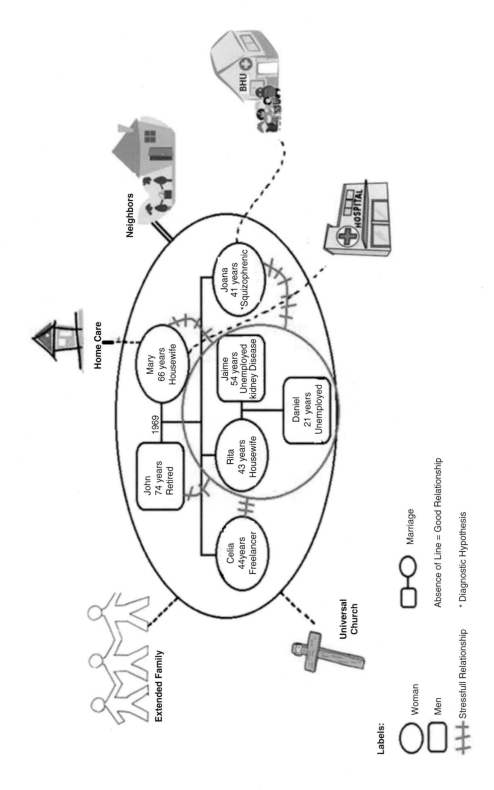

Fig. 71.3 Ecomap and genogram of Mary

more resolute, and welcoming to the demands of persons with skin lesions.

It is notable, however, that the organization of the work process by nurses requires consideration of the act of caring in terms of solidarity, with human relations, where flows of fondness happen between the professional and the user in a relationship of mutual responsibility to facilitate transfers inside the health care network [9]. It is also imperative to consider, and the case cited is plentiful in illustrating this, that care produces knowledge for everyone involved. In this case, a chronic skin lesion that does not react to the care procedures, it is stated that care is not always resolute and generates reactions in the group immediately surrounding the person requiring care. And these reactions, as well as those that permeate the way of life of the nuclear family and close relations with the user, make up the set of necessities that must be understood and managed by care professionals.

In the case of an articulated approach context among nursing, health professionals, and users, the organization of the processes that permeate the healthcare network can prove to be an excellent alliance. Nevertheless, the quality of care goes through many hands and implicates collective knowing and doing; in other words, there is a dependent association between all professionals [7]. Based on these considerations, it becomes a challenge to plan, implement, and evaluate the care for dermatologic health adopted or passed over, as the necessary interventions depend on the construction of interpersonal and professional relationships and the proper configuration of networks for care from the connections and linkages between the actors involved in the whole process. In the clinical case shown, the health needs related to comorbidity factors, besides the complexity of family relationships and territory, are also significant. There is no way to disregard the importance of the mastery of hard technologies (materials, supplies, and equipment) and moderately hard technologies (knowledge and protocols), but above all are the light technologies (relational) to congregate the health needs of people and to manage care [7] in situations of such complexity.

Therefore, the implementation and supervision of health interventions requires consideration of the risks to the population and the provision of care for people with dermatitis related to humidity, diabetic foot, vascular ulcers, myiasis, scabies, ostomy, minor burns, surgical dehiscence, abrasions and lacerations, bites, hanseniasis, pressure injury, skin tears, and care for the bedridden people in the context of their culture and their needs and preferences [1], considering also the existing resources.

The narrative that follows details another situation experienced by the authors, with the person called Emily, where although instigating reflections beyond the list of procedures, it also alerts for combined intervention strategies, fostering the creation of spaces built with life, motivation, confrontation, opportunities, and distinct social and collective contacts for nurses. This idea instills projective characteristics to the process of thinking and creating while retrieving desires, enabling new realities and new possibilities for the lives of those who live with the person with skin lesions.

Emily is 69 years old, black, currently single and Catholic, but believes in other religions. She has medical diagnosis of diabetes mellitus, hypertension, and anemia. For approximately 10 years she has had a venous ulcer on her left ankle, whose skin care was carried out in different services such as hospitals, ambulatory services, and specialized centers: a path guided by a precarious relationship with health professionals and short follow-up periods by these services. For example, in the Health Center, Emily disagreed with one of the vascular doctors from the service, and among comings and goings, decided to make the dressings by herself at home. In 2014, a teacher and her students met Emily in an academic activity of dispensing materials to affected users of skin lesions, and started to carry out home visits to assess the wound and execute dressing changes. After three months of follow-up, Emily agreed to consult with the nurse and the vascular doctor who supports the Basic Health Unit practice field of the group of students. In the same year she was diagnosed with uterine cancer that culminated in hysterectomy and radiotherapy. From this approach to the health service resulted the realization of a left saphenectomy at the hospital. After evaluation with the vascular surgeon, compressive treatment with an Unna boot was prescribed, with two changes per week, referring

Emily to a specialized center. Emily has a singular life history. When she was born, her father left her in a boarding school. During childhood, she went through several internships and only by 13 years old could she live with her father. From this coexistence, she suffered maltreatment by her stepmother, which led her to seek the juvenile court because of the frequency of the attacks. At this time she was 15 years old. As a preventive conduct, Emily moved into the house of the judge that took care of her case and there she had to perform housework in exchange for shelter and food. After a while, feeling exploited, Emily asked to return to the boarding school, and then another family assumed responsibility for her and took her to live with them. Again, Emily was required to perform household functions. Over time she followed as a domestic, living in the houses. In 2015, she is retired with a minimum income and has difficulty in maintaining and caring for the skin lesion. Emily did not marry but had two daughters with whom she doesn't have a good relationship. Her daughters don't forgive her for putting them into boarding schools when they were small. Emily repeated her story with her daughters, not knowing another way of looking after her children and believing that leaving them in the boarding school was something normal. Emily has shown quiet courage and adherence to the treatment, which is distinctively reflected in her injury that has been progressing for epithelialization. In the latest assessment by the nurse in the Specialized Center, it was recorded: "**Subjective**: Emily mentions to be well and believes that the wound is getting better. Complains about some irritation under the left foot. She says that the wound pain reduced and so she is avoiding taking painkillers. Reports that she will miss this pain when it disappears and did not remember how it is to live without it. Inform that she takes many drugs because of her diseases. **Objective**: Ambulating with difficulty and with help of crutches. After examination of the skin it is possible to observe calluses on the plantar region of the left foot, one near the hallux and one on the first metatarsal head. Noted dirt on nails, suggestive of fungal colonization. Skin adjacent to the wound with ocher dermatitis. No signs of inflammation. Ulcer with granulation tissue. Intact and irregular edges. Serosanguinous exudate in small quantities. **Measurements**: 18.5 cm × 15.5 cm. **Interpretation**: Impaired Ambulation, Impaired Tissue Integrity, Risk of Infection, Chronic Pain. **Conduct**: Execute dressing in Ulcer of Left Lower Limb with Hydrofiber impregnated with silver and bandaging with Unna Boot. Retreat excess calluses on the foot with a scalpel blade. Hydrate lower limbs. Keep bandage two times a week. Analyze laboratory tests performed. Refer user to dermatologist."

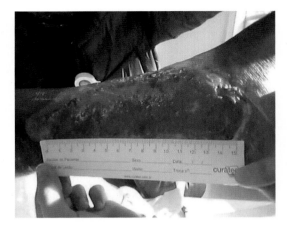

Fig. 71.4 Emily's wound: fabric with biofilm and fibrin. Macerated edges. Abundantly serous exudate, 2014

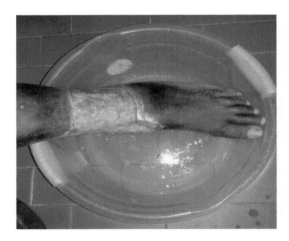

Fig. 71.5 Emily's wound: granulation tissue. Intact and irregular edges. Serosanguinous exudate in small quantities, in 2014

Figures 71.4, 71.5, and 71.6 show images of the evolution process of healing of Emily's Wound in the last 2 years of supervision.

Many situations, from both social as health systems, influenced this long and complex process of healing of Emily's wound, a complete and thorough medical history to evaluate all the factors that interfere in the healing of his wound having been fundamental.

Health has to be understood as an active condition against disease, linked to the state of being of the individual. For this reason it makes sense to ask Emily if she feels sick. To live with a skin lesion requires a redefinition of the confrontation

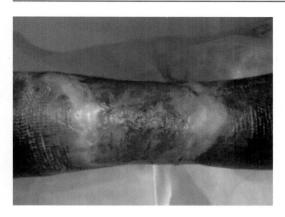

Fig. 71.6 Emily's wound: latest images, in 2015

to the constant visits to health services, the hospital admissions, laboratory and imaging examination, to the various evaluations of the skin lesion or dressing changes, not to mention the adverse effects such as pain, odor, discomfort, and therapy in their uniqueness, with the observation of all aspects in the process of becoming ill.

The care of the person with skin lesions is organized in a unique way in the relationship between the different sites of the network and health interventions, but a stable bond is necessary and it is desirable that this bond has been established in primary care. It is notable that the technical dimensions of care to people with wounds, being the main activities developed by the nurse such as the tissue repair process, the differential diagnosis of limb injuries and their care, prevention, evaluation, and treatment of skin lesions caused by pressure, or by neuropathy and angiopathy due to diabetes, and skin lesions can be performed in health care or in the user's home in a continuously and comprehensively routine manner. Therefore, the correct handling of the health conditions of the person with skin lesions has as one of its pillars support through self-care, which aims to prepare and empower people to manage by themselves their health and care [1]. All these situations are favored when the professionals have a good relationship with users and know their ways of life and the conditions under which they live and coexist.

The nurse's responsibility includes the important role of articulation of work organization to meet the needs of the users, integrating care activities with the skills and competence necessary for management and relational processes [9]. In complex cases, as health needs usually are, the ability to analyze the context and build therapeutic projects that transcend the logic of complaint-conduct that usually prevails when the professional uses only academic knowledge to take care of diseases (and not of a sick person) is essential. Therefore, home visits can be used as a care strategy, because besides planning the activity, assessing the conditions of individuals and family health to recommend conducts, the nursing professional develops enhanced mode of actions, including the individual cut in social longitudinal perspective, articulated with other network attention sites [6]. Given that no academic institution drains the supply of knowledge and technologies needed to care in the context of such complexity and to resolve this constant deficit, it is necessary to analyze, reflect, evaluate, seek new knowledge, and articulate knowledge with the other actors involved in the care scenario; in other words, it is necessary to learn continuously.

In the daily practice of nursing, care for people with skin lesions in different aspects of health care requires from the professionals the technical and scientific knowledge about nursing procedures, solutions, and techniques currently used to treat people with cutaneous conditions, seeking a way of care that it is not limited to the execution of dressing change but is also preventive and evaluative, accompanied by therapeutic activities through nursing consultations, home visits, and educational activities. An open attitude to continuing health education it also required [10], understood as the grounded learning on issues of daily work, where knowledge and user information about where he/she lives and circulates, the technical and scientific knowledge of the professional, the information on the network of care and the way of organizing services and the work inside them, besides the knowledge produced in relation with the user make up the inputs required for this method of learning.

Regarding the selection of the treatment for wounds, it must be considered that they are all different from each other, and the indication of care must be driven by particular characteristics of each lesion, such as necrotic tissue versus viable tissue, infected versus uninfected, amount of exudate, and pain, among others; relating this information to some important points that influence the healing process, such as control of the underlying disease, nutritional aspects, emotional state, infections, medications, immobility, and educational care associated with the treatment [11]. Moreover, it is necessary to remember that wounds are dynamic and change their characteristics when healing, requiring new modes of conduct, including changing the choice of topical therapy used.

Figure 71.7 summarizes the practice of the nurse in the care of a person with a skin lesion.

The nursing consultation is a space favorable to the development of care practices with the skin, as it gives nurses the opportunity to hear demands, evaluate the physical health and psycho-emotional conditions, get to know deeply the person, and initiate guidance, with the understanding of this person's socio-emotional context and family relations. Thus, this space favors a method of care that comprises an attitude of establishing constitutive relations to care for the other, strengthening the bond between professional and user for the best therapeutic decision [6]. It is important to remember that relational technologies can be also an excellent organizer of care, making it possible for the professional to establish the best conduct and offer the most appropriate treatment plan, unique to that user.

The educational activities are an important practice of care of nurses in the health care network, given that they relate mainly to the guidelines provided by them to various social actors. Educational activities, individual and group, compound the actions of care. This action runs through health promotion, prevention and control of diseases, self-care, and also the technical guidelines on performing procedures in dermatologic care. They are held by individual and collective consultations, lectures, and discussion groups [6], allowing the person to choose the best action. Educational activities are also produced by situations whereby the context in which the users live and the health problems are mobilized

are discussed and analyzed, including reciprocal learning for users and professionals. It is not only the transfer of information, which normally shows very low efficiency, the object that organizes the work of health professionals to educational activities, but also the exchange of knowledge, since, in addition to the knowledge available to the professional, situations are able to produce knowledge and practices that are appropriate by all the actors involved.

Final Considerations

Encompassing a discussion of the challenges that nursing professionals face in the care of the person with skin lesions is not considered a simple task, because in this specific scenario these professionals occupy key areas in the organization of the HCN, in which collective spaces of care require dialogue and evaluation of collaborative behavior, solidarity, criticism, and inter-subjectivity, whereby the ability to perform an accurate dynamic situational reading of the context in which the health system belongs is a unique and singular moment. As mentioned earlier, it does not seem possible to encompass the complexity that involves the health needs of people with skin lesions if there are no spaces of exchange in each service and between services; permanent education in health is a device of instruction and production of networks when it mobilizes different professionals involved in the care.

The complexity in discussing the various knowledge and skills that involve care is very large, requiring extensive and broad capabilities with high cognitive density. In this line of thought, viable proposals that help nursing professionals to answer to the particulars that skin care requires becomes necessary, considering the various sites of attention that are mainstreaming in HCN. This operates by the need of these professionals to reflect their ways of being in work, together with the consolidation of critical and purposeful pedagogic spaces that allow one to visualize more clearly the impact of the full skin care and, by extension, to be able to

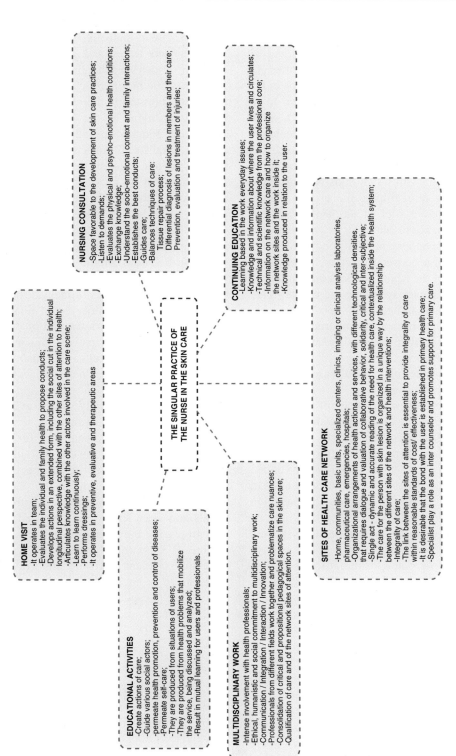

Fig. 71.7 The practice of the nurse in the care of a person with a skin lesion

build strategies and actions to promote the qualification of care and HCN.

There are many aspects of HCN, and all involve the reference and counter-reference relations. In this perspective the consolidation of referencing actions stands out, because if we do not have a consolidated network we have a veiled dispute of forces between tertiary, secondary, and primary health care. And underneath this confrontation of forces, gaps are created in the care of a person with skin lesions, leading to discontinuity in care, forcing the user to wander between different sites of the health care network. To enhance resoluteness it is mandatory to pursue the development of a good structure of communication between services, covering the uniqueness of the health services that must meet these users and strengthening the primary care. In this approach of approximation between network sites, nursing has an important interlocutory role to facilitate and qualify access to sites of SUS's attention, regardless of the level of complexity of the injury or disease that affects the person seeking care.

By contrast, a new viewpoint of nursing concerning integral care to persons with skin lesions is essential. It is necessary that the nursing professionals view themselves as protagonists of their strategies and actions, individual and collective, in the dermatologic care to be developed, participating in their formulation and execution. A leading role should be taken that highlights the participation of nurses in the care of the skin and included as assignment so they can expand, inside the services and institutions, their actions on the integral care of skin at every site of the HCN, from Basic Units of Health or Family Strategy, ambulatory services, emergencies, or specialized services, to hospitals or home care.

The care of the person with skin lesions in the network is recent and there are no experiences of large-scale or robust assessments. However, successful and local nursing practices in the care of users with skin lesions in different parts of the HCN can promote a more effective way for professionals to find ways and realize the challenges they face in daily life, with significant impact on the healthcare population. Since it is possible to produce effective care to the person with wounds, it may be able to mutually support nursing professionals and teams and produce synergetic effects in various sites that the network connects [12], enhancing benefits such as reduced cost of treatment, short-term improvements and more participatory logic in the execution of their actions and policies. In addition to the health, economic, and social impacts, effective and significant systemic action by the user also produces the feeling of good care and feeds a favorable conception of the health service and the work inside it, as can be seen in the reported cases.

By all of these considerations, it is recognized that the training of nurses in the care of people with lesions should be a challenge for the healthcare system, as it is characterized by an approach of various dimensions and in developing multidisciplinary care plans, with the establishment of various relationships that depend on user coparticipation. This will force changes, not only theoretical but also in practice. Here, we face a double challenge: to insert this topic in professional structures and to build learning capacity in daily work, as demonstrated at various times in this chapter. On the other hand, care is also a challenge for the person with the skin lesion, as this individual will only stabilize if he/she participates actively, in close collaboration with the health teams that follow its treatment. In such a way, both professionals and users should be supported in policies, programs, and management organizations capable of supporting this type of care. The process of treatment, recovery, and wound healing is much more consistent when the teamwork and self-responsibility of the person being cared for are strong.

Glossary

Health Network Care (HNC) The organizational arrangements of health actions and services of different technological densities, integrated through technical support systems, logistics, and management, which seek to ensure care with integrality.

National Primary Care Policy The result of the accumulated experience of several historical actors involved with the development and consolidation of the SUS, such as social movements, users, workers, and managers of the three levels of government (federal, state, and municipal) developed with a high degree of decentralization, capillarity, and closeness to people's lives.

Sistema Único de Saúde (SUS) *Unified Health System*, the name of the Brazilian National Health System.

References

1. Brasil. Conselho Nacional de Secretários de Saúde. A atenção primária e as redes de atenção à saúde Brasília: CONASS, 2015. 127 p.
2. Instituto Brasileiro de Geografia e Estatística (IBGE). Diretoria de Pesquisas Coordenação de Trabalho e Rendimento. Um Panorama da Saúde no Brasil: acesso e utilização dos serviços, condições de saúde e fatores de risco e proteção à saúde 2008. Rio de Janeiro: 2010. 250 p.
3. Ferla AA, Stedile NLR, Batista MV, Marcon SRA. Integralidade em saúde e envelhecimento: dobras, texturas e desafios à formação dos profissionais de saúde. Em: Heredia VBM, Ferla AA, Lorenzi DRS (Org.). Envelhecimento, saúde e políticas públicas. 1st ed. Caxias do Sul: EDUCS; 2007. 79–112 p.
4. Brasil. Ministério da Saúde. Secretaria de Vigilância em Saúde. Departamento de Análise de Situação de Saúde. Plano de ações estratégicas para o enfrentamento das doenças crônicas não transmissíveis (DCNT) no Brasil 2011–2022. Brasília: Ministério da Saúde; 2011. 160 p.
5. Brasil. Ministério da Saúde. Política Nacional de Atenção Básica. Brasília: Ministério da Saúde, 2012. (Série E. Legislação em Saúde). Disponível em: http://dab.saude.gov.br/portaldab/biblioteca.php?conteudo=publicacoes/pnab.
6. Acioli S, Kebian LVA, Faria MGA, Ferraccioli P, Correa VAF. Práticas de cuidado: o papel do enfermeiro na atenção básica. Rev enferm UERJ, Rio de Janeiro, 2014 set/out; 22(5):637–42.
7. Merhy EE. Um dos grandes desafios para os gestores do SUS: apostar em novos modos de fabricar os modelos de atenção. In: Merhy EE, Magalhães Jr HM, Rímoli J, Franco TB, Bueno WS, editors. O trabalho em saúde: olhando e experienciando o SUS no cotidiano. 3rd ed. São Paulo: Hucitec; 2006. p. 15–36.
8. Malaquias SG, Bachion MM, Sant'Ana SMSC, Dallarmi CCB, Lino Junior RS, Ferreira OS. Pessoas com úlceras vasculogênicas em atendimento ambulatorial de enfermagem: estudo das variáveis clínicas e sociodemográficas. Rev Esc Enferm USP. 2012;46(2):302–10.
9. Brandão ES. Enfermagem em dermatologia: cuidados técnico, dialógico e solidário. Rio de Janeiro: Cultura Médica; 2006. 400p.
10. Ceccim RB, Ferla AA. Educação e saúde: ensino e cidadania como travessia de fronteiras. Trab. Educ. Saúde. Rio de Janeiro. Nov.2008/Fev.2009;6(3):443–56. Disponível em: http://www.revista.epsjv.fiocruz.br/upload/revistas/r219.pdf.
11. Ferreira AM, Rigotti MA, Pena SB, Paula DS, Ramos IB, Sasaki VDM. Conhecimento e prática de acadêmicos de enfermagem sobre cuidados com portadores de feridas. Esc. Anna Nery. Junho de 2013 ;17(2): 211–19. Disponível em: http://www.scielo.br/scielo.php?script=sci_arttext&pid=S1414-81452013000200002&lng=en. http://dx.doi.org/10.1590/S1414-81452013000200002.
12. Gomes LB. A educação permanente em saúde e as redes colaborativas: conexões para a produção de saberes e práticas/Luciano Bezerra Gomes, Mirceli Goulart Barbosa, Alcindo Antônio Ferla, organizadores. Porto Alegre: Rede UNIDA, 2016. 272 p. Disponível em: http://www.redeunida.org.br/editora/biblioteca-digital/serie-atencao-basica-e-educacao-na-saude/a-educacao-permanente-em-saude-e-as-redes-colaborativas-conexoes-para-a-producao-de-saberes-e-praticas.

Care of Wounds: Dressings

Heloísa Cristina Quatrini Carvalho
Passos Guimarães, Sidinéia Raquel Bazalia Bassoli,
Regina Maldonado Pozenato Bernardo,
and Marcos da Cunha Lopes Virmond

Key Points Summary

- Wound and wound care – definition and context
- Evaluation of wound and its relevance for diagnosis and treatment
- Possible findings following evaluation of a wound
- The edge of the wound
- Etiology: arterial, venous, mixed, neuropathic wounds
- Evaluation of wounds: acute, chronic, complex; depth; infection; wound healing; phases of healing; the wound bed
- Treatment of wounds/types of coverage: dressings, ointments, and oils
- For the successful treatment of wounds, a complete assessment by a multidisciplinary team is necessary, leading to a comprehensive care plan for treatment and long-term monitoring of patients

H.C.Q.C.P. Guimarães • S.R.B. Bassoli
R.M.P. Bernardo • M. da Cunha Lopes Virmond (✉)
Lauro de Souza Lima Institute, Bauru, Brazil
e-mail: clinicapes@ilsl.br;
hpassoscarvalhoquatrini@hotmail.com;
e-mail: srbbassoli@ilsl.br;
e-mail: regis.maldonado@hotmail.com;
e-mail: mvirmond@ilsl.br

Concepts

The word *care* means "to pay attention," "take care of," "be responsible for," and denotes a dynamic action, thought, reflection. Thus, care has a connotation of responsibility and zeal, and the interactive care process includes actions, attitudes, and behaviors that are based on scientific knowledge, experience, and professional intuition, using critical thinking as its main tool. These behaviors are performed for and together with the individual needing care in order to promote, maintain, and/or restore their dignity and wholeness.

Concern in caring for wounds is ancient. Many civilizations evaluated and treated with existing resources and achieved results satisfactory for that time. The Egyptian civilization lent greater prominence to scientific and technical creations that even empirically treated wounds. It was they who concluded that infected areas closure with debridement healed rapidly and also classified the types of skin lesions and detailed treatment of each. Hippocrates in 300 BC suggested treatment with local heat, ointments, and removal of necrotic material. However, wound care has evolved, and in the late nineteenth century arose the concept that wounds should be kept dry and treated with antimicrobial substances to prevent contamination and infection. In the 1950s the first studies of wound healing in a moist environment appeared [1–3].

© Springer International Publishing Switzerland 2018
R.R. Bonamigo, S.I.T. Dornelles (eds.), *Dermatology in Public Health Environments*,
https://doi.org/10.1007/978-3-319-33919-1_72

For the successful treatment of wounds the patient should be assessed by a multidisciplinary team who should establish a comprehensive plan for the treatment and long-term follow-up of the affected person [4, 5]. The concept of the wound is shown in Box 72.1.

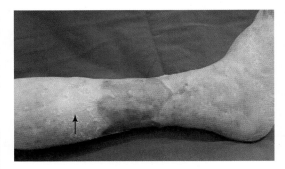

Fig. 72.1 Perilesional area with scaly skin (*arrow*)

> **Box 72.1 Wound**
> Wound is a disruption of skin integrity caused by physical, chemical, or biological agent, may reach the epidermis, dermis, subcutaneous tissue, fascia, muscle tissue, bones, organ cavities, and any other body structure [6, 7].

Clinical Presentation

Structured evaluation with clinical history, physical examination, collection of material for biopsy, culture, and log data is important to make the differential diagnosis and define systemic and local treatment, ensuring the proper selection of techniques and products to be used.

The evaluation of the perilesional area and the border is as important as evaluation of the wound bed. The perilesional area is the area that surrounds or encircles the wound. Its size depends on the etiology and the degree of compromise, as well as on the location of the wound. This area of the skin is exposed to exudative action resulting from both the wound itself and the application of products [8] (Fig. 72.1).

Particular findings are possible following evaluation of a wound:

Ocher dermatitis: Occurs due to extravasation of red blood cells in the dermis along the deposit of hemosiderin in macrophages, and presents as signs resulting from the confluence of purpuric spots, punctate, with hyperpigmented regions (gray-brown appearance) (Fig. 72.2).

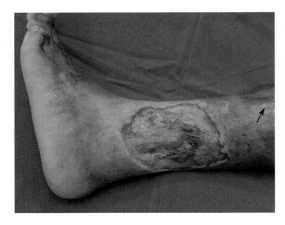

Fig. 72.2 Venous wound with ocher dermatitis (*arrow*) in perilesional area

Eczema: Skin injury resulting from inflammation that begins with erythema and edema. Fluids may accumulate in small vesicles. The secretion of a serous fluid may favor the formation of crusts [9].

Lipodermatosclerosis: Characterized as the concomitant presence of hard edema and slight pitting (sclerosis), diffuse pigmentation (ocher dermatitis), superficial scar areas, absence of hair, and hypohidrosis.

Maceration: Softening of the surrounding skin due to excess drainage or contact with fluids on intact skin. It can occur due to improper treatment or increased exudate due to changes in wound tissue.

Erythema: Redness of the skin due to increased blood flow in superficial capillaries; the color may range from pink to bright red that disappears by digital pressure. It can be due to irritation by exudate or substances resulting from covers and adhesives.

Excoriation: Superficial injury caused by trauma or skin erosion.

Scaling: Detachment of skin in scales resulting from local drying.

Itching: Can be due to drying of the skin in contact with chemicals [10].

The *edge of the wound* is its external limit. It may present as attached, detached, undermined, hyperkeratotic, or macerated.

- Edge bonded and flat: indicates good evolution of the wound.
- Detached: indicates the need to pack for healing.
- Undermined: worn, bumpy, lumpy, with friable tissue that may rupture spontaneously or by any friction.
- Maceration: softening of the surrounding skin due to excessive exudate or constant contact with fluids.
- Hyperkeratotic: when there is excessive production of keratin leading to thickening of the outermost layer of skin (stratum corneum and epidermis) forming hard whitish tissue, which is due to mechanical irritation or pressure, usually produced to protect the site [10].

Etiology

The most frequent chronic wounds are those with vascular or neuropathic origin. Vascular wounds can be of arterial or venous background.

Arterial wounds are the result of a chronic ischemic process. Usually the wound bed is not exudative; the surrounding skin is atrophic and has no hair. There are severe pain, numbness, and muscle stiffness due to lack of irrigation of the sensory nerves, as well low temperature in the extremities due to poor blood circulation in peripheral tissues. It represents 5% of vascular wounds [11].

Venous wound may occur from failure in the venous pump, valve incompetence or thrombophlebitis history, and chronic edema of the affected limb. The wound bed is red with presence of excessive exudate. It is usually superficial, multiple in number, and extensive in area. The surrounding skin shows changes such as atrophy, hyperpigmentation, and ocher-hardened cellulite. It accounts for 80–90% of extremity ulcers (Fig. 72.2).

Mixed wounds have venous and arterial components in the genesis of the process and for its treatment it is important to define the predominant factor [11].

Neuropathic wound is caused by peripheral neuropathy resulting from diseases such as leprosy, diabetes mellitus, or alcoholism. Many factors are associated with the development of neuropathic ulcers: altered skin sensation, continued unaware pressure, loss of autonomic fibers that are responsible for maintaining the sebaceous and sweat glands, allowing the inelastic skin and dryness, which may easily cause cracks and injuries [4, 5].

Etiologically, wounds can also be classified as:

- *Accidental or traumatic*: when it occurs unpredictably, being caused by sharp or, blunt objects, piercing, lacerating, inoculation of poisons, abrasions, crushing, bites, burns, and others.
- *Intentional or surgical*: when caused by a proposed therapeutic purpose.
- *Pathologic*: these are secondary injuries to a particular underlying disease (diabetes mellitus, hypertension, leprosy, gangrenous pyoderma, venous disease, arterial, oncologic, and others).
- *Iatrogenic*: inappropriate result from medical procedures or treatments.
- *External factors*: lesions that appears as a result of continuous pressure exerted by body weight, friction, shear, and moisture, such as pressure ulcers.

It is important to define the etiology of the wound because the treatment is an integrated and continuous process involving a multidisciplinary team [12]. In this connection, the reader is referred to the management chart that follows. Another important issue is to highlight the importance of the affected individual as a singular being who should not be addressed out of his/her familiar and

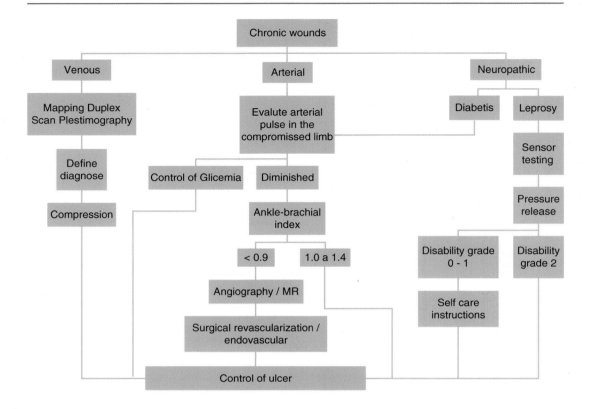

social context. As important as the etiology are the factors that slow the healing process, such as age, obesity, smoking, impaired nutrition, stress, anemia, hypertension, diabetes, and use of medications that interfere with coagulation, with platelet function, or in the immune responses [13].

Management Chart for Chronic Wounds

Diagnosis: Evaluation of Wounds

Taking into consideration the time span, wounds can be considered as acute and chronic.

Acute wounds originate from surgery or trauma, and repair occurs in a timely manner, without complications.

Chronic wounds are those that fail to progress through the orderly healing process, exceeding 3 months.

Complex wound is a new concept which aims to identify those chronic or acute wounds that are difficult to resolve using conventional and simple dressings. Complex wounds have high morbidity and mortality and have been identified as a serious public health problem in many centers, and must be approached by a multidisciplinary team [1, 14].

There are other aspects of the wound to be covered during the evaluation: depth, etiology, presence of infection, wound type, and phases of the healing process.

Depth

- Superficial: affects only the epidermis and dermis.
- Deep superficial: destroys the epidermis, the dermis, and the subcutaneous tissue (Fig. 72.3).
- Total deep: reaches the level of muscle tissue and adjacent structures.

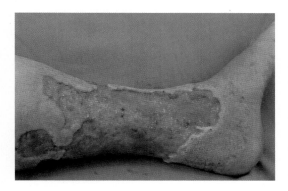

Fig. 72.3 Wound with superficial depth with silver impregnation points, indiscriminate use of silver coverage

Presence of Infection

- Clean or aseptic: free of pathogenic microorganisms; produced without glitches under aseptic conditions through an incision in sterile tissue or of easy decontamination, without evidence of signs of inflammation.
- Colonized or contaminated clean: the presence of microorganisms on its surface that proliferate due to a favorable environment, but do not trigger infection, which may or may not contribute to delay in the healing process. No obvious clinical manifestations.
- Contaminated: those recent accidental wounds that remain open for a period of time longer than 6 h and are invaded by considerable bacterial microbiota, although not virulent.
- Infected or septic: features over 100,000 colonies per gram of tissue or presenting an obvious infectious process, such as devitalized tissue, purulent exudate, and characteristic odor. They are potentially colonized by microorganisms such as parasites, bacteria, viruses, or fungi, due to reduced immune defenses.

An infection is the invasion and proliferation to deeper tissues layers of microorganisms from the wound bed, producing a reaction of the host as response of polymorphonuclear leukocytes causing local clinical symptoms (pain, heat, redness, odor, and purulent or seropurulent) and/or systemic (fever, loss of appetite, malaise).

The line that separates colonization and infection is not always clear, and in recent years the concept of bacterial load, defined as the concentration of microorganisms per gram of tissue of the wound, has been granted great importance.

The biofilm is a challenge in the treatment of chronic wounds. The biofilm is a community of microorganisms surrounded by a mucopolysaccharidic extracellular matrix creating a cohesive film in the wound bed that serves as a common defense strategy of these settler microorganisms.

Control of the biofilm is a fundamental part of the treatment of chronic wounds. Debridement, maintenance, and use of topical antimicrobials are more effective than systemic antibiotics. These should be reserved for the treatment of systemic infection (osteomyelitis, cellulitis, bacteremia, among others), because of the continuous increase of antimicrobial resistance to antibiotics [10, 11, 15].

Regarding the Type of Wound Healing

- First intention: occurs when the edges are rough, with minimal loss of tissue, absence of infection, and mild edema. Granulation tissue formation is not visible. Example: a surgical wound that is sutured.
- Second intention: occurs when there is excessive loss of tissue with the presence or absence of infection. The primary approximation of the edges is not possible. The wound is left open and closes by means of contraction and epithelialization.
- Third intention: occurs when there is an approximation of the wound edges (skin and subcutaneous) with suture after infection control and formation of granulation tissue, for better functional and aesthetic results.

Phases of the Healing Process [4]

- Hemostatic and inflammatory phase: vasoconstriction occurs shortly after the trauma; bleeding stops due to the presence of platelets; there are fibrin clots that activate the coagulation cascade, resulting in the release of substances forming the provisional extracellular matrix. This matrix is the support for the migration of inflammatory cells, followed by activation of protection mechanisms and tissue preparation for the development of healing. The clinical manifestations are pain, heat, swelling, redness, and loss of function. These signals can be minimal, transient, or lasting.

- Intermediate or proliferative phase: includes granulation tissue (neoangiogenesis, proliferation and migration of fibroblasts, collagen synthesis) and epithelialization (maturation of the extracellular matrix consists of basic elements of the basal membrane, such as structural and specialized proteins).
- Maturation or remodeling phase: starts with the formation of granulation tissue and the reorganization of collagen fibers. This phase can extend for months after the re-epithelialization.

Although these phases are clearly divided for pedagogic needs, on the histologic level they overlap, showing different wound bed phases simultaneously. The correct identification of the stages of healing leads to the accurate choice of coverage.

Tissues Found in the Bed of Wounds

There are two types of tissue that need to be considered in the evaluation of a wound bed.

Viable, which is composed of tissue formed in the healing process aiming at the epithelial reconstruction of the damaged area. These are:

- Granulation tissue: a granulose tissue, bright red, shiny, moist, richly vascularized (Fig. 72.4).
- Epithelialization fabric: new flooring, pink and fragile (Fig. 72.5).

Nonviable, which is the devitalized tissue composed of different organic materials. It can occur in different ways:

- Coagulation necrosis or dry necrosis (eschar): characterized by compressed layer of crusts of hard consistency; usually it can be dried and soft depending on the degree of hydration thereof (Fig. 72.6).

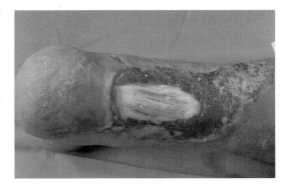

Fig. 72.4 Wound with granulation tissue and exposed tendon

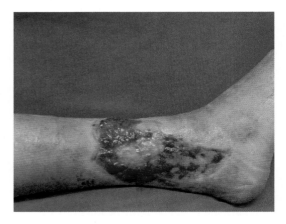

Fig. 72.5 Neuropathic wound with nonviable tissue, granulation tissue, and epithelialization

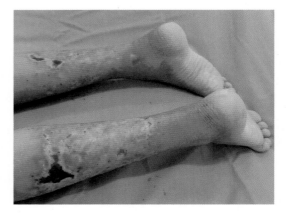

Fig. 72.6 Leprous wound (reaction) with necrosis

- Necrosis liquefaction or wet or crumbling necrosis: yellowish tissue, whitish, greyish, more slender, soft consistency, and can be tightly or loosely adhered to the bed and borders, presented as strings, crusting, or mucinous being formed by bacteria, fibrin, elastin, collagen, intact leukocytes, cellular debris, and large amounts of exudate DNA.

There are several instruments used to categorize these types of tissue. We will quote the RYB system, MEASURE, PUSH tool, TIME.

- RYB (Red/Yellow/Black), proposed in 1988 by Cuzzel, which reveals the condition of the tissues: viable and nonviable. Red means that the wound bed is red with a predominance of granulation tissue and new epithelium; the aim of the treatment is to favor the humid environment, protecting the tissue and preventing infection. Yellow: the bed is yellow in color due to the presence of fibrous exudate, devitalized soft tissue, which may be colonized. The goal is to identify the presence or absence of infection; if present institute systemic therapy and promote debridement and cleansing. Black: presence of necrotic tissue with thick eschar formation and requiring removal of this tissue quickly and effectively through debridement [16].
- The acronym MEASURE, where M stands for Measure (measure the length, width, depth, and surface area); E for Exudate (quantity and quality of exudate); A for Appearance (appearance of the wound bed type and amount of tissue); S for Suffering (type and intensity of pain); U for Undermining (presence or absence of detachment); R for Re-evaluation (periodic review of all parameters); E for Edge (conditions of the edges and the adjacent skin) [17].
- The PUSH tool scale (Pressure Ulcer Scale for Healing) is a tool developed in 1996 by NPUAP (National Pressure Ulcer Advisory Panel) that considers the following parameters for the assessment of pressure ulcer: area, amount of exudate, and appearance of the wound bed [18].
- TIME, the T assesses the viability/nonviability of the tissue in the wound bed; I relates to infection, colonization; M to the moisture imbalance; and E the edge of the wound [10].

Therapeutic Approach for Wounds

The care process is quite comprehensive, particularly when it comes to persons with chronic wounds, as they, most of the time, may feel fragile, embarrassed, and ashamed of his/her appearance, all of which goes beyond the physical aspect, affecting the psychological and social demeanor. Therefore, the type of reception the health team grants to these individuals as an attitude has a direct effect on treatment. In fact, a person properly hosted, to whom one pays attention to what they have to say, feels part of the care process. This sort of kindly approach should be used by all professionals working in the institution.

For the successful treatment of wounds, it is necessary for the person to be fully assessed by the multidisciplinary team. The nurse must establish a comprehensive care plan for the treatment and long-term monitoring of these patients [4].

After careful evaluation of the wound it must be cleansed using fluids to remove loosely adherent debris and necrotic tissue on the surface [19–21].

A fluid commonly used for wound cleansing is physiologic solution at 0.9%. Polyhexamethylene biguanide (PHMB) is one of the most advanced technologies for cleaning wounds. PHMB is an antimicrobial belonging to the group of chlorhexidines (biguanide), active against a large number of microorganisms, among them methicillin-resistant *Staphylococcus aureus* (MRSA), vancomycin-resistant *Enterococcus* (VRE), and the *Acinetobacter baumannii* that are responsible for multidrug-resistant infections. It is importantly to note that it is biocompatible, i.e., it has no toxicity on living tissues [22].

Other local antiseptics are not recommended. Usually they are chemical products with cytotoxic action that inhibits cell proliferation. Among them one can cite iodine-povidone, acetic acid, chlorhexidine, hydrogen peroxide, and hypochlorite solutions.

Debridement

The debridement consists of removing nonviable tissue, such as necrotic tissue, devitalized tissue, and colonized bodies and foreign matter, optimizing the healing process and preventing infection.

Types of Debridment (Fig. 72.7)

Enzymatic or chemical debridement is based on the use of proteolytic enzymes (papain, collagenase, fibrinolysin/DNase) which are capable of dissolving devitalized tissues. The choice of enzyme is dependent on the type of existing tissue in the wound.

The application of the selected enzyme should be restricted to the devitalized tissue, avoiding contact with the perilesional areas. For protection of these areas hydrocolloid powder, essential fatty acid oil, or creams that promote a protective barrier can be used. The wound should be covered with a bandage to retain the moisture needed for enzyme action.

Autolytic debridement is obtained by using hydrogels and hydrocolloids that act naturally and selectively. Through the maintenance of moisture, phagocytic cells and proteolytic enzymes are activated, promoting the degradation of nonviable tissue.

Surgical debridement is the method indicated for wounds with large amounts of devitalized tissues. Depending on the severity and extent of the wound, this procedure should be performed by surgeons in the operating room under anesthesia. In superficial wounds, which usually do not require anesthesia, it can be performed on an outpatient basis by medical professionals and trained nurses. Although aggressive, results are faster than with other methods.

Mechanical debridement is also indicated for wounds with large amounts of devitalized tissue. This technique consists in the removal of tissues by application of mechanical strength. This procedure, however, can damage the granulation tissue or already existing epithelialization, and

cause pain. Mechanical debridement methods include negative pressure therapy, wet–dry dressings, hydrotherapy, and irrigation.

Negative pressure therapy involves intermittent and continuous application of subatmospheric pressure at the wound surface. The mechanism of action in promoting the healing is by reducing the superficial edema; improvement of local blood circulation; reduction of excess exudate; stimulating the proliferation of fibroblasts, endothelial cells, and vascular smooth muscle cells; reduction of bacterial load; and favoring wound contraction.

Wet–dry dressings: moistened gauze with saline solution is applied to the wound bed and left until dry. The gauze when removed takes out necrotic tissue. It is a painful method that requires analgesia.

Hydrotherapy uses pulsed and pressurized irrigation. The water is delivered in a continuous or intermittent base under low, intermediate, and high pressure flow.

Irrigation is the steady flow of a solution across a wound bed with the use of a 40 × 12 needle in a 20 mL syringe or a 25 × 8 needle in a 20 mL syringe. The syringe must be positioned in a 45–90° angles and at a distance of 2.5–5.0 cm, which respectively ensure the pressure of 9.5 psi and 13.5 psi, capable of promoting the removal of cell debris, exudates with pathogens, and residues of topically applied creams and ointments which remain in the wound bed. The choice of pressure should vary according to the amount of debris to be removed. In the case of wounds with the largest amount of debris, one should use the 20 mL syringe and a 25 × 8 needle. It is also recommended to use a heated solution to prevent temperature reduction in the wound bed, since a constant temperature of 37 °C stimulates mitosis during granulation and re-epithelialization [23, 24].

Maggot or biological debridement therapy, or maggot therapy, requires the application in the wound bed of larvae reared in the laboratory. The larvae feed on necrotic/devitalized tissue and make selective debridement [10].

Based on the experience of the authors, topical therapy should be decided upon by evaluating the type of tissues, according to the algorithm that follows (Figs. 72.8 and 72.9):

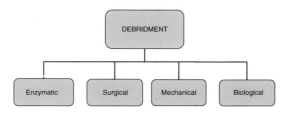

Fig. 72.7 Types of debridment

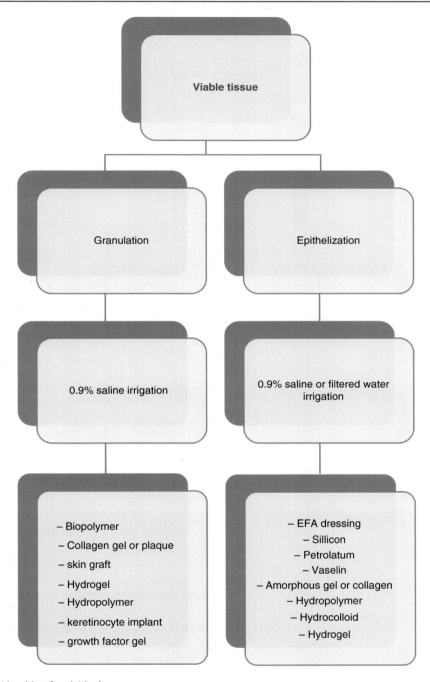

Fig. 72.8 Algorithm for viable tissue

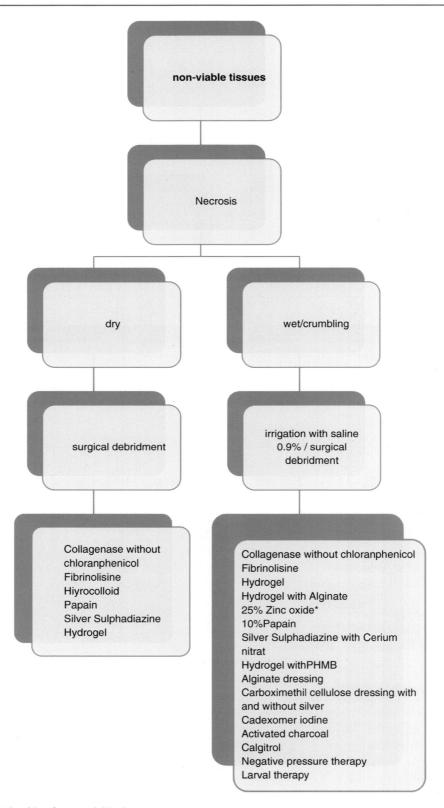

Fig. 72.9 Algorithm for non-viable tissue

Dressings: A Rapid Guide

EFA (Essential Fatty Acids)

Composition: polyunsaturated vegetable oils, linoleic acid, caprylic acid, capric acid, vitamin A and E, soybean lecithin, and lanolin.

Function: transporting materials across cell membranes, which ensures the life of the cell through balanced flow of nutrients and waste products in biological activity.

Indication: protection, hydration, skin restoration, and receiving area graft.

Contraindication: injury to tissue necrosis without debridement, sensitivity to the product.

Change frequency: every 24 h

AGin (Fatty Acids, Unsaturated)

Composition: oleic acid, vitamin A palmitate, DL-α-tocopherol, Vitamin E.

Function: antioxidant activity; protects the cell's DNA particularly in those who are in training; inhibits the free radicals produced by lymphocytes that hinder the process of tissue repair in chronic injuries.

Indication: maintain or restore normal skin characteristics; prevention of skin breaks; moisturizing dry skin.

Contraindication: sensitivity to product.

Change frequency: every 24 h

Hydrogel

Composition: deionized water, glycerin, sodium carboxymethylcellulose, allantoin (natural hydrocolloid).

Function: interacts with the exudate creating moist environment that favors the autolysis, pain relief by moistening the exposed nerve endings in the wound.

Indication: wounds with granulation tissue; with necrotic tissue, venous ulcers, arterial and pressure; second-degree burns of small extent; wounds with partial or total loss of tissue; post-traumatic areas.

Contraindication: patients with sensitivity to product.

Change frequency: 24 h to 3 days depending on the exudate

Hydrogel with Calcium Alginate and Sodium

Composition: calcium alginate and carboxymethylcellulose sodium in an aqueous, transparent, viscous excipient.

Function: keep moist medium, helps in autolysis.

Indication: soften and rehydrate necrotic and devitalized areas of pressure ulcers, stasis, burning of first and second grade, cut, abrasions, and lacerations.

Contraindication: sensitivity to the product, damage to infection and/or secretion.

Change frequency: 24 h for necrotic or very exudative lesions up to 3 days to clean lesions with granulation tissue

Silver Sulfadiazine with Cerium Nitrate

Composition: 0.4% cerium nitrate and silver sulfadiazine 1%.

Function: sulfadiazine (bactericidal and bacteriostatic acting on the bacterial cytoplasmic membrane) effective against Gram-positive and -negative viruses, dermatophyte fungi; cerium nitrate enhances the bactericidal effect.

Indication: devitalized tissue, burn, colonization prevention.

Contraindication: sensitivity to components.

Change frequency: daily in infected lesions and up to 3 days in fresh lesions.

Collagenase

Composition: collagenase, clostridiopeptidase A, and proteolytic enzymes.

Function: acts to selectively degrade the native collagen (necrolysis).

Indication: devitalized tissue: necrosis, fibrosis.

Contraindication: wound healing by first intention, hypersensitivity to enzyme.

Change frequency: every 12 or 24 h.

Fibrinolysin

Composition: bovine emollients, fibrinolysins, deoxyribonucleases, and 1% chloramphenicol.

Function: lytic action of fibrinolysin and deoxyribonuclease dissolve the exudate and necrotic waste.

Indication: devitalized tissue (necrosis, fibrosis).

Contraindication: hypersensitivity to bovine substances.

Change frequency: every 12 or 24 h.

Cadexomer Iodine

Composition: Cadexomer, polyethylene glycol, poloxamer, and iodine.

Function: Cadexomer beads are biodegradable, remove excess exudate and fibrin in the wound base, and reduce bacterial contamination on the surface.

Indication: topical treatment of chronic exuding wounds, infected wounds.

Contraindication: dry necrotic tissue or with known sensitivity to iodine or any of its components; pregnant women, breastfeeding women, children, people with diabetes insipidus, thyroid disorder.

Change frequency: fluid saturation; 72 h.

Zinc Oxide

Function: antiseptic, drying, and anti-inflammatory action, decreased odor and exudate, 25% concentration increases the mitotic index.

Indication: devitalized tissue, abundant exudation, fetid odor.

Contraindication: Hypersensitivity to the product and painful.

Change frequency: every 24–72 h.

Polyhexamethylene Biguanide

Composition: amorphous hydrogel polyhexamethylene biguanide 0.1%, pectin, cellulose.

Function: antimicrobial action (Gram-positive yeasts and fungi), autolytic, wound deodorization, promotes moist environment, facilitates mechanical debridement, stimulates epithelialization.

Indication: chronic wounds or acute, with devitalized tissue, exudative, infected.

Contraindication: none.

Change frequency: daily or up to 3–7 days

Biopolymer

Composition: glyceryl monostearate, cetostearyl alcohol, stearic acid, N-coconut acyl derivatives of L-glutamic acid, sodium acrylate copolymer, hydrogenated polyisobutene, phospholipids, polyglyceryl-10-esters, sunflower oil, hydrogenated olive oil, olive ester, phenoxyethanol, hydrogenated vegetable oil, behenyl alcohol, lecithin, soy sterols, shea butter, fatty acid triglycerides, of *Camelina sativa* oil, dimethicone, hydroxyethylcellulose, disodium EDTA, serum and water *Hevea brasiliensis*.

Function: Gel-cream for skin restoration, has angiogenic activity and accelerating the healing process.

Indication: skin ulcers of various pathologies: arterial, diabetic, mixed, venous, neuropathic, leprous, by pressure, in acute and chronic stages, little exudate.

Change frequency: daily or up to 3 days

Amorphous Collagen Gel

Composition: collagen hydrolysate in a hydrogel matrix.

Function: protective barrier against external contaminants preventing fungal and bacterial proliferation, accelerates healing, and promotes rapid regeneration of the skin after therapeutic and aesthetic dermatologic procedures.

Indication: beaten skin for dermatologic procedures (laser, peeling, or minor dermatologic surgery) or external factors.

Contraindication: sensitivity of formula.

Change frequency: up to 3 days.

Barrier Cream

Function: Protects, moisturizes, and restores the skin's pH, and against maceration.

Indication: perilesional skin for protection against excess moisture that can cause maceration and delayed wound-healing process.

Contraindication: not shown.

Change frequency: daily.

Hydrocolloid Powder

Composition: synthetic resin powder, microgranules, consisting of nonadherent hydrocolloids.

Function: Protects skin with exudate, absorbs moisture caused by chafing.

Indication: to be used in the peristomal skin. It is also indicated in bruised skin.

Contraindication: none.

Change frequency: daily.

Nonadherent Mash Dressing

Function: maintains moist environment, which prevents dehydration of the granulation tissue.

Indication: First- and second-degree burns, grafts, venous ulcers, pressure, eczema, surgical incisions.

Contraindication: sensitivity to components.

Change frequency: several days, depending on amount of exudate.

Sodium Alginate and Calcium

Function: calcium ions and sodium in the blood and exudates interact with the same ions found in the healing, inducing hemostasis, assists in autolytic debridement, promotes absorption of

exudate and maintains the humidity (gel formation).

Indication: pressure ulcers, venous, arterial, diabetic, donor area, and other skin lesions with no hemorrhagic bleeding.

Contraindication: dried injuries and sensitivity to product.

Change frequency: daily changes in infected lesions and lesions cleaned according to saturation.

Coverage Collagen and Alginate

Function: hemostatic properties, stimulates granulation tissue formation, epithelialization, makes healing occur faster.

Indication: treatment of wounds with low to high levels of exudate (pressure ulcers, venous, arterial, diabetic, donor area, and other skin lesions with no hemorrhagic bleeding).

Contraindication: dried injuries and sensitivity to product, and carcinomas.

Change frequency: daily change on exudative lesions and lesions cleaned according to saturation.

Hydrofiber

Function: retains the fluid forming a gel around the fibers, keeps the wound bed moist and warm.

Indication: chronic lesions (pressure ulcers, lower limb), acute injuries (lacerations, incisions, donor area, first- and second-degree burns, and control of small bleeding), highly exudative lesions requiring autolytic debridement.

Contraindication: sensitivity to the product.

Change frequency: up to 7 days.

Hydrofiber with Silver

Function: retain the fluid forming a gel around the fibers, keeps the bed of the wound moist, warm, free of bacteria and odors.

Indication: small abrasions, cuts, lacerations, superficial burns, infections.

Contraindication: sensitivity to the product.

Change frequency: up to 7 days

Activated Carbon and Silver

Function: carbon attracts bacteria and silver combats microorganisms and reduces bacterial colonization and infection control and odor.

Indication: chronic wounds, traumatic and surgical lesions, with or without infection, odor and fibrin.

Contraindication: necrosis, bone exposure.

Change frequency: 7 days.

Natural Biological Film

Function: retains moist environment, does not allow entry of microorganisms.

Indication: burns, wounds, skin graft donor sites.

Contraindication: infected wounds.

Change frequency: single use.

Hydrocolloids

Function: promoting moisture forming a gel that provides for autolysis debridement. It stimulates neogenesis, pH maintenance.

Indication: without infection lesions without exudate, necrosis, prevention of decubitus ulcer.

Contraindication: lesions with infection and/or exudate.

Change frequency: 7 days in clean lesions with granulation tissue.

Hydropolymers

Function: maintain moisture, absorb and retain excess exudate, adhered to the wound bed, preventing maceration, stimulates autolytic debridement.

Indication: no infected lesions, slightly exudative, in granulation tissue and for preventing decubitus ulcer.

Contraindication: lesions with infection and/or secretion.

Change frequency: up to 7 days and, in case of prevention, up to 10 days.

Hydropolymer with Silver

Function: antibacterial, releasing silver ions continuously; exudate is absorbed protecting perilesional area. It has selective permeability (water controls the output and input bacteria), minimizing the risk of infection.

Indication: wounds with moderate to high exudate with delayed healing, with risk or clinical signs of infection, such as leg ulcers, pressure ulcers, second-degree burns, diabetic ulcers.

Contraindication: individuals with allergic reactions to any component of the product.

Change frequency: up to 7 days.

Polyurethane Foam

Function: exchange of ions occurs between the ingredients and silver alginate matrix and wound exudate, leading to the presence of Ag^+ and Ca^{++} ions in the wound bed.

Indication: moist and thermal healing of wounds, infected or colonized; pressure ulcers, venous ulcers, and burns.

Contraindication: hypersensitivity known to alginate or silver, the presence of metals, ulcers due to infectious processes (tuberculosis, syphilis, deep mycoses or third degree burns).

Change frequency: up to 7 days.

Papain

Function: chemical debridement, bacteriostatic, bactericidal, and anti-inflammatory, provides alignment of collagen fibers.

Indication: chemical debridement and facilitator of the healing process, supporting systemic antibiotic treatment of infected wounds. Use concentration of 2% in wound granulation tissue; 4–6% when there is purulent exudate; and 10% when there is presence of necrotic tissue.

Contraindication: sensitivity to the substance or other component of the formulation.

Change frequency: every 12 h.

Growth Factor Gel

Function: acts on the cell membrane (activates the tyrosine kinase that comes into contact with DNA, stimulating cell division and proliferation).

Note: poorly healing ulcers with just partial damage, but with adequate blood supply.

Change frequency: daily, always at the same time.

Unna Boot

Function: reduces edema through the venous pump movement, facilitating venous return, aiding healing.

Indication: venous ulcers of the lower limbs.

Contraindication: arterial and mixed ulcers

Change frequency: every 7 days since there is no discharge or dirt.

Elastic Bandage

Function: reduces edema by means of pump action, making easier venous return and promoting healing.

Indication: treatment of venous leg ulcers and associated conditions where compression therapy indicated.

Contraindication: arterial ulcers and mixed ulcers, leg with circumference of 18 cm below the ankle.

Multilayer Compression Therapy

Function: promotes a recommended therapeutic pressure of 40 mmHg, facilitating venous return and reducing edema.

Indication: venous ulcer.

Contraindication: arterial and mixed ulcer.

Change frequency: up to 7 days.

Glossary

Iatrogenic Inappropriate result from medical procedures or treatments.

Biofilm Community of microorganisms surrounded by a mucopolysaccharidic extracellular matrix, creating a cohesive film in the wound bed that serves as a common defense strategy of these settler microorganisms.

Lipodermatosclerosis Concomitant presence of hard edema and slight pitting (sclerosis).

Maggot therapy Application in the wound bed of larvae of the species *Lucilia sericata* or *Phaenicia sericata* in order to selectively remove the necrotic/devitalized tissue.

Ocher dermatitis Extravasation of red blood cells in the dermis along the deposit of hemosiderin in macrophages.

Enzymes that promote protein breakdown.

References

1. Jorge AS, Dantas SRPE. Abordagem multiprofissional no tratamento de feridas. São Paulo: Atheneu; 2003.

2. Blanes L. Tratamento de feridas. In: Baptista-Silva JCC, editor. Cirurgia vascular: guia ilustrado. São Paulo; 2004. http://files.artedecuidar.webnode.com.br/200000015-0ad7c0b337/Tratamento%20de%20Feridas.pdf. Accessed 4 July 2016.

3. Santos AAR. O ensino da temática feridas no curso de graduação em enfermagem da Universidade Federal da Paraíba. [dissertação]. João Pessoa: UFP; 2012.

4. Ministério da Saúde (BR). Manual de condutas para tratamento de úlceras em hanseníase e diabetes. 2a ed. revisada e ampliada. Brasília: Ministério da Saúde; 2008. 92 p.

5. Puri V, Venkateshwaran N, Khare N. Trophic ulcers - practical management guidelines. Indian J Plast Surg. 2012;45(2):340–51. doi:10.4103/0970-0358.101317.

6. Oda RM, Galan NGA, Opromolla DVA. Úlceras de perna na hanseníase. In: Opromolla DAV, Baccarelli R, editors. Prevenção de Incapacidades e reabilitação em hanseníase. Bauru: Instituto Lauro de Souza Lima; 2003. p. 130–3.

7. Barros ALBL. Anamnese e exame físico: avaliação diagnóstica de enfermagem no adulto. 3rd ed. Artmed: Porto Alegre; 2016.

8. Fornells MG, González RFG. Cuidados de la piel perilesional. Espana; 2006. http://www.fundacionsergiojuan.org/pdf_gneaupp/libro_piel_perilesional.pdf. Accessed 4 July 2016.

9. Dealey C. Cuidando de feridas: um guia prático para as enfermeiras. 3a ed. Atheneu: São Paulo; 2008.

10. Malagutti W, Kakihara CT. Curativos, estomia e dermatologia: uma abordagem multiprofissional. 2a ed. São Paulo: Martinari; 2011.

11. Agredda JJS, Bou JET. Atenção integral nos cuidados das Feridas Crônicas. Petrópolis: EPUB; 2012.

12. Vries JCH, Groot R, van Brakel WH. Social participation of diabetes and ex leprosy -patients in the Netherlands and patient preference for combined self-care groups. Front Med. 2014;1(21). 10.3389/fmed.2014.00021.

13. Robb C. Module 1784: chronic wound management. Chem Drug. 2016;26:12.

14. Ferreira MC, Tuma P Jr, Carvalho VF, Kamamoto F. Complex wounds. Clinics. 2006;61(6):571–8.

15. Leaper D, Assadian O, Edmiston CE. Approach to chronic wound infections. Br J Dermatol. 2015;173(2):351–8. doi:10.1111/bjd.13677.

16. Cuzzel JZ. The new RYB color code. Am J Nurs. 1988;88(10):1342–6.

17. Keast DH, et al. MEASURE. A proposed assessment framework for developing practice recpmmedatios for wound assessment. Wound Rep Reg. 2007;51(12):S1–S17.

18. Santos VLCG, Azevedo MAJ, Silva TS, Carvalho VMJ, Carvalho VF. Adaptação transcultural do Pressure Ulcer Scale for Healing (PUSH), para a língua portuguesa. Rev Lat Am Enfermagem. 2005;13(3):305–13.

19. Joanna Briggs Institute. Solutions, techniques and pressure in wound cleansing. Nurs Stand. 2008;22(27):35–9.

20. Bee TS, et al. Wound bed preparation: cleansing techniques and solutions: a systematic review. Singap Nurs J. 2009;36:17–22.

21. Fernandez R, Griffiths R. Water for wound cleansing. Cochrane Database Syst Rev. 2012;(2):CD003861. doi:10.1002/14651858.CD003861.pub3.

22. Santos EJF, Silva MANCGMM. Tratamento de feridas colonizadas/infetadas com utilização de polihexanida. Rev Enf Ref [online]. 2011;serIII(4):135–42. http://www.scielo.mec.pt/scielo.php?script=sci_arttext&pid=S0874-02832011000200014&lng=pt&nrm=i&tlng=pt. Accessed 4 July 2016.

23. Martins PAE. Avaliação de três técnicas de limpeza do sítio cirúrgico infectado utilizando soro fisiológico para remoção de microrganismos [dissertação]. São Paulo: Escola de Enfermagem da Universidade de São Paulo; 2000.

24. Gall TT, Monnet E. Evaluation of fluid pressures of common wound-flushing techniques. Am J Vet Res. 2010;71(11):1384–6. doi:10.2460/ajvr.71.11.1384.

Physical Therapy in Leprosy

Lúcia Helena Soares Camargo Marciano,
Tatiani Marques, Cristina Maria da Paz Quaggio,
and Susilene Maria Tonelli Nardi

Key Points Summary

- For leprosy patients physical disabilities may lead to a reduction in work potential, restricted social life, and psychological disorders, and are responsible for discrimination against patients
- Early diagnosis, proper treatment, and prevention of disabilities impede the transmission of disease, and reduce disabilities including psychosocial impairment
- Physical rehabilitation and surgery are important tools to prevent disabilities, to improve functional capacity, aesthetics, and social life, and to alleviate pain

L.H.S.C. Marciano (✉) • T. Marques
C.M.P. Quaggio
Lauro de Souza Lima Institute, Bauru, Brazil
e-mail: lmarciano@ilsl.br

S.M.T. Nardi
Adolfo Lutz Institute, São José do Rio Preto,
São Paulo, Brazil

Introduction

Nerve damage in leprosy is responsible for a variety of physical injuries and can negatively affect the quality of life of patients [1, 2]. The presence of physical disabilities and the fear of contagion are the main factors responsible for the discrimination that still exists with respect to the disease [3].

Although multidrug therapy (MDT) is effective in the control of leprosy, the elimination of viable bacilli does not mean that patients will not suffer disabilities, including physical disabilities, as functional changes can be caused by reactions even after completing drug therapy. Several factors contribute to the appearance of disabilities, including delayed diagnosis, lack of patient adherence to treatment, and intermittent reactions [4, 5].

In Brazil, 6.5% of all patients diagnosed in 2014 had physical disabilities (grade 2) at the beginning of treatment, which indicates the importance of timely diagnosis of the disease [6]. This demonstrates that health care administrators and professionals need to reduce operational difficulties and investigate new cases in the population so as to minimize the problems caused by late diagnosis.

According to the Brazilian Ministry of Health, in order to prevent disabilities it is essential that the diagnosis is early, that patients receive MDT, and that the medical management and rehabilitation for leprosy reactions are carried out effectively. Moreover, guidance on self-care and

© Springer International Publishing Switzerland 2018
R.R. Bonamigo, S.I.T. Dornelles (eds.), *Dermatology in Public Health Environments*,
https://doi.org/10.1007/978-3-319-33919-1_73

psychosocial support must be provided. After completing MDT, care must be continued because reactions can occur before, during, and after MDT, often causing irreversible nerve damage and loss of function. These measures should be carried out throughout the healthcare network, from the simplest to the most complex levels, to ensure a good quality of care is provided by a multidisciplinary team acting in an interdisciplinary manner [7].

State of the Art

Pathophysiology of Nerve Damage in Leprosy

Mycobacterium leprae has an affinity for cells that envelop peripheral nerves, the Schwann cells, whose temperature is lower than that of the rest of the body. The most affected nerves in the face are the auricular, trigeminal, and facial nerves; in the upper limbs the ulnar, median, and radial nerves and the superficial branch of the radial nerve; and in the lower limbs the common peroneal and the tibial nerves.

Physical disabilities due to leprosy can be caused by neurogenic and non-neurogenic mechanisms. Neurogenic mechanisms are due to the direct action of the bacillus on the nerve, causing changes in the function of autonomic (hypohidrosis of the skin), sensory (loss of thermal and tactile sensitivity, and pain), and motor (paresis and muscle palsy) nerve fibers. These are considered primary lesions [8]. Secondary lesions are related to the aggravation of these injuries and can include retraction of the soft tissues, trophic and traumatic injuries, infections, burns, and cracks in the skin, among others. Non-neurogenic mechanisms include chronic and acute inflammation arising from leprosy reactions; this may affect the bones, joints, tendons, muscles, ligaments, and internal organs [9].

Face

In leprosy, eye injuries are observed in all clinical forms except the indeterminate form. The facial,

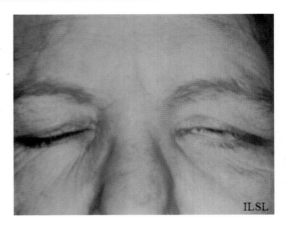

Fig. 73.1 Lagophthalmos

trigeminal, and auricular nerves are most commonly affected. Owing to the direct action of the bacillus, lepromatous leprosy is responsible for more disabilities of the face than the other types of the disease.

Facial Nerve

Motor fibers are responsible for innervations of the facial muscles. Injury to nerves may be complete, unilateral, or bilateral. Generally in leprosy, only the orbicularis oculi, the muscle that closes the eyelids, is affected; initially only paresis is felt by the patient but the condition evolves to paralysis of the muscle. In this case, the patient may experience an eyelid cleft due to lagophthalmos, the inability to close the eyelids completely (Fig. 73.1), which can be mild (up to 2 mm) or severe (≥ 2 mm). Other possible ocular manifestations are redness, itching, burning, a gritty feeling, and decreased visual acuity [10]. The autonomic fibers are responsible for the stimulation of the lacrimal, nasal, and salivary glands.

Trigeminal Nerve

The trigeminal nerve divides into three branches, the ophthalmic, maxillary, and mandibular branches, and is responsible for sensitivity of the cornea, nose, mouth, teeth, and tongue [11]. One feature of its injury in leprosy is diminished or complete loss of corneal sensitivity with complaints such as decreased or absent automatic blinking of the eyelids, decreased visual acuity, hyperemia, and corneal ulcers.

Nose

Involvement of the facial nerve is responsible for autonomic and motor abnormalities and damage to the trigeminal nerve causes the loss or reduction of nasal sensitivity. Primary changes to the nose may occur due to the replication of bacilli in the nasal mucosa resulting in obstructive infiltration, viscous secretion, crusts, and ulcerations. In more advanced stages, secondary injuries can occur such as destruction of the nasal cartilage, nasal septum perforation and collapse of the nasal pyramid. This disability can be one of the factors responsible for social exclusion of patients [12].

The Arms

The most affected nerve trunks of the upper limbs are the ulnar nerve followed by the median nerve and more rarely the radial nerve. Impairment of muscle strength and sensory afferent caused by damage to these nerves change grip patterns causing difficulties in using the hands, with limitations to perform activities of daily life and work and consequently restrictions in social participation [13].

Ulnar Nerve Injury

In the arm, the most commonly affected nerve in leprosy is the ulnar nerve with its point of greatest vulnerability being the elbow, where it is close to the surface, relatively fixed, and passes by a joint. The predisposing anatomy in this region associated with the biomechanics of the ulnar nerve, which is subjected to traction and friction during movements of the elbow, the most important factors that cause neural compression.

The clinical manifestations of this injury are changes to sensory, motor, and autonomic functions in the hypothenar region, the fourth (medial) and fifth fingers and the area of the back of the hand corresponding to these fingers. The dorsal cutaneous branch is found in the lower third of the forearm [14, 15].

The intrinsic muscles of the hand are innervated largely by the ulnar nerve and, as a morphologic characteristic, its paralysis causes flexion of the fingers and hyperextension of the metacarpophalangeal joints represented by palsy of the dorsal and volar interosseous muscles, medial lumbrical muscles (fourth and fifth digits), adductor pollicis and the deep portion of the short flexor of the thumb, and the opponens pollicis of the fifth digit, leaving the common extensor digitorum to function in an unbalanced manner; this results in the hand having a claw-like look [15].

This imbalance results in bending of the fourth and fifth digits with hyperextension of the metacarpophalangeal joints and flexion of the interphalangeal joints because of the isolated action of the flexor and extensor muscles due to intrinsic paralysis (Fig. 73.2). With the unbalanced forces, the medial edge of the hand loses the transverse and longitudinal radius, making it impossible to hold cylindrical objects in the hand. Precise pinch

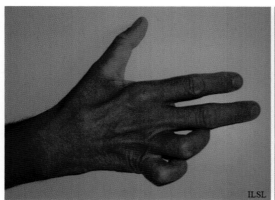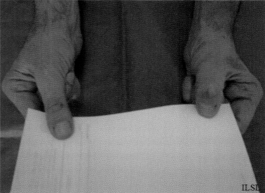

Fig. 73.2 Claw fingers (fourth and fifth) and atrophy of the first intermetacarpal space. Fig. 73.2 Froment's sign

grip is impaired with an inability to stabilize thin objects between the thumb and forefinger resulting from paralysis of the adductor and half of the short flexor muscle. Owing to the force applied when holding an object between the thumb and forefinger, there will be marked flexion of the distal phalanx of the thumb reflecting the instability of the metacarpophalangeal joint; this is known as Froment's sign (Fig. 73.2a) [13].

With the grip strength to hold cylindrical objects impaired and the lack of precision to grip small objects as a result of ulnar nerve injury, the strength of the hand is reduced by 40–70% [13].

As a result of the functional imbalance, the patient develops different ways to hold objects to become independent. However, often the individual uses areas of contact that were not designed to hold things, such as the back of the hand and the fingertips. The quest for independence using nonfunctional movements can affect the physical integrity of the individual in the future [13, 16].

Another important morphologic characteristic is the atrophy of the first dorsal interosseous muscle, which may cause social exclusion of the patient (Fig. 73.2).

Median Nerve Injury

Nerve compression occurs in the transverse and annular carpal ligaments [17]. This injury causes sensory, motor, and autonomic changes in the volar region, the thenar eminence, the thumb and the region of the palm corresponding to the second and third digits and the side of the fourth digit, as well as of the back of the hand in the region of the middle and distal phalanges of the second and third digits. The paralysis of this nerve in leprosy commonly occurs after ulnar nerve injury [18].

The characteristic of median nerve damage is the loss of opposition and abduction of the thumb caused by palsy of the short abductor, opponens, and short flexor (superficial portion) muscles which normally maintain the thumb on the same plane as the hand, making it impossible to grasp objects (Fig. 73.3). This paralysis results in serious disability, as the thumb is responsible for 50% of the hand functionality [18, 19].

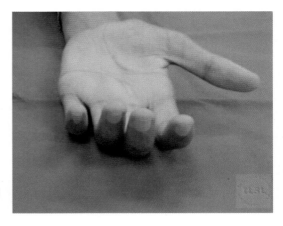

Fig. 73.3 Loss of opposition of the thumb

All the intrinsic musculature of the hand is affected by paralysis of the median ulnar, resulting in an imbalance of the extrinsic muscles causing functional disorders. In these cases, the function of the hand is reduced to that of a hook; objects are held with the fingers in adduction or between the fingers (interdigital) with practices unique to each patient.

Injury to the Radial Nerve

Compression of the radial nerve occurs in the humeral medullary canal, located in the middle third of the arm. Its sensory distribution corresponds to the central area of the back of the arm as far as the olecranon and posterior and central regions of the forearm. It is responsible for the innervations of the muscles of the arm and forearm used for extension and supination movements.

The morphology of radial nerve injury is drop wrist caused by paralysis of the extensor muscles of the wrist and fingers, which makes it difficult to hold objects [20].

This reaction occurs in only 1% of leprosy cases and generally occurs after injury to the ulnar and median nerves, a condition known as triple paralysis [18].

Injury of the superficial radial nerve branch causes loss of sensation in the posterior region of the thumb and the radial edge of the back of the hand.

Lower Limbs

The most affected nerve trunks of the lower limbs related to leprosy are the common peroneal nerve that branches out into the deep and superficial peroneal nerves, and the tibial nerve which subdivides in the plantar region of the foot as the medial plantar, lateral plantar, and calcaneal nerves. These two nerve trunks with their respective branches stimulate all the extrinsic and intrinsic muscles of the foot. Duerksen, after experience in Brazil and Paraguay, states that the most commonly affected nerve in the lower limb in leprosy is the tibial trunk [21].

Different levels of nerve damage result in changes in physiologic gait patterns from a slight reduction in sensitivity (the patient does not notice the loss of a slipper, for example) to paralysis resulting in foot drop gait, which is very susceptible to falls and traumatic injuries. The limitation in the ability to walk makes patients, apart from having a risk of further injury, restricted in their participation of social activities [13].

Common Peroneal Nerve

The common peroneal nerve is a branch of the sciatic nerve that runs down the side of the popliteal fossa and then winds around the fibula neck and passes through an osteofibrous opening known as the fibular tunnel, where it penetrates the superficial belly of the peroneal muscle. Inside this tunnel, the nerve divides into two branches, the deep and superficial branches. This section of the nerve is closer to the surface and susceptible to the installation of *M. leprae* causing nerve damage.

The common peroneal nerve muscle group is represented by the tibialis anterior muscle, the extensor digitorum longus and brevis, and the extensor hallucis longus, and the innervation of the superficial peroneal nerve is represented by eversion of the foot muscles. Regarding the sensory distribution, the area corresponding to the trajectory is the anterolateral region of the leg, foot, and toes, including the medial side of the hallux.

The clinical features of injury to the common peroneal nerve are sensory and autonomic loss in

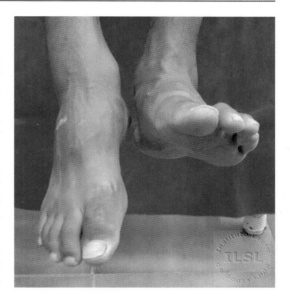

Fig. 73.4 Foot drop

the area of its distribution. An inability to perform dorsiflexion of the foot and extension of the toes, classically known as "foot drop," is observed in complete nerve lesions (Fig. 73.4).

The physiologic gait is represented by phases with each one having a key role in walking: the stance phase, when the heel touches the ground, the swing phase, the exchange stage, and the propulsive stage, when the forefoot produces leverage for the next step. With nerve palsy, the gait pattern becomes pathologic and the phases are changed with the forefoot being the first to touch the ground.

With changes in the gait, the patient is at risk of injury from loss of balance and falls, with twisting and shortening of the flexor unit leading to fixed deformities.

Tibial Nerve

The tibial nerve leaves the popliteal fossa similar to the common peroneal nerve, but its trajectory is deep in the gastrocnemius and soleus muscles. However, as it passes through the tarsal canal, it is close to the surface with an aggravating anatomic constriction.

The clinical characteristics of injuries to the tibial nerve are sensory and autonomic changes

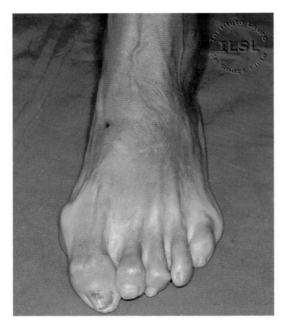

Fig. 73.5 Claw toes

in the plantar region of the foot. This trunk after going around the medial malleolus is divided into three branches: medial plantar, lateral plantar, and calcaneal nerves.

Motor alterations are apparent in the intrinsic muscles of the foot (interosseous and lumbrical). When paralyzed, the patient evolves with flexion of the interphalangeal joints and extension of the metatarsophalangeal joints (Fig. 73.5). Intrinsic paralysis associated with loss of sensitivity can cause the patient to develop severe trophic and traumatic injuries with devastating consequences, which may even lead to amputation after osteomyelitis.

Assessments and Preventive Measures

Instruments and measures to evaluate and monitor leprosy patients as recommended by the Brazilian Ministry of Health consist in the Simplified Neurologic Assessment (SNA), evaluation of the Degree of Disability (World Health Organization (WHO)), the Screening of Activity Limitation and Safety Awareness (SALSA)

scale, and the Participation Scale, as well as the application of basic prevention, control, and treatment strategies.

In leprosy, most of the problems resulting from injury to peripheral nerves can be avoided using the SNA to evaluate the situation of the nerve and neural function [22].

By means of this assessment, changes in neural function can be monitored, that is, routinely analyzed to identify neural inflammation early so as to prescribe the necessary treatment, monitor response to the treatment of neuritis, and determine the need for surgical intervention [22, 23].

The degree of disability, as proposed by Bechelli and Dominguez and standardized by the WHO, is a measure that indicates decreases or loss of sensation and muscle strength, and visible deformities; it is widely used in planning actions to prevent disabilities and as an epidemiologic indicator. The degree of disability related to injuries to the eyes, palms of the hands, and soles of the feet is assessed by this instrument because these are considered the areas that are most susceptible to injuries during daily activities [22].

According to Deepak, in addition to physical disabilities, 20% of patients with leprosy may also have psychosocial restrictions [24].

One screening instrument, the SALSA scale, was developed to assess how disabilities interfere with the activities of daily life of patients. This scale allows a measurement of the extent to which activities are limiting and the risk of worsening disabilities while carrying out activities. This scale is based on the International Classification of Functioning, Disability and Health (ICF) [10]. It was developed, tested, and validated in six languages, Chinese (Mandarin), English, Hausa, Hebrew, Tamil, and Portuguese (Brazil). The scale consists of 20 questions with the score ranging from 10 to 80. A low score indicates little difficulty, while higher scores indicate increasing limitations to perform activities.

The data collected using these instruments are part of the process of diagnosing, monitoring, treating, and preventing peripheral nerve injuries.

The Participation Scale (version 4.6), developed after anthropologic field work, aims to quantify restrictions in social participation experienced by people affected by leprosy and to assess the severity of the social needs of patients with disabilities.

The scale was subjected to psychometric tests of validity, reliability, and stability and was validated for use in India, Brazil, and Nepal after a multicenter study. It includes several domains of the ICF such as learning and applying knowledge, communication and self-care, mobility, domestic life, interpersonal interactions and relationships, major life areas, and community [25].

This scale consists of 18 items with scores ranging from 0 to 90 points, and takes about 20 min to apply. A score of from 0 to 12 points is considered unrestricted social participation, from 13 to 22 mild restriction, from 23 to 32 moderate restriction, from 33 to 52 severe, and scores from 53 to 90 completely restricted [25].

As rejection can begin in the family, in society, or even in the patients themselves, it is necessary to know the social participation of these patients and to determine the degree and nature of possible restrictions.

Simplified Neurologic Assessment

The SNA must be systematically carried out on a regular basis as part of leprosy control measures. This assessment is important because nerve damage can be very subtle and go unnoticed by the patient at the time of diagnosis, during treatment, and even after the end of treatment.

Neurologic assessments should be performed at diagnosis, that is, at the beginning of treatment, every 3 months during treatment if the patient does not complain, at discharge, and after completing MDT for up to 5 years. When neuritis or reactions are seen or suspected or when the patient complains, this assessment should be performed every month or more often if possible [22]. Additionally assessments should be performed at 15, 45, 90, and 180 days after neural decompression [26].

The minimum content of the SNA for the eyes, hands, and feet is based on the verification of the main complaint, inspection, evaluation of sensitivity, motor evaluation, nerve palpation, and evaluation of the degree of disability.

Patient complaints and the inspection conducted by the examiner are important, as they are correlated to the clinical picture and help to identify nerve damage early.

Investigation of the Main Complaint

Patients should be questioned about their complaints in relation to the nose, eyes, hands, and feet. The most frequent complaints in the nose are respiratory obstruction, dryness, crusts adhered to the nasal mucosa, and bleeding. In the eyes there are reports of a gritty feeling, burning, itching, watery eyes, decreased vision, redness, and pain. Complaints related to the hands and feet include pain, paresthesia, hypoesthesia, and paresis, or patients may report that they drop objects frequently or slippers fall off without them noticing.

Inspection

During the inspection of the outside of the nose, check the skin conditions and for the presence of lepromas, infiltration, hyperemia, ulceration, scarring, and collapse of the nasal pyramid.

During the examination of the eyes, look for hyperemia of the conjunctiva, lagophthalmos, ciliary and supraciliary madarosis, dryness and corneal ulcers, trichiasis, ectropion, entropion, and corneal opacity.

Edema, scars, skin cracks, sores, loss of hair, dry skin, cyanosis, atrophy, resorption, retractions, and morphologic characteristics of neural injury are investigated on the hands and feet.

Nerve Palpation

There is no laboratory gold standard for the diagnosis of leprosy, but a smear, which identifies the presence of *M. leprae* in lymph, and histopathology of tissue, support clinical findings which are still essential to arrive at a diagnosis. In the physical examination skin lesions, a decrease or complete loss of protective sensation, muscle strength, and thickening of peripheral nerves must be carefully investigated.

Early diagnosis of nerve thickening by palpation of the nerve trunks near the surface of the skin

Table 73.1 Palpation techniques

Nerve	Position	Local
Ulnar	Upper limb at 90–120° of flexion. The examiner supporting the patient's forearm in his hand	Proximal and distal trajectories of the nerve, in relation to the ulnar groove. (epicondylar groove) (Fig. 73.6)
Median	Position the patient's wrist at about 10° of flexion	Wrist between long palmar tendons and flexor carpi radialis (Fig. 73.7)
Radial	Position the shoulder with internal rotation and keep the elbow flexed with the forearm in pronation and supported by the examiner	Spiral canal in the rear middle third of the arm (Fig. 73.8)
Peroneal	Sitting with the knees flexed at 90° and feet flat on the floor	Back of the leg between the head and neck of the fibula (Fig. 73.9)
Tibial	Sitting with knees at 90° of flexion and inversion and passive plantar flexion	Medial malleolus, behind and below the bony prominence (Fig. 73.10)

Source: (Brazil, 2008; Baccarelli R, Marciano LHSC, 2003)

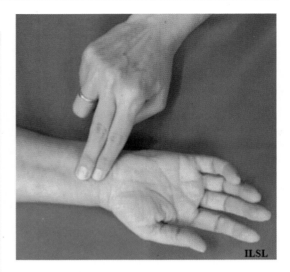

Fig. 73.7 Palpation of the median nerve

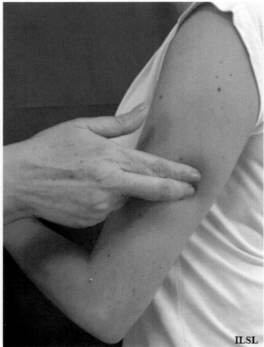

Fig. 73.8 Palpation of the radial nerve

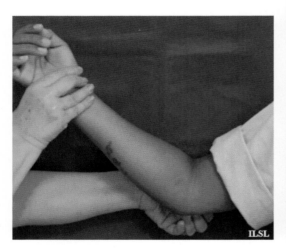

Fig. 73.6 Palpation of the ulnar nerve

allows the immediate institution of drug therapy and rehabilitative interventions (Table 73.1).

At the time of palpation the examiner should observe the patient's facial expression in relation to their pain threshold. Bilateral palpation is rec-

ommended in order to compare the left and right sides to identify nerve thickening, consistency, nodules, and Tinel's sign, a local tingling electric shock sensation [27].

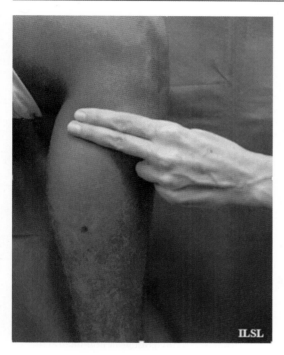

Fig. 73.9 Palpation of the common peroneal nerve

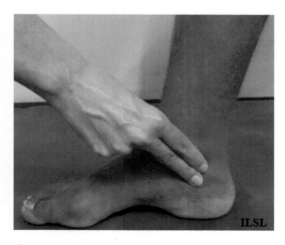

Fig. 73.10 Palpation of the tibial nerve

It is worth noting that the median nerve is rarely palpable, as it has a deep trajectory between the superficial and deep flexor tendons. The assessment of this nerve is conducted to verify the presence of pain on palpation, or a positive Tinel's sign. The radial nerve also passes along a deeper bed, and its palpation demands skill and experience of the examiner.

Sensitivity Assessment

In leprosy, the sensory evaluation can be limited to points representative of the sensory distribution of the ulnar, median, radial, peroneal, sural, and tibial nerves to diagnose and monitor nerve injury (Fig. 73.11).

Evaluation of Corneal Sensitivity

The sensitivity of the cornea should be tested to assess possible trigeminal nerve damage in leprosy. Therefore, we recommend the use of thin tasteless dental floss. The dental floss should measure 5 cm plus a length sufficient for the examiner to hold. The patient is asked to look at the forehead or the finger of the examiner. Then pull the dental floss in the temporal periphery of the cornea and observe whether blinking is immediate, delayed, or absent (Fig. 73.12).

Sensitivity Test for the Hands and Feet

The sensitivity test of the hands and feet is performed using Semmes-Weinstein (S-W) monofilaments. This is considered one of the most reliable tests and is valid for field work. It is a standardized and quantitative test adopted for the diagnosis of nerve disease by the International Society for Peripheral Neuropathy.

According to Moberg, the test is reliable in 84% of cases. Compared with other electrophysiologic studies, this test is a safe and inexpensive method of evaluation with high sensitivity, specificity, and reproducibility [28]. The S-W test is a subjective test, i.e., it depends on the concentration and cooperation of the individual being assessed, a condition that should be highlighted, given that it can be a factor in the accuracy and reliability of the test.

S-W monofilaments consist of 38-mm lengths of nylon yarn (No. 612) with different diameters. Commercially they are bought as kits of 5, 6, or 20 monofilaments.

Werner and Omer [29] found that clinically you can use a small number of monofilaments to evaluate peripheral sensitivity without affecting

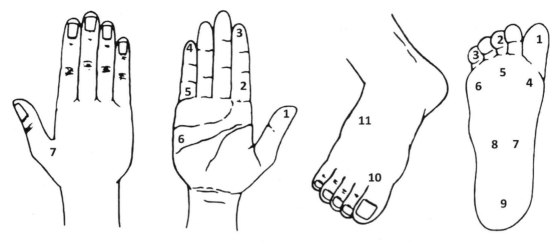

Nerves: 1,2,3- ulnar; 4,5,6- median; 7- radial   Nerves: 1-9 - tibial; 10- peroneal; 11- sural

Fig. 73.11 Points representative of the sensory distribution of the ulnar, median, radial, tibial, peroneal, sural nerves

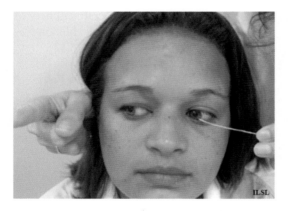

Fig. 73.12 Corneal sensitivity study

Motor Assessment

Voluntary muscle testing is reliable to evaluate neural function. It is valid to identify conduction blocks or larger axonal losses. Motor deficiency is identified after 30% of the fibers are affected [32, 33].

Daniels and Worthingham [34] recommend a muscle strength grading scale of 0–5 (Table 73.3).

The hand and foot muscles that must be evaluated for the SNA are described in Table 73.4. This assessment includes a muscle for each nerve that is generally affected by leprosy, but can be expanded depending on the needs of each individual.

Classification of the Degree of Disability (WHO)

The degree of disability is a measure that indicates the loss of protective sensation and visible deformities resulting from neural injury including blindness. It is an epidemiologic indicator used to evaluate leprosy control programs, determine early diagnosis of the disease, and compare the degree of disability at the start of treatment and at discharge to determine whether there has been an improvement or not [26].

Using the first physical evaluation and the sensory and motor assessment of the eyes, hands, and feet, it is possible to classify the degree of disability of the patient following the criteria of the WHO, as described in Table 73.5.

the outcome. In Brazil, the National Coordination of Sanitary Dermatology includes a set of six monofilaments as a source to assess sensitivity in leprosy.

On being applied perpendicularly to the skin, when the monofilament bends slightly, forces of 0.05 g, 0.2 g, 2.0 g, 4.0 g, 10.0 g and 300 g are exerted in the area being examined depending on the thickness of the thread (Fig. 73.13) [30].

Von Prince and Butler [31] conducted comparative studies of the S-W monofilaments and other tests such as temperature, static two-point discrimination, proprioception, stereognosis, pain and graphesthesia in patients with peripheral neuropathy. This comparison allowed the calculation of functional levels, as shown in Table 73.2.

Fig. 73.13 Semmes–Weinstein monofilaments

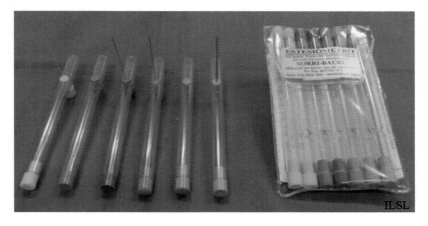

Table 73.2 Semmes–Weinstein monofilament, registration code, and functional level

Monofilament (grams)	Registration code	Functional level
0.05 g	●	Normal sensitivity of the hand and foot
		Conserved two-point discrimination, fine texture discrimination, stereognosis, thermoesthesia, feeling deep pressure and kinesthesia
0.2 g	●	Decreased sensitivity in the hand and normal in the foot
		Loss of graphesthesia
		Difficulty with two-point discrimination and fine texture discrimination
2 g	●	Decreased protective sensitivity in the hand
		Loss of two-point discrimination and fine texture discrimination
		Affected stereognosis and thermoesthesia
0.4 g	●	Loss of protective sensation in the hand and sometimes in the foot
		Loss of stereognosis and thermoesthesia
10 g	⊠	Loss of protective sensation in the foot
		Loss of thermoesthesia
300 g	○	Presence of the feeling of deep pressure on hand and foot
		Painful sensitivity may be present
		Preserved kinesthesia
Does not feel the touch of 300 g monofilament	●	Loss of sense of deep pressure on hand and foot
		Painful sensitivity and kinesthetic may be present

Simple Techniques to Prevent Disability and for Self-Care

The basic conducts and the procedures to treat changes in autonomic, sensory, and motor functions are shown in Tables 73.6, 73.7, and 73.8.

Exercises

In cases of paresis and paralysis, the prescribed exercises should be passive, assisted active, active, and active resistant, according to the degree of voluntary muscle strength. The exercises related to the muscles described are shown in Table 73.9.

Table 73.3 Degree of voluntary muscle strength and functional status

Degree of muscle strength	Functional description	Functional status
5	Full motion against gravity with maximum resistance	Normal
4	Full motion against gravity with partial resistance	Paresthesia
3	Full motion against gravity	
2	Partial movement	
1	Muscle contraction without movement	
0	Without evidence of muscle contraction	Paralysis

Source: Ordinance No. 3125, GM/Ministry of Health 7/10/2010

Table 73.4 Motor assessment of main muscles innervated by the facial, ulnar, median, radial and peroneal nerves

Nerve	Muscle	Action	Test
Facial	Orbicularis muscle of the eye	Eyelid occlusion	Ask the patient to close the eyes gently, while the examiner assesses whether the eyelids close completely or not with the help of a spotlight that should be placed at an inferior oblique angle
Ulnar	Abductor of the 5th finger	Abduction of the 5th finger	Position: forearm and palm down. Hold the 2nd to 4th fingers and ask the patient to move the 5th finger away as a counter force is applied, from the outside at the second phalanx, returning the finger to the plane of the hand. Ideally, the metacarpophalangeal joints should be at 30° of flexion (Fig. 73.14)
Median	Pollicis brevis	Abduction of the thumb	Position: forearm and palm facing up and resting on a table. The patient raises the thumb from the hand plane forming an angle of 90°, and then apply opposing force to the lateral edge of the base of the proximal phalanx forcing it down (Fig. 73.15)
Radial	Wrist extensors	Wrist extension	Position: forearm and palm down. The patient raises his wrist, leaving the fingers relaxed. After this movement, resistance is placed at the back of the hand in the direction opposite to the movement performed. (Fig. 73.16)
Peroneal	Extensor hallucis	Extension of the hallux	Position: patient sitting with the knee in flexion. The examiner, after stabilizing the foot and ankle in neutral, asks the patient to elevate the hallux as much as possible, applying counter resistance on the dorsum of the proximal phalanx of the toe (Fig. 73.17)
	Tibialis anterior	Dorsiflexion of the foot	Position: patient sitting with the knee in slight flexion. After stabilizing the leg, ask the patient to lift the foot, keeping the toes relaxed. Resistance should be applied on the medial side of the dorsum of the foot (Fig. 73.18)

Source: Brazil, Disability Prevention Manual, 2008

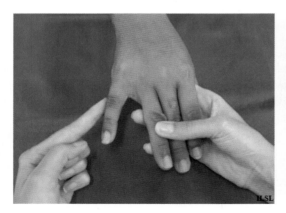

Fig. 73.14 Strength test for the abductor muscle of the fifth finger

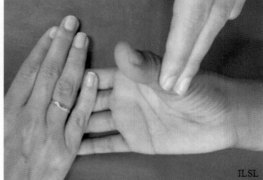

Fig. 73.15 Strength test for the abductor pollicis brevis muscle

In both paresis and paralysis, the muscles of the hand and foot may suffer muscle-tendon shortening and periarticular retraction resulting in joint limitations. These problems can be avoided or minimized by stretching exercises.

One of the techniques for stretching the flexor muscle tendon units of the wrist and fingers is that the patient supports the hand on a table and uses the other hand to keep the fingers in extension as far as possible. At the same time the patient must keep the elbow in extension. Thus, a gradual lengthening of these units will be produced (Fig. 73.26).

Stretching the muscle tendon units of the lower limbs should be carried out in the flexor

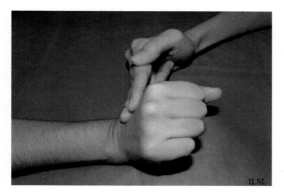

Fig. 73.16 Muscle strength test for the wrist extensors

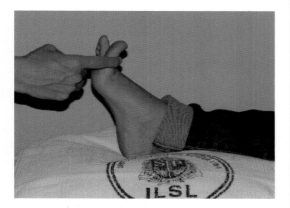

Fig. 73.17 Strength test for the extensor hallucis muscle

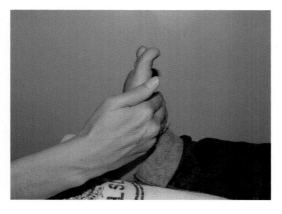

Fig. 73.18 Strength test for the anterior tibialis muscle

Table 73.5 World Health Organization disability grade

Degree	Characteristics
0	Eyes: muscle strength of the eyelids and corneal sensitivity preserved and patient can count fingers at 6 m or visual acuity ≥0.1 or 6:60
	Hands: muscle strength of the hands and palmar sensitivity preserved; can feel a 2 g monofilament (purple) or the tip of a ball point pen
	Feet: muscle strength of the feet and plantar sensitivity preserved; can feel a 2 g monofilament (purple) or the tip of a ballpoint pen
1	Eyes: decreased muscle strength of the eyelids but without visible disabilities or diminished or loss of corneal sensitivity: delayed or missing response to touch using dental floss or decrease/absence of blinking
	Hands: decreased muscle strength of the hand without visible disabilities or impairment of palmar sensitivity: does not feel a 2 g monofilament (purple) or the tip of a ballpoint pen
	Feet: decreased muscle strength of feet with no visible disabilities or altered plantar sensitivity: does not feel a 2 g monofilament (purple) or the tip of a ballpoint pen
2	Eyes: visible disability caused by leprosy, such as lagophthalmos, ectropion, entropies, and trichiasis. Central corneal opacity; iridocyclitis or cannot count fingers at 6 m or visual acuity <0.1 or 6:60, without other possible causes
	Hands: visible disability caused by leprosy, such as claw fingers, bone resorption, muscle atrophy, wrist drop, contracture and wounds
	Feet: visible disability caused by leprosy, such as claw toes*, bone resorption, muscle atrophy, foot drop, contracture, and wounds

Source: General Coordination of Leprosy and Diseases in Elimination-CGHDE/DEVIT/SVS/Ministry of Health

(Fig. 73.27a). Another option for stretching is shown in Fig. 73.27b.

Other measures may be necessary, such as the use of orthosis, adaptations, and reconstructive surgeries.

Assistive Technology

According to Bersch [35], assistive technology is an aid that will enable a desired function that has been prevented by circumstances such as disability or aging to be performed.

muscles of the ankle and foot. In this case the patient should stand facing a wall with the leg to be stretched behind with the knee in extension. The other leg must be placed in front of the body with the knee in flexion. From this position the patient should move the body forward flexing the elbows without taking the heels off the floor

Table 73.6 Signs and conducts in ocular changes

Signs	Conducts	Procedures	Objective
Dryness of the cornea	Artificial lubrication with eye drops and ointment	Keep the patient sitting and looking up. Retract the lower eyelid from the temporal portion and apply an eye drop, being careful not to touch the eye with the tip of the bottle	Eye lubrication
	Blink frequency	The patient should close the eyes gently for 30 s	
Trichiasis	Removal of lashes	Removal of upper eyelashes: patient sitting, looking down remove each lash facing the eyeball using eyebrow tweezers and a magnifying glass. Then lubricate	Prevent ocular lesions, in particular corneal ulcers
		Removal of lower lashes: Patient sitting, looking up. Follow the procedures above	
Initial lagophthalmos	Exercises to open and close the eyes	Ask the patient to gently close the eyes and then close with as much force as possible. Stay with the eyes closed for 5 s. Repeat 20 times the same exercise three times a day until complete recovery of the strength of the orbicularis oculi muscle	Strengthening of the orbicularis oculi muscle

Table 73.7 Signs and conducts in changes of the nose

Signs	Conducts	Procedures	Objective
Dry nasal mucosa	Hydration and lubrication	Put water in cupped hand or in a container, breathe in water and then let it drain (Fig. 73.19). Use cream or Vaseline at the entrance of the nostrils and gently massage the outer portion with the finger. The patient should be instructed not to blow the nose hard and not insert objects into the nostril to remove scabs, as this can damage the mucosa	Facilitate the removal of secretion, avoiding the accumulation, burning, dryness and crusting
Hypersecretion			
Crusts	Hydration and lubrication. Warn the patient not to remove crusts with the finger or objects such as cotton swabs, etc.		Remove the crust adhered maintaining the nasal cavity clean and free from ulcers
Ulcers	Clean to remove crusts and applying antibiotic ointment (provided by the doctor). Recommendation: repeat until healed		Prevent secondary infection

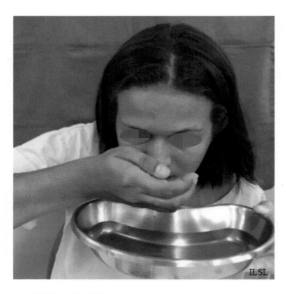

Fig. 73.19 Nasal hydration

Orthoses and Adaptations

Orthoses are devices externally applied to a limb to immobilize one segment, balance deforming forces, and assist manual function.

In leprosy, orthoses are indicated when paresis or paralysis is severe, and in cases of neuritis, leprosy reactions, injuries, infections, retractions of joints, postoperative neural decompression, and reconstructive surgeries. Some orthoses are shown in Figs. 73.28, 73.29, 73.30, 73.31, 73.32, 73.33, and 73.34.

The use of adaptations is recommended when sensory or motor disorders are present; these are simple modifications to personal working tools as well as insoles or adapted shoes. The objectives of these adaptations are to promote or facilitate functional independence, improve the grip or gait, and prevent or

Table 73.8 Signs and conducts in the skin changes of the hands and feet

Signs	Conducts	Procedures	Objective
Hyperkeratotic dry skin	Hydration lubrication massage	Immerse the limb in water at room temperature for 10 min. Then wipe off the excess of water and apply an oily or creamy substance to prevent the evaporation of water performing a sliding massage (Fig. 73.20)	To improve hydration and lubrication of the skin to avoid cracks and wounds
		This is not recommended when there are skin or nail lesions, or other dermatitis	
	Removal of calluses	After hydration, remove calluses using sandpaper being careful not to cause injuries. Remove only the surface layer of skin. Then lubricate the skin	Reduce points of over pressure
Loss of protective sensation	Training visuomotor Coordination	Guide the patient on how to use the vision to compensate for sensory impairment and reduce difficulties in manual skills	Improve functional performance
	Adaptations	Encourage the patient to use adaptations of tools for work and personal use, simple insoles in comfortable oversized shoes	Prevent secondary injuries

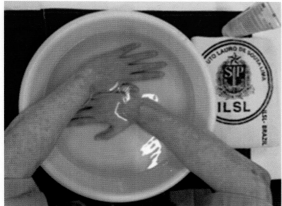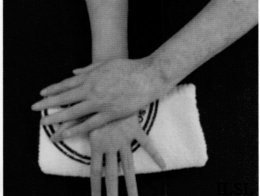

Fig. 73.20 Hydration, lubrication, and sliding massage

stop the worsening of disabilities (Figs. 73.35, 73.36, 73.37, and 73.38).

Self-Care

To prevent disabilities in leprosy it is necessary to change the behavior; this is difficult, especially in adults. Prevention is achieved by the professional winning over the patient's confidence and incorporating strategies to perform activities of daily life. Thus the professional needs to proceed with care, using the correct approach to preventive measures with the aim that they will truly be assimilated by the patient as a new conduct in daily life in order for them to become normal routine activities in day-to-day life. An essential feature is to adapt preventive measures to use available materials and

related to the patient's culture, as in this way success is facilitated [36].

To reduce the damage caused by leprosy, it is essential that patients develop the habit of caring for themselves day by day.

From the conditions of the patient and knowledge of individual problems of each member of the group, group interventions are geared to increase the patient's knowledge about the disease, clarify and advise on treatment methods and self-care practices, promote and/or restore functional performance in occupations that make up the daily lives of individuals, through dynamic actions, lectures, recreational activities, role playing, and strategies to follow at home, as well as to prescribe or create orthoses and adaptations of work and daily life instruments. All of these

Table 73.9 Exercises

Muscles	Resisted: grade 4	Active: grade 3	Assisted active: grade 2	Assisted active/ passive: grade 1	Passive: level 0
Abductor 5th finger	With the forearm resting on the table, palm facing down, put a rubber band around the 2nd and 5th fingers at the proximal interphalangeal joint for resistance. The patient should move the 5th finger as far from the 4th finger as possible. Hold for 10 s and return to the adduction position (Fig. 73.21)	With the forearm resting on the table, palm facing down, move the 5th finger as far away from the 4th finger as possible. Hold for 10 s and return to the adduction position	With the forearm resting on the table, palm facing down, move the 5th finger as far away from the 4th finger as possible. Using the other hand, the patient should complete the movement. Hold for 10 s or as long as they can and return to the adduction position	With the forearm resting on the table and the palm facing down, the patient should contract the abductor muscle of the 5th finger and with the help of the other hand, move the finger to its full range of motion, hold for 10 s and return to the adduction position	With the forearm resting on the table and the palm facing down, the patient, with the help of the other hand, should hold the abduction of the 5th finger in its full amplitude. Hold for 10 s and return it to the adduction position
Pollicis brevis	Forearm and hand resting on the table, facing up, put an elastic band of approximately 5 cm around the proximal phalanx of the thumb and forefinger forming a figure of eight. The aim is to raise the thumb perpendicular to the palm. Forming a 90° angle, hold for 10 s and return to the adduction position (Fig. 73.22)	Forearm and hand resting on the table facing up. Oppose the thumb to the other fingers to its full range of motion. Maintain the interphalangeal joint of the thumb in extension. The angle formed is 90° to the hand plane. Hold for 10 s and return to the starting position	Forearm and hand resting on the table facing up to oppose the thumb to the other fingers forming an angle of 90°.Use the other hand to complete the full range of motion, maintaining the thumb in this position and the interphalangeal joint in extension. Hold for 10 s and return to the starting position	With the forearm resting on the table and the palm facing up, the patient should contract the pollicis brevis. With the other hand move to the full range of motion. Hold for 10 s and return to the starting position	With the forearm resting on the table and the palm facing up, the patient, with the help of the other hand, should abduct the thumb to its full range of motion. Move the thumb in the perpendicular plane. Hold for 10 s and return to the starting position
Wrist extensors	Forearm resting on the table, palm down, hold an object with the maximum weight possible and lift the wrist. Hold for 10 s and return to the starting position (Fig. 73.23)	Forearm resting on the table, palm down, fingers semi-flexed, the patient should extend the wrist to its full range of motion. Hold for 10 s and return to starting position	With the forearm resting on the table, palm down and fingers semi-flexed, the patient should extend the wrist, as far as possible, completing the movement with the help of the other hand. Hold for 10 s and return to the starting position	With the forearm resting on the table and the palm facing down, the patient should contract the wrist extensors. With the other hand, move the wrist to its full range of motion. Hold for 10 s and return to the starting position	With the forearm resting on the table and the palm facing down, the patient should with the help of the other hand, extend the wrist to its full range of motion. Hold for 10 s and return to starting position

Table 73.9 (continued)

Muscles	Resisted: grade 4	Active: grade 3	Assisted active: grade 2	Assisted active/ passive: grade 1	Passive: level 0
Extensor hallucis	Sitting with the leg supported on a chair, ask the patient to extend the hallux as far as possible applying counter resistance to the dorsum of the proximal phalanx of that toe. The resistance may be with the patient's own hand or using an elastic band. Hold for 10 s and return to the starting position (Fig. 73.24)	Sitting with the leg supported on a chair, to ask the patient to extend the hallux to its full range while keeping the other toes relaxed. Hold for 10 s and return to the starting position	Sitting with the leg supported on a bench or with the legs crossed to facilitate assisted movement, ask the patient to extend the hallux as far as possible. Assist the movement with the hand. Hold for 10 s and return to the starting position	Sitting with the leg supported on a bench or with the legs crossed to facilitate assisted movement, ask the patient to contract the extensor hallucis. With the help of the hand, move the hallux to its full extent. Hold for 10 s and return to the starting position	Sitting with the leg supported on a bench or with the legs crossed to facilitate assisted movement, the patient should with the help of the hand, extend the hallux to its full range of motion. Hold for 10 s and return to the starting position
Tibialis anterior muscle	Sitting with the leg supported on a chair the patient should perform dorsiflexion with a resistance on the back of the foot. This resistance may be by using an elastic band or bag around the dorsum of the foot. Hold for 10 s and return to starting position (Fig. 73.25)	Sitting with the leg supported on a chair the patient should perform dorsiflexion of the foot to its full extent. Hold for 10 s and return to the starting position	Sitting with the leg supported on a bench or with the legs crossed to facilitate assisted movement, ask the patient to perform dorsiflexion as far as possible. With the help of hand, complete the range of motion. Hold for 10 s and return to the starting position	Sitting with the leg supported on a bench or with the legs crossed to facilitate assisted movement, ask the patient to contract the tibialis anterior muscle. With the help of hand, make full dorsiflexion. Hold for 10 s and return to the starting position	Sitting with the leg supported on a bench or with the legs crossed to facilitate assisted movement, the patient should perform with the help of the hand, full dorsiflexion. Hold for 10 s and return to the starting position

important resources attempt to improve the quality of life, interpersonal relationships, and the exchange of experiences in the social context. During consultations, problems, doubts, and the difficulties encountered in the implementation of care are discussed with the patient in an attempt to find the best solutions, always observing the feasibility of changes and patients' willpower to change their habits.

These experiences can occur individually or in groups with the participation of a multidisciplinary team trying to develop risk awareness, change attitudes, and increase autonomy.

Interventions can occur weekly or biweekly according to the availability of individuals and professionals.

Assessments and Measures for Surgical Rehabilitation

Reconstructive Surgeries

As a result of nerve damage, surgical rehabilitation aims to rebalance the action of deforming forces between agonists and antagonists to

Fig. 73.21 Resistance active exercise for the abductor muscle of the fifth finger

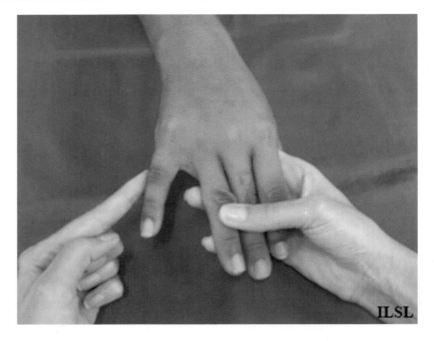

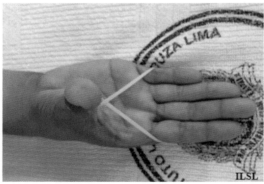

Fig. 73.22 Resistance active exercise for the abductor pollicis brevis muscle

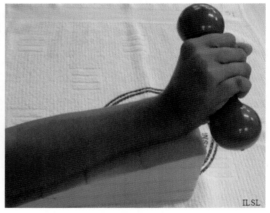

Fig. 73.23 Resistance active exercise for the extensor muscles of the wrist

minimize disabilities and improve the function of the eyes, hands, and feet. The most common surgeries are correction of lagophthalmos, neural decompression, and tendon transfer to correct claw hand, opposition of the thumb, claw toes, foot drop, and varus foot.

Reconstructive surgeries of the arm are often performed to recover the intrinsic hand position and abduction and opposition of the thumb.

In the first case the muscle most commonly used as the motor is the superficial flexor of the third finger, which upon removal from the palm is split into four slips. The Zancolli technique is indicated in cases of hypermobile hands where each of these slips is sutured over the A1 pulley of each finger, forming a loop. However, the Brand–Bunnell technique is indicated when the hand is rigid. In this case the four slips are inserted in the back of the fingers at the so-called tendon assembly. The superficial flexor of the fourth finger is used with the Brand–Bunnell technique in the second case for abduction and opposition of the thumb. This tendon is exteriorized on the forearm and tunneled through Guyon's canal to

Fig. 73.24 Resistance
active exercise for
extensor hallucis muscle

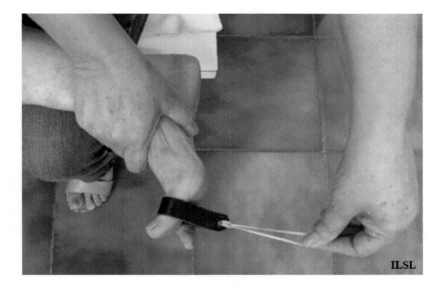

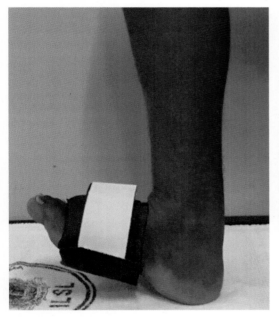

Fig. 73.25 Resistance active exercise for the tibialis
anterior muscle

the first metacarpal, where it is again exteriorized
divided into two slips and sutured on the back of
the thumb to the dorsal extensor tendon and the
adductor tendon on the radial edge of the thumb
[37, 38]. After correcting claw hand, use a circular plaster cast to position the wrist at 20° flexion,
the metacarpophalangeal joints at 90° flexion,
and interphalangeal joints at 0° flexion–extension

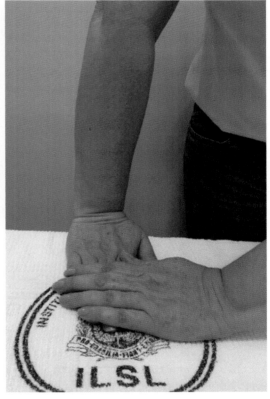

Fig. 73.26 Lengthening of the flexor tendons

(Fig. 73.39). To correct the loss of opposition of
the thumb, the wrist should be placed at 20° flexion and the thumb in abduction and opposition.

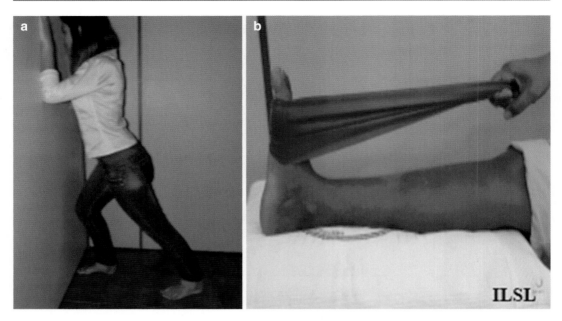

Fig. 73.27 (**a**, **b**) Lengthening of the gastrocnemius and soleus–calcaneal tendons

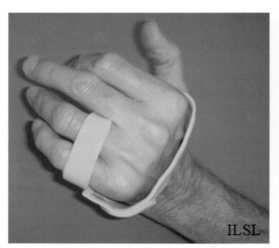

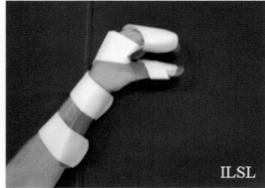

Fig. 73.29 Static orthosis for night use

Fig. 73.28 Static orthosis with lumbrical bar for fourth and fifth fingers

Reconstructive surgeries of the lower limbs are often performed to correct claw toes and foot drop. Normally the long flexor muscle of the toes is transferred to the extensors to correct claw toes. The tendon of the long flexor muscle of each toe is inserted into the extensor tendon at the proximal phalanx. The foot is immobilized using a plaster boot with heel for 6 weeks (Fig. 73.40). In the case of foot drop when the common pero-

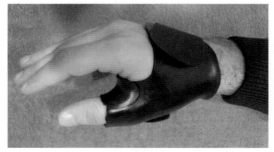

Fig. 73.30 Orthosis to reduce retraction of the first intermetacarpal space and position the thumb in palmar abduction and opposition

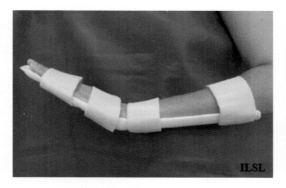

Fig. 73.31 Serial orthosis to stretch the flexor muscles of the fingers

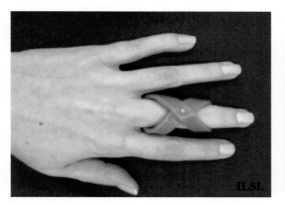

Fig. 73.32 Orthosis to reduce shortening of periarticular structures

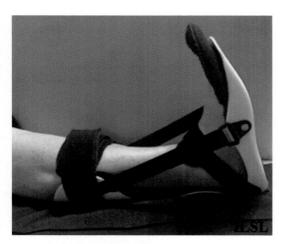

Fig. 73.33 Serial orthoses to stretch the flexor muscles of the foot

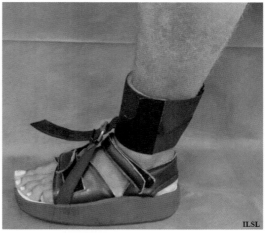

Fig. 73.34 Harris splint

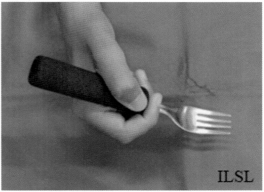

Fig. 73.35 Adaptations of household utensils to facilitate holding

neal nerve injury is complete, the posterior tibial muscle is divided into two slips and transferred to the dorsum of the foot where it is inserted into the extensor hallucis longus and extensor digitorum longus tendons. When the nerve injury is incomplete in foot drop, the tendon of the peroneus longus muscle is transferred to the dorsum of the foot and inserted on the side edge of the intertarsal ligament or the intermediate or lateral cuneiform [37, 38]. The foot is immobilized using a plaster boot without heel, with the ankle at 20–25° of dorsiflexion.

To obtain satisfactory results there are certain conditions that must be present preoperatively, such as:

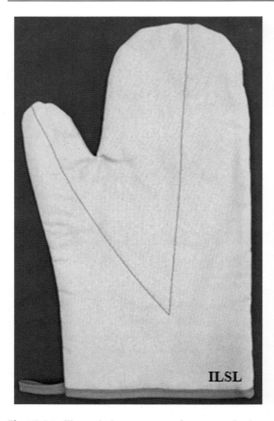

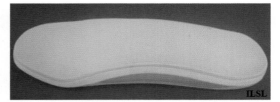

Fig. 73.38 Adapted in soles to improve plantar pressure distribution

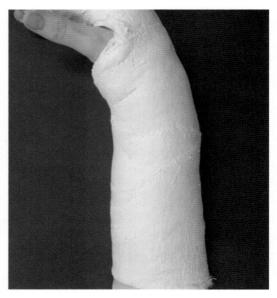

Fig. 73.36 Thermal glove to protect from excessive heat

Fig. 73.39 Plaster cast: wrist at 20° flexion, metacarpophalangeal joints at 90° flexion, and interphalangeal joints at 0° flexion–extension

- Completion of MDT for leprosy
- Be without leprosy reactions for more than 1 year
- Not have ulcers
- Have normal or close to normal muscle strength so that the transferred muscle can act properly in its new role
- Have functional passive joint mobility
- Capacity for contraction and individualized movement of the muscle being transferred
- Incorporate self-care practices

The objectives and conduct of the preoperative treatment [16, 38] are shown in Tables 73.10, 73.11, 73.12, and 73.13.

It is recommended to perform sensory, motor, and goniometric assessments, apply the Disabilities of Arm, Shoulder and Hand (DASH),

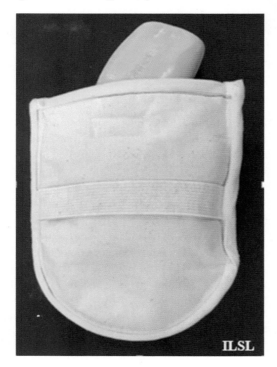

Fig. 73.37 Cloth to facilitate the use of soap

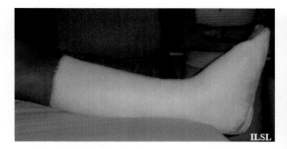

Fig. 73.40 Plaster cast with heel–ankle at 20–25° of dorsiflexion

Table 73.10 Objectives and preoperative rehabilitation conducts in tendon transfers

Objectives	Conducts
Maintain or restore the integrity and elasticity of the skin	Moisturize, lubricate and massage the skin (see Table 73.8)
Maintain or improve range of passive joint motion	Stretch muscle-tendon units of the hand/foot and first intermetacarpal space
	Perform passive exercises to stretch the tissue around joints
	Make static and progressively static orthoses
Isolate the muscle to be transferred	Active exercises to obtain individualized movement of the muscle to be transferred (Figs. 73.41 and 73.42). Avoid compensatory movements of the flexor and extensor muscles
Improve muscle strength	Perform exercises to strengthen the paretic muscles, especially the muscles that will function as the main motor after transfer
	Perform active resisted exercises to increase the muscle to be transferred (Fig. 73.43)

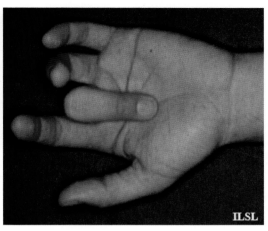

Fig. 73.41 Exercises to obtain isolated action of the superficial flexor muscle of the third finger

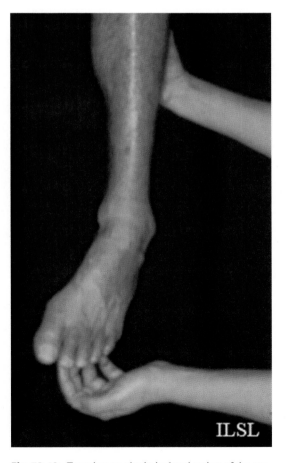

the SALSA scale, and the visual analog pain scale before and after surgery. In the case of tendon transfer in the hand, all the assessments above are applied with the exception of the DASH; however, the Jebsen–Taylor Hand Function Test should be added. The types of grip and support areas are also considered relevant to qualitatively assess the distribution of power and new patterns of grip acquired after surgery.

After surgery it is necessary to establish a motor rehabilitation program to regain motor control, aiming to recover the functional use of

Fig. 73.42 Exercises to obtain isolated action of the posterior tibialis muscle

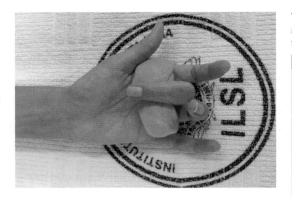

Fig. 73.43 Resistance exercises to increase the muscle to be transferred

Table 73.11 Postoperative rehabilitation in the treatment of lagophthalmus

Week	Postoperative conduct
1, 2 and 3	Avoid stretching the temporal fascia
	Control edema
4 and 5	Start the functional rehabilitation program
	Recover the strength of the temporalis muscle
	Stimulate the correct use of transfer (achieve eyelid closure by bringing the dental arches together)

the hand for activities of everyday life and the foot during gait.

To guarantee a functional outcome after transfer, it is essential to correctly activate the transferred muscles, and automate and integrate the new movement pattern until there is an engram in the motor cortex. Otherwise the patient will revert back to the old pattern while using the hands or walking.

The activities proposed in the postoperative period are selected and conducted for the transferred motor unit, but always respecting the healing phases of the transferred tendon [16, 37].

More detailed information about the procedures before and after surgery for transferring tendons in the hands and feet can be found in the Manual of Rehabilitation and Surgery in Leprosy [37].

Table 73.12 Postoperative rehabilitation of the hand after correction of claw fingers and opposition of the thumb

Week	Postoperative conduct
1–3	Immobilize the operated limb (plaster cast)
	Position the arm in a sling
	Mobilize the adjacent limbs
4	Remove surgical plaster cast
	Make an orthosis with wrist at 20° flexion and hand in an intrinsic position (Fig. 73.44)
	Skin care
	Minimize edema (lymph drainage, compression garment, etc.)
	Avoid stretching the transferred unit
	Prevent or reduce adhesions of the skin, subcutaneous tissue and tendons
	Controlled passive mobilization of the first intermetacarpal space, and metacarpophalangeal and interphalangeal joints individually and collectively extension and flexion
	Complete passive mobilization is contraindicated after the Bunnell–Brand technique due to the insertion in the extensor apparatus
	Active assisted exercises to activate the transferred muscle: reeducate the new movement pattern (intrinsic position and opposition of the thumb) (Figs. 73.45 and 73.46)
	Maintain the use of daytime and nighttime orthoses
5	Maintain the items described above, as necessary
	Maintain or increase the range of motion of fingers and wrist
	Active exercises to activate the transferred muscle: reeducate the new movement pattern (intrinsic position and opposition of the thumb), and gradually increase muscle strength (Figs. 73.47 and 73.48)
	From the intrinsic position, gradually start active flexion exercises of the fingers
6	Maintain the items described above, as necessary
	Use only nighttime orthosis
	Goniometric evaluation to ascertain retractions, if necessary use orthosis

Table 73.12 (continued)

Week	Postoperative conduct
7 and 8	Maintain the items described above, as necessary
	Recover the motor control in activities requiring strength using the transferred muscle correctly
	Develop motor skills in daily activities such as putting on clothes, eating, hygiene, and writing (Fig. 73.49)
	Suspend the use of nighttime orthosis in the 7th week
	Encourage carrying out daily activities to automate the transfer
	Wrist range of motion to its fullest extent with the fingers relaxed

Neural Decompression

Neural decompression can be performed in the acute or chronic phase of the inflammatory process. When performed in the acute phase, there is a reduction in the constrictive action of the nerve, decreasing the intraneural pressure. With decreased pressure, an improvement in vascularization is expected with varying degrees of recovery of the motor and sensory functions and pain relief. In the chronic phase after more than 1 year of injury, surgery significantly reduces pain symptoms, although the consensus is that there is no recovery of motor or sensory functions [39].

After surgery without nerve transposition, the arm and forearm can be immobilized using a sling for a week and the leg immobilized using a leg orthosis for 2 weeks. When the ulnar nerve is transposed, the sling is associated with the use of an axillopalmar orthosis for 2 weeks (Fig. 73.50).

The main complaints in the postoperative period are inflammation, pain, swelling, and muscle spasms. The conduct will be established gradually during the healing process, ranging from mobilization of adjacent structures, scar massage, and gentle joint and neural mobilization.

The return to daily activities should take place progressively after 4 weeks.

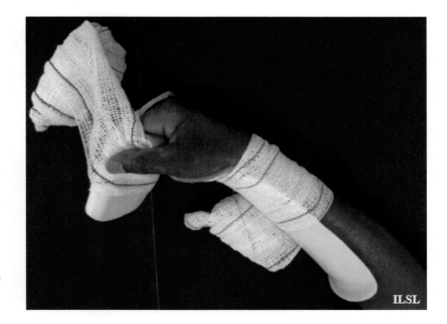

Fig. 73.44 Orthosis with wrist flexion of 20° and hand in intrinsic position

Fig. 73.45 Enable
transfer to obtain the
intrinsic position

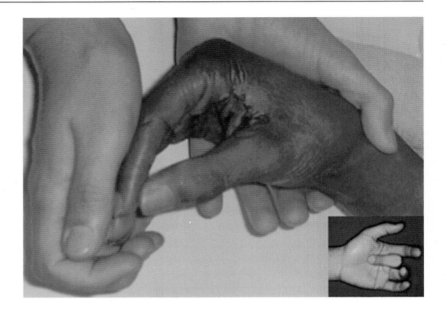

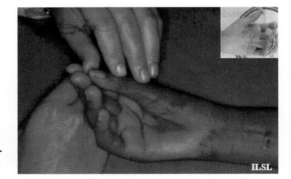

Fig. 73.46 Enable transfer for opposition of the thumb

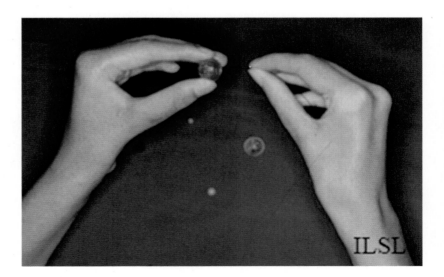

Fig. 73.47 Motor skill
training

Table 73.13 Postoperative rehabilitation after correction of foot drop

Week	Postoperative conduct
1–6	Immobilize the operated limb (plaster cast with heel)
	Mobilize the adjacent limbs
	Isometric exercises for the quadriceps
	Gait training with crutches (without putting weight on the operated foot) After 10 days put some weight on the operated leg
7	Remove plaster cast
	Make orthoses positioning the foot at a 20–25° angle of passive dorsiflexion (Fig. 73.49)
	Skin care
	Minimize edema (lymph drainage, compression garment, etc.)
	Avoid stretching the transferred unit. Do not perform goniometry of plantar flexion
	Passive dorsiflexion exercises of the ankle in a sitting or lying position
	Exercises to activate the transferred muscle remembering the isolation trained in the pre-op (Fig. 73.50)
	Gradually increase the muscle strength
	Isometric exercises for the quadriceps
	Maintain range of motion (avoid plantar flexion of the foot)
8	Maintain the items described above
	Avoid the pending position in the intervals between exercises
	Continue to use daytime and nighttime orthoses
9	Maintain the items described above
	Start gait rehabilitation using parallel bars
	Active dorsiflexion and plantar flexion exercises (lift the heel from the ground) in the sitting position
	Assess the need for insoles, adapted foot wear
10	Maintain the items described above as necessary
	Active dorsiflexion and plantar flexion exercises as necessary
	Stimulate gait training ensuring the automation of transfer out of the parallel bars

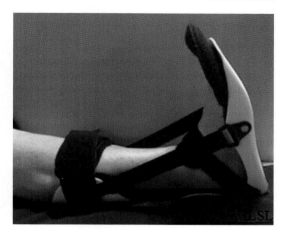

Fig. 73.48 Orthosis to position the foot at a 20–25° angle of passive dorsiflexion

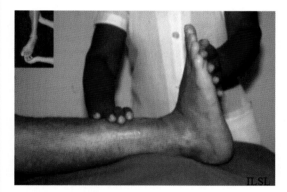

Fig. 73.49 Enable transfer to obtain dorsiflexion of the foot

Fig. 73.50 Axillopalmar orthosis for transposition of the ulnar nerve

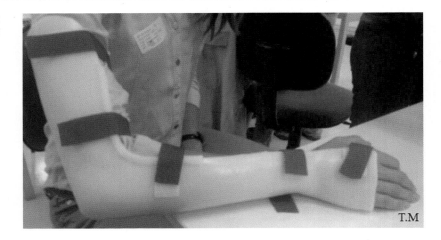

T.M

Future Perspectives

The reduction in the number of leprosy cases worldwide with the use of MDT is considerable, but curing the disease does not mean that disabilities are eliminated. Recent studies show that around 40% of patients have some type of deficiency. Early diagnosis is still the best strategy to avoid deformities; however, once the disease is in place, measures can only prevent further disabilities and rehabilitate patients.

Future perspectives for preventive actions are related to developing the professional's ability to assertively identify disabilities, and to perform further research seeking new technology and innovative rehabilitation practices.

Possibly the only way to achieve good results is through patients adopting changes in their activities of daily life.

Acknowledgement The authors wish to thank The Paulista Foundation against Leprosy for the financial support received, and the librarian Alessandra Carriel Vieira for assistance with the references.

Glossary

Bacilloscopy A complementary examination in the diagnosis of leprosy. It consists of an analysis by microscopy whereby *Mycobacterium leprae* are observed directly in smears of lymph and intradermal scrapings.
Corneal opacity The cornea has a white appearance throughout.

Disabilities Problems in the functions or body structure due to significant impairment or loss.
Ectropion A medical condition where the lower eyelid turns outward.
Engrams The neurologic organization of pre-programmed patterns of muscle activity. Once formed, the same pattern is produced every time the specific nerves are activated.
Entropion Inward folding of the eyelid, whereby in the eyelashes rub against the cornea.
Froment's sign A test used to evaluate paralysis of the ulnar nerve, specifically the action of the adductor muscle of the thumb. The test assesses whether the patient can pinch hold a sheet of paper by thumb adduction. Patients are considered Froment positive when they have sharp flexion of the distal phalanx of the thumb due to instability of the metacarpophalangeal joint.
Graphesthesia The individual's ability with closed eyes to recognize the writing of words or numbers on the skin.
Hypoesthesia Decreased sensitivity in a particular region of the body.
Infiltration Increased thickness and changed consistency of the skin with less evidence of skin creases. It consists in using an instrument specifically designed to apply one or two tactile stimuli using parallel metal points. The distance between the points varies from 2 to 20 mm.
Lagophthalmos Inability to close the eyelids.
Lepromas Prominent subcutaneous nodules resulting from an accumulation of Virchow cells.
Leprosy reactions Acute and subacute inflammatory episodes that intermittently occur in

the chronic course of both paucibacillary and multibacillary disease.

Madarosis of the eyebrows Loss of hairs of the eyebrows.

Mycobacterium leprae Known as the cause of leprosy, this bacterium has a rod shape. It is alcohol acid-resistant and so staining during biopsy must be carried out using Ziehl–Neelsen stain.

Palpation Process of semiologic observation that consists in exploring a particular region of the body with the fingertips and palm.

Paresis Dysfunction of movement of one or more limbs.

Paresthesia Subjective sensations of the skin that can be described by the individual as cold, hot, tingling, pressure, among others. It may occur due to neural lesions, either by the destruction or by disruption of the nerve endings.

Proprioception A sense or perception of the movement of the body, balance etc. provided by the bones, muscles, tendons, and joints.

Skin ulcers (ulceration) The generic name given to any superficial lesion in skin tissue. A complication related to neuropathy in leprosy.

Stereognosis The ability to recognize objects by touch, shape, and contour.

Tinel's sign A test to check irritation of a nerve. A tingling sensation is felt in the distal end of a limb when an injured nerve is struck.

Trichiasis Eyelashes growing toward the eyeball.

Two-point discrimination test A functional test that evaluates the ability of the digits to act as a sensory organ. The test determines the minimum distance at which the patient is able to discern that two nearby objects touching the skin are truly two distinct points.

References

1. Palande DD, Virmond M. Reabilitação social e cirurgia na hanseníase. Hansen Int. 2002;27(2):93–8.
2. Garbino JA. Neuropatia hanseniana, aspectos fisiopatológicos, clínicos, dano neural e regeneração. In: Opromolla DVA, editor. Noções de hansenologia. Bauru: Centro de Estudos Dr. Reynaldo Quagliato; 2000. p. 79–89.
3. Opromolla DVA. Aspectos gerais sobre hanseníase. In: Duerksen F, Virmond M, editors. Cirurgia reparadora e reabilitação em hanseníase. Bauru: Instituto Lauro de Souza Lima; 1997.
4. World Health Organization. Leprosy (Hansen disease): report by the secretariat [Internet]. Executive Board, 128th Session, Provisional Agenda Item 4.13, EB 128/16, December 2010. [Cited 2015 Oct 15]. Available from: http://apps.who.int/gb/ebwha/pdf_files/EB128/B128_16-en.pdf.
5. Lastória JC, Abreu MAMM. Hanseníase: diagnóstico e tratamento. Diagn Tratamento. 2012;17(4):173–9.
6. World Health Organization. Global leprosy update, 2014; need for early case detection. Wkly Epidemiol Rec [Internet]. 2015 Sept [cited 2015 Oct 15];90(36):461–76. Available from: http://www.who.int/wer/2015/wer9036.pdf?ua=1.
7. Ministério da Saúde (BR). Portaria n. 3125, de 7 de outubro de 2010. Aprova as Diretrizes para Vigilância, Atenção e Controle da Hanseníase [Internet]. Brasília; 2010. [citado em 22 dez 2013]. Disponível em: http://www.anvisa.gov.br/hotsite/talidomida/legis/portaria_n_3125_hanseniase_2010.pdf.
8. Goulart IM, Penna GO, Cunha G. Imunopatologia da hanseníase: a complexidade dos mecanismos da resposta imune do hospedeiro ao Mycobacterium leprae. Rev Soc Bras Med Trop [online]. 2002;35(4):365–75. Disponível em: http://dx.doi.org/10.1590/S0037-86822002000400014.
9. Opromolla DVA, Garbino JAA. Fisiopatologia das deficiências físicas em hanseníase. In: Opromolla DVA, Baccarelli R, editors. Prevenção de incapacidades e reabilitação em hanseníase. Bauru: Instituto Lauro de Souza Lima; 2003. p. 13–24.
10. Ministério da Saúde (BR), Secretaria de Vigilância em Saúde, Departamento de Vigilância Epidemiológica. Manual de prevenção de incapacidades. Brasília: Ministério da Saúde; 2008.
11. Dantas AM. Os nervos cranianos: estudo anatomo-clínico. Rio de Janeiro: Guanabara Koogan; 2005.
12. Warren G, Schwarz R. Surgery of the nose and other esthetic surgery. In: Schwarz R, Brandsma W, editors. Surgical reconstruction e rehabilitation in leprosy and other neuropathies. Kathmandu: Ekta Books; 2004. p. 271–302.
13. Duerksen F, Schwarz R. Ulnar nerve palsy. In: Schwarz R, Brandsma W, editors. Surgical reconstruction e rehabilitation in leprosy and other neuropathies. Kathmandu: Ekta Books; 2004. p. 47–64.
14. Dangelo JG, Fattini CA. Título. Nervos do membro superior. In: Anatomia básica dos sistemas orgânicos. São Paulo: Atheneu; 1998. Cap. XVIII, Membro superior; p. 328–40.
15. Tubiana R, Thomine JM, Mackim E. Exame da função dos nervos periféricos na extremidade superior. In: Diagnóstico clínica da mão e do punho. Rio de Janeiro: Ed. Interlivros; 1996. Cap.4; Exame da função dos nervos periféricos na extremidade superior; p. 269–383.
16. Marciano LHSC. Terapia ocupacional na reeducação motora após transferência de tendão na lesão dos nervos ulnar e mediano. In: Opromolla DVA, Baccarelli R, editors. Prevenção de incapacidades e reabilitação em hanseníase. Bauru: Instituto Lauro de Souza Lima; 2003. p. 106–8.

17. Brasil. Ministério da Saúde. Secretaria de Vigilância em Saúde. Manual de reabilitação e cirurgia em hanseníase. 2 ed., ver. e ampl. – Brasília:2008. 148p. Ministério da Saúde (BR), Secretaria de Vigilância em Saúde. Manual de reabilitação e cirurgia em hanseníase. 2a ed., rev. e ampl. Brasília: Ministério da Saúde; 2008.

18. Duerksen F, Virmond M. Fisiopatologia da mão em hanseníase. In: Cirurgia reparadora e reabilitação em hanseníase. Bauru: Instituto Lauro de Souza Lima; 1997. Mão; p. 199–220.

19. Tubiana R, Thomine JM, Mackim E. Anatomia funcional. In: Diagnóstico Clínica da mão e do punho. Rio de Janeiro: Ed. Interlivros; 1996. Cap. 1, Anatomia funcional; p. 1–159.

20. Schwarz R, Brandsma W. Surgical reconstruction e rehabilitation in leprosy and other neuropathies. Kathmandu: Ekta Books; 2004. p. 83.

21. Duerksen F. Comprometimento neural em hanseníase. In: Cirurgia reparadora e reabilitação em hanseníase. Bauru: Instituto Lauro de Souza Lima; 1997. p. 59–67.

22. Ministério da Saúde (BR), Secretaria de Atenção à Saúde, Departamento de vigilância epidemiológica. Manual de prevenção de incapacidades. 3a ed. Brasília (DF): Ministério da Saúde; 2008. p. 140p.

23. Last JM. A dictionary of epidemiology. New York: Oxford University Press; 1988.

24. Deepak S. Answering the rehabilitation needs of leprosy affected persons in integrated setting through primary health care services and community based rehabilitation. Indian J Lepr. 2003;75(2):127–42.

25. Nicholls PG, Bakirtzief Z, Van Brakel WH, Das-Pattanaya RK, Raju MS, Norman G, et al. Risk factors for participation restriction in leprosy and development of a screening tool to identify individuals at risk. Lepr Rev. 2005;76(4):305–15.

26. Ministério da Saúde (BR), Secretaria de Atenção à Saúde, Departamento de Vigilância das Doenças Transmissíveis. Diretrizes para vigilância, atenção e eliminação da hanseníase como problema de saúde pública. Brasília (DF): Ministério da Saúde; 2016.

27. Baccarelli R, Marciano LHSC. Avaliação dos membros superiores para a prevenção de incapacidades. In: Opromolla DVA, Baccarelli R, editors. Prevenção de incapacidades e reabilitação em hanseníase. Bauru: Instituto Lauro de Souza Lima; 2003. p. 72–81.

28. Villarroel MF, Orsini MBP, Lima RC, Antunes CMF. Comparative study of the cutaneous sensation of leprosy-suspected lesions using Semmes–Weinstein monofilaments and quantitative thermal testing. Lepr Rev. 2007;78(2):102–9.

29. Werner JL, Omer GE Jr. Evaluating cutaneous pressure sensation of the hand. Am J Occup Ther. 1970;24(5):347–56.

30. Lehman LF, Orsini MBP, Nicholl ARJ. The development and adaptation of the Semmes-Weinstein monofilaments in Brazil. J Hand Ther. 1993;6(4):290–7.

31. Prince KV, Butler B. Measuring sensory function of the hand in peripheral nerve injuries. Am J Occup Ther. 1967;21(6):385–95.

32. Naafs B, Dagne T. Sensory testing: a sensitive method in the follow-up of nerve involvement. Int J Lepr. 1977;45(4):364–8.

33. Lehman LF, Orsini MBP, Grossi MPF, Vilarroel MF. A mão na hanseníase. In: Freitas PP, editor. Reabilitação da mão. São Paulo: Ed. Atheneu; 2005. p. 311–8.

34. Hislop HJ, Montgomery J. Daniels e Worthingham: provas de função muscular: técnicas de exame manual. Rio de Janeiro: Elsevier; 2008.

35. Bersch R. Introdução à tecnologia assistiva [Internet]. Porto Alegre: Assistiva tecnologia e educação; 2013. [Citado em 17 dez. 2015]. Disponível em: http://www.assistiva.com.br/Introducao_Tecnologia_Assistiva.pdf.

36. Virmond M, Vieth H. Prevenção de incapacidades na hanseníase: uma análise crítica. Med , Ribeirão Preto. 1997;30:358–63.

37. Ministério da Saúde (BR), Secretaria de Atenção à Saúde, Departamento de vigilância epidemiológica. Manual de reabilitação e cirurgia em hanseníase. 2a ed. Brasília (DF): Ministério da Saúde; 2008. p. 140p.

38. Virmond M. Cirurgia da mão – indicações e técnicas. In: Opromolla DVA, Baccarelli R, editors. Prevenção de incapacidades e reabilitação em hanseníase. Bauru: Instituto Lauro de Souza Lima; 2003. p. 89–93.

39. Virmond MCL, Cury Filho M. Tratamento cirúrgico nos membros superiores e inferiores. In: Alves ED, Ferreira IN, Ferreira TL, editors. Hanseníase: avanços e desafios. Brasília: Universidade de Brasília; 2014. p. 305–32.

Suggested Literature

Cavalcanti A, Galvão C. Terapia Ocupacional: fundamentação & prática. Rio de Janeiro: Guanabara Koogan; 2007. p. 531.

Trombly CA, Radomski AV. Terapia ocupacional para disfunções físicas. 5a ed. São Paulo: Ed. Santos; 2005. p. 1157.

Pedretti LW, Early MB. Terapia Ocupacional: capacidades práticas para disfunções físicas. São Paulo: Roca; 2004. p. 1092.

Ferrigno ISV. Terapia da mão: fundamentos para a prática clínica. São Paulo: Ed. Santos; 2007. p. 157.

Teixeira E, Sauron FN, Santos LSB, Oliveira MC. Terapia Ocupacional na reabilitação física. São Paulo: Roca; 2003. p. 572.

Skirven TM, Osterman AL, Fedorczyk J, Amadio PC. Rehabilitation of the hand and upper extremity. 6th ed. Philadelphia: Mosby; 2011. p. 2096.

Organização Mundial da Saúde. Classificação Internacional de Funcionalidade, Incapacidade e Saúde. São Paulo: Edusp; 2003. p. 325.

Alves ED, Ferreira TL, Nery I. Org; Ramos-Junior NA, et al. Hanseníase: avanços e desafios. Brasília. NESPROM, 2014. p. 492.

Psychological Approaches in Treating Patients with Chronic Dermatoses

74

Luciana Castoldi, Fernanda Torres de Carvalho, and Daniel Boianovsky Kveller

Key Points

- Individual therapy: the treatment aims to work the patient's self-esteem and self-image, making effort to rescue their social, professional, and sexual interaction
- Family therapy: usually indicated for children and adolescents with psycho-dermatosis, the purpose is to share the responsibilities related to the presenting symptom and commit all members of the family to the treatment process
- Couple therapy: this therapeutic modality aims to share responsibilities about conflicts, even when symptoms are presented by only one partner
- Group therapy: this therapy assumes that participants have one common task and goal, and predicts a specific setting that meets the needs of space, frequency, and duration of meetings
- Psychodermatosis group with children: experience shows the importance of the participation of parents or substitute caregivers. For children, the group works as a setting to express feelings, anxieties, possible disabilities, and fears
- Psychodermatosis group with adults: the treatment aims to work with patients of both genders with different dermatologic diseases, more commonly psoriasis and vitiligo
- Psychoeducational group: group therapy for patients with atopic dermatitis: coordinated by a dermatologist and a psychologist, the group relies on the support of a multidisciplinary team, consisting of medicine, nutrition, psychology, nursing, and social work professionals.

Introduction

Cultural factors are known to influence directly the way each society expresses psychological distress. In diverse geographic locations and historical circumstances, feelings such as sadness, grief, and anxiety are represented differently, and may or may not be considered pathologic [1]. When treating the specific relationship between psychology and dermatology, it is necessary to underline one important element in our own popular culture that often leads us to associate what

L. Castoldi (✉) • F.T. de Carvalho
Psychology Service of Sanitary Dermatology Service of the Department of Health of Rio Grande do Sul State, Porto Alegre, Brazil
e-mail: lucianacastoldi@hotmail.com

D.B. Kveller
Federal University of Rio Grande do Sul, UFRGS, Porto Alegre, Brazil

© Springer International Publishing Switzerland 2018
R.R. Bonamigo, S.I.T. Dornelles (eds.), *Dermatology in Public Health Environments*,
https://doi.org/10.1007/978-3-319-33919-1_74

is on the "surface"—frivolity. When someone seems futile or simple-minded, for example, they are said to be "superficial." On the other hand, when a movie or work of art seems complex, interesting, and enigmatic, then we say it is "deep." In this sense, it is not unusual that patients presenting symptoms on the skin, the outermost and most superficial layer of the body, also underestimate the relationship that these pathologies have with "deep" issues in their lives, like the loss of loved ones, sudden changes in lifestyle, and other traumatic experiences.

The purpose of this chapter is to follow precisely the opposite direction, emphasizing the importance of the skin as a major somatic pathway of emotional expression, as well as to highlight the possible therapeutic approaches in Psychology. As the French poet Paul Valéry would say, "the most profound in the human being is the skin"; it is the organ that allows us tell the difference between the warmth of an embrace from the winter of solitude, the contours of happiness from the textures of sadness. The skin places us next to one another, approaches us to being human. Not accidentally, scars become symbols of one's life, and when important experiences do not leave physical marks spontaneously, they are translated on the skin through tattooed pictures or words. Our sufferings are no exception to this rule: their presence is expressed in paintings on this extensive screen called epidermis. The attempt to dispel the myth of "superficiality" related to skin symptoms and to provide a possibility to understand the existing intimacy between "skin labels" and "the deepest sufferings of the psyche" is common to all psychotherapy approaches related to dermatologic pathologies [2].

State of the Art

Psychology and Integrality

Dermatologic disorders are complex and multifaceted. They are usually related to emotional issues associated with important time periods in life, changes in family dynamics, or even traumatic past events. School issues, such as learning disabilities, and family matters, such as parental separation, may raise or exacerbate emotional disturbances. Adolescence is a time when one tends to leave the familiar context to experiment with new circles and is also one of the most vulnerable moments of the life cycle. The search for acceptance and other social demands that require maturity (still a developing issue for a teenager) are often associated with the high levels of anxiety and depression typical of this stage [3]. Maturity, in turn, is marked by several other emotional "challenges," such as building a career, getting married, and, later in time, the mourning process and the limitations of old age.

When such issues are addressed in public health services in Brazil, a country still frighteningly marked by social inequality and that only recently was consolidating its public policies, we must take into account the extreme influence that poverty, social vulnerability, and violence can have on health conditions, especially the mental health of individuals, families, and communities [4]. Racism [5], sexism [6], and homophobia [7], social forms of oppression quite widespread in Brazilian society, are factors that also influence considerably health conditions in women, afro-descendants, homosexuals, and transsexuals, and cause them to have problems accessing health services.

Therefore, to comprehend the various dimensions of a psychodermatosis, health services should offer, in addition to the medical view, the attention of a multidisciplinary team, capable of receiving and contextualizing people's distress in their social, affective, and family relations network. The more dynamic a team service is, the closer their different professionals work, the more comprehensive and complex will be the care provided by the health service. In collaboration, psychologists, social workers, medical doctors, nurses, nutritionists, and other health professionals will be able to understand the different dimensions of cutaneous disorders, taking into account physiologic, emotional, and social factors, and by doing so become able to indicate the best options for treatment [8] (Box 74.1). In addition, the principle of integrality in health care should be ensured, as it is proposed in the constitution of the Sistema Único de Saúde (SUS), the Brazilian health care system [9]. From this broad and multidimensional understanding, it is possible to think of a singular therapeutic project (Box 74.2). In the case of children, for example, who often come to the service because of the issue of atopic dermatitis, the singular therapeutic project, from an Integrality perspective, would contemplate the possibility of interventions with families, social network, and, of course, the school, as will be discussed further.

Box 74.1 Integrality
Among the different meanings of this polysemic term, "comprehensive care" can be found, which means to understand the person who is a user of the health service network as a whole individual, considering biological, psychological, and sociocultural aspects [1].

Box 74.2 Singular Therapeutic Project
A comprehensive treatment plan that contemplates the possibility of medication prescription, psychotherapy, and interventions by the family of the patient in their territory and with other institutions [1].

Skin and Psyche Interface

As with most chronic diseases, many skin problems tend to affect and be affected by patients' emotional and family life. A study carried out in a dermatology outpatient unit, based on document analysis of 103 Psychological Screening Forms, found that stressors related to losses and separations in different stages of life were responsible for triggering and/or worsening psoriasis and vitiligo. Psychological effects of episodes of loss and separation have been studied by Bowlby since 1969, after what he called the Attachment Theory [10]. The author considers the establishment of bonds of affection and care as key issues for one's physical and psychological survival. These bonds are established in early childhood,

from the very care devoted to the baby by the mother or a substitute caregiver. When a child's emotional needs are appropriately met, there is a secure attachment. However, when the child is threatened or at risk and does not rely on protection and emotional support on the part of the caregiver, he/she may develop insecure or anxious attachment. According to Bowlby [11], this relationship pattern may extend into adulthood. These situations of loss or separation can cause stress in some individuals, and can trigger physical illnesses such as psychodermatoses.

Some psychological interventions have been assessed considering their impact on the improvement of symptoms of psoriasis. A cognitive behavioral program of symptom management showed benefits in the frequency and severity of symptoms, the strength of belief in the severity of consequences of the illness, and patients' attributions to emotional causes of their psoriasis. The authors compared the group that participated in the program with a control group after 6 months of intervention [12]. Another group of researchers [13] evaluated a single educational intervention also focused on patients with psoriasis. Information on disease and treatment was given. A high level of satisfaction with the intervention, improvement in knowledge about the disease, and better attitude toward therapy was reported even after 6 months.

In our outpatient unit, patients with psychodermatosis are seen by the Psychology service in a host session. From this first contact, they are referred to the therapeutic modality that both the multidisciplinary team and the patient consider more appropriate. Individual therapy, family therapy, couple therapy, and group therapy are among the possibilities of psychotherapy. In the following section, clinical case samples are presented to illustrate each of these therapeutic modalities.

Therapeutic Modalities

Individual Therapy
Psychotherapy may be indicated when the person is unable to solve a psychological conflict.

The therapist, then, works as a facilitator of a process of change, enabling the patient to build new insights about him- or herself [14]. Whenever a patient identifies psychological distress associated with the onset or worsening of skin disease, he/she may benefit from psychological assistance. This approach is especially used with adult patients and female adolescents, to address issues related to low self-esteem or body image distortions. Capisano [15] defines body image as "body's picture in the individual's mind." A result of anatomic, physiological, and sociological contributions, among others, and organized subconsciously, body image can go changing in accordance with our emotional manifestations. When the perception that one has of his body does not match the actual body, there is chance of deviations or distortions of body image. This is what usually happens to the person suffering from skin lesions. Skin diseases generally refer to the idea that the skin is ugly or "dirty" and that, therefore, the injury must be hidden. In severe cases, it drives the patient to social and sexual isolation [16]. It is important to identify which areas of the body are affected by dermatosis and try to relate episodes of stress that can be associated with the onset and/or aggravation of lesions. The treatment aims to work the patient's self-esteem and self-image, making and effort to rescue their social, professional, and sexual interaction.

Case Report 6.1

A 45-year-old man, who lives with his ex-wife and two teenage children. He came to psychotherapy because of his psoriasis, with lesions in arms and legs. His symptoms started 8 years ago, having been triggered after an accident in which he drowned and almost died. Then, he went bankrupt. During the meetings, the patient brought low self-esteem issues and difficulty expressing feelings. Facing family conflicts, expressing positive and negative feelings, especially with his mother, older brother, and children were the issues approached. He was a motivated patient

who had insight regarding his family history and his relationship patterns. At the end of 4 months, his lesions had virtually disappeared. He was instructed to return in the case of new significant stress with recurrence of skin symptoms.

Family Therapy

Usually indicated in pediatric and adolescent psychodermatosis, Family Therapy assumes that the symptomatic patient or "identified patient" is merely the spokesperson of some family dysfunction, and its treatment strategy is to investigate the affective and emotional relationship in at least three generations [17]. The purpose of therapy is to share the responsibilities related to the presenting symptom and commit all members of the family to the treatment process [18]. Intervention can alternate sessions with the whole family group (system), with individual sessions or subgroups: siblings, parents, female members, etc. (subsystems). Minuchin, Nichols, and Lee [19] defended the need for a collaborative approach of the therapist: the changes should take place within the limits and possibilities of each family group.

Case Report 6.2

An 8-year-old girl, with learning difficulties and obesity disorder. She was brought by her mother to psychological care under the guidance of a dermatologist who treated her *alopecia*. The girl had been gradually losing her hair since her parents' separation, which occurred 2 years before. After the separation, mother and daughter moved to the house of the maternal grandparents. The father brought his new female partner and her 8-year-old child to live in the former family home. With the news of her stepmother's pregnancy, her alopecia intensified. She came to the first appointment completely hairless, wearing a cap to hide her head. The family showed good adherence to treatment, and followed all clinical and psychological recommendations. Family therapy consisted of alternating sessions with the girl and her mother, and with her father. Respecting the approach of the Singular Therapeutic Project, her teacher was included in the consultations, and there was a visit to the school for guidance for peers and teachers. The girl was revealing progress on school activities, could join a nutritional education program, lost weight, and improved her self-esteem. The family provided a natural hair wig, which negated the use of a hat. Despite all the efforts, the original symptom (alopecia), however, did not disappear. The benefit of treatment was to support the family, especially the mother, who came to accept her daughter's symptoms.

Couple Therapy

When dermatosis in an adult patient causes evident worsening in the couple's emotional and sexual relationship, the partner may be invited to participate in the therapeutic process. Couple therapy, as well as family therapy, does not imply that both partners are present in all meetings; couple meetings may be alternated with individual meetings with each one, but the emphasis of treatment is on the relationship [19]. This therapeutic modality aims to share responsibilities about conflicts, even when symptoms are presented by only one partner. It demands a collaborative, empathic, and committed attitude of the couple, with each other, and of the couple with the therapist.

Case Report 6.3
Male, 65 years old, presented symptoms of psoriasis and vitiligo, and sought psychological assistance due to marital issues especially on showing his lesions to his wife. Psoriasis-related lesions were more intense in legs and arms; vitiligo manifested on genitals exclusively. The patient reported a good social relationship of the couple. They used to travel a lot, have fun together, worked in the same place, and his wife was his boss. When asked about sexuality, he became surprised to realize it had been 6 years since they had their last sexual intercourse, precisely the time of appearance of the first lesions. The wife's presence was required and couple therapy recommended. Concomitant to clinical dermatologic assistance, couple therapy had to focus on issues of hierarchy, respect, and sexuality. The couple had good adherence to therapy, worked on the relationship, and recovered their sexual life. Lesions disappeared in a few months.

Group Therapy

Group therapy assumes that participants have one common task and goal, and predicts a specific setting that meets the needs of space, frequency, and duration of meetings. Although every group should respect the diversity of its members, it may be composed by age, gender, or symptoms of participants [20]. An intense therapeutic process, with affections, projections, and anxieties of so many people usually requires two therapists working together.

Psychodermatosis Group with Children

One possible approach for dermatologic manifestations in childhood is therapeutic groups with children and their caregivers. Experience shows the importance of the participation of parents in these groups, allowing separate spaces for working with children and also with their parents or substitute caregivers. For children, the group works as a setting to express feelings, anxieties, possible disabilities, and fears. Communication between therapist and children occurs by means of toys, play, and body language. It is all about creating a setting that makes it easier for children to access and communicate emotional issues using their playful world. For parents, it is to offer support in dealing with children's skin problems, understanding them as issues for the whole family, and attempting to provide an environment for help and expression of feelings and doubts.

At our outpatient unit, this intervention is offered in a 12-weekly-meeting program, whereby a therapist is responsible for the group with children and other therapist is responsible for the group of parents or caregivers. Other health professionals may be invited to participate in the adult group as needed. Families come to these groups after a previous contact and evaluation in the Psychology Service. This contact helps to assess families' motivations, the desire and openness to group work, and the availability of participation in a weekly fixed schedule; both child and adult caregiver need to commit to the intervention. The program may be extended into family therapy modality whenever necessary.

Groups always happen simultaneously to medical treatment, never replacing it. They are valuable for skin improvement because they help families to gain insights into the problem, reduce the level of stress and anxiety, support and extend the adherence to medical treatment, and, in many cases, enable the identification and management of psychodermatosis-triggering situations.

Case Report 6.4

A boy, 7 years old, living with his father and mother. He had vitiligo all over the body, with onset of the disease a year later, when the family was evicted from the house where they lived. His father was an alcoholic. In group meetings, the boy looked introverted and lonely at first. Gradually he started to play and showed intense fear of losing his mother, as well as his sadness for having lost the house. At the same time, in the parents' group, father and mother could write their own story and also told the story of their children. The patient's mother said that he was her fourth child. The first pregnancy was a miscarriage. The second baby was raised by the paternal grandmother, after she and her partner separated.

The same happened with the third baby. Our patient was the first child raised by mother and she would not consider leaving him. She was experiencing serious marital problems, which led to the loss of the house, but custody of him was not an issue. His siblings' story was unspoken but seemed to be alive to him, and he was afraid of being abandoned too. After these feelings were identified, the theme was approached with mother and child, separately, in group sessions. The expression of fears, anxieties, and frustrations was encouraged, to relieve him and minimize the manifestation of skin symptoms. Mother-and-child group session followed; communication and affection were stimulated. Gradually the symptoms of our patient decreased until they became almost unnoticeable.

Psychodermatosis Group with Adults

Groups with adults welcome people of both genders with different dermatologic diseases, more commonly psoriasis and vitiligo. Usually they are arranged according to age (20–40 years, for example) and psychological characteristics of patients. People with alcohol issues or other drug use or people with psychiatric commitment do not usually benefit from this approach. Intervention occurs weekly, lasting 1 h and 30 min for a period previously determined by the participants, usually 4 months. Coordination is typically performed by two therapists.

Case Report 6.5

Male, 36 years old, worked as a professional cleaner. Vitiligo on the face was very evident in his black skin. During a host interview in the Psychology service, he reported that the first episode of vitiligo occurred at age 6, after his mother's death. At that time, he responded well to dermatologic treatment. At 8 years of age, his teacher of the second grade died, victim of a car accident. The lesions returned, weaker, and he resumed dermatologic treatment for another year. He had been clear of lesions since 9 years old, but had lost his wife 1 year later, victim of breast cancer. His only daughter, 16, became pregnant immediately after. His current vitiligo condition was the most severe he had ever had. He resumed, on his own, using the former medication, with no effect. His current dermatologist referred him to immediate psychological assistance. He started individual psychotherapy and then was invited to join a group of patients living with psychodermatosis. Group work had an emphasis on patients' self-care and recovery of self-esteem. He was welcomed by the group, had support in his grief process, and was oriented due to caring for his pregnant daughter. As therapeutic work strengthened him, and with his good adherence to dermatologic treatment, the lesions disappeared. He was discharged from therapy with fully repigmented face; he was happy to regain his black identity.

Psychoeducational Group: Group Therapy for Patients with Atopic Dermatitis

Ferreira et al. [21] studied the dynamics of relationships of families facing atopic dermatitis and found that the frequency and intensity of symptoms are influenced by stressors, especially those linked to episodes of loss and separation. Staab et al. [22] assessed contributions from groups with children and adolescents with atopic dermatitis and their parents in an outpatient hospital in Germany. They had 6-week meetings, comparing the group with standard intervention. Group participants had a 12-month follow up and were significantly better when compared with the control group as to the severity of eczema, subjective severity, and quality of life of parents of affected children younger than 13.

To meet a proposition of the AADA (Association for Support of Atopic Dermatitis in Brazil), a group of patients and relatives living with this disease was created in the Ambulatório de Dermatologia Sanitária. This is an open psychoeducational group that gathered monthly on Saturday mornings for a nonstop period of 10 years. Coordinated by a dermatologist and a psychologist, the group counted on the support of a multidisciplinary team, consisting of medicine, nutrition, psychology, nursing, and social work professionals.

Group dynamics included three distinct stages: firstly, family members and patients were welcomed by the multidisciplinary team in a large auditorium. Presentations were made and general guidance on dermatosis was given. In a second stage, family members remained in the room while children and adolescents were moved to another room. At each meeting a common theme was proposed for discussion, including recreational resources for the children. Themes complied with participants' request, generally associated with care in different seasons of the year (e.g., attention to swimming pools and sun exposure in summer; hydration and use of cotton clothing in winter) or a related date (attention to diet at Easter, for example). At the end of the activities, children and family gathered one more time to exchange experiences. The group finished with a healthy snack, proposed by the nutritionist in the team [23].

Case Report 6.6

Girl, 6 years-old, participated in the Atopic Dermatitis Group for 2 years, always accompanied by her mother. She was an only child, both parents were health professionals; her mother had left the job to devote herself to the girl's care, who had been suffering severe attacks of atopic dermatitis since the age of 2. Alice had lesions all over her body and cried a lot when showering, scratched herself at night, and only accepted her mother to treat the injuries, although her father was a professional nurse and was willing to help. Initially, the girl remained absolutely silent during group sessions.

In the children group she was always alert, performed the activities proposed, but interacted little. She never talked. During the treatment, she would gradually become more participative. The girl enjoyed graphic and music activities, especially when one of therapists played the guitar to the group. The lesions that marked her face were decreasing. At school she became more independent, and even participated in the dance group. Her mother was supported in order to share the child's care with her father. The girl participated in the groups for 2 years, being discharged with great deal of autonomous care. The mother began to devote herself to other activities, and considered going back to work.

Perspectives and Final Considerations

An integral service of dermatology must offer a number of psychotherapeutic possibilities for the treatment of psychodermatosis. The wider range of treatments allows one to respond uniquely to each new case referred. The choice of an individual, family, or group approach should be made, however, only after a first contact of general acceptance and multidisciplinary assessment. Psychotherapy, regardless of the modality, reaches only one of the dimensions of an illness and can only be really effective if it is in tune with medical, nursing, nutritional, and social care.

Understanding that the "skin" communicates something with its symptom is of key importance in the psychological care of psychodermatosis. As Campos [24] says, "Body language is the first, the most primitive means of communication and defense of a human being. It is natural, therefore, to continue to use it throughout life, especially at times when other forms of communication and defense are locked (or have not been learned)." In this sense, a psychologist's first task is to help in a translation process: to help the patient to express in words the emotions, feelings, and distress that have been overloading their body so far.

Psychotherapy is not always able to provide a complete remission of skin symptoms. Sometimes it is all about changing the *relationship* the patient has with his symptoms, or the family's relationship with the patient, so that symptoms stop producing so much pain and can be given new meanings, subjectively [25]. One of the patients in the clinic, Ingrid, 16, illustrates how the process works. She says, "... broke up with my first boyfriend, began to work and help mother, and the stains increased. From then on, every speck (vitiligo) symbolizes a different problem. But I do not need stains to keep my problems. I have no reason to keep them because others will come. (Ingrid, 16 years old)".

Scars are permanent, but may no longer be horrific memories and become symbols of bravery. Skin stains, similarly, may be indelible; but to stop being just symptoms of a disease they can count on the help of psychotherapy.

Glossary

Multidisciplinary approach In collaboration, psychologists, social workers, medical doctors, nurses, nutritionists, and other health professionals will be able to understand the different dimensions of skin-related pathologies to indicate the best options for treatment.

Psychodermatoses Multifactorial dermatoses whose course is subject to emotional influence.

Psychological interventions Individual therapy, family therapy, couple and group therapy are among the possibilities of psychotherapy presented, besides psychoeducative interventions.

References

1. Canguilhem G. O normal e o patológico. Rio de Janeiro: Forense Universitária; 1943.
2. Silva AK, Castoldi L, Kijner LC. A pele expressando o afeto: uma intervenção grupal com pacientes portadores de psicodermatoses. Contextos Clínicos. 2011;4:53–63. doi:10.4013/ctc.2011.41.06.

3. Calligaris CA. Adolescência. São Paulo: Publifolha; 2000.

4. Neri M, Soares W. Desigualdade Social e Saúde no Brasil. Cad Saúde Pública. 2002;18(Suplemento):77–87.

5. Brasil. Secretaria de Políticas de Promoção da Igualdade Racial. Racismo como determinante social da saúde. Brasília: Presidência da República; 2011.

6. Villela W. Gênero, saúde dos homens e masculinidades. Cien Saude Colet. 2005;10(1):18–34.

7. Lionço T. Que direito à saúde para a população GLBT? Considerando direitos humanos, sexuais e reprodutivos em busca da integralidade e da eqüidade. Saúde Soc. 2008;17(2):11–21.

8. Campos GWS. Saúde pública e saúde coletiva: campo e núcleo de saberes e práticas. Ciênc Saúde Coletiva. 2000;5(Suppl 2):219–30.

9. Pinheiro R, Mattos R. Os sentidos da Integralidade na atenção e no cuidado à saúde. Rio de Janeiro: ABRASCO/UERJ, IMS; 2001.

10. Bowlby J. Perda, tristeza e depressão. São Paulo: Martins Fontes; 1998. (Original publicado em 1980).

11. Bowlby J. Formação e rompimento dos laços afetivos. São Paulo: Martins Fontes; 2001.

12. Fortune DG, Richards HL, Griffiths EMC, Main CJ. Targeting cognitive-behaviour therapy to patients' implicit model of psoriasis: results from a patient preference controlled trial. Article first published online: 24 Dec 2010. doi:10.1348/014466504772812977. 2004. The British Psychological Society.

13. Lora V, Gisondi P, Calza A, Zanoni M, Girolomoni G. Efficacy of a single educative intervention in patients with chronic plaque psoriasis. Dermatology. 2009;219:316–21. doi:10.1159/000250826.

14. Castro RC, Benetti S. Psicoterapia Psicanalítica com Adultos. cap.11. Em: Vera Regina Ramires & Renato Caminha. Práticas em Saúde no âmbito da Clínica-Escola: a Teoria. São Paulo, Casa do Psicólogo. 2006. p. 199–220.

15. Capisano HF. Imagem Corporal, cap.17. Em: Júlio de Mello Filho & Cols. Psicossomática Hoje. Porto Alegre: Artes Médicas; 1992. p. 179–92.

16. Müller MC. Psicossomática: uma visão simbólica do vitiligo. São Paulo: Vetor; 2005.

17. Bowen M. De la família al individuo. Buenos Aires: Paidós; 1991. (original 1979).

18. Castoldi L. Psicoterapia Familiar e de Casal. Cap 12. Em: Vera Regina Ramires & Renato Caminha. Práticas em Saúde no âmbito da Clínica-Escola: a Teoria. São Paulo, Casa do Psicólogo. 2006. p. 221–242.

19. Minuchin S, Nichols MP, Lee WY. Famílias e casais: do sintoma ao sistema. Porto Alegre: ArtMed; 2009.

20. Zimerman DE, Osorio LC, et al. Como trabalhamos com Grupos. Porto Alegre: Artes Médicas; 1997.

21. Ferreira VRT, Muller MC, Jorge HZ. Dinâmica das relações em famílias com um membro portador de dermatite atópica: um estudo qualitativo. Psicol Estud (Maringá). 2006;11:3.

22. Staab D, Diepgen L, Fartasch M, Kupfer J, Lob-Corzilius T, et al. Age related, structured programmes for the management of atopic dermatitis in children and adolescentes: multicentre, randomised controlled trial. BMJ. 2006;332. doi:http://dx.doi.org/10.1136/bmj.332.7547.933 (Published 20 April 2006) Cite this as: BMJ 2006;332:933.

23. Castoldi L, Labrea MGA, Oliveira GT, Paim BS, Rodrigues CRB. Dermatite Atópica: experiência com grupo de crianças e familiares do Ambulatório de Dermatologia Sanitária. PSICO. 2010;41:201–207.

24. Campos EP. O paciente somático no grupo terapêutico. Cap. 38. Em: Júlio de Mello Filho, Cols. Psicossomática Hoje. Porto Alegre: Artes Médicas; 1992. p. 371–85.

25. Carter B, McGoldrick M. As mudanças no ciclo de vida familiar: uma estrutura para a terapia familiar. Porto Alegre: Artes Médicas; 1995.

Index

© Springer International Publishing Switzerland 2018
R.R. Bonamigo, S.I.T. Dornelles (eds.), *Dermatology in Public Health Environments*,
https://doi.org/10.1007/978-3-319-33919-1

Printed by Printforce, the Netherlands